Undergraduate
Surgery

THIRD EDITION

Undergraduate Surgery

THIRD EDITION

AK Nan MS (Cal)

Retired Professor and Head
Department of Surgery
RG Kar Medical College
Kolkata

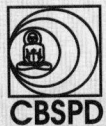

CBSPD

CBS Publishers & Distributors Pvt Ltd

New Delhi • Bengaluru • Chennai • Kochi • Kolkata • Lucknow • Mumbai
Gujarat • Hyderabad • Jharkhand • Nagpur • Patna • Pune • Uttarakhand

Undergraduate Surgery

THIRD EDITION

ISBN: 978-81-239-2930-9

Copyright © Authors and Publisher

CBS Edition: 2016
Reprint: 2017, 2019, 2021, 2022, 2023, **2026**
First Edition: 1978
Second Edition: 1987
Reprint: 1989, 1991, 1993, 1994, 1995
Third Edition: 1997
Reprint: 1998, 2000, 2001, 2003, 2004, 2007, 2008, 2011

Published by **Satish Kumar** Jain and Produced by **Varun Jain** for
CBS Publishers & Distributors Pvt Ltd
4819/XI Prahlad Street, 24 Ansari Road, Daryaganj, New Delhi 110 002, India.
Ph: 011-23266838, 23289259
Website: www.cbspd.com
e-mail: delhi@cbspd.com
Corporate Office: 204 FIE, Industrial Area, Patparganj, Delhi 110 092, India
Ph: 011-4934 4934   Fax: 011-4934 4935   e-mail: publishing@cbspd.com;
publicity@cbspd.com

Branches

- **Bengaluru:** Seema House 2975, 17th Cross, KR Road, Banasankari 2nd Stage, Bengaluru 560 070, Karnataka, India
  Ph: +91-80-26771678/79   Fax: +91-80-26771680   e-mail: bangalore@cbspd.com
- **Chennai:** 18/8B, Subbaraya Street, Shenoy Nagar, Chennai 600 030, Tamil Nadu, India
  Ph: +91-044-42032115, 044-26681266   e-mail: chennai@cbspd.com
- **Kochi:** 42/1325, 1326, Power House Road, Opp KSEB, Power House, Ernakulum Kochi 682 018, Kerala, India
  Ph: +91-484-4059061-65,67   Fax: +91-484-4059065   e-mail: kochi@cbspd.com
- **Kolkata:** 147, Hind Ceramics Compound, 1st Floor, Nilgunj Road, Belghoria, Kolkata-700056, West Bengal, India
  Ph: +033-25633055, 033-25633056   e-mail: kolkata@cbspd.com
- **Lucknow:** Basement, Khushnuma Complex, 7 Meerabai Marg (Behind Jawahar Bhawan), Lucknow-226001, UP, India
  Ph: +0522-4000032   e-mail: tiwari.lucknow@cbspd.com
- **Mumbai:** PWD Shed, Gala no 25/26, Ramchandra Bhatt Marg, Next to JJ Hospital Gate no. 2, Opp. Union Bank of India, Noorbaug, Mumbai-400009, Maharashtra, India
  Ph: 022-66661880/89   e-mail: mumbai@cbspd.com

Representatives

- Gujarat • Hyderabad • Jharkhand • Nagpur • Patna • Pune • Uttarakhand

For trade terms please contact customercare@cbspd.com
For general enquiries please contact info@cbspd.com

Printed at Mudrak, Noida, UP, India

to

_____

my parents
who fought hard against poverty
to bring me up
and
my teacher
Dr Amiya Kumar Sen
who taught me surgery

Preface to the Third Edition

The call for the third edition of this book has provided me with the opportunity to bring it up-to-date. With the publication of the current edition, the book has completed two decades of existence and it has served in its own way during this long span. In presenting this edition I have made every endeavour to keep in step with the march of surgical progress. The text has been revised. The same useful style of presentation has been retained as for the last edition because the students liked it. Some chapters have been completely rewritten or improved by addition, notably those dealing with 'shock', 'fluid and electrolyte balance', 'acid–base balance', 'healing of wounds', 'burns', 'blood transfusion', 'cysts', 'ulcers', 'arterial impairment and gangrene', 'abscess', 'gas gangrene', 'tetanus'. Intravenous fluid therapy, skin grafting and treatment and investigations of arterial impairment and gangrene have made great strides and the new material has been incorporated in this edition.

I would like to thank my students and friends, both at home and abroad, for their very helpful and constructive criticisms and I can assure them I have made full use of their suggestions.

In the preparation of this new edition, I owe a great debt of gratitude to Dr KK Chatterjee, Chief Assistant Editor, *Journal of the Indian Medical Association*, for the trouble he has taken in editing the revised chapters as well as going through the proofs. Sri Samar Chakraborty of *JIMA* helped me a lot and also gave assurance for the same courtesy to be extended for the future editions.

Finally, I wish to express my thanks to the printers of this book for their helpful cooperation.

AK Nan

Preface to the First Edition

This book is principally a compilation of the lecture notes that I have been delivering to my students over the last eighteen years. Essentially meant for the undergraduate students, the volume deals only with the basic aspects of the subject. While the more common diseases have been dealt with exhaustively, conditions not so important for undergraduate course have either been omitted or just touched upon.

While teaching the students, I have often found that, by the time they come to the clinical course, they forget the basic anatomy and physiology of the different organs, the knowledge of which is so essential in following the pathology, clinical features and treatment of the diseases. Emphasis has, therefore, been laid on the surgical anatomy and physiology of the organs, in the different chapters, as far as practicable. The knowledge of embryology is essential in understanding the congenital anomalies and so, wherever deemed necessary, the accent has been on this aspect. Chapters on instruments, splints and bandaging have been incorporated with a view to making the students conversant with the practical aspect of the subject and also to help them in the oral and practical examinations of the graduation course, where marks are specifically allotted to these items. The more common operations have been described in details either in the text or under the chapter on instruments.

I take this opportunity to express my reverence and gratitude to all my respected teachers. I feel I should make a social mention of the names of Dr Amiya Kumar Sen, FRCS (Eng), who taught me surgery and under whom I worked in different capacities, right from the internship to lecturership; of the late Dr Kalipada Das, FRCS (Eng & Edin), under whom I worked as a house surgeon; of Dr Binode Behari Roy, MS, DPhil, DSc, DSc, (Cal), FNA, who had been a constant source of inspiration to me while I was preparing this volume against all odds; and of Dr Bidhu Bhusan Roy, MB (Cal) who gave me valuable suggestions during the preparation of the book.

I possibly have no greater well-wisher than Sri Prafulla Kanti Ghosh and I take the opportunity of recording all my respects for him.

I really owe to my students and house surgeons who urged me to embark upon this virtue. Nothing can be of greater pleasure to me than to find the book meeting their requirements.

My friend, Sri Salil Kumar De, has assisted me in reading the proofs of the whole volume. Sri Atul Krishna Bose has drawn all the diagrams for the book. The entire photographic work of instruments and splints has been done by Sri Prafulla Mitra, with great care. Sri Chandi Charan Das, Sri Narayan Chandra Saha, Sri Sukumar Talukdar and Sri Sailen Bhattacharya have typed the manuscript. Sri Chittananda Rai Chowdhuri has helped me in different ways in the technical work. I find words insufficient to express my indebtedness and gratitude to all of them.

As regards printing, I shall fondly remember Sri NK Gossain, Chairman, Messrs NK Gossain & Co Private Ltd, the printers of the book, but for whose great affection it would have been virtually impossible for me to bring out this volume.

I extend my sincere thanks to Sri Bejoy Banerjee, Sri Santosh Banerjee, Sri Tuhin Basu Mallick and Sri Gour Hari Dutta of the press. It is unlikely that I would ever forget the help and co-operation received from them.

I am grateful to the Director of Health Services, and to the Department of Health, Government of West Bengal, for granting me permission to publish the book.

In the preparation of this volume I have utilised the knowledge of the authors of various publications, and I record my sincere gratitude to all of them. I hope to be excused for not being able to acknowledge the individual contributions.

Before concluding, I fondly acknowledge with thanks the encouragement, inspiration and help I have received throughout from friends and near ones, whose time I have often taxed.

AK Nan

Contents

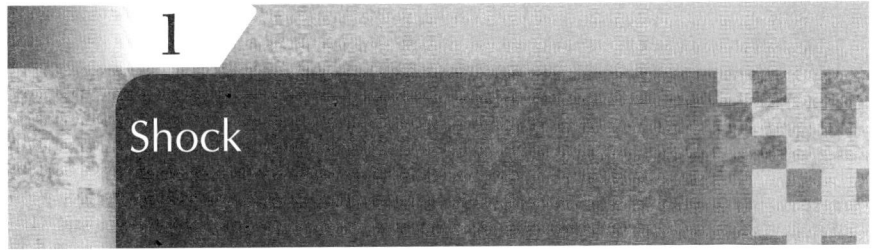

1

Shock

Definition.—Shock may be defined as a state of depression of the vital functions of the body due to inadequate tissue perfusion of the vital organs, resulting from insufficient microcirculation.

Basic Terminology: Microcirculation comprises that part of the vascular network which extends from the smaller arterioles to the venules, i.e. the terminal arterioles, capillaries and venules.

The terminal arterioles have thick muscle coat, the tone of which is controlled by the sympathetic nerves as well as some hormones. Thus, their calibre is altered as per need and they control the amount of blood flow through the capillaries. They make the peripheral vascular resistance, hence they are called *resistance arterioles.*

The venules are also lined by smooth muscles, though thin. The entire venous network, starting from the venules up to the major veins of the trunk and the limbs, comprises what is called the *capacitance veins.* The tone of the lining muscles of all the veins is also controlled by the sympathetic fibres. Their contraction evacuates the blood, reserved there in large *quantities* (*venous reservoir*) into the active circulation.

Types of Shock: Insufficiency of the microcirculation may be either due to inability of the central pump, i.e. the heart, to send blood at sufficient pressure to reach the microcirculation (*cardiogenic shock*) or because of a shortfall in the volume of blood available to the heart to be pumped out.

This latter condition may be due to either a reduction in the *body's total* blood volume (*haematogenic shock*) or a diminution of the actual *circulating* blood volume as a result of pooling of blood in the peripheral vessels (*vasogenic shock*). Basically, therefore, shock may be classified into three categories.

1. Haematogenic (*Syn* hypovolaemic, oligaemic)
2. Vasogenic
3. Cardiogenic.

The above is only a working classification and indicates the initial cause. Superimposition often occurs in any advanced case of shock. Septic shock is, from its onset, a combination of vasogenic and haematogenic shock.

Causes of Haematogenic (Hypovolaemic, Oligaemic) Shock

1. Haemorrhagic, i.e. Loss of Blood

    a. Blood lost from injured part—external or internal.

b. Blood lost into injured part—major fractures, big loops of strangulated gut, acute pancreatitis.

2. Non-haemorrhagic

a. Loss of plasma and fluid—burns

b. Loss of fluid:

    i. From and into the intestine—vomiting, diarrhoea, gut obstruction.

    ii. Into the peritoneal cavity—peritonitis, acute pancreatitis.

Causes of Septic Shock.—This is a sequela to severe systemic sepsis. The common sources of infection are the genito-urinary tract, respiratory tract, intra-abdominal sepsis, burns and indwelling monitoring catheters.

Causes of Vasogenic Shock.—The essential cause is pooling of blood in the terminal arterioles and capacitance veins, leading to gross reduction in the actively circulating blood volume:

1. NEUROGENIC SHOCK.—There is loss of sympathetic control of the peripheral vasculature:

a. Spinal cord injury.

b. Spinal anaesthesia.

2. PSYCHOGENIC SHOCK.—Also caused by loss of sympathetic control:

a. Sudden fright, apprehension, grief.

b. Acute pain, e.g. blow to the testis.

3. VASOVAGAL SHOCK.—Pooling of blood in the large venous reservoirs (limb muscles) and dilated splanchnic arterioles.

4. ANAPHYLACTIC SHOCK.—Massive peripheral vasodilatation caused by release of histamine and slow release anaphylactic substances (SRSA). The common agents are shellfish, penicillin, anaesthetic agents, equine serum.

Causes of Cardiogenic Shock

1. INTRINSIC CARDIOGENIC SHOCK.—The myocardial contractility is grossly impaired, e.g. myocardial infarction, myocarditis, cardiac arrhythmias.

2. CARDIAC COMPRESSIVE SHOCK.—There is compression of the cardiac chambers and/or great veins, e.g. cardiac tamponade tension pneumothorax.

3. CARDIAC OBSTRUCTIVE SHOCK.—There is obstruction either in the pulmonary or the systemic circulation:

a. Pulmonary embolism, pulmonary vascular disease.

b. Mechanical obstruction to aorta, systemic arteriolar constriction.

HYPOVOLAEMIC (OLIGAEMIC) SHOCK

Pathology.—With the onset of hypovolaemia, the body's compensatory mechanisms are set into action:

1. The first aim is to divert blood, as much as possible, from the relatively unimportant areas to the vital organs, of which the brain and the heart are the most important. This is primarily effected by stimulation of the sympathetic

nervous system and die adrenal medulla discharging adrenaline and noradrenaline (*adrenergic discharge*) which causes:

a. Contraction of the systemic venules and small veins (venous reservoir), pumping out the large volume of blood reserved therein, into the circulation.

b. Constriction of the arterioles, firstly, those of the skin, subcutaneous fat and skeletal muscles, thereafter the arterioles of the splanchnic organs including the liver and, finally, the arterioles of the kidneys, thereby maintaining blood flow to the heart and the brain. Angiotensin and vasopressin, released from the ischaemic kidneys, add to the constriction of the arterioles. The cerebral and cardiac arterioles are spared of this constriction because there are autoregulating mechanisms to conserve cerebral and cardiac blood flow.

2. Simultaneously, there are natural attempts to reinforce the total blood volume (intravascular fluid):

a. There is movement of fluid from the extracellular to the intravascular space through the capillary wall (capillary refill). This is effected by adrenergic discharge, vasopressin and angiotensin.

b. There is also shift of intracellular .fluid, via the extracellular space, into the intravascular space. Release of epinephrine, cortisol and glucagon,and inhibition of insulin secretion lead to high concentration of glucose in the extracellular fluid, causing its hyperosmolarity.

This draws water out of the cells into the extracellular space. The interstitial pressure rises, forcing water (with sodium and chloride) into the vascular space.

3. There are attempts to preserve whatever fluid is there in the vascular space by die kidney (*renal conservation of blood volume*). This is effected by:

a. Diminution of glomerular filtration rate.

b. Increased reabsorption of water (with sodium and chloride) by the distal renal tubules. This is effected by aldosterone (of adrenal cortex) as well as by angiotensin produced in the kidney when its blood flow is reduced. The chief stimulator to aldosterone secretion is also angiotensin itself.

4. The cardiac output is mechanically raised by traction on the great vessels and cardiac chambers. This is caused by the spontaneous hyperventilation due to metabolic acidosis resultant upon tissue anoxia.

5. There is an associated tachycardia in an attempt to, send blood more frequently to the tissues. This is induced by the adrenergic discharge as well as by depression of the vagal centre, caused by fall of pressure in the great vessels (Marey's reflex).

However, if the *hypovolaemia progresses,* the compensatory mechanisms gradually fail. Blood supply to the vital organs are progressively reduced and ultimately the organs start failing (*organ failure of shock*). To start with, the gastrointestinal system, pancreas and liver and, thereafter, the kidneys fail. Finally, there is a failure of the brain and the heart—the features of the former more manifest in the young and those of the latter in the elderly. The final event is cardiac arrest. Pulmonary failure, in the absence of chest injury, is a rate event in hypovolaemic shock (of septic shock).

Clinical Features: The features correlate with the structures and organs whose blood supply has to be curtailed. This starts with the least essential structures and ends with the most essentials:

i. Firstly the skin.

ii. Then the kidneys and other viscera, including the liver.

iii. Finally the heart and the brain.

The findings depend upon the degree of depletion of the blood volume:

1. In *mild shock* (less than 20 per cent volume depletion), features of adrenergic discharge to the skin are manifest as follows:

   a. The extremities, especially the feet, are pale and cold, and may be moist with sticky sweat (clammy).

   b. The subcutaneous veins collapse (making insertion of infusion needle difficult).

   c. The patient feels cold and complains of thirst (a constant feature).

   d. The temperature is subnormal, including the 'core' temperature (e.g. midoesophageal or tympanic membrane).

   The pulse and the blood pressure show little changes, especially in the supine position.

2. In *moderate shock* (20 to 40 per cent depletion) in addition to the skin features, the urine output is low (less than 0.5 ml/kg body wt/hour).

   The pulse and the blood pressure may still be near normal, particularly in supine position.

3. In *severe shock* (more than 40 per cent depletion), there is progressive rise of pulse rate and fall of blood pressure, and features of cerebral and cardiac ischaemia set in:

   a. Restlessness and anxiousness, gradually changing to apathy and exhaustion.

   b. The ECG shows depressed S-T segment and presence of Q wave. As the ischaemia progresses, there are arrhythmias, ventricular fibrillation and, finally cardiac arrest.

Treatment.—The principles of treatment for both haemorrhagic and non-haemorrhagic shock are basically the same, having two essential components, both equally important and demanding simultaneous attention-treatment of the cause and replacement of the depleted blood volume. The replacement must be equivalent to the loss, both quantitatively and qualitatively, i.e. blood for haemorrhage, fluids and plasma expanders for burns, and electrolyte-containing fluids for gastro-intestinal loss. The treatment of haemorrhagic shock, the commonest type encountered by the surgeon, is detailed as follows:

A. Arrest of haemorrhage.—The source of bleeding is quickly identified and steps taken for immediate control:

1. External bleeding should be primarily tamponaded by compression; surgical procedure may then be carried out.

2. In traumatic internal haemorrhage the source is to be surgically explored and bleeding controlled.

3. Bleeding from the gastrointestinal tract should have the source identified and treated with usual measures, e.g. decompression of the stomach by nasogastric suction in gastroduodenal ulcer haemorrhage.

B. Replacement of blood volume.—Intravenous infusion is started immediately. An amount approximating the amount of loss has to be infused and this must be done as quickly as possible without burdening the heart.

1. Whole blood is the best replacement for blood loss because the RBCs apart from their important physiological functions, serve as the biggest molecules in the fluid, providing high osmolarity that prevents extravascular escape of the transfused fluid.

2. An effective initial fluid regime, till type specific blood is available, is infusion of a non-sugar crystalloid solution. Sugar is avoided because it induces diuresis that reduces the blood volume. Lactated Ringer's solution is the best but acetated Ringer's solution or isotonic saline supplemented with sodium bicarbonate may be used instead. The lactate, acetate and bicarbonate are necessary to combat metabolic acidosis resultant upon tissue anoxia. However, the quantity of the transfused crystalloid fluid must be large (four times the estimated loss) and the rate of transfusion very rapid because three-fourths of the transfused fluid shall escape out of the capillaries into the interstitial tissues almost immediately (as per the normal intravascular: interstitial fluid distribution 1:3). This initial fluid therapy also serves as a *therapeutic trial*. It is often found that the blood pressure returns to normal and keep stable. If it happens so:

   a. the pre-existing blood loss is not severe, and

   b. the haemorrhage is not continuing.

   In these cases transfusion of whole blood may be avoided or minimised, thereby preventing depletion of blood bank and complications of blood transfusion.

   On the other hand, if the blood loss has been severe and/or the haemorrhage is still continuing, the rise of blood pressure is only transient. Blood transfusion has to be instituted. In these cases, if the patient can be operated upon promptly, transfusion of blood is withheld till the bleeding is surgically controlled, thereby avoiding drainage of the transfused blood.

3. In the absence of blood or as its part supplement, colloid solutions may be used. They are preferable to crystalloid fluids in that, by virtue of their high osmolarity, they prevent extravascular escape of the transfused fluid at least for several hours. However, in advanced cases of shock, there is a generalised capillary endothelial damage and the colloids may come out into the interstitial tissues, e.g. lungs, and this is dangerous.

The colloid fluids that may be transfused are:

a. Plasma, available as fresh frozen plasma (FFP).

b. Plasma substitutes:

    i. Natural: 4.5 per cent human albumin solution.

    ii. Synthetic: dextran, gelatin, hydroxyethyl starch, etc. (these have molecular weight more than 30,000).

Plasma transfusion is least preferred because its entry into the interstitial space causes serious problems and also because of the high risk of transmitting diseases like hepatitis.

C. OTHER SUPPORTIVE MEASURES:

1. *Posture.*—The time-old Trendelenburg head-down position, for bringing back the pooled blood from the capacitance veins into active circulation, is no longer advocated. Simple elevation of the lower limbs serves the purpose. Similarly, use of inflatable pneumatic garments round the lower limbs and abdomen (military anti-shock trousers, i.e. MAST) to compress these veins has been discarded for fear of compression of big vessels.

2. *Respiratory Support.*—In the absence of lung injury, respiration poses little problem. Simple oxygen inhalation with a face mask is sufficient. Only rarely ventilation with endotracheal intubation is required.

3. *Sedation.*—While no sedative is required in the absence of pain its use is imperative when pain is present (e.g. fracture, chest wall injuries, peritonitis) because pain aggravates shock. Morphine or pethidine for adults and barbiturates for children are advocated. The doses should be small and they should be administered only intravenously because peripheral collapse prevents absorption from intramuscular tissues making them useless and causing cumulative after-effects.

4. *Drugs:*

a. Inotropic drugs may have to be used to improve myocardial contractility, inefficiency of which is indicated by a rise in the CVP but fall in the arterial pressure. Drugs commonly used are dopamine and debutamine. Only small doses should be used to avoid systemic vasoconstriction and impaired renal blood flow.

b. Vasodilators, used at random in the past, with the idea of improving the peripheral circulation, are now generally discarded because vasodilatation in a hypovolaemic or dehydrated patient may result in disastrous fall in the arterial pressure.

c. Steroids are of no value unless the patient has adrenocortical deficiency, e.g. Addison's disease or under steroid therapy.

d. Digitalis is indicated in some elderly patients where the stress of shock induces or aggravates cardiac failure. Caution must be taken in its administration and dose regulation to avoid toxicity.

e. Sodium bicarbonate, available in ampoules, is administered intravenously if there is metabolic acidosis.

SEPTIC SHOCK

Pathogenesis.—Septic shock, to start with, is usually a combination of vasogenic and hypovolaemic components.

The vasogenic component consists of pooling of a large volume of blood in the skin, reducing the circulating blood volume.

The hypovolaemic component, the more predominant, is due to a generalised leakage of intravascular fluid into the interstitial tissue through the capillary walls,which suffer widespread damage due to bacterial toxins.

Except for occasional cases of Gram-positive infection, the causative organisms are Gram-negative (hence called *Gram-negative shock*). The commonest organisms are *Esch. coli* and then the Klebsiella and the bacteroids. However, most dangerous are the Gram-negative anaerobes.

The common sources of sepsis are:
  i. Genito-urinary system, especially after operations and instrumen-tations, and septic abortion.
  ii. Abdominal cavity, e.g. peritonitis, intra-abdominal abscess, strangulated gut, biliary tract infections.
  iii. Respiratory tract, especially after tracheostomy.
  iv. Monitoring catheters, left *in situ* for prolonged periods.

Pathology.—The sequence of events in septic shock is as follows:
1. With systemic sepsis there is a hypermetabolic state and heat production increases. Heat loss is accomplished by diversion of blood to the skin by diminution of arteriolar resistance and opening of cutaneous, arteriovenous shunts. As blood is pooled in the cutaneous vascular bed, the circulating blood volume is diminished and the blood supply to the other areas and vital organs are considerably reduced. This is how the state of shock is initially superimposed on simple systemic sepsis. At this stage, though other features of hypovolaemic shock are evident, the skin is red and hot (*stage of red shock*).
2. In the mean time, bacterial toxins cause an intravascular inflammatory process. There is release of inflammatory factors which produce an intense reaction that damages the lining wall of the capillaries and allows exit of fluid from the intravascular space into the interstitial tissues. This causes a sharp fall in the total blood volume and quick progress of the state of shock. At this stage, hypoperfusion of the vital organs activates the cutaneous pressor mechanisms, diverting blood from the less essential skin to the important vital organs. Now the skin becomes cold and pale (*stage of white or cold shock*).

    This sequence of red and white shock, however, occurs only when the patient is normovolaemic prior to the onset of systemic sepsis. In contrast, if systemic sepsis develops in a subject who is already hypovolaemic, the patient passes straightway to the stage of cold shock.
3. Another important pathological component of septic shock is marked oxygen desaturation of the tissues, effected by two factors:
    a. Progressive pulmonary dysfunction:
        i. The primary cause is leakage of proteinaceous fluid through the damaged capillary walls into the interstitial tissues of the lungs and

then into the alveolar spaces, causing gradual loss of alveolar functions.

ii. The condition is worsened by superimposed bacterial infection.

b. Decreased oxygen utilisation by the tissues resulting from:

i. Arteriovenous shunting—blood by-passes the tissues.

ii. Inability of the cells to utilise oxygen as a direct effect of sepsis.

In the terminial phase of septic shock, inadequate tissue perfusion due to extreme hypovolaemia causes gastrointestinal, pancreatic, hepatic and renal failure. To this is added the marked reduction in oxygen utilisation by the tissues, further hindering the functions of all organs, including the brain and the heart. The final event is cardiac arrest.

Clinical Features.—The *onset* of the symptoms and signs of septic shock may be coincident with those of systemic sepsis or there may be an interval of few hours to several days.

The features of septic shock are essentially those of hypovolaemia, with some modifications due to the sepsis itself.

A. Features of hypovolaemia:

1. Effects of adrenergic discharge to the skin:
   a. Pale, cold and clammy (sticky moist) skin, especially of the extremities.
   b. Empty subcutaneous veins.
2. Effects of renal ischaemia—low urine output (less than 0.5 ml/kg body wt/hour).
3. Effects of cerebral and cardiac ischaemia:
   a. Altered sensorium—restlessness and anxiety, gradually changing to apathy and exhaustion.
   b. Progressive tachycardia and fall of blood pressure with evidence of coronary insufficiency, e.g. arrhythmia, ventricular fibrillation and, finally, cardiac arrest.

B. Special features due to the sepsis:

1. *Skin.*—In the early stages the skin may be red and hot (cf hypovolaemic shock).
2. *Temperature.*—Primarily, with cutaneous hyperperfusion, the skin temperature rises. Thereafter, with reduced skin perfusion, the skin temperature falls, though the 'core' temperature (e.g. midoesophageal or tympanic membrane) may still be high. At this stage the patient feels a cold sensation and there may be shaking chills. The cutaneous vasoconstriction now disrupts the body's ability to dissipate heat and this may cause another rapid rise of body temperature.
3. *Respiration.*—Adult respiratory distress syndrome (ARDS) develops in many patients and at least some of them die of respiratory failure alone (cf hypovolaemic shock). The difference from classic respiratory failure is that the patient is hypocarbic instead of being hypercarbic.

Treatment.—Septic shock is best treated by *prevention,* i.e. prompt recognition of the presence of sepsis and institution of its proper treatment before the state of shock supervenes. This prevention necessitates:

1. Identification of the source of infection.
2. Administration of antibiotics as specific as possible.
3. Institution of surgical drainage, e.g. drainage of abscess, surgical debridement or removal of septic focus.

Once shock has set in, an early manifestation of which is increased fluid requirement to maintain the urine output, very rapid action has to be undertaken to save the patient. This consists of:

A. Treatment for the sepsis.

B. Treatment for the shock.

C. Other supportive measures.

A. TREATMENT FOR THE SEPSIS:

    1. Identification of the source.—In the majority of cases the source of infection is evident. If no source is apparent, the cause probably lies in the abdomen—USG, CT or MRI may be helpful to detect localised collections.

    2. Antibiotics:

        a. If previous culture-sensitivity tests are available, the specific antibiotic can be started immediately.

        b. In other cases, especially when gastro-intestinal tract organisms are suspected, combination of cefazolin, gentamicin/amikacin and metronidazole usually works well.

    3. Surgery.—Drainage of abscess or localised collections, surgical debridement, removal of products of abortion, etc.

B. TREATMENT FOR THE SHOCK.—Essentially the shock is hypovolaemic and the aim is restoration of the blood volume. Prompt correction of the pre-existing fluid deficit is necessary and large quantities of fluid are often needed. However, care must be taken that there is no overloading, because often the lungs are already damaged by the septic process. The types of fluid are:

    1. Usually crystalloid solutions, e.g. lactated or acetated Ringer's solution, or isotonic saline buffered with sodium bicarbonate, can effect resuscitation. As much as 10 to 15 litres may be necessary in the first 24 hours.

    2. In the absence of specific needs, colloid solutions (5% albumin in isotonic saline or synthetic plasma-expanders like dextran, gelatin or hydroxyethyl starch) are better avoided because of their escape into interstitium of the lungs, resulting from enhanced capillary permeability in septic shock, may be dangerous.

    3. Any deficit in RBC count should be corrected by blood transfusion because the damaged lungs must be properly oxygenated.

C. OTHER SUPPORTIVE MEASURES:

1. *Respiratory Support.*—Many patients develop pulmonary insufficiency. Endotracheal intubation with ventilation is necessary in such cases.

2. *Drugs:*

   a. Inotropic drugs may be necessary to improve myocardial contractility. An abrupt rise in the CVP but a fall in the arterial pressure indicates inability of the heart to contract properly. Drugs commonly used are dopamine and debutamine. Only small doses should be administered to avoid systemic vasoconstriction and impaired renal blood flow.

   b. Vasopressors.—Theoretically vasopressors are indicated because, in septic shock, there is peripheral vasodilatation and pooling of blood. Norepinephrine is the drug of choice. However, vasopressors are better avoided because the degree of constriction may be severe leading to tissue anoxia.

   c. Steroids are used in the cases where the blood pressure fails to rise with adequate fluid replacement. Use of steroids in the presence of infection is discouraged by many for fear of immunosuppression.

   d. Digitalis in small doses may have to be administered in elderly patient in whom the stress of shock may induce or aggravate cardiac failure.

Monitoring a Patient in Shock: While treating a patient of shock, frequent monitoring is essential to decide improvement or deterioration and to modify the treatment accordingly.

A. *In Less Severe and Uncomplicated Cases* the following observations are usually sufficient:

1. *Vital Signs:*

   a. *Pulse:* Progressive tachycardia and irregular pulse indicate deterioration.

   b. *Blood Pressure:* While systolic and diastolic pressures are important, the pulse pressure, i.e. the difference between the systolic and the diastolic, is a better indication of the cardiac output. Still better is the mean arterial pressure, i.e. diastolic pressure plus one-third of the pulse pressure.

   c. *Respiration:* Persistently rapid and deep respiration and presence of cyanosis are unfavourable signs.

   d. *Surface Temperature:* Warmth of the skin is a good sign while cold clammy skin is unfavourable. Hyperpyrexia in septic shock is dangerous.

2. *Sensorium.*—Restlessness indicates cerebral anoxia while alertness is a good sign.

3. *Urine Output.*—This is singularly the most reliable and easy guide. It reflects the renal blood flow which depends on the cardiac output. Urine output of less than 0.5 ml/kg body wt/hour is indicative of insufficient fluid transfusion.

B. *In Severe or Complicated Cases* additional investigations are necessary:

1. CVP (central venous pressure) measurement is necessary in the cases where the urine output is poor in spite of fluid transfusion. The best way is to raise the rate of transfusion till the CVP rises to 10–15 cm of water.

2. PCWP (pulmonary capillary wedge pressure) indicates the left ventricular function. In cases of severe shock and in patients with pulmonary dysfunction, there may be gross disparity between the left and right ventricular functions. A pulmonary artery floatation catheter is used for the purpose. The Swan-ganz type is the best because this can also record the cardiac output by a thermodilution technique.

3. ECG.

4. X-ray of the chest in patients with pulmonary complications.

5. Serum electrolyte estimations.—Sodium, chloride, potassium and calcium.

6. Blood gas analysis at regular intervals.

2

Fluid and Electrolyte Balance and Their Disturbances, Intravenous Fluid Therapy

BODY WATER IN HEALTH

Water accounts for 60 per cent of the body weight in the men and 50 per cent in the women. The body water is distributed in two main compartments—*intracellular* (i.e. within the cells) and *extracellular*. The proportion of intracellular water (ICF) to extracellular (ECF) is 2:1. The smaller extracellular compartment, again, comprises two components—*intravascular* (i.e. plasma) and *extravascular* or *interstitial* (i.e. tissue fluid and lymph). The proportion of interstitial to intravascular water is 3:1. Taking all these facts into account, the total body water in an adult male, weighing 70 kg is 42 litres and its distribution is as follows:

Total body weight	100 per cent	70 kg
Total body water	60 per cent	42 litres
a. Intracellular water	40 per cent	28 litres
b. Extracellular water	20 per cent	14 litres
i. Interstitial water	15 per cent	10.5 litres
ii. Plasma	5 per cent	3.5 litres

Water in these compartments continually interchange positions but this mutual interchange does not necessarily alter the net amount of water in each compartment. In fact, in health, this partition of water is remarkably constant.

However, body water is never stagnant as there are normal daily water losses (output) and allowances (intake). The daily turnover of water in health is about 2.5 litres, as follows:

A. WATER INTAKE:

1. Exogenous:
    a. Water taken as drinks—1200 ml.
    b. Water (moisture) in solid food—1000 ml.
2. Endogenous, i.e. water liberated during oxidation of food—300 ml.

B. WATER OUTPUT:

1. Urine— 1500 ml.
2. Faeces—100 ml.
3. Insensible loss:
    a. Drying of the skin (insensible perspiration)—500 ml.
    b. Drying of the respiratory epithelium—400 ml.

Several facts deserve special attention in this respect:

1. The amount of water taken as liquids and that as solids are, unknowingly, almost the same. Hence, a patient, kept on fluids only, should consume double the amount of his normal liquid intake.

2. In health and in the absence of visible sweating, a rough estimate of daily water turnover may be made by adding one litre to the urinary output.

3. Children require greater quantities of water in comparison to their body weight because of several reasons:

   a. They have a larger body surface area per unit of body weight.

   b. There is a greater metabolic activity because they are growing.

   c. Their immature kidneys (only the neonates) have poor concentrating ability.

4. About 8000 ml of fluid is secreted daily in the bowel lumen as digestive juices but almost the whole of this amount is reabsorbed from the gut, except a meagre amount of 100 ml, which is expelled in faeces (*see* intestinal obstruction).

It will follow from the description below *that fluid balance* in the body is effected by direct and indirect factors:

1. *Direct:*

   a. Regulation of water intake by sensation of thirst.

   b. Mechanisms that regulate the output of water by the kidneys— the ADH (antidiuretic hormone) of the posterior pituitary being the most important. ADH conserves water by increasing its reabsorption by the distal tubules and collecting tubules of the kidneys.

2. *Indirect.*—This is by way of mechanisms that regulate sodium balance. Sodium cannot be retained in the system without water, except under very abnormal circumstances (*see* metabolism of sodium, described elsewhere).

ELECTROLYTE BALANCE IN HEALTH

When inorganic salts are in solution (as in the body fluids) they dissociate into two types of *ions*—anions and cations, and these are collectively known as *electrolytes.* Ions are charged particles and they may be —(a) atoms (e.g. Na^+, Cl^-), (b) larger radicles (e.g. HCO_3^-, SO_4^-), or (c) molecules (e.g. protein). Cations are positively charged and anions are negatively charged and one positive charge is equivalent to one negative charge. Thus one Na^+ (monovalent) cation is equivalent to one Cl^- (monovalent) anion but one Ca^{++} (divalent) cation is equivalent to two Cl^- anions. The chemical reactivity of the various electrolytes in the body fluids cannot be evaluated when their concentrations in the fluid are expressed only by their weight in a given volume, e.g. mg/100 ml. Such expressions fail to allow a physiological comparison of the different solutes in a solution. They are, more or less, like specifying an electric motor by its weight rather than its work performance, i.e. horsepower. In expressing the physiological and chemical activities of the electrolytes three factors are of prime importance:

1. The number of electric charges per unit volume.
2. The number of particles present per unit volume.
3. The number of osmotically active particles per unit volume.

1. THE NUMBER OF ELECTRIC CHARGES PER UNIT VOLUME.—This is expressed as milliequivalents (mEq) per unit volume, e.g. mEq/litre. The term 'equivalent' refers to the chemical combining activity of the electrolyte. An equivalent of an ion is its atomic or molecular weight in grams divided by its valency. Milliequivalent is that figure expressed in milligrams. The mEq of Na^+ (atomic weight 23, valency 1) is 23 mg, of Cl^- (atomic weight 35.5, valency 1) is 35.5, of K^+ (atomic weight 39, valency 1) is 39, while that of Ca^{++} (atomic weight 40, valency 2) is 20 and of Mg^{++} (atomic weight 24, valency 2) is 12. To convert a concentration of an electrolyte from mg/100 ml to mEq/litre, the following simple formula is used:

$$\frac{mg/100\ ml}{mEq\ weight} \times 10 = mEq/litre$$

(The multiplication by 10 is required to convert 100 ml to 1000 ml, i.e. litre.)

Thus, if the plasma sodium is reported to be 322 mg/ml, the equivalent concentration is 140 mEq/litre, as calculated below:

$$\frac{322}{23} \times 10 = 140;\ 23\ \text{being the mEq weight of sodium.}$$

2. THE NUMBER OF PARTICLES PRESENT PER UNIT VOLUME.—This is important because the osmotic effect of solutes on a fluid is determined by the number of particles present in it—such particles in the body fluids may be ions (e.g. Na^+, K^+, Cl^-) or unionised molecules (e.g. glucose, urea). This is expressed as millimoles (mmol) per litre. The mole of a substance is its molecular weight in grams and mmol is that figure expressed in milligrams. Thus, one mmol of Na^+ is 23 mg, one mmol of Cl^- is 35.5 mg and one mmol of NaCl is 58.5 mg (23 mg + 35.5 mg). One mmol of Ca^{++} is 40 mg. One mmol of urea (molecular weight 60) is 60 mg and one mmol of glucose (molecular weight 180) is 180 mg.

To draw a relationship between (1) and (2) above, it may be remembered that in case of monovalent ions (Na^+, K^+, Cl^-) one mmol equals one mEq while in case of divalent ions (Ca^{++}, Mg^{++}) one mmol equals two mEq.

3. THE NUMBER OF OSMOTICALLY ACTIVE PARTICLES PER UNIT VOLUME.—The osmotic activity of an electrolyte depends upon its number of ions. For example, 58.5 mg of NaCl in one litre of water is converted into 23 mg of Na^+ and 35.5 mg of Cl^-; since the concentration of each ion is 1 mmol/litre of water, the osmotic activity of NaCl solution is 2 mmol/litre. Again, 111 mg of $CaCl_2$ in one litre of water is converted into 40 mg of Ca^{++} and 71 mg of Cl^- (35.5 × 2); since the concentration

of Ca^{++} is 1 mmol/litre and that of Cl^- is 2 mmol, the osmotic activity of the solution is 3 mmol/litre.

The osmotic activity of a fluid is expressed in two terms, viz. osmolarity and osmolality. *Osmolarity* denotes solute concentration (expressed in mmol) per kg of the solvent while *osmolality* means solute concentration per litre of the solution. When the solute concentration is low and the solvent is water, with a density of 1 g/ml (as in the biological system), there is practically no difference between osmolarity and osmolality. Thus, the plasma osmolarity and osmolality are 280–310 mmol/kg and 280–310 mmol/litre respectively.

Table 2.1: Chemical composition of body fluid components (mEq/litre)

		Plasma	Interstitial fluid	Intracellular fluid
A	Cl^-	103	114	—
N	HCO_3^-	27	30	10
I	HPO_4^{--} (as P)	2	2	100
O	SO_4^- (as S)	1	1	30
N	Organic acids	5	5	—
S	Proteins	16	1	60
	Total	154	153	200
C	Na^+	142	144	10
A	K^+	4	4	150
T	Ca^{++}	5	3	—
I	Mg^{++}	3	2	40
O				
N				
S				
	Total	154	153	200

It is evident from Table 2.1 that sodium and potassium are the predominant cations in the ECF and ICF respectively. The chief anions in the ECF are chloride and bicarbonate while in the ICF they are phosphate and proteins. The sum of concentration of cations (in mEq/litre) in each compartment, i.e. intracellular, interstitial and intravascular (plasma), equals the sum of the anions (in mEq/litre), making each compartment electrically neutral. This is called *Donnan's equilibrium.*

The mode of transport of water and electrolytes between the three compartments is noteworthy. The capillary endothelium which separates plasma in the intravascular compartment from the interstitial fluid *is freely* permeable to water, cations, anions and other soluble substances. On the other hand, the cell membrane, which separates the interstitial fluid from the intracellular, is freely permeable only to water and only *selectively* permeable to different ions. When there is an excess or deficit of water, its effects are maximum on the ICF volume, because water freely diffuses to and fro across the cell membrane. Changes in the sodium level, however, chiefly affects the interstitial fluid level because sodium carries water with it across the capillary endothelium (the intracellular fluid contains very little sodium).

METABOLISM OF SODIUM

The maintenance of the volume and distribution of body fluids, i.e. homeostasis, is essentially a function of the electrolytes, principally the salts of sodium and potassium, and body's primary aim is maintenance of the plasma volume. The sum total of body's sodium and potassium contents best signifies the total body water. Because sodium is the predominant electrolyte in the ECF, changes in the total body sodium or its distribution are immediately reflected as changes in the body water. A sodium depleted person must be dehydrated and he cannot be rehydrated unless sodium deficiency is simultaneously corrected. Conversely, retention of sodium is usually associated with overhydration, manifested as oedema, necessitating the use of diuretics to increase elimination of sodium salts in the urine.

The plasma concentration of sodium is 140 mEq/litre and the normal range is very narrow, i.e. 135 to 145 mEq/litre. In cases of sodium retention, the plasma level is seldom above 150 mEq/litre and in sodium deficiency, it is seldom below 120 mEq/litre. To keep the sodium concentration fairly so constant in the face of excess or deficit of sodium, the role of simultaneous retention or excretion of water is immediately apparent.

The total body sodium amounts to 5000 mEq, of which 44 per cent is in the ECF, only 9 per cent in the ICF and 47 per cent in the bones. Bone, therefore, is a large storehouse for sodium, ready to compensate its abnormal loss from the body. However, only a little more than half of the sodium in the bones is water-soluble and exchangeable.

The average daily intake of sodium is 100 mEq, available from 6 g of sodium chloride or, in the absence of oral feeding, from 570 ml of isotonic (0.9 per cent) saline solution. An equal amount is excreted daily, mainly in the urine, a little in the faeces. The loss in perspiration, under normal circumstances, is negligible. The daily urinary sodium output may be as little as 2 mEq or as high as 700 mEq in salt restriction and salt loading respectively. If sodium intake is stopped, kidneys stop excreting sodium (cf potassium).

It is evident from Table 2.1 that the level of sodium is the best index of the cationic concentration of plasma and this is balanced on the anionic side by the combined concentration of chloride and bicarbonate. This latter combined level is about 12 mEq less than that of sodium. Hence estimation of serum sodium is of great value in assessing the electrolyte pattern of a particular subject. Whenever possible, the serum chloride and the serum bicarbonate should also be estimated. The normal serum level of chloride is 95 to 105 mEq/litre, while that of bicarbonate is 25 to 30 mEq/litre: Variation in one is corrected by opposite effect in the other so that the sum of the two remains fairly constant, i.e. 120 to 135 mEq/litre.

Sodium (and chloride) balance in the system is effectively regulated by the kidney. There are three separate mechanisms:

1. Eighty per cent of the sodium excreted by the glomeruli is reabsorbed by the proximal convoluted tubules. This is believed to be under humoral control.

2. Regulation of the glomerular filtration rate is an important factor. If the rate is reduced, the amount of sodium excretion in the urine is diminished and sodium is retained. This occurs promptly whenever the blood volume falls, e.g. haemorrhage. The diminished blood volume works on the baroreceptors (in the carotid sinus and aortic arch). The effect is cast on the vasomotor centre and the sympathetics. The renal blood flow is reduced, the glomerular filtration is diminished and sodium is retained.

3. Reabsorption of sodium by the distal tubules. This is chiefly under control of aldosterone secreted by the adrenal cortex. The secretion of aldosterone, on the other hand, is related to the volume of extracellular fluid as well as its sodium content. The most important stimulator to aldosterone secretion is angiotensin, which again is produced when the renal blood flow is decreased. Apart from aldosterone, angiotensin itself has a direct effect in the regulation of sodium excretion by the kidney.

It is evident from the above description that the factors which act to conserve sodium (and chloride) in the system are inter-related.

METABOLISM OF POTASSIUM

The *total body potassium* amounts to approximately 3,500 mEq. It is the predominant cation of the intracellular fluid—98 per cent of the body potassium is intracellular and only 2 per cent is extracellular; 75 per cent of the potassium is in the muscles. When the muscle protein is used as a source of energy, both nitrogen and potassium are released. The released potassium passes to the extracellular fluid but the surplus is efficiently excreted by the kidneys, so that the plasma potassium concentration (3·5 to 5·3 mEq/litre) usually remains normal.

The average daily intake of potassium is about 75 mEq available from 5 g of potassium chloride. Dietary potassium is chiefly derived from animal and plant tissues as well as fruits and milk. An equal amount is excreted daily, mainly in the urine, very little in the faeces and sweat. Body cannot retain potassium in case of reduced intake (cf sodium), and hypokalaemia sets in. Hypokalaemia is commoner than hyperkalaemia.

Sudden loss of potassium from the cells into the plasma and then in the urine may occur under the following circumstances:

1. When cell protein is broken down. This is a normal response to trauma and operation. This may also occur during starvation. This is because, as has been stated, when the cell protein is used as a source of energy. both nitrogen and potassium are released.

2. When water is mobilised from cells, e.g. during water deprivation.

Potassium is actively excreted by the distal tubules of kidney. This is potentiated chiefly by aldosterone and, to a lesser extent, by cortisol.

Administration of glucose and insulin pushes potassium from the extracellular fluid into the cells, where it helps deposition of glycogen.

DISTURBANCES IN WATER AND ELECTROLYTE BALANCE

In deciding the causes, effects, and management of these disturbances, certain basic facts require attention:

1. Of the three body fluid compartments, viz. intravascular, interstitial and intracellular, body's primary aim is to maintain intravascular volume.
2. The intracellular fluid contains very little sodium but very high amount of potassium and the extracellular fluid (both intravascular and interstitial) just the reverse.
3. The levels of body water and sodium run hand in hand but potussium not so. Depletion of water (dehydration) is usually (but not always) associated with a fall in the sodium level and vice versa.

Taking into account all these facts, disturbances in water and electrolyte balance may be of the following types:

1. Total body water depletion.
2. Total body water excess.
3. Sodium depletion.
4. Sodium excess.
5. Potassium depletion.
6. Potassium excess

Total Body Water Depletion (Dehydration)

Causes.—This usually results from diminished water intake rather than from increased loss. Thus it may occur in:

1. Exhausted, depressed, apathetic or comatose patients, not taking water.
2. Severe nausea and vomiting, preventing drinking.
3. Painful lesions in the mouth or throat, or oesophageal obstruction making the patient unable to drink.
4. Diabetes insipidus, where there is defective absorption of water from the collecting tubules of the kidney and water is excreted in excess.

Effects.—The effect is an *intracellular dehydration*. This is because of the fact that the metabolic response to the stress results in potassium and nitrogen from the cell being extruded out of the cell, together with water, into the extracellular space. At the same time renal retention of sodium (due to increased aldosterone secretion) preserves this extruded water. Also, the water excretion in the urine is reduced to the minimum as a result of increased secretion of ADH of pituitary. Thus the extracellular water is not lost. Hence, pure water depletion leads to cellular dehydration but not to a circulatory failure from reduction in blood volume.

CLINICAL FEATURES:

1. Intense thirst.

2. Oliguria.

3. Weakness.—Though there is weakness, the patient remains capable of mental and physical exertion.

4. Fever.—This may be an important feature in the children.

PLASMA CHANGES:

1. The levels of plasma constituents, viz. sodium and proteins, are raised.

2. However, haemoglobin concentration and packed cell volume remain unchanged because of loss of water from the RBC.

3. The plasma urea level rises because of increased reabsorption of urea by the renal tubules (and not because of renal failure).

TREATMENT.—Non-saline fluids are given orally or parenterally. Plenty of water by the oral route is the best. If drinking is impossible, water is administered in 5 per cent solution of glucose by infusion.

RESULTS.—Recovery usually occurs. Only in long-standing cases hypotension and coma occur due to intracellular dehydration of vital organs.

Total Body Water Excess

This is also known as *overhydration* and *water intoxication.* Healthy individuals can safely take a large amount of water because they react by corrective diuresis, i.e. excreting water without electrolytes. This is done by the glomeruli increasing their rate of filtration and the distal tubules producing dilute urine.

CAUSES.—Overhydration, i.e. retention of water in the system without sodium retention, may occur as follows:

1. Overhydration with peripheral oedema.—Acute or chronic renal failure (especially acute), congestive cardiac failure, cirrhosis of liver with ascites.

2. Overhydration without peripheral oedema:
   a. Intravenous administration of large volume of electrolyte-free water. A common example is infusion of only 5 per cent dextrose solution for more than 24 hours in postoperative cases.
   b. Sudden absorption of large volume of water in the intravascular compartment, as in:
      i. Irrigating with plain water during transurethral resection.
      ii. Repeated colonic wash-out with plain water, especially in cases of megacolon, which has much higher capacity of absorbing water than normal colon.
   c. Impaired water excretion by the kidneys, as in:
      i. Syndrome of inappropriate secretion of antidiuretic hormone (SIADH).
      ii. Antidiuretic hormone-secreting tumours e.g. oat cell carcinoma of bronchus.

EFFECTS.—The primary effect of pure water excess is hyponatraemia.The plasma sodium level falls (135 mEq/litre), thereby reducing the plasma osmolarity. Water is drawn into the extracellular space from the plasma and this water is finally pushed into the cells. The final event, therefore, is intracellular overhydration, i.e. cellular oedema. This causes impaired cellular function, followed by cell damage.

CLINICAL FEATURES:

1. The features of impaired cellular function are most predominant with the brain cells. Features depend on the absolute plasma sodium concentration and its rate of decline. Initially there is apathy, dizziness and headache. With plasma sodium level below 120 mEq/litre, there is confusion and drowsiness. With further decline (< 110 mEq/litre), convulsions and coma set in.
2. Plasma sodium level below 100 mEq/litre causes cardiac arrhythmias and ventricular fibrillation.
3. Nausea and vomiting are important presenting features.

PLASMA CHANGES:

1. The plasma level of all electrolytes falls progressively because of dilution.
2. There is also reduction in plasma protein level.
3. The packed cell volume is reduced.

TREATMENT.—This consists in stopping water intake and, possibly, nothing more. Cases with severe CNS features are treated with hypertonic (5 per cent) saline at a slow rate, with close electrolyte level monitoring. Patients of SIADH may be benefited by administration of demeclocycline, which antagonises the effect of ADH on the distal renal tubules.

Sodium Depletion, i.e. Hyponatraemia

Because of the intimate relationship between salt and water balance, loss of sodium is usually associated with a reduction in the water content of the body.

CAUSES:

1. *Pure sodium depletion,* unattended by significant water loss, occurs only rarely when the person is losing both salt and water and is replacing only water by drinking salt-free liquids, e.g. diarrhoea, profuse sweating and Addison's disease.
2. More commonly the depletion is *mixed,* i.e. sodium depletion is attended by some degree of water loss. The condition is commonly called *salt depletion* because sodium and chloride are usually lost in equal proportions. In surgical practice this is most commonly encountered in conditions where there is rapid loss of gastric, biliary, pancreatic or intestinal secretions, e.g.
   a. Small intestinal obstruction, where these secretions are either vomited or are sucked out (this is the commonest cause encountered in surgical practice).

b. Duodenal, biliary, pancreatic or intestinal external fistulae.

c. Paralytic ileus, where these secretions are sequestrated in the dilated loops of intestine.

EFFECTS.—The effect of salt depletion is a reduction in the volume of *extracellular fluid* without cellular dehydration (cf pure water depletion). This is because sodium is predominantly extracellular and its depletion quickly reduces the volume of extracellular fluids.

CLINICAL FEATURES:

1. Dehydration.—Mental and physical lassitude, associated with features of extracellular dehydration in the form of dry tongue, wrinkled skin, sunken eyes with drawn face and depressed fontanelle (in infants).

2. Thirst is *not* predominant (cf pure water depletion).

3. The blood pressure tends to fall and the pulse rate rises.

4. The urine is scanty and dark with a high specific gravity.

5. The capacity of the body to get rid of urea diminishes so that uraemia sets in. In both water depletion and salt depletion, because of increased adrenal activity, there is gross dilution in the urinary output of sodium and chloride, and abundant increase in the urinary output of potassium and nitrogen.

6. Cramps in legs and abdomen are features of sodium deficiency.

PLASMA CHANGES:

1. Raised level of plasma protein due to reduced plasma volume.

2. Raised packed cell volume for the same reason.

3. A fall in the sodium level as the condition progresses.

4. A gradual rise in the urea level.

TREATMENT.—Intravenous infusion of isotonic saline or Ringer's solution, 500 to 2,000 ml, depending on the severity of the case, the volume required being the volume lost. Overdosage, leading to oedema because of hypoproteinaemia is prevented by monitoring the plasma protein level.

Sodium Excess, i.e. Hypernatraemia

In surgical practice this is encountered if an early postoperative or post-traumatic patient is infused large amounts of isotonic saline. This happens from ignorance of what is called the *'sodium excretion shut-down of trauma'*. During this period, the length of which is directly proportional to the degree of tissue damage, there is practically no excretion of sodium (less than 10 mEq/day). This is because of increased adrenocortical activity. This depression in sodium excretion cannot be overcome by administration of sodium. Rather, sodium administration at this stage leads to sodium intoxication.

Slight puffiness of the face is seen in early cases. Advanced cases may show generalised oedema, especially in the sacral region.

Treatment consists in stopping the infusion.

Potassium Depletion, i.e. Hypokalaemia

A low serum potassium is almost always an indication of true potassium depletion but there may be occasions where the serum level of potassium is kept normal even when there is intracellular potassium deficit. It should further be noted that, following trauma (including operations), there is a period when there is an increased excretion of potassium by the kidneys (*augmented potassium excretion of trauma*). This loss is maximum in the first 24 hours and its duration is proportional to the degree of tissue damage, sometimes continuing for 3 to 4 days (as after partial gastrectomy). However, the body's potassium reserve is so great that there is usually no need to replace the potassium during this period.

CAUSES.—Some common causes of hypokalaemia are as follows:

1. In postoperative cases, particularly after gastrointestinal surgery, when the patient is kept on infusions of potassium-free fluids for more than 3 days. This is because of two reasons:
   a. The patients are in negative caloric balance. Muscle protein is used as a source of energy and both nitrogen and potassium are released from the cells. The potassium is excreted in the urine, i.e. the augmented postassium excretion of trauma:
   b. All the gastrointestinal fluids are rich in potassium and major part of these fluids are aspirated out by nasogastric suction.
2. Diarrhoea of ulcerative colitis and large villous tumours of the rectum, where huge quantities of potassium-rich fluids are lost.
3. External fistulae of the intestinal tract (for the same reason).
4. Alkalosis favours potassium depletion, chiefly by increasing its excretion in the urine.
5. *Sudden hypokalaemia*, rather rare, may occur in patients of diabetic coma being treated with insulin and in cases of prolonged infusion of saline solution.

CLINICAL FEATURES

1. Apathy, drowsiness, slurring of speech and confusion.
2. Muscular weakness, sometimes paralysis.
3. Abdominal distension and paralytic ileus.
4. Tachycardia, sometimes gallop rhythms.
5. Rapid and shallow respiration (because of weakness of respiratory muscles).

SPECIAL INVESTIGATIONS

1. Estimation of serum potassium. The normal value is 3.5 to 5.3 mEq/litre. False negative results may be obtained (see above).
2. ECG.—The difficulty in estimating the serum potassium repeatedly and the possibilities of false negative indications have made ECG a standard guide. The characteristic findings in hypokalaemia are:
   i. Small or inverted T wave.

ii. Depression of the ST segment.

iii. Prolonged QT interval

iv. Prominent U wave.

TREATMENT.—This consists in administration of potassium:

1. Oral potassium is the safest and should be preferred wherever possible. Meat extracts, milk, fruit juices and honey are rich in potassium. Liquid KCl may be given six-hourly.

2. Intravenous potassium administration is reserved only for patients in whom oral feeding is contraindicated. The difficulty of parenteral potassium administration is that, unless rigidly controlled, this may easily lead to hyperkalaemia and cardiac arrest. A safe dose is 1.5 g KCl added to 500 ml of 5 per cent glucose solution, administered over a period of 4 hours and repeated as per serum potassium and ECG studies. Potassium should never be given intravenously in a patient of anuria. Also, as has already been stated, it is useless to administer potassium during the first 2 days after operation when there is migration of potassium from the cells to the serum.

Potassium Excess, i.e. Hyperkalaemia

CAUSES.—This commonly occurs under two circumstances:

1. Renal failure with severe oliguria or anuria (because of potassium retention).

2. Overdosage of potassium, administered intravenously, while treating case of hypokalaemia without proper monitoring.

CLINICAL FEATURES.—These are paradoxically, similar to those of hypokalaemia. However, there may be an irregular pulse and bradycardia due to heart block of varying degrees. The real danger of hyperkalaemia is ventricular fibrillation which is apt to occur when the serum potassium level is above 7.5 mEq/litre.

SPECIAL INVESTIGATIONS:

1. Estimation of serum potassium repeatedly.

2. The ECG changes are noteworthy. The T wave is tall, so much so that it may exceed the QRS complex in amplitude. There are atrioventricular and intraventricular conduction defects and, ultimately, ventricular arrest.

TREATMENT:

1. Immediate restriction of foods rich in potassium (e.g. fruit juice).

2. Treatment for renal failure. This is the usual cause and should be treated most effectively.

3. Sodium- or calcium-loaded ionic exchange resins, when given orally, abstract potassium from blood and intestinal contents; 30 g, in a small amount of water, is given 4 times a day. If there is vomiting, the same may be given as retention enema.

4. Administration of glucose and insulin to hasten entry of potassium into the cells from the extracellular fluids.

5. Calcium gluconate (10 ml of 10 per cent solution), given intravenously reduces the cardiotoxic effects of potassium.

INTRAVENOUS FLUID INFUSION

Commonly Used Intravenous Fluids

A. CRYSTALLOID SOLUTIONS:

1. *Dextrose (5 per cent)*—This is an isotonic solution which provides water and calories. This is the fluid of choice during the first 24 hours after operation, when only water should be administered and electrolytes are unnecessary, rather undesirable.

2. *Isotonic saline.*—This is 0.9 per cent NaCl in water. One bottle (500 ml) of the solution meets the patient's daily sodium requirement.

3. *Dextrose saline.*—This is a combination of 4.5 per cent dextrose and 0.18 per cent NaCl. This is isotonic. There is another solution, 5 per pent dextrose in normal saline, which is hypertonic.

4. *Ringer's lactate solution.*—This solution contains sodium, potassium and chloride in almost equal concentrations as they are in the plasma (Na^+130, K^+4, and Cl^-10 mmol/litre). It is most commonly used as the starting fluid for hypovolaemic shock, till blood is available for transfusion. The small amount of lactate (28 mmol/litre) is converted into bicarbonate by the liver immediately and this combats the metabolic acidosis of tissue anoxia. Direct inclusion of sodium bicarbonate would make the solution unstable. Ringer's acetate solution serves the same prupose as the lactate solution.

5. *Darrow's solution.*—This solution is specifically used to combat hypokalaemia as it contains as much as 36 mEq of K^+ per litre. It is safe to administer this solution than adding potassium chloride ampoules to other solutions, in the matter of preventing hyperkalaemia. However, the rate of administration should be slow and it should not be used in presence of alkalosis.

B. COLLOID SOLUTIONS.—In contrast to crystalloid solutions, which being rapidly excreted by the kidneys, cannot maintain the blood volume, colloid solutions can replenish and maintain the lost blood volume for a considerable period because they are excreted only slowly. The bigger the molecule, the slower is the rate of excretion. As they are used to restore the plasma volume, these solutions are also called *plasma substitutes* or *plasma volume expanders*. Plasma itself, available as fresh frozen plasma (FFP), is not preferred because of the risk of transmitting diseases and because of its type-specificity (grouping and matching). The available plasma expanders are:

1. *Human albumin (4.5 per cent).*—Prepared from FFP, this is safe in respect of transmission of diseases and does not require matching. One to two litres may be administered. This is especially indicated in cases of burns.

2. *Dextrans.*—These are polysaccharide polymers. According to their molecular weight, they are divided into two categories:
   a. Low molecular weight.—Dextran 40, i.e. molecular weight 40,000.
   b. High molecular weight.— Dextran 70 and Dextran 110 (molecular weight 70,000 and 110,000 respectively).

   Dextran 40 restores the plasma volume immediately but its effect is short-lasting because of quicker excretion by the kidneys as compared to the high molecular weight dextrans, which are long-acting (but they are not so effective in immediate restoration of plasma volume). Use of dextran is associated with some disadvantages:
   i. There is rouleaux formation of the RBC, which makes grouping and cross-matching of subsquent blood samples difficult.
   ii. A bleeding diathesis may develop because of interference with platelet functions.
      Not more than 1000 ml of dextran should be administered.
3. *Gelatin.*—Use of degraded gelatin (molecular weight 30,000) has gained popularity in recent years. One litre of a 3.5 per cent solution may be infused safely.
4. *Hydroxyethyl starch* is sometimes used. Not more than one litre should be administered.

Compartmental Distribution of Infused Fluid

A. WATER WITH SODIUM.—All the infused sodium remains in the ECF as sodium cannot enter the cells because of the 'sodium pump'.
   1 . When isotonic (0.9 per cent) NaCl is infused, it does not change the osmolarity of the ECF. So there is no exchange of water between ECF and ICF and there is volume expansion of ECF only.
   2. When hypotonic (0.18 per cent) NaCl is administered, the ECF osmolarity falls. Though the sodium is restricted to the ECF, fluid shifts from the ECF to the ICF.
   3. When hypertonic (1.8 per cent) NaCl is infused, the ECF osmolarity rises and fluid shifts from ICF to ECF, though the sodium is retained in the ECF.
B. WATER WITHOUT SODIUM.—Such fluids as 5 per cent glucose expands the total body water. Glucose enters the cells and is metabolised there to produce water and carbon dioxide. This water, together with the water in the solution, is redistributed to both ECF and ICF according to their natural proportion, i.e. ECF:ICF = 1:2.
C. COLLOID SOLUTION.—Colloid substances cannot pass through the capillary endothelium. They exert osmotic pressure to draw fluid into the intravascular compartment from the interstitial space.

When a fluid, containing electrolytes, is restricted to the ECF volume, it gets distributed between the two subdivisions of the ECF space, i.e. intravascular and interstitial, according to their natural proportion, i.e. intravascular:interstitial = 1:3.

Hence, in order to compensate for intravascular volume loss, if an electrolyte solution is used, its volume should be four times the estimated loss. But if a colloid solution is used, the lost volume can be replenished by just an equal volume of colloid solution.

Control of Flow of Intravenous Drip.—With an average PVC infusion set, 15 drops equals 1 ml. One litre of fluid can be infused:
1. In 8 hours if the rate is 30 drops per minute.
2. In 6 hours if the rate is 45 drops per minute.
3. In 4 hours if the rate is 60 drops per minute.

This is the usual maximum rate. A rate of up to 100 drops may be necessary in severely depleted patients but this rate should be cut down to 60 per minute after one hour.

Continuous intravenous infusion is also called *venoclysis*.

PERI-OPERATIVE FLUID AND ELECTROLYTE REGIME

This is usually required in cases of abdominal operations, where oral feeding has to be suspended for more than 24 hours and, often, nasogastric suction has to be employed. Oral feeding is commenced as soon as peristaltic sounds are audible.

The quantity of water and electrolytes to be administered is based on the following factors:
1. The daily maintenance need of a normal subject.
2. Pre-operative deficits.
3. Intra-operative loss.
4. Postoperative requirements in the first, second, third, and subsequent days.

Daily Maintenance Need.—An average normal adult needs:
1. Water: 2500 ml, which may be administered as 5 per cent dextrose.
2. Sodium: 100 mEq, which can be provided by a little more than 500 ml (one bottle) of isotonic saline.
3. Potassium: 65 to 75 mEq. This may be supplied by potassium chloride ampoules added to the infusion fluids (1 g potassium chloride provides 13 mEq of K^+).

The above schedule can be maintained by:
   a. either, 2000 ml (4 bottles) of 5 per cent dextrose + 500 ml (one bottle) isotonic saline + 1 g of KCl per each bottle of above solutions.
   b. or, 2500 ml (5 bottles) of 4.5 per cent dextrose with 0.18 per cent sodium chloride + 1 g of KCl per each bottle.

Pre-operative Deficits.—Losses may be due to vomiting, leakage from intestinal fistulae, or sequestration in the gut lumen and wall in intestinal obstruction (paralytic or mechanical). It is difficult to estimate the loss and close clinical observation and laboratory readings are necessary. Whenever possible, if time permits, these losses should be compensated pre-operatively since hypotension may promptly develop during induction of anaesthesia. If this cannot be done, the quantities of intra-operative and postoperative infusion have to be increased accordingly.

Intra-operative Loss.—There is either blood loss or loss of extracellular fluid in the form of what is termed as *third space loss* or *parasitic loss*. This is better called *sequestration of extracellular fluid* because fluid is not lost externally. It may be due to:

1. Oedema from extensive dissection.
2. Accumulation of fluid in the peritoneal cavity.
3. Accumulation of fluid in the wall and lumen of the gut.
4. Collection of fluid in the wound itself.

The first three of these are more or less assessable but the last, though usually small in volume, is very difficult to measure. Sometimes, this may be considerable, to the extent of 3 to 5 ml/kg/hour. This fluid is reabsorbed in the system after about 72 hours.

Intraoperative blood loss of more than 500 ml must be replaced by the same volume of blood during the operation. Loss below this quantity may be replaced by fluids like Ringer's lactate or isotonic saline, 0.5 ml to 1 ml per hour.

Post-operative Requirements

1. FIRST 24 HOURS.—During this period, due to increased secretion of ADH and aldosterone following trauma, there is retention of water and sodium in the system. So, the patient will require less water than daily requirement and no sodium. Also, exit of potassium from the injured tissues into serum makes administration of potassium unadvisable. Just two litres (4 bottles) of 5 per cent dextrose is sufficient for this period.

2. SECOND 24 HOURS.—The response to trauma diminishes. So, sodium and more water have to be provided—2 litres of 5 per cent dextrose and 0.5 to 1 litre of isotonic saline are advocated. No potassium is necessary even now.

3. THIRD 24 HOURS AND SUBSEQUENTLY.—Potassium is necessary towards the later part of the third 24 hours (otherwise paralytic ileus may set in). In 24 hours 65 to 75 mEq is necessary. Potassium chloride, 1 g (K^+ 13 mEq) ampoule, is inserted into each bottle of transfused fluid (total 5 bottles). Darrow's solution may be used instead (each litre provides 36 mEq K^+).

The above postoperative schedule may have to be modified:

1. To make for uncompensated pre-operative and intra-operative deficits.
2. High abnormal postoperative losses, e.g.
   a. gastroduodenal suction,
   b. exit from drainage site,
   c. sweating,
   d. fever (insensible loss increases by 12 per cent for each degree of rise in temperature).

3

Acid–Base Balance and its Disturbances

NORMAL ACID–BASE BALANCE

Life can continue only if the blood is kept within a range of alkalinity. In health, the physiological hydrogen ion concentration, i.e. pH, lies between 7.36 and 7.44, with a mean value of 7.4. The blood is alkaline because it contains strong bases like bicarbonate and phosphate, of which the bicarbonate is more important. Blood also contains acids like carbonic acid, acetoacetic acid and sulphuric acid, of which carbonic acid is the most important. In health, the balance between the acids and the bases is so maintained that the pH is kept at an average of 7.4. Further simplified, in order to keep the pH at 7.4, the ratio between carbonic acid (the chief acid) and bicarbonate (the chief base) must be kept constant, and this ratio is 1:20.

Plasma protein and ammonia deserve special mention as acids. The equations $NH_4 \rightleftharpoons NH_3 + H^+$ and H proteinate $\rightleftharpoons$ protein $+ H^+$ indicate that ammonia ions and plasma proteins act as acids because they are hydrogen donors.

The bases, viz. bicarbonate and phosphate, are conserved in the system by the renal tubular epithelium. This is essential because metabolism, on the whole, has a tendency to produce acids and these have to be balanced by the bases. However, the production of acid is so huge that these must be excreted out of the body. The bases are meant only to maintain the alkalinity of the blood till such time that these excess acids are excreted, that is only for that period when the acids, produced in the tissues, are carried in the blood to their sites of excretion. The routes of excretion are the lungs and the kidneys. By which of these two routes the acid will be excreted depends on whether or not the acid is capable of being oxidised completely to carbon dioxide (CO_2) and water. If it can, the route of excretion is the lung, by ventilation of the CO_2. Carbonic acid (H_2CO_3) is an acid of this type and this is the chief acid of the system. There is a continuous influx of CO_2 from the tissues because oxidation of all the components, viz. protein, carbohydrate and fat, gives rise principally to CO_2. This CO_2 is immediately mixed up with water to form carbonic acid ($CO_2 + H_2O = H_2CO_3$). Hence, H_2CO_3 is introduced into the blood in much more quantities than any other acid. However, metabolic processes may produce some non-volatile acids and these are excreted by the kidneys, e.g. uric acid from purines, sulphuric acid from sulphur-containing proteins (cystine, methionine), lactic acid from muscles (contracting anaerobically) and acetoacetic acid from fat (during starvation).

It may therefore be said that while the lungs and the kidneys must function properly to excrete this huge quantity of acids, the reaction of the blood has to be stabilised by some means when these acids, are being carried in the blood from their site of origin in the tissues to the lungs or the kidneys. Physiologically important buffer systems do exist in the blood in order to achieve this, and there are buffers both in the plasma and in the red blood cells.

The buffers in the plasma are weak acids paired with their sodium salts:

1. Carbonic acid and sodium bicarbonate—the *strongest* buffer pair.
2. Plasma protein and sodium proteinate.
3. Sodium dihydrogen phosphate (NaH_2PO_4) and sodium hydrogen phosphate (Na_2HPO_4).

The buffer activity in the red blood cells is carried out by the haemoglobin:

1. The haemoglobin in the venous blood is a weaker acid than oxyhaemoglobin of the arterial blood. In the tissues, haemoglobin (the weaker acid) can bear an excess load of acid, i.e. H_2CO_3 derived from the influx of CO_2 in the tissues. In the lungs, as haemoglobin is changed to oxyhaemoglobin (the stronger acid), it repels the excess of H_2CO_3, which is excreted as CO_2 by ventilation.
2. A small amount of CO_2 is transported from the tissues as a carbamino compound, reversibly bound to haemoglobin. This bond is detached in the lungs, wherefrom the CO_2 is excreted.

DISTURBANCES IN ACID–BASE BALANCE

The terms 'acidosis' and 'alkalosis' are used conventionally as synonyms of *acidaemia* and *alkalaemia (basaemia)* respectively. Gain or loss in the form of H_2CO_3 is described as 'respiratory acidosis' or 'respiratory alkalosis' respectively. Otherwise gain or loss of hydrogen ion is called 'metabolic acidosis' or 'metabolic alkalosis' respectively.

Any such disturbance passes through two phases:

1. The initial physicochemical or 'uncompensated' phase.
2. The secondary physiological or 'compensated' phase.

Methods of Measuring Acid–Base Disturbances.—The *Astrup apparatus* is extremely helpful in measuring the acid–base disturbances in clinical practice. It is helpful in rapidly calculating the following:

1. *Blood pH.*
2. *$PaCO_2$,* i.e. the tension or partial pressure of CO_2 in the blood. The normal *arterial* $PaCO_2$ is 31–42 mmHg.
3. *Standard bicarbonate,* i.e. the concentration of plasma bicarbonate after *fully oxygenated* blood has been equilibrated with CO_2 at 40 mmHg at 38°C. Simple estimation of plasma bicarbonate is only of limited value since, although the level is raised in metabolic acidosis and diminished in metabolic alkalosis, the actual degree of such acidosis or alkalosis is not indicated because the

bicarbonate level is also influenced to some degree by respiratory function (in respiratory alkalosis the bicarbonate is reduced and in respiratory acidosis it is increased). This is because the bicarbonate level is itself influenced by the H_2CO_3 level. Hence, if the blood is allowed to be equilibrated with CO_2, the respiratory causes and respiratory compensation of the ordinary bicarbonate level is eliminated, and the standard bicarbonate level is obtained. *The standard bicarbonate, therefore, is a true index of acidosis or alkalosis of metabolic origin.*

While it is easy to know the H_2CO_3 status simply by measuring the $PaCO_2$, there is no entirely satisfactory method of determining the bicarbonate level. It is calculated by using the popular Henderson-Hasselbalch equation:

$$pH = pK + \log \frac{HCO_3^-}{H_2CO_3}$$

The term pK is defined as the 'dissociation constant' of H_2CO_3. Though stated as constant, it rises with temperature—at 38°C it is 6.1, and at lower temperature its value is reduced.

The H_2CO_3 concentration, at body temperature is the product of $PaCO_2$ and the 'solubility coefficient', which is 0.30.

Thus the above equation comes to:

$$pH = pK + \log \frac{HCO_3^-}{\alpha PaCO_2}, \alpha \text{ denoting the solubility coefficient.}$$

As pK is constant, if the pH and $PaCO_2$ are known, the HCO_3^- (standard bicarbonate) is calculated out.

The *normal standard bicarbonate level* is 22–25 mEq/litre, and as has been stressed, it is altered only in *metabolic* acidosis and alkalosis.

4. *Base excess or base deficit.*—This is another index of metabolic alkalosis or acidosis. It denotes the total buffer ions present in blood, either in excess or deficit of normal. The normal mean is zero and the normal range is – 2.5 to + 2.5 mEq/litre. Alteration beyond these levels is excess or deficit. If this value is multiplied by 0.3 times the body weight (kg), the total extracellular base excess or base deficit of the body may be obtained.

From the discussions above, it may be summarised that pH indicates the acid–base status of body unqualified. Respiratory causes of disturbance in acid–base balance are indicated by changes in $PaCO_2$. Metabolic causes of such disturbances are indicated by standard bicarbonate level and base excess or deficit.

Respiratory Acidosis.—This occurs if CO_2, and consequently H_2CO_3, accumulates in the blood. In surgical practice this is encountered if there is inadequate ventilation during anaesthesia or if there is reinhalation of CO_2 from a faulty breathing circuit. Failure to reverse the effects of muscle relaxants at the end of an operation may also cause accumulation of CO_2. Depression of the respiratory centre by overdosage of morphine or other respiratory depressants may be the cause of acidosis (because of inefficient ventilation). Pre-existing lung lesions, e.g. pneumonia, emphysema, bronchitis, etc. enhance the risk of postoperative acidosis. This risk is further enhanced if a thoracic or upper abdominal incision is made because the patient prefers shallow respirations after the operation for fear of pain.

COMPENSATION.—Compensation for respiratory acidosis is brought about by the kidney. There is (a) increased tubular reabsorption of bicarbonate, and (b) increased excretion of hydrogen ion in the form of dihydrogen phosphate and ammonium salts. The ratio of carbonic acid to bicarbonate is thus restored to 1: 20 status, which is required to maintain the normal pH of blood.

TREATMENT.—*See* under metabolic acidosis.

Metabolic Acidosis.—This may occur in two ways:

1. Accumulation of acids in the system:
    a. If there is gross hypoxia, as in cases of severe shock. Tissue hypoxia results in accumulation of lactic acid and pyruvic acid due to anaerobic tissue metabolism. An extreme degree of such acidosis occurs in cases of cardiac arrest.
    b. If there is gross renal insufficiency resulting in retention of acid metabolites.
    c. Hyperchloraemic acidosis may occur in patients of ureterocolic anastomosis due to absorption of the urine by the colon.
    d. Formation of ketoacids in uncontrolled diabetes or in starvation.

2. Loss of bases from the system:
    a. Excessive loss of intestinal fluids, particularly from the small intestine, e.g. sustained diarrhoea, ulcerative colitis.
    b. Loss from small intestinal fistula, biliary or pancreatic fistula.
    c. Loss from prolonged *intestinal* aspiration.

COMPENSATION.—Compensation for metabolic acidosis is brought about both by the lung (*rapidly*) and the kidney (*slowly*):

1. Lung.—There is an increased rate of excretion of CO_2 by hyperventilation. Hyperpnoea is, therefore, a clinical sign of metabolic acidosis.

2. Kidney.—The excreted urine is highly acid—(a) the excretion of bicarbonate is stopped because of increased tubular reabsorption, and (b) there is an increased hydrogen ion excretion in the form of dihydrogen phosphate and ammonium salts (as in respiratory acidosis).

The natural aim is to bring the carbonic acid-bicarbonate ratio to 1: 20 in order to maintain the normal pH of blood.

TREATMENT OF ACIDOTIC STATES.—This primarily aims at eliminating the underlying cause. However, as an adjunctive immediate measure, alkaline solutions may be administered intravenously. Usually 8.4 per cent solution of sodium bicarbonate is used. A patient weighing 70 kg, having a base excess of –10 mEq/litre should get $10 \times 0.3 \times 70 = 210$ ml of the solution.

Respiratory Alkalosis.—This is rather unusual in clinical practice. It may be due to:
1. Excessive pulmonary ventilation in an anaesthetised patient who has received excess of muscle relaxants. Respiratory arrest may occur in extreme cases.
2. Hyperventilation due to hysteric states or at high altitude.

COMPENSATION.—Compensation is brought about by the kidney. The urine excreted is alkaline because (a) there is increased excretion of bicarbonate, and (b) diminished excretion of dihydrogen phosphate and no excretion of ammonium salts.

TREATMENT.—If there is respiratory arrest, CO_2 insufflation is instituted.

Metabolic Alkalosis.—There is either a base excess or a deficit of an acid other than H_2CO_3. This may be caused by:
1. Ingestion of excess of absorbable alkali, e.g. sodium bicarbonate.
2. Loss of acid from the stomach either due to repeated vomiting or gastric aspiration.
3. Excess of cortisone, either iatrogenic or due to Cushing's syndrome.

A combination of the first two factors is typically seen in a patient of pyloric stenosis. The term typically applied to these cases is *hypokalaemic alkalosis*. Due to repeated vomiting there is loss of potassium and acid. The serum (extracellular) potassium level falls. Intracellular potassium leaves the cells, and Na^+ and H^+ enter the cells. This shift of H^+ causes intracellular acidosis and extracellular alkalosis. The kidneys continue to excrete K^+. Also, the urine is acid because of the intracellular acidosis of the renal cells themselves (cf respiratory alkalosis, where the urine is alkaline).

The most striking *clinical feature* of metabolic alkalosis is Cheyne-Stokes' respiration. Tetany sometimes occurs.

COMPENSATION.—Compensation of metabolic alkalosis is achieved, both by the lung (*rapidly*) and the kidney (*slowly*):
1. Lung.—The rate of CO_2 excretion is lowered by slow and shallow respiration,
2. Kidney:
   a. There is increased excretion of bicarbonate.
   b. There is diminished excretion of dihydrogen phosphate and no excretion of ammonium salts.

TREATMENT:
1. Metabolic alkalosis without hypokalaemia requires no active treatment except removal of the cause and encouraging high urinary output.
2. If there is hypokalaemic alkalosis an infusion of 20 mEq of potassium chloride added to 500 ml of 5 per cent dextrose solution is given. A 10 ml ampoule of 15 per cent potassium chloride provides this amount.

4

Healing of Wounds

Terminology.—Two terms, viz. regeneration and repair are commonly used to describe the natural attempts effected to restore the structure and function of damaged tissues:

1. REGENERATION.—In human pathology, this term is used when dead or damaged cells are replaced by cells of the *same structure and function*. Human beings, during the course of evolution, have lost a valuable mechanism—the ability to regenerate *compound tissues* (cf axial regeneration of limbs in the amphibians and other lower species). *Cellular regeneration,* however, does occur in man:

    a. *Physiological regeneration.*—In some tissues aged cells are constantly shed and are replaced by new cells. Examples are the surface epithelium, blood cells, endometrium of the uterus, etc.

    b. *Reparative regeneration.*—Damaged cells are replaced by cells of the same structure and function. In human beings this is limited only to the epithelium and the liver cells.

2. REPAIR.—This term indicates replacement of lost tissue by granulation tissue, which later matures to form scar tissue. This is a far less valuable process than regeneration because the new tissue is devoid of the functions of lost tissue.

    The process of healing is functionally the same in all wounds but there are marked quantitative differences depending on the amount of tissue destruction. From this point of view it is convenient to consider wound healing under two headings:

1. *Healing by First Intention or Primary Union.*—This occurs in cases of clean incised wounds or when the wound margins have been apposed by immediate (primary) suture. The healing is quick and the scar minimum.

2. *Healing by Secondary Intention or Secondary Union.*—This happens when there is a gap between the margins either because of tissue destruction (due to the trauma or infection) or because the wound margins have not been apposed by suturing. A good quantity of new tissue has to grow. So the process is much slower and the amount of scar proportionately high.

Essential Components of Healing.—Whatever be the nature of the wound, there are four components in the process of healing:

1. Traumatic inflammation and dead tissue demolition.
2. Wound contraction, which reduces the size of the wound.
3. Epithelisation, which covers the surface of the wound.
4. Connective tissue formation, which fills the gap in the wound.

Traumatic Inflammation and Dead Tissue Demolition.—A process of controlled inflammation starts instantaneously after the trauma. Following a transient phase of vasoconstriction, all small vessels dilate and the capillary permeability increases under the influence of histamine liberated locally. Plasma and white blood cells escape into the site of injury. In a few hours, the wound space is filled with an inflammatory exudate consisting of red and white blood cells, plasma proteins and strands of interlacing fibrin (fibrin clot). The WBCs begin engulfing the cellular debris and injured tissue fragments. To start with, the polymorphonuclear leucocytes predominate but there is also a good number of monocytes. However, the short-living polymorphs die and lyse soon, so that the proportion of monocytes increases considerably by the fifth day. They are highly phagocytic (macrophages) and they ingest the tissue debris.

Wound Contraction.—There is always a mechanical reduction in the size of the defect. The process of contraction is slow for first 2 to 3 days (*the lag period*) but this is followed by a period of rapid contraction. Contraction is mostly completed by 14 days. The wound is reduced to about one-fourth its original size.

BENEFICIAL EFFECTS:
1. The time for healing is much shortened since only about one-fourth of the original amount of destroyed tissue has to be repaired.
2. The scar is smaller in size and this has both cosmetic and functional values.

ILL EFFECTS.—Contraction may lead to contracture and this may interfere with both cosmesis and function.

ASSESSMENT:
1. The end-result of wound contraction may be reasonably predicted by simply grasping the edges of a gaping wound and manually apposing them. The deformity and/or limitation of movements of neighbouring joint or joints, if any, manifested by such manoeuvre, are exactly the ones that will result from wound contraction.
2. If it is not possible to coapt the wound edges as described above, it is certain that the natural process will also fail to effect healing. A gap will persist in the form of an open granulating wound.

CAUSE.—The mechanism of wound contraction and the factors responsible for it are not definitely known. Majority of the workers believe that contraction occurs in the granulation tissue of the wound. However, the central mass of granulation tissue takes no share in wound contraction. The granulation tissue at the margins of the wound is believed to be the actual site of the contracting mechanism. This is a very limited zone of tissue just underneath the advancing dermal edges and is popularly known as the '*picture frame area*'. This granulation tissue is believed to contain a special type of fibroblasts. These fibroblasts have fibrillar components in their cytoplasm, resembling those found in smooth-muscle cells. Hence they are named 'myofibroblasts'. It is believed that these cells can exert migratory force of a magnitude necessary to mobilise the skin edges to effect the wound contraction.

INHIBITING FACTORS:

1. Contraction does not proceed normally in burn wounds.
2. Radiated wounds show delayed contraction.
3. Immediate skin grafting prevents wound contraction. Skin grafting during the course of healing of wound also stops the process of contraction. This is the basis of skin grafting in preventing occurrence of contracture. To achieve this, however, the graft must contain dermis.

Epithelisation—Within 24 hours of the injury, epithelial cells from the adjacent epidermis migrate and proliferate into the wound in an attempt to cover it:

1. MIGRATION.—There is active migration of sheets of cells from the epidermis just at the edge of the wound.
2. PROLIFERATION.—There is active mitosis in the basal layers of the epidermis at a little distance from the edge of the wound.

The exact mode of epithelisation varies according to the nature of the wound:

a. In a clean incised or a well-approximated wound, the epithelium, while proliferating and migrating into the wound, passes between the inert dermis and the accumulated blood clot. In 24 hours a continuous layer of epithelium makes a watertight cover for the whole wound surface overlying which there is a crust (the dried clot). During the next 24 hours the epithelial cells grow down the crevices of the wound so that the centre of the wound remains a little inverted. Connective tissue, growing inside the wound, subsequently pushes the epithelium back to the everted position. The regenerated ephithelium divides and differentiates, so that a multilayered strong epidermis is formed.

b. In wounds with edges separated, i.e. with tissue destruction, epithelium migrates and proliferates from all the edges. It proceeds below the clot, which has now dried to form a crust. The new epithelium not only passes below the crust but it also cuts through the fibrinous and fibrous tissue, now growing underneath. The epithelium multiplies and differentiates into multilayered epidermis. Whether the whole surface of the wound can be covered by epithelium (even after wound contraction) depends on the magnitude of the gap. Sometimes an area at the centre is left devoid of epithelium (with exposed granulation tissue) or is covered only by a thin layer of epithelium, the cells of which never multiply and differentiate to produce a multilayered epidermis and are damaged even by minor trauma.

Connective Tissue Formation.—This is a long-standing and complicated process and may be conveniently divided into four phases, as described below:

1. PHASE OF GRANULATION TISSUE FORMATION.—The capillaries at the base and sides of the wound put forth solid buds of endothelium, which grow into the fibrin clot. These buds unite with one another, become canalised and get filled with blood,

thereby forming a network of new *capillaries*. Simultaneously, connective tissue cells proliferate from the sides and base of the wound itself. These proliferating cells assume special characters and are called *fibroblasts*. These fibroblasts are embryonic in type, i.e. active, as compared to the resting adult fibrocytes. They support the capillaries. The fibroblasts and the capillaries (i.e. the granulation tissue) grow very rapidly and tend to fill up the cavity of the wound. The wound surface assumes a velvety appearance.

2. PHASE OF SYNTHESIS OF COLLAGEN AND GROUND SUBSTANCE.—The specially designed fibroblasts in the granulation tissue start synthesizing, from the fifth day, two very important substances and these are extruded outside the fibroblasts into the extracellular matrix:

   a. Collagen
   b. Ground substance

Collagen is a polypeptide and its two important amino acid components are hydroxyproline and hydroxylysine. The newly secreted collagen is soluble and it polymerises into fibrils. The collagen fibrils are laid down around the fibroblasts themselves. These fibrils, though soft and friable, are weaved in such a way that they give not only strength to the wound but also a fair amount of elasticity.

Ground substance liberated by the fibroblasts is believed to provide cementing action in the newly-growing tissue. It contains acid mucopolysaccharides, which are broadly divided into non-sulphated and sulphated groups. The non-sulphated group is the main component of the gel fraction of the ground substance while the sulphated group is closely associated with the fibrillar elements of connective tissue.

Although chemical linkages between the collagen and the mucopolysaccharides of the ground substance have not been established, chemical bonds must exist between the two and these may be of great importance in the development of strength and orientation of the collagen fibrils.

3. PHASE OF MATURATION AND SCAR FORMATION.—Three important changes now occur:

   a. The soft and friable collagen fibrils are converted into insoluble elastic fibres (fibrocollagen) by the chemical conversion of protocollagen to tropocollagen. The fibres are arranged in such a pattern that the tissue gains a great degree of mechanical strength.
   b. The active embryonic fibroblasts mature and get converted into adult resting fibrocytes.
   c. There is a phase of devascularization as the capillaries diminish in size and number.

This is how a pale avascular but strong scar is produced.

Strength of the Wound.—Two terms are in use to signify the strength.

Tensile strength denotes the strength necessary to rupture a unit of the wound while *burst strength* represents the load required to break the wound, regardless of its dimensions.

For the initial five days the strength of the wound is provided by the new blood vessels growing across the wound, the newly growing epithelial tissue and the adhesion of globular protein. The strength gained by this time is just sufficient to hold the wound edges together if they have been coapted and there is no tension.

The real gain in the strength of the wound starts with the collagen synthesis from the fifth day, increases rapidly for the next 17 days and, thereafter, slowly for another 10 days, proportionately with the amount of collagen synthesis. However, even long after this period, the strength of the wound continues to increase and this is believed to be due to cross-linkages between the collagen fibres. After the forty-second day there is no increase in the collagen content of the wound though collagen synthesis continues for many weeks thereafter, so there must be some device of proportionate collagen breakdown and removal. Presumably, this is effected by *collagenases.*

Factors Affecting Wound Healing.—Apart from the extent and depth of the injury, which are the sole factors in determining how long a wound will take to heal, there are various factors, local and systemic, which influence the rate of healing of a wound.

A. Local factors:

1. *Disposition.*—Skin wounds made in a direction parallel to the lines of Langer heal faster than those made at right angles to the lines. These tension lines of Langer are due to arrangement of collagen bundles in the dermis, the skin is less stretchable along the lines than across them. So, if skin incisions are made across these lines, they tend to gape and healing is delayed.

2. *Vascularity.*—The greater the *vascularity,* the quicker is the healing; Examples are wound of tongue, mouth, face and scalp. Wounds at sites having precarious blood supply (ischaemic limbs, irradiated tissues) show great delay or even failure in healing.

3. *Lymph and Venous Drainage.*—Impairment of lymphatic and venous drainage hampers the process of healing. Oedematous tissues are slow to heal. Elevation of wounded limbs greatly facilitates healing.

4. *Necrosis.*—Necrosis at the wound margin (due to trauma, lack of vascularity, tight suturing or infection) retards healing. This is because the 'phase of demolition' is unduly prolonged.

5. *Foreign Bodies.*—All foreign bodies induce tissue reaction which may vary from minimal inflammation to suppuration. This persists till the foreign body is extruded, removed or absorbed. The phase of granulation tissue formation cannot start till the tissue reaction ceases. *Suture materials* may be acting as foreign bodies, and in this respect catgut is the worst offender. The protein of the catgut initiates foreign body reaction, which antagonises collagen deposition. It is only

after catgut has been absorbed then only the collagen synthesis can progress smoothly. *Antiseptic materials,* particularly if strong, delay healing because of tissue damage caused by them.

6. *Infection.*—This is the *most important singular factor* that delays healing. As long as the process of destruction and active inflammation persists, granulation tissue cannot start forming. The fibroblasts have to compete with the bacteria and inflammatory cells for nutrition. Collagen synthesis is reduced and collagen breakdown is increased. The fibrous structure of non-absorbable sutures provide nidus for bacterial growth.

7. *Movements.*—While early mobilisation is desirable, but failure to provide rest to the wounded area retards healing. Movements damage the newly growing granulation tissue and epithelium. *Frequent change of dressings* (particularly dry dressings) may also have the same effect.

8. *Anchorage.*—Fixity to underlying structures impairs wound contraction and, therefore, healing (*see* wound contraction).

9. *Radiation.*—Radiated tissues heal very slowly, if at all.

B. SYSTEMIC FACTORS:

1. *Age.*—Wounds in young people heal quicker than those in the elderly. This is possibly because of a combination of factors, e.g. blood supply, nutrition and physiological tone.

2. *Nutrition:*
   a. Protein.—A high level of protein is necessary to facilitate wound healing. This is because of the following factors:
      i. All proliferating cells, concerned in healing, demand protein.
      ii. Collagen, which is the mainstay in wound healing, is actually a polypeptide, its chief amino acids being hydroxyproline and hydroxylysine. Hence, its formation requires supply of protein.
      iii. The protein loss of the catabolic phase, has to be made for sulphur-containing amino acids, e.g. methionine, are especially important as they are essential for synthesis of new protein.

   b. Vitamins:
      i. Vitamin C is essential for hydroxylation of proline and lysine to hydroxyproline and hydroxylysine and therefore, for wound healing. Failure of healing of wounds in patients of scurvy is well known due to vitamin C deficiency.
      ii. Vitamin A is essential for epithelisation.
      iii. Vitamin D is important for new bone formation.

   c. Minerals:
      i. Zinc is an essential component of many enzymes and also a cofactor in the enzyme systems involved in protein synthesis. Zinc deficiency inhibits healing, e.g. burns, intestinal fistulae.
      ii. Calcium, manganese, magnesium and copper are also important for wound healing.

3. *Diseases:*
   a. Anaemia.—If severe, adversely affects healing of wounds.
   b. Uraemia.—Clinically, wound healing is inhibited in uraemic patients. This is possibly due to inhibition of growth of the fibroblasts.
   c. Jaundice.—There is delay in formation of new vessels of the granulation tissue and also appearance of fibroblasts in the wound.
   d. Diabetes.—Sugar-laden tissues favour infection. Also the arteriosclerosis, associated with diabetes, causes lack of vascularity.

4. *Steroids.*—As traumatic inflammation is essential to start healing of wounds and as steroids have an anti-inflammatory action, their use retards healing of wounds. However, this is believed to occur only with their prolonged use in high dosage.

5. *Cytotoxic Drugs* retard healing of wounds.

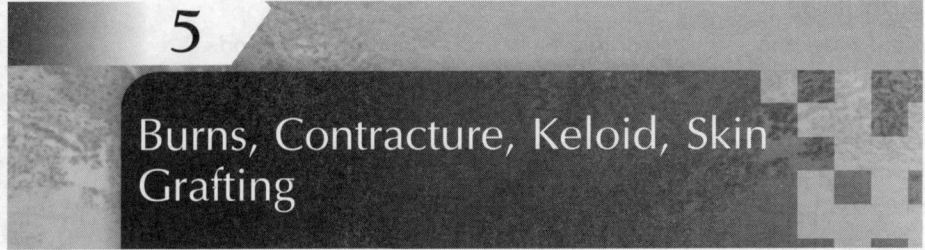

5

Burns, Contracture, Keloid, Skin Grafting

BURNS

Burns are caused by dry heat, mostly flames (ignition of clothings, house-fire) and hot metals.

Scalds result from moist heat, e.g. hot liquids or steam.

Electric burns are clinically evident at the point of entry and exit, the latter being more severe. The skin offers maximum resistance and, therefore, the visible burns are minimum. However, all tissues through which a high-voltage current passes are likely to be grossly damaged, e.g. nerves, vessels and muscles. Extensive muscle destruction causes release of haemochromogens which are excreted in the urine, giving it a typical 'port-wine' colour. There may be renal failure due to blockage of the tubules by myoglobin.

Chemical burns are caused by acids or alkalies. Initially they appear to be superficial, just as mild bronze discolouration of the skin. However, the burn is usually very deep and this is recognisable only after the slough separates. Immediate washing with water may minimise tissue destruction.

Radiation burns may be acute, subacute or chronic. Acute burns initially look superficial, like erythema. Ultimately they become quite deep, though slowly.

Pathology and Prognosis.—The chief problems in a patient with major thermal injury are:

1. The severe shock, mostly due to hypovolaemia.
2. The vast raw area that demands control of infection and skin coverage.

The magnitude of these problems is decided mainly by two factors:

1. The extent (surface area) of the burn.
2. The depth of the burn.

1. THE EXTENT OF THE BURN.—The area of body surface burnt is the major singular factor in deciding the immediate fate of the patient since this has a direct relationship with the severity of the shock. This is because of the highly important microvascular changes that occur at the site of the burn:

    a. There is dilatation of the vessels of the microcirculation, i.e. small arterioles, capillaries and venules.

    b. There is an increased capillary permeability, caused by various substances liberated at the site of the burn:

        i. by damaged tissues—histamine;

ii. by activation of coagulation system—complement, kinins;

iii. by activation of leucocytes and platelets—interleukin, kinins, histamine.

These microvascular changes allow escape of fluids and protein (plasma) from the intravascular compartment causing a sharp fall in the blood volume, i.e. hypovolaemic shock. This volume-loss is in direct proportion to the surface area of the burn.

For clinical purpose, the surface area of burn is estimated by *Wallace's 'Rule of Nine'*:

Head, neck and face	9 per cent
Front of trunk	18 per cent (9 × 2)
Back of trunk	18 per cent (9 × 2)
Upper limb (each)	9 per cent
Lower limb (each)	18 per cent (9 × 2)
External genitalia	1 per cent

In infants and children below 15 years, this proportion does not apply and estimation is guided by burn charts detailing site and age. Scattered burns are totalled by the *'palm of hand' rule*—the area of the patient's palm is taken as one per cent of burn.

2. THE DEPTH OF THE BURN.—This is especially important in determining the manner of healing. From this point of view, burns may be of two grades:

a. *Partial Thickness (Superficial) Burn.*—Only the superficial layer of the skin is involved (epidermis, with or without the superficial part of the dermis). Underneath the burnt tissues, there is sufficient amount of living epithelial element in the hair follicles, sweat glands and sebaceous glands, located at the depth of the dermis. This epithelium proliferates and gives a complete epithelial covering to the burnt surface. Thus spontaneous healing is expected.

b. *Full Thickness (Deep) Burn.*—The whole thickness of the skin, including the depth of the dermis, is injured. So, all local epithelial elements are destroyed and spontaneous epithelisation is impossible. Skin grafting is essential for healing.

Partial thickness burns usually appear red and moist (with blisters) while full thickness injuries are white and dry. Confirmation is sometimes made by *the pin prick test.* If, on firmly pressing a needle over the burnt surface, the patient can feel its tip, the burn is partial thickness because the nerve endings are intact.

Factors Worsening Prognosis

1. *Age.*—Patients at extremes of age (below 10 and above 50 years) tolerate bums poorly.

2. *Site.*—Burns of head, neck, face and external genitalia cause disproportionately severe shock. Burns on joint surfaces result in restricted movements and contractures.

3. *Associated Injuries and Pre-existing Illness*, e.g. renal, cardiovascular and metabolic (diabetes), worsen prognosis.

Causes of Shock in Burns

1. *Hypovolaemic Shock.*—This is the major cause.
2. *Psychogenic Shock* from the fright of burning and the severe pain. Superficial burns are more painful because of exposure of the intact nerve endings.
3. *Septic Shock.*—Next to hypovolaemic shock, this is the commonest cause of death. This usually occurs during the second and third weeks and is due to severe infection of the burn wound.

Treatment.—The immediate treatment in a patient of major burn is institution of resuscitative measures to overcome shock and to prevent fatal complications. The burn wound, even if extensive, is of secondary importance till haemodynamic stability has been established. The area is simply kept covered with sterile gauge sheets.

The management of burn patients may be conveniently described under three headings:

1. Immediate therapy.
2. Treatment for the burn wound.
3. Other supportive measures.

Immediate Therapy

I. EMERGENCY RESPIRATORY CARE:

1. Exposure to heavy smoke may lead to carbon monoxide poisoning. This gas immediately combines with haemoglobin, displacing oxygen. Treatment consists of administration of 100 per cent oxygen by ventilator through endotracheal tube.
2. Respiratory obstruction due to oedema of pharynx and vocal cords may occur in burns of head and neck. Endotracheal intubation, failing which, tracheostomy has to be done.

II. RELIEF OF PAIN:

1. The burnt area is kept covered with sheets to prevent irritation.
2. Exposure to cold is avoided as this induces pain.
3. Sedatives are administered intravenously and only in small dosage to ensure absorption and to prevent cumulative effects. For adults morphine or pethidine and for children barbiturates are advised.

III. INTRAVENOUS FLUID RESUSCITATION.—All adults with burns exceeding 15 per cent and children with burns above 10 per cent require fluid resuscitation. Gastrointestinal ileus is almost inevitable in major burns, so the fluid has to be given intravenously. A wide bore cannula is inserted either by subcutaneous puncture or by venesection.

The points to consider are the *quality* of the fluid (crystalloid or colloid), its *quantity* and rate of administration, in order to:

1. Restore the circulatory blood volume to a level adequate for tissue perfusion.

2. Replenish persistent plasma deficit
3. Provide the daily fluid requirement to maintain urinary output, cover evaporative (skin and lung) loss and meet metabolic needs.

During the first 24 hours, when the aim is to raise the circulating blood volume, crystalloid and colloid solutions are of equal value because the increased capillary permeability at this stage allows extravascular escape of the colloids as rapidly as the crystalloids. Further, escape of colloids into the interstitium, e.g. lungs, may pose serious problems. Crystalloid solutions are therefore preferred. A sugar-free balanced salt solution is used. Sugar is avoided because the patient is hyperglycaemic at this stage and also sugar induces diuresis that lowers the blood volume. Lactated Ringer's solution is the best but acetated Ringer's solution or isotonic saline supplemented with sodium bicarbonate ampoules may be used instead. The lactate, acetate combats the metabolic acidosis resultant upon tissue anoxia.

Various formulae have been introduced to guideline the quantity of fluid to be transfused. Almost all of them take into account die surface area of the burn and the weight of the patient. Whatever be their way of expression, in general, they advocate 2 to 4 ml of fluid/per cent of burnt surface/kg body weight. Whatever formula be followed, it acts just as an initial guide and the amount has to be modified according to the patient's response, for which close monitoring is necessary. A very valuable and easy guide is the urine output. In an average adult it should be 35 to 50 ml/hour and in a child 1 ml/kg body weight/hour. The amount of fluid has to be adjusted if the urine output is higher or lower by more than 33 per cent of the above rates.

In deciding the rate of transfusion, it is important to note that the increased capillary permeability (and therefore the extravascular escape of fluid) is maximum during the first few horns of injury and the capillary wall integrity is usually restored to normal by 24 hours. Hence the calculated quantity of fluid, intended to be transfused, is divided into two halves. One of these is rapidly transfused within the first 8 hours *from the time of the incidence* (not the. time of starting of transfusion) and the other half over the next 16 hours.

Additional fluid supplement to meet the patient's daily requirement is not necessary during this period since urine output is maintained by the above fluids and evaporative loss is negligible because of hypovolaemia and peripheral vasoconstriction.

During the second 24 hours the aim is to replenish any persistent plasma volume deficit and to provide the daily requirement.

The plasma volume deficit may be measured directly or estimated at 0.3 to 0.5 ml/kg body weight/per cent burns. which approximates to 250 ml for every 10 per cent burn above 20 per cent. Plasma itself (available as fresh frozen plasma) or plasma volume expanders (4.5 per cent human albumin, 5 per cent albumin in normal saline, dextrans, gelatin, pentastarch, etc.) may be used. Plasma itself is least preferred for its type-specificity, risk of transmitting hepatitis and causing pulmonary extravasation complications.

For burns involving more than 20 per cent of full thickness and especially when the total burnt surface exceeds 40 per cent, *whole blood* replaces a portion of plasma expanders, according to the case, to replace the burnt RBC.

The replacement for daily requirement is provided by infusion of a non-saline fluid, e.g. 5 per cent dextrose. A 70 kg person with 50 per cent burns requires about 4 to 5 litres. Hypernatraemia is thereby avoided. In children, there is a tendency for hyponatraemia, so 5 per cent dextrose in half-strength saline is infused.

IV. Tetanus prophylaxis:
1. Patients actively immunised within preceding 10 years should receive 0.5 ml of absorbed tetanus toxoid.
2. Others should, additionally, be given 250 units of TIG (tetanus immunoglobulin).

V. Antibiotics.—Burn wounds are always contaminated and topical chemotherapeutic agents must be applied in all cases in the form of ointments. Use of systemic antibiotics are discouraged to prevent development of bacterial resistance. However, if there is any indication of systemic sepsis or distal infection (e.g. pneumonia) or evidence of infection in the underlying unburnt tissues (invasive infection) systemic antibiotics have to be administered. Simple surface cultures cannot indicate the trend of bacterial growth and invasion underneath. These are best detected by repeated small but deep wound biopsies, i.e. *bacterial monitoring*. The specimens are subjected to histological examination and culture-sensitivity tests. Histology reveals spread of infection to the underlying tissues. If the culture shows huge number of bacteria initially or their very rapid proliferation within 24 hours, systemic antibiotics are necessary. The sensitivity test indicates the specific antibiotic to be used.

VI. Gastroduodenal care.—The inevitable paralytic ileus causes distension of the stomach, resulting in vomiting. The sedated patient may aspirate the vomitus, causing mortality and morbidity. Nasogastric suction with Ryle's tube is essential. Also, stress ulcers are common. The gastric aspirate may show presence of blood. Liquid antacids are introduced through Ryle's tube. Additionally, H_2-blockers, e.g. ranitidine, may be injected.

Treatment for the Burn Wound.—The aim is to control infection, obtain quick skin coverage, and prevent scarring and deformities.

1. Initial treatment.—As soon as the patient is resuscitated, the wound is attended. Adherent foreign bodies and loose skin tags are removed. The blisters are punctured and the overlying non-viable skin excised.

2. Wound-dressing.—Topical chemotherapeutic agents must be used to control infection of the contaminated raw surface. Water-soluble ointments are

applied, the commonly used are silver sulfadiazine or providone-iodine (betadine). In Pseudomonas infection, 0.5 per cent silver nitrate compress, once or twice a day, are useful. The wound is covered with sterile gauge and cotton, kept in position with bandages (*close method*). The dressings are usually changed on alternate days. For burns in head, face and neck and sometimes, for burns involving only one surface of the trunk, the wound, after application of ointment, is left uncovered, exposed to air (*exposure treatment*). This allows regular inspection of the wound. Burnt hand should be enclosed in a polythene bag and kept elevated, encouraging active finger movements.

3. WOUND EXCISION.—While superficial burns get spontaneous healing in absence of infection, the dead skin of deep burns forms what is called 'eschar'. This is very stiff and is tightly adherent to the underlying tissues. It has to be excised (*escharotomy*) to expose the living tissues under its cover. This procedure is better delayed till the eschar loosens (a matter of about 3 weeks), to make the process painless and non-haemorrhagic. Some surgeons advocate early escharotomy to reduce the chances of infection and the time of hospital stay. Escharotomy is done by sharp scalpel dissection, till a raw bleeding surface (living tissue) is reached. Alternatively, *tangential* escharotomy may by done, in which successive layers are removed by guarded skin knife or air-driven dermatome.

4. SKIN COVERAGE.—The raw area, after escharotomy, requires skin grafting at the earliest to prevent ugly scarring and development of contractures and keloids. Autogenous skin grafting is the ultimate aim. This can be done primarily if sufficient donor sites are available. If only partial coverage is possible, the hands, feet, face and joints should get the priority. Mesh grafts may be used advantageously to get wider coverage than available skin (*see* skin grafting).

If sufficient donor area is not available, instead of continuing with surgical dressings, temporary coverage with *biological dressings* may be done. These are better in that they minimise infection, prevent hypergranulation, reduce loss of evaporative water, heat, protein-rich exudate and RBC, protect the exposed nerves, vessels and tendons, and reduce pain to allow active movements. The commonly used materials are skin homografts, i.e. allografts (cadavers) or heterograft, i.e. xenografts (porcine, i.e. pig dermis). These have to be changed every 5 days. Amnion may be used instead but this requires changing every 48 hours. Recently synthetic skin substitutes are being used. They have silastic epidermal analogue and collagen gel dermal analogue, and do not require periodic changing. Autogenous grafting has to be done at the earliest opportunity, usually in phases.

Other Supportive Measures

1. NUTRITION.—Oral feeding is started usually after 48 hours. Patients with more than 30 per cent burns require especial nutritional support:

a. High protein with essential amino acids.

b. High-calorie (carbohydrates and fat).

c. Vitamins B-complex, C and B_{12} and minerals.

d. Repeated fresh blood transfusion to combat anaemia.

e. Fresh frozen plasma to supply antibodies and opsonins in cases of immunosuppression.

2. SPLINTAGE AND PHYSIOTHERAPY.—For burns involving the flexor surface of joints, the limb must be splinted in extension to prevent contractures. The shoulder should be kept abducted with the arm elevated.

Prolonged immobilisation has to be avoided. Physiotherapy is started immediately after the patient is resuscitated and continued till normal range of active movements return after wound healing. Early skin grafting allows early movements. Pressure garments made of elasticated materials are now available; applied during convalescence, they reduce formation of hypertrophic scar and, thereby, prevent contractures.

3. PSYCHOLOGICAL SUPPORT.—Burn patients are usually mentally depressed and need constant reassurance and encouragement.

KELOID

The term comes form the Greek word *Kele*, which means tumour. However, keloid is not a tumour and *it never turns malignant*. It is a self-limiting process and after a variable period, sometimes after several years, stops growing.

Keloid is an overgrowth of a scar but differs from an ordinary hypertrophic scar in two respects:

1. A hypetrophic scar stops growing after 6 months but keloid continues to grow, sometimes for many years.

2. Unlike hypertrophic scar, keloid spreads to neighbouring normal tissues not affected by the original injury or operation.

Predisposing Factors.—These may be systemic and local.

1. SYSTEMIC FACTORS:

a. Colour of skin and racial variation: Keloid is commoner in the coloured races, particularly the Negroes, than the whites.

b. Individual factors: Some persons have a tendency to form keloids (*keloid diathesis*).

c. Sex: Keloid is commoner in women. Repeated pregnancy may predispose keloid formation, suggesting possible influence of steroid hormones.

d. Tuberculosis: Tuberculosis patients are more prone to develop keloids.

2. LOCAL FACTORS:

a. There are some favourite sites, e.g. front of sternum (*butterfly keloid*), deltoid area, ear lobules, face and neck.

b. Infection in the wound undoubtedly predisposes to development of keloid.

c. Incisions along natural creases (Langer's lines) rarely develop keloids while those across the creases frequently do so.

d. Tuberculous scars are more likely to develop keloids, e.g. tuberculous sinus, operative scar of cold abscess.

Pathology.—The possible pathology is failure of normal maturation of the scar. This is evident from the presence of the active fibroblasts instead of inert fibrocytes and persistence of vascularity (in normal scars, the fibroblasts are converted into fibrocytes and there is a process of devascularisation). The hypertrophy is not from excess collagen formation but due to a defect in collagen breakdown.

Clinical Features

1. Any scar may become a keloid, e.g. burns, surgical wounds, vaccination marks, ear and nasal pricks, tuberculous sinuses, healed skin diseases and even insignificant pricks.
2. Some persons have keloid diathesis and many of them develop multiple keloids.
3. There are some common sites (*see* above).
4. Keloid has the appearance of a redundant scar, with the following features:
   a. Raised *from* the surface; at some sites, e.g. ear lobules, it may be pendulous.
   b. Shiny pink or red in the early stages (vascularity), hyperpigmented later on.
   c. Margins show 'crab's claw' like projections into the adjacent skin.
   d. Ulcers frequently develop on the surface and in the margins.
   e. Itching is a constant and diagnostic symptom.

Treatment.—Various methods have been tried but the results are uniformly poor. Simple excision is almost invariably followed by recurrence, and the recurrent keloids are larger and more distressing. Following are the different forms of treatment:

1. *Application of hydrocortisone ointment* may arrest the progress and diminish the itching in very early cases.
2. *Intrakeloid injections* of hydrocortisone are often helpful.
3. *Surgery.*—Two forms of surgery are available:
   a. Intrakeloid excision, i.e. excision, leaving behind the margins of the keloid, is the commonly practised procedure. Simple excision shall be followed by recurrence. So *adjuvant treatment is* necessary:
      i. Postoperative (sometime also pre-operative) *radiotherapy.* Surgery with radiotherapy was the standard procedure until recent past, but failure to obtain satisfactory results and ill-effects of radiation have gradually compelled surgeons to abandon the procedure.
      ii. Preoperative and postoperative injections of steroids are now gaining popularity.
   b. Shaving away the excess tissue over the keloid (particular care being taken not to encroach on adjacent healthy skin), followed by skin grafting, is on trial.

POSTBURN CONTRACTURE

Contractures *follow full-thickness* burns, commonly at the flexor creases and the shoulder, usually due to defective management.

Prevention

1. Preventing *infection,* which not only delays healing but also causes further tissue destruction that adds to scar formation.
2. Avoiding prolonged immobilisation. *Physiotherapy* must be started immediately after resuscitation of the patient and continued till normal range of active movements return after wound healing.
3. *Proper positioning* of the joints during bed rest and adequate *splintage* in anticontracture positions during sleep. These are easy for the lower limb but difficult for the upper, especially the shoulder.
4. Early *skin grafting*—delay in grafting predisposes contractures.
5. Fitting of *pressure garments,* made of elastic materials, during convalescence decreases the time of scar maturation (softening and flattening) and thereby prevents contracture.

Treatment.—The scar tissue has to be totally excised, releasing all tensions on the surrounding tissues. The new area is skin-grafted (skin and fat over the joints, and free skin on other raw areas).

Narrow bands of contracture can be lengthened by Y-V plasty. The tissues of a straight scar may be lengthened and positioned in the line of minimal tension by Z-plasty (transposition of two triangular skin flaps).

The release operation must be done as early as possible. If this is delayed, the underlying important structures like vessels, nerves and tendons are adaptable shortened and, at operation, may prevent release of the contracture. Preliminary traction may be required in such cases.

Types of Skin Graft.—Principally there are three types:

1. FREE GRAFTS.—These are detached totally from the donor site and transferred to the recipient area.

2. PEDICLE GRAFTS. —These maintain a vascular connection with the donor site by a pedicle either temporarily or permanently.

3. MICROVASCULAR GRAFTS.—These are detached totally from the donor site but their vessels are immediately anastomosed with those in the recipient area by microvascular technique.

Free Grafts:—Only skin, devoid of any other tissue, can survive temporary devascularisation. At the recipient bed, they live initially (48 hours) by imbibing plasma and, thereafter, gradually get revascularised from the underlying tissues in 5 to 10 days. The thinner the graft, the earlier is the vascularisation and, generally, better the prospect of *taking*. According to the thickness, these grafts are grouped into two categories:

1. *Partial-thickness or 'split-skin' grafts* (*Thiersch's*).—The epidermis with only part-thickness of the dermis is transferred. According to the amount of dermis included, the grafts are called thin, medium and thick.

2. *Full-thickness grafts* (*Wolfe's*).—The epidermis with the entire thickness of the dermis is grafted.

The grafts are raised either by Humby knife (having guarded disposable blades) or by electric dermatomes. They are either fixed at the donor site by marginal sutures or skin staples, or are retained in position, simply with pressure bandages. Movements prevent taking.

While free grafts are very widely used because large quantities are available and the technique is easy, they have certain limitations:

a. The recipient bed must be free of infection.

b. The receiving area must have adequate vascularity—a graft will survive on periosteum or peritenon but not on bare bone or tendon.

Partial-thickness and full-thickness grafts have their relative advantages and disadvantages, both at the receiving and the donor sites. The disadvantages of partial-thickness grafts are:

i. They have poorer cosmetic value because they have a tendency to be deeply pigmented (especially when exposed to sun rays) and to shrink; hence unsuitable for the face.

ii. They get damaged even with minor trauma; therefore unsuitable for the hands and feet.

The advantage is that the donor sites get spontaneous coverage by proliferation of the epithelial elements in the left-behind dermis, e.g. hair follicles. Also, if thin grafts are taken, the area is ready for re-donation by about 10 days on each occasion. This is of particular value where wide skin coverage is necessary, e.g. burns. Further, the donor site has better cosmetic appearance.

On the other hand, full-thickness grafts are cosmetically better and can stand trauma. However, the donor site has to be covered either by apposition of the margins or by split-thickness grafts taken from another site. Hence, the quantity of graft is limited and the donor site may have a poorer cosmesis.

The common donor sites for free skin grafts are the anterolateral aspect of the thighs, abdominal wall and buttocks, from where large quantities of grafts are available. Full-thickness grafts are best taken from the gluteal and inguinal folds because redundancy and mobility of the skin there allow approximation of the margins for wound closure.

Mesh Grafts, prepared from free skin grafts, are valuable for covering wide raw area, as in burns. The piece of graft, except at its margins, is subjected to multiple parallel incisions by especial devices. As tension is applied perpendicular to these incisions, they open and increase the size of the graft, sometimes up to six times. The created gaps get covered by epithelium proliferating from the incised margins.

Pedicle Grafts.—These grafts (flaps) are necessary when skin with some other underlying tissue is required to restore appearance and function at the recipient site. Subcutaneous fat is the most commonly incorporated tissue. Skin with fat flap was the original and even today, is the most commonly practised procedure. However, vast improvement have been made in the field and, along with skin and fat, deep fascia, muscles, etc. are being transferred.

1. LOCAL SKIN AND FAT FLAPS (ROTATIONAL FLAPS, TRANSPOSITION FLAPS).—These are used when the recipient site has redundancy of skin and subcutaneous fat in its immediate vicinity. Their advantages are the similarity of tissue texture and hair pattern, easy technique, and minimum expenditure and time-involvement. The graft is raised and then rotated on its pedicle to take it to the adjacent recipient gap, where it is sutured. The raw donor area is covered by split-skin grafts.

2. DISTANT SKIN AND FAT FLAPS.—The proposed graft, usually rectangular, is cut at its three margins, leaving one margin (pedicle) intact. The cut margins are sutured to the margins of the recipient gap. Initially the flap derives its blood supply from the pedicle. Subsequently new blood vessels grow into the flap from the sutured margins of the receiving area. The pedicle is then detached at a second operation. The aim is to fashion the flap in such a manner that the pedicle is as narrow as possible in comparison to its length, which should be sufficient to cover the defect. Such flap transfers may be of two types:

    a. *Direct pedicle graft (approximation flap).*—This method is applicable to those cases where the donor and the recipient sites can be apposed, e.g. abdomen to hand, one leg to the other (cross-leg flap), one finger to another. It is a two-stage procedure—approximation and detachment of the pedicle.

    b. *Indirect pedicle graft (tubed graft).*—In those cases where the donor and recipient sites cannot be approximated, the flap has to get an attachment to an *'intermediate carrier site'*. For instance, a graft from the abdomen gets an intermediate temporary attachment to the forearm, and then it is finally put on the face or the lower leg. This is, therefore, a multi-staged procedure and time-consuming. To eliminate the raw area in the flap, its margins are sutured to each other with the skin outwards. Hence this is also called 'tubed graft'.

3. ISLAND PEDICLE GRAFT.— The principle is to make the pedicle narrowest, comprising only the feeding artery, vein and, if possible, a cutaneous nerve, so that the graft can be drawn to a considerable distance. Examples are:

    a. Eyebrow reconstruction by transfer of a portion of the hair-bearing scalp, having temporal artery and vein pedicle.

    b. Deltopectoral flap based on second, third and fourth anterior perforating branches of the internal mammary artery.

    c. Groin flap surviving on the superficial circumflex iliac artery.

4. FASIOCUTANEOUS FLAPS.—Inclusion of the deep fascia with the skin and subcutaneous tissue offers greater vascularity to the flap because of the vascular

plexus contained in the deep fascia. A bigger flap can be made on a relatively narrow pedicle.

5. MYOCUTANEOUS FLAPS.—The fact that the underlying muscles provide abundant blood vessels to the overlying skin, a muscle mass together with the overlying fat and skin can be rotated as one unit on a relatively narrow pedicle containing blood vessels supplying the muscle. This type of flap is highly useful to cover gaps which are deep and wide, e.g. after excision of a malignant growth. They are also useful, for their vascularity, to cover bare bone. The commonly used flaps are pectoralis major, latissimus dorsi, gracilis and tensor fascia lata.

Microvascular Flaps.—Many of the musculocutaneous flaps have a single known constant vascular pedicle and the vessels have significant calibre. If the vessels have more than 0.8 mm internal diameter, they can be anastomosed microscopically with the vessels at the recipient site for immediate vascularisation of the flap. Such flaps can be totally detached from the donor site and taken as free grafts to a distant site. Muscle and skin or skin alone may be transferred in this way. For example, the latissimus dorsi with the overlying skin may be taken to the lower leg, anastomosing the thoracodorsal artery and vein with the anterior tibial vessels.

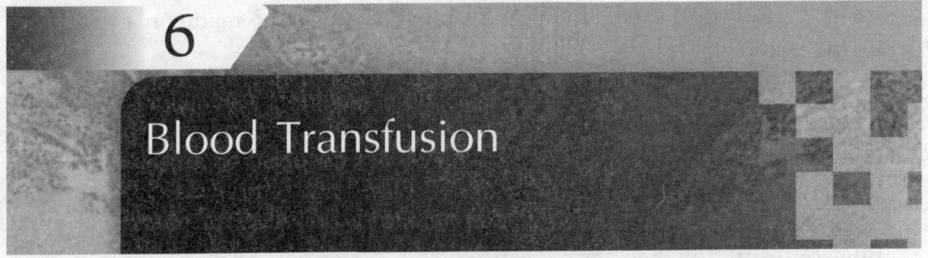

6

Blood Transfusion

BLOOD AND BLOOD PRODUCTS

1. WHOLE BLOOD:
   a. *Stored Blood.*—Blood from donors is mixed with an anticoagulant and stored at 4°C. The commonly used anticoagulants are CPP (citrate-phosphate-dextrose) and CPDA (citrate-phosphate-dextrose-adenosine) solutions; 450 ml whole blood is mixed with 63 ml of CPDA. The shelf-life of blood with CPD is 3 weeks. Addition of adenosine extends it up to 5 weeks. Heparin is sometimes used as an anticoagulant, e.g. exchange transfusion in infants and priming of heart-lung machine. The shelf-life is only 48 hours.
   b. *Fresh Blood*—This means blood transfused within 24 hours of collection. It is preferred to stored blood because the oxygen-releasing capacity in the tissues by the RBC suffers gradual setback after 24 hours.

2. RED BLOOD CELLS:
   a. *Packed Red Cells*, i.e. concentrated suspension of RBC, removing the supernatant plasma. It contains 70 per cent red cells by volume. Its advantages over whole blood are:
      i. Circulatory overloading is avoided, so especially useful in patients of chronic anaemia and enfeebled heart, and in the elderly and children.
      ii. Reactions secondary to allergens in the plasma are largely avoided.
   b. *Frozen Red Cells*, i.e. cells maintained frozen in a cryopreservative (glycerol), are still better because:
      i. They are thawed and washed before use, so there is further allergen elimination.
      ii. Viability of the cells are cent per cent as at the time of preservation, even after years.

3. PLATELETS:
   Selective platelet transfusion is indicated in thrombocytopenia:
   a. *Platelet-rich plasma,* prepared by centrifuging fresh blood.
   b. *Platelet concentrate,* obtained by centrifuging platelet-rich plasma.

4. PLASMA:—This is obtained by centrifuging whole blood. It may be processed and fractionised in various ways:
   a. *Fresh Frozen Plasma (FFP).*—Plasma, separated *from fresh blood*, is frozen and stored at 40°C. While this is a very good source of all the coagulation factors,

its special importance is in providing factors V and VIII because all the other factors, being stable, are available in stored blood.

b. *Cryoprecipitate.*—This is a white gelatinous preciptate obtained by thawing FFP. This is a source of factor VIII and vWF in moderately concentrated form. This is also a good source of fibrinogen, factor XIII and fibronectin.

c. *Concentrates.*—Almost all the coagulation factors are available in concentrated form, excepting factors I (bonned) and V. The most commonly used is factor VIII concentrate (also contains vWF).

d. *Human Albumin Solution* (4.5%).—Stored at 40°C in a liquid state. This is very useful for protein supplement (e.g. burns), without risk of transmitting diseases.

5. MODERN BLOOD PREPARATIONS:

For utilisation of coagulation factors separately, two methods of storage have been introduced recently:

a. *SAG-M Blood.*—The RBCs are separated from plasma which is utilised for preparation of haemostatic components. The separated RBCs are then mixed with 100 ml of a crystalloid solution, containing sodium chloride, adenine, glucose and mannitol (i.e. SAG-M), and very little citrate.

b. *Whole Blood, Modified.*—The RBCs and plasma are separated. Platelets and cryoprecipitate are removed for storage. The RBCs are then rejoined with the plasma.

Indications of Blood Transfusion

1. REPLACEMENT OF LOST VOLUME

a. Haemorrhage from trauma.

b. Haemorrhage from pathological lesions, e.g. from gastrointestinal tract, genito-urinary tract.

c. Major surgical procedures entailing blood loss, e.g. cardiovascular surgery, abdominoperineal resection, prostatectomy, etc.

2. FOR TREATING ANEMIA

a. Severe burns.

b. Severe infections that cause anaemia, e.g. gas gangrene, peritonitis, gut strangulation.

c. Postoperatively, in patients who become severely anaemic.

d. Pre-operatively in cases of chronic anaemia when early surgery is necessary and adequate time is not available for treating the anaemia with conventional therapy, e.g. bleeding piles, uterine haemorrhage, etc.

In all these cases blood transfusion should be considered on individual merit. Even when the haemoglobin level is only 50 per cent of normal patients who are stable and are unlikely to face increased demands or further significant blood loss, should be allowed to reproduce their own red cell mass, keeping in mind that blood transfusion has its risks and the transfused RBCs do not live long.

In treating anaemia concentrated RBC should be used.

3. REPLACEMENT OF CLOTTING FACTORS.—This may be necessary:
   a. To arrest haemorrhage.
   b. As a prophylactic measure prior to surgery in patients with haemorrhagic diseases.

Following is a list of some diseases and the suitable transfusing agents:
   i. Factor I (Fibrinogen).—Cryoprecipitate, FFP.
   ii. Factor II (Prothrombin).—Factor II concentrate, FFP.
   iii. Factor V (Parahaemophilic).—FFP.
   iv. Factor VII (Proconvertin).—Factor VII concentrate.
   v. Factor VIII (Antihaemophilic).—AHF concentrate, cryoprecipitate, FFP.
   vi. Factor IX (Christmas).—Factor IX concentrate, FFP.
   vii. Platelets.—Platelet concentrate, platelet-rich plasma,
   viii. Multiple coagulation defects (hepatic insufficiency, disseminated intravascular coagulation).—FFP.

Stored blood itself can supply all the coagulation factors, except factors VIII and V.

However, fresh blood is now believed to be an inadequate source of platelets and factor VIII.

4. OTHER INDICATIONS:
   a. To prime heart-lung machine. The quantity may be minimized by adding Ringer's lactate or dextran.
   b. For temporary improvement in case of thalassaemia, refractory anaemia or aplastic anaemia, Hodgkin's disease, leukaemia, etc.
   c. During chemotherapy for malignant diseases.

Autotransfusion.—The patient's own blood is transfused. There are two methods:

1. IMMEDIATE OR INTRA-OPERATIVE.—In cases of severe blood loss where the shed blood can be collected, e.g. ruptured ectopic, ruptured spleen, ruptured liver, etc. The blood is sucked from the peritoneal cavity and collected in a sterile container, to which transfusion tubings are attached. Clots or undesirable elements are eliminated by straining the blood through a piece of sterile gauge. Special autotransfusion apparatus is now available. This method is of particular value when stored blood is not available immediately.

2. DELAYED OR SELECTIVE.—The patient 'donates' his or her own blood within 3 weeks prior to the date of operation. This blood is stored and is transfused during the operation. By the period of 3 weeks the patient reproduces the major volume of red cells and plasma proteins. Obviously, this is the best matched blood.

Exchange (Replacement) Transfusion.—This is indicated in neonates suffering from erythroblastosis foetalis. Rh-negative blood is exchanged with the infant's blood, 5–10 ml at a time. The transfusion is made via the umbilical vein by a syringe fitted with a four-way adapter (one to the infant's body, one to the donor, one to citrated saline and the other to the waste). Replacement transfusion is also indicated in desperate cases of carbon monoxide poisoning.

Routes of Transfusion

1. *Venous Transfusion.*—This is the usual route:
   a. Almost always a peripheral vein is selected, usually in the upper extremity, sometimes in the long saphenous.
   b. Sometimes a central vein (jugular, femoral) has to be chosen, e.g. severe peripheral venospasm and obliteration of the peripheral veins by multiple previous transfusions.
   c. Umbilical vein in neonates, scalp vein or anterior fontanelle in infants.
2. *Arterial Transfusion* into the radial, femoral or carotid may have to be done in extremely quick massive bleeding.
3. *Intra-cardiac Transfusion* into the right auricle with the help of a cardiac catheter may be required in cases of extreme venospasm.
4. *Marrow Transfusion* into the sternum (above 3 years of age) or tibia (below 3 years) is a painful procedure and the rate of transfusion limited. This route is especially indicated for transplantation purposes, e.g. in leukaemia.

Blood Groups and Compatibility.—There are more than 20 antigens (agglutinogens) in the human RBC and corresponding antibodies (agglutinins) may be present in the serum. To avoid reactions, an antigen with the corresponding antibody is never present in the same individual. When a transfusion is made, if the antigens in the RBC of the donor blood meet with corresponding antibodies in the recipient's serum, a serious antigen–antibody reaction (agglutination) is likely to occur. The two bloods are, thus, incompatible. This is the basis of the compatibility tests that are essential before proceeding for a blood transfusion.

For practical proposes, these antigens in the RBC are divided into two classes:

I. *Antigens to which antibodies occur naturally.*—There are two such antigens— A and B (Landsteiner). Their presence or absence determines the popular "blood group" of the individual. Accordingly, there are four human blood groups:

Group A   : The red cells contain antigen A, and the serum contains anti-B.

Group B   : The red cells contain antigen B, and the serum contains anti-A.

Group AB : The red cells contain both antigens A and B, and the serum contains neither anti-A nor anti-B.

Group O : The red cells contain neither antigen A nor antigen B, and the serum contains both anti-A and anti-B.

It is obvious that, for transfusions to be devoid of agglutination reaction, the donor and the recipient should belong to the same blood group. Individuals belonging to group AB, who contain neither anti-A nor anti-B in their serum, should tolerate blood from any group, hence they are termed *universal recipients*. Similarly, individuals of group O whose red cells do not contain antigen A or B, and hence cannot be agglutinated, are called *universal donors*. However, these terms are not as accurate as they sound to be, since reactions may sometimes occur even with such donors and such recipients. Hence it is better that only the blood belonging to the same group as that of the recipient is transfused.

II. *Antigens to which there are no natural antibodies.*—There are some natural antigens in the RBC, to which there are no natural antibodies in the serum. There is only one such antigen—the antigen D, which is popularly known as the Rh-antigen or Rh-factor (this name comes from "Rhesus monkey", with whose RBC, the serum of rabbits showed reactions).

Those persons whose RBC contains the Rh-antigen are called Rh-positive, and persons in whose RBC this factor is absent are called Rh- negative; 85 per cent of the population are Rh-positive and 15 per cent are Rh-negative. Since this antigen cannot naturally produce antibodies, neither the Rh-positive nor the Rh-negative subjects have Rh-antibodies in their serum under usual circumstances. However, a Rh-negative person may sometimes produce Rh-antibodies in the serum. The circumstances under which this may occur and the results thereupon are as follows:

1. Rh-negative mother may acquire antibodies in the serum when she carries a Rh-positive foetus. The results may be:
   a. The mother's serum, with the antibody, crosses the placental barrier and may agglutinate the RBC of the foetus (erythroblastosis foetalis).
   b. The mother, if she requires blood transfusions, will not tolerate blood from Rh-positive donors.
2. Repeated transfusions of Rh-positive blood in a Rh-negative subject may produce antibodies in his serum, so that, while the earlier transfusions are tolerated well, a late transfusion may prove incompatible.

Incompatibility.—Transfusion of incompatible blood first causes agglutination and then haemolysis of the donated RBC. If the haemolysis is severe, there is acute renal tubular necrosis which may result in death from renal failure. Hence, before a transfusion is contemplated, the following points are to be ascertained:

1. The blood group of the recipient.—Transfusing only the same group of donor blood.
2. The Rh-status of the recipient.—Avoiding transfusion of Rh-positive blood in Rh-negative recipients.

3. Direct cross-matching of the recipient's serum with the donor red cells to be sure that no agglutination will occur with the particular transfusion.

Compatibility Tests

1. Blood grouping.—To determine the blood group of the recipient (the recipient's cells are tested against stock serum of known groups).

2. Rh-factor determination by Coomb's test.

3. Cross-matching.—In order to ensure absolute compatibility, the donor cells are directly tested against the recipient's serum.

Complications and Dangers of Blood Transfusion.—In view of the vast number of blood transfusions, complications are relatively rare. Also, complications arising out of haemolytic reaction are much rare than is apprehended, while other complications are relatively common. However, majority of the complications are preventable. In general, the reactions may be conveniently grouped as:

A. Haemolytic reactions.

B. Non-haemolytic reactions:
   1. Simple pyrexial reactions.
   2. Allergic and sensitisation reactions.
   3. Reactions caused by over-transfusion.
   4. Bleeding diathesis.
   5. Transmission of diseases.
   6. Other reactions.

Haemolytic Reactions

Causes:

1. Incompatible transfusion—ABO or Rh.

2. Transfusion of outdated blood.

3. Transfusion of blood already haemolysed by heating, over-freezing, shaking, or by infection.

Features.—The symptoms are variable and may not manifest themselves when the patient is under anaesthesia:

1. Fever with chill and rigor, flushing of the face, and tingling of the extremities.

2. Feeling of tightness in the chest with dyspnoea, sometimes cyanosis.

3. Sensation of heat and pain along the transfused vein.

4. Intense pain in the loin (blockage of renal tubules, i.e. the *transfusion kidney*) is the most characteristic feature.

5. Oliguria and haemolglobinuria, the latter is evident within two hours.

6. Continued hypovolaemia and anaemia despite adequate volume replacement.

7. Jaundice, appearing in 24 to 48 hours.

8. Abnormal bleeding, e.g. disseminated intravascular coagulation (DIC).

Prevention:

1. Perfect collection, storage, grouping, cross-matching and labelling.
2. Proper verification with the patient's papers before transfusion and noting the date of expiry.
3. Careful examination of each bottle to exclude haemolysis or degeneration.
4. Avoiding over-freezing, heating and rigorous shaking.
5. Maintaining strict asepsis in the set and the process.

Treatment:

1. Transfusion is stopped immediately on the appearance of the first symptom of suspicion.
2. All papers, the donor bag and the set are rechecked.
3. The donor bag with the remaining blood and the patient's blood samples are sent to the laboratory for re-examination.
4. Attempts are made to stimulate the 'transfusion kidney', i.e. preventing blockage of the renal tubules by:
   a. administration of intravenous fluids,
   b. making the urine alkaline by injecting sodium bicarbonate.
5. Antihistaminics and steroids often give beneficial results.
6. In desperate cases haemodialysis may be necessary.

Simple Pyrexial Reactions

Causes:

1. Presence of pyrogens in the donor apparatus and in the anticoagulant solution.
2. Infected blood.
3. Rapid transfusion.

Features.—There is fever (sometimes hyperpyrexia), with chill and rigor, headache and, sometimes, nausea and vomiting.

Prevention:

1. Using disposable plastic sets and maintaining strict asepsis.
2. Using antihistaminics routinely before starting a transfusion.

Treatment:

1. Stopping the transfusion temporarily and re-checking the papers.
2. Covering the body with blankets to overcome chill and rigor.
3. Injecting antihistaminics and calcium.
4. Inducing hypothermia by ice-bags, ice-sponging and antipyretics.
5. If everything goes all right, starting the transfusion again but with a separate set and at a slow rate.

Allergic and Sensitization Reactions

Causes:

1. Allergy to plasma proteins in the donor blood.

2. Production of antibodies to the donated WBC, platelets and other components related to the ABO and Rh-antigens. This occurs in patients receiving repeated transfusions.

3. Transfusion of antibodies from hypersensitive donors.

Features.—These appear a few hours after the transfusion and consist of urticarial rash, facial oedema and, sometimes, acute anaphylactic shock.

Treatment consists in administration of antihistaminics and, sometimes, steroids.

Reactions Caused by Over-transfusion.—These are likely to occur in patients with enfeebled heart (as in the elderly) and in the subjects of chronic anaemia. There is over-loading of the heart, resulting in congestive cardiac failure with pulmonary oedema, characterised by cough and dyspnoea.

A patient above 60 should not receive more than 300 ml at a time and a patient of severe anaemia is preferably transfused with packed cells.

Treatment consists in stopping transfusion, getting the patient in sitting position and administering diuretics. Rarely the patient has to be bled by venesection.

Bleeding Diathesis.—Bleeding from the field of operation and mucous surfaces, and petechial haemorrhages may occur. There are two causes:

1. Dilution of the clotting factors and/or platelets.

   This follows massive transfusion with stored blood because it is poor in platelets and factors V and VIII.

2. Disseminated intravascular coagulation (DIG) following ABO incompatible transfusions. Extensive coagulation causes consumption of the coagulation factors (I, II, V and VIII) and platelets.

   Treatment consists of administration of FFP, cryoprecipitate and platelet concentrate.

   Interestingly, heparin sometimes controls the bleeding.

   There is now a belief that DIC is largely due to persistent hypotension prior to the transfusion rather than the transfusion itself.

Transmission of Diseases

1. Hepatitis.—This is the commonest fatal complication. Almost always it is non-A, non-B (NANB) hepatitis. Fortunately B-hepatitis is rare. Symptoms appear after 3 months. Prevention is by careful verbal screening and test for hepatitis-related antigen in the donor blood.

2. AIDS.—There is now a test available for anti-HIV antibody, to be done at each donation.

3. Malaria.—Prevention is by careful verbal screening and testing the donor blood for parasites.

4. Syphilis.—Skin rash of secondary syphilis is the first manifestation. VDRL test is imperative for all donors' blood.

5. Bacteria.—Faulty storage and prolonged exposure to room temperature allows bacteria to multiply. Gram-negative organisms, e.g. *Esch. coli* and pseudomonas, are the commonest. Severe septic shock may occur on rare occasions, and may be fatal.

Other Complications

1. Thrombophlebitis.—Commoner in the lower limbs.
2. Air Embolism.—Very rare. The patient is turned to the left with head-down position.
3. Cardiac Arrest may occur if cold blood is transfused in large amount.

7
Cysts

Definition.—The term 'cyst' is Greek in origin, meaning 'bladder'. Cysts are defined as swellings containing fluid in a sac, usually, but not always, lined by epithelium or endothelium.

Classification.—Cysts may be classified as true and false or as congenital and acquired.

I. TRUE AND FALSE CYSTS:

    A. *True Cysts.*—These are usually lined by epithelium or endothelium though, if infections supervene, this lining may be replaced by granulation tissue. The nature of the content may be:

        1. Serous or mucoid, consisting of the secretions of the lining membrane. It may be colourless, or may be brownish because of altered blood. Cholesterol crystals are often present.

        2. Grey toothpaste-like, as a result of accumulation of desquamated epithelium in the fluid, e.g. sebaceous cysts, dermoid cysts.

    B. *False Cysts or Pseudocysts.*—These may be of the following types:

        1. Exudation cysts occurring in anatomical spaces already lined by endothelium, e.g. hydrocele, bursa, pseudopancreatic cyst.

        2. Degeneration cysts having no lining membrane, e.g. cystic degenerations in the centre of a malignant tumour, apoplectic cysts in the brain following ischaemia.

II. CONGENITAL AND ACQUIRED CYSTS:

    A. *Congenital Cysts*:

        1. Dermoid Cysts.

        2. Cysts of Embryonic Remnants.—Urachal cysts, intraperitoneal cysts arising from the central part of the vitello-intestinal duct (enteroteratoma), hydatid of Morgagni (from Muellerian duct).

    B. *Acquired Cysts*:

        1. Implantation Cysts.—Implantation dermoids.

        2. Retention Cysts.—Caused by retention of secretion of a gland resulting from blockage of ducts, e.g. sebaceous cysts, Bartholin cysts, cysts in parotid, breast, pancreas.

        3. Distension Cysts.—Resulting from dilatation of normal acini or follicles, e.g. thyroid cysts, ovarian follicular cysts, lymphatic cysts (including cystic hygroma).

        4. Exudation Cysts*.—Occurring from exudations in an anatomical space normally lined by endothelium, e.g. hydrocele, bursa, pseudopancreatic cyst.

5. Degeneration Cysts*.—Cystic degeneration in a malignant tumour due to haemorrhage or colliquative necrosis.
6. Cystic Tumours.—Cystadenomas of breast, thyroid, etc.
7. Traumatic Cysts.—To start with, these are the haematomas in muscles (e.g. loin, thigh, etc.). Thereafter they derive an endothelial lining and the fluid inside becomes brownish, containing cholesterol crystals.
8. Parasitic Cysts.—Hydatid cysts.
   (*These are examples of false cysts).

DERMOID CYSTS

These are epidermal cysts. This means that the lining membrane is epithelial and the contents are epithelial secretion. These contents are often pultaceous or grey toothpaste-like since they contain vast number of desquamated epithelial cells.

Types

A. *Congenital*:
   1. Sequestration dermoids.
   2. Tubulodermoids.
   3. Teratodermoid—in ovary, testis, etc.

B. *Acquired*: Implantation dermoids.

Sequestration Dermoids.—These are so named because they result from sequestration of dermal cells into the deeper tissues, during the process of fusion of embryonic segments. Thus they are found only in the midline and along the lines of embryological fusion.

The *common sites*, therefore are:
1. External angular, i.e. above the outer canthus of the eye.
2. Postauricular, i.e. behind the ear.
3. In the midline at the root of the nose.
4. On the skull, at the sites of fusion of skull bones.
5. In the neck, i.e. the site of fusion of branchial arches—branchial cyst.
6. Anywhere in the midline, particularly the neck.

Clinical features.—There is a painless, slowly growing swelling at a popular site described above. The skin over the swelling is free but the swelling is attached to the deeper tissues. At the depth, the underlying bone is usually felt to be indented. The consistency may be firm instead of cystic, because of the semisolid character of the contents.

X-ray.—This may show a gap or a depression in the bone underlying the cyst. In cases of external angular dermoids, a thick fibrous band may pass through this bony gap and connect the cyst with the underlying dura mater.

Treatment.—Excision of the cyst has to be performed. General anaesthesia is preferable since dissection of the cyst from the sensitive deeper structures (e.g. pericranium) may cause pain if local infiltration anaesthesia is used.

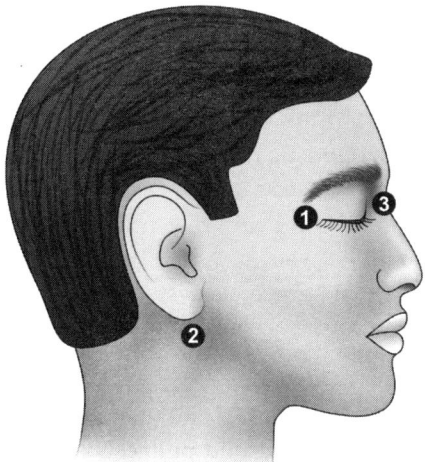

Fig. 7.1: The three common sites of sequestration dermoid; (1) External angular; (2) Postauricular; (3) Midline at the root of the nose

On cutting open the excised cyst, a grey pultaceous (sebaceous) material is found which often contains hairs (i.e. these secretions are all derivatives of the skin).

Tubulodermoids.—These are also known as *tubuloembryonic cysts* since they occur in developing ectodermal tubes:

1. The commonest of these is the thyroglossal cyst, developing in the thyroglossal duct.
2. Another not infrequent example is the postanal dermoid, developing in the postanal gut.
3. Ependymal cyst in the brain, developing in the infolding neuroectoderm.

Implantation Dermoids.—These are examples of acquired epidermal cysts.

They result from traumatic implantation of skin element into the deeper tissues, e.g. a needle prick which buries a little amount of surface tissues into the depth. They are, therefore, commonest in the pulp of fingers and palm of hand, particularly in people often getting pricks, e.g. tailors and gardeners.

They present as tense cystic (or firm) swellings. A suggestive history of trauma, sometimes an overlying scar, is diagnostic.

Treatment.—Excision of the cyst.

SEBACEOUS CYSTS

These are retention cysts resulting from obstruction to the opening of sebaceous duct (a sebaceous duct either opens into hair follicle or directly on to the skin surface). Like dermoids, they are also epidermal cysts.

The *common sites* are:

1. Scalp.—The characteristic feature is a baldness over the swelling (possibly caused by pressure-atrophy of the local hair follicles).
2. Face.
3. Scrotum, where the characteristic features of the cysts are as follows:
   a. They are usually multiple.
   b. They are often hard and solid, and the surface then looks yellowish; this is due to calcification in the cysts.

It is interesting to note that sebaceous cysts never occur on the palms or sole since these areas are devoid of sebaceous glands.

Clinical Features

1. The swelling may not have a cystic feel and (like the dermoids) it may be firm in feel because the contents are semisolid pultaceous material, i.e. the secretions of the sebaceous glands, rich in fat, together with the desquamated epithelium. Unlike dermoids, they do not contain hairs.
2. The swelling is free from deeper structures while it is fixed to the skin (cf dermoids).
3. The point of fixity to the skin is marked by a blue spot—the *punctum* of obstructed duct. In some cysts there may be multiple puncta. Sometimes sebaceous material is expressed from the punctum.

Treatment.—Excision of the cyst, usually under local anaesthesia. Excision may be performed by one of the following methods:

1. Dissection.—An elliptical incision is made on the skin surrounding the punctum, and the intact cyst is dissected out.
2. Incision-avulsion.—The cyst is incised and the contents are squeezed out. The cyst wall is then seized with a forceps and avulsed out. This method is particularly suitable for infected sebaceous cysts.
3. For scrotal sebaceous cysts:
   a. If it is solitary—excision of the cyst.
   b. If the cysts are multiple, a part of the scrotal skin, including the cysts, is excised.
   c. If the cysts are multiple and scattered widely, the whole scrotal skin has to be excised. The testes are placed in pockets made in the subcutaneous tissue on the medial side of the respective thigh.

Complications

1. *Infection.*—The cyst may convert into an abscess. Unless the inflammation subsides with early antibiotic treatment, it has to be incised. The material that comes out is semiliquid and highly foetid. Following the incision:
   a. The cyst may disappear due to fibrosis of the wall (rare)
   b. The cyst may again fill up
   c. There may be a persistent ulceration at the opening made (*see* below).

If possible, avulsion of the cyst wall should be done with the incision, to avoid these complications.

1. Ulceration.—This occurs when an infected cyst ruptures or is incised, following acute inflammation. The ulcer is covered by a mass of granulation tissue. In sebaceous cysts of the scalp this granulation tissue is often excessive, resembling a fungating epithelioma. This condition is known as Cock's peculiar tumour, which usually has an offensive discharge.

2. Sebaceous Horn.—Sometimes the sebaceous material comes out slowly from the orifice of the duct and dries up in successive layers, resembling a horn.

3. Calcification.—This is particularly common in sebaceous cysts of the scrotum.

4. Malignancy.—An adenocarcinoma may develop very rarely.

HYDATID CYST

Etiology.—Hydatid disease in man is caused by the larval stage of *Taenia echinococcus* (*T granulosa*). This cestode completes its life-cycle in two hosts. The definitive host is dog in whose intestine the adult worm is found. The intermediate host is usually sheep, occasionally man, in whom the egg enters the intestine either by contact with infested dog or from contaminated food.

Pathology

A. DEVELOPMENT OF HYDATID CYST.— In the duodenum the egg ruptures and liberates the hexacanth embryo (with six booklets). The embryo penetrates the intestinal wall and is carried to the liver by portal circulation. The embryo is caught in the liver-filter and here it changes into a cystic larva. This cystic larva is called hydatid cyst. If the embryo escapes the liver-filter, it is arrested in the lung capillaries, where it may form a cyst. When the pulmonary capillaries are escaped, the embryo enters the systemic circulation and reaches any organ where it may form cysts. Thus, cysts may occasionally form in brain, kidney, muscles and bones.

In order of frequency, therefore, the sites for hydatid cysts are liver (80 per cent) and lung (15 per cent) and then the brain, kidney, muscles and bones.

B. STRUCTURE OF THE CYST:

1. Wall of the cyst.—The actual living layer in the wall is the germinal epithelium, which secretes externally a fluid that is converted into the laminated membrane and internally the hydatid fluid. From outside inwards, the layers of the wall are:

    a. Adventitia (*pseudocyst*).—This is formed by reactive fibrosis in the surrounding healthy tissue. It is thick and tough but elastic.

    b. Laminated membrane (*ectocyst*).—It is multilayered and is impervious to noxious agents.

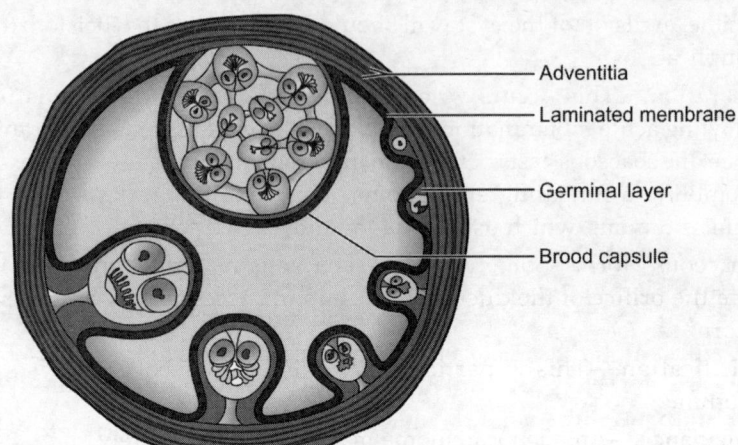

Fig. 7.2: Hydatid cyst

 c. Germinal epithelium (*endocyst*).—This is thin and translucent, consisting of a single layer of cells. Proliferation of the cells internally produces the brood capsules, which keep attached to the germinal layer by pedicles. The brood capsules have no covering of the ectocyst (cf daughter cysts). Within the wall of each brood capsule develop 5 to 20 scolices (head of future worms).

2. *Contents of the Cyst:*

 a. Hydatid fluid, secreted by the germinal layer. It is watery. The fluid may produce severe anaphylactic reactions if it escapes into the tissues (either by spontaneous rupture of the cyst or at operation).

 b. Hydatid sand, formed by disintegrated brood capsules which get detached and fall into the cavity of the cyst.

 c. Daughter cysts.—A daughter cyst is a replica of the mother cyst, inside which it develops. It has all the layers of the mother cyst, including the ectocyst. It develops from a brood capsule that gets detached from the wall and falls into the cavity of the mother cyst, which has undergone degeneration, following damage of the laminated membrane.

C. COMPLICATIONS:

1. Rupture:

 a. A liver cyst may rupture into bile ducts (commonest), peritoneal cavity, gastrointestinal tract or one of the pleural cavities.

 b. A lung cyst may rupture into the pleural cavity or a bronchus.

2. Infection and Suppuration.—Repeated infections cause adhesions between the adventitia and the cyst wall, making enucleation difficult. An infected hepatic cyst may rupture directly into the lung tissue through adhered subphrenic and pleural spaces, causing *hepatobronchial fistula*.

3. Calcification, following death of the parasite.

4. Anaphylactic reactions (urticaria and fever), sometimes severe.

Special Investigations

1. Imaging:
   a. Straight X-ray may show a round calcified shadow.
   b. Ultrasonography is the commonest aid to diagnosis—a round reticulated shadow is seen with calcified wall.
   c. CT scan may be useful if ultrasonographic findings are inconclusive. Details of the cyst are shown.
   d. ERCP may be necessary to detect communication of the cyst with bile duct.

2. Allergic Test (*Casoni's intradermal test*).—A wheal formation on the skin following intradermal injection of a small amount of hydatid fluid. This is positive in 75 to 80 per cent of patients.

3. Serological Tests.—These are positive in 85 per cent of cases:
   a. Indirect agglutination test.
   b. Complement fixation test.

4. Blood Count.—Eosinophilia, though a diagnostic aid, is absent in many cases.

Clinical Features

1. SILENT CYSTS.—Many cysts pass unrecognised and are detected either accidentally or at postmortem. In fact, many of the cysts are clinically detected years after their origin.

2. CYSTS PRODUCING SYMPTOMS:
   a. Swelling is often the only presenting feature of liver and kidney cysts. It is palpable and sometimes visible. A typical 'hydatid thrift' is occasionally noted on percussion. History of contact with dogs is an important aid to diagnosis. Renal cysts may be clinically mistaken for hepatic cysts.
   b. Jaundice may occasionally occur in cases of liver cysts. This may be either due to pressure by the cyst on bile ducts or rupture of the cyst into the ducts.
   c. Cysts in the lung present with chest pain.

Treatment.—Small cysts are kept under observation and treated medically (see below). Large cysts have to be enucleated. In performing this, the intact cyst, together with the true wall, has to be dissected from the adventitial lining—there is a relatively easy plane of cleavage here.

Care must be taken that the cyst does not rupture during the operation, because the liberated scolices may form new cysts. For this purpose:

   a. The cyst is aspirated carefully to reduce the tension inside.
   b. The surrounding structures are kept separated with packs soaked with hypertonic saline (25 per cent) or sodium hypochlorite solution (0.5 per cent). These kill the escaping scolices, if any, during aspiration or enucleation.

The overlying tissues including the adventitia, are incised and the cyst is enucleated. In case of a lung cyst, positive pressure respiration after liberal incision of the adventitia, expresses the cyst out rather spontaneously.

A course of mebendazole, 400 to 600 mg thrice daily, has to be administered for 3 to 4 weeks in all cases, and repeated as necessary in the cases being treated conservatively.

CYSTS IN THE MOUTH

1. Sublingual Dermoid.
2. Ranula.
3. Mucous Cyst.

Sublingual Dermoid.—This is a dermoid cyst under the tongue. The cyst may be:
1. Above or below the mylohyoid muscle.
2. Median or lateral, i.e. located in the midline or laterally.

Most commonly it is a median cyst, above the mylohyoid, in the floor of the mouth.

CLINICAL FEATURES:
1. A *cyst above the mylohyoid* has to be differentiated from a ranula. A dermoid in this situation has an opaque white appearance (because of its thick wall and sebaceous contents), as compared to the transparent bluish appearance of a ranula.
2. A *midline cyst below the mylohyoid* gives the appearance of a double chin and has to be differentiated from a suprahyoid thyroglossal cyst (a dermoid does not move up with protrusion of tongue).
3. A *lateral cyst below the mylohyoid* presents as a cystic swelling in the region of submandibular salivary gland.

DEVELOPMENT:
1. A median cyst is derived from inclusion of ectoderm at the midline fusion of mandibular processes.
2. A lateral cyst is derived from the second branchial cleft.

Sublingual dermoids differ from other dermoid cysts in that they never contain hairs.

TREATMENT.—Excision of the cyst is done. The approach, for all types of sublingual dermoids, is by an incision on the skin under the mandible.

Ranula.—A ranula is a cystic swelling in the floor of the mouth. The term has come from the word *Rana* which means frog, because the cyst looks like the belly of a small frog.

CLINICAL FEATURES:
1. The cyst is usually found in the childhood.
2. It is usually situated on one side of the frenum linguae, either on the floor of the mouth or on the under surface of the tongue. A big cyst may encroach on to the other side of the floor of the mouth, deep to the frenum linguae. The duct of the submandibular salivary gland is found to cross on its surface.

3. The mucous membrane is freely mobile on the cyst.
4. The cyst is bluish in colour.
5. It is brilliantly transilluminant.
6. A big ranula may dissect its way downwards, between the mylohyoid muscles of the two sides, in which cases the swelling may be visible or palpable under the mandible. This is *called a plunging* or *dissecting ranula*. A cross fluctuation by bimanual palpation may be elicited between the two parts of the swelling—that located at the neck and that situated intrabuccal.

NATURE:
1. The wall is lined by epithelium (cuboidal, columnar or ciliated) or by fibrous tissue.
2. The fluid inside is jelly-like and colourless. There are no salivary ferments in it.

ORIGIN.—There are different views:
1. These are retention cysts in relation to the mucus-secreting glands of the sublingual mucous membrane (glands of Blandin and Nuhn).
2. These are retention cysts in relation to sublingual salivary glands.
3. The plunging variety may be due to a forward prolongation of an unobliterated part of the cervical sinus.

TREATMENT:
1. Total excision is ideal. The difficulty is that the cyst, because of high tension inside it, easily bursts during dissection. Aspiration of some of the contents may overcome this difficulty, but aspiration often fails as the contents are too thick to pass through the needle.
2. Partial excision with *marsupialization*.—This is the usually possible procedure. The dome of the cyst, together with the overlying oral mucosa, is excised. The cut margins of the cyst wall are then sutured to the cut edges of the mucosa, so that the remaining cyst cavity becomes a part of the floor of the mouth. During excision, care must be taken to preserve the Wharton's duct.
3. A plunging ranula has to be approached from the neck, dissection carried between the mylohyoids.

Mucous Cyst.—These are retention cysts of buccal mucous glands.

CLINICAL FEATURES:
1. There is a small cyst, smaller than a pea, located usually on a lip, sometimes inside the cheek.
2. Occasionally there may be more than one cyst.
3. The cyst may have a little bluish colour like a ranula.
4. It is translucent to light.
5. It may be abraded or ulcerated by bite of the teeth.

TREATMENT.—Excision under local anaesthesia. Further cysts may develop later.

MESENTERIC CYSTS

Classification

1. DEVELOPMENT OR EMBRYOLOGICAL CYSTS.—These make most of the cases. They may be of the following types:
   a. Chylolymphatic.
   b. Enterogenous.
   c. Urogenital.
   d. Dermoid (i.e. teratomatous).

2. TRAUMATIC CYSTS.—These arise from encapsulated haematoma (rare). The fluid inside is serosanguineous.

3. INFLAMMATORY CYSTS.—These are tuberculous in origin and are rare. Either there is a tuberculous abscess of the mesentery or a mesenteric tuberculosis heals with cyst formation.

4. PARASITIC CYSTS.—Hydatid cysts, usually secondary to cysts in the liver (rare).

Chylolymphatic Cysts.—These are believed to arise from embryologically misplaced lymph-vessel network in the mesentery, that fails to develop communications with the lymphatic system, very much comparable to cystic hygroma in the neck. They are commoner in relation to the ileum. The cyst wall, which is thin and translucent, is made of fibrous tissue lined with flattened endothelium. The content may be clear lymph or milky chyme. The blood supply to the cyst is independent of that to the adjacent intestine. Therefore the cyst can be enucleated out without damaging the blood supply to the gut, and there is no necessity for intestinal resection.

Enterogenous Cysts.—Compared to chylolymphatic cysts, these are much rare. As their name signifies, they are related to developmental anomalies in the adjacent gut. They may originate in either of the following ways:
  i. Duplication of the gut (more commonly).
  ii. Diverticulum arising from the mesenteric border of the gut, which thereafter loses continuity with the gut.

The commonest site is the neighbourhood of the ileocaecal region. The cyst wall, which is always very thick, consists of fibrous tissue lined by mucus-secreting epithelium. The content, therefore, is mucoid. The cyst wall has a common blood supply with the related intestine (the origin of the cyst explains this). Hence, removal of the cyst always necessitates resection of the related portion of the gut.

Urogenital Cysts.—As their name signifies, these cysts originate from the sequestrated rudiments of the developing urogenital system, especially the Wolffian body. They are as common as the chylolymphatic cysts. The wall of the cyst may be thin or thick, and the content is watery. They can be enucleated out easily.

Complications of Mesenteric Cysts.—About 30 per cent of the cysts develop complications, which may be as follows:

1. *Intestinal Obstruction.*—This may be caused by any of the following factors:
   a. Development of adhesions, usually secondary to infection in the cyst.

b. Pressure by the cyst on surrounding coils of intestine.

c. Impaction of the intestinal contents in a segment of gut that has been narrowed by the cyst. In these cases the obstruction is temporary and recurrent.

d. Torsion of the mesentery. Here also the obstruction is temporary and recurrent.

2. *Torsion* of that part of the mesentery which contains the cyst.—The patient presents with features of an acute abdominal catastrophe.

3. *Haemorrhage* in the cyst.—There may be a bout of severe hemorrhage or there may be repeated small haemorrhages. In the first instance, the patient develops an acute abdominal catastrophe. In the latter event, there may be prolonged anaemia.

4. *Rupture* of the cyst.— This may sometimes be caused by insignificant trauma. The patient presents with features of severe intra-abdominal haemorrhage and peritoneal irritation.

5. *Infection* in the cyst.—Infection usually reaches the cyst from the bowel. The cyst becomes painful. It loses its mobility and acquires the features of an intra-abdominal abscess.

Clinical Features.—Three groups of cases are encountered.

A. Silent cases.—A good number of cases belong to this group. The cyst, causing no symptoms, is found at laparotomy or autopsy.

B. Usual group.—The patient usually presents with a painless swelling in the abdomen. The swelling is characterised by *Tillaux's triad:*

1. It is fluctuant and located near the umbilicus.

2. It is freely mobile at right angles to the line of attachment of the mesentery, but not so along that line.

3. There is a zone of resonance around the cyst (the neighbouring intestinal coils) and, characteristically, a band of resonance across the cyst (the intestine related to the cyst).

C. Cases with complications:

1. Recurrent attacks of intestinal colic, with or without vomiting, caused by:

   a. Impaction of the intestinal contents in the segment of the intestine narrowed by the cyst.

   b. Torsion of the mesentery.

2. Acute abdominal catastrophe, which may be due to:

   a. Torsion of that part of the mesentery which contains the cyst.

   b. Haemorrhage in the cyst.

   c. Rupture of the cyst.

3. Pain and features of intra-abdominal abscess due to infection in the cyst.

Special Investigations

1. Ultrasonography reveals an well outlined, sonolucent and transonic swelling.

2. CT scan may be necessary in cases of inconclusive ultrasonographic findings. An unenhancing near-water density mass is characteristic.

3. Intravenous urography is an alternative procedure to ultrasonography (to exclude renal swelling).
4. Barium meal X-ray shows displacement of the loops of gut around the mass and, sometimes, narrowing of the adjacent loop. A good straight X-ray may also reveal this by the displacement of the shadows of gas in the gut.
3. Injection of a contrast medium (water soluble) into the cyst, after partially aspirating it, and taking an X-ray is only rarely done now.

Treatment.—The cyst has to be removed:

1. In cases of chylolymphatic and urogenital cysts, enucleation is usually possible. If the major part of the cyst is dissectable but one part of its wall is closely adherent to the intestine or to major blood vessels, this part of the wall may be left behind and the rest of the cyst wall removed after partially aspirating it. The lining of the left-out wall is destroyed by diathermy.
2. In cases of enterogenous cyst, excision of the cyst entails resection of the related part of the gut.

8

Ulcers

Definition.—An ulcer is a breach in continuity of an epithelial surface—skin or mucous membrane. There is destruction of the surface tissue and the destruction is cell by cell, i.e. microscopic (cf gangrene, where tissue death is *en masse*, i.e. macroscopic).

Classification

A. NON-SPECIFIC

1. *Traumatic:*
   a. Mechanical.—Dental ulcers (caused by ill-fitting dentures, pressure-sores (*by* splints or plaster).
   b. Physical.—Burns and scalds.
   c. Chemical.—Burns caused by acids or alkalies.

2. *Inflammatory:* Usually resulting from secondary infection in traumatic ulcers, caused by non-specific pyogenic organisms like Staphylococcus, Streptococcus, etc.

3. *Nutritional* or *Trophic* (Greek *Trophe* = nutrition): These are results of impairment of nutrition and may be due to:
   a. Poor arterial supply.—Buerger's disease, arteriosclerosis, etc.
   b. Venous stasis.—Varicose ulcer, post-thrombotic ulcer.
   c. Lymphatic stasis, i.e. following lymphoedema.
   d. Neurogenic.—Due to loss of sensation, e.g. bedsores, perforating ulcers.
   e. Associated with malnutrition.—Tropical ulcer, diabetic ulcer (the sugar-laden tissues favour infection), ulcers in severe avitaminosis, ulcers over deposits of gout, etc.

B. SPECIFIC

1. *Due to specific infections:*
   a. Tuberculous ulcers.
   b. Syphilitic ulcers.—Hard chancre (primary stage), snail-track ulcers, mucous patches (secondary stage), gummatous ulcers (tertiary stage).
   c. Soft chancres.
   d. Actinomycotic ulcers.

2. *Due to specific internal causes:*
   a. Peptic ulcer.
   b. Ulcerative colitis.

C. MALIGNANT

1. Rodent ulcer.

2. Epithelioma.
3. Malignant melanoma.
4. Any malignant growth fungating through skin.

Examination of an Ulcer

A. EXAMINATION OF THE ULCER ITSELF

1. *Inspection:*
   a. Site.—This is often typical, e.g. varicose ulcer, rodent ulcer, peptic ulcer.
   b. Number, shape, and size.
   c. Margin.—This is often diagnostic, e.g.
      i. Thin overhanging margins in tuberculous ulcers.
      ii. Punched out margins in gummatous ulcers.
      iii. Rolled out everted margins in malignant ulcers.
      iv. Rolled out or rampart margins like motor car tyres in rodent ulcers.
      v. Stepping margins in varicose ulcers.
   d. Relationship to the surface:
      i. Below the surface level.—Non-malignant ulcers.
      ii. Above the surface level, i.e. raised from surface.—Malignant ulcers.
   e. Floor.—This signifies the surface of the ulcer, i.e. that part which can be seen. This may show:
      i. Necrosed granulation tissue, i.e. slough, which may be typical— watery or apple-jelly in tuberculous ulcers, wash-leather in gummatous ulcers.
      ii. Healthy granulation tissue, as seen in healing non-specific ulcers.
      iii. Malignant tissue.
   f. Discharge.—This may be small or profuse. The type of discharge may be typical, e.g. sulphur-granules in actinomycotic ulcers.

2. *Palpation:*
   a. Local rise of temperature.
   b. Tenderness.
   c. Base.—This signifies the area on which the ulcer rests. The base is palpated for:
      i. Induration.—A little induration may be felt at the base of any chronic ulcer but marked induration is almost diagnostic of a malignant ulcer. Hard chancres also show induration at the base.
      ii. Mobility over the underlying structures.
   d. Friability.—Too much friability is often diagnostic of malignancy.
   e. Bleeding to touch is again suggestive of malignancy (sometimes also found in healthy granulating ulcers).

B. EXAMINATION OF THE SURROUNDING AREA.—This may show important features, e.g. pigmentation in varicose ulcer (due to haemosiderin pigments), melanotic halo in malignant melanoma.

C. EXAMINATION OF REGIONAL LYMPH NODES.—The nature of the enlarged nodes may often indicate the type of the ulcer.

D. EXAMINATION FOR IMPAIRMENT OF CIRCULATION
   1. Absence of arterial pulsation.
   2. Varicosity of veins.

E. EXAMINATION FOR NERVE LESIONS

Special Investigations
1. Examination of urine for sugar.
2. Examination of blood:
   a. Sugar (diabetes).
   b. ESR (tuberculosis).
   c. VDRL, WR and Kahn tests (syphilis).
3. Examination of the discharge from the ulcer:
   a. Smear examination.
   b. Culture (and sensitivity test, if there is growth on culture).
4. Biopsy:
   a. Cutting biopsy.—Removing a wedge from the margin of the ulcer. The central part of the ulcer is not chosen because it contains only necrotic material.
   b. Excision biopsy.—The whole of the ulcer may be excised and examined.
5. X-ray:
   a. Of the underlying bone.
   b. Chest, in cases of tuberculous or malignant ulcers.

Life-history of an Ulcer.—This consists of three phases:
1. *Stage of Spreading:*
   Floor—covered with slough.
   Margins—sharply defined.
   Base—indurated.
   Discharge—profuse, purulent, sometimes blood-stained.
   Surrounding area—inflamed.

2. *Stage of Transition:*
   Floor—cleaner, with sloughs separating, and small reddish areas of granulation tissue appearing.
   Base—induration diminishing.
   Surrounding area—signs of inflammation regressed.

3. This stage may either show signs of healing or characters of a callous ulcer:
   a. *Stage of Healing:*
      Floor—the granulation tissue is converted into fibrous tissue which later contracts to form a scar.

Margins—become more shelving, and epithelium from here gradually extends on to the floor of the ulcer to cover it up (one mm per day).

b. *Change to Callous Ulcer:*

This means that the ulcer has no tendency to heal by itself—

Floor—unhealthy pale granulation tissue.

Base—indurated.

Margins—thickened, oedematous, indurated, and often discoloured.

Surrounding area—oedematous and indurated.

Tuberculous Ulcers.—These may result from bursting of cold abscesses—

a. in relation to tuberculous nodes (commonest),

b. from tuberculous bone or joint lesions,

c. from submucous lesions, e.g. intestine, tongue.

CHARACTER

Number—often multiple.

Pain—may be present.

Depth—usually shallow.

Margins—overhanging with thin bluish margins (Fig. 8.1).

Floor—pale granulation tissue with variable amount of discharge.

Base—may be a little indurated and attached to the pathological lesion, e.g. nodes.

Syphilitic Ulcers.—Syphilis may manifest itself as ulcer in all its three stages.

PRIMARY STAGE.—A hard chancre (*Hunterian chancre*) usually appears 3 weeks after contact. It develops at the site of contact, i.e. usually genitalia, but occasionally at extragenital sites, e.g. lip, tongue, etc.

Number—single (usually).

Base—indurated (hence the ulcer feels like a *button*).

Discharge—serous, in which *Tr pallida* may be demonstrated.

Lymph nodes—enlarged, discrete, firm, painless, and non-suppurating.

SECONDARY STAGE.—The lesions are usually manifested at the mucocutaneous junctions, e.g. mouth, anus, or vulva. The types of lesion are:

1. *Mucous Patches.*—White patches of thickened and sodden epithelium.

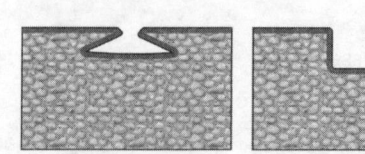 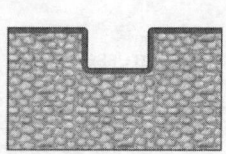 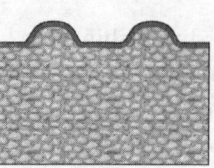 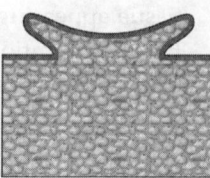

Tuberculous   Gummatous   Rodent   Carcinomatous

Fig. 8.1: Characters of different types of ulcers

2. *Condyloma.*—White patches of hypertrophic epithelium which are raised from the surface as fungating sessile masses, but their surfaces flat. The surface is moist and sodden.

3. *Snail-track Ulcers.*—Usually multiple, narrow, shallow, and curved ulcers.

With the above lesions, a generalised enlargement of lymph nodes is usually found; the suboccipital and epitrochlear nodes are almost always involved.

TERTIARY STAGE.—A gummatous ulcer may be found:

1. Over subcutaneous bones (e.g. skull, sternum, tibia, ulna).

2. Over the scrotum—in relation to testis.

3. Rarely over the tongue.

    Number—solitary.

    Pain—absent.

    Margin—clean, punched out (Fig. 8.1).

    Floor—wash-leather slough.

    VDRL, WR and Kahn tests—positive.

Soft Chancres.—These are also known as *soft sores* or *chancroids.* They are also called *Ducrey's ulcers* as they are caused by Ducrey's Streptobacillus. They appear on the genitalia 2 to 5 days after the infection.

Number—always multiple.

Pain—present.

Margins—oedematous.

Floor—yellowish slough, discharging profusely, and often bleeding to touch.

Base—no induration.

Lymph nodes—acute lymphadenitis with tendency to suppurate.

Rodent Ulcer.—This is a tumour arising from the basal cells of the skin or from cells of similar origin, as in hair follicles and sweat glands. It is called an ulcer because the tumour has a tendency to break on the surface, causing ulceration. It is called rodent because it has a tendency to erode any tissue, including cartilage and bone, in contact of which it comes (Rodent = rat).

Though in the majority of cases it makes an ulcer, the tumour may be macroscopically of other types as well.

The *macroscopic types* are:

1. Ulcerative, with typical rolled edge (not necessarily everted), often beaded (like a motor car tyre), and the floor showing scabbing over some areas and breaking at others. This is the usual type (Fig. 8.1).

2. Nodular.

3. Cystic.

4. Linear fissure.

5. Field-fire.—So named because it has a tendency to heal over some areas while breaking over fresh areas.

MICROSCOPIC FEATURES.—There are solid columns of darkly-staining epithelial cells that grow down into the dermis. There are no cell-nests and only few prickle cells (cf epidermoid carcinoma). Rarely the tumour may change into an epidermoid carcinoma (*baso-squamous carcinoma*).

CLINICAL FEATURES.—Commonly starting at or above the middle age, it has a tendency to occur in people more exposed to sunrays. More than 90 per cent of the cases occur in the skin of the face, above a line joining the angle of the mouth and the ear lobule. The commonest site is near the inner canthus of the eye (hence called *tear cancer*).

SPREAD.—The tumour is locally malignant, without a tendency to spread to nodes or distally (cf epithelioma). However, its local infiltrative power is very strong, and it not only spreads peripherally but also infiltrates through skin, subcutaneous tissues, deeper structures and even cartilage and bone, producing severe disfigurement.

TREATMENT.—There are two methods of treatment:

1. *Surgery.*—Excision of the growth with healthy tissue at circumference and at depth (tridimensional wide excision). The gap may have to be covered with split-skin or full-thickness grafts. Biopsy, after excision, must be done to confirm the diagnosis and ensure tumour-free margins.
2. *Radiotherapy.*—This gives a better cosmetic result than excision. The eye has to be shielded properly from radiation. Repeated small doses over several weeks are better than large single dose to minimise necrosis and scarring. Radiotherapy is ideal for recurrence after excision but is contraindicated if cartilage or bone is involved.
3. *Cryosurgery* is ideal for small superficial lesions, especially in the elderly, because it can be done under local anaesthesia.
4. *Cautery and Curettage* is also advocated for small superficial tumour in the elderly and done under local anaesthesia.

Marjolin's Ulcer.—Formerly known as 'chronic scars', these are actually low-grade malignant epithelial tumours (epithelioma) developing on scars, usually of burn. To start with, and for a long time:

1. It grows slowly—since the scar is relatively avascular.
2. It is painless—since there are no nerves in the scar.
3. There is no lymph node metastasis—since the lymphatics have been destroyed and occluded.

Later however, when the ulcer spreads to the surrounding healthy skin, it grows more rapidly and may metastasise to nodes.

Treatment.—Wide tridimensional excision, followed by split-skin or full-thickness grafts.

Trophic Ulcers.—A trophic ulcer is due to an impairment of nutrition—either an inadequate blood supply or absence of properly functioning nerve supply (*see* classification).

The neurogenic variety of trophic ulcer, which is due to impaired sensory nerve supply, i.e. anaesthesia, is often called *perforating ulcer*. Such ulcers may be found in diabetic neuritis, peripheral nerve injury, spina bifida, leprosy, tabes dorsalis, etc.

A perforating ulcer is most commonly found to start beneath the head of the first metatarsal but may also be found on the heel, i.e. the *pressure points* under the foot. The condition usually starts as a corn or callosity, under which suppuration occurs. The pus is discharged out through a small central opening. This opening gradually deepens in the form of a tunnel, which burrows through the fascial planes, and may involve the bones and joints. The cavity becomes filled with offensive material and, spreading upwards along the fascial planes, it may even come up to the calf. Later, the track becomes lined by skin, and then healing becomes impossible.

Bedsores (Dccubitus Ulcers).— These are of two types—acute and chronic.

Acute bedsore (*the trophic variety*) is associated with disease or injury of the spinal cord. An acute bedsore differs from a chronic one in two points:

a. It develops and spreads with alarming rapidity in spite of every care and attention.

b. Occasionally it does not develop at one of the usual points of pressure.

As regards the causes of acute bedsores, there are two views:

i. They are due to disturbances in the trophic centres of the spinal cord (there are doubts whether such centres exist).

ii. They are due to capillary stasis from injury to the vasomotor nerves.

Chronic bedsore (*the postural variety*) is predisposed by several factors:

1. Pressure.—It develops over the pressure points, e.g. sacrum, buttocks, heels.

2. Devitalised condition of the tissues:
   a. Malnutrition, particularly protein deficiency.
   b. Anaemia.
   c. Old age or prolonged illness.

3. Oedema and moisture:
   a. Hypostasis from feeble circulation.
   b. Oedema due to anaemia.
   c. Maceration of the skin by sweat, urine, or pus.

4. Injury.—This may be of a chronic nature, e.g. folds of bedsheets, rubber clothes.

Treatment:

A. Prophylactic Treatment.—This is of utmost importance. A bedsore is apprehended if there is an erythema over a pressure point which does not change colour on pressure. The prophylactic treatment consists of:

1. A suitable soft smooth bed of foam. Water beds, ripple beds and airless beds are now used.
2. Alteration of posture every 2 hours as far as practicable.
3. Maintaining the parts dry and clean.
4. Hardening of the skin on the pressure points, by cleansing with rectified spirit.
5. Correction of malnutrition and anaemia.

B. Established Cases:

1. Turning the patient away from over the pressure point or using air cushions under the sores.
2. Correction of malnutrition and anaemia. Repeated blood transfusion often work miraculously.
3. Antibiotics.
4. Dressing of the sore with lotions or ointments, and hardening the surrounding skin with rectified spirit. The surrounding skin must be kept dry and clean.
5. In selected cases the dead tissues are excised and the raw area covered with rotational or sliding skin grafts.

9

Erysipelas, Cellulitis, Boil, Abscess, Carbuncle

ERYSIPELAS

Organism.—*Streptococcus pyogenes.*

Pathology.—The condition is commoner in debilitated subjects, usually at the extremes of life. There is a spreading cuticular lymphangitis with varying degrees of cellulitis, in the neighbourhood of a scratch or abrasion. A varying degree of toxaemia occurs.

Clinical Features

1. The skin over the involved area shows a rose-pink rash, which disappears on pressure. This rash is raised from the surface (better felt than seen). The margins are well-demarcated. The area is irritable and stiff. The face is the commonest site—'butterfly lesions' occur on the nose and cheeks.
2. Vesicles then appear, burst, and discharge serum.
3. A variable amount of oedema occurs and this may be considerable in lax tissues, e.g. eyelids, scrotum.
4. The rash gradually fades away but a brown discolouration of skin remains for a few weeks (due to pigments set free by disintegrated RBC).
5. Fever and other constitutional symptoms of varying degrees occur.

Treatment.—Injection penicillin or erythromycin tablets completely controls the condition.

Complications

1. Sloughing or gangrene may rarely occur in grossly debilitated or diabetic patients, particularly in areas with lax subcutaneous tissue, e.g. scrotum.
2. Lymphoedema may rarely occur due to lymphatic obstruction, caused by fibrosis of the lymph vessels and glands, in severe infections. This is more likely to occur in lax tissues, e.g. eyelids.

CELLULITIS

Definition.—This is a spreading inflammation of the subcutaneous tissues and fascial planes, usually ending in suppuration. Sometimes it may lead to sloughing or even gangrene, particularly in the diabetics.

Pathology.—Any organism may cause a cellulitis but it is particularly due to *Streptococcus pyogenes* which has the inherent property of causing diffuse inflammation.

Thus, cellulitis has a pathological similarity to erysipelas, from which it is clinically differentiated by the following points:

1. The rose-pink rashes are not seen.
2. The edges are indefinite and not raised up.
3. In case of the face, while erysipelas may spread to the pinna (being a cuticular infection), cellulitis cannot do so because it is a subcutaneous infection (the skin here is closely adherent to the underlying cartilage).

Clinical Features

1. There is a varying degree of fever and toxaemia.
2. The affected part is swollen and painful, hot and tender. There is a pitting oedema and a brawny feel (other features have been described above).
3. The regional lymph vessels may be seen as red streaks and the draining nodes may show features of acute lymphadenitis.

Treatment

1. Rest to the part.
2. Keeping the part elevated, to reduce oedema.
3. Antibiotics, preferably broad spectrum.
4. Investigations and treatment for diabetes.
5. When there is localisation of pus, free incision along the long axis of the limb.

BOIL (FURUNCLE)

Definition.—This is an acute infection of a hair follicle with associated perifolliculitis, caused by staphylococcal infection.

It appears as a painful swelling, which is indurated for the first 2 to 3 days. Thereafter central softening occurs and a small pustule appears on the summit of the swelling. This pustule ruptures, discharging a little pus and a small slough. The resulting cavity quickly heals by granulation and fibrosis.

A *blind boil* is one which subsides without suppuration.

Treatment

1. Usually, only local hot fomentation is sufficient.
2. If the condition is very painful, a small incision may be required.
3. Antibiotics are generally not required. If the boils are multiple or recurrent, erythromycin may have to be administered.
4. If the boils are recurrent, particularly in an elderly person, diabetes should be excluded.

ABSCESS

An abscess is a collection of pus. There are three types of abscess:

1. Pyogenic abscess.
2. Pyaemic abscess.
3. Cold abscess.

While a pyogenic abscess shows all evidences of acute inflammation, the pyaemic and cold abscesses are usually non-reacting in nature, i.e. they do not show all evidences of acute inflammation.

Pyogenic Abscess

This is a collection of pus, resulting from infection by pyogenic organisms. This pus is formed by liquefaction of tissues, caused by a proteolytic enzyme derived from the polymorphonuclear leucocytes which infiltrate at the site of the inflammation.

The commonest *precursors* of pyogenic abscess are cellulitis and acute lymphadenitis.

Fate:

1. Tension inside the abscess cavity gradually rises owing to exudation of plasma, and the abscess spreads along the paths of least resistance to:
   a. the surface of the body, or
   b. a hollow viscus, into which it ruptures.
2. Occasionally, body resistance, aided by antibiotics, may kill the bacteria before the abscess finds its way to the surface. The fluid is then gradually absorbed and
   a. either fibrosis occurs, or
   b. the cavity persists and contains thick, sterile pus (*antibioma*).

Clinical Features:

1. The cardinal features of acute inflammation are all present, viz.
   a. *Calor* (heat).—The inflamed area is hot due to hyperaemia.
   b. *Rubor* (redness).—There is redness over the area due to hyperaemia.
   c. *Dolor* (pain).—A throbbing pain is characteristic of pus under tension and is due to pressure on the surrounding nerves by the exudates. There is tenderness.
   d. *Tumour* (swelling).—Due to inflammatory exudates.
2. The presence of pus is detected by:
   a. Fluctuation, when the pus is superficial.
   b. A brawny oedema, pitting under pressure, together with induration, when the pus is deep-seated (e.g. breast, parotid, ischiorectal).
3. Fever and other constitutional features of varying degrees.

Treatment:

1. In very early cases, where pus is still to form, a conservative treatment is advised—rest and elevation of the part, together with antibiotics.
2. As soon as presence of pus is diagnosed, a liberal incision with dependant drainage has to be instituted. It should be remembered that fluctuation is late or never to appear in deep-seated abscesses and, in these cases, the induration and the pitting brawny oedema should be the indications for immediate incision. In this respect, breast, parotid, and perianal abscess and those associated with hand infections, including whitlow should be especially remembered.

Drainage of Abscesses

A. ANAESTHESIA: Superficial abscesses may be drained with surface anaesthesia (ethyl chloride spray). Deep abscesses require general anaesthesia. Local infiltration anaesthesia should not be used because it helps spread of infection to the neighbouring tissues.

B. INCISION: There are two methods of opening abscesses:

1. *Free or liberal incision.*—A liberal incision is made usually over the most prominent part of the abscess, thus causing minimum damage to the surrounding healthy tissues. The principles of the incision should be as follows:

   a. It should be liberal to ensure adequate drainage.

   b. It should be parallel to important vessels, nerves and tendons.

   c. If the pus has to be drained from a part deep to a muscle, the muscle fibres should be split rather than cut through.

2. *Hilton's method.*—This method is preferred for abscesses underlying which there are important structures that might be damaged by bold free incisions, e.g. neck, axilla, groin. A small incision is made over the most prominent part of the abscess, cutting through the skin, subcutaneous tissue and deep fascia. A sinus forceps, with its blades apposed, is now thrust into the abscess cavity through this incision and the blades are separated. This enlarges the opening on the surface without causing damage to important structures underneath. The forceps is withdrawn with its blades still open and this process further enlarges the opening.

C. EXPLORATION: A finger is introduced into the abscess cavity:

   i. to define its limits,

   ii. to break any septum inside, thus making all loculi into one cavity, for complete drainage.

D. COUNTER-INCISION: An abscess will always drains better if there is a counter-incision. Counter-incision is obligatory for those abscesses in which the most prominent part (where the original incision is put), is not the most dependant part; here the counter-incision helps drainage by gravity.

A sinus forceps is passed through the original incision, along the abscess cavity, to its most dependant part, and is made prominent on the skin there. A small nick is made on the skin over the forceps to make the counter-opening.

E. DRAINAGE: This may be provided by:

1. A corrugated rubber drain or a wick of gauge.

2. Where the wall of the abscess is very vascular, a tight packing of the cavity; this is required to achieve haemostasis.

F. POST-OPERATIVE CARE:

1. Rest to the part.

2. Antibiotics, preferably chosen by culture-sensitivity test.

3. Regular dressings. If the cavity has been packed, the packing should gradually be make lighter, enabling the cavity to heal.

Axillary Abscess
Causes:
1. Suppurative lymphadenitis.
2. Extension of infection from hair follicles or sweat glands.

Incision.—The pus is usually located behind the pectoralis major. The abscess is opened by Hilton's method, with the arm fully abducted. The incision is placed half an inch behind the anterior axillary fold (there is no important structure in this situation).

Inguinal Abscess (Bubo)
Causes.—This is due to suppuration of the inguinal nodes. There are two types:
1. Suppuration of the vertical and lateral horizontal chain of nodes. This is usually secondary to infection in the lower limb.
2. Suppuration of the medial horizontal chain of nodes, usually secondary to infections in the genitalia.

Incision:
1. In the first variety, the incision is made vertical:
    a. to avoid cutting across the femoral vessels.
    b. to afford better drainage, since the opening widens when the hip is flexed.
2. In the second variety, the incision is a transverse one, along the inguinal ligament.

Popliteal Abscess
Causes:
1. Suppurative lymphadenitis.
2. Acute osteomyelitis of lower femur or upper tibia.
    (The condition should be carefully diagnosed from a popliteal aneurysm).

Incision.—The abscess is opened by Hilton's method. The incision is placed on the lateral side of the popliteal space, by the side of, and parallel to, the biceps tendon. The lateral popliteal nerve should be taken care of.

Gluteal Abscess
Causes:
1. Injections.—In older days quinine was a common cause. It has been found that even injections of antibiotics may cause abscess formation.
2. Infected haematoma.

Incision.—A liberal incision is made over the most prominent part, along the fibres of the gluteus maximus, i.e. downwards and laterally.
A counter-incision must be made.

Thigh Abscess
There are two types—superficial and deep.

Causes:
1. Superficial:
   a. Subcutaneous infusion of saline.
   b. Extension of infection from hair follicles, sweat glands, etc.
2. Deep:
   a. Infected haematoma in muscles.
   b. Acute osteomyelitis of femur.

Incision.—A liberal incision is made on the lateral side of the thigh. If the abscess is deep, the deep fascia must be incised.

A counter-incision should always be employed.

Deltoid Abscess
Causes:
1. Injections (as for gluteal abscess).
2. Infected haematoma.

Incision.—A liberal incision is made over the most prominent part of the abscess. The incision is along the direction of the muscle fibres.

A counter-incision is obligatory.

Sole Abscess and Heel Abscess
Causes:
1. Foreign body prick.
2. Acute osteomyelitis of calcaneum.

Incision.—A liberal incision is made along the lateral or medial margin of the sole or heel, according to the prominence of the swelling. This avoids scar on the weight-bearing areas.

A counter-incision on the other side (medial or lateral) is preferred. It must be sure that the plane of the abscess has been reached. Sometimes the abscess is collar-stud and wrongly the superficial part (prominent under the cuticle only) is incised, the main abscess cavity being spared.

Pyaemic Abscess
These are metastatic abscesses, caused by infective emboli in cases of pyaemia.

Pyaemia is a condition in which infective emboli, consisting of clumps of organisms, infected clot, or vegetation, circulate in the blood stream. They are commonly associated with conditions like acute osteomyelitis, infected compound fracture, acute inflammation of an intracranial sinus, acute bacterial endocarditis, etc. Acute appendicitis may cause pyaemia in the portal venous system, i.e. *portal pyaemia.*

Bacteriaemia is a state where organisms circulate in the blood stream.

Septicaemia is a condition in which organisms not only circulate in the blood stream but also proliferate therein and produce toxins which cause toxaemic illness.

Toxaemia is a state in which toxins, bacterial or chemical, circulate in the blood stream and produce characteristic toxaemic symptoms.

PYAEMIC ABSCESSES are characterised by the following features:

1. They are multiple.
2. Some of them occur on the surface and here they are commonest in the subfascial plane. They are non-reacting in nature—usually presenting as swellings with little pain and little or no sign of acute inflammation.
3. Some may occur in the viscera, particularly in the spleen and kidneys. Death may be caused by such abscesses developing in the vital organs like heart or brain.

Treatment:

1. Treatment of the source, if detectable.
2. Antibiotics, preferably chosen by culture-sensitivity test.
3. Incision of the abscesses located on the surface.

Cold Abscess

These denote tuberculous abscesses, most commonly arising in lymph nodes, bones or joints. As their name signifies, they are non-reacting, i.e. not presenting with the cardinal features of acute inflammation, as seen in pyogenic abscesses. Nevertheless, some of them may be associated with considerable evidence of acute inflammation.

The abscesses in relation to the nodes are diagnosed by their characteristic positions where important sets of nodes are located, e.g. neck, axilla, or groin. The underlying nodes may show, on palpation, characteristic features of tuberculous lymphadenitis, i.e. soft and matted nodes.

Cold abscesses from bone or joints also have certain characteristic situations. They are most commonly found in caries spine which is the commonest form of bone tuberculosis. These cold abscesses have a peculiar tendency to travel to long distances along definite anatomical planes, usually tracing a nerve, sometimes a vessel.

Special Investigations:

1. Blood examination.—TC, DC, and ESR.
2. X-ray chest.
3. Mantoux test.
4. ELISA test.—False positive results are common.
5. Aspiration of the abscess, followed by smear and culture examinations. Special staining is required to show the acid-fast bacilli. The pus is usually sterile on ordinary culture. Special culture media (e.g. Lowenstein's) may be necessary. Guinea-pig inocculation test may be confirmatory.

Treatment:

1. Full antituberculosis treatment.
2. Treatment for the primary focus.
3. For the abscess itself:
   a. Repeated aspiration with local instillation of INH solution.
   b. Some surgeons advocate complete excision of the abscess with its wall, together with the focus of origin, e.g. a group of nodes.

4. An incision should not be made on a cold abscess, since it invariably invites secondary infection, leading to a persistent tuberculous sinus.

CARBUNCLE

Pathology.—This is a superficial infective gangrene, involving the subcutaneous tissue, caused by staphylococcal infection. The points of importance are:

1. It is not a simple inflammatory process but a gangrene. However, the gangrene only involves the subcutaneous tissue.
2. Very often the patient is a diabetic subject.
3. Most commonly it occurs over the nape of the neck. Here the skin is coarse and ill-nourished. Also, the skin is closely adherent to the underlying deep fascia and so the inflammatory exudates are under high tension in the subcutaneous tissues. These factors, together, lead to loss of vascularity of the skin and subcutaneous tissues, causing a superficial gangrene. Other relatively common sites are the back and shoulders, the cheek and the upper lip, and the dorsum of fingers.

Clinical Features.—The patient complains of pain and stiffness over the area which, on palpation, reveals an induration of the skin and subcutaneous tissues. This area gradually increases in size considerably.

The skin over the area is red and dusky. Subsequently, multiple vesicles appear on it and are transformed into pustules which burst on the surface one after another, bringing out a purulent discharge. Thus the surface looks *sieve-like*. Thereafter the central openings coalesce to make a big crateriform ulcer, surrounding which there are the 'rosette' of the smaller openings. At the base of the ulcer lies a greyish slough.

If healing is favourable, the slough separates and the cavity gradually fills up with healthy granulation tissue.

Treatment

1. Adequate treatment for diabetes, if present.
2. Antibiotics.—Erythromycin is usually the best.
3. Hot compresses, preferably with SS Mag Sulph and local application of osmotic pastes, e.g. Mag Sulph, are often helpful in earlier cases, reducing the oedema.
4. Infrared or shortwave diathermy are believed to be helpful.
5. *Operation.*—This has to be undertaken only when the carbuncle has softened. Severe pain, toxaemia, and a big size are the special indications for operation. A cruciate incision, liberally extended to the margins of the carbuncle, is made. All sloughs are removed either with gauge swabs or by sharp cuts with scissors, care being taken not to encroach on the living tissues. The apices of the four skin flaps are now cut, making the opening circular and large.

   Post-operatively, antibiotics must be continued.

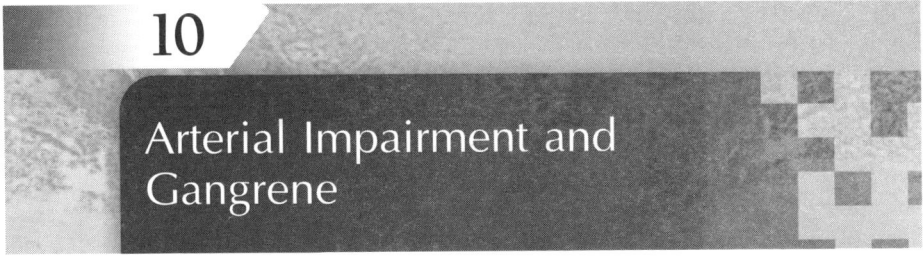

10

Arterial Impairment and Gangrene

The following are the effects of interruption of blood supply to any part of the body:

I. Opening up of collateral circulation.

II. Ischaemic pain.

III. Ischaemic ulceration and gangrene.

COLLATERAL CIRCULATION

There is always a natural attempt for collaterals to develop. Efficient opening of the collaterals may *not* occur:

1. If the obstruction is sudden.
2. If the area of obstruction has anatomically a poor collateral distribution, e.g. coronaries, popliteal, etc.
3. If the tissues have a poor vascular network—as in areas round the joints that are not covered by muscles.
4. If there are pre-existing cardiovascular disorders, e.g. atherosclerosis, heart failure, etc.

To stimulate opening up of collateral circulation, in an attempt to prevent gangrene, 'various vasodilator methods' are used (*see* page 96).

ISCHAEMIC PAIN

Almost all cases of arterial impairment are associated with some form of pain. The pain is acute in cases of sudden obstruction and chronic in cases of gradual obstruction. The cause of pain is due to ischaemia of the muscles and the nerves, but the presentation of pain resulting from ischaemia of these two tissues are different. Ischaemia of the muscles causes intermittent claudication while ischaemic neuritis gives rise to rest pain.

Intermittent Claudication.—This is believed to be due to accumulation of irritant metabolites in the ischaemic muscles. The pain is in the form of a cramp and is particularly noticed in the calf muscles during exercise (walking or cycling). The distance that a patient can walk before the onset of the cramp is called *the claudication distance* and this is often a good index of the level and the severity of the obstruction.

Usually intermittent claudication passes through *three stages* (Boyd):

Grade I: The patient feels pain just as he starts walking and the pain passes off after a little walk (it is presumed that, with exercise, the accumulated irritant metabolite is pumped out of the muscle).

Grade II: The patient feels pain after walking for some distance but can manage to proceed further with effort.

Grade III: The pain, on walking for some distance, is so severe that the patient has to take rest. This distance is the claudication distance.

Rest Pain.—The pain, which is due to ischaemic neuritis, is mostly felt in the forefoot and toes (cf claudication in the calf). To start with, it is noticed at night, gradually getting more severe, and ultimately occurring day and night. Unlike claudication, it is reinless.

GANGRENE

Definition.—Gangrene means macroscopic death of tissue with putrefaction superadded (cf ulcer, where the tissue death is microscopic).

While gangrene is clinically seen in the limbs, particularly the toes and feet, it may be found at operation or at postmortem in the appendix, intestines, gall bladder, pancreas, and testis. Bedsore and carbuncles, which are also variant forms of gangrene, are often seen on the trunk.

The term *'necrosis'* applies to death of a group of cells including the bone (sequestrum). A *'slough' signifies* a piece of necrotic soft tissue.

Causes of Gangrene

I. *Secondary* to:

   A. Arterial obstruction:

      1. Atherosclerosis (senile gangrene).

      2. Embolism (embolic gangrene).

      3. Vasospastic conditions

         a. Raynaud's disease.

         b. Other conditions—cervical rib, ergot poisoning, etc.

      4. Buerger's disease.

      5. Diabetic gangrene in the elderly.

      6. Syphilitic gangrene (due to endarteritis obliterans).

   B. Venous obstruction.—Deep vein thrombosis.

   C. Nerve diseases.—Syringomyelia, tabes dorsalis, peripheral neuritis (including diabetic), hemiplegia, leprosy, etc.

II. *Traumatic:*

   A. Direct:

      1. Physical.—Crushing of tissues, pressure sores, bedsores.

      2. Thermochemical

         a. Heat.—Burns and scalds.

         b. Cold.—Frostbite.

         c. Chemicals.—Acids and alkalies.

         d. Irradiation.

         e. Electricity.

   B. Indirect.—Injury to the main artery of the limb. The gangrene occurs at some distance from the site of arterial injury, e.g. gangrene of the foot due to injury of the popliteal artery.

III. *Infective:*
1. Boils and carbuncles.
2. Diabetic gangrene.
3. Gas gangrene.
4. Gangrene of the scrotum (Fournier's gangrene).

Signs of Gangrene
1. Loss of temperature.—The area becomes cold.
2. Loss of arterial pulsation (and loss of venous return with lack of response to pressure, i.e. loss of colour return).
3. Loss of sensation.
4. Loss of function.
5. Change of colour.—To start with, the colour of the part may be pale, purple, mottled, dusky, or grey, but finally it takes a typical greenish-black or black appearance. This black colour is due to formation of iron sulphide—the iron from disintegrated haemoglobin mixing up with atmospheric H_2S.

Clinical Types of Gangrene
1. *Dry Gangrene.*—This occurs:
    a. When the arterial obstruction is gradual.
    b. When the arteries are obstructed but the veins are still open.
    c. When the gangrenous area was not primarily infected.
    d. When the gangrenous area was not primarily oedematous.
    e. When the gangrenous area is exposed to evaporation, e.g. toes. The best example of dry gangrene is senile gangrene. The gangrenous area is dry, wrinkled, and greasy to touch.

2. *Moist Gangrene.*—This occurs:
    a. When the arterial occlusion is sudden.
    b. When the main arteries and veins are simultaneously obstructed.
    c. When the area was infected prior to arterial occlusion,
    d. When the area was oedematous prior to arterial occlusion.
    e. When the gangrenous area is not exposed to evaporation (e.g. bedsores, scrotal gangrene).

The best example of moist gangrene is diabetic gangrene in the younger ages. The affected area is swollen, discoloured, foul-smelling, and the epidermis may be raised in blebs. Intestinal gangrene gives the ideal picture of moist gangrene.

Separation in Gangrene.—There is always a natural attempt for the dead tissue to be separated from the living tissues. This is achieved by granulation tissue which grows at the cost of living tissues. The formation of this granulation tissue is possible provided:
a. there is a fairly good blood supply in the proximal part of the limb.
b. there is no gross infection in the gangrenous area.

1. WHEN DEMARCATION IS NOT POSSIBLE, the gangrene either spreads upwards along the limb (spreading gangrene) or produces skip areas of gangrene up the limb.

2. WHEN THE FACTORS FAVOUR DEMARCATION:

   a. A *line of demarcation* appears between the living and the dead tissues. This is the area of granulation tissue, grown at the cost of the living tissue. This area, which may be of variable width, appears reddish-blue in colour and is hyperaemic as well as hyperaesthetic. The depth of the line of demarcation is variable—it may be skin, muscle, or bone-deep.

   b. A *line of separation* may finally develop as the granulation tissue completely cuts off the living tissue from the dead, and the dead tissue falls off. Obviously the line of separation will be distal to the line of demarcation. Since bone can stand impairment of blood supply better than other tissues, the loss of bone is minimum and the stump (after the dead tissue is separated) is conical with the bone projecting at the apex of the cone.

Special Investigations in Cases of Arterial Impairment and Gangrene

1. *Urine Examination* for sugar (diabetes).
2. *Blood Examination and Serological Tests:*
   a. Estimation of blood sugar (diabetes).
   b. Estimation of serum cholesterol and triglycerides (arteriosclerosis)
   c. VDRL, WR and Kahn tests (syphilis-endarteritis is rare nowadays).
3. *Straight X-ray* may show:
   a. calcification in big arteries (arteriosclerosis),
   b. calcification and flecks of calcium (aneurysm),
   c. gas bubbles (gas gangrene),
   d. cervical rib.
4. *ECG.*—A grossly abnormal ECG may be a contra-indication to a major direct arterial surgery under general anaesthesia.
5. *Investigation for Venospasm.*—In Raynaud's disease and early cases of Buerger's disease, vasospasm plays an important role in causing obliteration of blood supply to the distal limb. Later however, organic obliteration of the vessel becomes increasingly predominant. As long as vasospasm is an important factor in vascular obstruction, sympathectomy has a role to play in improving the circulation because the vasospasm is expected to pass off with sympathectomy. In any case of arterial obstruction and gangrene, therefore, before a sympathectomy is undertaken, it is desirable to know what proportion of the arterial interruption is due to spasm—the more the proportion, the better is the effect of sympathectomy. This is estimated by calculating *Brown's vasomotor index.*

The body temperature (mouth temperature) and also the temperature of the skin over the affected area are first recorded. Attempts are now made to overcome the vasoconstrictor effect of the sympathetic on the affected limb. This may be done by:

a. Heating the other healthy limbs—either by hot bags or cradles, or better by immersing in hot water at 110°F.

b. By inducing fever with an injection of typhoid vaccine.

c. By regional nerve block with local anaesthetics.—injection of the posterior tibial nerve behind the medial malleolus or high spinal anaesthesia for the lower limb, and injection of the ulnar nerve at the back of elbow for the upper limb.

After this has been done, the mouth temperature and the local skin temperature are again noted, and the rise in each is estimated. The rise in the local skin temperature is partly due to that effected by sympathetic withdrawal and partly due to the general rise in the body temperature. So, if the rise in mouth temperature is deducted from the rise in skin temperature, the actual rise in the skin temperature due to the sympathetic withdrawal is obtained. Hence,

$$\text{Brown's Vasomotor Index} = \frac{\text{Rise in skin temperature} - \text{Rise in mouth temperature}}{\text{Rise in mouth temperature}}$$

i.e. the proportion of elevation of the local temperature as compared to that of general body temperature. It is believed that, unless the index is more than 3.5, sympathectomy does not give effective results.

6. *Arteriography.*—This is the most reliable method of studying the arterial circulatory state of the limb including the level, extent and nature of obstruction and the condition of the collaterals. Hypaque (45 per cent) or Diodone (35 per cent) solution may be used as the contrast medium.

The dye may be introduced in two ways:

a. Direct puncture of the artery,

   i. Femoral artery at the groin for lower limb vessels.

   ii. Carotid artery at the neck for intracranial and extracranial vessels.

   iii. Abdominal aorta with long needle passed by translumbar route.

b. Retrograde Percutaneous Catheterisation by polythene catheter.

   The Seldinger catheter with needle and a guide wire, which is malleable and can be moulded into any shape, is best for the purpose:

   i. Introduced through the femoral artery and passed upwards (retrograde) into the abdominal aorta to visualise the abdominal aorta and iliacs. Malleability of the catheter allows its tip to be introduced into any branch of the aorta under X-ray control and a *selective arteriography* of the artery to be performed.

   ii. Introduced via the brachial artery, for subclavian, innominate, thoracic aorta and vertebral arteriograms.

7. *Digital Subtraction Venous Angiography.*—This is a method of obtaining an arteriogram with (a) venous injection of the dye and (b) deduction of other misguiding images from the X-ray to get a real picture of the artery. A preliminary X-ray is taken and is computerised. The contrast medium is injected intravenously and this passes via the heart to the artery under study. A series of X-rays are now taken (arteriograms). One with small amount of contrast medium in the artery is selected and is computerised. The first image is subtracted from the second and a good arteriogram is obtained.

8. *Blood Velocity Detection by Doppler Ultrasound.*—When a narrow ultrasound wave is beamed on an artery, it passes through the moving red blood cells within it and is reflected therefrom. The reflected beam undergoes a change in frequency. This is called *Doppler shift* or *Doppler effect.* The degree of frequency change depends on the velocity of blood flow, which is indicative of stenotic or destructive lesion in the artery.

   The Doppler apparatus has a probe, which is placed on the skin overlying the artery, for the purpose of introduction and reception back of the ultrasound waves. Within the apparatus, the source of the ultrasound wave is a electrically stimulated piezoelectric crystal. The reflected beam is converted into audible signals for easy studying.

   Further, analysis of the sound shows that it has three phases (triphasic) when reflected from a normal artery. When the Doppler probe is made to travel down the artery, as it crosses an obstruction in the artery the sound becomes biphasic, and further distally (with more severe obstruction) it turns uniphasic.

   If *laser beam* is used instead of the ultrasound beam, the instrument provides special information about the cutaneous vascularity.

9. *Measurement of Specific Arterial Pressure by Doppler Ultrasound.*—The probe of the instrument is used as a sensitive stethoscope placed over an artery distal to an appropriately sized sphygmomanometer cuff in order to record the blood pressure not only accurately but also at site where the arterial pulse is not palpable. Two investigations are possible:

   a. Measuring the *'pressure index'* (PI) which is the ratio of blood pressure in the posterior tibial artery at the ankle (with the cuff placed just above the ankle) to the pressure in the brachial artery. At rest, the PI is greater than 1.0 in a normal subject. Values less than 0.9 indicate arterial obstruction in the limb. Re-assessment after exercise is important—the PI will rise in the absence of obstruction.

   b. Measuring segmental blood pressures by placing the cuff on the midthigh, on the calf, and just above the ankle to indicate the site of obstruction.

10. *Duplex Imaging.*—The two units of the duplex imaging are visualisation of the structure of the artery and detection of the nature of blood flow within it. Thus it is a combined study of the anatomy and functional details of an artery. The structure visualisation is done by a β-scan ultrasound unit (producing two

dimensional images) detailing the site and nature of the arterial obstruction. The abnormalities of blood flow (stenotic jets, just distal to a stenotic site and turbulence due to vessel wall irregularity) are obtained by a Doppler ultrasound, as described above. The two units may be separate or may be incorporated in one apparatus. The structural aspects are now better detailed by the utilisation of colour mapping.

11. *Plethysmography.*—This records the changes in the volume of a limb that occur with each myocardial contraction and serves as an index of blood supply to the limb, i.e. whether ischaemia is present. Measuring the same before and after vasodilatation of a limb (as for detecting Brown's vasomotor index), it also signifies the proportion of vasospastic fraction in the ischaemia. The measurement may be done by one of four equipment—water-filled volume recorder, air-filled volume recorder, mercury in rubber strain gauge and mercury in silastic strain gauge. However, this does not provide any clue to the site and nature of arterial obstruction.

Segmental plethysmography, done by placing cuffs at the three sites mentioned under Doppler segmental arterial pressure recording, may provide some idea about the level of the obstruction.

12. *Oscillometry.*—The cuff of the instrument is applied on the limb and the needle of the galvanometer, connected to it, shows deflection with each pulsation. As the cuff is gradually brought down the limb, where the level of obstruction in the main artery is crossed, the wide deflections of the needle, seen so long, will be missing and only fine deflections due to the patent collaterals will be present. Finally, at the level where efficient collaterals are also absent, the needle will stop showing any deflection.

13. *Isotope Clearance Tests.*—Xe_{133} or Technetium is injected into the calf muscles and their rate of clearance studied to assess vascularity of the muscles.

14. *Electromagnetic Flowmetry.*—Electromagnetic electrodes are placed on the *exposed* artery. The electric potential produced by the flowing blood in the artery as it passes through the magnetic field, is directly proportional to its velocity. This is fed back to an electronic amplifier for studying. As the electrodes are gradually moved distally on the artery, there is reduction in electric potential as the site of obstruction is reached.

General Outline of Treatment in Cases of Arterial Impairment and Gangrene.—This may be conveniently discussed under the following headings:

    I. Symptomatic and general treatment.

    II. Conservative methods to effect vasodilatation (vasodilator methods).

    III. Indirect surgery to effect vasodilatation (sympathectomy).

    IV. Direct arterial surgery.

    V. Minor adjunctive surgery.

    VI. Care of the ischaemic parts.

    VII. Amputations.

Vasodilator Methods.—These are methods to overcome vasospasm and to stimulate opening of collaterals in the ischaemic limb. It is doubtful whether the blood supply to the muscles is improved but it is definite that blood flow to the skin is increased and this may minimise, if not prevent, gangrene:

1. *Buerger's Position.*—The foot end of the bed is lowered by six inches for a few hours daily. This aims at increasing the blood flow by congestion.

2. *Buerger's Exercise.*—The limb is elevated for two minutes and then lowered below the bedside for two minutes, and the process is repeated several times at a stretch. This exercise is performed twice or thrice daily.

3. *Reflex Stimulation.*—This is done by heating the healthy limbs and the trunk, with hot bags, cradles, etc. This process may achieve considerable vasodilatation in the affected limb.

4. *Vasodilatation by Drugs:*
   a. Systemic vasodilator drugs (*see* under symptomatic and general treatment).
   b. Paravertebral injection of the sympathetic chain.—For the lower limb the injection is made by the side, of $L_{2,3,4}$ vertebrae, and for the upper limb by the side of $T_{2,3,4}$ vertebrae, One per cent lignocaine (10–20 ml) is safe but the effect is short-lasting (2 to 3 days), and has to be repeated. Injection of 5 per cent phenol (5 ml) gives a more permanent effect (*chemical sympathectomy*).

Care of the Ischaemic Parts

1. Protection of the part from:
   a. heat or excessive cold,
   b. pressure (e.g. skin over heel, malleoli, etc.),
   c. trauma (including nail-cutting).

2. Exposure of the part to ambient temperature (including cool breeze from a fan) assists in desiccation, diminishes tissue metabolism (so lessens chances of gangrene), and reduces pain.

3. Avoiding excess of muscular activity, e.g. walking at slower pace, restricting walking at a stretch, stopping cycling. A little elevation (1 cm) of the shoe-heel diminishes the effort of the calf muscles during walking.

4. Minor surgical toileting, e.g. lifting a crust, removing a slough, may release pus and relieve pain.

Minor Adjunctive Surgery.—These are performed to reduce muscular activity in the ischaemic limb:

1. Tenotomy (division) of the tendo Achilles diminishes the effort of the calf muscles during walking and thereby relieves pain.

2. Division of the nerves to gastrocnemius and soleus muscles, in the popliteal fossa, may improve claudication by defunctioning the muscles.

Indirect Surgery to Achieve Vasodilatation (Sympathectomy).—This is employed for the treatment of vasospasm. Its indications, therefore, are:

a. Raynaud's disease and other vasospastic conditions.
b. Buerger's disease (the result is likely to be significant provided the Brown's vasomotor index is 3.5 or more).
c. Senile gangrene or diabetic gangrene in the elderly (the result is unpredictable since vasospasm has only little role to play, but the operation is done just because direct surgery on the vessels rarely produces better results).

It has been found that, for sympathectomy to have any effect, the preganglionic fibres have to be severed. To achieve this, sympathetic ganglionectomy has to be performed. Postganglionic sympathectomy, as may be done by stripping of the tunica adventitia containing the periarterial sympathetic fibres, though technically easy, does not produce effective vasodilatation. This is because the sympathetic fibres reach the vessel segmentally throughout its length from the peripheral nerves, and scraping of the adventitia at one segment does not desympathise the entire limb. In order to cut the preganglionic sympathetic fibres, sympathetic ganglionectomy has to be done.

For the lower limbs lumbar sympathectomy and for the upper limbs cervicodorsal sympathectomy have to be performed.

Lumbar Sympathectomy.—This is most commonly done for Buerger's disease. Even if the symptoms and gangrene are unilateral, a bilateral lumbar sympathectomy has to be done since (i) the sympathetic supply to any limb comes from both sides, and (ii) the disease being generalised, is very likely to affect the other limb sooner or later, and so a prophylactic sympathectomy is beneficial. The first, second, third and fourth lumbar ganglia are to be excised, together with the intervening sympathetic chain. Since excision of the first lumbar ganglion on both the sides leads to impotency, the first lumbar ganglion of one side is spared.

In performing bilateral lumbar sympathectomy there are two approaches:

i. *Extraperitoneal.*—This is the usual approach. Each side is operated by a separate incision and the two sides are usually done at one sitting. The patient is placed in a semirecumbent position. The incision starts from the tip of the 12th rib and is directed towards the midpoint between umbilicus and symphysis pubis, but stops at the lateral border of the rectus. The muscles are divided along the line of incision, and the peritoneum is raised forwards and medially. On the right side, the sympathetic chain is overlapped by the inferior vena cava and on the left side by the aorta. The second ganglion is easily identified by its size. The first ganglion may be hidden under the crus. The chain is cut above the first ganglion and below the fourth ganglion, and the intervening part is removed. On the right side, the lumbar veins, crossing superficially, may have to be ligated. The muscles are sutured in two layers and the skin wound closed. The patient is then tilted to the other side and that side is operated on. (This is also the approach for the middle third of the ureter—the ureter is raised along with the peritoneum when the latter is stripped forwards and medially).

ii. *Intra-peritoneal.*—The two sides may be operated by one incision—lower midline, paramedian, or transverse. On opening the abdomen, the sympathetic chains are reached by incising the posterior peritoneum. This approach is only rarely advocated.

Cervicodorsal Sympathectomy.—This is most commonly performed for Raynaud's disease or other allied conditions. It is sometimes done for Buerger's disease, affecting the upper limb. The second and the third thoracic ganglia are removed. The stellate ganglion, lying above the second thoracic ganglion, has to be left intact in order to prevent development of Horner's syndrome (ptosis, myosis, and enophthalmos).

The operation may be done by either of the following methods:

i. Anterior approach (supraclavicular).

ii. Posterior approach (resecting part of the third rib).

iii. Axillary approach (via the second intercostal space).

iv. Transthoracic approach (via fourth intercostal space with a posterolateral thoracotomy).

Direct Arterial Surgery

1. *Repair of Injured Artery:*
   a. A punctured wound may be sutured with 5/0 atraumatic silk.
   b. A through and through clean cut may be sutured end-to-end.
   c. A lacerated or contused segment has to be excised. If the two fresh ends can be apposed without tension, an end-to-end anastomosis is done. If this is not possible, a vein graft (reversed) may be used to bridge up the gap. The long sapheous vein in the lower limb and the cubital vein in the upper limb may be conveniently used.
   d. Where no repair is practicable, the cut ends of the vessel are ligated and attempts are made to stimulate opening up of collaterals.

2. *Surgery for Arterial Embolism.*—The operation to be performed is *embolectomy with thrombectomy,* because it removes the embolus with the thrombi, which form (due to stasis of blood) both distal and proximal to the embolus, either in continuity with it or as separate pieces. Introduction of *Fogarty balloon catheter* has vastly minimised the magnitude of the operation of thrombus removal which can be performed under local anaesthesia with minimal surgical exploration. This is of special importance because these patients usually have badly damaged heart (myocardial infarction, atrial fibrillation, etc.).

For example, an embolus located at the aortic bifurcation can be removed with small incision placed on the femoral arteries at the groin, instead of performing a laparotomy. The balloon catheter is pushed upwards till it passes above the thrombus. The balloon is inflated thereafter and as the catheter is slowly withdrawn, it drags the clot down. The process is repeated till the whole thrombus is removed and bleeding starts. For other arteries, the incision is made directly just at the upper limit of the thrombus and the catheter is passed downwards and thereafter upwards for removal of distal thrombi.

3. *Surgery for Atherosclerotic Arterial Obstruction.*—The bigger the artery the better is the result of surgery. For the lower limbs, the best results are with aorto-iliac obstruction and than the fempropopliteal. Surgery for tibioperoneal occlusions is seldom beneficial and usually avoided. The available methods are—direct arterial reconstruction by bypass, arterial disobliteration, i.e. reboring (thrombo-endarterectomy), indirect revascularisation by extra-anatomic bypass and balloon dilatation with percutaneous balloon catheters.

a. *Bypass Grafting.*—Aorto-iliac occlusions are bypassed with knitted Dacron prosthesis of inverted Y-shape, anastomosing it proximally with the aorta and distally with the two femoral arteries (better than common iliacs), ends of the prosthesis anastomosed to opening made on the sides of the vessels. For femoropopliteal bypass reversed (to overcome valve effects) long saphenous vein acts as a much better prosthesis. If suitable vein (4 mm wide) is not available either PTFE (polytetrafluroethylene) or umbilical vein graft is used.

b. *Thrombo-endarterectomy.*—This operation, also known as 'disobliteration' and 'reboring' entails removal of the atherosclerotic tunica intima with the adherent thrombus, along the whole length of the affected segment, carefully separating it from the tunica media. Different types of metal 'strippers are available for this dissection. The artery is exposed along the whole length of obstruction and is opened by proximal and distal incisions (e.g. aorta and the two common iliacs). Blunt dissection, performed very carefully, enables the whole length of the affected segment to be opened out. The operation is time consuming and requires specialist skill but is associated with lesser incidences of reocclusion, false aneurysm and infection than the bypass operations. In case of femoropopliteal occlusion, however, the whole length of the affected segment has to be slit open longitudinally and, after removing the atherosclerotic core, the arterial open roof is closed with a vein patch (to prevent stenosis). Alternatively, multiple small incisions are made on the affected artery and multiple vein roof patches are used for closure.

c. *Extra-anatomic Bypass.*—These are reserved for poor-risk, debilitated and aged patients.

   i. Femoro-femoral bypass is done when one common iliac artery is occluded while the other is patent. A donor graft, placed subcutaneously above the pubis, is anastomosed end to side to the two femoral arteries.

    ii. Axillofemoral bypass is done for bilateral iliac obstruction, with one limb in the pregangrenous state. With a long PTFE graft placed subcutaneously, the axillary artery is connected to the femoral artery of the affected side.

d. *Balloon Angioplasty.*—Short segment arterial stenoses can be dilated by passing a balloon catheter (Griintizy) percutaneously and inflating it. The catheter is introduced on a guide wire passed through the stenosis. Best results are seen in iliofemoral stenoses. The process may be repeated for recurrences.

e. *Laser* drill holes through short segment stenoses are now being employed.

In cases of direct arterial surgery, errors can be detected before closure of the wound by on-table ultrasound or arteriography or flowmetry.

In all cases of direct arterial surgery, judicious use of heparin *perioperatively*, both systemic and local (intra-arterial), is imperative.

The above description relates especially to lower limb ischaemia but the principles of surgery are basically the same for the neck and the upper limbs as well.

General and Symptomatic Treatment.—While rest pain and ulceration demand surgery, as is feasible, two-thirds of the patients with intermittent claudication only can be managed by medical treatment alone:

1. Stopping smoking and abstinence from any form of tobacco are mandatory. This applies not only to Buerger's disease but also in atherosclerosis (arrests progress of the disease and reduces incidence of arterial graft failure).

2. Encouraging walking up to claudication distance. This is not at all harmful. Rather it is beneficial in that the collateral circulation improves and claudication distance gradually increases.

3. Control of diabetes and hyperlipidaemia:

    a. Diet control and standard drugs for diabetes.

    b. Low cholesterol diet, weight reduction and use of cholestyramine.

4. Analgesics.—Non-addictive drugs should be used. Short-acting barbiturates are preferred as they have an additional effect of vasodilatation.

5. **Drugs:**

    a. In arteriosclerosis, drugs preventing clot formation by reducing platelet aggregation (aspirin in small dosage, prostacycline, etc.) or by reducing blood viscosity (trental) may be used.

    b. In vasospastic conditions, e.g. Raynaud's disease, Buerger's disease, *vasodilator drugs* are used with benefit. Methyldopa, calcium antagonists like nifedipine, prostaglandin E, prostacycline may be used orally. Intra-arterial reserpine, if available, give the best and prolonged results.

    c. In all cases of ischaemia, praxiline may be effective because it allows tissue metabolism in the presence of oxygen deficit.

Amputations

1. *Conservative Amputation.*—This is the present day trend, especially for gangrene in cases of Buerger's disease and arteriosclerosis, as compared to high-up amputations advocated in the past.

The important points about conservative amputation are:

a. The extent of amputation can be grossly minimised by improving the circulation by direct arterial surgery or lumbar sympathectomy.

b. As long as the gangrene is limited to a toe, the amputation should be delayed to allow the toe to mummify and get auto-amputated. Surgical amputation may cause extension of the wound to the foot. Uncontrollable infection and severe rest pain, however, may demand an early amputation of the toe. In cases of small vessel occlusion (e.g. Buerger's disease), relatively good blood supply to the surrounding tissues usually allows wound healing.

c. When several toes are gangrenous and irreversible ischaemia has extended to the forefoot transmetatarsal amputation has to be performed. It is important to note that a foot remains useful for bearing weight only when its posterior half, including the heel, is intact. Loss of more than half of the sole makes the foot useless for weight bearing. High-up amputations have to be performed in these cases because the skin flap of a Syme's amputation almost always fails to heal in an ischaemic limb.

d. In diabetic gangrene the infection tends to pass proximally along the tendon sheaths. In the cases where the metatarsophalangeal joint-region is involved, transmetatarsal amputation is supplemented by cutting the tendons back (*ray amputation*).

2. *High-up Amputation.*—For the lower limb this means either a below-knee or an above-knee amputation. Preservation of the knee greatly facilitates wearing of a prosthesis. In the presence of popliteal pulsation the decision is easy. In its absence, preoperative segmental arterial pressure measurements, isotope clearance tests of the calf muscles, and laser Doppler study, and peroperative degrees of skin bleeding are useful guides.

The indications for high-up amputation are:

a. Spreading moist gangrene, i.e. gangrene without line of demarcation.

b. Gangrene of Buerger's disease or arteriosclerosis where more than half of the foot has to be sacrificed making it useless for weight bearing.

RAYNAUD'S PHENOMENON AND RAYNAUD'S DISEASE

Raynaud's phenomenon is essentially due to spasm of digital arteries, sometimes affecting the normal vessels and sometimes vessels which are the seat of some organic disease.

Phases.—The attack is usually precipitated by cold (abnormal sensitivity of the arterioles to cold) and consists of three phases:

1. As the arterioles go into spasm, the part is blanched and is incapable of movements (*stage of blanching*).

2. As the hand is warmed, the arterioles relax and the capillaries are slowly filled up with blood. This blood is very quickly deoxygenated and so the part becomes cyanosed (*stage of cyanosis or dusky anoxia*).

3. As the arteriolar spasm completely passes off, blood enters more quickly, and so the part becomes scarlet red and swollen (*stage of red engorgement*). There is a burning sensation and pain which is due partly to irritation caused by the local metabolites and partly to increased tissue tensions.

Causes

A. *Primary or Idiopathic (Raynaud's Disease)*.—There is no definite cause for the phenomenon. The peripheral pulsations are normal. There is no generalised vascular disease. Arteriography, done between attacks, shows absolutely normal digital circulation. The condition is possibly due to an exaggeration of the normal process of arteriolar spasm in response to cold.

   The patient is almost a girl at adolescence and in 50 per cent of cases there is a family history. Almost always it is the fingers that shows the phenomenon and typically the condition is *bilateral*.

   If the attacks are oft-repeated, organic obliterative changes may gradually occur in the peripheral vessels, leading to superficial necrosis and dry gangrene at the finger tips. At this stage the condition is called Raynaud's disease. Thus, Raynaud's disease is characterised by *bilateral symmetrical superficial* gangrene at the finger tips in young girls, preceded by repeated attacks of Raynaud's phenomenon.

B. *Secondary*.—Raynaud's phenomenon may sometimes occur in other pathological conditions, e.g.

   1. Obliterative arterial diseases.—Buerger's disease, atherosclerosis.
   2. Cervical rib and scalene syndrome.
   3. Thrombosis or embolism of axillary artery.
   4. Atrophic changes in the limb—following poliomyelitis, trauma, frostbite, etc.
   5. Ergot poisoning.

Treatment

1. Prevention of exposure to cold.
2. Vasodilator drugs:
   a. Oral—Methyldopa (the earliest effective drug), calcium antagonists (nifedipine), prostaglandin E.
   b. Intra-arterial reserpine (if available) produces prolonged vasodilatation and freedom from symptoms.
3. Cervicodorsal sympathectomy (*see* page 98).

BUERGER'S DISEASE

This disease is characterised by low grade inflammation and obliteration of the arteries and veins of a limb simultaneously. The alternative name *thromboangiitis obliterans* is very appropriate.

Etiology.—The cause of the disease is unknown but is now believed to be either of the following:

1. A low grade infection.

2. A low grade toxaemia.

3. Primarily a vasospastic condition, and a long-continued vasospasm leading to organic obliteration of the vessels. The beneficial results obtained by sympathectomy, in the early cases, supports this view.

4. Smoking is definitely a predisposing factor since the disease is almost unknown in the non-smokers.

Pathology.—The disease is almost limited to the males (rarely women may suffer) and the patient is usually aged between twenty and forty. The lower limbs are always the first to be involved but subsequently the upper limbs may be affected. There may be simultaneous involvement of both lower limbs but more commonly one is affected earlier than the other.

The disease primarily starts in the small and medium sized arteries (e.g. plantars, tibials, palmars, radial, ulnar, etc.), but later it may involve the bigger arteries (e.g. popliteal, femoral, etc.). There is a mild chronic inflammatory change in the arterial wall but the lumen of the artery is occluded by thrombosis. Simultaneously there is a thrombosis, associated with mild infection, in the veins as well—both superficial and deep. The chronic infection results in fibrosis in the vessel walls. The fibrosis ultimately spreads outside the vessel (perivascular) and, in a late case, may be so extensive as to bind the artery, the vein and the nerve together, in it. The strangling of the nerve may cause unbearable pain in the limb.

Since the arterial occlusion is gradual, collaterals tend to open up. The second ill-effect of the disease is a spasm occurring in the collaterals. A sympathectomy at this stage may overcome this spasm and the limb may be saved.

Ultimately obliterative changes also occur in the collaterals and gangrene supervenes.

Clinical Features

1. Usually a male patient between 20 and 40 years of age.

2. Usually the complaints are in the lower limbs—one or both. Later, the upper limbs may be affected.

3. Intermittent claudication (described on page 89).

4. Rest pain (described on page 90).

5. Sometimes there may be attacks of Raynaud's phenomenon, i.e. stages of blanching, dusky anoxia, and red engorgement.

6. Ultimately gangrene sets in. The gangrene is usually dry and slowly progressing. A minor trauma may precipitate the gangrene.

Special Investigations.—Details have been described earlier, under general considerations of gangrene.

The characteristic features of arteriography are:

1. The large arteries, e.g. femoral and popliteal are smooth and normal (cf arteriosclerosis).
2. Arteries of the size of the tibials show abrupt areas of occlusion. There may be a *corkscrew appearance* due to partial recanalisation following occlusion.
3. Evidence of extensive collateral circulation.—Grossly tortuous vessels giving a *spiderlike* or *two root* appearance.

Treatment

1. Symptomatic and general treatment.
2. Vasodilator methods.
3. Lumbar sympathectomy.
4. Minor adjunctive surgery.
5. Care of the ischaemic parts.
6. Amputations.

All the above points have been discussed earlier, under general considerations of gangrene.

Direct arterial surgery are usually avoided because results are uniformly unsatisfactory.

Causes of Death

1. Hepatic failure from long-continued use of sedatives.
2. Coronary or cerebral thrombosis (as a part of Buerger's disease).
3. Toxaemia from gangrene.
4. Exhaustion from pain.
5. Suicidal deaths (to get rid of pain).

AINHUM

This is a disease of unknown etiology, most commonly affecting adult males who walk barefooted. It is uncommon in women and in children. It starts as a transverse groove in an interphalangeal joint, usually of the 5th toe and frequently bilaterally. In diminishing order of frequency, the 4th, 3rd, 2nd, and great toes are affected. Often more than one toe are involved. Rarely a finger may be involved. The groove gradually deepens and simultaneously enlarges in length, ultimately encircling the whole circumference of the toe. It causes swelling of the toe, often painful. Finally, the toe distal to the band, may fall off. The arterial pulsations are normal.

Treatment

1. Longitudinal incisions through the constricting band, one on the medial and another on the lateral side, often arrest progress of the disease.
2. Alternatively, a Z-plasty may be done.
3. In late cases, an amputation through the constricting band has to be performed.

DIABETIC GANGRENE

A diabetic gangrene is due to three factors:

1. Diminished resistance of the sugar-laden tissues to trauma and infection—the sugar serves as a medium for the bacteria to grow.
2. Atherosclerosis, resulting in circulatory impairment.
3. Trophic changes due to peripheral neuritis. Sensation is impaired and so minor trauma is not appreciated by the patient or is neglected.

Clinically the cases belong to two distinct groups:

1. *Moist gangrene,* usually superimposed on a trauma or infection in an uncontrolled diabetic, often at the younger age group. The first factor mentioned above plays the more important role in these cases. The gangrene is of spreading type.
2. *Dry gangrene,* usually occurring in an elderly diabetic. The second and third factors mentioned above play the more important role in these cases. The gangrene is slowly progressing and there is usually a line of demarcation.

Special Investigations.—Described earlier, under general considerations of gangrene.

Treatment

A. In the *first group of cases* the principles of treatment are:
   1. Active control of diabetes.
   2. Broad spectrum antibiotics.
   3. Rest with the limb elevated.
   4. Liberal incisions.
   5. High-up amputation in uncontrolled spreading cases.

B. In the *second group of cases:*
   1. Vasodilator methods (described on page 96).
   2. Care of the ischaemic limb (described on page 96).
   3. Symptomatic and general treatment, including active treatment for diabetes (discussed earlier).
   4. Indirect surgery to effect vasodilatation, i.e. sympathectomy.
   5. Amputations:
      a. High-up amputation.—When the ischaemic factor is predominant (peripheral pulsations absent).
      b. Conservative amputation.—When the trophic factor predominates (peripheral pulsations present).

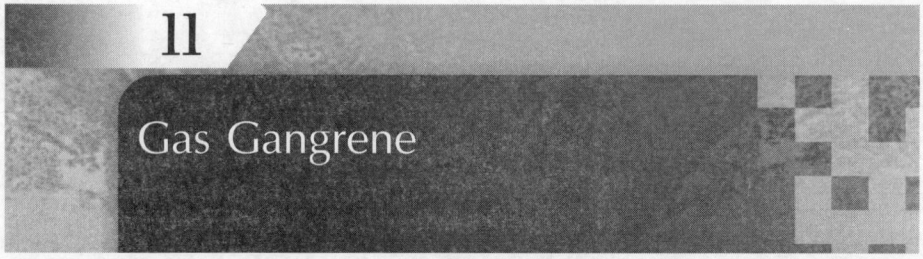

11

Gas Gangrene

Definition.—This is a quickly-spreading infective gangrene, consequent upon clostridial myositis and myonecrosis, and characterised by collection of gas in the muscles and subcutaneous tissues.

Etiology and Pathogenesis

A. Predisposing factors:

1. Lacerated and crushed injuries *involving muscles.*
2. Inadequate wound excision and poor drainage of wounds.
3. Impairment of circulation due to (a) vascular damage, (b) tight bandaging or plastering, (c) prolonged use of tourniquets.
4. Presence in the wound of (a) devitalised tissues and blood clots, (b) soils, particularly those rich in calcium, (c) foreign bodies, especially torn pieces of garments.
5. Presence of non-clostridial anaerobes and aerobic bacilli, e.g. streptococci, *Esch. coli,* pseudomonas, staphylococci, in the wound.
6. Diabetes and pre-existing occlusive arterial diseases.

B. Infective organisms and their biological characters:

The clostridia are large Gram-positive and spore-bearing organisms. There are several species, some of them highly pathogenic and others less so. The first group comprises *Cl. perfringens* (welchii), *Cl. septicum* and *Cl. novyi* (oedematiens). The low pathogenic group includes, amongst others, *Cl. histolyticum* and *Cl. sporogenes. Cl. perfringens* is the most dangerous pathogen and, unfortunately, the most frequent (70 to 80 per cent).

The damaging effects of the clostridia are due to *toxins* and *enzymes.* Several toxins are liberated by each strain. Of these, the alpha toxin is the most dangerous and this is most abundant in *Cl. perfringens.* The toxins cause, on one hand, severe toxaemia (often leading to death) and, on the other, extensive tissue necrosis, especially of muscles. The alpha toxin is also responsible for haemolysis, resulting in marked anaemia and, sometimes, haemoglobinuria and jaundice. Among the damaging enzymes, one is hyaluronidase (*the spreading factor*), responsible for quick and extensive spread along the tissues, especially the muscle fibres.

Pathology.—Several strains of clostridia enter the wound simultaneously but their merepresence does not initiate gas gangrene. There are two prerequisites for the pathology to start:

1. Necrotic tissues, especially muscles.
2. An anaerobic atmosphere that may be caused by:
   a. Presence of aerobic bacilli in the wound, which consumes the oxygen available in the locality.

b. Closed wound, not allowing air-entry.

c. Low oxygen tension in the tissues because of crushing, vascular damage, and pressure on the capillaries by extravasated blood.

The chief pathology is muscle necrosis, resulting in glycogen and protein breakdown. The glycogen is broken into organic acids, carbon dioxide and oxygen. Breakdown of muscle proteins results in gross putrefactive changes in the area and formation of NH_4, H_2S and other noxious gases. Large amounts of fluids are also produced (especially by *Cl. oedematiens*—hence the name). These gases and fluids collect in the muscles, spread along their fibres, spread to the subcutaneous tissues, and are emitted through the wound, very foul-smelling.

The disease should have been arrested because of formation of organic acids from glycogen breakdown, which would inhibit further growth of the bacteria. Unfortunately, this cannot happen because:

i. part of the acid is lost in the profuse discharge from the wound, and

ii. rest of the acid is neutralised by ammonia derived from protein breakdown, by the alkaline inflammatory exudates and by the calcium salts present in the soil that has entered to the wound.

Thus, there is rapid progress of the myonecrosis, aided by the spreading factor, proximally and distally along the limb as well as circumferentially along its whole girth (*massive type*). In some cases, especially those with *Cl. perfringens* predominance, the pathology progresses proximally to the trunk (*fulminating type*). Sometimes with low virulence organisms, or with prompt detection and treatment, the disease may be limited. There may be involvement of only one group of muscles, e.g. glutei, adductors or extensors in the thigh, flexors in the leg (*group type*) or, rarely, involvement of one muscle only (*single muscle type*).

Occasionally, there is no involvement of the muscles and the infection is limited to the subcutaneous tissue and fascial planes. These cases, caused by low pathogenic clostridia, have to be carefully differentiated from anaerobic cellulitis (*subcutaneous gas abscess*), caused by *Esch. coli* and streptococci:

The overall effects of clostridial myositis are:

1. Severe muscle necrosis with putrefaction, resulting in formation of offensive smelling gases and fluids.

2. Severe toxaemia and shock, often leading to death. Autopsy often reveals gas in the vital organs, especially the liver (*the foaming liver*).

3. Profound anaemia.

Clinical Features

A. INCUBATION PERIOD.—This usually ranges between 24 and 72 hours. Occasionally this may be less than 12 hours (with *Cl. perfringens*) and sometimes prolonged, rarely up to 6 weeks.

B. GENERAL FEATURES:

1. The patient is conscious often highly alert. Delirium and coma occur just before death.

2. The pulse is rapid (out of proportion to the temperature) and there is quick fall of blood pressure.

3. There is rise of temperature but this is seldom high. In fact, severe cases may have subnormal temperature.
4. There is marked anaemia, rarely jaundice and haemoglobinuria.
5. There may be oliguria and anuria from renal failure.

C. LOCAL FEATURES:

1. The patient complains of local pain.
2. There is swelling and gross oedema, and the stitches often give way.
3. There is profuse discharge from the wound which is frothy and foul-smelling. The discharge may also form blebs on the skin.
4. The skin is pale yellow (*khaki*), greenish, or black with putrefactive changes (*dermatonecrosis* of alpha toxin).
5. Crepitus, due to gas, is often palpable and sometimes audible with the stethoscope.

Special Investigations

1. A swab with the wound exudate is sent for confirmation of clostridial infection and identification of the predominant species.
2. X-ray may show gas shadows.

Treatment

A. PROPHYLAXIS.—This is the mainstay in the treatment and consists of the following:
1. Meticulous wound excision, removing:
   a. all foreign bodies,
   b. all devitalised tissues and blood clots,
   c. all dead and damaged muscles.
2. Avoiding use of tourniquets during wound excision, avoiding primary closure of the wound, and establishing proper drainage.
3. Antibiotics—Penicillin in large and frequent doses is advised for all gas gangrene-prone wounds. A dose of 10 lac units, every 3 hours, is advocated. For patients allergic to penicillin, chloramphenicol, 2 to 4 g per day, may be used. However, in view of coexistence of other anaerobic and aerobic infections, broad-spectrum antibiotics are often preferred. A combination of metronidazole, gentamicin/amikacin and cefazolin is commonly used.
4. Passive immunisation is attempted with intramuscular injection of *anti-gas gangrene serum,* containing 25,000 IU of polyvalent antitoxin. This contains 10,000 units *Cl. perfringens*, 10,000 units *Cl. novyi* and 5,000 units *Cl. septicum*. Because of doubtful efficacy and considerable risk of hypersensitivity reactions of equine serum, this is avoided in many centres.

   Active immunisation with toxoids, claimed to be highly effective in experimental animals, still awaits clinical application.
5. Treatment for diabetes in known diabetic subjects.

B. TREATMENT IN ESTABLISHED CASES.—Surgery is the treatment and this has to be supplemented by adequate supportive measures.

1. *Surgery.*—This should be undertaken immediately after clinical diagnosis is made. The principle is to remove all muscles involved in the process. The affected muscles:
   a. Show change in nature; they are dull, opaque, friable, defluent and crepitant due to gases.
   b. Show change in colour; to start with, they are brick-red, then yellowish, and finally, black in colour, due to deposits of iron sulphide.
   c. Loose power of contractility.
   d. Do not bleed to touch.

The nature of surgery depends upon the extent of muscle involvement:
   i. In the usual massive type, where the muscles along the whole girth of the limb is involved, amputation has to be performed. The principles of amputation are:
      a. It must be at a sufficiently high level, where the muscles are free from infection. If necessary, the muscles at the stump have to be slit open to exclude involvement.
      b. It should be preferably of guillotine type, so that the stump can drain itself and receive atmospheric oxygen.
      c. Tourniquet should not be used, so that anoxia is avoided and bleeding from muscles can be seen.
   ii. In the group type, the whole group of muscles, irrespective of its anatomy, is excised. The excision has to be done piecemeal, till healthy muscles, identified by their colour, contractility and bleeding capacity, are encountered. If total clearance is impossible, amputation is undertaken.
   iii. In the rare single muscle type, excision of the particular muscle is sufficient.
   iv. In the cases where the infection is limited to the subcutaneous tissue and fascial planes, multiple liberal incisions are made. Careful search for muscle involvement must be done.
   v. In the fulminating type, the patient usually succumbs before surgery can be undertaken.

2. *Supportive Treatment:*
   a. Antibiotics, as described under prophylaxis.
   b. Antiserum.—Three ampoules of polyvalent anti-gas gangrene serum are administered intravenously, and then repeated every 6 hours. Serum treatment has been discarded in many centres for its doubtful efficacy and high risk of anaphylactic reactions. Some surgeons advocate local infiltration of the serum into the exposed muscles during the surgery.
   c. Blood transfusion to combat anaemia and shock, and adequate fluid infusion.
   d. Hyperbaric oxygen.—The limb may be placed in chamber of hyperbaric oxygen, where available. This effectively reduces muscle necrosis and toxin production, so that the chances of survival are enhanced and excision may be made less drastic.

12

Tetanus

Tetanus is a local infection that causes a general toxaemia and a selective effect upon the motor centres in the spinal cord and medulla.

Etiology

A. ORGANISMS.—The causative organism *Clostridium tetani* is a Gram-positive slender rod with a terminal spore, thus having a 'drum-stick' appearance. A normal inhabitant of the intestines of cattle, the organism is found frequently in soil manured with their excreta.

B. TYPES OF WOUND.—The bacillus being an obligatory anaerobe, its growth in an wound is dependent on the presence of other pyogenic or aerobic bacilli that are introduced into the wound simultaneously. These organisms utilise the local oxygen, making an anaerobic field for the *Cl. tetani* to grow. Thus tetanus is not an ordinary wound infection but an infection of infected wounds. Tetanus is likely to develop:

1. In deep and infected wounds, including infected compound fractures, particularly when the injury was primarily contaminated with soil.
2. In wounds with devitalised tissues and foreign bodies—the foreign body often carrying the bacteria.
3. In wounds of operation, where imperfectly prepared catgut may be the source of the bacteria.
4. Sometimes in a trivial wound which the patient cannot even recall.

C. INCUBATION PERIOD.—This ranges from 2 to 21 days. The shorter the incubation period, the worse is the prognosis.

If ATS is given as prophylaxis and yet the patient develops tetanus, the incubation period may be prolonged to 8 weeks or more. Occasionally, spores introduced with foreign bodies may remain dormant for many months till they are disturbed and activated by a subsequent operation, e.g. removal of the foreign body (late tetanus).

Pathogenesis.—Tetanus clostridia do not invade or damage the local tissues (cf, gas gangrene). All the pathology is caused by the exotoxin liberated by the bacteria. This exotoxin, known as *tetanospasmin,* is highly damaging for the central nervous system (CNS). The toxin reaches the CNS by either of the following routes:

1. Entering the blood stream, either directly or by way of the lymphatics. This explains why the earliest effects such as trismus, difficulty in deglutition, rigidity of neck muscles, etc. are all well away from the wound.
2. Bound to the motor nerve endings and, passing retrograde along the respective axis cylinders, reaches the spinal cord. This explains local tetanus (mentioned under 'Special Types of Tetanus').

Whatever be the route, as soon as the toxin reaches the cord, it is fixed to the motor cells in the anterior horn. Once the toxin gets fixed to the motor cells, no amount of ATS or TIG can neutralise it. For the reason of fixation, again, the toxin cannot be detected in the CSF.

Pathology.—Exotoxin has two-fold effects on the nervous system:

1. It causes an imbalance between the acetylcholine and cholinesterase levels at the peripheral motor end plates. There is inhibition of cholinesterase and the acetylcholine preponderance produces a sustained state of hypertonicity, i.e. *tonic* muscular spasm.
2. It causes an extreme hyperexcitability of the anterior horn motor cells. The result is manifested as violent and widespread reflex *clonic* muscular spasms in response to even minor stimuli.

   Hence, the muscles are in a continuous state of hypertonicity and also exhibit violent spasms in response to minor stimuli. These effects are purely physiological because there are no organic changes in the cord or the brain.

Clinical Features

A. Stiffness of the muscles of mastication, particularly the masseters, producing the condition of 'lock-jaw', is the first difficulty noticed by the patient. The first reflex spasm appears somewhat later. The interval between these two phases is known as the *'period of onset'*. This serves as a prognostic index—if it is less than 48 hours, death is very likely to occur.

B. Constitutional symptoms—malaise, rise of temperature, tachycardia.

C. Sustained hypertonicity of muscles:
   1. Lock-jaw—muscles of mastication.
   2. *Risus sardonicus* or 'sardonic smile'—facial muscles.
   3. Pain and rigidity in the neck, back and abdominal muscles. The limbs are relatively spared.
   4. Difficulty in swallowing—muscles of pharynx.
   5. Reduction in breathing capacity—respiratory muscles.

D. Reflex muscular spasms, i.e. clonic contractions, which may be mild, moderate or severe, depending upon the amount of toxin fixed. These spasms may be brought on by the slightest stimulation or even without any stimulation. Hypertonicity of the muscles, as described above, remains although (cf, strychnine poisoning) and the reflex clonic spasms are superimposed at variable intervals—occurring almost ceaselessly in severe cases. The effects of the spasms may be:
   1. Generalised convulsions.
   2. Opisthotonos, i.e. bending of the body forwards like an arc, with convexity anteriorly, caused by spasm of the muscles of the back.
   3. Further difficulty in swallowing due to spasm of pharyngeal muscles.
   4. Asphyxia, as a result of spasm of respiratory muscles. Aspiration of the pharyngeal contents into the lungs may occur in between the attacks of spasm.
   5. Rupture of some muscles due to vigorous contractions may rarely occur, e.g. rectus abdominis, psoas, pectoral.

Special Types of Tetanus

1. *Tetanus Neonatorum* occurring in newborn infants, the infection gaining entry along the raw stump of the umbilical cord.
2. *Latent Tetanus.*—Where the wound of entry remains unrecognised.
3. *Local Tetanus.*—This is a milder form of the disease. The hypertonicity as well as the clonic spasms are limited to the muscles in the neighbourhood of the wound. This may be explained by the fact that the tetanus exotoxin is absorbed from the motor nerve endings and passes along the axis cylinders to the cord; and in these cases, involves only the segmental anterior horn cells of the cord.
4. *Cephalic Tetanus.*—This follows wounds on the face or head, and the manifestations are convulsions and paralysis in relation to the third, fourth, sixth, or seventh cranial nerves. Probably this is a type of local tetanus but is much more dangerous. This type may be mistaken for meningitis because of the associated hyperpyrexia.
5. *Bulbar Tetanus.*—This form, which is highly dangerous, is characterised by extensive spasm of the muscles of deglutition and respiration. This may be wrongly diagnosed as hydrophobia.
6. *Late Tetanus.*—Here the incubation period is considerably prolonged (vide etiology).

Prognosis

1. The lesser the incubation period, the worse is the prognosis. A period of less than 5 days is really dangerous.
2. The lesser the 'period of onset', the worse is the prognosis—death is almost inevitable when this period is less than 48 hours.
3. The extremes of age bear poor prognosis.
4. Tetanus neonatorum, bulbar tetanus and postoperative tetanus are almost always fatal.

Treatment

I. PROPHYLACTIC TREATMENT.—Tetanus prophylaxis has three components:
   1. Care of the wound.
   2. Antibiotics.
   3. Immunisation—active and passive.

1. *Care of the Wound.*—This is the most effective measure. All foreign bodies, dead tissues and blood clots are removed. Primary closure is avoided. There can be no better method in prophylaxis than not allowing tetanus bacilli to have a condition favourable for growth.
2. *Antibiotics.*—Penicillin acts as a bacteriostatic for *Cl. tetani* and prevents production of exotoxin. Moreover, it acts on the pyogenic organisms, whose presence in the wound is more disastrous. A dose of 5 lac units twice daily, should be administered till the wound heals. Alternatively, a single dose of long-acting depot penicillin, e.g. penidure LA 12, is used. For persons hypersensitive to penicillin, erythromycin, and, for wounds grossly infected broad-spectrum antibiotics are advocated.
   Antibiotics have no effect on the toxins and cannot replace immunisation, to which they act only as useful adjuncts.

3. *Immunisation:*
   a. *Active Immunisation.*—The population at large should be actively immunized against tetanus because this is the only way to prevent the disease occurring with unrecognised or unattended minor injuries, in which it is fairly common. This is done with formal toxoid (tetanus vaccine) of which two varieties are available—plain (soluble) and adsorbed. The adsorbed toxoid, which is purified toxoid adsorbed on aluminium phosphate, known as Tet Vac/PTAP, is a better antigen and is generally used. This can well be administered in the childhood along with the toxoids of diphtheria and whooping cough (triple antigen). The dose for tetanus toxoid is 0.5 ml to start with, repeated after 6 weeks, and again after 6 months, followed by a 'booster' dose every 10 years.

   As per this dose schedule, a person's immunity status is categorised as follows:
   - i. Immune.—All three initial doses and boosters taken.
   - ii. Partially immune.—Only two initial injections taken.
   - iii. Non-immune.—Only one or no injection taken.
   - iv. Unknown.—Toxoid history not available.

   b. *Passive Immunisation.*—This is unnecessary for the fully immunized patients. When tetanus toxoid is administered to a non-immune person, it takes at least 7 days' time to produce sufficient antitoxin. Passive immunisation with horse antitetanus serum (ATS) or human tetanus hyperimmuneglobulin (TIG) provides immunity during this period. Either of these has, therefore, to be administered simultaneously with the toxoid. This is injected at a separate site from that of the toxoid injection with a separate syringe (two deltoids are generally chosen).

Equine ATS, prepared from horse serum, is administered subcutaneously or intramuscularly. The dose is 1500 International Units, irrespective of the age of the patient. A preliminary sensitivity (skin) test must be done. ATS provides protection against tetanus for 7 to 10 days. Being a foreign protein, ATS has three distinct disadvantages:

- i. It is almost completely eliminated from the body by the end of 2 weeks, which, at least in some cases, may not cover the tetanus incubation period and prevent tetanus developing.
- ii. Hypersensitivity reactions are fairly common and may be severe.
- iii. There is stimulation of formation of antibodies to it, so that a person, who had received ATS previously, eliminates the present dose rapidly. For this reason of rapid excretion, persons developing tetanus despite prophylactic ATS injection, shall require much higher and frequent dosage of ATS as a therapeutic measure.

For these major disadvantages, use of prophylactic ATS is gradually being discarded. However, it should be appreciated that ATS not only reduces the incidence of tetanus but also, by prolonging the incubation period, reduces severity and mortality of the disease.

Human TIG is progressively replacing ATS as a prophylaxis. The dose is 250 IU, administered intramuscularly or intravenously. It establishes *immediate* immunity. However, it is expensive and, being prepared from human volunteers, its availability is limited.

Tetanus prophylaxis, which depends on the nature of the wound and the immunity status of the patient may be summarised as follows:

Immunity status		Nature of the wound	
	Clean	Contaminated	Infected
* Immune	None	None	Antibiotics
Partially immune	One toxoid	One toxoid + TIG + Antibiotics	One toxoid + TIG + Antibiotics
Non-immune or Unknown	Three toxoids	Three toxoids + TIG + Antibiotics	Three toxoids + TIG + Antibiotics

* Patients receiving the booster more than 3 years back should be treated as "Partially immune".

II. TREATMENT IN ESTABLISHED CASES.—This aims at eliminating toxin production (wound excision and antibiotics), neutralising the circulating toxin (TIG or ATS), preventing muscle spasms (sedatives and muscle relaxants) and providing respiratory and general support.

A. *Treatment in* GENERAL:

1. Isolation.—The patient should be kept in an absolutely quiet, dark, well-ventilated room. Isolation is necessary only for protection from noises (which provoke painful spasms). The disease is not infectious and man to man spread does not occur.

2. TIG or ATS.—These can only neutralise the circulating toxin. TIG, in doses of 6,000 to 10,000 units, is given intravenously after suitable dilution. If given intramuscularly, divided doses have to be used because it is voluminous.

   ATS is administered when TIG is not available. ATS 100,000 units, is given half intravenously and half intramuscularly. Care must be taken of hypersensitivity reactions. Because of chances of these reactions and doubtful efficacy, use of ATS has been discarded in many centres.

3. Antibiotics.—Penicillin in high dosage, 5 lac units every 6 hours, is administered. Erythromycin, 500 mg thrice daily, is used for persons allergic to penicillin. Badly infected wounds require broad-spectrum antibiotics and metronidazole.

4. Care of the wound.—The wound should be handled only after a few hours of administration of TIG or ATS. All stitches are cut, blood clots and foreign bodies removed, and pus drained. Radical wound excision need not be attempted.

5. Toxoid.—An attack of tetanus does not provide future immunity against the disease. All three injections are to be given if the patient survives.

B. *Further treatment in* MILDER *cases:*

These are the cases where there is hypertonicity of the muscles but no difficulty in swallowing or respiration, and no clonic spasms.

These cases require sedation with diazepam or barbiturates in suitable dosage, repeated as necessary. Promazine, in repeated doses, is given intramuscularly as a muscle relaxant, to prevent spasms.

C. *Further treatment in* MODERATELY SERIOUS *cases:*
These are the cases where there is difficulty in swallowing, some clonic spasms but no major asphyxial episodes. Treatment includes the following:
1. Sedatives like diazepam and barbiturates are administered in higher and more frequent doses.
2. Muscle relaxants like promazine are also to be used more frequently and in higher doses.
3. Dysphagia is managed by Ryle's tube feeding with liquid balanced food.
4. Irritation by full bladder and incarcerated stools are controlled by continuous catheterisation and suppositories, respectively.
5. If there is difficulty in respiration, a tracheostomy is performed gently. Regular suction and humidification are essential.

D. *Treatment in the* MOST SERIOUS *cases:*
These are the patients who have a major cyanotic convulsion. In addition to the treatment advocated for the moderately serious cases, the following measures are to be taken:
1. A strong muscle relaxant, curare, has to be administered *(curarisation)*. Repeated injection of 20 to 40 mg are given, intravenously to start, and intramuscularly thereafter, as necessary, to achieve continuous relaxation. This drug paralyses all the muscles, including those of respiration.
2. As the respiratory muscles are paralysed, intermittent positive pressure respiration has to be provided through a cuffed tracheostomy tube.

Causes of Death
1. Lung Complications.—These are the commonest causes of death. The complications may be:
   a. Lack of ventilation of lungs due to spasms of muscles of respiration.
   b. Aspiration of pharyngeal contents into the lungs because of absence of swallowing, due to spasms of pharyngeal muscles.
   c. Sudden loss of air entry either due to laryngeal spasm or due to vigorous spasm of the muscles of respiration.
   d. Pulmonary embolism—emboli being carried from stagnant limbs resulting from excessive sedation.
2. Hyperpyrexia, due to associated septicaemia or as a result of direct action of the exotoxin on the brain.
3. Toxic Myocarditis.

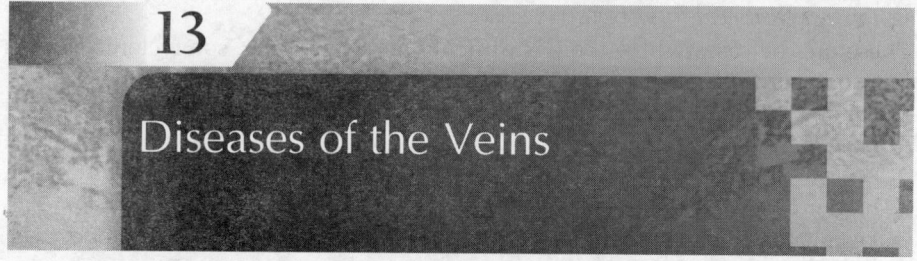

13

Diseases of the Veins

VENOUS DRAINAGE OF THE LOWER LIMBS

The consideration of the anatomy and physiology of the venous drainage of the lower limbs essentially aims at explaining the frequent occurrence of two pathological conditions in these veins. One of these is varicosity and the other is inflammation with thrombosis (phlebothrombosis and thrombophlebitis).

Anatomy.—The veins consist of three groups:

I. Deep veins.
II. Superficial veins.
III. Perforating or communicating veins, i.e. veins connecting the superficial to the deep veins.

I. Deep Veins.—These lie amongst, and are well supported by powerful muscles. The veins are—tibial, peroneal, popliteal, and femoral. Their characteristic features are as follows:

a. The veins are valved, the valves directing the flow of blood upwards.
b. The veins in the soleus muscle, which is the most powerful of the calf muscles, are of the nature of wide venous sinuses. They have no valves. They empty segmentally into the posterior tibial and peroneal veins. Some perforating veins enter the posterior tibial vein just opposite to the sites where the venous sinuses from the soleus enter this vein. These facts are of importance because of the following points:

   i. If the calf muscles are in complete rest for a long period (as in postoperative patients) the blood-flow through the venous sinuses is very slow. In this condition there is every possibility for the blood to form clot (thrombus), and this may be the starting point of a deep vein thrombosis.

   ii. Inflammation in these sinuses may easily spread to the posterior tibial vein (deep vein inflammation). It may also spread to the perforators that open into the posterior tibial vein in this situation. This may damage the valves in the perforators and that may be the starting point of varicose veins.

II. Superficial Veins.—These lie in the fat between the skin and the deep fascia. There are two sets:

1. Long saphenous vein ⎫
2. Short saphenous vein ⎭ with their tributaries

LONG SAPHENOUS VEIN.—This is the longest vein in the body. It starts on the inner side of the foot, passes in front of the medial malleolus straight to the posteromedial aspect of the knee, then upwards to the fossa ovalis, i.e. the saphenous opening in the deep fascia. It passes through this opening, thus coming deep to the deep fascia, and immediately ends in the femoral vein.

There are many no-return valves along the course of the vein, the strongest being located at the sapheno-femoral junction. These valves prevent downward flow of blood and the sapheno-femoral valve prevents back-flow of blood from the femoral to the saphenous vein.

Tributaries

1. In the leg:
   a. Posterior arch vein.
   b. Anterior vein of leg.
   c. A communicating twig from the upper part of the short saphenous vein.
2. In the thigh:
   a. Posteromedial vein of thigh.
   b. Anteromedial vein of thigh.
3. Near the fossa ovalis:
   a. Superficial external pudendal vein.
   b. Superficial epigastric vein.
   c. Superficial circumflex iliac vein.
   d. Deep external pudendal vein. (Fig. 13.1)

Importances

   i. The posterior arch vein is made up of a series of small venous arches behind the leg. These venous arches receive delicate venules which drain the skin of the ankle and the heel.

      Dilatation of these venules may occur in venous incompetence and this gives rise to a swelling with a haemangiomatous appearance that obliterates the hollow behind the ankle. This is called 'ankle flare'.

  ii. Anatomical communications between the long saphenous and the short saphenous veins may cause spread of varicosity from one system to the other.

 iii. In operations for varicose veins, when a ligature is applied to the sapheno-femoral junction, the veins draining into the long saphenous vein near the fossa ovalis must be ligated and cut since otherwise these small veins may get the back-pressure from the incompetent sapheno-femoral junction and produce big varicosities.

Short saphenous vein.—This vein starts on the lateral side of the foot, passes behind the lateral malleolus, ascends along the lateral border of tendo Achillis, and then along the midline on the back of the leg. It pierces the deep fascia at the popliteal fossa and opens into the popliteal vein.

There are no-return valves along its length and particularly one at the sapheno-popliteal junction.

III. Communicating or Perforating Veins.—These are the communicating vessels between the superficial and the deep veins. There are of two types:

A. Indirect perforators.—There are innumerable small vessels which start from the superficial venous system, pierce the deep fascia, and communicate with a vessel in an underlying muscle, the latter vessel in turn being connected to a deep vein. In the ankle region there is very little muscle, so only few such indirect perforators.

B. DIRECT PERFORATORS.—These veins, piercing the deep fascia, directly connect the saphenous veins (or their tributaries) to the deep veins. These direct veins are more or less constant in their number and situation:

1. In the thigh—between the long saphenous and the femoral vein in the adductor canal.
2. Below the knee—between the long saphenous and the posterior tibial vein.
3. Above the ankle (*ankle perforating veins*)—
   a. On the *medial side* there are three perforators—one behind and below the medial malleolus, one at the junction of the middle and lower third of the leg, and the other in between these two (Fig. 13.1).
   b. On the *lateral side* there is one perforator at the junction of the middle and lower third of the leg.

The communicating veins are all valved. These valves allow the flow of blood only in one direction, i.e. from the superficial to the deep veins.

Physiology.—The return of blood from the dependent lower limbs to the heart, against the gravity, is effected by several factors:

A. *General Factors:*
   1. Negative pressure in the thorax.
   2. Vis-a-tergo produced by arterial pressure.
B. *Local Factors:*
   1. Muscular
   2. Fascial
   3. Valvular

In the lower limb the muscles surround the deep veins and act as strong pumps for the blood in these veins. Of these, the calf muscles (*calf pump*) is the most effective. These muscles are surrounded by dense unyielding deep fascia and so

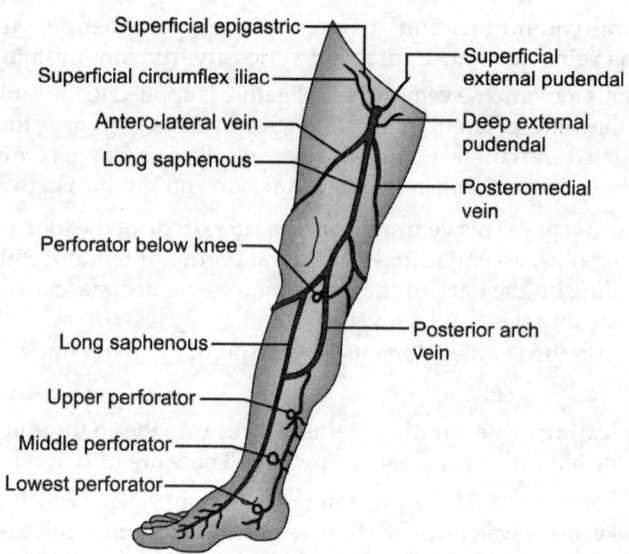

Superficial epigastric
Superficial circumflex iliac
Antero-lateral vein
Long saphenous
Superficial external pudendal
Deep external pudendal
Posteromedial vein
Perforator below knee
Long saphenous
Posterior arch vein
Upper perforator
Middle perforator
Lowest perforator

Fig. 13.1: The long saphenous vein

the muscular contractions can be effective on the veins. The valves in these veins force the blood to flow only in an upward direction.

The saphenous veins have to carry long columns of blood and since they are not well supported (being situated in the lax subcutaneous tissues), there was every possibility for these veins to become dilated. This difficulty is overcome because of the presence of the communicating veins which drain the saphenous veins segmentally into the deep veins. So, no segment of the superficial venous system, under normal conditions, has to carry any long column of blood. Further, the valves in the superficial veins prevent downward flow of blood. Since the valves are placed segmentally and since there is a segmental drainage of superficial venous blood into the deep veins, none of these valves has to bear weight of a long column of blood.

The communicating veins along the whole length of the limb are therefore of great importance. The valves in these veins allow the flow of blood only from the superficial to the deep system. This again is highly essential. The pressure in the deep veins is higher than that in the superficial veins and becomes much higher during muscular contractions. In the absence of the valves, blood would flow from the deep to the superficial veins, which would be hazardous.

It is interesting to note that the long saphenous and the short saphenous veins are also actually communicating veins. They are long no doubt but in all other respects they are similar to the communicating veins. The valves at the sapheno-femoral and sapheno-popliteal junctions prevent back-flow from the deep to the superficial veins.

VARICOSE VEINS

Definition.—A vein is said to be varicose when it becomes dilated, elongated, and, therefore, tortuous.

Sites.—Varicosity is common with the superficial veins of the lower limbs. It is also frequent in some other situations, e.g. haemorrhoidal veins (piles), spermatic veins (varicocele), and oesophageal veins (oesophageal varix).

Etiology

1. Morphological Factor.—Varicosity is a penalty that man pays for his erect posture, the veins having to drain against gravity. The superficial veins, having a little tissue to support them, have to suffer.
2. Secondary varicose veins are usually the results of venous obstruction or of conditions which hamper venous return, e.g.:
   a. Pregnancy and tumours in the pelvis.
   b. Thrombosis of the deep veins.
   c. Congenital arterio-venous fistula (occurs below the age of 20).
3. Primary varicose veins, which are much the commoner, are due to defects of the valves. The valvular defects may be congenital or acquired (due to infection in the veins). The defect may be:
   a. In the sapheno-femoral valve—causing varicosity of the long saphenous system.
   b. In the sapheno-popliteal valve—causing varicosity of the short saphenous system.
   c. In the valves of the communicating veins—causing a patchy varicosity in the neighbourhood of the communicating veins.

    d. Usually, a combination of the third with either of the first two. In long standing cases, there may be a combined varicosity of the long saphenous and the short saphenous systems.

Complications

1. *Thrombophlebitis*, i.e. infection of the varicose veins.
2. *Pigmentation*.—The skin, particularly that in the lower part of the leg, shows brownish black pigmentation. This is due to haemosiderin deposits resulting from break down of RBC, that had migrated out of the thin-walled veins.
3. *Eczema* (chronic dermatitis).—Occurring over the areas of pigmentation. The haemosiderin causes itching that results in scratching and abrasions, giving rise to the eczematous condition.
4. *Ankle Flare*.—Discussed under anatomy of the veins.
5. *Varicose Ulcers*.—These are chronic ulcers associated with varicose veins. They are usually found on or near the medial malleolus. This is a common site because of the following factors:
    a. There being very little soft tissue on the bone here (and so, little blood supply), any ulcer fails to heal and tends to become chronic.
    b. There are three direct perforating veins in the locality, and incompetence of either of these veins causes a venous regurgitation. This results in stasis of venous blood in the tissues with consequent tissue anoxia and lymphatic obstruction. Any ulcer on such tissues is apt to become chronic.
6. *Periostitis*.—May occur in the tibia at the base of a long-standing varicose ulcer.
7. *Haemorrhage*.—Brisk haemorrhage, either externally or as subcutaneous extravasation, may occur from rupture of some veins. Simple elevation of the limb and a firm bandaging easily controls the haemorrhage. Tourniquets should never be applied as they are likely to cause pressure on the veins, leading to further engorgement and more bleeding.
8. *Talipes Equinus*.—With long-standing chronic ulcers, the patient feels it easier to walk on the toes and, if this turns into habit, it may lead to talipes equinus.
9. *Saphena Varix*.—This denotes an extensive localised bulging of the wall of a varicose vein, making a sac for venous blood, and thus appearing as a bluish swelling. This occurs if there is a segmental thinning of the wall of the vein (the varicose veins usually become thick-walled), which yields under internal pressure. Since the pressure is maximum in the long saphenous vein just proximal to the sapheno-femoral junction (in cases of incompetence of this valve), saphena varix is commonest and most well-manifested in this situation.
10. *Calcification*.—This may rarely occur in the wall of the veins in long-standing cases.

Popular Clinical Tests.—These tests aim at localising the valve or valves, whose incompetence has led to the varicose condition in a particular case.

1. *Site*.—In general, a varicosity of the long saphenous system is manifested on the medial side of the leg and thigh, while that of the short saphenous system is seen on the posterolateral aspect of the leg. In a long-standing case, however, because of liberal communication between the two systems, varicosity in one may spread to the other. In cases of incompetency of a perforator, a localised varicosity may be seen. The majority of cases belong to a combination of incompetency of the sapheno-femoral valve and many perforators.

2. *Trendelenburg Test.*—With the patient lying, the limb is elevated to drain out the veins. A tourniquet is applied on the sapheno-femoral junction at the fossa ovalis (4 cm below and lateral to the pubic tubercle), sufficiently tight to occlude the vein (in clinical practice, pressure by the thumb is often used instead). The patient is now made to stand. The tourniquet (or pressure) is now released. If there is a rapid filling of the veins from above, the Trendelenburg test is positive, which means that the sapheno-femoral valve is incompetent. If this does not occur, the valve is competent and the test is negative.

A further modification of this test may be applied. With the tourniquet (or the pressure) on, the patient stands for a minute. If there is quick filling of the veins at different levels, it indicates incompetency of the communicating veins at these levels. If this does not occur and the veins fill up only slowly, the communicating veins are working normally.

A positive Trendelenburg test is an indication for operative interference.

3. *Morrissey's Test.*—This is applied for sapheno-femoral incompetence. The limb is elevated to empty the veins and the patient is asked to cough forcibly. If there is an expansile wave in the veins, the valve is incompetent.

4. *Schwartz Test.*—In an advanced case of varicosity, a thrill can be felt by a finger placed over the fossa ovalis when the most prominent part of the varicosity is tapped with another finger.

5. *Perthe's Test (modified).*—*This* test is especially helpful in determining whether the deep veins are patent or not. A tourniquet is applied round the upper thigh, sufficiently tight to occlude the long saphenous vein. With the tourniquet in position, the patient is asked to walk for a few minutes. If the deep veins and the communicating veins are normal, the superficial veins shrink. If the superficial veins get dilated or remain unchanged, either the deep vein is blocked or the perforators below the tourniquet are incompetent.

Treatment for Varicose Veins

A. PALLIATIVE TREATMENT.—Support by elastic stockings or elastocrepe bandages and, as far as practicable, avoiding standing. A palliative treatment is indicated for:

1. Varicosity associated with pregnancy.

2. Patients awaiting operation.

3. Patients unwilling or unfit for operation.

B. INJECTION TREATMENT.—This is done by careful injections of sclerosing agents into the dilated veins. It aims at intimal destruction followed by fibrosis and occlusion of the veins. 5 per cent ethanolamine may be used. The injection should be made only at one site in one sitting, and not more than 2 ml of the agent should be injected. Following the injection, a firm strapping of the limb is obligatory.

This treatment is effective in small patchy areas of varicosity—either in an original case or in one having small remnants following an operation.

C. OPERATIVE TREATMENT.—A positive Trendelenburg test is an indication for operation. There are two types of operation:

1. Ligation.

2. Ligation with stripping.

1. *Ligation.—*
   a. For sapheno-femoral incompetence.— A *'flush'* sapheno-femoral ligation is done at the fossa ovalis, and the long saphenous vein is divided. This means that the ligature has to be put right at the sapheno-femoral junction. Particular care must be taken to see that between the ligature and the sapheno-femoral junction there is no intervening tributary of the saphenous vein. For this purpose, the superficial epigastric, the superficial external pudendal, and the superficial circumflex iliac veins must be ligated and cut. Unless this is done, all the back-pressure from the femoral vein, via the incompetent valve, will be transmitted to these tributaries and cause tremendous varicosities in them.
   b. For sapheno-popliteal incompetence.—A 'flush' ligature is applied at the junction of the short saphenous vein with the popliteal vein at the popliteal fossa, and the short saphenous vein is divided.
   c. For incompetency of a communicating vein.—The particular vein has to be exposed, ligated, and divided.
2. *Ligation with Stripping.*—This is particularly useful for those cases where incompetence of either of the saphenous veins is associated with that of perforators as well (i.e. majority of cases). After 'flush' ligation as above, a vein-stripper (Meyer's) is passed through the saphenous vein and the whole length of the vein is stripped out, tearing all its tributaries and perforators. Haemostasis is easily achieved by firm bandaging of the limb.

Treatment of Varicose Ulcers

1. CONSERVATIVE METHODS.—Almost all ulcers can be made to heal by elevation and bandaging of the limb, together with proper exercises and massage *(Bisgaard method)*. Special methods of bandaging are practised, whereby selective pressure is applied on the ulcer-bearing area to minimise its oedema. Different ointments are advocated for protection and healing of the ulcer.

2. OPERATION FOR THE VARICOSE VEINS:
   a. Ligation, or ligation with stripping, as described above.
   b. Subfascial ligation.—As majority of these ulcers are due to incompetence of the perforating veins on the medial side of the ankle, these defective veins may be exposed at the lower part of the leg and ligated. These veins are better ligated *under* the deep fascia (subfascial).

3. OPERATION FOR THE ULCER.—While majority of the ulcers are likely to heal by the methods described above, some of them may fail to do so. These are more often cases of venous ulcers due to deep vein thrombosis. These ulcers have to be treated by excision and skin grafting.

HAEMANGIOMA

Definition.—Originally believed to be tumours of the blood vessels, haemangiomata are now regarded as developmental malformations (i.e. hamar-tomas) in relation to the vessels. This idea is based on the following observations:

a. The lesions are congenital, and during childhood they grow at the same rate as that of the surrounding tissues, after which they cease to grow and may even regress.

b. They are always benign.

Origin.—Haemangioma may arise from capillary, vein, or artery, and accordingly it is named:

From capillary.—Capillary haemangioma.

From vein.—Venous or cavernous haemangioma.

From artery (very rare).—Arterial or plexiform haemangioma *(cirsoid aneurysm).*

While haemangiomata may occur in any tissue of the body, they are much commoner in the skin and subcutaneous tissues.

Capillary Haemangioma

Clinical characters:

i. They are present since birth.

ii. They appear merely as coloured areas—bright red, purple, or violet in colour.

iii. The colour diminishes or disappears on pressure, to reappear immediately on release of the pressure.

iv. They are flat, i.e. not raised above the surface.

v. They are non-pulsatile.

Types.—There are several types of capillary haemangioma:

1. *Salmon Patch.*—On the midline of the forehead, disappearing by one year of age.

2. *Port-wine Stain.*—The commonest variety, keeping unchanged throughout life.

3. *Strawberry Angioma.*—This differs from an ordinary capillary haemangioma in that it is raised from the surface and forms a sessile, lobulated, localised, red tumour. It has a natural tendency to regress when the child grows to the age of seven or eight years.

Treatment.—Ordinarily no treatment is required, unless demanded for cosmetic reasons. The different methods of treatment are:

a. Excision with skin grafting—the best method.

b. Injection of sclerosing agents for strawberry angioma.

c. Application of carbon dioxide snow.

d. X-ray therapy.

Cavernous Haemangioma.—This consists of dilated venous spaces containing blood, making spongy masses.

Clinical characters:

i. They are always raised from the surface as circumscribed swellings.

ii. They show partial compressibility on pressure, refilling on release of the pressure.

iii. They are bluish in colour, containing venous blood.

iv. They are non-pulsatile.

v. Like capillary haemangioma, they are present since birth but unlike capillary haemangioma, they do not show tendency to spontaneous regression. In fact, they may get bigger to a troublesome degree. Unlike capillary haemangioma again, they may show complications like ulceration, bleeding, calcification and rarely, malignant change to haemangio-endothelioma (this is doubtful).

SITES:

1. Skin—face, cheek, ears.
2. Mucous membrane—lips (a very common site), mouth, tongue.
3. Brain, kidney, liver, or other organs.

Combination of external and internal haemangioma may occur.

TREATMENT:

1. *Sclerosing Treatment.*—This is done with the idea of coagulating the blood and damaging the endothelial lining of the venous spaces, to be followed by fibrosis and obliteration of the spaces. This procedure diminishes the size and checks further growth of the swelling. This may be done by:

    a. Injection of sclerosing agents, e.g. boiling water, hypertonic saline, 3 per cent sodium morrhuate, etc. The injection is made once a week, and repeated 5 to 6 times.

    b. Cautery.—A needle is passed through the swelling and its end is touched with a diathermy knob.

2. *Excision.*—The whole mass has to be carefully excised, which often proves difficult. Excision with a diathermy is technically easier since haemorrhage is minimised.

A preliminary treatment with sclerosing agents diminishes the size of the swelling, and makes its walls tough and more readily identifiable at operation (as with cystic hygroma). Recurrence, however, is fairly common (as with cystic hygroma).

Plexiform Haemangioma.—This is a type of congenital arteriovenous fistula, usually found on the scalp. The vessels in it, therefore, consist of arteries and *arterialised veins*—dilated, tortuous, and pulsatile—feeling like a bag of pulsating earthworms. This is also known as *cirsoid aneurysm*.

14

Lymphatics and Lymph Nodes

Lymphoedema means oedema due to lymphatic stasis. To start with there is a pitting oedema, but in a long-standing case this oedema becomes solid (due to myxomatous tissues). The subcutaneous tissues are grossly thickened, and the overlying skin thickened and coarse. The condition thus resembles elephant's skin and so it is known as Elephantiasis.

Types and Causes

A. PRIMARY LYMPHOEDEMA.—This is due to congenital malformations of the lymph vessels of the subcutaneous tissues, e.g.

   a. Aplasia—failure of development of the vessels.

   b. Hypoplasia—underdevelopment of the vessels.

   c. Dilatation and varicosity of the lymph vessels in association with congenital arteriovenous fistula.

   d. Reflux of chyle back from the cisterna chyli downwards, causing dilatation of the lymph vessels (chylous reflux).

     Primary lymphoedema is usually hereditary (familial) and is known as *Milroy's disease*. It may:

     i. Start at birth.—Lymphoedema congenita.

     ii. Start at puberty.—Lymphoedema praecox.

     iii. Start in adult life.—Lymphoedema tarda (i.e. late).

B. SECONDARY LYMPHOEDEMA.—This is due to acquired obstruction to the flow of lymph—obstruction either in the vessels or in the glands. The causes may be:

   1. *Traumatic,* e.g. removal of axillary nodes in radical mastectomy.

   2. Inflammatory.—Filariasis, tuberculosis, and fungal disease.

   3. *Neoplastic.*—Obstruction by malignant diseases.

In this country filariasis is the commonest cause of lymphoedema. Whatever be the cause, a vicious cycle is set in:

   Obstruction → Stasis → Infection → Fibrosis → Further obstruction.

Influence of gravity and preponderance of infection make the lower limbs and the scrotum the commoner sites for lymphoedema.

LYMPHANGIOMA

Types.—There are two types:

1. CAPILLARY LYMPHANGIOMA.—Found on the skin as small brownish papules which, on examination with a lens, show small vesicles. These congenital lesions are composed of a network of lymph vessels.

2. CAVERNOUS LYMPHANGIOMA.—These are of two types:

   a. Consisting of masses of lymphatic cysts—*cystic hygroma*. This is most commonly found in the neck. This is much the commoner type (*see* Chapter 26).

   b. Dilated lymph spaces, comparable to cavernous haemangioma, may occur on the lip or tongue. The lip or the tongue becomes bulky and the conditions are known as macrochelia (lip) and macroglossia (tongue). Extensive cavernous haemangioma may also cause macrochelia and macroglossia. Lymphangioma differs from haemangioma in that it lacks the bluish colour of a haemangioma.

ANATOMY OF THE IMPORTANT GROUPS OF LYMPH NODES

Cervical Nodes.—There are three chains:

A. Circular chain—some superficial and some deep.

B. Vertical chain of deep cervical nodes.

C. Supraclavicular chain.

A. CIRCULAR CHAIN.—These glands are located in the upper part of the neck, some of them superficial and some deep to the deep fascia. From before backwards, the glands are:

1. Submental.
2. Submandibular (submaxillary)—deep to the deep fascia, some of them in close relation with the submandibular salivary glands.
3. Preauricular, parotid (both superficial and deep to the parotid fascia), facial (some superficial and some deep).
4. Post-auricular or mastoid (on the mastoid process).
5. Suboccipital.

The efferent vessels from all these nodes drain into the deep cervical nodes.

B. VERTICAL CHAIN.—There are a large number of glands closely related to the jugular vein, under cover of the sternomastoid. These are the nodes popularly known as deep cervical nodes. There are two groups:

1. *Jugulo-digastric.*—At the junction of the jugular vein and the digastric muscle (also known as *upper deep cervical* nodes).
2. *Jugulo-omohyoid.*—At the junction of the jugular vein and the central tendon of omohyoid (also known as *lower deep cervical* nodes).

C. SUPRACLAVICULAR CHAIN.—Located in the supraclavicular fossa, these glands are:-

1. Medial set.
2. Intermediate set.
3. Lateral set.

The medial set of nodes are situated between the two heads of the sternomastoid and these are the glands popularly known as the *Virchow's nodes*.

The efferent vessels from the deep cervical and the supraclavicular nodes merge into one trunk on each side of the neck. This is called the *jugular lymph-trunk*. On the left side this trunk ends in the thoracic duct while on the right side it directly enters the junction of the internal jugular vein and the subclavian vein.

Axillary Nodes.—The axilla is a pyramidal space and the axillary nodes are located on the three walls, the floor, and the apex of the pyramid:

1. *Anterior Group.*—Situated on the anterior wall of the axilla, behind the pectoralis major. Hence they are also called *the pectoral group*.

2. *Posterior Group.*—On the posterior wall of the axilla, i.e. in front of the subscapularis muscle. Hence called the *subscapular group.*

3. *Lateral Group.*—On the lateral wall of the axilla, i.e. on the humerus, in close relation to the axillary vein. Hence called *humeral group.*

4. *Central Group.*—*Situated* on the floor of the axilla, in the fat there.

5. *Apical Group.*—These glands are situated at the apex of the axilla just under the clavicle, i.e. *infraclavicular group.* Some of these glands are located in the deltopectoral groove.

Drainage

1. ANTERIOR GROUP:

   Afferents from:
   i. Major part of the lymphatics of the breast.
   ii. Anterior abdominal wall, above the umbilicus.

   Efferents to:
   i. Central nodes.
   ii. A major part directly to apical nodes.

2. POSTERIOR GROUP:

   Afferents from:
   i. Some of the lymphatics of the breast.
   ii. The back, corresponding to the thoracic vertebrae.

   Efferents to:
   Central nodes.

3. LATERAL GROUP:

   Afferents from:
   The upper limb.

   Efferents to:
   Central nodes.

4. CENTRAL GROUP:

   Afferents from:
   Anterior, posterior, and lateral groups.

   Efferents to:
   Apical nodes.

5. APICAL GROUP:

   Afferents from:
   i. Central nodes,
   ii. Anterior nodes.
   iii. The deltopectoral group receive some lymph from the upper limb, along vessels running with the cephalic vein.
   iv. Directly from the breast.

   Efferents to:
   A single trunk, known as the subclavian trunk, emerges on each side and drains at the junction of the subclavian vein and the internal jugular vein.

Inguinal Nodes.—According to their location in relation to the deep fascia, these nodes are:

A. Superficial.

B. Deep.

SUPERFICIAL INGUINAL NODES.—These again consist of two sets:

1. *Proximal (Horizontal) Set.*—Below and parallel to the inguinal ligament, in three groups—medial, intermediate, and lateral. They drain:

   a. Anterior abdominal wall below the umbilicus.

   b. Penis, scrotum, vulva, perineum.

   c. Buttock.

   d. Anterior urethra, anal canal, vagina.

   e. Lymphatics along the round ligament of uterus.

2. *Distal (Vertical) Set.*—Lying alongside the termination of the long saphenous vein. They receive the lymph from the superficial tissues of the whole lower limb (excepting a small portion consisting of the posterolateral part of foot and leg, whose lymphatic run along the short saphenous vein to drain into the popliteal nodes).

   The efferents from the superficial inguinal nodes drain into the deep inguinal nodes.

DEEP INGUINAL NODES.—These are only 4 to 5 in number, lying close to the upper part of the femoral vein. The uppermost of them is constant in position, lying in the femoral canal, and known as the *gland of Cloquet*. The deep nodes drain deeper tissues of the whole of the lower limb and receive the efferents from the superficial inguinal nodes.

The efferents from the deep inguinal nodes drain into the external iliac nodes.

Acute Lymphadenitis.—The nodes are highly tender and soon get fixed. The overlying skin is red and hot. A primary focus is almost always evident. Early institution of antibiotics may cause resolution; otherwise suppuration occurs, and this requires incision.

Flow Chart 14.1: Enlargement of lymph nodes

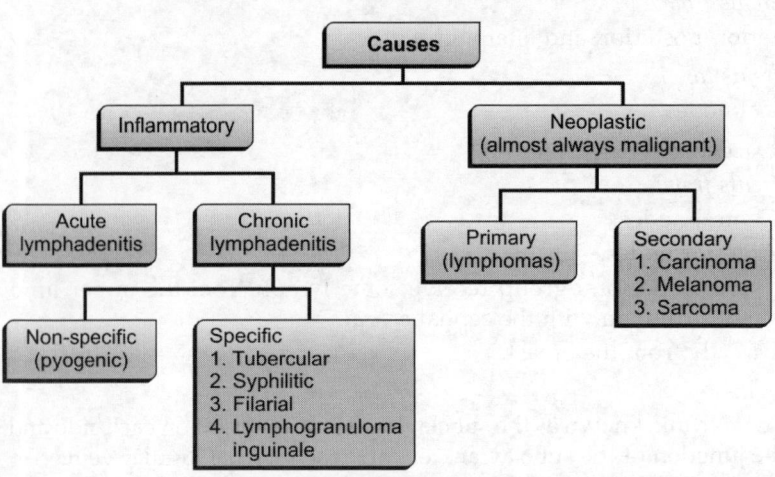

Chronic Septic Lymphadenitis.—This condition is fairly common in the cervical and inguinal nodes. For the cervical nodes the primary focus is usually in the oral cavity, including gums and tonsils, or in the scalp. For the inguinal nodes infected skin on the genitalia or the lower limb is the usual cause.

The nodes are moderately enlarged, firm, and elastic in feel, with little tenderness. In absence of a demonstrable primary septic lesion, the condition may be difficult to be diagnosed from tubercular lymphadenitis.

Such nodes may also occur in relation to malignant ulcers and it may be difficult to confirm clinically whether the involvement of the nodes is due to malignancy or only due to sepsis, the ulcer being almost always infected.

Syphilitic Lymphadenitis

1. *Primary stage:*
   a. With genital chancres, the nodes are moderately enlarged, not painful and not tender, firm, discrete and shotty.
   b. With extragenital chancres, the nodes are considerably enlarged, usually painful and tender, and may be matted.

2. *Secondary stage.*—Generalised lymph node enlargement, particularly involving epitrochlear and occipital groups.

3. *Tertiary stage.*—Lymph node involvement is rare.

Filarial Lymphadenitis.—The inguinal nodes in the males are usually involved. Typically, there is a history of periodic fever (particularly during the full moons and new moons), associated with pain, swelling, and tenderness, simultaneously involving the scrotum, epididymis, spermatic cord, and the inguinal nodes. Often there is evidence of a chronic filarial scrotum.

Special Investigations:
1. Blood—shows eosinophilia.
2. Thick blood film drawn at night—may show microfilaria.
3. Biopsy of the nodes—may reveal adult filaria.

Lymphogranuloma Inguinale.—This is a type of venereal disease due to a filterable virus, which causes suppurative lymphadenitis of the inguinal nodes. Following suppuration, there is extensive ulceration, sinus formation, and fibrosis.

A positive *Frei reaction* is confirmatory. This is an allergic reaction induced by intradermal injection of extracts of a fresh infective material.

Lymphatic Leukaemia.—This condition is of a little *surgical* importance. There is a generalised involvement of the nodes, associated with enlargement of the spleen. Examination of the blood shows a very high lymphocytic count and presence of lymphoblasts. This is a form of reticulosis, the origin being the primitive mesenchymal cells.

Lymphosarcoma.—This form of reticulosis has its origin in the lymphoid tissues of the lymph nodes. It is characterised by rapid growth and a high degree of local malignancy. The patient is usually young, and the cervical nodes are the most commonly involved. The mediastinal and the abdominal nodes or any other collection of lymphoid tissue may also be the site of the pathology. The nodes rapidly increase in size, loose their individual outlines, and make a big mass, firm in feel. This quickly gets fixed to the deeper structures. Involvement of the skin and fungation may occur, but much less commonly than with nodes of secondary carcinoma. Subsequently distant glands may be affected and metastases may develop in the liver, spleen, or other organs.

Reticulosarcoma.—The clinical presentation is usually like lymphosarcoma. The differentiation is done under microscope, when big reticulum cells and reticulum fibres are seen instead of the lymphocytes and lymphoblasts.

Burkitt's Tumour.—Found usually in the African children *(African Lymphoma)*, this form or reticulosis is characterised by widespread involvement of the lymph nodes and other lymphoid tissues of the body, and particularly the jaw. The disease has a very rapid course but may respond very well to chemotherapy and radiotherapy.

LYMPHOMAS

This term denotes primary lymphoreticular neoplasms. The lymphoreticular cells develop from the primitive mesenchymal cells. From these primitive cells two types of tissues are differentiated, viz. the lymphoid tissue (consisting of the lymphoblasts and the lymphocytes) and the reticulum cells (belonging to the reticuloendothelial system). Lymphomas or lymphoreticular neoplasms may arise in the lymphatic cells, the reticulum cells or the primitive mesenchymal precursor cells.

The lymphoreticular cells are located in:
1. The lymph nodes.
2. The spleen, liver and thymus.
3. The bone marrow.
4. The submucosa of the gastrointestinal and the respiratory tracts.

The lymphomas, which are almost always malignant, and predominantly solid tumours and are broadly divided into two histological groups:
1. Hodgkin's lymphoma or Hodgkin's disease, which is regarded as a malignant neoplastic process of the *haemopoetic tissues.*
2. Non-Hodgkin's lymphomas, which are monoclonal neoplastic process of the *lymphoid cells* (usually 'B' cells, occasionally 'T' cells). These lymphomas, therefore, merge with lymphocytic and lymphoblastic leukaemias with which they have many features in common.

HODGKIN'S DISEASE

Pathology.—In this form of lymphoma, which is also known as *'Lymphadenoma'*, both the lymphoid tissue and the reticulum have their share.

The disease is characterised by glandular enlargement, enlargement of the spleen and sometimes the liver, and an anaemia of secondary type. The lymphoreticular tissues in other parts of the body may also be involved (see above).

Glandular enlargement, which is the commonest feature of the disease, is usually to start with, unifocal. Most commonly it starts either in the supraclavicular nodes or in the jugulo-digastric group. While in some cases only one group of nodes is thus involved, usually the node involvement becomes fairly generalised, though at a variable interval. The glands, on *macroscopical* section, show a typical fish-flesh appearance. *Microscopically*, proliferation of all cells, that take part in the formation of lymph glands, including the reticular cells, are seen. Different types of giant cells are found, of which the characteristic is the *Sternberg-Reed* cell. Thus the histology is characterised by cellular pleomorphism. However, the histological picture varies so widely from case to case that Hodgkin's lymphoma is divided into 4 main *histological types*. In order of frequency, these are:

1. Nodular sclerosis—there is fibrosis in the glands.
2. Mixed cellularity—there is cellular pleomorphism as stated above.
3. Lymphocyte predominant.
4. Lymphocyte depleted.

   The nodular sclerosis and the lymphocyte predominant cases bear rather good prognosis. The lymphocyte depleted variety has worst prognosis. The mixed cellularity type usually denotes changing or transitional phase of the disease which ultimately settles into one of the other three types.

Clinical Features

1. The patient is usually an young adult, more commonly a male. However, children are also frequent sufferers.
2. There is a painless swelling consisting of mass of lymph nodes—usually either the supraclavicular or the jugulo-digastric. Subsequently, other cervical nodes and other nodes in the body show similar enlargements. In the swelling, the glands are all felt discrete, i.e. they are not matted together since there is no periadenitis (cf tubercular nodes). They have a typical elastic India-rubbery feel. Softening and suppuration are absent. There is no tenderness.
3. The spleen may be enlarged and sometimes the liver also.
4. There is a secondary anaemia.
5. In some cases there is an irregular temperature which may sometimes be of the *Pel-Ebstein type* (i.e. recurrent attacks of remittent fever).
6. In some cases big glandular lumps may cause pressure symptoms as follows:
   a. Air passages—dyspnoea.
   b. Superior vena cava in the mediastinum—oedema and venous engorgement in the head and neck.
   c. Abdominal nodes—intestinal obstruction, portal vein obstruction, obstructive jaundice, etc.
7. Bone lesions may cause bone pain, pathological fracture, paraplegia, root-pain, etc.

Clinical Staging.—The extent of the disease may vary widely and it is necessary to stage the disease clinically in order to express the extent of involvement as well as to decide the prognosis and treatment.

Stage I.—Involvement of single group of nodes above the diaphragm (e.g. neck or axilla or mediastinum).

Stage II.—Involvement of two groups of nodes above the diaphragm.

Stage III.—Involvement of groups of nodes both above and below the diaphragm (e.g. inguinal, retroperitoneal).

Stage IV.—Generalised disease affecting nodes, organs and/or bones.

Each stage is subdivided into 'a' and 'b' categories according to the absence or presence of systematic symptoms, e.g. loss of weight, fever, night sweats, anaemia, bone pain, etc.

The disease falls in the 'a' category when these are absent and in 'b' category when they are present.

Special Investigations

1. Blood examination—secondary anaemia and slight eosinophilia.
2. Biopsy confirms the diagnosis.
3. X-ray Chest—may show enlargement of mediastinal nodes.

Treatment.—Two forms of treatment are advocated—radiotherapy and chemotherapy—according to the stage of the disease:

Radiotherapy—Stages I, II and IIIa

Chemotherapy—Stages IIIb and IV

The patients are anaemic and radiotherapy or chemotherapy make them further anaemic. So *blood transfusion* has usually to be supplemented.

RADIOTHERAPY.—Supervoltage therapy allows wide areas to be treated. The therapy is given in divided doses over several weeks, with a total of 3500–4000 rad. Normal tissues are protected with lead shields. In cases of localised lesions in the neck glands, radiotherapy often acts miraculously.

CHEMOTHERAPY.—Combination chemotherapy is advocated—cytotoxic and antimitotic drugs are combined together with prednisolone.

SURGERY.—Surgery is only indicated for biopsy.

NON-HODGKIN'S LYMPHOMAS

As has already been said, in this variety of lymphoma there is proliferation of lymphoid cells. These lymphomas are broadly divided into two groups:

1. *Nodular.*—The nodular structure can still be seen.
2. *Diffuse.*—The nodular structure is replaced by diffuse sheets of cells. Each variety has 4 *histological types*:
   1. Well-differentiated lymphocytic type.
   2. Poorly differentiated lymphocytic type.
   3. Mixed lymphocytic and histiocytic type.
   4. Histiocytic type.

Treatment

1. For the rather benign types, e.g. nodular lymphocytic type—no treatment is usually necessary except periodic follow-up.
2. The disease is usually diagnosed in stage III and stage IV (the staging principle is the same as for Hodgkin's lymphoma) and so combination *chemotherapy* is the treatment of choice.
3. If there are pressure effects local *radiotherapy* has to be added.

TUBERCULAR LYMPHADENITIS

Routes of Infection

1. Most commonly the bacilli reach the node via lymphatics—tubercles then first form in the cortex.
2. Sometimes the bacilli reach the node by blood stream—tubercles then first form in the medulla.

Glands involved.—The bacilli usually enter the body via the tonsil, pharynx, lungs and small intestine. Consequently the glands in these territories are first affected:

a. The cervical nodes are most commonly involved (via tonsil and pharynx).

b. The mesenteric nodes and the mediastinal nodes are next in order of frequency (via small intestine and lungs respectively).

c. The axillary nodes are also fairly commonly involved (usually as a spread from mediastinum).

d. The inguinal nodes are involved rather frequently.

Pathology.—The disease runs in 3 stages:

1. Tubercles form and coalesce in the gland substance and, unless early treatment is instituted, there is caseation in the central part of the gland. At this stage the glands are enlarged, discrete, firm and elastic in feel, and only little tender. If they remain in this stage for long period they may be mistaken for Hodgkin's disease (*lymphadenoid type*).

2. A periadenitis usually supervenes, which means that the capsule of the gland is involved in the inflammatory process. The inflammatory plastic exudate of the periadenitis binds the adjacent nodes together and causes *matting* of the glands that is evidenced clinically. Since in the majority of cases, the tubercular process usually starts in the cortex of the gland, i.e. towards the periphery, periadenitis occurs early and matting is an early clinical feature.

3. The disease may now either spread further or be arrested:
   a. If it is arrested, healing occurs by fibrosis and particularly if caseation has occurred by calcification as well.
   b. If progress occurs, the caseation extends and forms a cold abscess

This abscess, coming out of the gland, pierces through the overlying structures including the deep fascia. to come under the skin. Thus there is a small rent in the deep fascia and part of the abscess is superficial and part of it deep to the deep fascia, i.e. there is a "collar-stud" abscess. The skin at first cold and white, later becomes red, breaks down, and forms a sinus. A sinus may persist for a long period and may subsequently heal with much scarring.

Clinical Features

1. The disease is much commoner in the children and young adults, particularly in the poorer people

2. The patient presents with enlargement of lymph nodes in either of the stages, viz.
   a. glands discrete and firm elastic (lymphadenoid type)
   b. glands typically matted.
   c. glands with cold abscess or sinus.

   With the common cervical gland involvement. two distinct types are recognised
   i. In some patients the adenitis is a manifestation of widespread primary infection in the chest—often in an ill-nourished child. The node involvement is bilateral and multiple, mainly those in the lower part of the neck, i.e. in the posterior triangles. However, the glands are neither greatly enlarged nor caseous.
   ii. In others, usually a healthy child or an adult without any evidence of other tubercular lesions, only one group of glands, most commonly the jugulo-digastric, is involved. Often it is evident that one gland is grossly diseased, surrounding which there are a few glands involved to a lesser extent, with typical matting. Cold abscess formation is rather frequent.

3. Constitutional features of tuberculosis, e.g. evening rise of temperature, loss of weight, night-sweating, etc. may or may not be present.

Special Investigations

1. Blood examination.—DC (Imphocytosis), and ESR.
2. Urine examination for sugar (and blood sugar estimation) for elderly patients.
3. Mantoux test, particularly in children.
4. X-ray chest
5. Biopsy in doubtful cases.

Treatment

A. GENERAL TREATMENT

1. Good nutritions diet.
2. *Antitubercular drugs.*—To start with, three antitubercular drugs are used *(triple attack)*. There are two popular combinations:
   i. Streptomycin, ethambutol and INH (isoniazid).
  ii. Rifampicin, ethambutol and INH.

Rifampicin, INH and streptomycin are bactericidal, while ethambutol is bacteriostatic.

When streptomycin, INH and ethambutol are used, streptomycin is given intramuscularly 1 g daily, usually up to a maximum of 90 g. In the later stages the drug may have to be used on alternate days if the patient cannot tolerate daily administration. INH is given 300 mg daily as a single dose. Ethambutol is administered 20 mg/kg body weight, i.e. 800 to 1200 mg per day in a single dose. While streptomycin is omitted after administration of 90 g, INH and ethambutol have to be continued for at least 18 months or till clinical cure occurs, whichever is later.

Rifampicin, INH and ethambutol is a better combination because rifampicin is much more bactricidal than streptomycin. However, it is costlier. It is particularly indicated for elderly patients who cannot tolerate streptomycin because of vestibular damage. The advantage of rifampicin is that, when it is used, INH and ethambutol can usually be discontinued after 9 months' therapy. Rifampicin is administered 450 to 600 mg daily orally (commonly in single dosage), usually for a period of three months.

B. LOCAL TREATMENT

1. No local treatment is necessary for glands without cold abscess or sinus formation.
2. In cases with cold abscess—repeated aspiration with instillation of INH solution locally, till the abscess resolutes.
3. *Surgery* is indicated under the following circumstances:
   a. For biopsy in confirming the diagnosis in doubtful cases.
   b. Block dissection of the nodes which become stationary in size and do not regress further after antitubercular treatment.
   c. Block dissection with excision of sinuses where sinuses have formed.
   d. Block dissection in those cases where cold abscess had formed—thereafter the abscess has either resoluted or has failed to resolute.

In the last two groups, surgery has to be undertaken because the antitubercular drugs will not reach the organisms in the avascular caseous material.

Also, surgery is not dangerous because the pus of cold abscess is usually sterile.

SECONDARY CARCINOMA

There are three groups of cases:

1. The patient presents with a primary growth, and during examination, the regional nodes are found to be involved.
2. The patient presents with a secondary node, and during examination, the primary growth is discovered.
3. The patient presents with a typical secondary node, but in spite of all clinical examinations and special investigations, the primary growth cannot be discovered. These cases are called *'obscure primary'*.

The Nodes.—The nodes are irregularly enlarged, discrete, and typically *stony hard* in consistency. To start with, they are painless but later pain of a variable intensity appears. Very quickly the nodes get fixed to the deeper structures. Later they get fixed to the skin and may ultimately fungate out.

Special Investigations

1. All investigations for and to find out the primary growth.
2. X-ray chest.
3. In cases of doubt, biopsy for confirmation of the diagnosis.

Treatment.—The patients may be divided into 4 groups:

GROUP 1: The nodes in relation to a primary growth are not palpable. Treatment for the primary is done and the nodes are kept on a periodic check-up.

GROUP 2: The nodes are enlarged and significant (that means, they are characteristically malignant). Block dissection of nodes is done.

GROUP 3: The nodes are enlarged but clinically it is not sure whether the enlargement is due to secondary deposits or to secondary infection from a fungated primary growth. In these cases two courses may be adopted:

   a. Treatment for the primary is done and the patient is kept on a course of antibiotic treatment, usually for three weeks. If the nodes subside, they were possibly infective, and the patient belongs to group 1 and treated as such. If they fail to subside, they are taken as malignant and treated as in group 2, i.e. a block dissection is advised.
   b. Alternatively, a biopsy may be done to ascertain the nature of the nodes and the patient treated accordingly.

GROUP 4: The nodes are malignant but have become fixed. Surgery cannot, therefore, be undertaken. Palliative treatment with radiotherapy, chemotherapy, or in suitable cases, hormone therapy is the only recourse. Secondary nodes are usually not so much radiosensitive and hence many surgeons discourage radiotherapy.

SURGERY FOR LYMPH NODES

1. *Excision:* This is done where there is a solitary node enlargement, particularly for the purpose of biopsy.
2. *Block Dissection: This* means en bloc (i.e. in one mass) removal of all the nodes of a particular region. This is the type of operation done for tubercular or malignant nodes. If the nodes are excised separately instead of in one mass, the lymph vessels connected to the nodes are severed. These vessels usually contain tubercle

bacilli or malignant cells, and as they are cut, these materials fall on the surrounding tissues, causing spread of the pathology. To avoid this, the nodes together with their communicating lymphatics are excised in one mass. Since the lymph vessels cannot be dissected out as such, all the nodes, together with the surrounding subcutaneous tissues and the attached deep fascia, are removed en bloc.

Block dissection of the Neck Nodes

1. *Crile's Block Dissection.*—This method is particularly used for malignant nodes. It is also known as *radical neck dissection* because the operation aims at radical removal of the whole of the lymphatic bearing tissues on the affected side of the neck. Thus the following structures are removed en bloc:

a. All lymph nodes of the side.

b. The internal jugular vein on which the all important vertical chain of deep nodes are located (the vein is ligated above and below, and the central part is excised).

c. Deeper fibres of sternomastoid, if adherent to the nodes.

d. Parts of omohyoid and digastric muscles, if the nodes infiltrate into them.

e. All fat and fascia over the region.

If a bilateral block dissection is required, the two sides are operated at an interval of about three weeks. It is preferable that the internal jugular vein on one side is left intact in order to avoid an obstructed cerebral venous flow (this idea is debatable).

One incision below and parallel to the lower border of the mandible and another above and parallel to the clavicle are made. The centres of these two transverse incisions are joined by a vertical incision. By reflecting the two skin flaps, wide exposure is obtained.

2. *Suprahyoid Block Dissection.*—This is done when the nodes only in the upper part of the neck have been involved in the pathology. A long transverse incision is made, parallel to the lower border of the mandible, across the midline. The advantage of this procedure is that both sides of the neck can be attended at one operation.

EXAMINATION OF A PATIENT WITH ENLARGED CERVICAL NODES

1. A complete examination of the nodes with which the patient presents—particularly their consistency, fixity, matting, tenderness, etc.

2. Examination of all the cervical lymph nodes of both the sides.

3. Examination of the drainage area as far as practicable, viz. the oral cavity including the floor of the mouth, tongue and cheek, the face, the scalp, the back, and the neck.

4. Examination of other lymph nodes of the body (to exclude generalised lymphadenopathy, e.g. Hodgkin's disease).

5. Examination of the abdomen.—Spleen (Hodgkin's disease), liver (secondary metastasis, Hodgkin's disease), ascites (malignancy), stomach (if there are enlarged Virchow's nodes).

6. Clinical examination of the chest and breasts.
7. Examination of the testes, if the patient presents with enlarged Virchow's nodes.
8. The patient is advised:
   a. Laryngoscopic examination to visualise the larynx, upper part of pharynx, and posterior part of tongue.
   b. X-ray chest.
   c. Bronchoscopy, oesophagoscopy, if required.
   d. Barium swallow examination of the oesophagus and barium meal examination of stomach, if required.

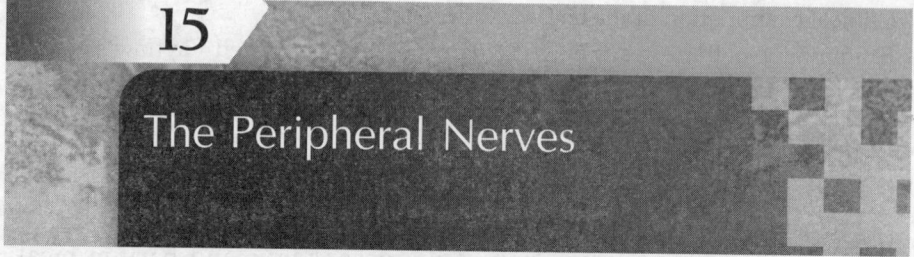

15

The Peripheral Nerves

INJURIES OF NERVES

Structure of a Nerve Trunk.—Each nerve trunk consists of a large number of nerve fibres.

Each nerve fibre consists of central axon which is enclosed in a myelin sheath, and outside this there is a continuous syncytium of cells making the *sheath of Schwann (neurilemma sheath)*.

The nerve fibres are embedded in a connective tissue reticulum known as the *endoneurium*. Several nerve fibres, running parallel to each other cable-like, are enclosed in a condensation of connective tissue, called the *perineurium*. The nerve trunk itself has a strong sheath to enclose it, known as the *epineurium*.

Changes after Division.—There are two phases—degeneration and regeneration.

DEGENERATION

1. The nerve fibres *distal* to the division undergo what is called *Wallerian degeneration*. This degeneration occurs along the whole length of the distal fibres and consists of:
   a. disintegration and disappearance of the axons,
   b. fragmentation of the myelin sheath,
   c. proliferation of the neurilemmal cells. This proliferation gives rise to a globular swelling—the *distal glioma* (false neuroma). These proliferating neurilemmal cells grow proximally, towards the plane of division, being drawn by chemotaxis.
2. The nerve fibres *proximal* to the division also undergo (retrograde) degeneration but this extends only to the next node of Ranvier, i.e. for only about a centimeter. After a short interval, the axons begin to regenerate and spread out in search of the distal cut end. If it can reach that, regeneration of the nerve is likely to occur. If this is not possible, the proliferating axons together with the proliferating neurilemmal cells produce a swelling—the *proximal neuroma*. This is usually tender and often palpable.

When a nerve trunk has been completely divided, retraction of the two cut ends takes place and the gap between the two is usually filled up by fibrous tissue.

After incomplete division affecting only one side of a nerve trunk, a *lateral neuroma* often develops. Similarly, if only the central fibres of a nerve trunk are injured (as in contusion), a *central neuroma* may develop.

REGENERATION

1. *Successful.*—This is likely to occur in any of the following conditions:
   a. The cut ends are united by suture.

b. The sheath (epineurium) is intact.

c. Only a small gap is present between the cut ends.

In these cases the neurilemmal sheaths, proliferating from the proximal and distal cut ends towards each other, meet together. If this has occurred, majority of the axons regenerating in the proximal end will grow downwards into the sheath of the distal stump.

As this regeneration is taking place, it is essential that, for functional recovery to occur, the sensory fibres proliferating from the proximal stump grows down a sheath that was previously occupied by a sensory fibre, and the same is true for motor fibres. Otherwise, even if structural regeneration occurs, functional recovery is impossible. A regenerated motor fibre can have no effect on a sensory end-organ and similarly a regenerated sensory fibre will have no control on a motor end-plate. In nerve suturing therefore, all care must be taken to avoid axial rotation of either cut end so as to ensure full anatomical continuity.

2. *Unsuccessful.*—All attempts at regeneration fail if:

a. A wide gap exists between the cut ends.

b. There is a considerable degree of fibrosis (as in wounds complicated by infection).

Changes after Closed Injuries.—Nerve trunks may undergo contusion, compression, stretching, etc. These are injuries where the epineurium is left intact and there is no loss of anatomical continuity. Degeneration occurs (as after division of a nerve trunk), but regeneration is usually the rule since the neurilemmal sheaths are intact. However, due to intraneural fibrosis, regeneration may be incomplete.

Rate of Regeneration.—Regeneration occurs initially at the rate of 2 mm a day but the rate diminishes as time passes—after about three months it is only about 1 mm a day. On arrival at their endings, there is a further delay of three weeks before the end organs are activated.

The rate of regeneration may be calculated clinically as follows:

1. *Tinel's Sign.*—The course of the nerve is lightly percussed with a patella-hammer from below upwards. A tingling sensation is experienced by the patient as the hammer hits the level of regeneration. This is due to the heightened threshold of the freshly regenerated axons.

2. Measuring the rate at which pain and touch sensations return.

3. Noting the times at which the function of the muscles at different levels from the injury returns.

Recovery occurs first in the muscle groups nearest to the site of injury and last in the peripheral skin areas, where the anaesthetic areas begin to decrease steadily from the margin inwards.

Secondary Pathological Changes Accompanying Nerve Injury

1. SKIN.—It becomes thin and may develop trophic ulcers as a result of unrecognised (due to anaesthesia) minor trauma.

2. MUSCLES:

a. Paralysed and flaccid.

b. Overstretched by unopposed action of the antagonist group of muscles.

  c. Reaction of degeneration:
    i. The fibres no longer respond to faradic stimulation (in which there is rapid make and break) but they still respond to galvanic stimulation (slow make and break); this is because of increase in the duration of chronaxie.
    ii. There is a change in the polarity, i.e. ACC becomes greater than KCC.
    The reaction of degeneration appears in about 4 days and becomes fully established in about a fortnight after the injury.
  d. If nutrition of the muscles is not maintained by galvanic stimulation, the muscle fibres degenerate and they are gradually replaced by fibrous tissue. This makes recovery impossible.

3. Joints.—These being immobile, develop periarticular adhesions and are fixed in contracted position.

4. Bones.—These are decalcified due to disuse.

Prevention of Secondary Pathological Changes

1. Skin.—Should be protected by warm padding to prevent injury.

2. Muscles:
  a. The limb should be so splinted that the paralysed muscles are kept relaxed, prevented from over-stretching.
  b. Muscle movements are maintained by regular galvanic stimulation of all the paralysed muscles.
  c. Physiotherapy.

3. Joints.—All joints are subjected to gentle passive movements daily, in order to prevent contracture.

Gradation of Muscle Power.—According to the Medical Research Council of London, power of a particular muscle is graded as follows:
0 = Complete paralysis.
1 = Flicker of contraction.
2 = Contraction with gravity eliminated.
3 = Contraction against gravity alone.
4 = Contraction against gravity and some resistance.
5 = Contraction against powerful resistance (i.e. normal power).

Nature of Nerve Injury.—Whatever be the mode of injury (tear, laceration, contusion, compression, or stretching), the lesion in the nerve may be of three types:
1. Neurapraxia.
2. Axonotmesis.
3. Neurotmesis.

Neurapraxia.—There is only a transient physiological block. The condition may be compared to concussion of the brain and is the result of stretching or distortion of the nerve without any organic rupture. Some people believe that it is due to a transient ischaemia at the point of injury. The axons are intact, there is only a degeneration of the myelin sheaths. The larger motor fibres are mainly affected, the smaller sensory fibres to a lesser extent; hence complete sensory loss is unusual. Complete and spontaneous recovery is the rule.

Axonotmesis.—This consists of intrathecal rupture of nerve fibres. The internal architecture of the nerve is preserved because the neurilemmal sheaths are kept intact. However, the axons are so badly damaged that Wallerian degeneration occurs in the distal portion of the broken axons, leaving empty neurilemmal sheaths. The regenerating axons grow down into these empty sheaths. Complete and spontaneous recovery can be expected since there is very little maldistribution because the relative position of the axons and the respective distal tubules is preserved by the intact sheath. Some degree of intraneural fibrosis may however occur and recovery may be incomplete in these cases. If there is extensive scarring at the site of trauma, axons cannot regenerate through it and recovery does not occur.

NEUROTMESIS.—The normal architecture of the nerve is lost. This may be of two types:

a. *Complete neurotmesis.*—When the nerve is divided across its whole thickness.
b. *Partial neurotmesis.*—When the nerve is partly cut through, some portion remaining undivided.

Unless nerve suture is performed, recovery is impossible after neurotmesis.

NERVE SUTURE

Whether to Suture?

1. Neurotmesis, partial or complete, must be sutured.
2. Axonotmesis, if not associated with neurotmesis, does not require suturing unless regeneration is prevented by extensive perineural scarring.
3. Neurapraxia, unaccompanied by any other type of lesion, needs no suturing. The clearest indications for suturing are:
   a. A nerve already seen divided during wound excision.
   b. A tender swelling on the course of the nerve (i.e. palpable neuroma) at the site of the injury, associated with motor and sensory loss in the distribution of the nerve.

When To Suture?

There are two types of suturing:

1. Primary (or immediate) suture.
2. Secondary suture. *Primary suturing* is indicated:
   a. When the wound is clean-cut and there is relative freedom from bruising and contamination so that with the administration of antibiotics, infection is unlikely and healing is likely to occur by first intention.
   b. When a digital nerve is injured.

Secondary suturing is obligatory in all cases where the wound is bruised or contaminated. This is because healing is unlikely in the presence of even slightest infection and because bruising causes extensive fibrosis along the length of the nerve. The *advantages of a secondary nerve suture* over a primary suture are as follows:

1. Primary suturing usually requires enlargement of the wound by further incisions in order to mobilise the nerve ends in performing suture without tension. As the wound is contaminated, such interference may lead to spread of contamination to tissues which were unaffected prior to the handling. This can only be prevented if exploration is undertaken after the infection has been controlled.
2. The sutures on the nerve should not be taken in the presence of even the slightest infection.

3. The epineurium (nerve sheath) is a very delicate structure, having a tendency to give way during suturing. In addition, it undergoes longitudinal slitting or tears, making repair further difficult. After about three weeks of the injury, epineural fibrosis occurs, making the sheath tough and thick, capable of retaining sutures.
4. The neuroma at the ends of the injured nerve is well-localised after about three weeks, so that the level upto which the fibres are living is well demonstrated.

The optimum time for secondary suture is, therefore, after three weeks of the injury or after infection has been overcame, whichever is later. If the wound is explored, it is best to keep the two cut ends approximated to each other either with black silk or with fine wire to prevent their retraction and for ease of later identification (when wires are used, X-rays are helpful).

Technique of Suturing

A. Methods of overcoming shortening.—Except when a primary suture is undertaken, there is usually a variable amount of retraction of the two cut ends. Moreover, trimming of the cut ends is obligatory in nerve suturing. These factors almost always lead to certain amount of shortening of the nerve and this has to be overcome. This is usually achieved by the following methods:
1. Mobilisation of the two cut ends by carefully dissecting them from surrounding structures.
2. Stripping of branches.—During the process of mobilisation, it may be found that a nerve is relatively anchored by its branches to surrounding structures. Branches which arise proximal to the lesion can be elongated by carefully incising the sheath. Mobilisation of the parent nerve is then possible.
3. Sacrifice of branches may be done to facilitate mobilisation, provided such branches are relatively unimportant.
4. Positioning the limb.—Usually it is found that flexion of joints, over which the nerve passes, facilitates approximation of the cut ends. The exceptions to this are—the sciatic nerve (where the hip has to be extended to obtain relaxation), and the ulnar nerve (where the elbow has to be extended).
5. Transposition of the nerve to a new bed may shorten its course, e.g. ulnar nerve brought to the front of the medial epicondyle, radial nerve brought to the front of the humerus.

B. Trimming of the ends.—This procedure is essential in allowing approximation of healthy nerve fibres and that is the only way to encourage regeneration. In a primary suture, only the ragged ends of the nerve are trimmed. In secondary suturing, all fibrous tissues present at the nerve ends have to be trimmed, till healthy nerve bundles are seen at either end. A very sharp knife or a razor blade held on a forceps is used. Only short segments are cut at a time (trial section) so as to conserve as much length as is possible.

C. Positioning the ends.—Prior to suturing, the trimmed fresh ends have to be so positioned that there is no twist along their course. Only by this means it is possible to allow the proximal nerve fibres join their corresponding distal fibres, thus avoiding 'shunting'.

D. Suturing.—An end-to-end anastomosis is carried out. The suture material picks up only the epineurium (nerve sheath) without traumatising, in any way, the underlying nerve fibres. Non-irritating material should be used for suturing, in order to avoid fibrosis; fine black silk or tantalum wire is used (catgut encourages fibrosis). Suturing must be without tension.

E. EMBEDDING.—The sutured area must be embedded in a muscle or fascial sheath to prevent the nerve from being entangled in fibrosis or from being traumatised. A layer of tantalum foil wrapped round the suture prevents epineural fibrosis.

F. CLOSURE OF THE WOUND.—Perfect haemostasis must be obtained prior to closure in order to prevent fibrosis and infection.

G. POST-OPERATIVELY:
1. The limb must be adequately splinted in order to prevent:
    a. any strain on the sutured nerve.
    b. over-stretching of the paralysed muscles.
2. The tone of the muscles is maintained by physiotherapy and galvanic stimulation.

Where Approximation of the Cut Ends is Impossible.—Various procedures have been advocated as follows:
1. *Bulb Suture.*—When it appears that the shortening of the nerve is such that it will not allow approximation of the ends after trimming, the untrimmed nerve ends may be sutured to each other with overlapping of the scarred parts (bulbs), and the joints are kept flexed. When union occurs, the joints are extended gradually. This causes elongation of the nerve so that, at a subsequent date, trimming and anastomosis can be undertaken.
2. *Bone Shortening.*—This is justifiable if nerve injury is associated with an ununited fracture which also needs operative treatment, e.g. facilitating repair of the radial nerve in cases of ununited fracture of the humerus.

Irremediable Injury.—If suturing is impracticable because of loss of tissue or gross separation of the cut ends, one or a combination of the following procedures may be adopted:
1. *Nerve Anastomosis,* e.g. part of the hypoglossal nerve or the phrenic nerve is sutured to the distal cut end of the facial nerve.
2. *Nerve Grafting.*—Only autogenous grafting (i.e. the patient's own nerve) is successful. The graft may be as follows:
    a. Cutaneous Nerves.—Medial cutaneous nerve of the forearm at the arm, sural nerve in the lower leg, saphenous nerve in the thigh, or superficial branch of the radial nerve in the forearm may be conveniently used as a graft. Single strands may be used for the repair of small nerves (e.g. digital) while three to four strands combined in the form of a *cable graft,* may be used for larger nerves.
    b. Main Nerves.—A segment of a main nerve may be used as a graft in a case where two main nerves have been extensively damaged. A segment from the relatively less important nerve (e.g. ulnar) is used to bridge the gap in the relatively more important nerve (e.g. median). If the blood supply of the grafting nerve (i.e. ulnar) is conserved, it is known as *pedicle nerve graft* (comparable to pedicle skin graft).
3. *Tendon Transplantation,* carefully fashioned, is often helpful.
4. *Arthrodesis* of the flail joints to give them rigidity.
5. *Amputations* for persistent sores or ulcers.

Neurolysis.—This term implies art operation in which a nerve is freed from scar tissue, callus, or other abnormal structures. This may be necessary because simple entanglement of a nerve in fibrous tissue or callus may result in its palsy.

AURICULOTEMPORAL NERVE

Exploration of this nerve, just above the parotid, is sometimes required to perform its avulsion in the treatment of parotid fistula.

Anatomy.—The nerve arises from the mandibular nerve by two roots that encircle the middle meningeal artery. It runs first backwards and then laterally, behind the temporomandibular joint. Thereafter it courses upwards, lying just *behind* the superficial temporal vessels. In its lower part it is in the substance of the parotid.

Avulsion.—A vertical incision 1″ long is made just in front of the tragus, with its centre on the zygoma. Just as the skin and the subcutaneous tissues are incised, the nerve lying behind the superficial temporal vessels is seen.

The secretomotor nerve of the parotid is derived from the glossopharyngeal nerve and passes through the otic ganglion to the auriculotemporal nerve, with which it is carried to the parotid gland. As the auriculotemporal nerve passes through the parotid, the secretomotor nerve leaves it to supply the gland.

The site where the auriculotemporal nerve is exposed, as described above, only contains its sensory fibres because the secretomotor fibres have already left it in the substance of the parotid. Simple division of the auriculotemporal nerve here will, therefore, have no effect on the parotid. In order to destroy the secretomotor fibres, the nerve has to be avulsed, i.e. pulled and torn.

Frey's Syndrome.—*see* Chapter 27.

PHRENIC NERVE

Exploration of this nerve at the neck is sometimes required to perform its avulsion, in the treatment of pulmonary tuberculosis.

Anatomy.—The nerve arises from the anterior rami of C3, 4 and 5 respectively. As it comes down, it crosses in front of the scalenus anterior from its lateral to its medial side, bound down to it by the fascia covering the muscle (prevertebral layer of deep cervical fascia). The left phrenic nerve is more obliquely situated than the right, so that it crosses the scalenus anterior at a higher level and then passes over the first part of the subclavian artery. The contribution of C5 may join the main trunk of the phrenic at a lower level (in the thorax), usually reaching it as a communicating branch from the nerve to subclavius. This communication is known as the *accessory phrenic nerve.*

The nerve is crossed in front by the omohyoid and two arteries, viz. the transverse cervical and suprascapular. It is overlapped by the internal jugular vein. Superficial to these structures it is covered by the clavicular head of the sternomastoid.

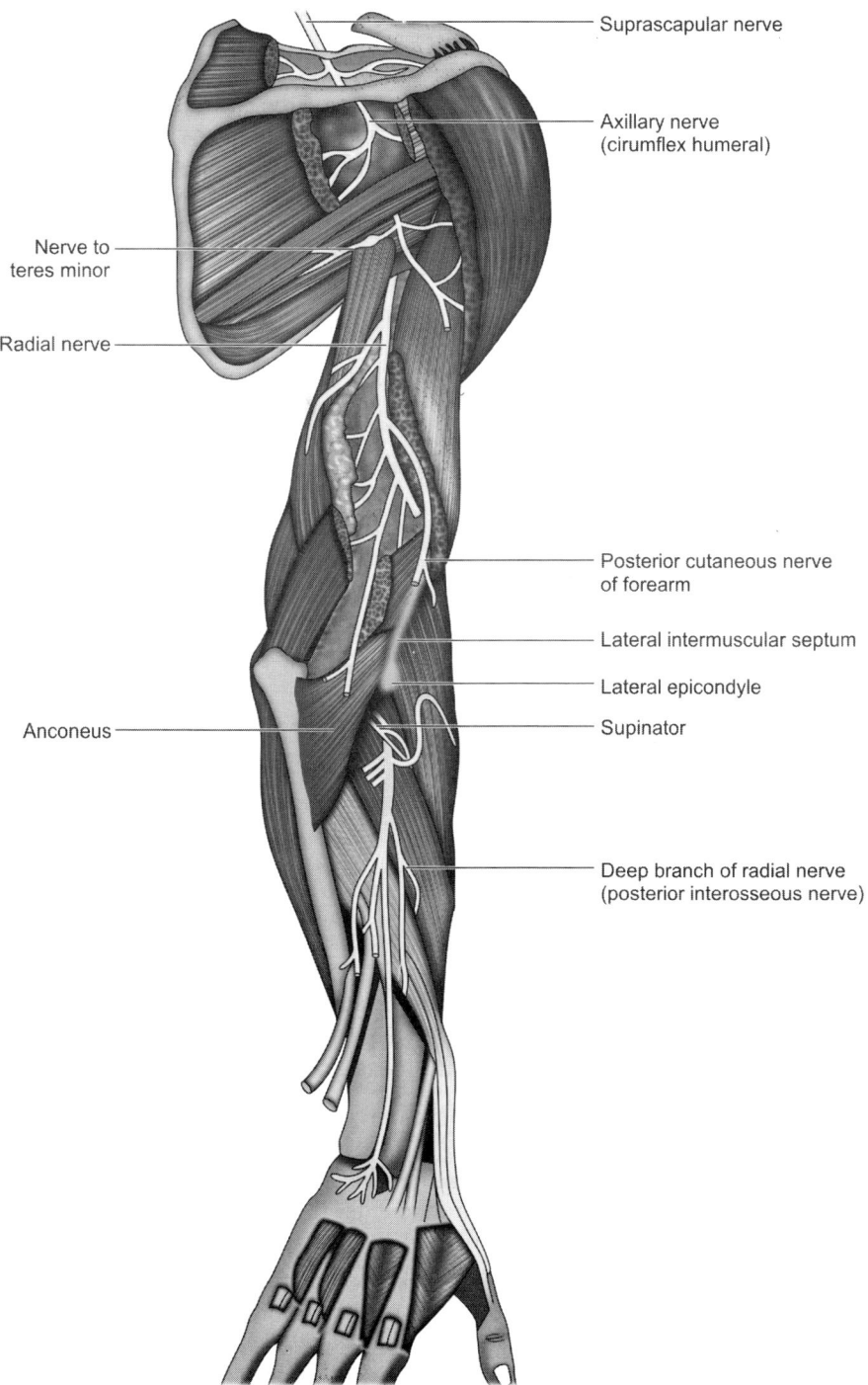

Suprascapular nerve

Axillary nerve
(cirumflex humeral)

Nerve to
teres minor

Radial nerve

Posterior cutaneous nerve
of forearm

Lateral intermuscular septum

Lateral epicondyle

Anconeus

Supinator

Deep branch of radial nerve
(posterior interosseous nerve)

Fig. 15.1: Radial nerve

Avulsion.—The neck is extended by placing a sandbag between the scapulae, and the head is turned to the opposite side. The operation may be done with local anaesthesia, but a general anaesthesia is usually preferred.

A transverse incision 2" long is made just above the clavicle, with its centre at the lateral border of the sternomastoid: Skin, superficial fascia, platysma, and deep fascia are cut in the line of incision, taking care of the external jugular vein. The lateral border of the sternomastoid and the internal jugular vein are retracted medially, while the omohyoid is retracted upwards. The scalenus anterior can now be felt getting inserted into the first rib. It is however still invisible being covered by fat, fascia and lymph nodes. These are cleared and the phrenic nerve is seen crossing the muscle under cover of the prevertebral layer of deep fascia covering the muscle (on the left side identification of the nerve may be a little difficult as it has often crossed the muscle higher up and lies on its medial side, in front of the subclavian artery).

The nerve is raised on a hook and a local anaesthetic agent is injected into it. It is clamped with a forceps below this level and divided at the site of infiltration. The nerve is now winded on the forceps and by steady traction, a considerable length (about 10 cm) can be avulsed.

Avulsion is preferred to simple division because only by this means the C5 component, if it joins the main trunk at a lower level (accessory phrenic nerve, described above), can be torn out at the same time.

Risk.—One risk of this operation is the rare chance of tearing the subclavian vein. This may occur only when there is an accessory phrenic nerve that crosses in front of the subclavian vein while the main trunk of the nerve passes behind the vein. The vein is then encircled by the nerves and may be torn during the process of avulsion.

RADIAL NERVE

The radial (musculospiral) nerve is commonly injured—classically at the axilla and sometimes within the radial groove of the humerus.

Anatomy.—Figure 15.1. The radial nerve is the direct continuation of the posterior cord of the brachial plexus (C5, 6, 7, and T1). It descends behind the axillary artery. It crosses the back of the arm, from the medial to the lateral side, within the spiral (radial) groove of the humerus, along with the profunda brachii artery. In its upper part it lies between the long and medial heads of the triceps. While in the radial groove it is under cover of the lateral head of the triceps between it and the medial head.

On reaching the lateral side of the humerus in the lower third of the arm, it pierces the lateral intermuscular septum to enter the anterior compartment of the arm. Now it lies on the lateral side of the brachialis, between this muscle and the brachioradialis above and the extensor carpi radialis longus below. As it descends to the front of the lateral epicondyle of the humerus, it gives off the important *posterior interosseous branch*.

The main trunk of the nerve, now purely sensory (also known as the *superficial branch* of the radial nerve), crosses the capsule of the elbow joint and enters the forearm under cover of the brachioradialis. This muscle covers the nerve in the upper two-thirds of the forearm. In the middle third of the forearm the nerve lies close to the lateral side of the radial artery. In the lower third of the forearm the nerve leaves the artery and emerges on the posterior border of the brachioradialis. Thereafter it descends over the abductor pollicis longus, extensor pollicis brevis and extensor pollicis longus, to come to the dorsum of the hand. Here it supplies the skin on the dorsal aspect of the thumb, index, middle and lateral half of ring fingers (i.e. three fingers and a half). The tips of these fingers at the dorsum are however supplied by the ulnar nerve.

The main trunk of the radial nerve supplies the following muscles:

Triceps (all three heads) and anconeus.

Brachioradialis, extensor carpi radialis longus and a part of the brachialis.

The posterior interosseous branch of the nerve (which is purely motor) passes to the back of the forearm by winding round the lateral side of the upper third of the radius, where it lies in the substance of the supinator muscle. Thereafter, it runs down between the superficial and deep muscles on the back of the forearm, to end at the wrist joint. This branch supplies the supinator and all the extensor muscles at the back of the forearm, together with the abductor pollicis longus.

Surface Marking.—A line drawn from just below the posterior axillary fold to the lateral side of the humerus at the junction of its middle and lower thirds.

From this point a vertical line to the front of the lateral epicondyle.

Thereafter a line to the lateral border of the radius at the junction of its middle and lower thirds.

From this point, on the back of the forearm, across the radius, to the wrist.

Sites and Causes of Injury

A. *At the axilla:*
1. Pressure of a crutch (*crutch palsy*).
2. Fractures and dislocations at the upper end of the humerus.

B. *In the radial groove:*
1. Fracture of the humeral shaft (injury of the nerve or its entanglement in the callus).
2. Pressure by a tourniquet or plaster.
3. Pressure on the edge of an operating table or compression during heavy sleep (*'Saturday night' paralysis*).
4. Overstretching during operations on the humerus.

C. *At the elbow* (posterior interosseous nerve):
1. Fracture of the neck or head of the radius, or dislocation of the radius.
2. Accidental injury during excision of the head of the radius.

Clinical Features

I. INJURY AT THE AXILLA

A. *Motor Paralysis and Wasting:*
1. Extensors of the elbow (i.e. triceps).—Extension, however is carried out by the weight of the forearm.

2. Extensors of the wrist (i.e. extensor carpi radialis and ulnaris), resulting in the characteristic *wrist drop,* which is diagnostic of radial nerve lesions.
3. Extensors of the metacarpophalangeal joints of the fingers (i.e. extensor digitorum communis). The patient however is able to extend the interphalangeal joints with the help of the unaffected interossei (which are supplied by the ulnar nerve).
4. Extensors of all the joints of the thumb (extensor pollicis longus and brevis).
5. Supinator and brachioradialis are paralysed but supination is ably performed by the biceps.

B. *Sensory Loss:* A sensory loss would be expected over the lateral side of the dorsum of the hand and the dorsum of the lateral three fingers and a half (including the thumb). In practice, however, it is found that sensory loss is much less (usually only over the base of the thumb and the first interosseous space), there being an overlapping by other two nerves, viz. the posterior cutaneous and the lateral cutaneous nerves of the forearm. These two nerves together with the superficial branch of the radial nerve supplies a wide area on the dorsolateral aspect of the forearm and the hand. If any two of these escape injury, the sensory loss is minimum.

C. *Trophic Changes:* Minimum.

II. INJURY IN THE RADIAL GROOVE
1. *Motor Paralysis:* Same as above except that the patient can extend the elbow since the triceps and anconeus escape paralysis. This is because the branches supplying all the three heads of the triceps (and the anconeus) originate at a level higher than the radial groove.
2. *Sensory Loss:* Very little, usually only over the ball of the thumb.
3. *Trophic Changes:* Minimum.

III. INJURY AT THE ELBOW (i.e. posterior interosseous nerve injury):

Same as in II excepting that there is no sensory loss, this nerve being purely motor.

Exposure

1. *In the infra-axillary part.*—With the upper limb abducted and externally rotated, a longitudinal incision is made along the medial border of the biceps. The skin, subcutaneous tissue, and deep fascia are divided in the same line, care being taken to preserve the basilic vein which pierces the deep fascia here. The biceps is carefully mobilised and retracted laterally. The nerve lies behind the brachial artery. Very close to these structures lies the median nerve. A little medially lies the ulnar nerve.

2. *In the radial groove.*—An oblique incision is made in the line of the radial groove, i.e. downwards and laterally across the arm, a finger's breadth behind the posterior border of the deltoid. In the upper part of the incision, the interval between the lateral head and the long head of the triceps is opened up, while at a lower level, the lateral head of the muscle is divided carefully in the line of incision. The fascia roofing the radial groove is seen, and this is incised to expose the nerve. Here the nerve lies in company with the profunda artery, partly on the naked bone and partly on the medial head of the triceps.

3. *In the lower third of the arm.*—The incision in (2) above is prolonged downwards. The interval between the brachialis and brachioradialis muscles is opened up, and the nerve is seen.
4. *At the upper end of radius* (posterior interosseous nerve).—An oblique incision, starting from the head of the radius and running infero-medially to the posterior surface of the bone, is made. The gap between the extensor carpi radialis and the extensor digitorum profundus is opened up and the supinator muscle is seen. The nerve lies in the substance of this muscle. The superficial fibres of the muscle are carefully divided to display the nerve.

MEDIAN NERVE

The median nerve is classically injured at the wrist, and (less commonly) at the elbow.

Anatomy.—Figures 15.2 and 15.3. The median nerve (C5, 6, 7, 8 and T1) arises by two roots, one each from the median and the lateral cords of the brachial plexus.

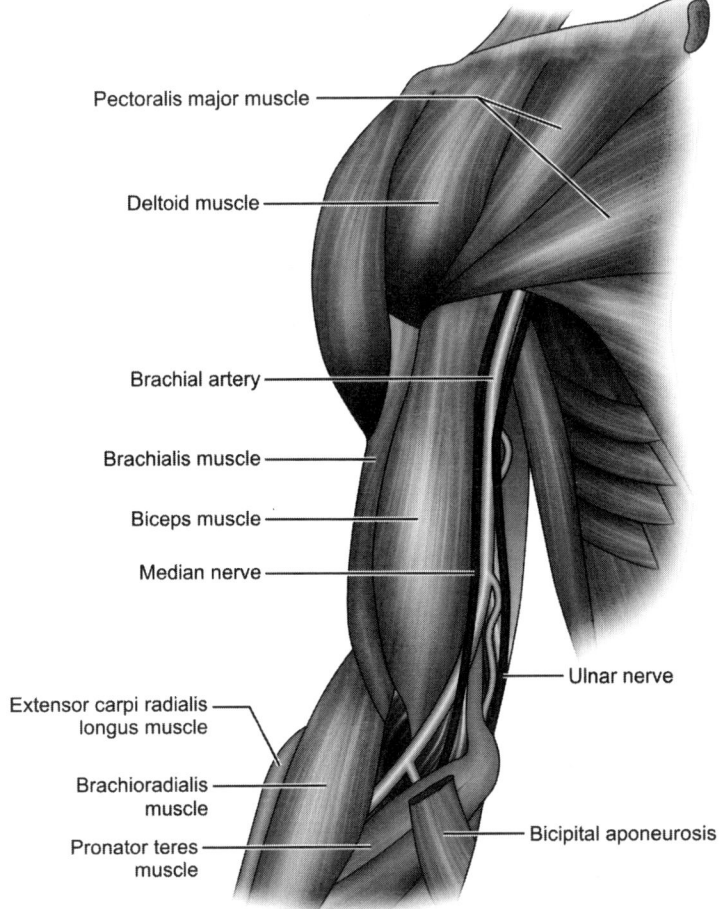

Pectoralis major muscle

Deltoid muscle

Brachial artery

Brachialis muscle

Biceps muscle

Median nerve

Ulnar nerve

Extensor carpi radialis longus muscle

Brachioradialis muscle

Pronator teres muscle

Bicipital aponeurosis

Fig. 15.2: Nerves and arteries on the anterior aspect of the arm

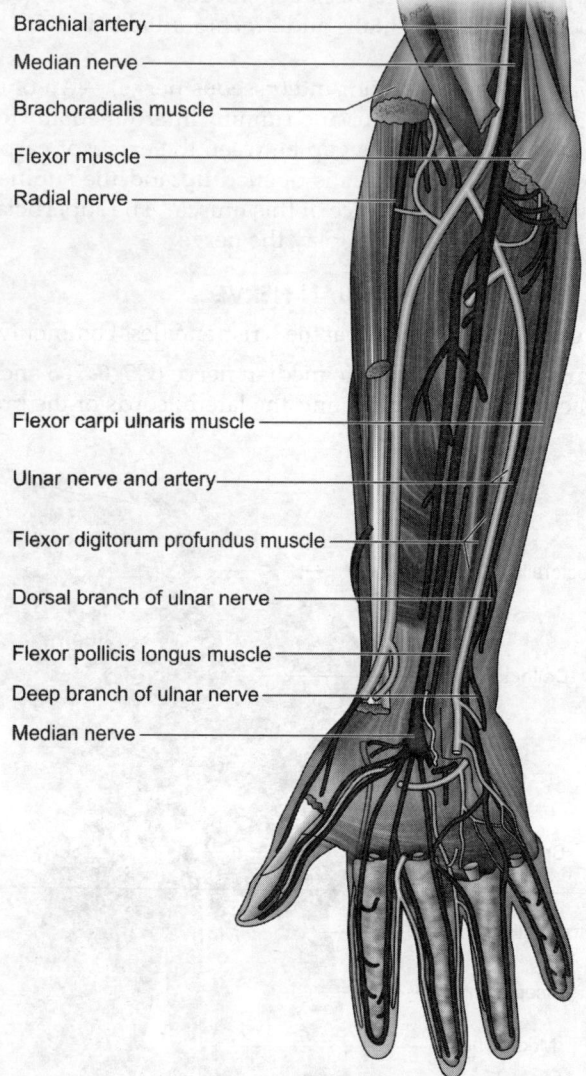

Brachial artery

Median nerve

Brachoradialis muscle

Flexor muscle

Radial nerve

Flexor carpi ulnaris muscle

Ulnar nerve and artery

Flexor digitorum profundus muscle

Dorsal branch of ulnar nerve

Flexor pollicis longus muscle

Deep branch of ulnar nerve

Median nerve

Fig. 15.3: Nerves and arteries on the front of the forearm and hand.

In the arm it is closely related to the brachial artery—lying lateral to the artery in the upper third, in front of it in the middle third, and medial to it in the lower third (i.e. at the cubital fossa).

It enters the forearm between the two heads of pronator teres, the deep head of which separates the nerve from the ulnar artery. Thereafter, it descends between the flexor digitorum sublimis and the flexor digitorum profundus. In the lower third of the forearm the nerve becomes superficial by emerging on the lateral side of the flexor sublimis. Just above the wrist it lies between the palmaris longus (on the medial side) and the flexor carpi radialis (on the lateral side). The palmaris longus often lies in front of the nerve.

It enters the palm, passing deep to the flexor retinaculum, where it lies in the carpal tunnel in association with the flexor tendons. At the lower border of the flexor retinaculum it ends by dividing into two branches—lateral and medial.

Supply

1. In the forearm.—The nerve supplies all the superficial muscles in front of the forearm, excepting flexor carpi ulnaris (supplied by the ulnar nerve). Thus it supplies—pronator teres, flexor carpi radialis, flexor digitorum sublimis and palmaris longus.
2. Its volar interosseous branch supplies some deep muscles in the forearm, viz. flexor pollicis longus, lateral half of the flexor digitorum profundus (medial half is supplied by the ulnar nerve), and pronator quadratus.
3. The lateral terminal branch gives a twig to supply the thenar muscles (i.e. abductor pollicis brevis, opponens pollicis, and superficial head of flexor pollicis brevis). Thereafter it gives off three digital branches. Two of these supply the two sides of the thumb while the third gives a twig to the first lumbrical and supplies the lateral side of the index finger.
4. The medial terminal branch divides into two branches. One runs to the second cleft to supply the adjacent sides of the index and middle fingers, and also supplies the second lumbrical. The other runs to the third cleft to supply the adjacent sides of the middle and ring fingers.

Surface Marking.—In the arm the line of the nerve is from a point at the junction of the anterior and middle thirds of the line joining the anterior and posterior axillary fold at the base of the axilla, to a point midway between the medial epicondyle and the biceps tendon at the elbow.

In the forearm the course is from the point at the elbow mentioned above to the midpoint in front of the wrist. The palmaris longus is an important landmark at the wrist, the nerve lying either deep or just lateral to it.

Sites and Causes of Injury

A. *At the elbow:*
   1. Supracondylar fracture (by the projecting lower end of the shaft).
   2. Dislocation of the elbow.

B. *In front of the wrist:*
   1. Cuts (particularly glass-cut injuries).
   2. Colles' fracture or dislocation of the lunate (rare).
   3. Compression:
      a. Carpal tunnel syndrome.
      b. Compound palmar ganglion.

Clinical Features

I. INJURY AT THE LEVEL OF THE ELBOW
   A. *Motor Paralysis and Wasting:*
      1. The patient is unable to clench the fist when he is asked to do so. This is because the thumb and the lateral two fingers have no power of

flexion (flexion of the medial two fingers, however, is preserved because of the function of the flexor profundus and the lumbricals

2. When the patient is asked to flex the wrist against resistance, the hand deviates to the ulnar side (because of the unaffected flexor carpi ulnaris).

3. Paralysis of the thenar muscles:

   a. Abductor pollicis brevis.—The patient is unable to move the thumb at a plane perpendicular to the palm. To test for this paralysis, *the pen test* is useful. The patient is asked to lay his hand supine and flat on the table, and asked to touch with the thumb, a pen placed in front of the hand. He is unable to do so.

   b. Opponens pollicis.—There is inability to touch the ends of the fingers with the tip of the thumb.

   c. Wasting of the thenar muscles leads to flattening of the thenar eminence so that the metacarpal bone of the thumb is apparently in the same plane as the other metacarpals—the *'ape-like'* or *'Simian' hand.*

4. The patient is unable to bend the terminal phalanx of the thumb while the proximal phalanx is steadied firmly by the surgeon to eliminate the short flexors. This is because of paralysis of the flexor pollicis longus.

5. *Clasping test.*—When the patient is asked to clasp the hands, the index finger on the affected side fails to flex, i.e. there is a *'pointing index'.* This is because of paralysis of the flexor sublimis and lateral half of flexor profundus. It should be noted that in injuries of the median nerve, the only digits which lose *all* flexion are the thumb and the index finger.

6. Pronation is feeble and completed only by the weight of the forearm (because of paralysis of both the pronators—teres and quadratus).

7. Wasting of the major bulk of forearm muscles in the front.

B. *Sensory Loss:* There is a variable amount of sensory loss on the palmar aspect of the lateral three and half fingers (including the thumb) together with the corresponding part of the palm.

The tip of these fingers (including the thumb), on their dorsal aspect, is also supplied by the median nerve and may not lose sensation.

The area of sensory loss gradually reduces due to overlapping from adjacent nerves.

C. *Trophic Changes:* These are obvious in the hand and the affected fingers. The tip of the index finger suffers most commonly.

II. INJURY AT THE LEVEL OF THE WRIST

A. *Motor Paralysis:* The long flexors escape paralysis so that the diagnosis is less easy. However, there is paralysis and wasting of the thenar muscles, leading to:

1. A positive 'pen test'.

2. Inability to oppose the thumb.

3. 'Ape-like' or 'Simian' hand.

B. *Sensory Loss:* As in injuries at the elbow.

C. *Trophic Changes:* Same as in injuries at the elbow.

Exposure

1. *At the elbow (cubital fossa).*—A 2" long incision is made along the medial border of the biceps tendon at the cubital fossa. The basilic vein is retracted medially. The

bicipital aponeurosis is now seen. The deep fascia and the bicipital aponeurosis are incised vertically. The biceps tendon is then retracted laterally to display the contents of the cubital fossa. Here the brachial artery lies in the centre, with the median nerve on its medial side and the biceps tendon on its lateral side.

2. *At the wrist.*—A longitudinal incision 1″ in length is made along the lateral border of the tendon of palmaris longus. The nerve is very superficial, lying either just on the lateral side or under cover of the palmaris longus. Owing to its flattened shape it may be mistaken for a tendon.

ULNAR NERVE

Like the median nerve, the ulnar nerve is also classically injured at the elbow and at the wrist.

Anatomy.—*See* Figures 15.2 and 15.3. The ulnar nerve (C7, 8 and T1) is the main continuation of the medial cord of the brachial plexus. In the upper arm the nerve descends along the medial side of the brachial artery as far as the middle of the arm. Here it deviates medially and (together with the ulnar collateral artery) pierces the medial intermuscular septum to gain the back of the arm.

In the lower arm, therefore, the nerve lies in the posterior compartment in front of the medial border of the triceps. At the elbow it lies closely applied to the back of the medial epicondyle.

The nerve enters the forearm between the two heads (humeral and ulnar) of flexor carpi ulnaris. In the upper two-thirds of the forearm it descends under cover of this muscle, running between it and the flexor digitorum profundus. Thereafter it becomes superficial and lies between the flexor carpi ulnaris and the medial border of flexor digitorum sublimis. In the lower two-thirds of the forearm and at the wrist the ulnar artery is closely related to the lateral side of the nerve.

The nerve courses down to the palm, passing *superficial* to the flexor retinaculum at the wrist. Opposite the hook of the hamate, it divides into two terminal branches—superficial and deep.

Supply

1. In the forearm.—The nerve supplies the flexor carpi ulnaris and the medial half of the flexor digitorum profundus (lateral half is supplied by the median nerve).
2. The superficial terminal branch is mainly sensory, supplying the skin on the medial side of the palm, both sides of the little finger, and the medial side of the ring finger (i.e. medial one and a half fingers) on their palmar surfaces. This branch also supplies the palmaris brevis muscle (supplying the muscle from its depth).
3. The deep branch is motor. It passes through the muscles of the hypothenar eminence along with the ulnar artery. It supplies the three hypothenar muscles (viz. abductor digiti minimi, flexor digiti minimi brevis, and opponens digiti minimi), all the interossei (dorsal and palmar), third and fourth lumbricals, two heads of adductor pollicis, and the deep head of flexor pollicis brevis.
4. The dorsal cutaneous branch, which arises from the nerve about 2 inches above the wrist, supplies the dorsum of the medial one and a half fingers and the corresponding part of the dorsum of the hand.

Surface Marking.—In the upper arm the line of the nerve is from the point of junction of the anterior and middle thirds of the line joining the anterior and posterior axillary folds at the base of the axilla to a point on the medial surface of the middle of the arm.

From this point the nerve descends to the back of the medial epicondyle.

A line from the medial epicondyle to the lateral side of the pisiform bone represents the course of the nerve in the forearm.

Sites and Causes of Injury

A. *At the elbow:*
1. Fracture of the medial epicondyle:
   a. Injury to the nerve by the displaced fragment.
   b. Friction of the nerve in the roughened bony groove (friction neuritis).
2. Cubitus valgus deformity resulting from old fracture of the lateral condyle of the humerus. The nerve is stretched because the carrying angle is increased. Continuous friction occurs in the groove behind the medial epicondyle which acts as a pulley for the nerve now (friction neuritis).
3. Accidental injury during excision of the elbow joint.
4. *'Entrapment neuropathy'.*—Fixation of the nerve in the groove behind the medial epicondyle by adhesions complicating osteoarthritis.
5. *'Ulnar tunnel syndrome'.*—Compression of the nerve in between the heads of the flexor carpi ulnaris.

Causes 1 (a) and 2 above lead to *'tardy ulnar palsy'*, i.e. a late palsy. The paralysis occurs at a later date than the injury.

B. *At the wrist:* Glass cut injury.

Clinical Features

I. Injury at the elbow

A. *Motor Paralysis, Wasting, and Deformity:*
1. There is an *'ulnar claw hand'. Typical claw-hand* or *main-engriffe* is a condition in which the metacarpophalangeal joints are hyper-extended and the interphalangeal joints are flexed. This results from paralysis of the lumbricals (which are the sole flexors of the first phalanx) and the interossei (which are the sole extensors of the middle and distal phalanges). Extension of the proximal phalanx only is done by the extensor digitorum (this action is opposed by the lumbricals). A typical claw-hand results when both the median and the ulnar nerves are paralysed. The lumbricals being paralysed, there is an overaction of the extensor digitorum communis which results in hyperextension of the metacarpophalangeal joints. At the same time, the interossei having been paralysed, the interphalangeal joints are kept flexed.

   In ulnar claw-hand, the deformity is not so typical because the first two lumbricals, which are supplied by the median nerve, escape paralysis and so the deformity is minimum in the index and middle fingers.
2. There is wasting of the small muscles of the hand, including the hypothenar muscles but excluding the thenar muscles.
3. Flattening of the inner border of the forearm due to wasting of the flexor carpi ulnaris.
4. The tendon of the flexor carpi ulnaris, which is normally palpable just above its insertion in the pisiform bone when the wrist is flexed is no more palpable.

5. Paralysis of the interossei:
   a. The patient cannot fan out (abduct) and close the fingers (adduct) to each other. The palmar interossei are the adductors and the dorsal interossei are the abductors of the fingers.
   b. The patient cannot extend the distal and middle phalanges while the proximal phalanx is steadied by the surgeon.
   c. The patient is asked to grip a card in the cleft between two fingers (requiring adduction of the fingers). He is either unable to grip it or offers only poor resistance to its withdrawal. This is the *card test.*

6. Paralysis of the adductor pollicis.—The patient is unable to grip a card between the thumb and the palm (which requires adduction of the thumb).

7. Paralysis of the adductor pollicis and first palmar interosseus.—The patient is asked to grasp a book firmly between the thumb and other fingers of both hands together. Normally he can do so with both the thumbs straight. In ulnar palsy, it will be found that there is an automatic flexion of the terminal phalanx of the thumb of the affected side. The two said muscles being paralysed, the flexor pollicis longus in its attempt to grip the book causes flexion of the terminal phalanx.

B. *Sensory Loss:* There is a variable amount of sensory loss over both palmar and dorsal surfaces of the medial one and a half fingers and the corresponding part of the hand.

   This area of sensory loss gradually reduces due to overlapping from adjacent nerves.

C. *Trophic Changes:* These are usually well marked.

II. Injury at the wrist
   A. *Motor Paralysis*: Paralysis and wasting of the small muscles of the hand as described above (all the points except 3 and 4).
   B. *Sensory Loss*: Since the dorsal cutaneous branch of the ulnar nerve leaves the main trunk about 2 inches above the wrist, loss of sensation is confined only to the palmar aspect of the medial one and a half fingers, and the corresponding part of the palm.
   C. *Trophic Changes*: This occurs corresponding to the area of sensory loss.

Exposure

I. *In the infra-axillary part* (*upper arm*).—The exposure is the same as for the radial nerve here.

II. *At the bend of the elbow.*—The arm is carried across the chest and held in such a position that the point of the elbow looks upwards. A curved incision, is then made along the line of the nerve (which can be felt here), with its centre at the back of the medial epicondyle. The nerve is covered by a fascia which is carefully incised to expose it. The nerve is accompanied by the superior collateral artery.

III. *At the wrist.*—An incision about 2" long is made along the lateral border of the tendon of the flexor carpi ulnaris. The nerve, being superficial here, is seen immediately on incising the skin and fasciae. The ulnar artery lies on its lateral side.

Anterior Transplantation of the Ulnar Nerve.—This means placing the ulnar nerve in front of the medial epicondyle.

Indications:
1. To prevent friction neuritis, e.g. tardy ulnar palsy following fractured medial epicondyle or cubitus valgus deformity.
2. To overcome shortening at nerve suturing which involves trimming and resection.
3. After any operative treatment on the nerve, including nerve suture, it is advisable to transplant the nerve anteriorly where it will be less subject to stretching and friction.

Operation.—The arm is put across the chest with the elbow pointing upwards.

An incision about 5" long is made with its centre behind the medial epicondyle. The incision is concave anteriorly. Such a long incision is required because the nerve has to be mobilised considerably so that it can be slipped forwards to the front of the epicondyle.

On incising the covering fascia, the nerve is easily seen. It has now to be mobilised. In the upper part, mobilisation is simple. In the lower part, as the nerve is elevated from its bed, five branches may be encountered—an articular twig to the elbow joint (this may be sacrificed), two branches to the flexor carpi ulnaris and two branches to the flexor digitorum profundus (these four have to be preserved).

The nerve is then brought to the front of the medial epicondyle. As for the new bed for the nerve, there are two procedures:
  a. Some surgeons prefer to bury the nerve in the muscle bulk in front of the medial epicondyle. An incision 1/2 inch deep is made in the common flexor origin in front of the epicondyle, the nerve is inserted in the gap, and the muscles overseen.
  b. Others prefer to leave it in the superficial fascia (believing that the above procedure may lead to fibrosis).

The Brachial Plexus

Roots	Trunks	Divisions	Cords	Main Branches
C5 C6 }	Upper	{ Anterior / Posterior	Lateral ----→	Median
C7	Middle	{ Anterior / Posterior	Posterior ──→	Radial
C8 T1 }	Lower	{ Anterior / Posterior	Medial (Inner)	Ulnar

Upper Brachial Plexus Lesion (Erb-Duchenne Paralysis)

Involvement.—The injury occurs usually where the C5 and C6 roots join to form the upper trunk. This is known as the *'Erb's point'*. Usually the contribution from C5 is affected, only occasionally that from the C6 as well.

Causes.—The injury occurs as a result of excessive displacement of the head to the opposite side, or excessive depression of the shoulder, or a combination of the two, e.g.
1. Birth Injury.—Traction on the head while the shoulder of the foetus is still obstructed. This cause is so common that paralysis of this type is known as *'obstetrical palsy'*.

2. A fall on the shoulder, causing hyperabduction of the arm.
3. Fall of a weight on the shoulder with the head moving away, resulting in an increase in the neck-shoulder angle.

Paralysis and Deformity:
1. The arm hangs by the side of the body (adducted) with the shoulder internally rotated. This is because of paralysis of the abductors and external rotators of the shoulder (deltoid, supraspinatus, and infraspinatus).
2. The elbow is extended, and the forearm fully pronated. This is due to paralysis of the flexors and supinators of the elbow (biceps, brachialis and brachioradialis).
3. The hand is normal.

The above deformities, together, produce the position of *'policeman receiving a tip'* and is due to paralysis of the C5.

Lower Brachial Plexus Lesion (Klumpke's Paralysis)

Involvement.—This paralysis is due to either of the following causes:
a. Injury of the lower trunk (C8 and T1) of the brachial plexus.
b. Injury of the inner cord of the brachial plexus.
c. Avulsion of the nerve roots (C8 and T1) from the spinal cord.
The contribution from T1 usually suffers, that from C8 only rarely.

Causes:
1. Above the clavicle—by inclusion in a ligature with the subclavian artery.
2. At the axilla—by an unreduced dislocated head of humerus.
3. Sudden hyperabduction of the shoulder (nerve roots are torn from the spinal cord).

Paralysis and Deformity:
1. There is typically a claw-hand.
2. There is wasting of the small muscles of the hand.
3. The features are those of combined median and ulnar nerve palsy.
4. There is sensory loss over the medial three and a half fingers in front and medial one and half fingers behind.
5. Rarely there may be an associated Horner's syndrome if the cervical sympathetic is involved.

Horner's Syndrome

1. Narrowing of the palpebral fissure due to partial ptosis of the upper eyelid, resulting from incomplete paralysis of the levator palpebrae superioris.
2. Enophthalmos (recession of the eyeball backwards), due to paralysis of Muller's muscle.
3. Myosis, i.e. contraction of the pupil, due to unopposed action of the oculomotor nerve.
4. Anhidrosis, i.e. absence of sweating in the face, on the affected side.

Claw-hand.—Claw-hand or *main-en-griffe* is a condition in which the metacarpophalangeal joints are hyperextended and the interphalangeal joints are flexed. This may occur under the following conditions:
1. True and typical claw-hand is caused by paralysis of the lumbricals (which are the chief flexors of the first phalanx) and the interossei (which are the sole extensors of the middle and distal phalanges). Extension of the proximal phalanx

only is carried out by the extensor digitorum (this action is opposed by the lumbricals) The interossei and lumbricals are supplied by the T1 segment of the spinal cord by way of the ulnar and median nerves. Paralysis of these muscles, resulting in a claw-hand may occur in:

a. Combined lesions (e.g. injury, leprosy) of the ulnar and median nerves (simple ulnar nerve lesion causes an ulnar claw-hand—*see* under ulnar nerve).

b. Klumpke's paralysis.

c. Friction of the lowest trunk of the brachial plexus against a cervical rib.

d. Progressive muscular atrophy, including amyotrophic lateral sclerosis, syringomyelia, etc.

The lumbricals being paralysed, there is hypertension of the metatarsopha-langeal joints, caused by the uninterrupted action of the extensor digitorum. The interossei being paralysed, the interphalangeal joints are kept flexed.

2. Imitation of a claw-hand may occur in:

a. Volkmann's ischaemic contracture (with or without associated nerve damage).

b. Post-burn contracture.

c. Dupuytren's contracture.

d. Fibrosis secondary to suppurative tenosynovitis.

Muscle Action on the Fingers

PHALANX	FLEXED BY	EXTENDED BY
First	Lumbrical	Extensor digitorum
Second	Flexor sublimis	Interossei
Third	Flexor profundus	Interossei

The small muscles of the thumb are abductor, adductor, flexor brevis, and opponens.

The small muscles of the little finger are abductor (no adductor), flexor brevis, and opponens.

Summary of Nerve Supply of the Muscles in the Forearm and Hand

I. *Radial Nerve:*

1. Supinators (i.e. supinator and brachioradialis) on the back of the forearm.

2. Extensors on the back of the forearm.

II. *Median Nerve:*

1. Pronators of the forearm (teres and quadratus).

2. Flexors on the front of the forearm except the medial one and a half muscles, viz. flexor carpi ulnaris and medial half of flexor digitorum profundus.

3. Muscles of the thenar eminence and the first two lumbricals in the hand.

III. *Ulnar Nerve:*

1. Only the medial one and half flexor muscles on the front of the forearm.

2. All small muscles in the hand excepting the thenar muscles and the first two lumbricals.

LATERAL POPLITEAL NERVE

Causes of Injury.—This nerve is classically injured at the neck of the fibula. The causes may be:

1. Fracture of the neck of the fibula.

2. Accidental injury during excision of the upper end of the fibula.
3. Cut at the site.
4. Pressure from plaster.

Clinical Features

A. *Motor Paralysis and Deformity:*
   Complete paralysis of the extensor and peroneal groups of muscles, resulting in talipes equinovarus and *'foot drop'*.

B. *Sensory Loss:*
   1. Lateral side of the lower two thirds of the leg.
   2. Dorsum of the foot, excepting the area near the cleft between the great toe and the second toe (which is supplied by the anterior tibial nerve).
   3. Dorsum of all the toes excepting the lateral side of the little toe (which is supplied by sural communicating nerve).

TUMOURS OF THE PERIPHERAL NERVES

Terminology.—The broad term that designates peripheral nerve tumours is 'neuroma'. True neuromas which actually arise from the nervous tissue and consist of their proliferation are rare, and are found only in connection with the sympathetic system. False neuromas arise from the connective tissues making the nerve sheaths and thus they are really neurofibromas; they are much the commoner and are frequently encountered.

Classification and Types*

A. FALSE NEUROMAS (NEUROFIBROMAS):
1. Solitary neurofibroma
2. Neurofibromatosis
3. Traumatic neuromas
4. Glomal tumours
   (*All these tumours are described below).

B. TRUE NEUROMAS:
   1. *Ganglioneuroma.*—This tumour consists of ganglion cells and nerve fibres. It is a benign tumour. It is found in connection with the sympathetic trunks in the mediastinum and the abdomen. In the abdomen the tumours therefore lie in the retroperitoneal tissues in close relation to the suprarenal glands.
   2. *Neuroblastoma.*—These tumours arise from immature cells of the sympathetic nervous system. They are highly malignant, metastatising widely, particularly to bones. They are commonly found in relationship to the suprarenal glands. A variant form of this tumour originates in the developing retina and is known as *'retinoblastoma'*.

Solitary Neurofibroma.—It has now been established that this tumour arises from the sheath of Schwann, i.e. neurilemma sheath. Hence it is also known as *neurilemmoma or Schwann cell tumour*. There is no proliferation of the nervous tissue itself.

Sites:

1. Most commonly it occurs in relation to a cutaneous nerve. Almost any nerve may be affected but commonly those of the extremities.

2. It may arise from the cervicodorsal sympathetic within the thorax.
3. It may occur intraspinally, presenting the features of an intradural extramedullary tumour.
4. It may arise intracranially. Any cranial nerve may have it, but classically it arises in relation to the eighth nerve (*acoustic neurofibroma*).
5. It may be found within bones and very rarely intramuscularly.

Clinical Features of Peripheral Neurofibroma:
1. Majority are symptomless, the tumour presenting as a slow-growing swelling which may be moved from side to side but is otherwise fixed by the nerve from which it arises.
2. Some present as 'painful subcutaneous nodules'.
3. Occasionally there is paraesthesia or referred pain, caused by pressure of the tumour on the nerve fibres which are spread over the surface of the tumour.

Complications:
1. Cystic degeneration.
2. Malignant change to a neurofibrosarcoma. The incidence is rare but may occur after partial removal and local recurrence of a simple tumour. Acoustic neurofibroma is an exception. It virtually never turns malignant, even after partial removal (which is its standard treatment).

Treatment.—Excision of the tumour without damaging the affected nerve. As the tumour is encapsulated by the perineurium, it may be easily dissected from the nerve, without damaging it.

Neurofibromatosis.—This condition is a developmental disorder of the fibrous sheaths of the nerves and represents a form of hamartoma. It is a defect with the gene. The disorder often runs in families.

Some people believe that solitary neurofibroma is also a form of malformation as neurofibromatosis.

The condition may present itself in different manners as follows:
1. Generalised neurofibromatosis
2. Cutaneous-neurofibromatosis
3. Plexiform neurofibromatosis
4. Elephantiasis neuromatosa

GENERALISED NEUROFIBROMATOSIS (VON RECKLINGHAUSEN'S DISEASE)
1. There are multiple subcutaneous swellings on the limbs, face, and trunk, each representing a neurilemmoma (arising from the sheath of Schwann).
2. There is often a pigmentation of the skin.
3. There may be associated tumours in relation to the cervicodorsal sympathetic, intraspinal, intracranial (including acoustic), intraosseous, intramuscular, and visceral.
4. Only occasionally the swellings produce symptoms (*see* below).

Complications:
1. Cystic degeneration.
2. Malignant change to a neurofibrosarcoma.
   Both the complications are commoner than they are with solitary neurofibroma.

Treatment.—The swellings are so numerous that excision of all of them is impossible; nor it is usually required.

In case of neurofibromatosis, one of the swellings may require excision:
1. If it is very large, causing mechanical discomfort.
2. If it is painful.
3. If it is causing pressure symptoms.
4. If there is a suspicion of malignancy.

In other instances no surgery is advocated. Even biopsy may be followed by a malignant change.

CUTANEOUS NEUROFIBROMATOSIS.—This is also known as *molluscum fibrosum.*

There are multiple subcutaneous sessile or pedunculated swellings over the breast, back, and abdomen. They may be abundant on the scalp (turban-tumour).

It is a form of generalised neurofibromatosis but there are no internal tumours. There is usually associated pigmentation of the skin.

Treatment.—The large and unsightly swellings may be excised.

PLEXIFORM NEUROFIBROMATOSIS.—This rare condition is characteristically found in connection with the branches of the trigeminal nerve, though they may be found in the extremities and the scalp.

The pathology is a fibromyxomatous degeneration of the nerve sheaths, occurring in the terminal branches of the cutaneous nerves. In 50 percent of cases it is found in association with von Recklinghausen's disease.

There is a big swelling, in and around which the thickened nerves are felt like thrombosed veins. The overlying skin may be pigmented.

A variant form of this condition is *pachy dermatocele.* The swelling is huge and pendulous, and the overlying skin is thickened. It is typically found at the neck, where coils of soft tissues hang around the root of the neck.

ELEPHANTIASIS NEUROMATOSA.—This is virtually a severe form of plexiform neurofibromatosis, affecting the subcutaneous nerves of the lower limbs. The subcutaneous fat is replaced by fibrous tissue which is thickened and oedematous (non-pitting oedema). The overlying skin is coarse, resembling that of an elephant.

Other causes of elephantiasis are:
a. Filariasis.
b. Brawny arm, following radical mastectomy.
c. Nodular leprosy (*elephantiasis graecorum*).

Traumatic Neuromas

1. *Stump Neuroma.*—This occurs in the amputation stumps in relation to the divided nerves. It consists of proliferating axons, together with proliferating neurilemmal cells.

   While stump neuroma is a constant feature of an amputation stump, it is usually symptomless. Sometimes, however, the neuroma is painful (*painful neuroma*), often because of irritation by a misfit artificial limb.
2. After division of nerves:
   a. Proximal neuroma, occurs in relation to the proximal cut end of the nerve.
   b. Distal glioma, occurs in relation to the distal cut end of the nerve.

Glomus Tumour.—This rare tumour arises in relation to cutaneous glomus, which is a specialised arteriovenous anastomosis, regulating the temperature and maintaining the circulation in the parts exposed to cold.

The tumour is small but produces pain, out of proportion to its size. It is compressible.

Microscopically, it is an angiomyoneuroma, consisting of cavernous blood spaces, muscle tissues (derived from vessel walls), and nerve tissues. Large cuboidal cells, called *'glomal cells'*, are characteristic.

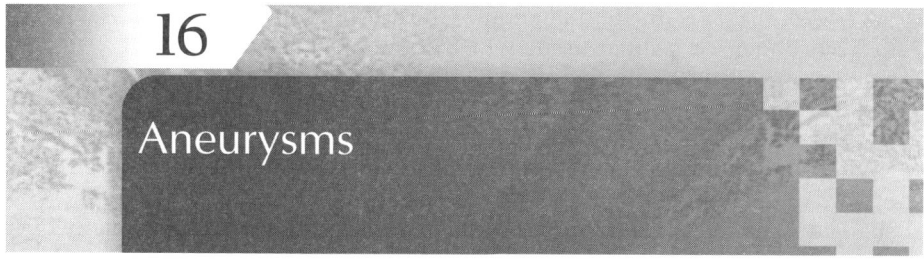

16
Aneurysms

Definition.—An aneurysm is a blood-filled space or sac, formed by the widening or extension of the lumen of an artery, caused by the weakness of the arterial wall that may be congenital, traumatic, or pathological.

Causes.—As has been said in the definition, there must be a defect or weakness in the arterial wall for an aneurysm to occur. Such weakness may be as follows:

A. CONGENITAL
1. Arterial aneurysm from developmental defect occurs in one situation only, i.e. the cerebral arteries (rupture causes subarachnoid haemorrhage).
2. Congenital arteriovenous aneurysm.

B. ACQUIRED
1. *Due to trauma*:
   a. Usually a penetrating wound to the artery.
   b. Occasionally a closed injury causing aneurysm of the aorta.
   c. Rarely damage by a fracture, e.g. internal carotid artery.
   d. Arteriovenous aneurysms, when acquired, are always due to trauma.
2. *Due to disease*:
   a. Arteriosclerosis.—This is by far the commonest cause of aneurysm nowadays; the arterial wall is weakened by severe atheroma or hypertension.
   b. Syphilis.—A common cause in older days, now rare; the tunica media is weakened by endarteritis of the vasa vasorum.
3. *Due to infection* (*mycotic aneurysms*):
   a. As an occasional complication of subacute bacterial endocarditis—the arterial wall becomes weak either because of an abscess formation or because an infected embolus rests there (brain or limbs).
   b. In an artery traversing tubercular cavities in the lung.
   c. In an artery located at the base of a peptic ulcer.

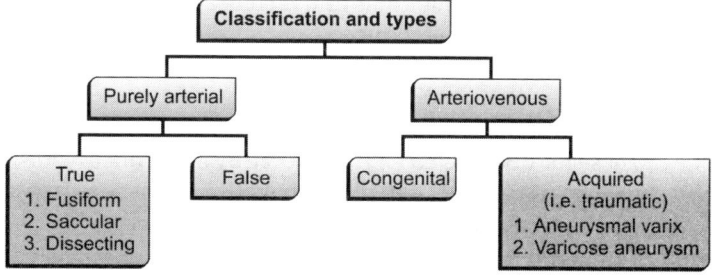

A *true aneurysm* is due to dilatation of the artery itself. A *false aneurysm* is a sac lined by condensed cellular tissue which communicates with the artery through an opening somewhere in its wall.

When the dilatation of the artery involves its whole circumference to give it a spindle-shaped enlargement, it is called a *fusiform aneurysm* (the commonest type).

When only a small part of the circumference of the arterial wall stretches outwards as a rounded bulbous mass, it is called a *saccular aneurysm*. These are usually traumatic. A penetrating wound in the artery does not close spontaneously as retraction of the intima keeps it patent. A *pulsating haematoma* develops, which is partly enclosed by peripheral clot. Later, the saccular cavity becomes walled in by fibrous tissue and is partly lined by endothelium derived from the intima. This is how a saccular aneurysm develops.

A *dissecting aneurysm* occurs when a path of tunica intima ruptures (usually beneath an atheromatous plaque) and blood is forced through the intima to collect and expand between the inner and outer coats of the tunica media (as if dissecting the arterial wall).

Mycotic aneurysm has been already described.

In *arteriovenous aneurysm* (*or fistula*), there is a communication between an artery and a vein. This may be due to:

a. Congenital malformation.—Mostly in the extremities.
b. Acquired.—Usually as a result of a penetrating wound injuring simultaneously an artery and a vein, lying close to each other; during the process of healing, communication develops between the artery and the vein:
    i. The artery and the vein may communicate directly through a short wide channel—*aneurysmal varix*.
    ii. The anastomosis may be indirect through an intermediate sac lying in the soft tissues—*varicose aneurysm*.

Pathological Effects and Clinical Features

A. INTRINSIC:
1. The essential feature is a swelling along the line of the artery.
2. The swelling shows an expansile pulsation.
3. The pulsation ceases and the swelling reduces if the artery is compressed at the proximal point.
4. A thrill may be palpable over the swelling.
5. On auscultation, a systolic bruit may be audible over the swelling.

B. EXTRINSIC.—These are either due to pressure effects on adjacent structures or due to distal arterial occlusion caused by emboli that are formed in the aneurysmal sac and are carried distally:

1. *Artery:*
    a. The distal pulse is smaller than that of the contralateral side and the pulse-pressure in the distal vessel is reduced.
    b. Gangrene due to embolism.
2. *Nerves:*   Altered sensation or paralysis.
3. *Veins:*   Distal oedema.
4. *Bones:*   These may be eroded (e.g. vertebrae by aortic aneurysms; the more resilient structures like the inter-vertebral discs escape).
5. *Tubes:*   Trachea, oesophagus, etc. may be compressed.
6. *Skin:*   The overlying skin may be stretched or even necrosed.

Complications

1. Pressure effects, as described above.

2. Diffusion into cellular planes.

3. Rupture:

   a Into a serous cavity—pleura, peritoneum.

   b. Into hollow viscera.

   c. On the skin surface.

4. Suppuration followed by rupture.

5. Embolism as described above.

Spontaneous Cure.—This may rarely occur in a saccular aneurysm due to gradual clotting in the sac.

Treatment.—This is always surgical. The nature of the operation depends on the size and position of the artery involved:

1. *Arterial Ligation.*—Simple ligature of the arteries that enter and leave an aneurysm prevents embolisation and rupture. The operation, however, has the disadvantage of producing intolerable distal ischaemia. On the other hand, if there is sufficient collateral circulation to prevent distal ischaemia, the aneurysm fails to close as sufficient blood again reaches it. The procedure is, however, suitable in some situations, e.g. splenic artery, intracranial aneurysms, etc. There are different types of ligation, e.g.

   a. Anel's method.—The ligature is applied just *proximal* to the sac.

   b. Hunter's method.—The ligature is proximal as above, but is applied immediately *above a branch* of the artery.

   c. Brasdor's method.—The ligature is applied just *distal* to the sac.

   d. Wardrop's method.—The ligature is distal but applied immediately *below a branch* of the artery.

   e. Antylus' method.—Two ligatures are applied, *one proximal and another distal* to the sac.

2. *Aneurysmorrhaphy (Matas').*—(Figure 16.1).—This is particularly suitable for saccular aneurysms which are small-mouthed—the diseased sac can be totally excised and the defect in the arterial wall closed by lateral suture of the healthy arterial wall (Fig. 16.1).

3. *Wiring.*—This operation is valuable for poor-risk patients with difficult aneurysms. Random coils (200 to 1000 feet) of very fine stainless steel wire are introduced into the aneurysm via a stout hypodermic needle that pierces the

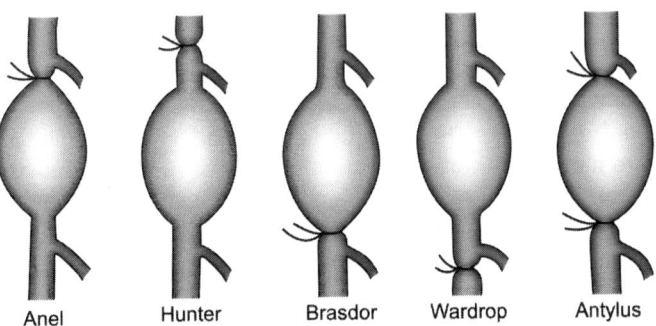

Anel Hunter Brasdor Wardrop Antylus

Fig. 16.1: Ligation of aneurysms.

wall of the aneurysm. The wire causes clotting of blood within the sac except for a central channel which remains open. The wire itself, as well as the thrombus, strengthens the aneurysmal wall.

4. *Reinforcement.*—Wrapping the aneurysm with fascia or plastic material is seldom helpful. Its only indication is for intracranial aneurysms that may be reinforced with a coating of rapidly-setting plastic to strengthen the wall and prevent haemorrhage.

5. *Excision and Artery Grafting, i.e. Reconstruction.*—This is the most recent operation, particularly for aortic aneurysms (specially abdominal ones). The part of the artery involved in the aneurysm, together with the aneurysm itself, is excised and the gap replaced by a prosthesis as shown in Fig. 16.2 (e.g. dacron graft).

6. *Exclusion, i.e. By-pass Grafting.*—Excision of the aneurysmal part of the artery is sometimes undesirable as neighbouring vital structures (e.g. the vena cava in aortic aneurysm) may be damaged. The artery is ligated above and below the aneurysm, and a graft is put in between the proximal and distal segments of the artery. The circulation is thus kept intact while the aneurysm thromboses and shrinks into a fibrous mass (Fig. 16.2).

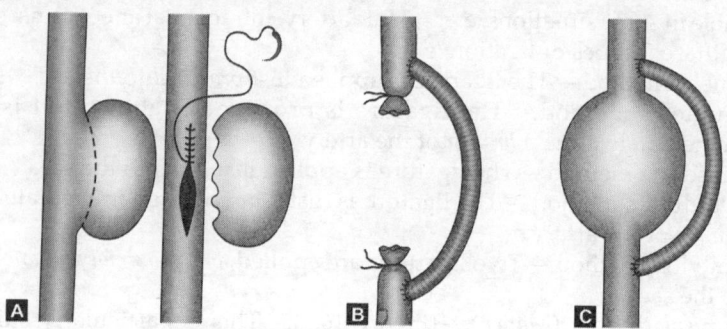

Fig. 16.2: Operations for aneurysms. (A)—Aneurysmorrhaphy (Matas'), (B)—Excision and grafting, (C)—By-pass grafting.

Arteriovenous Aneurysms.—As has already been stated, they may be congenital or acquired (traumatic).

The veins involved in the aneurysm become arterialised, i.e. thick-walled, and get dilated and tortuous.

The *congenital* lesions are stationary and seldom require intervention. The *acquired* lesions are progressive and often demand surgical treatment. The types of surgery may be:

1. *Quadruple Ligation.*—This is suitable for smaller vessels. The artery and the vein are ligated both above and below the communicating fistula (i.e. four ligatures).

2. *Reconstruction.*—The vessels are separated and any intervening sac is excised. The defects in the vessel walls are repaired. It may be necessary to reconstruct the artery at the expense of the vein. The vein is simply ligated above and below, and the intervening part is utilised in arterial repair.

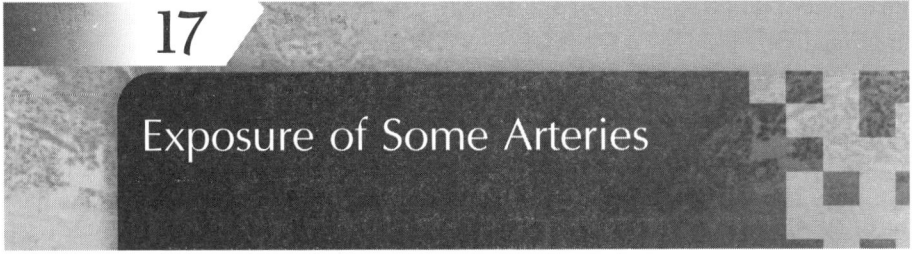

17

Exposure of Some Arteries

Indications

1. To arrest haemorrhage from a bleeding artery.
2. To investigate into the possibility of occlusion of an artery by pressure or constriction, e.g. brachial artery in supracondylar fracture.
3. To diminish haemorrhage in certain operations (as a preliminary step), e.g. the external carotid artery prior to hemimandibulectomy, the femoral or axillary artery before disarticulation of hip or shoulder.
4. To diminish circulation, e.g. lingual artery in bleeding haemangioma or carcinoma of tongue.
5. For elective operations on the arteries.—Arteriography, embolectomy, reconstruction, ligation (for aneurysms), etc.

COMMON CAROTID ARTERY

Anatomy.—On the left side the artery arises directly from the arch of the aorta (the vessels arising from the arch are the innominate, left common carotid, and left subclavian; rarely the arteria thyroidea ima). On the right side, it arises from the innominate artery (the other branch is right subclavian).

In the neck the artery starts behind the sternoclavicular joint. It passes upwards, towards the lobule of the ear. Opposite the upper border of the thyroid cartilage it ends by dividing into external and internal carotid arteries.

It lies within the carotid sheath together with the internal jugular vein and the vagus nerve. The vein lies lateral to it, and the nerve in the groove behind and between the artery and the vein.

Superficial relations are skin, subcutaneous tissue, platysma, deep fascia, sternomastoid, sternohyoid and sternothyroid. It is crossed in front by the superior and middle thyroid veins, as well as the ansa hypoglossi. The omohyoid muscle crosses the artery obliquely at the level of the cricoid cartilage. The lateral lobe of the thyroid partly overlaps the artery.

Branches.—It has *no* branch.

Surface Marking.—A line is drawn from the sternoclavicular junction to a point midway between the angle of the mandible and the trip of the mastoid process. The lower part of this line up to the upper border of the thyroid cartilage represents the common carotid artery while the upper part corresponds to the external carotid artery.

Indications for Exposure

1. For cerebral arteriography.
2. For ligating the artery in the treatment of intracranial aneurysms.

Exposure.—The neck requires hyperextension, and to achieve this, a sandbag is placed under the *shoulders*. The head is turned to the opposite side.

The artery is more easily exposed above the omohyoid because here it lies more superficially.

A transverse incision is made along the line of the skin crease at the level of the cricoid cartilage, with its centre at the anterior border of the sternomastoid (in the cadaver where the tissues are stiffened, it is better to make an incision in the line of the artery—about 3 inches in length with its centre at the level of the cricoid cartilage). The skin, superficial fascia, platysma, and deep fascia are divided in the line of incision, taking care of the external jugular vein on the sternomastoid. The sternomastoid muscle is retracted laterally. At the lower part of the wound the omohyoid is seen and it is retracted downwards. The carotid sheath is now seen with the superior and middle thyroid veins crossing in front of it. These veins may have to be divided between ligatures. A valuable guide to the common carotid artery is the prominent transverse process of the sixth cervical vertebra, which lies behind the artery. This is also known as the *Chassaignac's tubercle* and it corresponds to the level of the lower border of the cricoid cartilage.

The carotid sheath is now incised carefully along its medial side (to avoid injury to the internal jugular vein and the decendens hypoglossi nerve). The internal jugular vein is gently separated from the artery and then an aneurysm needle is passed from the lateral side inwards, behind the artery, to pass the ligature round the artery (this avoids injury to the vein). Care must be taken of the vagus nerve which lies behind.

Establishment of Collateral Circulation Following Ligature

A. *Inside the skull:*
1. Between the branches of the internal carotid artery of the two sides.
2. Through the *Circle of Willis* (vertebral arteries and internal carotid arteries).
3. Retrograde flow along the external carotid artery.

B. *Outside the skull:*
1. Between the branches of the external carotid and those of the subclavian, e.g.
   a. Superior thyroid (external carotid) and inferior thyroid (subclavian).
   b. Descending branch of the occipital (external carotid) and deep cervical and transverse cervical (subclavian).
2. Between the branches of the external carotid of the two sides.
   However, ligature of the common carotid artery is not without danger to the cerebral circulation, particularly in the elderly. In more than 25% of cases there is impairment of cerebral circulation and softening of the brain.

EXTERNAL CAROTID ARTERY

Indications for Exposure
1. As a preliminary step, to minimise haemorrhage, during parotidectomy, linguectomy, maxillectomy, mandibulectomy, etc.
2. To arrest haemorrhage from carcinoma or haemangioma of the tongue.

Anatomy.—The artery begins at the bifurcation of the common artery, opposite the upper border of the thyroid cartilage. It runs upwards in the carotid triangle and then passes deep to the posterior belly of digastric, to lie in a groove on the deep surface of the parotid gland. Here it ends behind the neck of the mandible by dividing into two branches, viz. superficial temporal and maxillary arteries.

Superficial relations in the carotid triangle are two nerves (cervical branch of the facial nerve and the hypoglossal nerve), and numerous veins (lingual, common facial, superior thyroid, etc.) which cross the artery to end in the internal jugular vein.

Branches.—(1) Superior thyroid (2) Ascending pharyngeal (3) Lingual (4) Facial (5) Occipital (6) Posterior auricular (7) Superficial temporal (8) Maxillary.

Surface Marking.—*See* under the common carotid artery.

Exposure.—The patient is positioned as for exposure of the common carotid artery.

A transverse incision is made along the skin crease 1 inch below the angle of the mandible (in the cadaver where the tissues are stiffened, an incision about 3 inches long is made along the anterior border of the sternomastoid, with its centre opposite the greater cornu of the hyoid bone). The skin, superficial fascia, platysma, and deep fascia are all divided in the same line, taking care of the external jugular vein. The sternomastoid muscle is retracted laterally and the posterior belly of the digastric is retracted upwards to expose the carotid sheath. Several veins, e.g. common facial, lingual, etc. have to be secured before the carotid sheath is incised to expose the artery. Care must be taken of the hypoglossal nerve which crosses the artery superficially, just above the level of the greater cornu of the hyoid.

The artery is distinguished from the internal carotid artery by the presence of branches (the internal carotid has no branch in the neck). The internal jugular vein is carefully separated from the artery. An aneurysm needle is passed behind the artery from outside inwards (to avoid injury to the vein), and a ligature is passed round the artery.

Establishment of Collateral Circulation Following Ligature

1. Between the branches of the artery and those of the opposite side.
2. Between the branches of the external carotid and those of subclavian, e.g.
   a. Superior thyroid (external carotid) and inferior thyroid (subclavian).
   b. Descending branch of the occipital (external carotid) and deep cervical and transverse cervical (subclavian).

INTERNAL CAROTID ARTERY

Indications for Exposure

1. Ligation for intracranial aneurysm.
2. Endarterectomy for atheroma.

Anatomy.—The artery begins at the bifurcation of the common carotid artery opposite the upper border of the thyroid cartilage. At its commencement the artery is actually external (i.e. lateral) to the external carotid artery. However, it soon slopes up posteriorly to occupy a medial and deeper plane. The internal jugular vein lies posterolateral to the artery and the vagus nerve lies deep to the interval between them, inside the carotid sheath.

The artery enters the skull through the carotid canal which lies at the level of the lower border of the external auditory meatus. Inside the skull artery makes half a dozon bends (seen in an arteriogram), and ends in the anterior perforated substance.

The artery has no branch in the neck.

The *carotid body* is a small yellowish-grey structure lying behind the bifurcation of the common carotid artery. Its cells are chemoreceptors.

Surface Marking.—From the termination of the common carotid (*see* under the common carotid artery) a line is drawn upwards to the posterior border of the neck of the mandible.

Exposure.—Same as for the external carotid artery (*see* above).

Establishment of Collateral Circulation Following Ligature

1. Between the branches of the internal carotid artery of the two sides.
2. Through the *Circle of Willis* (vertebral arteries and internal carotid arteries).
3. Retrograde flow along the external carotid artery. However, impairment of cerebral circulation may sometimes occur.

FACIAL ARTERY

This is a branch of the external carotid artery.

The artery may be easily exposed at the lower border of the mandible, where it lies at the anterior border of the masseter muscle. A small incision is made along the lower border of the mandible here and the artery is immediately seen.

SUPERFICIAL TEMPORAL ARTERY

Anatomy.—This is a terminal branch of the external carotid artery (the other terminal branch is the maxillary artery).

The artery begins in the parotid gland, behind the neck of the mandible. It runs up behind the temporomandibular joint and crosses over the zygomatic process, in close relation to the auriculotemporal nerve which lies immediately behind it. About 2 inches above the zygoma it divides into two branches—frontal and parietal.

Branches.—(1) Transverse facial (2) Anterior auricular (3) Zygomaticoorbital (4) Middle temporal (5) Frontal (6) Parietal.

Exposure.—An incision 1 inch long is made in front of the upper part of the ear. On little dissection of the dense subcutaneous tissues, the artery is readily seen. The auriculotemporal nerve lies just behind the artery.

SUBCLAVIAN ARTERY

Indications for Exposure

1. As a preliminary step to a forequarter amputation.
2. To arrest uncontrollable haemorrhage from the axilla.
3. Rarely for the treatment of aneurysm.

Anatomy.—The left subclavian artery arises directly from the arch of the aorta while the right is a branch of the innominate artery. Each artery runs from the sternoclavicular joint to the outer border of the first rib, where it becomes the axillary artery. The artery is convex upwards, with its summit reaching to a level of about ½ inch above the clavicle (when the shoulder is depressed).

The scalenus anterior muscle crosses in front of the artery and arbitrarily divides it into three parts. The first part lies medial and the third part lies lateral to the muscle. The second part is behind the muscle. The subclavian vein lies in front of the muscle here but at a lower level, i.e. behind the clavicle.

It is the third part of the artery which is usually selected for ligature since it is the most accessible.

Superficial relations of the third part are (a) the skin, superficial fastia and platysma, supraclavicular nerves, and the deep fascia; (b) the external jugular vein with its tributaries, viz. transverse cervical, suprascapular, and anterior jugular veins; (c) the suprascapular artery; (d) the nerve to subclavius.

Branches.—It is only the first part of the artery which gives off branches. These are: (1) Vertebral (2) Internal mammary (3) Thyrocervical trunk (4) Costocervical artery.

Surface Marking.—The artery is represented by a thick line, convex upwards, extending from the sternoclavicular joint to the lower border of the middle of the clavicle. On the left side, this line is extended proximally to about the middle of the manubrium sterni.

Exposure.—As has already been stated, it is the *third part* of the artery which is most easily exposed.

The arm is placed at the side and is drawn downwards, in order to depress the shoulder as strongly as possible. This procedure elevates the artery to the neck. The head is turned to the opposite side.

An incision, about 3 inch long, is made 1/2 inch above and parallel to the upper border of the clavicle. It extends from the sternal end of the clavicle to about the anterior border of the trapezius. The skin, superficial fascia and platysma are divided. While incising the deep fascia, care must be taken not to cut the external jugular vein or its important tributaries, before securing them (as the circumference of the external jugular vein is fixed to the deep fascia, the vein cannot undergo natural collapse after a cut and this may lead to sucking in of air, causing air embolism).

The omohyoid muscle is retracted upwards and the lateral border of the scalenus anterior is defined. The artery is identified as it emerges from behind the scalenus anterior. The suprascapular artery, crossing in front of the subclavian, should be carefully preserved since it forms an important channel for collateral circulation following ligature of the subclavian. The upper and middle trunks of the brachial plexus are found lateral to the artery while the lower trunk is behind the artery. The lower trunk should be carefully isolated before passing an aneurysm needle round the artery so that it is not included in the ligature. If the needle is passed *from above downwards*, this complication is less likely to occur.

Establishment of Collateral Circulation Following Ligature

1. *Scapular Anastomosis.*—The suprascapular and (deep branch of) the transverse cervical arteries from the subclavian anastomosing with the subscapular artery from the axillary.

2. *Axillary Anastomosis.*—Small unnamed branches from the subclavian and the axillary anastomosing with each other.

3. *Intercostal Anastomosis.*—The internal mammary artery from the subclavian anastomosing with the superior intercostal, lateral thoracic, and subscapular arteries from the axillary.

INTERNAL MAMMARY ARTERY

Anatomy.—This is a branch of the first part of the subclavian artery. It passes downwards over the apex of the lung, where the phrenic nerve crosses it in front, from the lateral to the medial side. On entering the thorax, the artery passes vertically downwards, a finger's breadth lateral to the border of the sternum up to the sixth intercostal space. Here it divides into two branches—the musculophrenic and the superior epigastric arteries. It gives off two anterior intercostal artery in each intercostal space.

The artery is covered in front by the pectoralis major and the upper six costal cartilages together with the intervening anterior intercostal membranes and internal intercostal muscles. It is crossed in front by the upper six intercostal nerves. Posteriorly the artery is separated from the parietal pleura by the transversus thoracis muscle.

Along the sides of the artery lie the important internal mammary chain of nodes and the venae comites.

Exposure.—A small transverse incision is made at the anterior end of the intercostal space concerned. The skin, subcutaneous tissue, pectoralis major, anterior intercostal membrane, and internal intercostal muscle are divided in the line of incision. The artery is readily seen. Care must be taken not to injure the parietal pleura.

AXILLARY ARTERY

Anatomy.—It is the continuation of the third part of the subclavian artery. It starts at the outer border of the first rib (behind the midpoint of the clavicle) and ends at the lower border of the posterior axillary wall (teres major), from where it continues as the brachial artery. The pectoralis minor muscle, which crosses the artery in front, divides it into three parts. The first part lies above, the second part behind, and the third part below the muscle.

The second part of the artery is clasped by the three cords of the brachial plexus. To its lateral side is the lateral cord, behind is the posterior cord, and on the medial side is the medial cord.

Branches

1. The first part has *one* branch—the superior thoracic.
2. The second part has *two* branches—the acromiothoracic and the lateral thoracic.
3. The third part has *three* branches—the subscapular, the anterior circumflex humeral, and the posterior circumflex humeral.

Surface Marking.—The artery is represented by a line starting from the mid-point of the clavicle to a point which marks the junction of the anterior with the middle third of a line joining the anterior and the posterior axillary folds, at the base of the axilla.

Exposure.—It is usually the third part of the artery which is exposed.

The patient lies supine with the shoulders raised and the arm abducted to a right angle and externally rotated. An incision 3 inches long is made along the lower part of the line representing the artery (*see* surface marking). On incising the skin and subcutaneous tissues, the medial border of the coracobrachialis muscle is defined. This muscle, together with the musculocutaneous nerve (running along the medial margin of the muscle), is retracted laterally. The median nerve, the medial cutaneous nerve of the forearm, the ulnar nerve, and the axillary vein are all carefully retracted laterally. The artery is now seen in the gap so made and an aneurysm needle is passed from within outwards (to avoid injury to the axillary vein which lies medial to the artery).

Establishment of Collateral Circulation Following Ligature

1. After ligature of the first part of the artery, the development of the collateral circulation is the same as that after ligature of the subclavian artery (*see* subclavian artery).
2. After ligature of the third part of the artery, collateral circulation develops as it does after ligature of the brachial artery above the origin of the profunda brachii (*see* below).

BRACHIAL ARTERY

Indications for Exposure
1. For ligature in uncontrollable haemorrhages of the upper limb.
2. For investigation into possible occlusion of the artery in cases of supracondylar fracture.

Anatomy.—*See* Figs 15.2 and 15.3. It is the continuation of the axillary artery, starting at the lower border of the posterior axillary wall (teres major). The artery is superficial throughout its course in the arm, lying immediately deep to the deep fascia. It runs downwards and slightly outwards, at first medial to the humerus and then in front of it. In the cubital fossa, at the level of the neck of the radius, it ends by dividing into radial and ulnar arteries.

Important Relations
1. The medial nerve is lateral to the artery above, then crosses it in front very obliquely, and thereafter lies on its medial side.
2. The ulnar nerve is posterior to the artery in its uppermost part and then lies medial to the artery. However, in the lower arm it diverges from the artery and passes backwards through the medial intermuscular septum.
3. The artery lies successively on the long and medial heads of the triceps, the coracobrachialis, and the brachialis muscle.
4. The biceps overlaps the artery on its lateral side.
5. In the cubital fossa, the tendon of the biceps lies on the lateral side of the artery while the medial nerve lies on its medial side. All these structures lie on the brachialis muscle (which forms the floor of the upper part of the cubital fossa). These structures are roofed over by the deep fascia, re-inforced by the bicipital aponeurosis which stretches medially from the tendon of the biceps.
6. In the lower part, the artery is accompanied by venae comites and in the upper part by the venae comites as well as the basilic vein.

Branches
1. Profunda brachii, which arises near the commencement of the artery and accompanies the radial nerve along the spiral groove of the humerus.

2. Ulnar collateral, which accompanies the ulnar nerve.
3. Supratrochlear.
4. Nutrient, to the flexor muscles.
5. Terminal, i.e. radial and ulnar arteries.

Surface Marking.—The line of the artery starts from a point which marks the junction of the anterior and middle third of a line joining the anterior and the posterior axillary folds at the base of the axilla. It is continued along the medial border of the biceps to 1 inch below the midpoint of the line joining the two epicondyle.

Exposure

I. *In the Middle of the Arm.*—The limb is abducted and laterally rotated while the forearm rests on a small table. The upper arm must not be supported on a table as this process pushes the triceps forwards and this muscle is likely to be mistaken for the biceps.

An incision about 2 inches long is made along the medial edge of the biceps. The skin, subcutaneous tissue, and deep fascia are divided in the same line, taking care of the basilic vein which pierces the deep fascia here. The biceps is retracted laterally and the artery is readily seen with its two vanae comites. The medial nerve is seen to cross the artery in front.

II. *At the Bend of the Elbow.*—The arm is abducted and laterally rotated and is supported on a table, with the elbow extended.

An incision about 2 inches long is made on the cubital fossa along the medial border of the biceps tendon. The superficial veins are secured. The deep fascia which is reinforced here by the bicipital aponeurosis is incised vertically. The biceps tendon is now retracted laterally. A little flexion of the elbow at this stage easily brings into view the brachial artery, with the median nerve lying on its medial side.

Establishment of Collateral Circulation Following Ligature.—The collateral circulation is maintained by the *anastomosis around the elbow joint.* Recurrent branches from the radial, ulnar, and common interosseous arteries ascend upwards both anterior and posterior to the elbow joint. They anastomose with the descending articular of the profunda brachii, ulnar collateral and supratrochlear arteries (branches of brachial).

RADIAL ARTERY

Anatomy.—*See* Fig. 15.3. This is a terminal branch of the brachial artery. From its commencement, at the neck of the radius, it runs along the radial side of the front of the forearm to the wrist. It lies successively on the biceps tendon, supinator muscle, tendon of insertion of pronator teres, radial origin of flexor digitorum profundus, origin of flexor policis longus, proaator quadratus and the lower part of the radius itself. In the upper part of the forearm the artery is covered by the brachioradialis; in the rest of the forearm it is superficial, covered only by skin and fasciae. The radial nerve lies close to it only in the middle third of its course, being lateral to the artery.

From the front of the wrist the artery winds round the outer side of the carpus (the trapezium) passing under cover of the abductor pollicis longus and extensor pollicis brevis tendons. It now slopes across the anatomical snuff box and reaches the proximal end of the first inter-metacarpal space on the back. The *anatomical snuffbox* is a triangular space bounded laterally by the abductor pollicis longus and extensor pollicis brevis tendons, and medially by the extensor pollicis longus tendon; its apex is formed by the meeting of these tendons; its base is the lower margin of the radius; the floor is formed by the trapezium and the scaphoid.

Having reached the back of the hand, the artery passes between the two heads of the first dorsal interosseous muscle to come to the palm, where it forms the deep palmar arch by anastomosing with the deep branch of the ulnar artery (the proximal border of the outstretched thumb indicates the level of the deep palmar arch).

Branches

1. *In the cubital fossa.*—Radial recurrent.
2. *In front of the wrist:*
   a. Palmar carpal.
   b. Superficial palmar, which unites with the ulnar artery to form the superficial palmar arch (the distal border of the outstretched thumb indicates the level of the superficial palmar arch).
3. *In the anatomical snuff box.*—Dorsal Carpal.
4. *In the first intermetacarpal space:*
   a. First dorsal metacarpal.
   b. Arteria radialis indicis (supplying the radial side of the index finger).
   c. Arteria princeps pollicis (supplying the thumb).

Exposure

I. *In the Forearm.*—The forearm is rested completely supinated. An incision about 2 inches in length is made along the course of the artery (in the upper, middle, or lower third, as is required). The gap between the brachio-radialis and the flexor carpi radialis is carefully opened and the artery is radially seen. In the middle third of the forearm the radial nerve lies close to the lateral side of the artery.

II. *In the Anatomical Snuff Box.*—The tendon of the extensor pollicis longus is made prominent and thus the outline of the snuff box is defined. A longitudinal incision is made over the centre of the space, parallel to the tendon of the extensor pollicis longus. The origin of the cephalic vein, which crosses the space, is secured. The artery, which lies rather deep here, is dissected out of the fatty tissue occupying the space.

ULNAR ARTERY

Anatomy.—*See* Fig. 15.3. This is a terminal branch of the brachial artery. Commencing at the neck of the radius where the brachial artery bifurcates, the artery at first runs downwards and medially to reach the medial border of the forearm, along which it descends to the wrist. Here it passes superficial to the flexor retinaculum into the palm, where it forms the superficial palmar arch by anastomosing with the superficial palmar branch of the radial artery.

In its upper part the artery is located deeply under cover of the obliquely lying muscles here, viz. pronator teres, flexor carpi radialis, palmaris longus, flexor digitorum sublimis, and flexor carpi ulnaris (from above downwards). The artery rests on the brachialis above, and the flexor digitorum profundus below. The median nerve crosses the artery in front, from the medial to the lateral side, but is separated from the artery by the ulnar head of the pronator teres.

In the lower half the artery is situated superficially, covered only by skin and fasciae. It lies in the gap between flexor carpi ulnaris (medially) and the flexor digitorum sublimis (laterally). It rests on the flexor digitorum profundus. The ulnar nerve is close to the medial side of the lower two-thirds of the artery.

Branches

1. Ulnar recurrents—anterior and posterior.
2. Common interosseous, the main branch, which divides into the anterior and posterior interosseous arteries.
3. Carpals—dorsal and palmar.
4. Deep branch, which forms the deep palmar arch.

Exposure.—The artery is very deeply situated in the upper third of the forearm and is therefore rarely exposed there.

I. *In the Middle Third.*—An incision, about 3 inches long, is made along the line of the artery in the forearm. On dividing the skin and subcutaneous tissue, search is made for a white line which indicates the gap between the flexor carpi ulnaris and flexor digitorum superficialis. Great care should be taken to identify this line because it is on this that the success of the operation depends. When the line is defined, the deep fascia is incised along the whole length of the line. The two muscles are then separated and the artery is seen, with the ulnar nerve lying on its medial side.

II. *In the Lower Third.*—An incision about 2 inches in length is made along the lateral border of the tendon of the flexor carpi ulnaris. After the deep fascia is divided, the tendon is retracted medially. The artery is readily seen, with the ulnar nerve on its medial side.

EXTERNAL ILIAC ARTERY

Indications for exposure.—For arresting haemorrhage from the femoral vessels at the groin, resulting from:

a. Injury, i.e. primary haemorrhage.
b. Secondary carcinoma of inguinal lymph nodes or severe infection in the groin causing secondary haemorrhage.

Ligature of the external iliac artery is a safer procedure than that of the femoral artery above the origin of the profunda femoris in as far as the viability of the limb is concerned because of the abundant collateral circulation. For the same reason, however, such ligature is less effective in arresting haemorrhage from the lower thigh in which case, therefore, it is advisable to ligate the femoral artery.

Anatomy.—The artery starts at the pelvic brim from the bifurcation of the common iliac artery (the ureter crosses in front of the bifurcation). It runs downwards to the mid-inguinal point where, behind the inguinal ligament, it is continued into the thigh as the femoral artery.

Posterior to the artery is the psoas major muscle. Anteriorly the artery is in contact with the peritoneum above, while below the peritoneal reflection it is directly related to the anterior abdominal flat muscles, viz. transversus, internal oblique, and external oblique. Medial to the artery lies the femoral vein. Lateral to the artery and a little away from it is the femoral nerve, while the genitofemoral nerve lies in the gap between the two.

Branches.—These arise near the termination of the artery and are two in number:
1. Inferior epigastric.
2. Deep circumflex iliac.

Exposure.—The artery should be ligated as high as possible so that the ligature is above its two branches. This allows the development of an effective collateral circulation.

There are two approaches, viz. extraperitoneal and intraperitoneal, of which the former is usually preferred. For an extraperitoneal approach, an incision is made 1/2 inch above and parallel to the middle three-fourths of the inguinal ligament. The skin, superficial fascia (two layers), and the external oblique aponeurosis are cut along the line of incision, as in the operation for an inguinal hernia, and the inguinal canal is thus exposed. The spermatic cord is retracted upwards and medially. A finger is then passed behind the arched muscular fibres of the internal oblique arising from the inguinal ligament and the muscle is divided laterally for about an inch. The fascia transversalis is divided (both medial and lateral to the deep inguinal ring), taking care not to injure the peritoneum and the inferior epigastric vessels (these vessels play an important role in-the establishment of collateral circulation). The peritoneum is now peeled off carefully forwards and upwards, and the external iliac vessels are seen behind it. As the vein lies medial to the artery, the aneurysm needle should be passed from inside outwards behind the artery to avoid injury to the vein.

Establishment of Collateral Circulation Following Ligature

I. *On the Anterior Abdominal Wall:*
  1. The superior epigastric (from the internal mammary) anastomosing with the inferior epigastric (from the external iliac).
  2. The lumbar (from the aorta) and the iliolumbar (from the internal iliac) anastomosing with the deep circumflex iliac (from the external iliac).

II. *Over the Gluteal and Pudendal Areas:*
  1. The superior and inferior gluteal arteries (from the internal iliac) anastomosing with the medial circumflex and perforating branches of the profunda femoris (from the femoral).
  2. The internal pudendal (from the internal iliac) anastomosing with the superficial and deep external pudendal arteries from the femoral).

FEMORAL ARTERY

Indications for exposure
1. Penetrating injuries in the thigh (injury to the femoral artery is one of the common vascular lesions encountered).
2. Secondary haemorrhage from the stump of an above-knee amputation.

Anatomy.—Figure 17.1. The femoral artery starts at the mid-inguinal point as the continuation of the external iliac artery. It runs downwards to the junction of the middle and lower thirds of the thigh, where it passes backwards through an opening in the adductor magnus, to be continued as the popliteal artery.

In its course, the artery has two parts—one in the femoral (Scarpa's) triangle and the other in the subsartorial (Hunter's) canal.

1. *In the Femoral Triangle.*—This triangle is bounded laterally by the medial border of the sartorius and medially by the *medial* border of the adductor longus. The apex is the point where these two muscles meet, while the base is formed by the inguinal ligament. The femoral artery and vein, encased in the femoral sheath, pass through the triangle. The anterior layer of the sheath (in front of the vessels) is derived from the fascia transversalis while the posterior layer (behind the vessels) is derived from the iliopectineal fascia. Inside the sheath, the vein is medial to the artery above, but gradually passes behind the artery near the

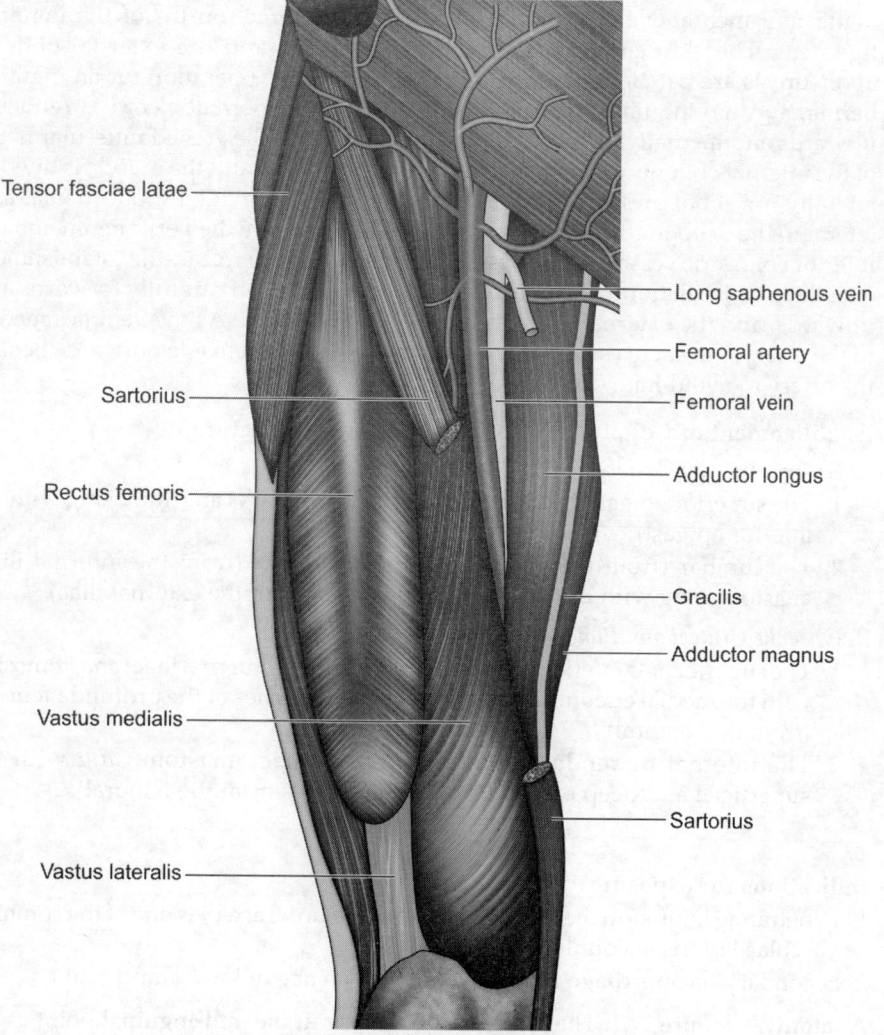

Fig. 17.1: Right femoral vessels

apex of the femoral triangle. The femoral nerve which is lateral and a little away from the artery is outside the femoral sheath. In the femoral triangle, the femoral vessels lie successively on the psoas, pectineus, and adductor longus muscles, from above downwards.

2. *In the Subsartorial Canal.*—This canal is bounded posteriorly by the adductor longus (above) and adductor magnus (below), and anterolaterally by the vastus medialis. It has a fibrous roof anteromedially, and this is covered by the sartorius (hence it is called subsartorial). Inside the canal the femoral vein is at first behind the artery but gradually comes to its lateral side in the lower part of the canal. The saphenous nerve crosses the artery in front, from the lateral to the medial side.

Branches

A. *At the commencement of the artery:*
   1. Superficial epigastric.
   2. Superficial circumflex iliac.
   3. Superficial external pudendal.
   4. Deep external pudendal.
B. About 1½ inches below the inguinal ligament, the profunda femoris artery arises from the lateral side of the femoral artery. The branches of the profunda femoris are (i) the medial circumflex (ii) the lateral circumflex (iii) four perforating branches and (iv) the descending genicular.

Surface Marking.—The artery is represented by the upper two thirds of a line drawn from the mid-inguinal point to the adductor tubercle (with the hip flexed and laterally rotated).

Exposure.—For efficient collateral circulation to develop, the artery should always be ligated below the origin of the profunda femoris. If this is impossible, it is preferable to ligate the external iliac artery instead of the femoral.

I. *At the Base of the Femoral Triangle.*—An incision 2 inches long is made along the line of the artery, starting from the mid-inguinal point. The skin, superficial fascia (two layers), and deep fascia are divided along the line. The anterior layer of the femoral sheath is then carefully incised. An aneurysm needle is passed from within outwards behind the artery (this avoids injury to the femoral vein which lies on the medial side.

II. *At the Apex of the Femoral Triangle.*—The apex of the triangle is about 5 inches below the inguinal ligament. Centering this point, a 3-inch long incision is made along the length of the artery. The skin, superficial fascia, and deep fascia are divided. The sartorius muscle is then retracted laterally. The artery is carefully isolated from the neighbouring important structures, viz. femoral vein posteriorly, saphenous nerve laterally, and the medial cutaneous nerve anteriorly.

III. *In the Subsartorial Canal.*—An incision, 3-inch long, is made along the line of the artery at the middle of the thigh (*see* surface marking). The skin, superficial fascia, and deep fascia are divided, and the sartorius muscle is identified (its fibres run downwards and medially). As the muscle is retracted medially, the fibrous roof of the canal is seen. This is divided along the line of incision and the artery is found. It is carefully isolated from the neighbouring structures, viz. femoral vein and saphenous nerve.

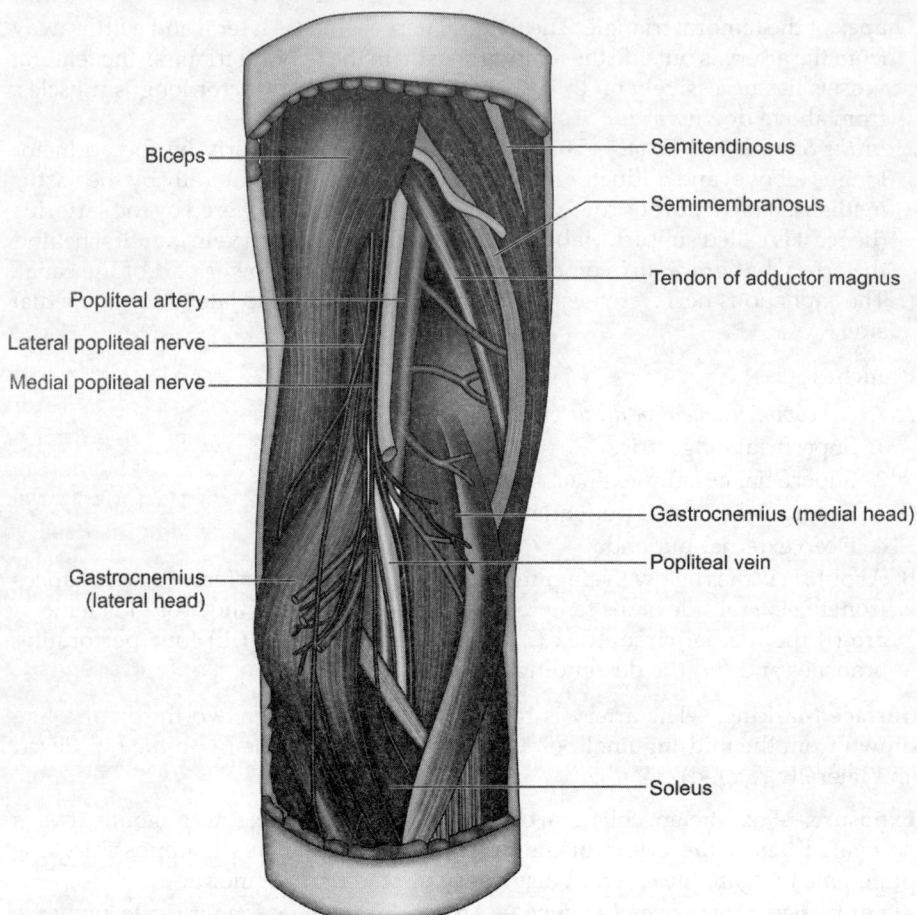

Biceps

Semitendinosus

Semimembranosus

Tendon of adductor magnus

Popliteal artery

Lateral popliteal nerve

Medial popliteal nerve

Gastrocnemius (medial head)

Popliteal vein

Gastrocnemius
(lateral head)

Soleus

Fig. 17.2: Left popliteal fossa

Establishment of Collateral Circulation Following Ligature.—As the artery is
ligated only below the origin of the profunda femoris, efficient collateral circulation
usually develops. This is done chiefly by a chain of anastomosis on the back of the
thigh, in which the following arteries take part from above downwards:

1. Superior and inferior gluteal (branches of internal iliac).
2. Medial circumflex (branch of profunda femoris).
3. The four perforating arteries (branches of profunda femoris).
4. Muscular branches of the popliteal.

POPLITEAL ARTERY

Indications for Exposure

1. For ligature in uncontrollable haemorrhages in the lower limb.
2. For investigation into possible occlusion of the artery in cases of dislocation of
   the knee.
3. For the treatment of aneurysms.

Anatomy.—Figures 17.2 and 17.3. The popliteal artery starts as the continuation of the femoral artery at the opening of the adductor magnus muscle. It descends vertically through the popliteal fossa and ends at the lower border of the popliteus muscle by dividing into two branches—the anterior tibial and the posterior tibial arteries.

The *popliteal fossa* is a diamond-shaped space behind the knee. The upper part of the diamond is bounded laterally by the biceps femoris, and medially by the semimembranosus and semitendinosus. The lower part of the diamond is bounded medially and laterally by the medial and lateral heads of the gastrocnemius respectively. The roof of the fossa is made by the fascia lata, reinforced here by some strong transverse fibres (the roof is pierced by the short saphenous vein and the posterior cutaneous nerve of the thigh). The floor is made, from above downwards, by the popliteal surface of the femur, the capsule of the knee joint, and the popliteus muscle covered by its fascia.

The contents of the fossa are the popliteal artery, popliteal vein, medial and lateral popliteal nerves, popliteal lymph nodes and popliteal pad of fat. The artery is situated most deeply, next to the floor. The vein is the next superficial structure; it is situated lateral to the artery in its upper part, then crosses behind it, and comes to the medial side of the artery in the lower part of the fossa. The medial popliteal nerve is situated mote superficially. It crosses the vessels posteriorly from the lateral side above to the medial side below. The lateral popliteal nerve is well away from the vessels on their lateral side.

Branches

1. Genicular branches—superior, middle and inferior.
2. Muscular.
3. Cutaneous.

Surface Marking.—The line of the artery starts at a point at the junction of the middle and lower thirds of the thigh on the back, one inch medial to the midline. It passes through the middle of the back of the knee joint and ends at the level of the tibial tubercle.

Exposure.—With the patient in the prone position and the knee extended, a vertical midline incision is made over the popliteal fossa. The skin and subcutaneous tissue are divided. The short saphenous vein is cut between ligatures and the sural nerve is protected. The strong deep fascia making the roof of the fossa is divided. The muscles making the boundary of the fossa (i.e. the hamstrings and the gastrocnemius) are retracted to their respective sides and the contents of the fossa are seen. It should be remembered that the artery is the deepest structure here.

Establishment of Collateral Circulation Following Ligature.—Following ligatures of the popliteal artery, development of collateral circulation is often inadequate and there is a serious risk of gangrene of the lower part of the limb. This is because the branches of the artery are small. It is therefore often advised that, instead of ligating the popliteal artery, the femoral artery should be ligated just below the origin of the profunda femoris (blood is diverted downwards through this big artery.)

However, circulation may be maintained after ligature of the popliteal artery by way of the anastomosis around the knee joint. This anastomosis is made by the following vessels:

1. *From above:*
   a. Superior medial and superior lateral genicular (branches of popliteal).
   b. Descending genicular (branch of femoral).
   c. Descending branch of the lateral circumflex femoral (branch of profunda femoris).
2. *From below:*
   a. Inferior medial and inferior lateral genicular (branches of popliteal).
   b. Anterior recurrent branch of anterior tibial.
   c. Circumflex fibular branch of posterior tibial.

POSTERIOR TIBIAL ARTERY

Anatomy.—Figure 17.3. This artery arises at the lower border of the popliteus as one of the two terminal branches of the popliteal artery. It passes under the fibrous arch of the soleus muscle. It then runs in the gap between the flexor digitorum longus (laterally) and flexor hallucis longus (medially). Thus the upper part of the artery is situated at considerable depth, under cover of the gastrocnemius and soleus. The lower part of the artery however is situated superficially, covered by the skin and fasciae only. The artery ends under the flexor retinaculum, by dividing into the medial and lateral plantar arteries.

The posterior tibial nerve is situated on the medial side of the artery in the upper part of the leg. It then crosses behind the artery and, in the lower part, lies on the lateral side of the artery.

[The structures passing under cover of the flexor retinaculum (which extends from the medial malleolus to the medial margin of the calcaneum) are, from the medial to the lateral side, arranged as follows—tibialis posterior tendon, flexor digitorum longus tendon, posterior tibial artery with one venae comites on either side, posterior tibial nerve, flexor hallucis longus tendon.]

Branches

1. Circumflex fibular.
2. Nutrient (to the tibia).
3. Muscular.
4. Peroneal (the biggest branch)
5. Terminal—medial and lateral plantar.

Surface Marking.—The line of the artery starts in the midline of the calf at the level of the tibial tubercle. It ends at a point midway between the medial malleolus and the prominence of the heel.

Exposure.—It is difficult to expose the artery in the upper part of leg where it is situated very deep. The artery is therefore exposed either in the lower part of the leg or under the flexor retinaculum.

I. *In the lower part of the leg.*—A longitudinal incision, 2 inches long, is made midway between the tendo Achilles and the medial margin of the tibia. On dividing the skin and fasciae, the artery is seen lying on the flexor digitorum

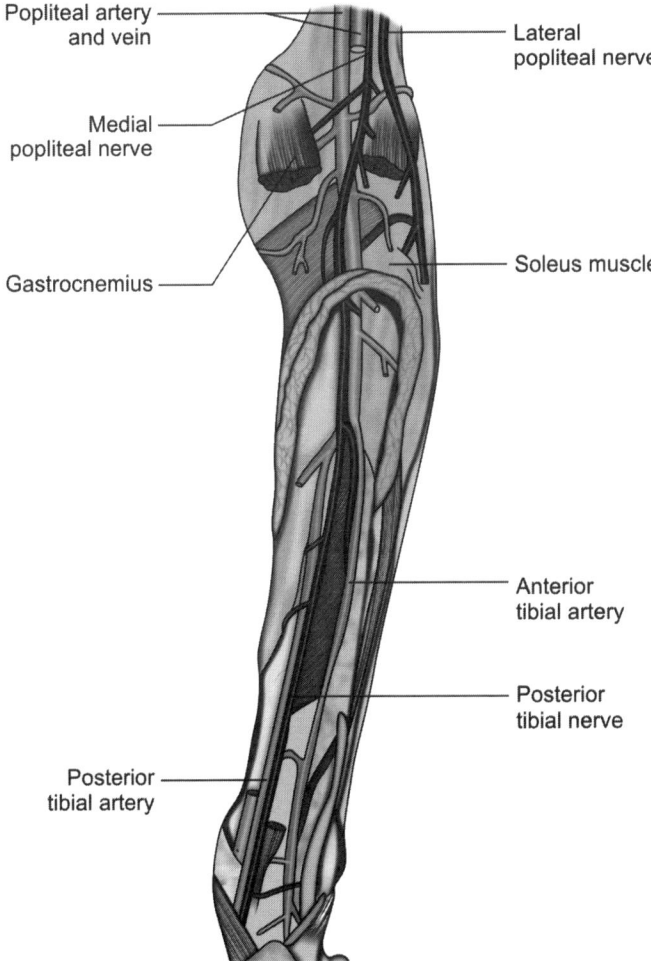

Popliteal artery
and vein

Lateral
popliteal nerve

Medial
popliteal nerve

Gastrocnemius

Soleus muscle

Anterior
tibial artery

Posterior
tibial nerve

Posterior
tibial artery

Fig. 17.3: The main arteries at the back of the knee and the leg

longus. As the posterior tibial nerve is on the lateral side to the artery, the aneurysm needle is passed round the artery from the lateral to the medial side.

II. *Under the flexor retinaculum.*—A curved incision, 2 inches in length, is made parallel to the medial malleolus, midway between the malleolus and the heel. The skin, superficial fascia, and the flexor retinaculum are divided in the same line. The artery is seen between the tendons of the flexor digitorum longus (medially) and the flexor hallucis longus (laterally), with the posterior tibial nerve on its lateral side.

ANTERIOR TIBIAL ARTERY

Anatomy.—Figure 17.3. This artery starts at the lower border of the popliteus (under the calf) as one of the terminal brandies of the popliteal artery. Immediately after its origin, it comes to the anterior compartment of the leg by passing forwards above the upper border of the interosseous membrane. Thereafter, it runs vertically downwards on the interosseous membrane and then crosses the lower end of the tibia, midway between the two malleoli. From here it is continued on to the dorsum of the foot as the dorsalis pedis artery.

Relations.—The tibialis anterior is medial to the artery throughout its course. The extensor digitorum longus and the peroneus tertius are lateral to the artery throughout its length. The extensor hallucis longus is lateral to the artery in the upper part but crosses in front of the artery at the ankle, to come to its medial side. The anterior tibial nerve (also known as the deep peroneal nerve) lies at first lateral to the artery, then in front of it, and thereafter again on its lateral side (the nerve is, as if, hesitating to cross the artery, and so it is often called a 'hesitating nerve').

Branches

1. Tibial recurrents—anterior and posterior.
2. Muscular.
3. Anterior malleolars—medial and lateral.

Surface Marking.—The line of the artery starts at a point 1 inch below the medial side of the head of the fibula. It ends in front of the ankle midway between the two malleoli.

Exposure

I. *In the Upper Third.*—A 3-inch long vertical incision is made along the length of the artery in its uppermost part (*see* surface marking). On incising the deep fascia, the cleft between the tibialis anterior and the extensor digitorum longus is identified. This cleft is opened up and the artery is seen lying on the interosseous membrane. The anterior tibial nerve lies on its lateral side.

II. *In the Middle Third.*—A 3-inch long vertical incision is made along the length of the artery in its middle part (*see* surface marking). On incising the deep fascia the cleft between the tibialis anterior and the extensor hallucis longus is identified, and opened up. The artery is seen lying on the interosseous membrane with the anterior tibial nerve lying in front of it.

III. *In the Lower Third.*—An incision, 3 inches long, is made vertically along the line of the artery (*see* surface marking). The tendons of the tibialis anterior and extensor hallucis longus are identified. The thick deep fascia is divided in the gap between these two tendons. The two tendons are retracted, one on either side, and the artery is found in the gap, lying on the tibia. The anterior tibial nerve lies on its lateral side.

DORSALIS PEDIS ARTERY

Anatomy.—This is the continuation of the anterior tibial artery. It starts at the lower end of the tibia, midway between the two malleoli, and runs to the base of the first inter-metatarsal space. Here it passes between the two heads of the first dorsal interosseous muscle, to reach the sole. In the sole it joins the lateral plantar artery (a terminal branch of the posterior tibial artery) to complete the *plantar arch.*

On the dorsum of the foot the artery is situated very superficially, being covered only by skin and fasciae (and so its pulsation can be easily felt). It is crossed superficially by the tendon of the extensor hallucis brevis. The tendon of the extensor hallucis longus lies on its medial side, and the first tendon of the extensor digitorum longus lies on its lateral side. Between the latter tendon and the artery (i.e. just lateral to the artery) runs the medial terminal branch of the anterior tibial nerve.

Branches

1. Lateral tarsal.
2. Arcuate.
3. First dorsal metatarsal.

Surface Marking.—The line of the artery starts at the midpoint between the two malleoli in front of the ankle. It ends at the base of the first inter-metatarsal space (this is why, in palpating the pulsation of the artery, the fingers should be placed close to the ankle and not in the distal part of the inter-metatarsal space, because the artery does not reach to that extent).

Exposure.—An incision, 1 inch in length, is made along the line of the artery. The skin and fasciae are divided. The artery is easily found between the tendons of extensor hallucis longus and extensor digitorum longus. The tendon of extensor hallucis brevis is seen crossing the artery. The medial terminal branch of the anterior tibial nerve lies on its lateral side.

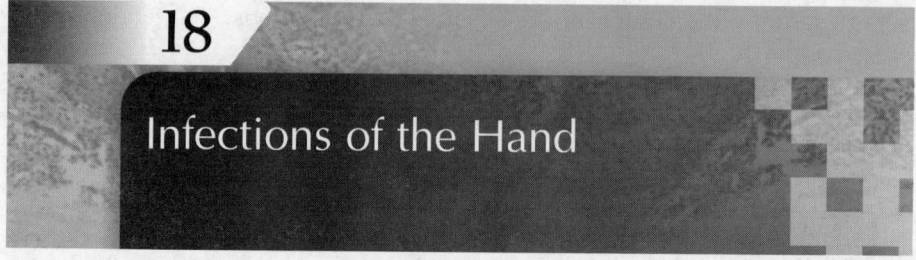

18

Infections of the Hand

ETIOLOGICAL FACTORS

1. In about 70 per cent of cases the infection follows some form of injury, including minor ones like 'hang nail' or careless nail paring. In the remaining 30 per cent there is no known injury; in these cases it is presumed that an epithelial crack from chapping or a forgotten prick serves the portal of entry for the organisms.
2. In 80 per cent of cases the causative organism is *Staph. aureus*, which by its powerful exotoxin causes early death of the tissues, resulting in sloughing. This is particularly likely to occur in the fibro-fatty subcutaneous tissue of the pulp space of the fingers and in the palm.
3. Infections are fairly common in the diabetic subjects.

Classification

I. DIFFUSE SUBCUTANEOUS INFECTIONS
   1. Lymphangitis.
   2. Cellulitis.
   3. Erysipeloid

II. LOCALISED INFECTIONS

A. *Infection of the fingers (whitlow):*
   1. Subcuticular whitlow, including paronychia and carbuncle.
   2. Subcutaneous whitlow, i.e. infection of the pulp spaces:
      a. Distal pulp space.
      b. Middle pulp space.
      c. Proximal pulp space and web-space.
   3. Thecal whitlow (i.e. infection of tendon sheath (tenosynovitis).
   4. Subperiosteal whitlow, i.e. osteomyelitis of a phalanx.
   5. Apical space infection

B. *Infection of the cellular (i.e. fascial) spaces of the hand:*
1. Palmar aspect:
   a. Superficial palmar space
   b. Deep palmar space
      i. Middle palmar space (midpalmar space), ii. Thenar space
2. Dorsal aspect:
   a. Subcutaneous space
   b. Subaponeurotic (i.e. subtendinous) space.

C. *Infection of the Peroria's space in the forearm.*

DIFFUSE SUBCUTANEOUS INFECTIONS

Lymphangitis—This may be:
1. Superficial—Commoner.

2. Deep.

The organisms (usually streptococci) enter through an abrasion.

The hand is painful hot, and swollen. There is considerable oedema particularly on the dorsum. Characteristically, red streaks are seen coursing up the arm (these may not be seen in deep lymphangitis). The axillary and, often, the supratrochlear nodes are enlarged and tender.

Treatment consists in rest to the limb and antibiotics.

Cellulitis.—This is a spreading inflammation of the subcutaneous tissue and fascial planes, usually ending in suppuration.

This is the initial lesion in all the fascial space infections described below.

In the majority of cases this initial lesion localises into an abscess. In some cases, however (particularly in the loose subcutaneous spaces), there is resolution of the inflammation.

Treatment consists in rest to the limb and antibiotics. It is dangerous to go for incision at the stage of cellulitis as this procedure causes further spread of infection. Only when localisation to an abscess has occurred that incision is advisable.

WHITLOW

The term 'whitlow' is applied to any acute inflammation of the finger. According to the plane of tissue in which the inflammation occurs, whitlows are classified as follows:
1. Subcuticular whitlow (including paronychia and carbuncle).
2. Subcutaneous whitlow.
3. Thecal whitlow.
4. Subperiosteal whitlow.
5. Apical space infection.

Subcuticular Whitlow.—Here the pus collects within the layers of the skin, the epidermis being elevated in the form of a purulent blister.

It is common on the palmar surface of the fingers and in the webs.

There are two types:
   a. Simple—without any internal communication.
   b. Collar-stud—this superficial abscess communicates, through a narrow track, with a deep abscess (usually subcutaneous).

Treatment.—The raised epidermis (which is insensitive) is removed with a scalpel or scissors. If the abscess is simple nothing else is required. If it is a collar-stud abscess, the deeper abscess has to be drained properly. In such cases again, if the communicating channel between the two parts is wide, this itself will serve for drainage.

Acute Paromychia.—This denotes an infection of the nail fold with or without extension deep to the nail. This is a type of subcuticular whitlow because the infection is located entirely within the epidermis in which the nail is developed.

This is the commonest infection of the hand (30 per cent), usually resulting from a 'hang nail' or careless nail paring. There is pain, redness, and swelling around the side and base of the nail. Often the pus is visible through the skin.

Treatment
1. The pus is liberated by pushing back the nail fold away from the base of the nail.
2. To provide adequate drainage, a small wedge of nail fold directly over the pus is excised. This also removes the loose cuticle.
3. In the majority of cases the pus is found to extend deep to the nail. If there is such an extension:
   a. When the extension occurs beneath half or more of the width of the nail, the whole width of the proximal one third of the nail is removed.
   b. When the extension is limited to under a corner of the nail, some surgeons advise excision of only the 'floating part' of the nail while others advocate excision of the whole width of the proximal part of the nail (because, if only the corner of the nail is excised, an irregular and fissured nail grows).

Chronic Paronychia.—This should not be included under whitlow as this is not an acute inflammation and also it is not a sequela to acute paronychia. It classically affects women who do much washing. The history is for weeks or months, and often several fingers are affected. The infection may be bacterial or fungal.

Treatment.—Antibiotic treatment is of a little or no help. Fungicidal drugs, systemic and local, are sometimes, beneficial. In the majority of cases operative treatment, has to be undertaken. The operation is in the same line as for acute paronychia and the whole nail may have to be removed.

Carbuncle of the fingers and Hand.—Like carbuncle elsewhere, these result from staphylococcal infection of the hair follicles. So they are commoner in males and usually on the dorsum of the proximal segment of a digit or the dorsum of the hand.

Treatment.—Same as for carbuncle elsewhere.

Subcutaneous Whitlow.—These are infections of the pulp (i.e. the subcutaneous tissues in the volar aspects) of the fingers and thumb. These pulps are subjected to more pricks than any other part of the body and so pulp space infection is so common. Infection may occur in the terminal, middle, or proximal pulp space, but terminal pulp space infection hugely outnumbers the others. It accounts for 25 per cent of all infections of hand, being second only to paronychia.

TERMINAL PULP SPACE INFECTION.—This is also known as 'Felon'.
Surgical Anatomy.—The terminal pulp is a closed space because proximally the deep fascia is attached superficially to the thin skin of the distal flexion crease and in the depth to the periosteum of the distal phalanx just distal to the insertion of the flexor digitorum profundus. This closed space, therefore, has tough walls. The space is transversed by fibrous strands which extend from the skin down to the periosteum, and carry the terminal branches of the digital artery to supply the bone. Inflammatory exudates in the pulp space are therefore in high tension. This not only causes severe pain but also occludes the blood vessels going to supply the distal phalanx through the fibrous septa. This may lead to an osteomyelitis with necrosis of the distal four-fifths of the bone (the proximal one-fifth escapes because it is supplied by a twig which enters the bone without traversing the pulp space).

Sometimes the abscess becomes 'collar-stud'—presenting as a subcuticular whitlow.

Treatment.—As soon as the pus has localised, it should be incised. This is not only to relieve the patient of the intense pain but also to prevent osteomyelitis of the phalanx.

The different *types of incision* used are:

a. A transverse incision over the point of maximum tenderness (some surgeons avoid this incision as the scar may be painful) (Fig. 18.1: 1a).
b. A 'hockey stick' incision with the angle over the distal end of the space (this is the classical incision) (Fig. 18.1: 1b)'
c. A 'horseshoe' incision with its curve over the distal end of the space (Fig. 18.1: 1c).
d. Two lateral incisions, one on either side of the finger, made through and through in order to cut through the fibrous septa, making the cavity into one (Fig. 18.1: 1d).

Complications
1. Osteomyelitis of the terminal phalanx (see above).
2. Pyogenic arthritis of the distal interphalangeal joint
3. Spread of infection to the tendon sheath—usually as a result of an incision extended wrongly into the sheath proximally.

INFECTIONS OF MIDDLE AND PROXIMAL PULP SPACES.—These are much less common than terminal pulp space infection. Also, the pus is under less tension because the fibro-fatty tissue here is loosely packed.

An infection of the proximal pulp space often extends to a web space because the proximal pulp space freely communicates with the web space.

Treatment. Either a transverse incision over the point of maximum tenderness or two lateral incisions, communicating with each other, are made.

WEB SPACE INFECTION.—There are three web spaces between the four fingers. There are triangular spaces between the dorsal and volar skin. In between, there is loose fat which bulges between the divisions of the palmar fascia, and this fat is a favourite site for the development of abscess.

Infection of an web space gives rise to a swelling of the web which extends to the base of the adjacent finger as well as to the dorsum of the hand. The maximum tenderness is in the web and often also in the proximal pulp space (these two spaces communicate with each other).

The pus in the web space straddles the deep transverse ligament So, although the major part of the pus is volar, the abscess points dorsally.

The web space communicates proximally with the deep fascial spaces in the palm via the lumbrical canals and so the infection may extend proximally to these spaces. Here lies the danger of web space infection.

Treatment.—A transverse incision is made on the palmar surface about 1 cm. proximal to the web margin. If the incision is less than 7 to 8 mm, the digital vessels and nerves are not injured. The pus is drained by careful plunging in of a sinus forceps.

Thecal Whitlow.—This means infection of the tendon sheath, i.e. acute suppurative tenosynovitis.

SURGICAL ANATOMY.—Each finger has a fibrous sheath and a synovial sheath which cover its flexor tendons.

The *fibrous sheath* for the thumb is occupied by the tendon of flexor pollicis longus alone. In the case of the four fingers the sheaths are occupied by the tendons of superficial and deep flexors, the former splitting to spiral around the latter within the sheath. These sheaths are strong and dense over the phalanges, weak and lax over the joints. They keep the flexor tendons in apposition to the bones when the fingers are flexed.

The *synovial flexor sheaths* cover the tendons throughout their course in the fingers. Thus, distally the sheaths of all the fingers (including the thumb) extend to the distal digital crease. Proximally the sheaths of the index, middle, and ring fingers end at about the level of the metacarpophalangeal joint. The sheath of the little finger is proximally continuous with the ulnar bursa, while that of the thumb is continuous with the radial bursa (Fig. 18.2).

The *ulnar bursa* is the name given to the synovial sheath which encloses all the flexor tendons passing to the fingers (but not the thumb). Hence it is also called the common flexor sheath. Its proximal blind end extends to a level of about one inch above the wrist While its main part, enclosing the tendons of the index, middle, and ring fingers, end at about the middle of the palm (i.e. just distal to the flexor retinaculum), the medial part is prolonged to become the digital sheath of the little finger. There is a constriction where the ulnar bursa becomes continuous with the digital sheath of the little finger (Fig. 18.2).

The *radial bursa* is the upper continuation of the digital synovial sheath of the thumb, in the palm and wrist regions. Proximally it extends to the same level as the ulnar bursa, and here it may have a communication with the ulnar bursa in more than 80 per cent of cases (Fig. 18.2).

It therefore stands that while the flexor tendons of the thumb and the little finger are covered with synovial sheath from the level of the wrist to their insertion, those of the index, middle, and ring fingers lack the sheath between the proximal end of their digital sheaths and the lower end of the ulnar bursa.

PATHOLOGY.—The tendon sheaths may be infected in two ways:

a. Organisms gaining entrance with the point of a needle or other sharp objects penetrating the sheath.
b. Extension of infection into the sheath from the terminal pulp space. The organisms are usually *Staph. aureus* or *Strepto. haemolyticus*.

According to the extent of involvement, acute suppurative tenosynovitis may be of the following types:

1. Localised Suppurative Tenosynovitis.—Only one segment of the sheath is involved.
2. Acute Fulminating Tenosynovitis.—The whole length of a digital sheath is involved.
3. Infection of the Ulnar Bursa.—Usually an upward spread from tenosynovitis of the little finger. The anatomical constriction in the course of the bursa may prevent such spread.
4. Infection of the Radial Bursa.—Usually an upward spread from tenosynovitis of the thumb.
5. Infection of both Ulnar and Radial Bursae.—This may sometimes occur because of the anatomical communication that exists between the two bursae in about 80 per cent of people.

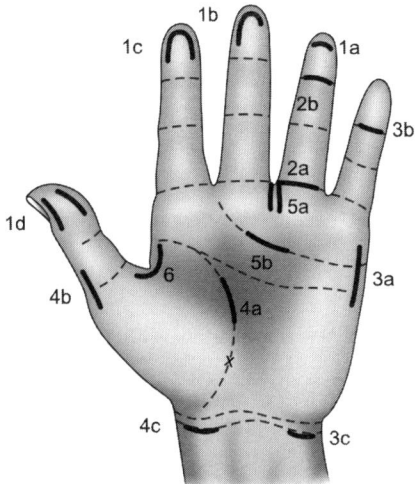

Fig. 18.1: Incisions for hand infections. 1a, 1b, 1c or 1d—for distal pulp space. 2a and 2b—for tendon sheath. 3a, 3b and 3c—for ulnar bursa. 4a, 4b and 4c—for radial bursa. 5a or 5b—for middle palmar space. 6—for thenar space. 'X' indicates the site of that branch of the median nerve which supplies the thenar muscles

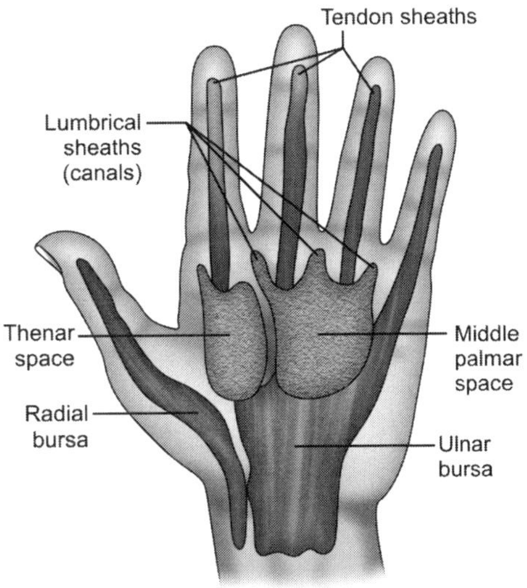

Fig. 18.2: The tendon sheaths and the deep palmar spaces. Note that the lumbrical canals are, as if, the diverticula from the middle space and thenar space

CLINICAL FEATURES

A. *Localised Suppurative Tenosynovitis* usually presents the features of a subcutaneous whitlow from which it is difficult to be differentiated prior to operation.

B. *Acute Fulminating Tenosynovitis,* which is the usual type, presents with the following features:

1. Symmetrical swelling of the entire finger, excepting the terminal phalanx (because the sheath ends at the distal digital crease).
2. Persistent flexion attitude of the finger (the *'hook' sign*), with severe pain on attempts of passive extension. In this flexed position the sheath attains maximum capacity, hence this is the position that the finger assumes.
3. Tenderness along the sheath, usually maximum at the proximal end (metacarpophalangeal joint).
4. No movement is possible in the interphalangeal joints; some movement is present in the metacarpophalangeal joint.

C. *Infection of the ulnar bursa is characterised by:*

1. Swelling:
   a. Oedema of the whole hand, especially the dorsum (due to lymphatic spread).
   b. Moderate swelling of the palm.
   c. Sometimes a swelling just above the flexor retinaculum in the wrist.
2. Flexion of fingers, with pain on extension—maximum in the little finger and minimum in the index.

3. Tenderness, maximum over that part of the ulnar bursa which lies between the two transverse palmar creases (Kanavel's sign).

D. *Infection of the Radial Bursa usually presents the following features:*
   1. Swelling:
      a. In the thumb.
      b. Sometimes in the wrist, just above the flexor retinaculum.
   2. Flexion of the thumb, with pain on attempted extension.
   3. Tenderness along the tendon of flexor pollicis longus.

TREATMENT

I. Antibiotics, preferably erythromycin, should be started immediately.
II. Rest and elevation of the limb.
III. Incision should be considered only under cover of the antibiotics, when the infection has localised.

INCISION

For the index, middle, or ring finger.—The proximal end of the sheath should be opened through a short transverse incision on the flexion crease at the root of the finger. The pus is expressed out from the distal part of the sheath by pressure on the finger (Fig. 18.1: 2a).

If the collections are extensive, a counter-incision should be placed on the distal crease in the finger, i.e. the distal end of the sheath. The sheath may be washed out with an antiseptic solution by the help of a ureteric catheter introduced through the two incisions (Fig. 18.1: 2b).

For the ulnar bursa:

1. An incision is made along the medial border of the fifth metacarpal. A gap is made between the abductor and the flexor digiti minimi; through this gap the opponens digiti minimi is cut close to the bone. The ulnar bursa is now seen the incised (Fig. 18.1: 3a).
2. If required, a counter-incision may be put on the distal digital crease of the little finger (Fig. 18.1: 3b).
3. If there is extensive collection, a third incision may be required to open the upper end of the bursa. This is a transverse incision, 1 cm above the distal crease of the wrist (medial side). If required, the flexor retinaculum has to be slit longitudinally for effective drainage (Fig. 18.1: 3c).

For the radial bursa:

1. An incision is made along the medial border of the thenar eminence on the palm (Fig. 18.1: 4a). This incision must be at least one finger's breadth distal to the flexor retinaculum in order to avoid injury to that branch of the median nerve which supplies the thenar muscles (Fig. 18.1: X).
2. A counter-incision is made along the lateral border of the proximal phalanx of the thumb (Fig. 18.1: 4b).
3. If required, a third incision is made on the upper end of the bursa. This is a transverse incision, 1 cm above the distal crease of the wrist (lateral side), if required, the flexor retinaculum has to be slit longitudinally for effective drainage (Fig. 18.1: 4c).

For localised tenosynovitis, the incision is the same as for subcutaneous whitlow over the digit where the tenderness is maximum. Care must be taken to open the sheath (cf subcutaneous whitlow where the sheath should never be opened).

Formerly it was customary to drainage tenosynovitis with extensive longitudinal incision along the finger. This invariably leads to adhesions between the tendon and the sheath, resulting in crippling. Hence such incisions are no longer advised, and these have been replaced by small transverse incisions as described above.

Apical Space Infection.—This is also known as *apical abscess* and is caused by a prick.

It is small abscess located at the tip of the finger, under the free margin of the nail. Though the abscess is very small, it is highly painful and tender.

Tenderness consists in evacuating the pus with a small incision over the most tender part. If the collection of pus under the nail is considerable, a V-shaped portion of the nail, from its free end, has to be excised.

INFECTION OF THE CELLULAR (FASCIAL) SPACES OF THE HAND

Surgical Anatomy.—The *superficial palmar space* is situated just deep to the palmar aponeurosis and is superficial to the flexor tendons. It is situated in the centre of the palm. It contains the superficial palmar arch and the digital branches of the median and ulnar nerves.

Deep palmar spaces are two in number—the *middle palmar space* and the *thenar space* (the hypothenar space is not important surgically since it contains no long flexor tendons and encloses only the hypothenar muscles).

The (deep) *middle palmar* space (Fig. 18.2) lies under the inner half of the hollow of the palm. It is triangular in shape. Its relations are as follows:

Anteriorly	1. Flexor tendons of the little, ring, and middle fingers within the ulnar bursa.
	2. The lumbrical muscles related to the tendons of the ring and little fingers, i.e. 3rd and 4th lumbricals.
Posteriorly	The 3rd, 4th and 5th metacarpals, and their related interossei.
Medially	The hypothenar muscles.
Laterally	The fibrous partition between this space and the thenar space.
Proximally	1. It reaches the level of the distal margin of the transverse carpal ligament.
	2. Sometimes this space is continuous with the Perona's space in the forearm through a small tunnel behind the flexor sheaths at the wrist.
Distally	It reaches the level of the distal palmar crease.

The *thenar space* (Fig. 18.2) lies under the lateral half of the hollow of the palm. It is also triangular in shape. Its relations are as follows:

Anteriorly	1. Flexor tendons of the index finger with their sheath.
	2. The lumbricals related to the index and middle fingers, i.e. 1st and 2nd lumbricals.
Posteriorly	The adductor pollicis.
Medially	The fibrous septum between this space and the middle palmar space.
Laterally	1. The flexor pollicis longus tendon within the radial bursa.
	2. The thenar muscles.
Proximally	It reaches the distal border of the transverse carpal ligament
Distally	It reaches the level of the proximal transverse palmar crease.

In considering the distal limits of the middle palmar and thenar spaces the following points are of importance:

1. The upper ends of the digital flexor sheaths of the middle and ring fingers extend into the midpalmar space. Similarly, the upper end of the digital flexor sheath of the index finger extends into the thenar space. Hence suppurative tenosynovitis in these sheaths may result in infection of the middle palmar and thenar spaces respectively (Fig. 18.2).

2. The lumbrical muscles have fascial sheaths which are so thin and so intimately related to the palmar spaces that infection of a space invariably spreads to the related lumbrical sheath. In other words, the lumbrical sheaths may be looked upon as diverticula of the palmar spaces. Thus the third and the fourth lumbrical sheaths are, as if, the diverticula of the middle palmar space. Similarly the first lumbrical sheath is a diverticulum from the thenar space. The second lumbrical sheath may be a diverticulum either of the thenar or of the midpalmar space (Fig. 18.1). This is the reason why abscesses in the midpalmar space are drained through incisions on the finger-webs, opening the lumbrical sheaths there.

The *dorsal spaces* contain areolar tissue which is much looser than that in the palm. Moreover, the lymphatics of the palm pass over the dorsal aspect of the palm. This is why, in all infections of the palm, there is considerable swelling and oedema of the dorsum. The palm cannot swell to this extent because its areolar tissue is not that lax.

The extensors of the fingers are connected to each other by fibrous tissue. This tissue, together with the tendons, create an aponeurotic partition which divides the dorsum of the hand into two spaces:

1. The dorsal subcutaneous space which is superficial.
2. The dorsal subaponeurotic (i.e. subtendinous) space which is deep to this partition.

Both these spaces are triangular in shape, with the base at the knuckles and the apex at the wrist.

Etiology.—Infection of these spaces may be caused by:

1. Penetrating wounds.
2. Infection in haematoma in these situations.
3. As a complication of acute suppurative tenosynovitis in case of midpalmar and thenar space infections.

Presenting Feature.—All cases present with:

1. Acute pain.
2. Constitutional symptoms.
3. Swelling.—As has already been mentioned (under surgical anatomy), any inflammation in the palm is almost always accompanied with swelling and oedema of the dorsum of the hand. This should not be wrongly diagnosed as abscess in the dorsal spaces. Only when there is persistent tenderness, redness, induration, and fluctuation on the dorsum, that an abscess of the dorsum should be thought of.

Physical Signs.—These vary according to the location of the abscess:

Infection of the Superficial Palmar Space:

1. Local tenderness.
2. The overlying skin is usually whitened and often desquamated.
3. The epidermis may be raised by a collar-stud abscess, the pus having tracked through a small opening in the palmar aponeurosis.
4. Swelling of the dorsum (oedema).

Infection of the Midpalmar Space:

1. Obliteration of the normal hollow of the palm. A bulging is usually prevented by the strong palmar aponeurosis. For the same reason fluctuation is often difficult to elicit
2. An accompanying swelling of the dorsum (oedema). In midpalmar space infection dorsal swelling is usually maximum *(frog-hand).*
3. The fingers are in flexed position (because the palmar aponeurosis is relaxed in this position).
4. Extension of the metatarsophalangeal joints is very painful but that of the interphalangeal joints is free (cf suppurative tenosynovitis).
5. If the pus bursts through the palmar aponeurosis, the palmar swelling becomes more prominent, fluctuation appears, but pain diminishes.
6. The abscess may point on a web—either between the middle and the ring finger, or between the ring and the little finger.

Infection of the Thenar Space:

1. Marked swelling on the web of the thumb and on the thenar eminence.
2. The thumb is held in abduction and flexion.
3. Extension of the thumb is painless (cf tenosynovitis).
4. The pus may point at the web of the thumb.

Treatment
  I. Antibiotics, preferably erythromycin.
 II. Rest and elevation of the limb on a sling.
III. Incision when the abscess has localised under antibiotic coven

INCISION

Superficial Palmar Space.—The incision is placed over the point of tenderness, or where there is evidence of a subcuticular collection. Wherever possible the incision is made on a palmar crease.

Middle Palmar Space:

1. The incision is placed on the free margin of the web either between the ring and the little finger, or between the middle and the ring finger. The incision is deepened to open up the lumbrical canal but must *not be carried proximally* beyond the distal palmar crease (Fig. 18.1: 5a).
2. Some surgeons make the incision on the middle third of the distal palmar crease (Fig. 18.1: 5b).

Thenar Space.—The incision is placed on the free margin of the web of the thumb and then a sinus forceps is thrust in *front* of the adductor pollicis (Fig. 18.1: 6).

Dorsal Spaces.—The incision is made over the point of maximum tenderness, or at a site where the abscess points.

INFECTION OF THE PERONA'S SPACE IN THE FOREARM

Surgical Anatomy.—This space is located in the lower part of the forearm, deep to the flexor tendons and superficial to the pronator quadratus.

Etiology.—Infection in this space usually an extension from the hand, passing through the transverse carpal ligament. Thus it is usually an extension from:
1. Suppurative tenosynovitis.
2. Middle palmar or thenar space infection.

Clinical Features
1. Brawny induration.
2. Pitting oedema.
3. Fluctuation is difficult to elicit as the abscess is situated deep.

Incision.—The pus has a tendency to travel towards the ulnar side along the ulnar vessels and nerves. Hence the incision is placed longitudinally on the medial side in front of the ulna. If required, a longitudinal counter-incision may be made in front of the radius.

STENOSING TENOVAGINITIS

Types.—This is a condition where the fibrous sheath of a tendon undergoes thickening so as to entrap the tendon. Naturally it occurs at sites where the fibrous tendon sheath is strong. The common sites of occurrence are as follows:

1. The common sheath enclosing the tendons of abductor pollicis longus and extensor pollicis brevis where they cross the radial styloid (De Quervain's disease).
2. The finger flexors at the metacarpophalangeal joints (trigger finger).
3. The flexor pollicis longus at the metacarpophalangeal joint of the thumb (trigger thumb).
4. The peroneal retinaculum enclosing the peronei, behind and below the lateral malleolus.

Deouervain's stenosing tenovaginitis

Etiology.—Not definitely known. Possibly it is due to excessive friction from over-use, e.g. wringing clothes, typing, etc.

Women are affected ten times as often as men. Middle-aged women are the commonest victims.

Pathology.—The common fibrous sheath enclosing the tendons of abductor pollicis longus and extensor pollicis brevis undergoes thickening where these tendons cross the tip of the radial styloid. The sheath is thickened to a firm nodule of the size of an orange-pip. The tendons themselves are normal.

Clinical Features

1. Middle aged women usually suffer.
2. Pain on using the hand, especially when movement tenses the abductor pollicis longus and extensor pollicis brevis.
3. There is tenderness, and often a palpable nodule, where the tendons cross the radial styloid.
4. Passive adduction of the wrist or thumb causes the patient to wince with pain (*Finkelstein's test*).

Treatment

1. *Conservative Treatment* with:
   a. Rest.
   b. Physiotherapy.
   c. Local hydrocortisone injection.
   These are usually without avail.
2. *Operative Treatment* is simple and effects complete cure. The affected part of the sheath is exposed through a transverse incision on the overlying skin. The diseased sheath is then longitudinally slit throughout the length of constriction. If the operation is done under local anaesthesia, unrestricted movements can be ascertained at operation immediately after the slitting.

Trigger finger

Etiology—Unknown. Middle-aged women are the usual sufferers. Excessive friction due to overuse may be the cause.

Pathology.—The fibrous sheath of the flexor tendon of a finger is thickened and constricted opposite the metacarpo-phalangeal joint, i.e. near the base of the finger. This results in constriction of the contained tendons at this level with swelling distal to this. Since the flexor tendons are strong, the swollen part of the tendon can be forced through the constricted sheath during flexion, without interference. But during extension, the swollen segment of the tendon enters the mouth of the constricted sheath only with difficulty, because the movement of extension is less powerful. Hence, as the finger is extended actively from the flexed position it becomes arrested at a point (the swollen tendon reaching the mouth of the constricted sheath). It has then to be passively extended a little when there is a snapping sound (*snapping finger*). Thereafter full active extension is possible.

Clinical Features

1. The patient is usually a middle-aged woman.

2. History and demonstration (by the patient herself) of locking and snapping, as described under pathology.
3. Tenderness at the base of the affected finger.
4. Occasionally a nodule (the thickened sheath) may be palpable at the base of the finger.

Treatment.—This consists in longitudinal division of the constricted and thickened part of the sheath. The approach is through a transverse incision placed on the distal palmar crease.

TRIGGER THUMB.—The features are all the same as for trigger finger but the patient is usually an infant (*contracted thumb of infants*).
Treatment is the same as for a trigger finger.

GANGLION

A ganglion is a localised, tense-cystic swelling, containing clear gelatinous fluid (resembling the white of an egg).

Origin
1. The etiology is unknown. They are sometimes predisposed to, by injury.
2. Majority of people believe that they arise from mucoid degeneration of the connective tissues in the capsule of a joint or a tendon sheath.
3. Others believe that they occur as a consequence of leakage of synovial fluid through the capsule of a joint or a tendon sheath.

Sites
1. The commonest site is the dorsal aspect of the wrist (the common *dorsal ganglion).*
2. The front of the wrist.
3. The dorsum of the foot.
4. Occasionally small ganglion develops on the flexor aspects of the fingers.

Clinical Features
1. Though the condition is usually painless, often there is considerable aching pain and tenderness when the ganglion starts developing. Ganglia on the fingers are exquisitely painful and tender.
2. The swelling is often mistaken for an exostosis because of its hard feel (tense-cystic) and close attachment to the bone. The popular site, and presence of a little mobility on the bone, confirm the diagnosis.
3. It is transillumination-positive.

Treatment
1. Sometimes *no* treatment is advocated. This is because the condition is self-limiting and, not infrequently, there is a spontaneous regression.
2. *Conservative Treatment* is gradually gaining popularity because of the chances of recurrence after operation. This may be of the following types:
   a. A blind strike on the cyst that causes its rupture (traditionally the family Bible was used in the West).
   b. *Seton method.*—The ganglion is transfixed with a stout silk suture, which is tied loosely in position and left *in situ* for a week. This allows gradual escape of the contents and simultaneously causes obliterative fibrosis.
   c. Aspiration of the cyst contents an injection into it of sclerosing agents (3 per cent sodium murrhuate) or hydrocortisone. The process has to be repeated. Immediately after the injection an elastocrepe bandaging is done.

3. *Operative Treatment,* i.e. excision of the ganglion. The ganglion must be removed completely by a careful dissection. Hence application of a tourniquet is essential in order to provide a bloodless field that allows meticulous dissection. Thus the operation should be done under general or regional block anaesthesia (instead of local infiltration). In spite of all care, recurrence is common.

COMPOUND PALMAR GANGLION

Pathology.—This means a tubercular infection (or rarely rheumatoid affection) of the ulnar bursa (cf ordinary ganglion).

It is so named because there are two swellings, one on the hollow of the palm (obliterating the normal concavity here) and another in front of the wrist. There is a constriction between the two, caused by the flexor retinaculum. That the two swellings are continuous is proved by the presence of cross-fluctuation between the two.

The contents inside are some amount of glairy fluid in which there are melon-seed bodies (resulting from fibrinous deposits). The lining membrane contains tubercular granulation tissue.

Clinical Features

1. To start with, the condition is painless; later pain supervenes.
2. In the beginning, the finger movements are only little hampered Later, as the tendons get matted, movements are grossly restricted.
3. An hour-glass swelling with cross-fluctuation, as described above, is present.
4. In some cases, the median nerve may be compressed inside the flexor retinaculum (with added features of carpal tunnel syndrome—see below).
5. In some cases, cold abscess may result from suppuration.

Treatment

1. *Conservative Treatment* is the usual rule and consists of:
   a. Immobilisation in a plaster east.
   b. A complete course of anti-tubercular treatment.
   c. Aspiration and local installation of INH solution, if required.
   Cure is not expected in less than a year.
2. *Operative Treatment.*—If no improvement occurs with conservative treatment for 3 to 4 months. With a meticulous dissection, all the diseased synovia have to be excised.

CARPAL TUNNEL SYNDROME

Pathology.—This is caused by compression of the median nerve inside the carpal tunnel. This tunnel is formed by the flexor retinaculum anteriorly and by the distal row of carpal bones posteriorly. The flexor tendons (with their covering sheaths) and the median nerve pass through this tunnel. The nerve may undergo compression in two ways:

1. Chronic inflammatory thickening of the tendon sheaths of the flexor tendons, increasing their bulk, that compresses the nerve.

2. Sometimes there is no obvious increase in the bulk of the tendons and their sheaths. In these cases probably there is a stenosing tenovaginitis of the flexor retinaculum itself.

The condition may occur in otherwise normal subjects but may be associated with:

a. Myxoedema.

b. Rheumatoid arthritis.

c. Malunited Colles' fracture.

d. Pregnancy.

Clinical Features

1. The patient is usually a female.
2. Pain, classically localised along the distribution of the median nerve. The pain is usually worse at night and often the patient notices that the pain is relieved by hanging the hand over the edge of the bed (this is diagnostic). Pain is increased if the fingers and wrist are kept fully flexed for some time.
3. Paraesthesia and numbness along the distribution of the median nerve.
4. Incoordination and, thereafter, frank weakness in the hand.
5. The fingers may feel stiff, particularly in the morning (possibly due to compression of the flexor tendons themselves).
6. All features of median nerve lesion at the wrist.
7. Slight tenderness over the flexor retinaculum.

Treatment.—Simple decompression of the tunnel, by incising the flexor retinaculum longitudinally, gives excellent results.

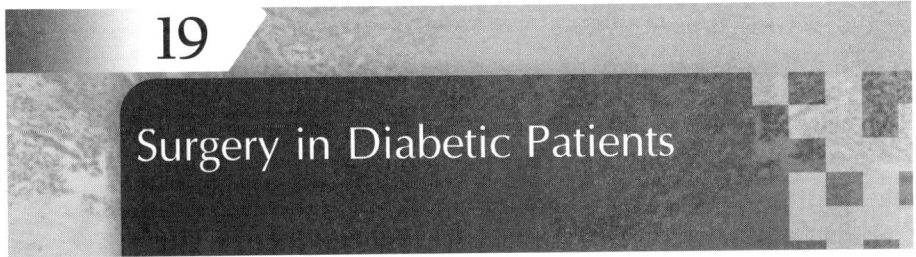

19
Surgery in Diabetic Patients

THE PRINCIPLES OF TREATMENT IN DIABETES

1. **Diet**
   a. Some carbohydrate restriction is necessary, and the amount of carbohydrate varies from patient to patient according to:
      i. the caloric requirement of the individual;
      ii. whether increase or reduction in weight is desired.
   b. In diabetics of normal weight, protein and fat intake do not need control.

2. **Weight**
   a. Elderly fat diabetics (*maturity onset diabetes*) often have much insulin in their blood but they are resistant to its action. They develop ketosis only rarely. Often the glycosuria ceases when the weight is reduced.
   b. Young patients with diabetes (*growth onset diabetes*) are often underweight. They need insulin to restore normal weight. Their blood contains no insulin (they are sensitive to its action) and they readily develop ketosis.

3. **Drugs**
   a. Insulin:
      i. *Soluble Insulin*, which is an aqueous solution of insulin. It is given subcutaneously 2 to 3 times a day, half an hour before meals. The onset of its action is after an hour, the maximum effect is reached in 2 to 3 hours, and the action lasts for 6 to 8 hours.
      ii. *Insulin Zinc Suspensions* are depot preparations, the duration of action of which is more (long-acting), depending on the size of the particle, e.g. semilente=amorphus, ultralente = crystalline, lente = a mixture of the two. Lente insulin starts working in 2 to 4 hours, has its maximum effect between 8 and 12 hours, and the duration of action is 18 to 24 hours.
      iii. *Isophane Insulin* and *Globin Zinc Insulin* are similar in action to lente insulin.
      iv. *Protamine Zinc Insulin* is also a depot preparation, being a combination of insulin with protamine and zinc, making it less soluble. It starts working in 3 to 6 hours, has its maximum effect between 14 and 20 hours, and the duration of action is 24 to 40 hours.
   b. Oral Hypoglycaemic Drugs:
      i. *Sulphonylureas*, e.g. tolbutamide (Rastinon).
      ii. *Clorpropamide* (Diabenese).
      iii. *Biguanides*, e.g. phenoformin (DBI), metformin (Glycophage).

Selection of Therapy for Diabetes—Diabetic patients may be treated in three ways:
1. Only control of diet—specially if the patient is overweight.

2. Control of diet + hypoglycaemic drugs.

3. Control of diet + insulin.

Broadly speaking, the cases may be divided as follows:

1. Diabetics *under* 30 years of age: Control of diet + insulin.

2. Diabetics *over* 30 years of age.—On an average:
   a. One third—only control of diet.
   b. One third—Control of diet + oral hypoglycaemic drugs.
   c. One third—Control of diet + insulin.

PRINCIPLES OF MANAGEMENT OF DIABETIC PATIENTS UNDERGOING SURGERY

1. Surgery and anaesthesia temporarily aggravate the state of diabetes. Therefore:
   a. For patients controlled by insulin, the dose of insulin may have to be increased to cover up effectively the stress during the pre-operative, operative, and immediate post-operative periods.
   b. For patients controlled by diet alone, insulin may have to be administered.

2. Patients controlled by long-acting insulin or by oral hypoglycaemic drugs have to be converted to soluble insulin if a major operation has to be performed

3. Injuries, especially fractures, aggravate the diabetic state similarly and require same considerations.

4. While diabetes calls in infection (excess of sugar in the tissues serves as a medium for the bacteria to grow), pent up collections of pus aggravate the state of diabetes. In such cases, while the insulin need of the patient increases, it is equally important to see that the pus is drained early.

5. In diabetic gangrene, control of infection and control of diabetes must always precede amputation, if it is necessary.

6. While operating on diabetic subjects, both ketosis and hypoglycaemia are to be carefully avoided. While hypoglycaemia is dangerous, hyperglycaemia, if not severe and prolonged, matters a little.

Operations in Diabetic Subjects.—This should be considered under three headings:

1. Planned operations.

2. Emergency operations.

3. Operations for sepsis or gangrene which develop as complications of diabetes.

PLANNED OPERATIONS

I. **General Principles**
   1. The patient should be admitted at least 3 days before the operation so that the line of control of diabetes can be adjusted according to the blood sugar estimations and urine tests.
   2. If a major surgery is proposed, the patient has to be changed from oral hypoglycaemic agents or long-acting insulin to soluble insulin.
   3. Operation should be fixed up only when the patient gets insulin controlled.

4. Glucose by mouth, or any other food, should be avoided from at least 4 hours before the operation in order to avoid post-anaesthetic vomiting.

5. The case should be fixed as the first one in the day's list, so that the pre-operative fasting and the metabolic disturbances are minimum.

6. An indwelling catheter is helpful to make urine available for examination as and when necessary.

7. Oral feeding is commenced as early as possible after the operation. Similarly, the pre-operative antidiabetic regime should be restored at the earliest opportunity (including reversion to oral hypoglycaemic drugs or to long-acting insulin).

II. **Actual Management.**—This depends on how the patient's diabetes has so long been controlled:

A. DIABETICS CONTROLLED BY DIET ONLY

1. *Pre-operative.*—As the patient is in bed rest, the diet is altered to one containing 250 calories less than his usual diabetic diet. If glycosuria of over 0.75% persists or if the blood sugar is high, a suitable dose of insulin has to be supplemented.

2. *For Minor Operations.*—Neither glucose nor insulin is necessary before, during, or after the operation if the patient has not been kept fasting for more than a few hours.

3. *For Major Operations.*—If a prolonged fasting is necessary (e.g. abdominal operations), and intravenous drip of 5% dextrose solution is started in the morning, and continued throughout the operation and postoperatively, as long as is considered necessary. The urine is tested for sugar and ketones every 3 hours. If there is ketonuria or persistent glycosuria, soluble insulin in suitable dosage is given every 4 to 6 hours.

B. DIABETICS CONTROLLED BY DIET PLUS INSULIN

1. *Pre-operative.*—As in (A) above, the diet is reduced by 250 to 500 calories. If the patient was on long-acting insulin, he is converted to only soluble insulin.

2. *For Minor Operations.*—As the patient is not allowed to take anything in the morning and for a few hours after the operation, the morning dose of insulin is omitted. In the evening, normal diet and normal dose of insulin are administered.

3. *For Major Operations:*

   a. Intravenous drip of 5% dextrose solution is started in the morning, and is continued during the operation and postoperatively as long as it is necessary, i.e. till the patient gets to oral feeding.

   b. Half of the usual morning dose of insulin is administered in the morning subcutaneously. The post-operative doses of insulin are adjusted according to the blood sugar level, and urine analysis for sugar and ketones. It should be kept in mind that ketonuria and hypoglycaemia must be cautiously avoided while a little hyperglycaemia, if short-lasting, is of a little concern.

   c. Oral feeding is commenced as early as possible. Even then the dosage of insulin is adjusted on the blood sugar level, till the patient recovers completely. Thereafter the patient is put back to his usual diet and usual insulin doses.

C. Diabetics controlled by diet plus oral hypoglycaemic drugs

1. *For Minor Operations.*—The oral hypoglycaemic drug is omitted on the day of operation.

2. *For Major Operations:*
   a. The patient has to be changed to soluble insulin and the operation is fixed only after the patient gets insulin-controlled.
   b. The management on the day of operation and postoperatively, till the patient gets to normal diet and till the wound heals, is on the same lines as in patients controlled by insulin, described in (B) above.
   c. Thereafter the patient may revert to oral hypoglycaemic drugs.

EMERGENCY OPERATIONS

1. In a Controlled Diabetic.—The operation may be undertaken immediately as in cases of planned operations described above. An additional dose of insulin may be necessary to cover up the actual operation.
2. In an Uncontrolled Diabetic.—The operation may be undertaken immediately, giving small doses of soluble insulin every 2 to 4 hours together with a 5% dextrose drip, keeping the blood glucose level between 150 and 300 mg/100 ml, but carefully avoiding ketonuria.
3. In a Case Complicated with Diabetic Ketosis.—Attempts should be made to control the ketosis before undertaking the operation. Thereafter the management is the same as in an uncontrolled diabetic.

OPERATIONS FOR DIABETIC SEPSIS AND GANGRENE

A diabetic gangrene is due to *three factors*:
1. Diminished resistance of the sugar-laden tissues to trauma and infection: The sugar serves as a medium for the bacteria to grow.
2. Atherosclerosis, resulting in circulatory impairment.
3. Trophic changes due to peripheral neuritis; sensation is impaired, so minor trauma is not appreciated by the patient or is neglected

Clinically the cases belong to two distinct categories:
1. **Moist Gangrene,** usually superimposed on a trauma or infection in an uncontrolled diabetic, often at the younger age group. The first factor, mentioned above, plays a more important role in these cases. The gangrene is of spreading type.
2. **Dry Gangrene,** usually occurring in an elderly diabetic. The second and third factors play the more important role in these cases. The gangrene is slowly progressing and there is usually a line of demarcation.

Treatment

A. *In the first group of cases:*
   1. Active control of diabetes.—Diet plus insulin.
   2. Broad spectrum antibiotics.
   3. Rest with the limb elevated.
   4. Liberal incisions to ensure drainage.—It is often found that, with drainage established, the insulin requirement comes down.

5. High-up amputation in uncontrolled spreading cases. In very toxic cases, amputation (or incisions) may have to be done with refrigeration anaesthesia.

B. *In the second group of cases:*
   1. Vasodilator methods.—Buerger's position, Buerger's exercise, vasodilator drugs.
   2. Care of the ischaemic limb.—Protection from heat or cold, pressure or trauma; reduction of muscular activity.
   3. Active control of diabetes.—Diet plus insulin.
   4. Indirect surgery to effect vasodilatation.—Sympathectomy.
   5. Amputations:
      a. *High-up amputation* when the ischaemic factor predominates (peripheral pulses absent).
      b. *Conservative amputation,* when the trophic factor predominates (peripheral pulses present).

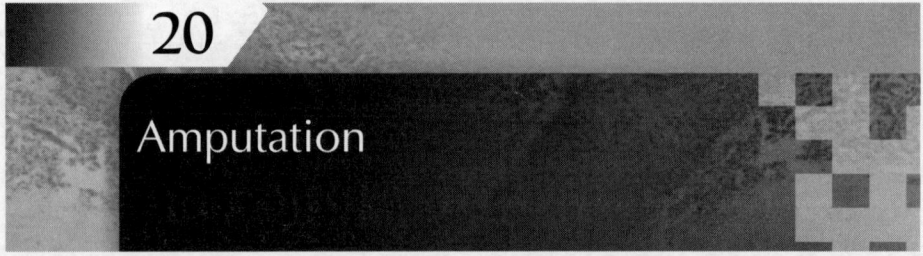

20

Amputation

Indications

A. *Congenital:*
 1. Supernumerary digits (polydactylism).
 2. Gross congenital deformity making the limb flail and useless, so much so, that an artificial limb works better.

B. *Traumatic.*—This makes the commonest indication for amputation:
 1. Grossly lacerated or gun-shot injuries of limbs, associated with irreparable damage to the main artery as well as the main nerve (all cares must be taken to see whether the artery and the nerve can be repaired).
 2. Even when the main vessel is intact, if there is such a gross laceration that uncontrollable infection is inevitable or crush syndrome (renal failure) is apprehended.
 3. Death of a limb or part of it, following ligation or repair of its main vessel after injury.
 4. Gas gangrene.
 5. Severe secondary haemorrhage, uncontrollable by other means.
 6. Incarcerated limb.
 7. Charred limb, as may occur in epileptic or unconscious patients.

C. *Vascular:*
 1. Gangrene resulting from Buerger's disease, arteriosclerotic gangrene, diabetic gangrene, or gangrene following embolism. In these cases amputation is performed as the last procedure, when sympathectomy, embolectomy, adrenalectomy, etc. fail. Even then the amputation is often conservative as compared to the high-up amputations advocated in the older days.
 2. In some cases of aneurysm where conservative surgery or reconstruction fails.

D. *Inflammatory:*
 1. Acute Inflammations, e.g.
    a. Spreading cellulitis with toxaemia, e.g. diabetic.
    b. Acute osteomyelitis or acute suppurative arthritis associated with severe toxaemia and pyaemia (rarely).
 2. Chronic Inflammations, e.g.
    a. Actinomycosis of foot, i.e. Madura foot.
    b. Deformities in fingers or toes following chronic inflammation.
    c. Chronic osteomyelitis of foot associated with gross arthritis and long-standing sinuses.

E. *Neoplastic.*—Malignant tumours in the limbs, particularly those of mesodermal origin, e.g. osteogenic sarcoma.

F. *Paralytic.*—Gross deformity and a very flail lower limb following paralysis, which makes normal work impossible, and it is thought that an artificial limb will be better. In these cases amputation should be thought of only when other reconstructive operations, e.g. muscle transplants, fail (for the upper limb the selection must be far more rigid).

The *commonest indication* for amputation is a grossly injured limb. Other rather common indications are gangrene and malignant mesodermal tumours.

Site of Election.—This indicates the level of a limb at which a stump is most suitable for an artificial limb. This is because the muscles at the stump get maximum leverage of work on the artificial limb at this level. The sites of election are as follows:

Above-knee amputations—11″ from tip of greater trochanter.

Below-knee amputations—5½″ from level of knee joint.

Above-elbow amputations—8″ from tip of acromion.

Below-elbow amputations—7″ from tip of olecranon.

The Scar.—The scar in the limb should always be transverse. A sagittal scar is painful as it has a tendency to be drawn up, particularly in the gap between two bones, e.g. forearm and leg. In older days *terminal scar*, i.e. a scar at the end of the stump, was avoided since the artificial limbs were end-bearing and would press on the scar. In those days *posterior scars* (by making longer anterior flaps) were therefore preferred. The modern artificial limbs are side-bearing so that they do not cause pressure at the end of the scar; hence a 'terminal scar' is preferred nowadays. A terminal scar has also the advantage that a long flap, with the danger of lack of vascularity, is avoided. For the upper limb, the stump, which is not weight-bearing, should ideally have a terminal scar.

Criteria for an Ideal Stump
1. It should be located at the 'site of election'.
2. It should be conical in shape having:
    a. no projecting bony spur;
    b. no redundant muscle mass.
3. It should heal by primary intention so that:
    a. the skin is not adherent to the underlying structures and therefore movements of the artificial limb on the stump do not cause pain;
    b. the skin is not in folded;
    c. neither is the skin parchment-thin, so that it might tend to break and ulcerate.
4. The joint above the stump should have full range of mobility.
5. The stump should be free from any tenderness.
6. The scar should be transversely placed and not exposed to pressure, particularly by the socket of the artificial limb (*see* above).

Methods of Amputation.—Basically, there are two methods:

A. *Guillotine Method*—Here all tissues, from the skin to the bone, are cut through at the same level. There is nothing to cover the stump, which slowly heals by granulation. Thereafter, either skin grows from the margins to cover it or a skin graft is necessary. Its disadvantages are:
    1. It takes a long time to heal.
    2. The scar is adherent to the underlying structures and, therefore, often painful.

3. The stump is not conical.
4. The cut bone end often gets infected, and may form a sequestrum (*ring sequestrum*).

Thus guillotine amputation is usually not favoured. However, it is often done (a) in presence of infection, e.g. street injuries, cellulitis, gas gangrene, etc.; in these cases, if the stump is covered with flaps, organisms particularly those of the anaerobic type get a good chance to grow under their cover, (b) where the amputation has to be performed rapidly, e.g. gas gangrene.

B. *Flap Method*—Here skin flaps are so designed that they cover up the stump, i.e. the skin is cut at a lower level than the bone. For efficient covering, on an average, the combined length of the two flaps should be 1½ times the diameter (or half the circumference) of the limb, at the level of bone section.

Since the scar is usually made transverse, the skin flaps are one anterior and one posterior. The flaps may either be made equal (*terminal scar*) or the anterior flap longer (*posterior scar*). The shape of the flape varies—circular for the arm, oval for the thigh, semicircular for the forearm and leg, and racquet for the fingers and toes.

Amputation in Presence of Infection.—When amputation is performed in presence of infection, as in street injuries, gas gangrene, etc. it should be done by guillotine method and at as much a lower level as permissible. This is called *primary amputation*. Later, when infection in the stump is overcome, the *final amputation* should be performed by the flap method and at the site of election.

Technique of Amputation.—A tourniquet is usually used to minimise the bleeding. Tourniquets should not be used in the cases where blood supply to the limb is precarious, e.g. Buerger's disease. In these cases digital compression of the main artery to the limb, by an assistant, may be conveniently used. When there is no available space for a tourniquet to be tied, the main vessels may be ligated primary at a proximal site, e.g. external iliac, subclavian, etc.

The skin flaps are planned and made; their thickness should consist of skin and subcutaneous tissue only. Thereafter, all soft tissues down to the periosteum are cut through, preferably in one sweep, with a *Syme's amputation knife*. It is better not to care for the individual structures in order to cut them separately, e.g. vessels and nerves; also there is no necessity for injecting the nerves with local anaesthetics. The periosteum is elevated just a little from the bone so that the amputation saw can work, and the bone is cut through. The sharp margins of the cut bone-end are made blunt with a bone-nibbler.

The main and anatomically known vessels are picked up and ligated. Thereafter the tourniquet is released and other bleeding points secured.

It is preferable that the muscle mass from either side be drawn over the bone-end, and sutured. This will (a) prevent pulling of the stump towards the stronger muscle, (b) make the stump more firm, and (c) prevent pressure on the skin against the bone by the artificial limb. The skin is sutured separately from the deep fascia to prevent the scar getting attached to the bone. A rubber drain should be kept under the skin at the stump. A moderately tight bandage is applied to serve for haemostasis.

Post-operatively, the stump, together with the proximal joint, must be kept immobilised for a few days. This is done either by encasing the limb in plaster of Paris or by the use of a splint.

Complications of Amputation Stump

1. *Haemorrhage.*—Reactionary or secondary.

2. *Infection.*—(a) in soft tissues; (b) at the bone end.

3. *Necrosis* of the skin flap due to loss of vascularity; later, *ulceration.*

4. *Adherent scar,* making the scar painful.

   This may be due to:

   a. infection,

   b. necrosis of skin flap,

   c. suturing the deep fascia and skin together.

5. *Stump Neuroma.*—This results from proliferation of the nerve fibres at their site of division, and occurs in all amputations. Only when a neuroma is *painful* that it is a complication.

6. *Phantom Limb.*—The patient feels that he still possesses the limb that has been amputated.

7. *Painful Phantom.*—This is more distressing. The patient has not only a false sensation of possessing the amputated limb but also feels severe pain into.

8. *Causalgia.*—There is pain, tenderness, and redness at the end of the stump. This is fairly common with finger amputations.

9. *Jactitation.*—Intermittent distressing spasms in the stump.

10. *Stiffness* of the proximal joint.

AMPUTATIONS IN THE FINGERS

Anatomical Considerations

SURFACE MARKING OF THE JOINTS

Joints	Palmar Surface	Dorsal Surface
1. Distal interphalangeal	1/4 inch distal to the crease.	1/8 inch distal to the knuckle, with the finger flexed.
2. Proximal interphalangeal.	Opposite the distal of the two creases here	1/4 inch distal to the knuckle, with the finger flexed.
3. Metacarpophalangeal	3/4 inch proximal to the crease at the finger web	1/2 inch distal to the knuckle, with the finger flexed.

INSERTION OF TENDONS

Tendon	Insertion
1. Flexor digitorum sublimis	Base of middle phalanx.
2. Flexor digitorum profundus	Base of distal phalanx.

3. Extensor digitorum	Tripartite insertion into both middle and distal phalanges.
4. Interossei	Base of proximal phalanx.
5. Lumbricals	Joins the extensor expansion on the dorsum of the proximal phalanx.

FLEXION AND EXTENSION OF THE PHALANGES

Phalanx	Flexed by	Extended by
Proximal	Lumbrical	Extensor digitorum
Middle	Flexor sublimis	Interossei
Distal	Flexor profundus	Interossei

THE INTEROSSEI.—The anatomical characteristics of the interossei are the same in the hands and feet. They are as follows:

1. Number.—There are seven interosseus muscles in each hand and each foot— 4 dorsal and 3 palmar.

2. Origin.—Each dorsal interosseus arises from two adjacent bones (metacarpals or metatarsals) while each palmar interosseus arises from one bone only (metacarpal or metatarsal).

3. Insertion.—The interossei are inserted into the dorsal extensor expansion and the base of the proximal phalanx.

4. Actions:

   a. All the interossei are the extensors of the middle and distal phalanges (by virtue of their insertion into the dorsal extensor expansion).

   b. The dorsal interossei are the abductors of the fingers while the palmar interossei are adductors of the fingers.

5. Nerve Supply.—In the hand all the interossei are supplied by the deep branch of the ulnar nerve. In the foot all are supplied by the lateral plantar nerve.

THE LUMBRICALS.—The anatomical characteristics are more or less the same in the hands and feet, and are as follows:

1. Number.—There are 4 lumbricals in each hand and each foot.

2. Origin.—From the tendons of the flexor digitorum profundus in hand, and the tendons of the flexor digitorum longus in the foot.

3. Insertion.—Into the dorsal extensor expansion and the base of the proximal phalanx.

4. Course.—In the hand they wind round the thumb side (lateral side) of the fingers while in the foot they wind round the big-toe side (medial side) of the toes.

5. Action.—They flex the proximal phalanx.

6. Nerve Supply:

   a. In the hand.—1st and 2nd supplied by the median; 3rd and 4th supplied by the ulnar.

   b. In the foot.—1st supplied by the medial planter; 2nd, 3rd, and 4th supplied by the lateral planter.

STRUCTURE OF THE JOINTS.—The capsule of the metacarpophalangeal joint and that of the interphalangeal joint is strongly reinforced on the palmar aspect by the tough palmar ligament. On the dorsal aspect the capsule is deficient, its place being taken by the dorsal extensor expansion. So during the process of disarticulation, the joints are opened from their dorsal surface.

ARTERIAL SUPPLY.—There are four palmar digital arteries, arising from the superficial palmar arch. The most medial of them supplies the medial side of the little finger. The other three run towards the subsequent webs, and each divides into two branches which supply adjacent sides of the fingers. The lateral side of the index finger is supplied by the arteria radialis indicis (branch of radial artery). The arteria princeps pollicis (branch of radial artery) supplies one branch to each side of the thumb.

General Principles in the Amputation of Fingers

1. Ordinarily, the aim of the surgeon is to conserve as much tissue as is possible. Thus, instead of aiming at standard amputations, each case should be judged on its own merit The exceptions to this rule are:

   a. In the index finger.—A stump having less than one and a half phalanges is not only useless by itself but also prevents the middle finger from taking up the functions of the index finger. Thus, if it is impossible to preserve at least one and a half phalanges, it is better to remove the index finger as a whole.

   b. In the little finger.—A short stump is useless and so, instead of performing amputation through the proximal phalanx, disarticulation through the metacarpophalangeal joint is preferred.

   c. While performing disarticulation of the metacarpophalangeal joints, many surgeons advocate removal of the metacarpal head as well. Its advantage is that it makes the deformity, resulting from the loss of a finger, less conspicuous. Its disadvantage is that it reduces the gripping power of the hand because the integrity of the metacarpal arch is destroyed. Thus, for manual workers, the metacarpal heads must be preserved.

2. Wherever possible, amputation through a phalanx is preferable to disarticulation. This preserves the attachment of the flexor and extensor tendons at the base of the phalanx, and thus maximal power is retained in the stump.

3. After amputation, the flexor and extensor tendons should never be sutured to each other across the stump, because this procedure limits the movements of the other fingers.

4. The skin flaps should be comparatively long because the bones of the fingers are wide and the surrounding soft tissue scanty. Whenever possible the scar should be placed on the dorsal aspect by making a long palmar flap (a scar on the palmar, i.e. tactile surface, is subject to pressure and, if painful, it interferes with the grip).

Amputation Through the Terminal Phalanx.—As has already been said, amputation through the phalanx distal to the insertions of the flexor and extensor tendons is always preferable to removal of the whole phalanx, i.e. disarticulation through the distal interphalangeal joint.

The distal interphalangeal joint is flexed by holding the tip of the finger. A transverse incision is made on the dorsal surface about ¼ inch distal to the knuckle. This extends to the lateral border of the finger on each side. A long palmar flap is now made with two lateral incisions, each commencing from either end of the dorsal incision and extending to near the tip of the finger. The ends of the these two lateral incisions are joined by another transverse incision on the palmar end of the finger. The vascularity of the long palmar flap is maintained if:

a. The two lateral incisions are placed behind the position of the digital vessels.
b. The flap is raised with the fatty pulp, i.e. keeping the knife close to the phalanx.
c. The end of the flap is rectangular in shape, and not pointed.

The bone is cut distal to the attachment of the tendons at its base. The palmar and dorsal skin flaps are sutured on each on the dorsal surface of the finger.

Disarticulation through the distal Interphalangeal Joint.—The distal interphalangeal joint is flexed by holding the tip of the finger. A transverse incision is made on the dorsal surface about 1/8 inch distal to the knuckle (this is the level of the joint). The palmar flap is fashioned in the same way as for amputation through the distal phalanx.

The dorsal incision is deepened and, as this is done, the knife goes through the joint after cutting the flattened extensor tendon. The phalanx is now pulled out and the knife is made to cut distally along the palmar aspect of the phalanx, thus making the palmar flap. The phalanx is removed, and the skin flaps sutured.

Amputation through the Middle Phalanx.—A racquet-shaped incision is made with the handle along the middle of the dorsum of the finger. The blade of the racquet is so made that there is a long palmar flap, sufficient to cover the stump and to meet the dorsal flap on the dorsal surface of the amputated finger. (Fig. 20.1: 1).

The bone is cut distal to the insertion of the tendons at its base. The digital vessels should be secured.

Disarticulation through the Proximal Interphalangeal Joint.—The technique is the same as for amputation through the middle phalanx (Fig. 2.1: 1), The joint is

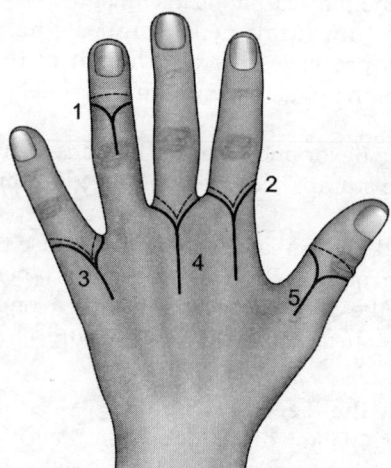

Fig. 20.1: Incisions for amputations in the fingers. 1. Amputation through the middle phalanx or disarticulation through the proximal interphalangeal joint; 2 and 3. Disarticulation through the metacarpophalangeal joint of the index and little fingers respectively (in these fingers this is preferred to amputation through the proximal phalanx; 4. Amputation through the proximal phalanx, which is preferred to metacarpophalangeal disarticulation in the middle and ring fingers; 5. Removal of the thumb.

opened from the dorsal surface where the capsule is deficient and the phalanx is removed. The digital vessels should be secured.

Amputation through the Proximal Phalanx.—As has already been said, this is seldom advisable for the index and little fingers, where disarticulation through the metacarpophalangeal joint is preferred instead. For this middle and the ring fingers however this is preferably to disarticulation because, however short the stump may be, it prevents deviation of the other fingers towards the amputated finger.

A racquet-shaped incision is made with the handle of the racquet placed along the midline of the dorsum of the metacarpal. The blade of the racquet is made with a long palmar flap, sufficient to cover the stump (Fig. 20.1: 4).

The bone is cut distal to the insertion of the tendons at its base. The digital vessels should be secured.

Disarticulation through the Metacarpophalangeal Joint.—A racquet-shaped incision is made with the handle of the racquet placed along the midline on the dorsum of the metacarpal. The blade of the racquet is made with a long palmar flap, sufficient to cover the stump (Fig. 20.1: 2 and 3).

The joint is opened from the dorsal surface (where the capsule is deficient) and the finger is removed. The digital vessels are secured.

Whether the metacarpal head should be excised is a matter of controversy (see above).

Amputations in the Thumb.—The thumb is functionally as valuable as all the other fingers taken *together*. Therefore, all attempts should be made to preserve the thumb or maximum part of it. Even a very short stump, composed of the metacarpal (or its part) alone, is a valuable asset to the patient. Thus, every case should be judged on its individual merit, and no formal amputation should be advocated.

The techniques of amputation and disarticulation are the same as for the other fingers (Fig. 20.1: 5).

AMPUTATIONS IN THE TOES

Anatomical Considerations
SURFACE MARKING OF THE JOINTS

Joint	Site
Distal interphalangeal	1/8-inch distal to the joint prominence on the dorsum.
Proximal interphalangeal	1/4-inch distal to the joint prominence on the dorsum.
Metatarso-phalangeal	1 inch proximal to the free border of the web.
Interphalangeal joint of the great toe.	Midway between the base of the nail-fold and the joint prominence.

STRUCTURE OF THE JOINT.—The capsules of the metatarsophalangeal and interphalangeal joints are strongly reinforced on their plantar aspect by the tough plantar ligament (in the case of the first metatarsophalangeal joint the ligament is replaced by two sesamoid bones). On the dorsal aspect, the capsule is deficient, its place being taken by the expanded extensor tendon.

THE INTEROSSEI AND THE LUMBRICALS.—*See* amputations in the fingers.

General Principles in the Amputation of Toes

1. Ordinarily, the aim of the surgeon is to conserve as much tissue as is possible and so, instead of aiming at standard amputations, each case should be judged on its own merit. The great toe is of particularly importance in this respect.
2. The head of the first metatarsal is of great importance in weight bearing and no effort should be spared to save it.
3. Whenever possible, amputation through a phalanx is preferable to disarticulation. This preserves the attachment of the flexor and extensor tendons at the base of the phalanx, and thus maximum power is retained in the stump.
4. The skin flaps should be comparatively long. The scar should be placed on the dorsum, by making a long plantar flap.

Amputation through the Distal Phalanx of the Great Toe.—The incision and the making of flaps are the same as they are for the fingers. A long plantar flap is made, and while cutting the flap, the knife is kept close to the bone thus avoiding injury to the plantar digital arteries which provide blood supply to the flap. The bone is cut distal to the insertion of the tendons at its base.

Disarticulation (i.e. Removal) of the Distal Phalanx of the Great Toe.—The incision is the same as above. The joint is opened from the plantar surface (cf the fingers).

Amputation through the Proximal Phalanx of the Great Toe.—A racquet-incision is made. The handle, about 1/2 inch long, is placed well to the lateral side of the midline of the metatarsal, on the dorsum. The blade of the racquet encircles the toe obliquely, making a long medial flap, whose summit extends almost as far distally as the interphalangeal joint. This procedure provides a scar, free from pressure.

The digital arteries are secured. The long tendons are divided. The phalanx is divided just distal to its base.

Disarticulation of the Proximal Phalanx of the Great Toe.—The incision is the same as above. The joint is opened from the plantar surface. The sesamoid bones are preserved.

Partial Amputation in the Other Toes.—These are carried out in the same way as in the great toe. Amputation through a phalanx is always preferable to disarticulation, since the tendon insertions are preserved.

Some surgeons advocate complete removal of a toe in preference to partial amputation, with the idea that the stump is useless for weight bearing, and tends to become dorsiflexed and come in the way. This view is generally discarded. The stump at least acts as a spreader, and keeps the adjacent toes in normal alignment. Dorsiflexion of the stump can easily be prevented by tenotomy of the extensor tendon.

Disarticulation (i.e. Complete Removal) of the Lateral Four Toes.—A racquet-shaped incision is made in each case.

In case of the middle three toes, the handle of the racquet is in the midline on the dorsum of the metatarsal concerned and the blade is so made that there is a long plantar flap.

In case of the little toe, the handle of the racquet is placed well medial to the midline of the metatarsal on the dorsum, and the blade is so made that there is a long lateral flap. This procedure provides a scar, free from pressure.

The metatarsophalangeal joints are opened from their plantar surface. It should be noted that these joints are located much more proximally than one would expect.

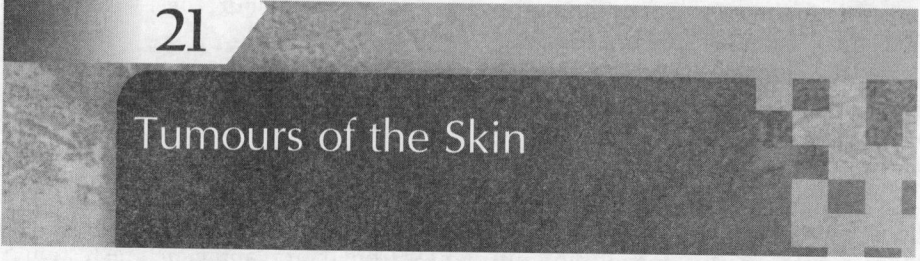

21

Tumours of the Skin

The different tumours that may arise from the skin are as follows:
1. Papilloma.
2. Squamous cell carcinoma.
3. Basal cell carcinoma.
4. Melanoma—benign and malignant.
5. Preinvasive carcinoma, i.e. carcinoma *in situ*.
6. Tumours of the dermis:
    a. from blood vessels,
    b. from muscles.
7. Tumours of dermal appendages:
    a. from sweat glands,
    b. from sebaceous glands,
    c. from hair follicles.

PAPILLOMA

Although essentially an epithelial structure, this benign epithelial tumour always includes connective tissue element that forms a core of blood vessels and lymphatics, on which the epithelium is laid down. A papilloma may arise in any situation from an epithelial surface, and the epithelium contained in it is of the same histological character as that of the epithelial surface from which it arises:

1. From the epidermis.—Papilloma of the skin, i.e. cutaneous papilloma (squamous cell or basal cell type).

2. From mucous membrane:
    a. From mucous membrane of squamous cell type.—Tongue, mouth, larynx, oesophagus, vagina.
    b. From mucous membrane of transitional cell type.—Bladder, renal pelvis.
    c. From mucous membrane of columnar cell type.—Colon and rectum (commonest), stomach, small intestine, gall bladder.
3. From the wall of ducts, as in breast.
4. From the wall of cysts, as in breast or ovary.

Papilloma of the Skin.—A cutaneous papilloma may arise:

1. From squamous cell.
2. From basal cell.

SQUAMOUS: CELL PAPILLOMA.—There are four types
1. *Infective Papilloma* or *Infective Wart*—the common wart (discussed).
2. *Congenital Papilloma*—single or multiple, seen at or immediately after birth.
3. *Soft Papilloma*— that is sometimes seen on the eyelids of elderly people.
4. *Keratin Horns*—also seen in the elderly people; there is excess of keratin formation.

The commonest of these squamous papillomata is the infective wart. This is a disease principally of the children or adolescent and is caused by a virus. It affects especially the fingers and palm, and the sole. Those in the sole *(plantar warts)* usually occur on the pressure points, particularly under the head of the second metatarsal, and may be mistaken for a corn.

The infective wart has a tendency to regress by itself but equally a tendency to recur after removal. The outlines of treatment are:
a. Change of shoes, the shoes being disinfected with formalin vapour.
b. Change to cotton socks which can be boiled.
c. Nightly application of formaldehyde on the wart may cure it.
d. Curettage of the wart is a more sure treatment, but there may be a relapse.

BASAL CELL PAPILLOMA.—These are also known as *seborrhoeic warts or senile warts* and occur in persons past middle age.

WARTS

There are 3 types of warts:
1. Infective Warts of children and adolescents.
2. Senile Warts.
3. Venereal Warts or *papilloma acuminata* or *moist warts.*

Infective warts and senile warts have been discussed above, under papilloma. Venereal warts are caused not by gonococci but by a superadded virus. They occur most commonly in the coronal sulcus of the penis, but may occur anywhere on the penis, as well as in the anal region, scrotum, and perineum. Characteristically, they are multiple and moist, with an offensive serous discharge. They are treated:
a. By fulguration with a diathermy.
b. By podophyllin.—A 10 to 20 per cent solution in tinct. benzoin is used.

CORN

(French *corn* = grain)
This is a localised hyperkeratosis of the skin, clinically characterised by the following features:
a. A horny induration of the cuticle with a hard centre.
b. Occurring at sites of undue pressure—usually the sole and toes, and the occupational pressure-points.
c. Sometimes painful.
d. A notorious tendency to recur after excision.

Treatment
1. Change to shoes with elastic-covered sole.
2. Prevention of infection, particularly in diabetic patients.

3. Application of salicylic acid in collodion on successive nights may be beneficial
4. Excision may have to be performed but recurrence is very common. Proper care must be taken to remove the central core.

A callosity is a localised hardened skin due to hyperkeratosis, caused by friction, often occupational, e.g. gardener's hand.

SQUAMOUS CELL CARCINOMA

The tumour is also known as epidermoid carcinoma and *epithelioma*.

Origin

1. Some tumours grow *de novo,* on healthy skin.
2. Others grow on skin that has been exposed for a long period to some form of irritation—mechanical, chemical, thermal, bacterial or X-ray:
   a. Chronic skin lesions, e.g. eczema, wart, lupus vulgaris.
   b. Chronic ulcers, e.g. Marjolin's ulcer following burn.
   c. Areas exposed to irradiation.
   d. Prolonged irritation by chemicals, e.g. dyes, tar.
3. Some develop from a basal cell carcinoma (*baso-squamous carcinoma*).

Site.—The tumour may occur anywhere on the skin but the favourite sites are the mucocutaneous junctions, e.g. lip, penis, vulva, etc.

Pathology.—The tumour starts as a small nodule which soon breaks to form a typical malignant ulcer—raised from the surface, with rolled out everted margins, and induration at the base.

Microscopically, solid clumps of epithelial cells are seen growing irregularly downwards into the dermis. In the centre of many of these clumps, the cells degenerate and are converted into a hyaline structureless mass of keratin. At the periphery of the clumps, the cells often take the characteristic 'prickle cell' appearance. These peculiar masses, composed of central keratin and peripheral prickle cells, are known as *cell nests* or *epithelial pearls*. Presence of these structures indicates cellular differentiation and, therefore, a low grade of malignancy.

Spread.—The spread is generally slow:
1. Direct Spread.
2. Lymphatic Spread.
   The rate varies with the site of the primary lesion. It is earlier with the cancers of foot, face and neck, as compared to those of the hand of an old person.
3. Venous Spread.—Very rare (usually never occurs).

Special Investigations
1. Biopsy, to confirm the diagnosis and to ascertain the degree of differentiation.
2. Local X-ray, to find if the underlying bone has been involved.
3. X-ray chest.

Treatment
A. Treatment for the primary growth:
   1. *Surgery.*—Wide excision with skin grafting.
   2. *Radiotherapy.*—Particularly indicated for growths not invading the bone.
B. Treatment for the regional lymph nodes.—*See* Chapter 14.

BASAL CELL CARCINOMA (RODENT ULCER)

Discussed under ulcers (*see* Chapter 11).

THE MELANOMAS

Melanomas are tumours containing melanin pigment. It is necessary to remember that there are certain pigmented lesions of the skin which should be distinguished from melanoma:

1. The common 'blue naevus' which is a smooth, hairless, rounded, dark-blue nodule, typically seen to the face or the back of hand, is not a melanoma. It consists of masses of spindle cells, possibly neurogenic in origin.
2. Squamous cell papilloma (wart).
3. Pigmented basal cell papilloma.
4. Pigmented basal cell carcinoma.
5. Sclerosing angioma.

The **Physiology of Pigmentation**—The pigment melanin is normally found in:

a. Skin (the whole body in the coloured people, and the nipple, areola, perineum and axilla in the whites).
b. Choroid coat of the eye.
c. Mucous membranes close to the skin surface.
d. Substantia nigra.
e. Telachoroidea.

Melanin is derived from the essential amino-acid tyrosine. Tyrosine is first converted into a colourless substance DOPA (dihydroxy phenylalanine). HOPA reaches the pigment-forming cells (*see* below), wherein it is converted into melanin by the action of an enzyme *dopa-oxydase, which these cells contain.*

The pigment-forming cells are the melanoblasts and melanocytes (the mature form of the melanoblasts). There are two views about their origin:

a. *The Epithelial Theory.*—The cells are derived from the surface epithelium, i.e. epidermis.
b. *The Neurogenic Theory.*—The cells are derived from the neuroectoderm of the neural crest (this view has more supporters).

Melanoblasts and melanocytes are capable of producing pigment, as they contain dopa-oxydase. They are located in the epidermis. The cells are dendritic so that, though they are apparently separate, they actually communicate with each other via these dendritic processes. They lie intercalated between the basal cells of the epidermis.

The melanin, produced by these cells, is partly contained in the melanoblasts and melanocytes, and is partly transmitted to:

i. the adjacent basal cells.
ii. the dermal macrophages (phagocytes).

These basal cells and macrophages only carry melanin which they cannot produce because they do not contain the enzyme dopa-oxydase. They are called *melanophores.* Thus, while melanoblasts and melanocytes are dopa-positive, melanophores are dopa-negative.

The production of melanin is controlled by the hormone, MSH (melanocyte-stimulating hormone) of pars intermedia of the pituitary.

BENIGN MELANOMAS

The other terms applied to benign melanoma are mole, naevus, and simple melanocytic tumours.

Histogenesis.—In normal skin the melanoblasts and melanocytes are located in the epidermis. In melanotic conditions the first and constant change is an increase in number of these cells (tumour cells), but they still keep limited within the epidermis. Depending on the nature of further proliferation of these tumour cells, the benign melanomas are classified as follows.

Types

1. Lentigo.—When the cells proliferate throughout the epidermis.
2. Junctional Naevus.—When the cells proliferate only in the deepest layers of the epidermis against the basement membrane.
3. Intradermal Naevus.—When the cells proliferate down into the dermis and then completely get detached from the epidermis. They are, therefore, totally located in the dermis.
4. Compound Naevus.—When the cells proliferate into the dermis but still keep their attachment to the epidermis. They are, therefore, partly located in the epidermis and partly in the dermis. Most of the melanomas of the childhood belong to this variety. As puberty is reached, these tumours either get limited to the dermis, or to the deepest layers of the epidermis against the basement membrane. In other words, at puberty, a compound naevus changes either to an intradermal naevus or to a junctional naevus, the former being much the commoner. Thus, compound naevus may be stated to be just representing a transitional phase.

Intradermal Naevus.—This is the commonest melanoma in the adults. Though distributed widely over the body, and intradermal naevus is seldom found in the palm, sole, or external genitalia. They may be:

a. Flat or raised from the surface.
b. If raised—smooth or warty.
c. Hairless or hairy.

In the tumour the melanoma cells are located completely inside the dermis.

This variety virtually never turns malignant because:

 i. Only the epidermal component of a naevus can undergo malignant change and there is no epidermal component in this variety.
 ii. The melanoma cells here gradually loose the property of proliferation and melanin synthesis (they are called *naevus cells*).

Junctional Naevus.—The melanoma cells are located in the deepest layers of the epidermis at its junction with the dermis, so the tumour is called 'junctional'. The points of importance in a junctional naevus are:

1. It is common on the palm, sole, or external genitalia, at which sites an intradermal naevus only rarely occurs.
2. This variety may change to malignancy, although majority of them remain benign throughout.

3. Malignant change, if any, in a junctional naevus almost invariably occurs in the adults and is an utmost rarity before puberty. Sometimes a junctional mole may show rapid progress before puberty and then it may be mistaken for a malignant change. This type, which is termed 'juvenile melanoma', is actually not a malignant melanoma, and differs from it in the following respects:

a. It occurs at or before puberty, while malignant change in a melanoma is an utmost rarity at this age.

b. Its progress is arrested after some time, when it either becomes static or regresses.

c. Microscopically, there is no irregular proliferation of the melanocytes into the dermis and there is considerable amount of round cell infiltration.

4. Occasionally, at the margin of the junctional mole, small coloured spots are seen. These are the 'skip areas', possibly representing involvement of peripherally placed cells that form part of the melanocyte dendritic network.

Compound Naevus.—The melanoma cells are partly located in the deepest layers of the epidermis and partly in the dermis. Majority of moles in childhood belong to this variety. At puberty, almost all of them change to intradermal naevus and only a few to junctional type. Compound naevus is only rarely found in the adults but these are the cases which hold the greatest risk of malignancy.

Treatment for Benign Melanomas.—No treatment is necessary for any of the above varieties, including the junctional. Treatment, which always means surgical excision, may be required:

1. If the mole is exposed to repeated trauma, e.g. cut when shaving.

2. For cosmetic reasons;

3. If malignant change is suspected (*see* below).

MALIGNANT MELANOMA

Origin

1. May arise '*de novo*' in an area of skin which, to the naked eye, was normal.

2. More commonly, arises as a secondary malignant change in a benign melanoma. It should be remembered that only the epidermal component of a naevus can change to malignancy and this is one reason why an intradermal naevus virtually never turns malignant. Malignant changes, therefore, may occur in a naevus which has epidermal component in it, viz.

a. Junctionai naevus.

b. Lentigo.

c. Compound naevus persisting in an adult.

Features Suggesting Malignant Change in a Benign Mole

1. Rapid increase in size.

2. Increase in the intensity of pigmentation.

3. Appearance of a halo of pigment in the surrounding skin. This is called the *Melanotic halo* and is due to spread of the tumour peripherally. The spread occurs through the epidermis, along the junctional layers.

4. Itching, which results in erosion and then ulceration.
5. Oozing or bleeding from the surface and crust formation.

Etiological Factors

1. *Sunlight.*—Exposure to sunlight has been incriminated most. The UV_c component of ultraviolet of the sunlight is held responsible. It causes nuclear damage and collagen disruption in the skin, favouring malignancy.
2. *Race.*—Common in the white races, especially those of them who live in hot climates.
3. *Family.*—Only occasionally hereditary.
4. *Sex.*—Equal distribution in the two sexes.
5. *Sites:*
   a. Lower limb, trunk, upper limb, head and neck, and genitalia in that order of frequency.
   b. Mucosal melanoma may occur in the mouth, anal canal, vagina and urethra.
   c. Subungual melanoma is a streak of dark pigmentation under the nail.
   d. Melanoma may arise in the choroid coat of the eye.
   e. Occult melanoma may sometimes be encountered when the patient presents with secondary lymph nodes or haematogenous dissemination while the primary site remains undetected.
6. *Site and Sex.*—There is a predilection for the trunk in the males and the lower limb in females.

Microscopic Features

1. The melanoblasts and melanocytes proliferate in the deeper layers of the epidermis and also grow down very irregularly into the dermis.
2. There is usually an increased pigmentation in the cells.
3. There is round cell infiltration in the dermis.

A. Usual types.—Three main types are encountered:

1. *Superficial Spreading Melanoma (SSM).*—Flat, irregular, black, spreading pigmentation of the skin. There is a tendency for *lateral spread*. Lymph node metastasis is rare unless nodules appear in the primary lesion. Intermittent itch occurs but pain and bleeding are uncommon.
2. *Nodular Melanoma.*—A rapidly growing black lump. There is more a tendency for *vertical spread* than lateral. Early lymph node metastasis is usual. Itching, pain, bleeding and ulceration are commoner than SSM.
3. *Hutchinson's Melatic Freckle (HMF).*—This is an irregular flat pigmented lesion found in the skin of the cheek or temple of elderly people. After more than ten years a blue or black nodule develops in some part of the lesion and this is the malignant change. The lesion is slow-growing, and lymph node metastasis is rare and late.

B. Uncommon types:

1. *Amelanotic Melanoma.*—The typical black colour of a melanoma is not seen and this may cause difficulty in diagnosis. However, on closer examination, traces of pigment are usually seen.
2. *Ring Melanoma.*—There is a central depigmented zone. The tumour is slow-growing and usually does not form metastasis.
3. *Ulcerating Melanoma.*—There is a rapidly growing, fleshy ulcerated tumour.

4. *Tumour with Satellites* (*see below*).

5. *Multiple Primary Tumours* may rarely be found.

Spread

1. DIRECT SPREAD:
   a. From their original site the tumour cells grow peripherally through the epidermis (in the junctional layer), and thus produce the melanotic halo.
   b. The deep fascia acts as a strong barrier against infiltration for some period
   c. Melanoma has a special tendency to form satellite nodules in and under the skin around. The satellites develop at progressively greater distances from the primary tumour. These may be of two types:
      i. *Epidermal.*—Caused by involvement of the cells lying at more and more peripheral parts of the melanocytic dendritic network, in the basal layer of the epidermis.
      ii. *Lymphatic.*—Caused by lymphatic permeation. The tumour cells grow along the lymphatics in the dermis and subcutaneous tissues, and form nodules at distances. These nodules come to the surface.

2. LYMPHATIC SPREAD.—This is a dreadful route of spread and usually occurs early. The regional nodes are involved in two ways:
   a. By *embolism*.
   b. By *permeation*.—The spread by permeation is important in two senses:
      i. It is a cause for the formation of satellite tumours.
      ii. It makes surgery difficult. To make the operation radical, the standard surgery in the past was *en bloc* removal of the tumour, the regional nodes and, *in continuity*, a wide connecting strip consisting of the skin, subcutaneous tissues and deep fascia (containing these lymphatic channels). However, this procedure has now been abandoned.

3. HAEMATOGENOUS SPREAD.—This is also frequent, and the structures involved are:
   a. Skin of an area, outside the area of lymphatic drainage of the primary (commonest).
   b. Lung.
   c. Liver.
   d. Brain.
   e. Bones.
   f. Breast.
   The secondary tumours may sometimes be amelanotic.

Clinically Staging.

Stage I: Primary lesion only; no metastatic nodes.

Stage II: Primary lesion with clinically significant nodes.

Tumour Thickness.—Breslow introduced measurement of tumour thickness to denote the extent of the growth and this is now believed to be of utmost importance in the classification and management of melanomas. A simple vertical measurement through the centre of the tumour is done. There is definitely a close relationship between the tumour thickness and the prognosis.

Special Investigations

1. X-ray chest.

2. Biopsy.—75% of the cases can be diagnosed clinically. Even then a biopsy is essential. It is always an excision biopsy. Incision biopsy and needle biopsy are dangerous in that there is the risk of transfer of melanoma cells to the subcutaneous fat, converting a superficial melanoma into deep melanoma. Scrap biopsy from the surface often provides false negative results. While doing the excision biopsy, a margin of at least 2 mm of healthy skin on all sides must be included. Facilities of freeze section are always beneficial since the definitive treatment can be instituted immediately in the biopsy-positive cases, thus minimising risks of dissemination (melanoma cells have a notorious tendency to grow rapidly in the subcutaneous fat). If freeze-section is not available, the definitive surgery must be undertaken at the earliest.

Treatment

I. SURGERY.—This is the mainstay of treatment. Surgical management of melanoma consists of:

1. Biopsy of suspected lesions.
2. Adequate excision of the primary tumour.
3. Block, dissection of the nodes:
   a. Prophylactic
   b. Therapeutic
4. Excision of troublesome metastatic lesions.

1. *Biopsy.*—Already discussed.

2. *Adequate excision of the primary: lesion.*—The extent of excision is made out on the tumour thickness:

   a. If the tumour thickness is less than 0.75 mm—a margin of 2 mm clearance on all the sides is sufficient. In practice, therefore, excision biopsy has done the definitive excision.

   b. If the tumour thickness is more than 1 mm, a wider excision, with an all-round clearance of 3 cm has to be done. A primary closure of the gap has to be done and this is done either by rotation flap or by split-skin graft. The graft should always be taken from the contralateral limb. The donor area may show recurrences if the skin is taken from the same limb. This is possibly because of diversion of the tumour cells, contained in the injured lymphatics, to the raw surface, where they proliferate.

3. *Block dissection of the nodes.*—This may be prophylactic and therapeutic:

   1. In Stage I cases (no signifiant nodes) if the tumour thickness is more than 2 mm a prophylactic node dissection is advisable since this procedure definitely increases the 5-year survival rate. In these cases the standard inguinal block dissection is sufficient (axillary block dissection has to be done for the upper limb).

   2. In Stage II cases (with significant nodes) block dissection is obligatory. However, in these cases, the dissection has to be more radical. Apart from the inguinal nodes, the iliac nodes have to be resected (up to the bifurcation of the common iliac vessels). This is done by dividing the inguinal ligament.

   Only where the primary lesion is close to the lymph nodes, e.g. on the face or neck, near the axilla or groin, that a block dissection is performed *in continuity* with the primary growth. Otherwise it is not necessary to resect the lymphatics in the intervening part between the primary growth and the nodes.

4. *Excision of troublesome metastatic lesions:*
   a. A painful or ulcerated subcutaneous metastasis may be excised.
   b. Isolated pulmonary or cerebral metastasis may be excised.
   c. A very big lesion may be excised just to remove the tumour bulk prior to radiotherapy or chemotherapy.

II. RADIOTHERAPY.—Malignant melanoma is usually radio-resistant. However, in inoperable cases radiotherapy may be tried. It has been found that response is better if large dose fractions (400–800) radians) are used instead of the standard 200 radian fractions. Radiotherapy is especially beneficial in the treatment of bone and cerebral secondaries.

III. CHEMOTHERAPY.—This is of very limited value. The standard chemotherapeutic agent for malanoma is dimethyl-triazine—imidazole+carboxamide (DTIC). Only 20 per cent of the cases respond and even then the duration of remission is very short.

IV. IMMUNOTHERAPY.—This is still in the experimental stage. Interferon and interleukins are being tried. Up till now the results are not encouraging.

LIPOMA

This is a benign tumour made of fat cells of adult type. This is the commonest tumour of the body and, because of its wide distribution, it is *sometimes* termed *universal tumour*.

Macroscopic Types

1. Encapsulate.—The vast majority of lipoma are of this variety.
2. Diffuse (*pseudo-lipomal*).—Occasionally occurs in the subcutaneous and intermuscular tissues of the neck. It is not a true tumour but a localised overgrowth of the fat in this region and therefore it possesses no capsule. It gives rise to a bulky collar-like swelling.
3. Multiple.—Occasionally lipomas are multiple (*lipomatosis*). Sometimes these are painful and in these instances they often contain nerve tissue in them (*neurolipoma*). Dercum's disease (*adiposis dolorosa*), a condition in which there are tender lipomatous swellings, especially on the trunk and hips, possibly belongs to the group of neurolipoma.

Combinations.—Sometimes a lipoma may contain considerable amount of other tissues, e.g.

1. Fibrous tissue—fibrolipoma.
2. Vascular element—Naevolipoma or haemangiolipoma.
3. Nerve tissue—neurolipoma (described above).
4. Myxomatous, cartilagenous, or xanthomatous element.

Sarcomatous change in a lipoma is exceedingly rare but primary liposarcoma (i.e. *de novo*) is not so uncommon.

Liquefaction or calcification may sometimes occur in lipoma of long duration.

Classification according to Anatomical Situation.—The encapsulated lipomas are classified according to their anatomical situations as follows:

1. Subcutaneous.—This is the commonest variety. It may occur anywhere but the usual sites are the shoulder, back, buttock, and supraclavicular regions. The characteristic features of the swelling are:
   a. Lobulated and well-demarcated.

    b. Freely mobile in both axes.

    c. The overlying skin is often loosely attached at one or more points, thus showing dimplings.

    d. Soft in feel and this soft feel may give a false impression of fluctuation—*pseudo-fluctuation.*

    e. The margin tends to insinuate under the examining finger.

    f. A big lipoma may become pedunculated.

2. Subfascial—under the palmar or plantar fascia.

3. Intermuscular—in between muscle planes.

4. Submucous—in the gut or respiratory tract.

5. Subserous—on the gut, under the pleura, retroperitoneal.

6. Subsynovial.

7. Intra-articular—often termed *lipoma arborescens.*

8. Subperiosteal.

9. Intramedullary, in the bone.

10. Extradural—on the spinal cord (there is no fat within the skull and so intracranial lipoma does not occur).

11. Intraglandular—pancreas, breast, etc.

Treatment.—Excision is indicated on account of site (cosmesis), size, and symptom (pain).

22

Prognosis and Principles of Treatment in Cancer

PROGNOSIS

Factors, on which the prognosis of a case of cancer depend, include the followings:

1. *Differentiation of the tumour cells.*—The more undifferentiated the cells are, the worse is the prognosis. Broder's grading is a valuable guide in this respect (*see* below).
2. *Extent of the disease* as regards local infiltration, node involvement, and distant metastasis. The TNM classification is based on these points (*see* below).
3. *Biology of the cancer.*—Some cancers have very rapid growth leading to death, e.g. squamous cell carcinoma of the lung. On the other hand, some cancers are definitely slow growing, e.g. papillary carcinoma of thyroid. Others have an unpredictable course, e.g. malignant melanoma.
4. *Age of the patient.*—In general, the younger the patient is, the worse is the prognosis.
5. *Host factor.*—Like infection, cancer is also resisted by the host with marked individual variations.
6. *Tumour location.*—Cancers involving unpaired organs, e.g. liver, brain, etc. bear a worse prognosis for obvious reasons.
7. *Institution of treatment.*—Early and correct treatment not only prolongs the life of the patient, but may also actually cause a 'cure'.

Broder's Grading.—This is the histological method of assessing malignancy. It is based on the degree of differentiation, as shown by the component cells of the tumour. The more the cells are undifferentiated the more malignant is the tumour. Accordingly, the tumours are divided into four categories:

Grade I : Up to 25 per cent cells are undifferentiated.

Grade II : 25 to 50 per cent cells are undifferentiated.

Grade III : 50 to 75 per cent cells are undifferentiated.

Grade IV : More than 75 per cent cells are undifferentiated.

TNM Classification.—This is a clinical method of assessing malignancy. In determining the extent of the disease, three points are considered:

T = The extent of the primary tumour.

N = The involvement of the nodes.

M = The presence of distant metastasis.

T expresses the size of the tumour (e.g. breast) or the amount of involvement of the thickness of the wall of hollow viscera (e.g. stomach, bladder, etc.)—from the mucous membrane to the peritoneum or adjacent organs. For breast carcinoma, T is expressed from T_1 to T_4, T_1 = less than 2 cm; T_2 = 2 to 5 cm; T_3 = 5 to 10 cm; T_4 = more than 10 cm. For smaller organs or areas (e.g. cheek) smaller tumours have relatively bigger T-gradations in comparison to those of the breast.

N is expressed according to the absence or presence of regional or distal nodes as N_0 to N_3. N_0 = no significant nodes; N_1 = significant but mobile regional nodes; N_2 = significant and fixed regional nodes; N_3 = significant distant nodes.

M is expressed according to the presence or absence of distant metastasis as M_0 or M_1.

For example, a breast cancer expressed as $T_2 N_1 M_0$ denotes that the primary tumour is 2 to 5 cm in diameter, there are significant but mobile axillary nodes, and no distant metastasis.

PRINCIPLES OF TREATMENT IN CANCER

The aim of treatment in cancer varies according to its extent. There are distinctly two groups of patients. In one group the cancer is believed to be reasonably limited, and here the aim is to eradicate the cancer totally with the purpose of achieving cure. To the other group belong the cases where the cancer has spread beyond the bounds of local cure, and in these cases the only aim is palliation. By palliation is meant maintaining control on the spread and manifestations of the malignant process, so that the patient can live with the maximum possible comfort and activity, for the longest possible period.

Up to the present day, the available methods of treating cancer are surgery, radiation, and chemotherapy (including hormone treatment), and each of these has its role to play in both curative and palliative therapy. These methods are used singly or in various combinations, and in the latter instance, in varying sequences.

Surgery

I. RADICAL SURGERY.—This aims at combining wide local excision with block dissection of the regional nodes. The local excision is made through normal tissue surrounding the growth. The regional nodes are removed with the idea that the carcinoma cells, spreading along the lymphatics, are likely to be arrested in these nodes. Usually the nodes are not resected unless they show evidence of malignant involvement. As regards resection of the nodes, there are two principles:

   a. Where the nodes are in close proximity to the primary growth, the resection of the primary growth and the nodes are done *in continuity*, e.g. radical mastectomy for carcinoma of breast.

   b. Where the nodes and the primary growth are at some distance from each other, resection of the two are performed separately, sparing the intervening lymphatics. In these cases the block dissection of the nodes is either performed at the same operation or at a second stage. Many surgeons prefer the two stage operation with the belief that, in the intervening period, the carcinoma cells, which are locate in the lymph vessels (or were pushed into them at the time of the first operation), get a chance to float up to the nodes and thus come within the field of the second operation.

II. PALLIATIVE SURGERY.—Palliative surgery aims at local removal of a primary or, sometimes, a metastatic growth with the following ideas:

   1. Relieving obstruction in a hollow viscus, e.g. gut.

   2. Controlling pain.

   3. Prolong life.

   4. Restoring function, e.g. excision of a mass which interferes with movements.

   5. Controlling infection.

   6. Preventing disfigurement, i.e. for cosmesis.

Radiation

I. CURATIVE.—The choice and effect of curative radiation is solely dependent on the susceptibility of the cancer to total destruction by irradiation. In this respect, the tumours with least differentiation of the cells are, in general, the most radiosensitive. Unfortunately, these least differentiated tumours mean the most malignant ones and they kill the patient because of their grave biological characters.

As a curative treatment for cancer, surgery and radiation closely resemble each other in that:

    a. Both can work only when the cancer is localised to an accessible organ or locality.

    b. Both can achieve only a local control.

With these features in common, surgery and radiation work with different efficiency on different tumours, e.g.

    i. Cancers of the gastrointestinal tract are better treated surgically than by radiation.

    ii. Tumours like seminoma and Hodgkin's disease are better treated by radiation.

    iii. Some cancers, such as those on the skin and lip, respond almost equally to surgery and radiation.

II. PALLIATIVE.—Palliative radiation is advocated with the ideas of:

    1. Slowing down the rate of growth of uncontrolled cancers, thus prolonging life.

    2. Relieving pain, thus making life bearable and more useful.

The principles and methods of radiation are discussed in details later in this chapter.

Combined Surgery and Radiotherapy.—Up to the present day, this form of treatment is the commonest advocated for a cancer. Usually radiation is applied post-operatively. In some cases a pre-operative course of radiation is advocated by some surgeons, e.g. Wilms' tumour.

Chemotherapy

I. CURATIVE—At present there are two tumours in which chemotherapy works as a curative measure—choriocarcinoma in females and Burkitt's lymphoma.

II. PALLIATIVE—Chemotherapy usually reserved for palliation. In general palliative chemotherapy is indicated in:

    1. Malignancy of systemic origin, e.g. leukaemias, lymphomas, etc.

    2. Locally uncontrolled cancers.

    3. Cancers with systemic metastatic spread

The result of chemotherapy as a palliative measure in the different types of malignancy may be briefly summarised as follows:

    1. EXCELLENT—Hodgkin's lymphoma, non-Hodgkin's lymphoma, acute lymphoblastic leukaemia in children, Wilms' tumour, testicular malignancy.

    2. GOOD.—Acute leukaemia in adults, chronic leukaemia, myeloma, breast carcinoma, ovarian carcinoma.

    3. POOR.—Head and neck tumours, thyroid carcinoma, bronchial carcinoma and cancers of the gastro intestinal tract, cervix and bladder.

The principles and methods of chemotherapy, together with the chemotherapeutic drugs, are discussed in details, later in this chapter.

Hormone Treatment.—There are certain cancers which are hormone-dependent. This means that the cancer cells grow at the influence of some hormones. If these hormones are antagonised or their production in the body is stopped, the cancers stimulated by them may be controlled for a considerable period. This is the basis of hormone treatment.

There are principally three cancers in the body that are often hormone-dependent, viz. cancers of breast, prostate, and thyroid. The prostatic cancers may be controlled by oestrogen treatment. The breast cancers of premenopausal women respond well to anti-oestrogen treatment. Thyroxin is often used in the treatment of thyroid cancers.

Hormone treatment may be instituted in three ways:

1. By administration of an antagonising hormone, e.g. oestrogen in prostatic cancers, androgens in breast cancers.
2. By surgical removal of the endocrine glands that produce the stimulating hormones, e.g. oophorectomy adrenalectomy, and hypophysectomy for breast cancers.
3. By radiation ablation of the endocrine glands, e.g. ablation of the pituitary by yttrium 90, in cancers of breast or prostate.

THE PRINCIPLES OF RADIOTHERAPY

Radiation treatment may be effected either with X-rays (generated in electrical machines) or with the radioisotopes (radioactive isotopes).

RADIOISOTOPES

All the 104 known elements can be obtained in radioactive form. Of these, some exist only in the radioactive form, e.g. radium Ra_{226} and technetium $Tc_{99}m$. Others exist in a stable form, from which the radioactive form is prepared. Iodine is the best example of this latter group. The stable iodine, i.e. I_{127}, can be converted into different radioactive forms, e.g. I_{131}, I_{132}, I_{123}, etc. These radioisotopes have all the chemical properties of the stable element, and when introduce into the body behave just like the stable element. For example, I_{132} behaves in all respects like ordinary iodine, being taken up by the thyroid for conversion to thyroxin. Its added advantage is its radioactivity, by which it acts as a tracer (it can be traced, i.e. found out after introduction) and also as a radiotherapeutic drug. It is not used routinely in place of ordinary iodine because it will cause radiation hazards.

The radioisotopes are useful from the medical point both for diagnostic and therapeutic purposes:

I. **Diagnostic Uses.**—The diagnostic applications of radioisotopes can be described under two major headings:

   A. Measurements *in vivo*, i.e. procedures in which the radioactive isotope is administered to the patient.

   B. Measurements *in vitro*, i.e. procedures in which no radioactivity is administered to the patient, but samples obtained from the patient are analysed by techniques that involve the use of isotopes.

    a. MEASUREMENT *IN VIVO*: A tracer dose (i.e. a very small dose used for the purpose of tracing, i.e. following it) is used for the purpose of diagnosis:

       1. *Dilution Studies:*

         Volumes and spaces.

         Turnover rates.

         Loss of the tracer from the body, e.g. gastrointestinal blood loss, gastrointestinal protein loss.

       2. *Dynamic Function Studies:*

         Absorption tests.

         Uptake tests.

         Clearance tests.

         Blood flow to organs.

         Cardiac output

         Pulmonary ventilation.

       3. *Organ Scanning.*—That is pictorial representation of distribution of the radioisotopes in an organ. Such pictures are called 'scans' or 'scanti graphs'. This may be done for the thyroid, brain, lung, liver, kidney, spleen, bone, bone marrow, placenta.

    b. MEASUREMENT *IN VITRO*: Because of the accuracy and ease of measuring the tracer substances, they are often used for assays in different biological specimens in the laboratory.

II. Therapeutic Uses.—The radioisotopes have a wide use in the therapy of malignant tumours (and some non-malignant conditions as well), and this is discussed below in details.

THE BASIC PRINCIPLES: The nuclei of the isotopes are unstable and, when they disintegrate, they emit three types of rays—alpha, beta, and gamma. It is by virtue of these rays that the isotopes are useful either in diagnosis or in treatment. Of these, the alpha and beta rays are particles (alpha consists of two protons and two neutrons, and beta is a high-speed electron), while gamma rays are not particles but are electromagnetic waves like X-rays.

The alpha rays are biologically so much damaging that they are never used. Radium is the only isotope, used medically, that emits rays. Hence, when radium is used, it has to be covered with such materials which shield the alpha rays and do not allow them to come in contact with the tissues. Fortunately, alpha rays have very little penetrating power (only a few-tenths of a millimeter of tissue or water), so that they can be easily shielded (e.g. platinum sheaths used for shielding radium).

The beta rays have the power of penetration of a few millimeter or less, of the tissues or water:

a. The beta rays of some of the isotopes are very dangerous for the system and they are not allowed to come in contact with the tissues. When these isotopes are introduced into the system (for their gamma rays to work), they are covered with such materials which cut off the beta rays (e.g. platinum sheaths for radium, platinum plating for gold grains or tantalum wires, plastic for cobalt beads, stainless steel for cobalt needles).

b On the other hand, the beta rays of some isotopes are used for the purpose of radiotherapy (e.g. I_{131}, P_{32}, etc.). These beta rays, having very small penetrating power, can produce their effect on the desired tissues without producing any ill-effect on other tissues. They may be used in two ways:

  i. Direct introduction into the tissue that is required to be damaged, e.g. yttrium-90 rods implanted into the pituitary to ablate the gland.

  ii. Systemic introduction, and because of selective affinity of an organ for the element, it is taken up by the particular organ in high concentration. Here it produces its desired effect of destruction. Examples are I_{131} for thyroid, given orally (either in carcinoma or thyrotoxicosis) and P_{32} for bone marrow, given orally or intravenously (in polycythaemia vera).

Since beta rays have very little penetrating power, they cannot be traced from outside after being introduced into the system. So they cannot be used for the purpose of diagnosis, i.e. as a tracer.

The gamma rays have high penetrating power like X-rays. They are used for purposes of both diagnosis and therapy, and are thus the most useful of all the rays.

Half-life $(T_{1/2})$.—The nuclei of the radioisotopes are unstable, and as they emit the above rays, they gradually become stable. When they get stable they loose their radioactivity. The period, within which the initial radioactivity of an isotope is reduced to halt is called the half-life of the isotope. For example, the half-life of I_{131} is 8.1 days, which means that an initial activity of 100 microcurie will be reduced to 50 microcurie after 8.1 days. In the same way, it will be reduced to 25 microcurie after 16.2 days (2 half-lives), to 12.5 microcurie after 24.3 days (3 half-lives), and so on.

Some of the isotopes have very short half-life, e.g. gold grains (16.2 days), radon seeds (3.8 days). These may, therefore, be allowed to remain permanently in the body after introduction. Other isotopes have long half-life and must be removed after a calculated time-interval (usually a week). Examples of this group are radium needles, tantalum wires, etc.

Curie and Rad.—A quantity of radioactivity equal to one curie (C) contains radioactive atoms which are disintegrating at the rate of 3.7×10^{10} per second. The terms millicurie (one thousandth of a curie) and microcurie (one thousandth of a millicurie) are, thus, often used. In one millicurie there are 3.7×10^{7} atomic disintegration per second and in one microcurie 3.7×10^{4} disintegration per second.

Gamma rays deposit some of their energy in the tissues. Beta rays dissipate all their energy in the tissues. The unit of radiation is rad (r), which is a measure of the energy absorbed per gram of tissue.

RADIOTHERAPY

This can be instituted in two ways:

  I. External sources or external beams.

  II. Internal sources.

  I. External Sources.—The tumour tissue is attacked by a beam of radiation from outside the patient's body:

    1. *The original X-ray Therapy:* The X-ray are generated in electrical machines.

2. *Teletherapy:* The gamma rays of the radioisotope, Cobalt-60, are used in the form of a beam from an external source, which is directed on to the treatment area of patients with deep-seated cancer. It is better than the ordinary X-ray treatment in several respects:

   a. A small dose rate of radiation is required.
   b. There is much greater penetration into the tissues. Also, soft tissues and bones are penetrated almost equally. Therefore, deep-seated cancers receive a good dose and are well radiated.
   c. There is a substantial skin-sparing effect, so that the skin and superficial tissues are least damaged while the deep-seated growths get maximum radiation effect.

   Caesium-137 is also used like cobalt-60 but its skin-sparing effect is lesser.

II. **Internal Sources.**—The tumour tissue is attacked by radiation from inside the body:

   A. *Local Introduction:*
      1. Interstitial implantation of needles, beads, seeds, wires, or cylinders, containing the isotope. Examples are radium needles, cobalt needles, cobalt beads, radon seeds, tantalum wires, gold grains, etc. These are implanted into the substance of the tumour.
      2. Surface application as ointments.
         Skin—P_{32}
         Eye—Yttrium-90

   B. *Systemic Introduction.*—For example, oral I_{131} for thyroid, oral or intravenous P_{32} for polycythaemia vera.

   C. *Regional Introduction:*
      1. Endolymphatic.—I_{131} injected into the subcutaneous lymph trunks to irradiate the regional nodes in melanoma.
      2. Intra-arterial—Injections of Au_{192} or yttrium-90.
      3. Serous cavities.—Intraperitoneal introduction of colloidal suspensions of yttrium-90, etc.

   From what has been described above, it may be seen that radioisotopes are used for therapeutic purposes to irradiate:

   1. Malignant tumours.
   2. Normal glands, e.g. pituitary.
   3. Abnormally high-working normal tissues, e.g. in thyrotoxicosis, polycythaemia vera.

CHEMOTHERAPY

The original principles of cancer chemotherapy was based on assumption that the problem of eradicating cancer cells is similar to that of eradicating bacteria, where great success has been achieved with chemotherapy. Unfortunately, there are wide fundamental differences between the two problems.

In bacteria infections, the chemotherapeutic drugs mainly work by blocking the metabolic pathway essential for the survival of the bacteria and while they do so, they exercise little or no effect on the cells of the host. On the other hand, the tumour cells originate from normal cells and fundamentally there are no differences between the metabolic processes of the normal cells and those of the tumour cells. Thus the chemotherapeutic agents have basically the same damaging effects on the normal cells as on the tumour cells.

The encouraging point, however, is that these agents tend to attack rapidly-dividing cells more powerfully than the ordinary cells, and in this respect the malignant cells are more susceptible to these drugs than the inert cells of most normal tissues.

Here again, there are certain normal cells which, even under normal physiological conditions, divide more actively than the cells of even the most malignant tumours. Examples are the marrow cells, the precursors of lymphocytes, the cells of the gonads, etc.

The practical problem of chemotherapy, therefore, is how to determine a dose of the drug that will be sufficient to destroy the malignant cells while causing minimum harm to these important normal-tissues.

The chemotherapeutic drugs available up to the present day may be. classified under four broad groups—antimetabolites, alkylating agents, antibiotics and antimitotic agents.

Antimetabolites.—These are substances which are sufficiently like a normal metabolite to combine with the same enzymes, but sufficiently different to prevent the usual metabolic reaction. Thus there is a concept of 'competition'—these substances competing with normal metabolites that are essential for cellular reproduction. More precisely, they exert their effect on the nuclear metabolism.

Deoxyribonucleic acid (DNA) is an essential constituent of cell nucleus and is thus very important in cell reproduction. DNA is derived from ribonucleic acid (RNA) which is synthetised in the microsomes of the endoplasm in cell. RNA is made up of hundreds of nucleotides. Each nucleotide consists of a nitrogenous base (purine or pyrimidine), combined with a sugar, ribose, and a phosphate.

Antimetabolites work by blocking the nucleotide formation (and thereby RNA and DNA synthesis) in different ways:

1. Interfering with purine or pyrimidine synthesis (*folic acid antagonists*).—In the synthesis of purine and pyrimidine, folic acid is an important ingredient. Folic acid has to be converted into folinic acid for this purpose. This conversion of folic acid to folinic acid is prevented by drugs which are termed 'folic acid antagonists'. The principal member of this group is methotrexate. These drugs are so powerful that even administration of folic acid cannot overcome their action, which can only be combated by administration of folinic acid (*citrovorum factor*). This countering effect may be clinically utilised by giving methotrexate by regional intra-arterial injection into the tumour, while folinic acid is given intravenously to protect the vulnerable cells in the rest of the body.

2. Competing with purine in the formation of the nucleotide, i.e. *purine analogues*—mercaptopurine.

3. Competing with pyrimidine in the formation of the nucleotide, i.e. *pyrimidine analogues*—5-fluorouracil.

Alkylating Agents.—These drugs produce intranuclear tissue-damage. Alkylating agents are substances which are capable of transferring an alkyl group in exchange of a hydrogen atom in another compound. They thus react with many cell components, including the nucleoprotein, and exert specific effect on the cell nucleus. These effects are very similar to those of the X-rays and gamma rays.

This group includes nitrogen mustard (which resembles mustard gas chemically but with nitrogen in place of sulphur—hence the name), cyclophosphamide (endoxan), chlorambucil (leukeran), melphalan (alkeran), busulfan (myleran), thiotepa, etc.

Antibiotics.—These drugs cause destruction of DNA directly. The. cancericidial antibiotics are actinomycin D, adriamycin. bleomycin, mitomycin C etc.

Antimitotic Agents.—These are drugs which arrest cell-division. Plant alkaloids, e.g. vincristine (oncovin) and vinblastine (velban), belong to this group.

Administration of Chemotherapeutic Drugs.—These may be administered in two ways:
1. Systemic Administration.—By oral or parental route. This is the most commonly practised procedure.
2. Regional Intra-arterial Infusion.—The advantage of this method is that, while the drug is allowed to produce maximum damaging effect on the tumour area, its systemic ill-effects are kept at a minimum. In this respect tumours of the head and neck give the best results, better than those in the limbs. The drug is directly injected into the appropriate artery after exposing the artery.
   a. Alkylating agents, like nitrogen mustards, are given by single injection. Their activity lasts for a few minutes, and further injections, usually on alternate days, may be made.
   b. Antimetabolites, like methotrexate, may be administered by a continuous infusion, lasting over two to three weeks.

Combination Chemotherapy.—In the present days cancer chemotherapy is conducted usually by a combination of several drugs. The advantages of using multiple drugs are:
1. To prevent development of drug resistance.
2. To minimise the toxicity of a high dose of a single drug.
3. To attempt to interrupt the cell cycle at various stages.

The classical examples of combination chemotherapy are the CMF (cyclophosphamide, methotrexate and 5-flourouracil) combination for breast carcinoma and the MOPP (mustard, oncovin, procarbazine and prednisolone) protocol for Hodgkin's disease. The latter combination has led to an 80 per cent complete response rate in disseminated Hodgkin's disease as compared to only 25 per cent response with any single drug.

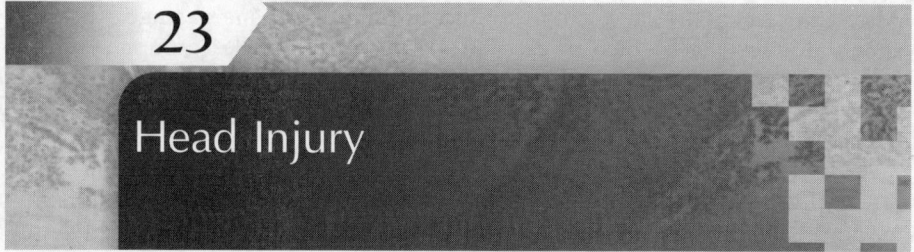

23

Head Injury

Definition.—Head injuries are injuries of composite nature, in which injury to the brain, the intracranial vessels, and the skull bones occurs either singly or in different combinations. Almost always injury to the brain is a constant factor and the other injuries may or may not be associated with it.

INJURY TO THE BRAIN

The injury to the brain occurs instantaneously with the infliction of the trauma. This injury is due to sudden vigorous movement of the brain inside the skull box. Such movements are possible because the brain is loosely fitted inside the cranial cavity. The midline septum of the falx prevents much side-to-side movement of the brain, so that, generally speaking, a trauma inflicted on the front or the back of the head is more dangerous than one inflicted on the side.

The injury to the brain is primarily one of deformity due to sudden vigorous shaking (as the brain is soft), and this goes by the name of cerebral concussion. However, contusion of the brain substance or its laceration may occur if the trauma is severe. Depending on the severity, therefore, brain injuries may be:

1. Cerebral concussion.
2. Cerebral contusion.
3. Cerebral laceration.

The site of injury in the brain depends on the line of force setup by the cerebral distortion:

1. In a good proportion of cases, the injury is in the region of the third ventricle, hypothalamus, and brain stem (medulla and pons)—the cerebral hemispheres being displaced in relation to these structures. Such lines of forces are usually set up as a result of *posterior* displacement of the *two* hemispheres.
2. In some cases, one cerebral hemisphere moves against the other, so that the junctional tissues of the commissures and corpus callosum are damaged. Such lines of forces are usually set up by an *anterior* displacement of *one* hemisphere.
3. In severe cases (contusion and laceration), the grey matter of the cortex moves over the white, causing tear of nerve cells and axon fibres in the locality.

Whatever be the nature of the brain injury, the immediate result is unconsciousness, and this is why almost all cases of head injury develop an immediate unconsciousness.

In analysing the cases of brain injury there are two distinct categories:

1. Cerebral Concussion, where there is no macroscopic pathological changes in the brain.

2. Cerebral Contusion and Laceration, where pathological changes in the brain are well-marked.

Cerebral Concussion.—This clinical state is characterised by three essential features:

a. Sudden loss of consciousness.

b. Widespread motor and sensory paralysis.

c. Complete recovery without any intervening period of imperfect consciousness.

In the majority of cases, the unconsciousness is short-lasting, usually from half a minute to half an hour. In some rare cases, however, it may be prolonged for hours, day, or weeks.

The state of cerebral concussion occurs when the injury to the brain is minimum. There is no gross pathological change in the brain. There is only a temporary suspension of the physiological functions of the brain. There are different views as regards the cause of concussion:

a. There is a molecular disturbance, which quickly returns to normal, affecting particularly the hypothalamus and the brain stem.

b. There is a transitory anaemia of the brain.

c. There is a wave of pressure transmitted by the CSF through the ventricles, and the wave impringes on the floor of the fourth ventricle.

d. There is an abrupt stretching (and associated spasm) of the delicate anterior and posterior perforating arteries, causing immediate or sustained ischaemia of the diencephalon.

Cerebral Contusion and Laceration.—In *cerebral contusion* the stretch on the brain substance is severe and some fibres are actually torn. In some cases there is a sliding movement of the grey matter in relation to the white, and this results in damage to nerve cells and axons. Contusion may occur:

a. at the site of impact of the blow.

b. at a part of the brain, which is located diagonally opposite to the site of trauma; this results from percussion of the brain against the skull at this point (this is called 'contre-coup' injury).

Cerebral laceration, which means actual tearing of the brain substance, occurs when the delicate brain strikes against a stiff dural fold or a bony prominence on the inner aspect of the skull. Occasionally, laceration may be caused by a depressed fracture fragment. Laceration, therefore, is commoner on the inner aspect of the cerebral hemispheres, on the under surface of the frontal lobe, at the tip of the temporal lobe, etc.

In both contusion and laceration, the stretch on the brain is more severe and the unconsciousness more prolonged than with concussion. When the patient recovers from unconsciousness, there is an intervening state of imperfect consciousness. Irrespective of any other associated factor, a severe contusion or laceration in the region of the brain stem *may kill* the patient.

In cases of cerebral contusion laceration, as the patient is unconscious he looks pale, having rapid and feeble pulse, rapid shallow respiration, a generalised flaccid paralysis and bilateral dilated pupils (but reacting to light).

Unless quick death occurs from severe contusion or laceration involving the brain stem, one or more of the following features may be seen in cerebral contusion or laceration:

1. Since there is damage and degeneration of some of the brain tissue, there is often headache, photophobia, nausea and vomiting and sometimes, confusion, irritability, or delirium (indicating damage to the cortical or hypothalamic levels of the brain) when the patient recovers to consciousness. This is called *post-contusional syndrome.*

2. In severe contusion or laceration the grey matter may move in relation to the white, causing rupture and degeneration of some axon fibres in the locality. This may lead to what is called the *post-contusional state* characterised by change in personality and defective memory. The patient often suffers from *post-traumatic amnesia,* the duration of which varies according to the severity of the injury. There is often a *retrograde amnesia,* the patient forgetting events from some period prior to the injury to the actual time of injury.

3. A localised oedema often occurs around the area of contusion or laceration in the brain, and this may lead to the state of *cerebral irritation.* This may occur at variable intervals from the time of injury but usually reaches its maximum after 48 hours. The patient curls up on his side, avoids light, and resents all interference. The mental state varies from drowsiness or irritability to delirium.

4. A contusion or laceration located at some important focal centre of the cerebral cortex may lead to permanent damages, e.g. anosmia in tip of temporal lobe lesion, hemianopia and blindness in occipital lobe lesion.

5. The damaged brain tissue may become sclerotic from neuroglial proliferation, and this sclerosis may cause epilepsy in the future.

6. If the haemorrhage and oedema around the contused or lacerated area is considerable, the patient develops features of *cerebral compression.*

Cerebral Compression.—Following head injury, the brain may be compressed by either of the following:

1. Intracranial haematomas from haemorrhages (discussed below).
2. Accumulated fluid:
   a. Oedema around contused or lacerated brain tissue.
   b. Retention of CSF in the lateral ventricles.
   c. Failure of absorption of CSF by the basal cisterns and arachnoid granulations, which are blocked by effused blood.

Unless the patient dies of severe contusion or laceration involving the brain stem, death in head injury is usually due to unrelieved cerebral compression.

INTRACRANIAL HAEMORRHAGES

These may be of three types:

1. Intracerebral.
2. Sudural.
3. Extradural.

It is often difficult to distinguish between subdural and intracerebral haematomas and the two are often combined. Therefore, all haematomas inside the dura should better be regarded as *intradural haematoma.* In the majority of these cases there is a subdural haematoma associated with contusion, laceration, haemorrhage and oedema of the adjacent brain. This combination is sometimes called '*burst lobe*'.

Also, in some cases extradural and subdural haematoma co-exist.

INTRACEREBRAL HAEMORRHAGE

This is haemorrhage under the pia-arachnoid mesh in the brain substance.

This type of haemorrhage is usually associated with cerebral laceration, but occasionally the bleeding may occur from a central artery.

The *effects* of intracerebral haemorrhage are seldom of much importance except when the haemorrhage ruptures into the ventricles and kills the patient of intraventricular haemorrhage characterised by hyperthermia.

EXTRACEREBRAL HAEMORRHAGE

This is a common component and a major cause of death in head injuries. The bleeding occurs between the dura mater and the skull. The source of bleeding is usually a meningeal artery, rarely a vein. Almost always it is a sequela to fracture of the skull.

Sources

1. In vast majority of the cases the bleeding is in the middle cranial fossa, the source being a torn middle meningea artery. The main trunk of the middle meningeal artery, or more commonly, one of its branches—anterior or posterior—is injured The anterior branch is much more commonly injured than the posterior (5 : 1).
2. Occasionally the bleeding may occur in the anterior cranial fossa and the source may be:
   a. Anterior branch of the middle meninpal artery.
   b. Anterior meningeal artery over the frontal lobe.
   c. Internal maxillary artery.
3. Rarely, the bleeding may occur in the posterior cranial fossa, and the source is a torn posterior meningeal artery over the occipital lobe.
4. Still rarely, the bleeding may be of venous origin as a result of tear in one of the venous sinuses—superior sagittal sinus (anterior or middle fossa) or transverse sinus (posterior fossa).

Mechanism.—The injury to the middle meningeal artery (which is responsible for the majority of cases of extradural hemorrhage) occurs as a result of trauma inflicted on the lateral side of the skull on the thin plate of the temporal bone in that area. Such a trauma causes not only fracture of the thin temporal bone but also a sudden medial shift of the underlying cerebral cortex with its covering dura away from the bone. In this region the anterior branch of the middle meningeal artery, coming out of the bony canal in the pterion (lower anterior angle of the parietal bone) transverses the potential extradural space to gain attachment to the underlying dura. The sudden shift of the dura from the bone may cause the artery to be torn in its free part, i.e. in the extradural space (the artery is fixed at one end to the pterion and at the other to the dura).

The escaping blood has three ways to go:
1. Part of it comes out through the fracture line in the temporal bone and collects as a haematoma under the temporal muscle, causing a boggy swelling there.

2. Part of the blood gravitates downwards, to the base of the middle cranial fossa.

3. Clots start collecting over the underlying motor cortex, gradually extending upwards.

Clinical features

A. *Unconsciousness:*

1. In a typical case, the cerebral concussion, associated with the trauma produces an instantaneous unconsciousness, from which the patient recovers quickly and completely. By this time, blood is collecting, but its quantity is not sufficient to cause pressure on the cortex (particularly if there is considerable shock following the injury). When the pressure of the clot becomes sufficient, cerebral compression sets in. Now the patient passes to unconsciousness again, but this time *gradually,* with a period of confusion preceding it. So, in these cases, there are two periods of unconsciousness, with an intervening period of full consciousness, and this intervening period is called the *lucid interval.*

2. In many cases, however, the phase of lucid interval is not seen and the patient is unconscious throughout. This occurs:

   a. If concussion is considerably prolonged, by which time sufficient blood clots collect, to set in cerebral compression.

   b. If the bleeding is rapid arid produces sufficient blood clots to cause compression before the patient recovers from concussion.

B. *Other Features* (Fig. 23.1):

1. In the meantime, the temporal haematoma develops, and this is a very important clinical sign.

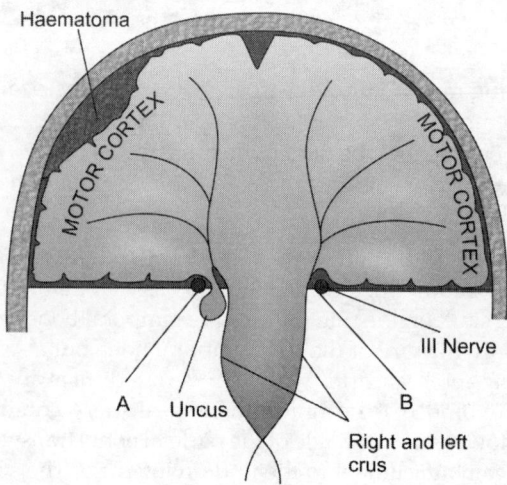

Fig. 23.1: The effects of middle meningeal haemorrhage on the right side. The haematoma presses on the motor cortex, which represents the other half of the body upside down. Note the uncus. 'A' points at the site where the III nerve (oculomotor) of the same side is affected just above the tentorial margin. 'B' points at the site where the opposite crus is pressed against the opposite tentorial margin.

2. The blood, collecting from below upwards on the motor cortex, causes compression of the cortex, resulting in anoxia. The motor cortex of the side represents the other half of the body, and here the body is represented upside down. Thus, paralysis occurs (following a short phase of twitching) in the other half of the body and in a descending order—face, arm, and then leg.
3. Simultaneously, pressure of the blood clot causes the temporal lobe of the same side to be displaced medially. The inner part of the lobe causes stretching of the oculomotor nerve, which in this situation, runs just above the edge of the tentorium. The nerve is first irritated and then paralysed This results in a short period of constriction followed by dilatation of the pupil of the same side.
4. Further pressure by the blood clot causes the cerebral hemisphere to be displaced more inwards, and with it, the brain stem is pushed to the opposite side. The opposite crus is pressed against the opposite tentorial margin. So a paralysis now develops suddenly on that side of the body on which the trauma on the head was inflicted, i.e. the side of the haemorrhage (because the opposite crus contains motor fibres for this side of the body).
5. Simultaneously, the opposite oculomotor nerve is pressed above the opposite tentorial margin. The nerve is first irritated and then paralysed. Hence there is constriction followed by dilatation of the *opposite* pupil now. These characteristic pupillary changes on the two sides are known as *Hutchinson's pupils*. In addition, various degrees of palsy of the fourth and the sixth cranial nerves may be present.
6. Still unrelieved, the pressure of the clot forces the inferomedial part of the temporal lobe (the part known as the 'uncus') down through the tentorial orifice, so that there is impaction of a midbrain cone at the tentorial orifice. This results in decerebrate rigidity with bilateral fixed dilated pupils.
7. The midbrain ischaemia causes a slowing of the pulse rate and this is of special significance. Slowing of the pulse with a rise of blood pressure is strong evidence of mounting intracranial pressure.
8. Another important feature of increased intracranial pressure is augmentation in the depth of breathing rather than its rate. In a late case, the breathing is of Cheyne Stokes type.

Treatment.—As soon as the diagnosis has been reached, immediate exploration must be made to remove the clot and arrest the haemorrhage. The whole of the head must be shaved. The side to be explored is determined by:
a. the side of the temporal haematoma,
b. the side of the skull fracture,
c. the side on which the pupil first got dilated,
d. the side from which a calcified pineal gland has been shifted in the X-ray.

To expose the middle meningeal artery and to deal with the extradural clot, one of the following two procedures may be adopted:
1. A low temporal *osteoplastic flap* is raised. This gives a very adequate exposure and provides easy handling of the condition. However, this requires a good neurosurgical practice (Figs. 23.2A and B).
2. Alternatively, an *exploratory burr-hole* is made on the skull, right at the site of the artery. The surface marking of the anterior division of the middle

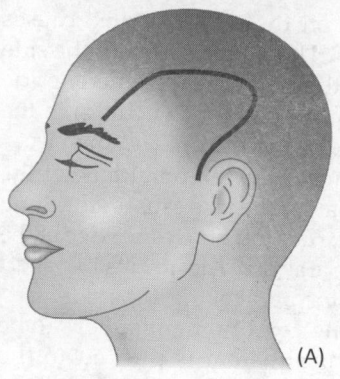 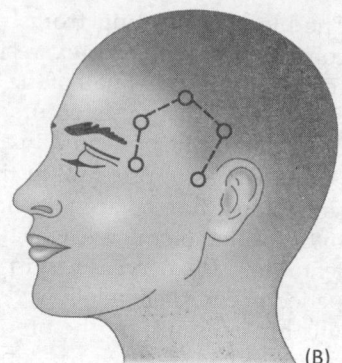

(A)   (B)

Fig. 23.2: Raising a temporal osteoplastic flap: (A) the scalp incision; (B) burr holes and wire-saw cuts on the skull.

meningeal artery is at a point 2 inches behind the external angular process and 2 inches above the zygomatic process. The standard incision of a temporal burr-hole is a vertical incision placed just above the zygomatic arch, midway between the external angular process and the external auditory meatus (Fig. 23.3). While all soft tissues including the temporal muscle are divided, the temporal haematoma is evacuated. A burr-hole is made in the skull at the abovementioned point. Immediate finding of blood clots confirm the diagnosis. The incision is extended and the *burr-hole is enlarged* with a bone nibbler, as required (*craniectomy*).

All clots are removed and the bleeding point is detected. If it is from the bony canal in the pterion, the canal is plugged with Horsle's bone wax. If the bleeding is from the dural surface, the bleeding point is secured either by underrunning with a fine needle or by diathermy. Venous oozing is carefully controlled thereafter, and the wound is closed. If required, a drain is put up to the extradural space.

If, on opening, the blood is found to come from the back, it is the posterior division of the artery which is bleeding. A second incision and a second burr-hole are made a little posteriorly and the bleeding is secured.

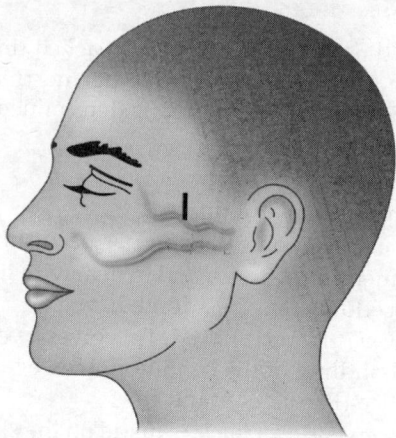

Fig. 23.3: Incision for standard temporal burr-holing.

SUBDURAL HAEMORRHAGE

This is also a common component and a major cause of death in head injuries. It is at least six times commoner than extradural haemorrhage because it can be caused by relatively minor trauma Subdural haematoma may form in two ways:

1. Laceration of the cortex associated with venous or arterial haemorrhage—the haematoma collecting under the dura.

2. Rupture of one or more superior cerebral veins. These veins run from the superior surface of the cerebral hemisphere, on either side, in rows, and pierce the dura mater lining the superior sagittal sinus, to end in the sinus. Thus the veins are fixed on one side to the arachnoid (on the surface of the hemisphere) and on the other side to the dura (lining the sinus). If there is a shaking of the cerebral hemisphere inside the skull, some of these veins (which are actually keeping the hemisphere hanging from the sinus) may be torn. This tear occurs in the free part of the veins, lying between two fixed points (arachnoid and dura), i.e. in the potential subdural space. In the elderly people, as the brain atrophies, there is more space for the brain to move within the skull, so that subdural haemorrhage is much *commoner in the elderly.*

In about 50 per cent cases, the veins on both the sides are torn, and the subdural haemorrhage is *bilateral.*

Clinical Features.—While the presenting features of subdural haematoma may be similar to those of extradural haematoma, there may be certain differences:

1. The unconsciousness may be persisting without any lucid interval. This occurs if there is severe primary brain contusion or laceration. Also, the patient deteriorates more quickly than in extradural haematoma.

2. There is no temporal fracture or temporal haematoma.

3. In cases of bilateral haemorrhage, the pupillary changes and the paralysis may be mixed on the two sides.

4. In some cases the presentation is less acute and delayed by several days. These cases are known as *subacute* subdural haematoma (cf *acute* subdural haematoma being discussed here). The role of the haematoma and that of the underlying brain damage in causing deterioration of the patient is a matter of controversy in these cases. Some of the cases show a variation in the level of consciousness—sometimes improving and sometimes deteriorating—and the patient continues to live with a moderately fair general condition for weeks. These are the cases of *chronic* subdural haematoma.

Treatment.—Effective surgical treatment involves wide craniotomy (Burr-holes are of no value), because, in spite of all investigations, it may be very difficult to localise the site of the haematoma. Even with wide exposures, the haematoma may elude detection. Even if the haematoma is detected and removed, the patient may succumb to the widespread brain damage associated with the haematoma.

FRACTURE OF THE SKULL

Fracture may occur either at the base or at the vault of the skull.

Basal Fractures

1. These are produced:
   a. by compression of the skull,
   b. by extension of fissures radiating from the vault.
2. They are always crack or fissure type.
3. They may be simple or compound. Compound fractures may occur through the middle ear, accessory air sinuses, and cribriform plates.

Vault Fractures

1. These are produced:
   a. by compression of the skull,
   b. by local indentation,
   c. by tangential injuries.
2. They may be of the following types:
   i. Cracks or fissures
   ii. Comminuted
   iii. Depressed (pond, gutter).
3. They may be simple or compound (i.e. associated with scalp injury).

Importances of Skull Fractures in Head Injuries

1. Medicolegal.—In many cases, the fractures are of little importance except for medicolegal reasons.
2. Vault fractures at special sites may be associated with characteristic intracranial vascular injury, e.g. temporal bone fracture associated with injury to the middle meningeal artery.
3. Compound fractures may result in infection of the meninges and the brain.
4. Escape of cranial contents in basal fractures:
   A. CSF:
      i. Anterior Cranial Fossa.—CSF escaping through nose (*cerebrospinal rhinorrhoea*).
      ii. Middle Cranial Fossa.—CSF escaping from the ear.
   B. Blood:
      i. Anterior Cranial Fossa.
         a. Epistaxis, if there is fracture of the cribriform plate.
         b. Effusion of blood into the orbit.
      ii. Middle Cranial Fossa.
         a. Epistaxis, if the fracture involves the nasal sinuses.
         b. Bleeding from the ear.
      iii. Posterior Cranial Fossa.
         a. Boggy swelling at the nape of the neck.
         b. Patch of ecchymosis over the mastoid process (*Battle's sign*).
5. In basal fractures of the anterior cranial fossa, air may enter the cranial cavity, producing *intracranial aerocele*.
6. Depressed fractures of the vault may cause cerebral laceration.
7. Injury to cranial nerves may sometimes occur with basal fractures.

Any of the cranial nerves *excepting the* hypoglossal may be injured:
a. Laceration of a nerve by the fracture line causes immediate and permanent paralysis.
b. Compression of a nerve by blood clots produces paralysis after a few days, and this is usually temporary.
c. Involvement of a nerve in scar or callus produces paralysis after a few weeks, and this is permanent.

MANAGEMENT OF HEAD INJURY

I. **Proper History Taking**
   1. Nature and site of trauma on the head.
   2. History of unconsciousness and whether there is a history of lucid interval.
   3. Bleeding from nose, mouth, or ear.

II. **Careful Clinical Examination.**—This is done with the idea of drawing a base line as regards the condition of the patient, so that onset of complications, particularly features of cerebral compression, can be detected early:
   1. Level of consciousness.—This is the *most important singular criterion* for assessing the injury on the brain.
   2. Pulse, respiration, blood pressure, and temperature.
   3. Paralysis, if any.
   4. Pupils—size, and reaction to light.
   5. Escape of blood (or CSF) from nose, mouth, ear, etc.
   6. Injuries on the scalp and any clinical evidence of vault fracture.
   7. Any injury to cervical vertebrae.
   8. Any other important injury in the body chest, abdomen or pelvis, or fractures of long bones.

III. **Special Investigations**
   1. X-ray of the skull.—Anteroposterior and lateral views are taken as well as a 35° half-axial plate. The X-rays may indicate important diagnostic features:
      a. Fracture of the skull. Position of the fracture may be a valuable guide in some cases, e.g. temporal bone fracture indicating extradural haemorrhage. Also the presence and nature of the fracture may give an indication as to the severity of the head injury.
      b. A depressed fracture may demand surgery for elevation.
      c. Demonstration of a calcified pineal gland and its position relative to the midline. Subsequent change in position in repeat skiagrams may indicate intracranial haemorrhage, pushing the brain in opposite direction.
   2. X-ray cervical vertebrae in doubtful cases.
   3. Carotid arteriography.—This may establish the diagnosis of intracranial haemorrhage and cerebral compression by showing characteristic displacements of the known vessels (middle cerebral artery and anterior cerebral artery).
   4. Echo-encephalogram may indicate intracranial haemorrhage and cerebral compression, suggested by a shift of the midline structures to the opposite side. The introduction of automated machines has made diagnosis of the shift easier.

5. Computerised axial tomography (CAT Scan).—When available, this provides the best diagnostic and therapeutic guidelines in case of head injury. There is no necessity for carotid arteriography, or echo-, encephalogram, none of which can always provide correct diagnostic information and guidelines for treatment. The head is scanned from above downwards in a series of planes (tomography). The findings are computerised. The computer records the brain substance grey; bone, clot or tumour white; areas of oedema mottled dark; and ventricular fluid black. Taken all together, the scanner gives a complete picture of the pathology—haemorrhage (with its plain and extent), swelling of the brain (contusion, laceration and oedema) and shifting of the brain to one side. The nature of treatment is made out rather easily on the report of the scan. Unfortunately, such facilities are available only in a few specialised centres. However, the patients who are not in the need of an immediate surgery for decompression may well be sent to a centre having the facility of CAT scan, where the management becomes much more rational.

6. Intracranial pressure monitoring.—A high intracranial pressure (ICP) has two-fold importances:

   a. An extremely high ICP can shut off the cerebral blood flow and may cause damage to the brain which was otherwise healthy after the trauma.

   b. A very high ICP is an indication of the presence of an intracranial haematoma.

   The development of methods of measuring ICP which do not require ventricular catheterisation has encouraged its application in the diagnosis and management of head injuries.

IV. **General Nursing Care**

1. *Posture*.—This is maintained as demanded by the condition of the patient, e.g.

   a. An unconscious patient is treated in lateral position.

   b. If the blood pressure is very low, the head end is kept low.

   c. A delirious or restless patient is kept on a railed bed.

   d. Elderly patients, particularly those with associated chest injury, are kept in propped-up position.

   e. A conscious patient is kept propped-up or flat, as he likes (according to high- or low-pressure headache, respectively).

2. *Care of the Airway:*

   a. An unconscious patient must have an airway tube to prevent the tongue falling back.

   b. All secretions must be repeatedly sucked out to prevent aspiration.

   c. A tracheostomy has to be performed:

      i. If there is prolonged unconsciousness and reflexes are lost (as in brain stem lesions).

      ii. If there is profuse bleeding from a basal fracture

      iii. If there are profuse secretions.

3. *Bladder* requires continuous catheterisation in unconscious patients. A full bladder induces restlessness.

4. *Nutrition* must be adequately maintained. For unconscious patients a nasogastric tube feeding has to be instituted. To start with, intravenous infusions may be necessary.

V. Supportive Treatment

1. *Medicines:*
   a. Antibiotics, to combat infection.
   b. Sedatives for restless patients. The patient must not be allowed to be restless but, at the same time, sedatives should be minimum. Paraldehyde, 8–10 ml intramuscularly, is very useful. Bromides and barbiturates should be avoided, particularly in the elderly. Morphine should *never* be administered as it depresses respiration.
   c. Aspirin for headache.

2. *Hypothermia.*—This is beneficial in severe brain stem lesions:
   a. to restrict rise of temperature, especially hyperthermia, as often occurs in brain stem lesions,
   b. to improve the prognosis by diminishing the oxygen-requirement of the damaged brain tissue.
   Hypothermia may be ordinarily induced by cold sponging, ice bags, and ice blankets.

3. *Maintenance of Systemic Blood Pressure.*—As there is always the risk of ischaemic brain damage, the normal cardiac output has to be maintained and blood loss from other injuries, if any, has to be adequately replaced. The lost blood has to be replaced by blood. Other intravenous fluids must be isotonic.

4. *Hyperventilation.*—In unconscious patients this may be beneficial in lowering the intracranial pressure since it washes out CO_2 which is a vasodilator and therefore raises the intracranial pressure.

VI. Monitoring of the Patient.

Monitoring of the Patient.—A close watch is kept on the patient to find out if features of cerebral compression are setting in. In an unconscious patient it is often difficult to decide whether the patient is suffering from cerebral contusion or cerebral compression but this differentiation is highly important because active treatment has to be instituted immediately in cases of compression. The following points may be helpful in reaching at the diagnosis:

Cerebral Concussion	Cerebral Compression
1. Unconsciousness from the time of injury.	1. Two periods of unconsciousness, with a lucid interval in between.
2. Patient looks pale, with quick shallow respirations.	2. Patient looks dusky, with slow deep respirations, which later become irregular and stertorous, often Cheyne-Stoke's type.
3. Pulse quick and weak.	3. Pulse slow and bounding.
4. Blood pressure normal or lowered.	4. Blood pressure raised.
5. Pupils dilated, equal, and reacting.	5. Pupils show typical changes (Hutchinson's pupils).

VII. Treatment for Cerebral Compression.—As soon as there is evidence of cerebral compression, active treatment has to be instituted:

1. If the compression is due to haemorrhage (extradural or subdural), immediate exploration has to be undertaken.

2. If the compression is due to oedema or raised CSF tension, *dehydration therapy* has to be instituted. The idea behind this treatment is to raise the osmotic tension of blood so that it can absorb more CSF and thereby reduce the intracranial tension. The following methods may be used:

   a. The daily fluid intake is reduced to less than 2 pints.

   b. Osmotic agents:

      i. Mannitol is the most commonly used osmotic agent. It is administered as a 20% solution in IV drip. A volume of 250 ml is given over a period of 30 minutes. This may be repeated every 6 to 8 hours but after being sure that diuresis is taking place and that electrolytes are being used simultaneously for replacement

      ii. Diuretics such as furosemide are sometimes used. They may have two fold effects—increasing the plasma osmolarity as well as a direct effect on the transport mechanisms of the brain itself. Furosemide is administered intramuscularly, 40–80 mg.

   c. Steroids.—Corticosteroids in high doses (up to 24 mg, daily) are widely used, largely on the belief that they would reduce cerebral oedema as they do in cases of brain tumours. Their value in cases of head injury is, however, debated.

   Though dehydration therapy is very effective, it should not be continued for more than 3 days as this may cause gross sodium-potassium imbalance in blood. If the patient's condition does not improve by this time, bi-temporal trephining is done in an attempt to reduce the intracranial tension.

24

The Spine

SPINA BIFIDA

Definition.—This denotes a gap in the posterior wall of the vertebral arch.

Embryology.—In the mesoderm on each side of the developing neural tube (the future spinal cord), develops a cartilaginous bar. This bar extends backwards to meet its fellow of the opposite side in the midline, behind the neural tube. The two, together, make the vertebral arch, which encloses the neural tube. Between the vertebral arch and the neural tube, the thin layer of mesodermal tissue differentiates into the dura mater. The pia and the arachnoid, however, develop from the neural ectoderm.

If the cartilaginous bars from the two sides fail to meet each other, a gap forms, and there is failure of development of the laminae and the spinous process behind the neural tube. This condition is known as spina bifida. As fusion of the bars begins at the cephalic end of the foetus and proceeds caudally, the incidence of spina bifida is greatest in the lumbosacral segment of the vertebral column. Occasionally it may be found in the cervico-occipital region. As a rule, only one vertebra is affected.

The condition is frequently associated with developmental anomalies of the spinal cord and its membranes, and these make the different types of spina bifida.

Types—There are two broad types:

A. *Spina Bifida Cystica*, where there is a protrusion of the meninges, and sometimes of the cord, through the gap.

B. *Spina Bifida Occulta*, where there is no such protrusion.

SPINA BIFIDA CYSTICA.—There are four types:

1. Meningocele.
2. Meningomyelocele (myelomeningocele)
3. Syringomyelocele (syringocele or myelocystocele)
4. Myelocele.

Meningocele

1. Through the vertebral defect only the meninges protrude, and the sac contains only CSF.
2. The swelling is covered completely by healthy skin (cf meningomyelocele).
3. The swelling is brilliantly transilluminant.
4. There may or may not be features of nerve paralysis—affecting the lower limb, the bladder (incontinence), the rectum (incontinence), or all three.

5. A transmitted impulse from the swelling to the anterior frontanalle may be elicited in some cases.
6. Hydrocephalus may be associated, and this combination is known as *Arnold-Chiari malformation*.

Meningomyelocele
1. This is the commonest variety found in the living children.
2. Through the vertebral defect not only the meninges but the spinal cord or cauda equina bulges out.
3. The spinal cord and cauda equina are, however, normally developed.
4. There is failure of development of normal skin at the summit of the swelling and here the meninges are uncovered. To this part of the meninges the spinal cord and the nerves are attached. The swelling may burst through this weak spot.
5. As the swelling shows a positive transillumination, the nerves running on its wall are found as contrast dark shadows.
6. Associated paralysis of the lower limbs, bladder (incontinence), and rectum (incontinence) are much commoner than with meningocele. In the lower limbs, talipes and trophic ulcers are the commonest manifestations.
7. The other features are like meningocele.

Syringomyelocele.—The central canal of the spinal cord is dilated. Through the vertebral gap not only the meninges but also the central canal of the cord, together with the overlying ill-developed posterior part of the spinal cord, protrudes. There are gross paralytic manifestations.

Myelocele.—This is the gravest of all. In addition to the vertebral defect, the neural groove has failed to close, so that the posterior part of the spinal cord also is not developed. There is an elongated fissure, at the bottom of which the anterior part of the spinal cord is seen. As the central canal is opened out, CSF is discharged on the surface. Infection sets in and the infant dies shortly after birth.

SPINA BIFIDA OCCULTA.—This is so named because the spina bifida is hidden. There is no protrusion of the meninges or the cord through the vertebral gap, and so there is no swelling. The manifestations may be:
1. A patch of hair or a naevolipoma in this situation.
2. A dimpling on the skin.
3. Weakness, or even paralysis, of the lower limbs; incontinence of urinary and anal sphincters.

The last two features, mentioned above, are due to the *membrana reuniens*. The spinal cord and the skin never loose their primitive connections completely, and a band of fibrous tissue extends from the skin, through the vertebral defect, to the dura mater. This fibrous tissue, called the membrana reuniens, can neither stretch nor grow and remains stationary in length, while the cord and the vertebrae grow. Thus it pulls on the skin at one end (causing the dimpling on the skin) and the spinal meninges and nerve roots at the other end, causing the paralytic features.

Treatment of Spina Bifida
1. Myelocele and syringomyelocele are incompatible with life.
2. For meningocele and meningomyelocele, operation should be undertaken at the earliest opportunity—often within a few days of birth. The skin and the sac

are opened with incisions perpendicular to each other (this cris-crossing minimises the chances of post-operative CSF leakage). The redundant part of the sac is excised. In cases of meningomyelocele, meticulous care must be exercised to replace all nerve tissues into the vertebral canal. The margins of the excised sac are then apposed to each other. In order to strengthen the weak spot, a part of the erector spinae muscles and the overlying fasciae are approximated over the gap by lateral release incisions. The skin wound is closed.

3. For spina bifida occulta, operation should be undertaken if there are symptoms. On proper exposure, the membrana reuniens is excised in its whole length from the skin, through the vertebral gap, to the spinal meninges. Any lipomatous tissue, encountered during the process of dissection, is also excised since this also may be the cause of the pressure on the cord.

SPINAL DEFORMITIES

1. Scoliosis
2. Kyphosis
3. Lordosis

SCOLIOSIS

Definition.—The term 'scoliosis' denotes lateral curvature of the spine.

Types.—Broadly, there are two types:

I. Mobile scoliosis.
II. Fixed scoliosis.

I. Mobile Scoliosis

FEATURES

a. The deformity is essentially temporary and may correct completely.
b. There is no associated rotation of the vertebrae.
c. The scoliosis diminishes or disappears when the patient bends forwards.
d. There is a single curvature.

CAUSES

1. *Postural.*—Found in school-going children. When the child is asked to bend forward, the curvature disappears.
2. *Compensatory.*—Due to a cause that is usually obvious, e.g.
   a. Cervical Spine—in torticollis.
   b. Thoracic Spine—pulmonary scoliosis, i.e. when the chest wall is drawn to one side due to pulmonary diseases or operations (pneumonectomy, thoracoplasty).
   c. Lumbar Spine—where one leg is short or there is a deformed hip.
3. *Sciatic.*—This is due to protective spasm conditions, e.g. prolapsed intervertebral disc impinging upon a nerve root

II. Fixed Scoliosis (Structural Scoliosis)

FEATURES.

a. The deformity tends to be permanent and never disappears spontaneously. Correction with treatment, including operations, is also difficult.
b. There is always an associated rotation of the vertebrae—the vertebral bodies rotate towards the convexity, while the spinous processes rotate towards the

concavity. In case of the thoracic spine, this rotation is very evident on the ribs. The ribs make a prominent *hump* on the convex side. This is because the rotation of the vertebral bodies causes the ribs to be displaced posteriorly.

c. When the patient is asked to bend forwards, the scoliosis, as well as the rib-hump, become more prominent.

d. There are usually three curves. The middle one is the original or *primary*. Above and below this, there are two curves to the opposite side—the *compensatory* curves.

CAUSES

A. *Idiopathic Structural Scoliosis.*—This is the commonest form of scoliosis, shows the maximum deformity, and is the most difficult to be treated. The cause is not known, hence it is called idiopathic. It starts at about the age of ten, and progresses rapidly till growth is complete.

B. *Secondary Structural Scoliosis.*—There is an attributable cause for the scoliosis:
   1. Congenital—This is due to the presence of a hamivertebra.
   2. Paralytic.—Inequal pull of the muscles of the two sides. This usually follows poliomyelitis.
   3. In neurofibromatosis (von Recklinghausen's disease).

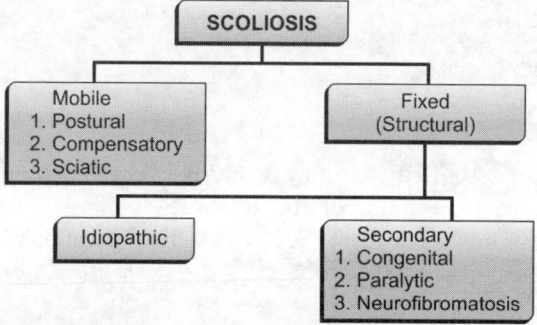

KYPHOSIS

This denotes an excessive posterior convexity (i.e. anterior bending) of the spinal column. Since there is a natural posterior curvature in the thoracic part of the vertebral column, kyphosis is most prominent in this region. On the other hand, the cervical and lumbar regions, having a normal lordosis, seldom show evidence of kyphosis.

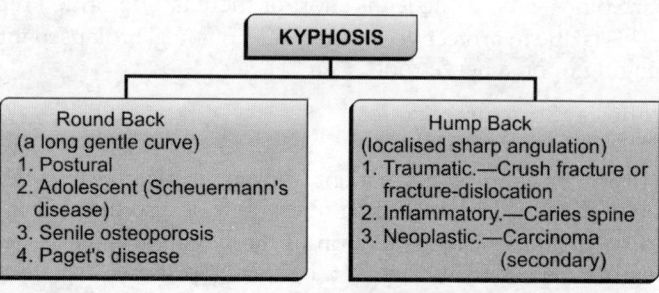

LORDOSIS

This denotes an excessive anterior curvature of the spine. In practice, the condition is only seen in the lumbar region, where there is a natural lordosis. There is an exaggeration of this natural lordosis.

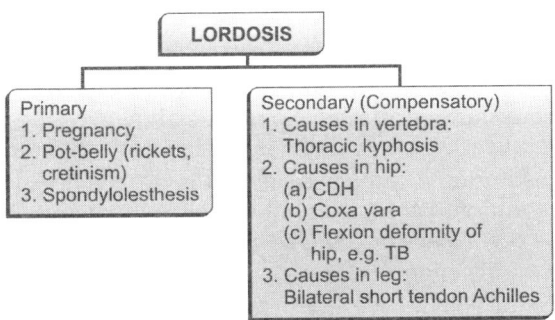

CARIES SPINE

Tuberculosis of spine, also known as Pott's disease, accounts for more than half of the cases of bone tuberculosis.

The disease may occur at any age, but is commonest in children below 5 years.

Though no pan of the vertebral column is immune, the lower three thoracic and upper two lumbar (T_{10} to L_2) are much the commoner to be affected. This susceptibility is usually attributed to the great range of mobility in and the considerable amount of weight-bearing by this region of the spine.

Almost always it is the body of a vertebra that is involved. Only exceptionally the spinous process, the lamina, the transverse process, or the articulating process is the site of a tubercular lesion.

Pathology.—Tuberculosis of the spine (like all bone and joint tuberculosis) is always secondary and the disease reaches the spine by way of blood stream. As the blood supply to the vertebral body comes chiefly from two sources, two types of lesions are essentially noted:

1. If the infection comes by way of the nutrient artery of the vertebra (a branch of the posterior spinal), which enters the vertebral body from its posterior surface and supplies its major part, the process of tuberculosis starts in the centre of the bone and affects its major part. Softening and destruction of the major part of the vertebral body makes it unable to bear the weight of the vertebrae above, and it collapses. This results in spinal deformity (given below). This type is commonly encountered in children in whom blood supply to the vertebral body comes almost exclusively by way of the nutrient artery.

2. An additional supply to the vertebral body is derived from the branches of intercostal or lumbar arteries, and this supplies a limited area on the anterior aspect of the body. As age advances, this supply gradually gets abundant with relative diminution in the supply from the central nutrient artery. In adults, therefore, this is often the route of tubercular infection to the vertebra. In these

cases, the process of tuberculosis starts in the anterior periphery of the vertebral body, keeping its major weight-bearing central part undamaged. So, the vertebrae do not collapse, and a little or no spinal deformity results.

Characteristically, the process of tuberculosis has a tendency to start near the upper or lower surface of the vertebral body rather than at its centre. Very early in the course of the disease, therefore, the adjacent intervertebral disc is involved. Whether the disease may actually start in an intervertebral disc is a matter of dispute. Weight of the vertebral column compresses tubercular caseous material into the adjacent lower vertebra which is thus involved. In this way several consecutive vertebrae may be affected. Sometimes, however, the disease may start separately in several vertebrae—either consecutive or at different levels.

A very early institution of proper treatment in a patient with good resistance may result in resolution. More often, however, the progress of the disease is aggravated by the occurrence of collapse of bodies of the affected vertebrae, and this may lead to complications as follows:

1. Deformity of the spinal column.
2. Formation of cold abscess and its spread.
3. Onset of paraplegia (Pott's paraplegia).

Deformity of the Spinal Column.—As has already been discussed, this occurs only with a central type of lesion, and so it is seen commonly in the children. The deformity is usually one of kyphosis, because the collapse is limited to the vertebral bodies the back being held by the unaffected neural arches. The manifestation of the deformity, however, varies according to the level of the spine involved. In the cervical region, the transverse processes are just lateral to the vertebral bodies and tend to prevent or minimise any deformity. In the lumbar region, the vertebral column is so broad and deep, and is supported by so strong ligaments and muscles, that the deformity may, at the most, cause a diminution of the normal lordosis existing there. In the thoracic region, there is a normal kyphotic curvature in the vertebral column so that even a little kyphosis makes itself evident. This kyphosis may be in the form of a gradual bend or of an acute angulation (known as *gibbus*). When the angulation is acute, the spinal canal may be narrowed considerably.

In some cases, the destruction of the vertebral body is limited or is more advanced in its one lateral half, keeping the other half more or less intact. In these cases, the deformity is a scoliosis rather than kyphosis.

Formation of Cold Abscess and its Spread.—The collapse of the affected vertebrae squeezes out, from inside, the caseous material which may:

a. infect the adjoining disc and vertebra (thereby increasing the deformity),
b. be expressed backwards into the spinal canal, pressing on the cord (thereby causing paraplegia).
c. be expressed forwards and on the sides of the vertebrae (thereby forming pre-vertebral and para-vertebral abscesses).
d. escape into the neighbouring soft tissues forming cold abscess (which spreads).

This last one, viz. the spread of the abscess, varies widely according to the level of vertebral involvement, and this is described below in details.

A. *In the Cervical Region:*
1. A paravertebral abscess may bulge into the pharynx (in case of upper cervical), or press on the oesophagus or trachea (in case of lower cervical). The abscess is situated in the midline and is considerably deep-seated, lying deep to the prevertebral fascia (c.f. an acute retropharyngeal abscess which is situated on one side of the midline and is superficial).
2. Such an abscess, therefore, seldom bursts into the pharynx but tracks laterally, behind the prevertebral fascia, into the posterior triangle of the neck and appears on the surface at the posterior border of the sternomastoid.
3. The abscess may track downwards behind the prevertebral fascia and come to the posterior mediastinum.
4. Occasionally, the abscess, lying behind the prevertebral fascia, may track backwards and, on entering the open mouth of the axillary sheath, gain entrance into the axilla; thereafter it may come down to the arm.
5. The abscess may follow the course of the posterior division of the spinal nerve and appear on the back of the neck on one side of the midline.

B. *In the Upper Dorsal Region:*
1. Very often the abscess remains paravertebral in the posterior mediastinum.
2. The abscess may trace a thoracic nerve and follow one of the following courses:
    a. Extends along the intercostal nerve, and
        i. either, follows the anterior cutaneous branch—thus presenting itself on the surface by the side of the midline at the anterior end of the intercostal space,
        ii. or, follows the lateral cutaneous branch and presents itself on the surface in the midaxillary line.
    b. Extends along the posterior division of the thoracic nerve and presents on the side of the back:
        i. either, 1 cm from the spine—if it follows the medial division of the nerve,
        ii. or, 3 cm from the spine—if it follows the lateral division.
3. The abscess may gravitate downwards and behave as an abscess originating in the lower dorsal region (given below).

C. *In the Lower Dorsal Region:*
1. The abscess may remain paravertebral
2. It may follow the course of a thoracic nerve as above (the only difference is that, when it follows the intercostal nerve and comes to the surface along its anterior cutaneous branch, it presents itself in the rectus sheath).
3. The paravertebral abscess, as it gravitates downwards and reaches the lower end of the posterior mediastinum, finds three openings, into either of which it may enter:
    a. Lateral lumbocostal arch
    b. Medial lumbocostal arch
    c. Median arcuate ligament
    a. If it passes deep to the lateral lumbocostal arch, it courses down between the quadratus lamborum muscle and its fascia. Under such conditions:
        i. it may remain inside the quadratus lamborum behind the kidney,

    ii. it may follow the course of one of the three nerves which lie in this situation, viz. subcostal, iliohypogastric and ilioinguinal, and extend along the abdominal wall on to the iliac fossa.

  b. If it gains entrance behind the medial lumbocostal arch, it enters the psoas sheath (this arch is the open upper end of the psoas sheath) and forms a psoas abscess. The psoas abscess may be huge and may come to the surface over a variety of places:

    i. It may come to the surface over the lumbar region,

    ii. It may extend to the iliac fossa.

    iii. It may pass down behind the inguinal ligament and come as far down as the insertion of the psoas to the lesser trochanter. It thus points in the region of the groin where it is apt to be mistaken for a femoral hernia (the abscess pushes the femoral artery forwards).

    iv. Rarely, it may extend further down along the inner side of the thigh, to appear in the popliteal fossa.

  c. When the abscess passes behind the median arcuate ligament, it lies in contact with the aorta. It may, therefore, pass into the abdomen along the aorta and may follow the branches of the abdominal aorta.

4. In case of the lowest three thoracic vertebrae, the abscess, coming out of the vertebral body, gains direct entrance into the psoas sheath since the sheath is attached internally to the bodies of these vertebrae. It then forms a psoas abscess, described above.

D. *In the Lumbar Region:*

1. The abscess may remain paravertebral.

2. It may gain entrance into the psoas sheath and form a psoas abscess (as above).

3. It may gain entrance into the quadratus lamborum (vide above).

4. It may extend along the aorta and its branches and, on some occasions, follow the internal pudendal artery to appear as an ischiorectal abscess, or follow the superior gluteal artery to appear as a gluteal abscess.

5. It may extend between the flat muscles of the abdomen and present itself in the lumbodorsal triangle of Petit.

6. It may follow the course of a lumbar nerve and

  a. either, point on the back,

  b. or, follow the course of the femoral or obturator nerve and appear in the thigh.

Pott's Paraplegia.—The cause of the paraplegia varies from case to case. One or a combination of the following factors may be responsible for the paraplegia:

1. Soft inflammatory materials may compress the cord. These may be:

  a. Cold abscess emerging from the back of the vertebral body (usual).

  b. Tubercular granulation tissue.

  c. Caseous mass.

    Inflammatory material can shrink with healing; so spontaneous recovery is possible. Therefore, simple taking off the weight from the spine often cures the paraplegia. If operation proves necessary, simple evacuation of the abscess (at the most with a costotransversectomy) is sufficient.

2. Solid material may compress the cord, or the cord may be stretched on it. This may be:

a. Bony ridge at the kyphos.

b. Sequestreted bone, or disc, or both.

c. True pathological dislocation (rare).

Such solid materials cannot shrink, and so recovery is impossible without full-scale decompression (e.g. anterolateral decompression).

3. Thrombosis of the vessels of the cord.

4. Fibrosis:

a. Fibrous tissue may strangle the cord transversely.

b. After many years, the cord may shrink longitudinally.

Clinical Types of Pott's Paraplegia.—*Seddon and Weedon-Bulter* classify the cases as follows:

A. EARLY ONSET PARAPLEGIA.—This occurs during the active phase of the disease and there is a dramatic onset of the paraplegia. The paraplegia is always complete. These cases may be of two types:

Type I paraplegia.—Here the paralysis recovers within 6 months of institution of active treatment. The cause of such paraplegia is compression by soft inflammatory material.

Type II paraplegia.—Here the paraplegia does not recover within 6 months of institution of ordinary treatment. The cause is either (a) compression of the cord by solid material, or (b) thrombosis of the vessels of the cord.

B. LATE ONSET PARAPLEGIA.—These are called Type III paraplegia. Here the paralysis occurs much late, often after many years of the active disease. The cause of such paraplegia may be:

a. Fibrosis affecting the cord.

b. Extensive thrombosis of the vessels of the cord.

c. Reactivation of the tubercular lesion in the spine.

The paralysis in these cases is usually incomplete, but tends to be *permanent.* These cases are sometimes subdivided into two groups, viz.

Type III a—recovering with antitubercular treatment (reactivated cases).

Type III b—persisting, irrespective of whether antitubercular treatment is instituted or not (fibrosis or thrombosis).

Clinical Features of Caries Spine

1. The Usual Group.—The patient presents with back pain, aggravated during movements. There may be referred pain along the nerve-roots. Constitutional symptoms of tuberculosis may be present, viz. temperature, night-sweating, loss of weight. Sometimes there is a history of pulmonary or other form of tuberculosis, or a family history of the disease.

The earliest clinical sign is a restricted flexion of the spine. Tenderness on the affected spines is elicited either by direct pressure or by the 'Anvil test' (sudden jerk on the head causes pain in the spine).

2. Some patients present with cold abscess.

3. Often a child is presented with a 'gibbus'. Otherwise, a gradual kyphosis may be the presenting feature in a child.

4. Some patients may present with Pott's paraplegia.

Special Investigations

1. Local X-ray:
   a. A lateral view will show very early diminution of the intervertebral disc space. The affected vertebrae show evidence of rarefaction due to tubercular destruction.
   b. The AP view may show a paravertebral abscess, which is occasionally calcified.
2. X-ray Chest
3. Blood Examination.—DC, ESR.
4. Mantoux Test, particularly in children.
5. Aspiration of suspected cold abscess for bacteriological examination and culture. A cold abscess is usually sterile on ordinary culture.
6. If an elderly patient presents with a suspected cold abscess, examination of the urine and blood for sugar.

Treatment.—This has to be considered under four headings:
1. Management of uncomplicated cases.
2. Treatment for cold abscess.
3. Treatment for spinal deformity.
4. Treatment for Pott's paraplegia.

Management of Uncomplicated Cases.—The treatment has to be considered in 3 stages.

I. *Stage of Recumbency and Rigid Immobilisation.*—This has to be done when the patient is in the active stage of the disease. In any case, the vertebral body should not be allowed to bear weight and so the patient is put to recumbency.

Movements of the affected vertebrae have to be restricted and this requires an external immobilisation. The best immobilisation is obtained by a *plaster jacket* and the areas of immobilisation must include a good number of healthy vertebrae above and below. When the lesion is above the mid-thoracic level, the head should be fixed, so a 'minerva jacket' has to be applied. In lesions of lower thoracic and lumbar vertebrae, the hips should be immobilised as well This is because the psoas major muscle originates from these vertebrae and movements of the hip joints cause movements of the vertebrae. A bilateral 'half-pant' plastering has to be done in these cases.

Such rigid immobilisation may be difficult in some cases. In these cases a little relaxation may be allowed in the form of immobilisation in a *plaster bed.*

Immobilisation has to be continued till the disease has been arrested and this is confirmed when 3 consecutive monthly X-rays do not show any evidence of further destruction. The local clinical condition, absence of complications, improvement in the general health, absence of pulmonary or other lesions, and diminution of ESR are the other factors to act as guideline.

With the immobilisation, a complete antitubercular regime has to be instituted. Preferably a combination of three drugs is used—either streptomycin, INH and ethambutol or rifampicin, INH and ethambutol. Streptomycin or rifampicin is withdrawn after 3 to 4 months but INH and ethambutol have to be continued till signs of healing set in, but for a minimum period of 18 months. If rifampicin is used, these drugs may be discontinued after 9 to 12 months.

II. *Stage of Ambulation with Support.*—When the disease has been arrested, the patient may be allowed to bear weight and to move, but the spine must be supported. This is efficiently done with a posterior *spinal brace.* If the brace also braces back the shoulders, the kyphotic tendency is prevented. In the cervical region a padded *collar* prevents kyphosis.

The support has to be continued till:

a. either, the operation of spinal fusion is undertaken.

b. or, the spine shows absolute healing.

III. *After Treatment.*—Tuberculosis of the spine is the only example of bone and joint tuberculosis where healing occurs by bone and not by fibrous tissue, even in absence of secondary infection. Thinking in this line, a healed caries spine requires no further treatment. However, though it theoretically sounds strong, in the majority of cases healing is never so perfect. So, after the disease has reached the healed stage, the operation of spinal fusion has to be undertaken in order to achieve complete and permanent immobilisation of the affected segment of the spine. This has two-fold effects:

1. It prevents pain in the future that may occur if movement between the affected vertebrae remain.

2. It prevents flaring up of the dormant bacilli, some of which always keep concealed in the affected area, even after healing. Such chances of flaring up are more likely if movements between the vertebrae do occur.

Various types of spinal fusion operation are available. In all the operations however, at least five vertebrae should be fused—two above and two below the affected vertebra. The two principle types of spinal fusion operation, commonly practised, are as follows:

1. The spinous processes, together with the supraspinous and interspinous ligaments, are split vertically. A conical graft, taken from tibia, is placed in the gutter between the split spinous processes (*Albee's method*).

2. The entire posterior surface of the vertebrae, to be fused, are exposed and cleared of all soft tissues. The spinous processes are excised. The posterior surfaces of the laminae are made raw. The raw area is now grafted. A tibial graft is taken and is divided longitudinally into two halves. Each of these is placed on the raw laminae, on either side of the excised spinous processes. Additional chip grafts from the iliac crest may be put into the different hollows, to make the fusion more solid.

After a spinal fusion, six months' recumbency in a plaster bed is essential.

Treatment for Cold Abscess

1. In the majority of cases, repeated aspirations with local installation of INH is advised.

2. Since administration of antitubercular drugs together with systemic antibiotics prevent secondary infection and sinus formation, some surgeons advocate incision of the abscess, drainage of the contents, and primary closure of the wound. Majority of surgeons, however, discourage incision for fear of secondary infection and sinus formation.

3. If the abscess is associated with Pott's paraplegia, a more drastic type of drainage, e.g. costotransversectomy or anterolateral decompression has to be undertaken.

Treatment for Spinal Deformity.—In some children, the kyphotic deformity cannot be dealt with by simple immobilisation. Different types of corrective extension apparatus are available and these may be used to serve the dual purpose of immobilisation and correction of the deformity.

Treatment for Pott's Paraplegia

1. In the majority of cases of early onset paraplegia, simple stoppage of the weight-bearing of the spine (i.e. recumbency and immobilisation), together with antitubercular treatment, causes gradual improvement.
2. Otherwise, the paravertebral abscess has to be drained, and if the paralysis is due to compression by soft inflammatory material, costotransversectomy should be sufficient for the purpose of drainage.
3. If, however, the compression on the cord is by solid agents, an anterolateral decompression has to be undertaken and the compressing agent removed.
4. In cases of late onset paraplegia, before the operation of anterolateral decompression is undertaken, it must be ascertained that the paraplegia is not due to reactivation of the tubercular process in the spine.

FRACTURES AND DISLOCATIONS OF THE SPINE

Surgical Anatomy.—The vertebral column serves the dual purpose of supporting the trunk with transmission of the body weight and affording protection to the spinal cord within the vertebral canal Flexibility and mobility are served as the column is composed of a series of individual and movable segment that are separated by soft tissue pads, i.e. the intervertebral discs.

The upper and lower surface of each vertebral body is composed of modified spongy bone which is covered by a plate of hyaline cartilage (vertebral end-plate). This cartilage is directly related to the intervertebral disc. The vertebral bodies are also joined by the powerful anterior and posterior longitudinal ligaments which lie in front and behind the bodies respectively and are firmly attached both to the discs and to the bones.

The superior and inferior articular processes of the adjacent vertebrae articulate with each other by means of synovial joints which have loose articular capsules. These are called interarticular joints.

While the anterior and posterior longitudinal ligaments hold the vertebral bodies together, the spinous processes of the vertebrae are held together by the interspinous and supraspinous ligaments. The interspinous ligaments extend between adjacent spinous processes (from base to tip). The supraspinous ligaments are attached to the tips of the spinous processes.

Stability in Spinal Injuries.—Spinal injury, which denotes fractures and dislocations of spine, has its main importance in that it may be associated with injury to the spinal cord, at least in some proportion of cases. Fortunately, in about 80 per cent of the cases there is no injury to the spinal cord or its nerve roots, and these cases are as simple as uncomplicated fractures in other parts of the body. In the remainder, however, injury to the spinal cord occurs, and this results in either death or a permanent disability, too severe for the patient to bear.

It is from this point of view that spinal injuries are divided into two broad groups—*stable* and *unstable*. For practical purposes, this depends on whether the posterior ligaments (i.e. the interspinous and supraspinous) are intact. When these ligaments are intact, one vertebra cannot slip forwards in relation to the adjacent vertebra so as to damage the cord. The spine is then said to be stable—the cord is not likely to have been damaged nor will subsequent movements endanger it. When, however, the posterior ligaments are ruptured, the spine is unstable—the cord has either been damaged or, even if it has escaped, subsequent movements may damage it

It is readily understood that this is the singular factor of importance in all cases of spinal injuries. In subsequent discussion it will be found that the spinal cord may suffer damage under some other conditions, even when the posterior ligaments are intact. Such occurrences are, however, uncommon.

Types of Trauma.—The vertebral column is so well-supported by muscles and ligaments, and its architecture is so perfect that, excepting on rare occasions, only trauma of severe nature can cause its injury. The types of trauma may be as follows:

1. *Flexion:*
   a. In the cervical and lumbar regions, where there is natural lordosis of the vertebral column, local hyperflexion is the cause.
   b. In the thoracic spine, where the natural curve is one of flexion, vertical compression force tends to increase the flexion and cause the injury (*see* below).
2. *Vertical Compression.*—This is caused by a vertical force acting through the long axis of the vertebral column. This force may act from above (by fall of a heavy weight, e.g. fall of a roof) or from below (by a heavy fall of the person from a height, either on the feet or on the buttocks):
   a. In the thoracic spine, this causes hyperflexion of the naturally existing flexion of the vertebral column in the locality.
   b. In the cervical and lumbar regions, such a force can cause injury only when the vertebral column is in the straight position instead of in the natural lordosis.
3. *Rotation (usually combined with flexion).*—This type of trauma often causes the most dangerous type of injury.
4. *Extension.*—The cervical spine is the commonest site where a hyperextension of the spine may be the cause of the injury.
5. *Avulsion.*—The spinous and the transverse processes, which serve for the attachment of muscles, may be avulsed by muscle traction.

Types of Injury

A. *Fractures:*
1. Vertebral Body:
   a. Wedge compression fracture $\Big\}$ These are described below.
   b. Burst fracture
2. Transverse Process.—These injuries are almost confined to the lumbar region.
3. Spinous Process.—The seventh cervical or the first thoracic is most commonly involved. The spinous process is avulsed by uncoordinated muscle action, e.g. while lifting a heavy shovel. This is why the fracture is often called *clay-shoveller's* fracture.

4. Lamina

B. *Subluxations.*—These occur only in the cervical region. There are two types:

1. Extension Subluxation.—The anterior longitudinal ligament is ruptured by a severe extension force and the bodies of the adjacent vertebrae are forced apart from each other anteriorly. The cord may or may not escape injury. The spine is unstable in extension, but is stable in flexion or neutral position of the neck.

2. Flexion Subluxation.—This occurs in the joint between the articular processes. There is forward displacement of one vertebra on the other but the displacement is not so great as to cause overriding of the articular processes. Cord injury is very unlikely unless the neutral canal has been narrowed by osteophytes due to gross osteoarthritis.

C. *Dislocations.*—Simple dislocation of the joint between the articular processes, without fracture of the vertebral bodies, is possible only in the cervical region where the articular processes have horizontal disposition. In the thoracic and lumbar regions this is impossible because of the vertical disposition of the articular processes. The characteristic features of dislocation are as follows:

1. There is overriding of the articular processes either on one side or both, i.e. *unilateral* or *bilateral dislocation.* The inferior articular process of the upper vertebra slips to the front of the superior articular process of the lower vertebra.

2. Dislocations are commonest at the sites of maximum mobility, viz. C_5–C_6 and C_6–C_7.

3. Dislocation of the atlanto-axial joint sometimes occurs. The normal atlanto-axial joint depends upon the odontoid process (dens) of the axis and the transverse ligament which keeps it in position to the anterior arch of the atlas. Dislocation of the joint may be caused either by rupture of the transverse ligament or by fracture of the dens. The dens fragment moves with the axis. The displacement is forwards in flexion injuries and backwards in extension injuries. If the violence is severe (as in hanging) cord injury occurs and injury of the cord at this level is instantaneously fatal. With milder forces the cord escapes injury.

D. *Fracture Dislocations.*—The articular surfaces are out of contact and there is overriding of the articular processes. This is the dislocation element. The associated fracture may be:

1. A fracture of the vertebral body, usually occurring in the upper part of the lower vertebra. Typically, the fracture line is horizontal and, on the X-ray, the appearance is as if the vertebral body has been sliced.

2. A fracture of the neural arch, usually the lamina.

Fracture-dislocations occur most commonly at the sites of maximum mobility of the spine, viz. C_5–C_7 and C_3–C_5.

Types of Vertebral Body Fracture

1. *Wedge Compression Fracture.*—A severe flexion or vertical compression force crushes the cancellous bone of one or more vertebral bodies. The compression is always more marked at the front of the vertebral body, which consequently becomes wedge-shaped. The fracture is stable and there is no associated

cord injury. Pathological fractures, due to osteoporosis in the elderly, or due to rarefying bone diseases including secondary carcinoma, belong to this group.

2. *Burst Fracture.*—This is caused by a vertical compression force acting when the spine is straight at the moment of the injury (if the spine is fixed at the time of the injury, a similar trauma causes a wedge compression fractured. The force fractures one of the vertebrae and the intervertebral disc is forced into the body of the fractured vertebra. This results in a *comminuted,* fractured of the vertebral body and it appears as if the fragments have burst out peripherally in all directions. In at least some cases the spinal cord may be damaged by the posterior fragments of the vertebral body which may be driven back into it. This fracture is, therefore, more dangerous than wedge compression fracture.

Relationship of Trauma to the Nature of Injury

1. Fractures of spinous processes and transverse processes are caused by muscle traction (avulsion).
2. Fractures of the vertebral bodies are caused by severe flexion or vertical compression force.
3. Fracture-dislocations are caused by a combination of flexion and rotational forces.
4. Extension subluxation of the cervical spine is caused by extension.

Level of Injury.—Injury is more likely to occur at those sites where a relatively mobile part of the spine joins a relatively fixed part, viz. the flexible lumbar segment joining the relatively fixed thoracic and sacral segments, i.e. the dorsolumbar and lumbosacral junctions. In the lumbosacral junction prolapse of the intervertebral disc is commoner, while in the dorsolumbar region fractures and fracture-dislocations are commoner.

In the *cervical region* the articular processes of the vertebrae have horizontal disposition and the intervertebral discs are large. So the spine has a high degree of mobility associated with relatively minor strength. Thus, forces of milder nature may cause injury at this level The spinal cord often escapes injury because the neural canal is large in relation to the spinal cord and because the injuring force has relatively little 'follow through'. However, injuries of more severe nature may cause damage to the cord, and cord injury at this level often proves fatal.

In the *thoracic region* the articular process have a vertical disposition and the spine is very well supported by muscles. The spine possesses great strength and less mobility. Only major forces can injure the vertebrae. The follow through of such forces causes displacement, and cord injury is highly probable. This chance is further increased because there is only a little space round the spinal cord in the neural canal of the thoracic region.

In the *lumbar region* the articular processes are vertical. The spine possesses great strength but also enjoys a good amount of mobility, particularly flexion and extension. Only major forces can injure the spine at this level. As the spinal cord ends at the level of the first lumbar vertebra, injury of the roots of the cauda equina can only occur. However, there is a large space round the cauda equina in the neural canal. Thus, nerve injury is often absent or is limited only to a few roots of the cauda.

Spinal Cord Injury

CAUSES

1. Long axis stretch of the cord occurring at the moment of acute flexion.
2. Crushing of the cord, as it is nipped between the lamina of the upper vertebra (which has slipped forwards) and the posterior edge of the body of the lower vertebra.
3. Compression of the cord by (a) the backward protrusion of an intervertebral disc at the moment of acute flexion, (b) vertebral body fragment which has been displaced backwards, in case of comminuted fracture, (c) the ligamenta flava (from behind).

TYPES

1. *Concussion of the Cord*—There is a temporary suspension of function without actual destruction of nerve fibres or nerve cells in the cord. The condition closely resembles cerebral concussion occurring in head injuries, and is probably caused by momentary displacement of the vertebrae, or of the discs or ligaments.

   The clinical state is known as *spinal shock,* which is characterized by a flaccid motor paralysis, sensory loss, and visceral paralysis, below the level of the cord lesion.

   There is always an evidence of some recovery within a few hours, and recovery is always complete by 48 hours. If, even after a few hours of the injury, there is still total loss of sensation, motor paralysis, and loss of vibration sense, it is sure that the case is not one of simple concussion—there must be some destruction of the cord as well.

2. *Transection (Crushing of the Cord).*—There are definite anatomical lesions in the cord. There is a transverse zone of bruising (hence called *cord contusion)* either along the whole girth of the cord or a part of it. Accordingly, cord transection is *complete* or *partial*. At this site the cord has been crushed. Above and below this level there is an area of petechial haemorrhage. Later, oedema develops at these areas of haemorrhage. Only occasionally the haemorrhage may be massive (*haematomyelia)*. Any damage inflicted on the cord is permanent since the cord has no power of regeneration.

   The clinical state typically passes through two stages:

   a. There is an initial phase of spinal shock, characterized by flaccid motor paralysis, complete sensory loss, and visceral paralysis, below the level of the lesion. Reflexes are absent and, since there is no reflex activity of the bladder, there is retention of urine with overflow incontinence (*atonic neurogenic bladder)*. This stage lasts for a few days or sometimes weeks, in contrast to cord concussion where it lasts only for a few hours.

   b. Thereafter, the phase of spinal shock gradually passes off and the cord below the level of transection acts as an independent structure without control of higher centres. The characteristic features are as follows:

      i. The motor paralysis now becomes spastic.

      ii. Minor stimuli tend to cause widespread spastic movements—the *mass reflex*. Such stimuli may be caused by light touch or pressure, by irritability of bed sores, or by distended bladder or rectum. The characteristic feature of mass reflex is that the adductor muscles overpower the other muscles of the hip, the hamstrings overpower the extensors of the knee, and the calf muscles overpower the extensors of the ankle.

iii. As a result of spastic imbalance of the muscles, contractures tend to develop in the adductors of the hip, flexors of the knee, and plantar-flexors of the ankle.

iv. If the lesion is above the T_{12} cord segment, i.e. above the bladder centre, an *automatic bladder* develops, which means that the function of the bladder becomes entirely reflex. This is because the bladder centres in the cord are intact but work uninhibited of high control, a condition similar to that seen in early infancy. The bladder evacuates itself when the intravesical pressure rises and the detrusor muscle contracts reflexly—usually every one to four hours.

From what has been stated above, it is evident that, if the cord has been transected in the mid-thoracic area, there is sensory and motor paralysis, and lack of normal control of the bladder and rectum. However, irregularly distributed the sensory and motor loss may be persistence or reappearance of mass reflex in the lower limbs indicates that there has been a cord transection. There are three other reflexes which are very important in the diagnosis of interruption of the spinal tracts:

Anal reflex.—A stimulus to the perineum causes contraction of the anal muscles.

Penile reflex.—A stimulus to the glans penis causes contraction of the bulbocavernosus muscles in the perineum.

Plantar response.—Extensor in type.

In other words, it is usually possible to know within a few hours, by the combination of the sensory and motor paralysis with the mass reflexes and the special reflexes, that the spinal cord has undergone transection.

3. *Crushing of the Nerve Roots and the Cauda Equina.*—The spinal cord ends at the lower level of the L_1 vertebra. Below this level the neural canal contains only the roots of the cauda equina. Vertebral injuries below the level of L_1 can cause injury only to these roots, i.e. *root-transection.* There are two factors which make root-transection a much rarer condition than cord-transection, even with the same severity of bony injury:

a. There is much room in the lumen of the lumbar spinal canal.

b. The roots are much more resistant to injury than the spinal cord itself.

If is for these factors again, that root transection, even if it occurs, is often incomplete.

If however, the nerve roots of the cauda equina are severed, the results is loss of sensation, motor paralysis of flaccid type, and abolition of reflexes. The bladder becomes isolated, an *autonomous bladder* results, because of paralysis of the detrusor muscle (supplied by the third and fourth sacral segments). Emptying of the bladder is now dependent only upon the precarious and inefficient control by the nerve plexus situated between the strata of the bladder wall. The result is a continual dribbling. However, as the muscles in the upper abdominal wall are not paralysed (being supplied by T_7 to T_{10}), the patient learns to evacuate the bladder by voluntary contraction of these muscles and also by pressing the hypogastrium with hands. The passage may be made easier by diminishing the resistance at the bladder neck by a transurethral 'V' resection of the internal sphincter. At night, the patient has to wear a receptacle. However, residual urine and hydronephrosis almost always result.

The nerve roots, in contrast to the non-medulated nerve tracts of the spinal cord, are capable of complete regeneration, so that there may be complete recovery just as it occurs in other peripheral nerves.

4. *Crushing of Both the Cord and the Nerve Roots.*—This occurs typically at the thoracolumbar junction of the vertebral column. This again is the commonest site of vertebral injury associated with nerve injury. The L_1 cord segment is at the level of the T_{10} vertebra and the spinal cord ends at the lower border of the L_1 vertebra. Hence, between the T_{10} and L_1 vertebrae, all the lumbar and sacral segments of the cord are crowded together. The nerve roots, emerging from these segments of the cord also, lie side by side with the spinal cord up to the lower border of the L_1 vertebra, below which level there are only the nerve-roots and no spinal cord.

Vertebral injuries at the thoraco-lumbar junction (T_{10} to L_1), therefore, may cause:

a. Transection of the cord, leaving the nerve roots intact.

b. Transection of the cord together with injury to some of the nerve roots.

c. Transection of the cord together with injury to all the nerve roots.

Injury only to the nerve roots, keeping the cord intact, seldom occurs because the nerve roots are much more resistant to injury than the cord itself.

Escape of regeneration of the lumbar nerve roots in the presence of spinal cord injury is a great boon to the patient. Important muscles that control the movements of the hip and the knee may escape paralysis, and the patient may even walk well. *Lumbar root escape* is of vital importance in injuries of the thoracolumbar spine, a patient of cord transection with root escape being much more fortunate than one of cord transection with root transection. It follows, therefore, that a patient with an injury at this level presenting with lumbar root escape must be handled, with great precaution, lest injury to these roots occurs subsequently during transport or nursing.

Characteristic Features of Cord Injury in the Cervical Spine

The segmental level of the cord transection corresponds more or less to the level of the vertebral injury:

1. In cervical lesions above C_4, all the respiratory muscles (including the diaphragm, which receives its motor nerve supply from the phrenic nerve, mainly C_4) are paralysed, and the injury is fatal.

2. In lesions of C_3 segment, the patient only breaths with his diaphragm. There is isolation of the lower cervical cord (with paralysis of the upper limbs), the thoracic cord (with paralysis of the trunk) and the lumbar and sacral cord (with paralysis of the lower limb and the viscera).

3. In lesions of C_6 segment, the quadriplegia mentioned above, is modified a little. The deltoid escapes, so that abduction of the shoulder is paralysed.

Management of Spinal Injuries.—This will be discussed under two headings:

I. Management of injuries of the cervical spine.

II. Management of injuries of the thoracic and lumbar spine.

Management of Injuries of the Cervical Spine

A. FRACTURES.—For simple fractures, i.e. wedge compression fractures and burst fractures, no reduction is necessary. A simple support to the neck for 2 months is all that is required. This is done with a collar of plaster of Paris, applied from the crown of the head to the middle of the sternum, encasing the brow, head, neck, and upper thorax, but leaving the face exposed. This is known as *Minerva jacket* (Minerva—the Goddess of Wisdom and Arts). Alternatively, a stiff collar, made of polyethylene, may be used, and this is more convenient for the patient.

B. SUBLUXATIONS

1. *Extension Subluxation.*—The neck is supported in little flexion, with a Minerva jacket, for 2 months.

2. *Flexion Subluxation:*
   a. Reduction.—It is necessary to reduce the subluxation. This is done by extending the cervical spine over the edge of a table on which the patient is lying supine.
   b. Immobilisation.—Redisplacement is prevented by a Minerva jacket.

C. DISLOCATION OR FRACTURE DISLOCATIONS

1. *Conservative Treatment.*—Damage to the spinal cord is common with these types of injuries. A very careful handling is necessary to prevent occurrence or aggravation of injury to the spinal cord. Reduction is urgently required and may be done either by manipulation under anaesthesia or by traction. Manipulation is quicker but traction is safer and is therefore preferred. Traction is applied through skull calipers (*skull traction*). The tip of the calliper, on either side, is engaged in a small hole made in the parietal region. A weight of 20 lb is usually sufficient to achieve reduction within a few hours. Frequent X-rays are taken to see that reduction is complete. Subsequent treatment depends on the particular case:
   a. If there is no paraplegia and there seem to be no risk of redisplacement, immobilisation in a Minerva jacket for 2 to 3 months is all that is necessary.
   b. If there is paraplegia or if there is any risk of redisplacement, a light traction with about 10 lb of weight has to be maintained for another 3 weeks. Thereafter, a Minerva jacket is applied and kept for 3 months. General management for paraplegia, if it is present, has to be instituted (see below, under management of spinal injuries with paraplegia).

2. *Operative Treatment.*—The indications for operative treatment are:
   a. Irreducible locking of the articular processes.
   b. Persistent instability.
   c. As a method of preference by some surgeons, particularly in the cases associated with paraplegia.
   d. If paraplegia is due to compression of the cord, caused by a protruded intervertebral disc.
   a. Irreducible locking of the articular processes.—This is indicated if reduction cannot be effected even after one week's skull traction. Operative excision of the obstructing articular process has then to be undertaken. Simultaneously, the affected segment of the spine is fused with bone grafts.
   b. Persistent Instability.—In the cervical region there are several factors that favour re-displacement:
      i. The horizontal disposition of the articular processes.

ii. Imperfect healing of the torn ligaments.

iii. Absence of good muscular support.

iv. In cases of dislocation without fracture—absence of new bone formation.

If gradual redisplacement tends to occur after traction and plaster immobilisation, operative treatment, to effect an internal fixation, has to be undertaken. This spinal fusion may be done in two ways:

i. Posterior Fusion.—Bone grafts are placed to bridge the spinous processes of the affected vertebrae. Simultaneously the spinous processes are wired together with stainless steel which provides fixation during the period that the grafts take to become incorporated.

ii. Anterior Fusion.—A slot is cut in the front of the affected vertebrae and an inlay bone graft is put in it.

c. As a method of preference to conservative treatment.—Many surgeons prefer operative fusion to conservative treatment in cases of cervical fracture-dislocations. Two reasons are put forward:

i. Frequency of late redisplacement following conservative treatment.

ii. Easier nursing management of a paraplegic patient after operative fusion.

Fusion may be undertaken immediately after the injury (reduction being done at operation), or after reduction has been achieved by skull traction.

d. Protruded Intervertebral Disc.—If there is gross paraplegia in the absence of bone displacement, a myelography should be done. If this suggests compression of the cord by a protruding disc, operative excision of the disc has to be undertaken.

Management of Injuries of the Thoracic and Lumbar Spine

A. FRACTURES.—Simple fractures, i.e. wedge compression fractures and burst fractures, are always stable, unassociated with damage to the cord. There are two schools of thought as regards the management of these cases:

1. *Orthodox Method.*—The fracture has to be reduced and immobilised. Hyperextension of the spine achieves reduction, and this is best done by the Watson-Jone's method. The prone patient is stretched between two tables with the manubrium sterni and the symphysis clear of them. Immobilisation is done with a plaster jacket extending from the manubrium to the symphysis, with the spine in the hyperextended position. The plaster is worn for 3 months. The back muscles are exercised actively within the plaster and thereafter as well.

2. *Recent Method.*—The fracture is disregarded, only the soft tissues are treated, and attempts are made to early restoration of function. As soon as the pain subsides, the patient is advised active muscle exercises, especially of the erector spinae. He is allowed up after 3 to 4 weeks. Thereafter, effective physiotherapy is instituted to strengthen the spine and to restore mobility.

B. FRACTURE DISLOCATIONS.—These injuries are always unstable. In the majority of cases there is paraplegia, but in some cases the cord may escape damage.

1. *Fracture dislocations without Paraplegia.*—Further displacement must be prevented in order to save the cord. Treatment depends upon the state of the

articular processes sharing in the dislocation—in some cases the articular processes are fractured and in the others they are overridden:

a. If the articular processes are fractured.—Conservative treatment is instituted. Reduction can be done by gently extending the spine. Immobilization is done with a plaster jacket, extending from the manubrium sterni to the symphysis pubis, for a period of 3 to 6 months. Thereafter, the patient should wear a back-brace because healing is usually slow.

b. If the articular processes are overridden.—Operative treatment has to be undertaken since reduction cannot be achieved by closed method (by extension of the spine). The fracture is exposed and reduction is done under direct vision, if necessary by doing a facetectomy. An internal fixation is done—two vertebrae above and two below the level of the dislocation being fixed. Fixation is done by strong metal plates or cortical (tibial) bone grafts. Two such plates or grafts are used, one placed on either side of the spinous processes. Over and above this internal fixation, external immobilisation with and plaster jacket is maintained for 3 months.

2. *Fracture-dislocations with Paraplegia.*—This is discussed below in details.

Management of Traumatic Paraplegia.—This is discussed under four headings:

A. First-aid treatment.
B. The diagnosis.
C. The actual management.
D. Rehabilitation.

First-aid Treatment

1. All care must be taken to avoid unnecessary movement or examination that might increase the cord damage.
2. Sedatives.—Morphine or pethidine should be given to relieve pain and anxiety.
3. Transport.—In cervical injuries, the patient should be transported supine with the head supported between sandbags on either side, care being taken not to flex the neck. Patients with injuries of thoracic or lumbar spine should have the spine hyperextended during transport. This is done by placing them prone on the stretcher and placing pillows under the pelvis and shoulders. The stretcher should be so supported that there is no bending or torsion of the spine.

The Diagnosis

1. *Clinical.*—In the stage of spinal shock, it may be difficult to ascertain the nature of the cord damage—whether it is concussion or transection. In all cases the patient says that he 'feels dead' below certain level. Some examinations are important:

a. Sensation to pin prick on the trunk which indicates the segmental level of the cord lesion. Also, if some sensation is present below the affected level, the possibility is that the cord has undergone only concussion, in which case recovery has almost always begun by the time the patient reaches the hospital.

b. Test for joint sensations.—Whether the patient can appreciate the movements of the foot or knee. If he can do this, the case is possibly one of concussion and not transection.

c. If sensation is absent but penile and anal reflexes are present, the cord has been transected.

d. Absence of sensation and power along the distribution of segments above the cord-lesion indicates cord-transection *with root-transection*. Presence of some sensation or power, on the other hand, denotes cord transection *with root escape.*

e. Though there is a deformity of the vertebral column, it is not advisable to do a clinical examination of the back to search for it, because neurological disturbance denotes an unstable fracture.

2. *Radiological.*—Only a lateral view of the spine, at the affected level, is taken without disturbing the patient.

The Actual Management.—The aim of treatment is:

1. Prevention of bed sores in the anaesthetic skin.
2. Care of the paralysed bladder.
3. Care of the paralysed bowel.
4. Care of the paralysed muscles and joints.
5. Treatment of the bone injury itself.
6. Care of the depressed mental condition.

1. *Prevention of Bed Sores:*

a. The patient is placed on a very soft bed (dunlopillow) and soft pillows must be reinforced under the pressure points.

b. The pillows also aim at maintaining the appropriate position of the patient—slight extension of the spine, extension with little abduction of the hips, extension of the knees, and dorsiflexion of the ankles.

c. The skin is subjected to scrupulous drying and powdering.

d. The patient is turned regularly at 2-hourly intervals throughout the day and night.

Plaster immobilisation increases the risk of sores and is therefore avoided. This is particularly so when the cord has undergone complete transection because nothing can be gained by immobilisation. Plastering is only of value in those cases where the cord lesion is incomplete and there is a chance of neurological recovery.

Immediate internal fixation of the spine enables the nursing of the skin to be carried out much more easily and without discomfort to the patient. This is, therefore, preferred by many surgeons. This again is of particular value in cases with incomplete cord lesions because moving the patient while nursing may further damage the cord.

2. *Care of the Paralysed Bladder.*—In the initial stages all patients suffer from spinal shock when there is retention of urine with overflow incontinence (*atonic neurogenic bladder*). In this stage continuous catheterisation of the bladder is done with an indwelling Foley's catheter, passed per urethra. A tidal drainage is advocated by some surgeons. Strict asepsis must be maintained in passing the catheter. However, some degree of infection is inevitable, and so antibiotics are administered. A high fluid intake is advocated.

In cases of cord transection, *an automatic bladder* results and this automatically is usually established within one to three months of the injury. If, from the level of injury (above T_{12} cord segment), it appears that an automatic bladder is likely to develop, bladder training is commenced very early. The catheter is clamped and released at regular intervals, finally four times a day. Later, the catheter is removed and the patient passes urine himself. He knows when the bladder is distended and thus gets sufficient time to make himself ready for the act.

In cases of cauda equina injury with bladder involvement, an *autonomous bladder* results. Micturition is no longer governed by the reflex centres and therefore the mechanism is less reliable. If the patient can use his hands, manual expression of the bladder is advocated; if the abdominal muscles are not paralysed, their contraction also helps evacuation of the bladder. Otherwise, the patient has to have a permanent suprapubic cystostomy, or a life-long urethral catheter, or else a urinal has to be worn permanently.

3. *Care of the Paralysed Bowel.*—If the paralysed bowel is neglected the difficulties are two-fold:

a. Dirty beds and dirty linen result.

b. The loaded rectum may initiate mass reflexes.

The patient should not be allowed to remain constipated for more than three days. Laxatives and enemas are used judiciously in the earlier days. Thereafter, every effort should be made to establish regular periodic evacuation, initiated by a habit reflex and aided by abdominal straining.

4. *Care of the Paralysed Muscles and Joints.*—As the patient has lost active control of the joints of the lower limb, the only way to preserve the range of movements of the paralysed joints is assisted passive movements. This is done by moving the joints passively, through their full range, twice daily. In doing these movements, particular care should be taken so that the toes are flexed, the ankles are dorsiflexed, the knees flexed to beyond the right angle, and the hips extended and abducted. This is done in order to counteract the muscle contractures (secondary to spastic imbalance) that tend to develop in the adductors of the hip, flexors of the knee, and plantar-flexors of the ankle.

5. *Treatment of the Bone Injury itself:*

a. In injuries of the cervical spine, reduction is achieved and maintained with skull traction for 3 weeks. Thereafter, the neck is immobilised with a Minerva jacket. Internal fixation may be necessary or more reliable in some cases. In some cases again, operation may be necessary to achieve the reduction.

b. In injuries of the thoracic and lumbar spine, conservative treatment is often discouraged because:

i. If the articular processes are overridden and not fractured, the dislocation can only be reduced by operation—no amount of hyperextension of the spine can achieve reduction by the closed method.

ii. If plaster is used for immobilisation, sores inevitably develop in the anaesthetic skin.

iii. Operative treatment with internal fixation makes nursing, i.e. regular turning of the patient, much easier with much less discomfort to the patient. Moreover, fixation of the spine also gives a support to the damaged roots, if any, and helps in their regeneration.

Internal fixation is therefore the ideal treatment for traumatic paraplegia at the thoracic and lumbar levels. Two vertebrae above and two below the level of the dislocation are fixed. Fixation is done by strong metal plates or cortical (tibial) bone grafts. Two such plates or grafts are used, one placed on either side of the spinous processes.

6. *Care of the Depressed Mental Condition.*—Constant enthusiasm and encouragement are of great help in boosting up the morale of the patient, who is apt to lose self-confidence. The unpleasant smells, associated with bed sores, dirty linens, and urinary infection, add seriously to the mental depression and all cares should be taken to avoid them.

Rehabilitation.—In cases of complete transection of the cord, despite the severe permanent paralysis, some patients may be enabled to live a reasonably independent and useful life. Though some can walk for short distances with calipers and crutches, for the major part they are to use wheelchairs. Calipers are used during walking to keep the knee straight and the foot plantigrade. All attempts are made to over-develop the muscles above the site of the injury, so that they may move the pelvis. The pelvis, in its turn, moves the lower limbs fitted with calipers. At the same time, the upper limbs are so trained that they develop sufficient power to enable the patient to use crutches and wheelchair. In lesions below the cervical cord, the patient should be up within 3 months.

In cases of cauda equina injuries, the prospects of rehabilitation are much better. Even in the absence of regeneration in such cases, the patient can usually move about with crutches, and sometimes only with sticks together with the use of calipers.

25

Tumours of the Jaw

Types.—The jaw bones may develop the same types of tumours as the other bones of the body but they may also be affected by tumours arising in relation to the alveolar processes (epulis) and those originating in the embryological components of developing teeth (odontomes). Thus, tumours of the jaw may be divided into 4 broad groups:

1. Epulis.
2. Odontomes.
3. Benign tumours of jaw bones.
4. Malignant tumours of jaw bones.

Structure of a Tooth.—Each tooth has a central soft core known as the pulp, which is surrounded by the hard shell known as *dentine*. The exposed part of the tooth (crown) is covered by a layer of enamel. The embedded part (root) is covered by a sheath of *cement substance*. The tooth is held in its socket (alveolar process) by the *periodontal membrane (alveolar periosteum)* that surrounds the root of the tooth.

Development of Tooth.—Embryologically, tooth is a part of the skin—the enamel organ of the tooth representing the epidermis, while the pulp, dentine and cement substance representing the dermis.

The epidermal element of the tooth, i.e. the enamel is derived from the surface ectoderm of the mouth. A thick plate of epidermal tissue grows inwards from this surface ectoderm into the underlying mesoderm of each jaw. This is called the *primary dental shelf (lamina)* or *common dental rudiment*, and this is destined to give origin to the epidermal element of all the teeth developing in the jaw. The epidermal element for the individual tooth, known as the *tooth bud*, develops from this shelf. Thus, each shelf produces 10 tooth buds for the milk teeth and 16 for the permanent teeth. The tooth buds of the permanent teeth appear later than those of the milk teeth and are located at a posterior plane. The smart remnants of the primary dental shelf, which do not take part in the formation of the tooth buds, are called the *paradental epithelial debris*.

Each tooth bud gets cup-shaped and, into the hollow of the cup, it incorporates some of the mesenchyme of the jaw. This incorporated mesenchyme is termed the *dental papilla*. The central part of the papilla remains soft and forms the pulp of the tooth while the peripheral part turns ivory-hard to form the dentine.

The deeper (basal) layer of the tooth bud contains the ameloblasts. These are the cells which produce the enamel substance. The superficial layer of the tooth bud persists as a fine membrane. This is known as the *Nasmyth's membrane*, and it covers the crown of the developing tooth before that erupts. When the tooth erupts, this membrane degenerates and disappears.

Each developing tooth, lying within the mesenchyme of the jaw, becomes surrounded by a specialised vascular fibrous tissue, derived from the mesenchyme. This specialised part, which surrounds the tooth like a sac, is called the *dental sac*. The developing tooth, together with the dental sac is termed the *tooth follicle* or *dental follicle*. The fate of the dental sac is important. The part of the sac around the future crown of the tooth is destroyed when the tooth erupts. The part of the sac around the future root of the tooth splits into two laminae. From the inner lamina develops the cement substance (*crusta petrosa*). From the outer lamina develops the periodontal membrane, i.e. the alveolar periosteum, that anchors the tooth to the alveolus.

EPULIS

The word 'epulis' literally means *'situated on the gum'*. In fact, a wide variety of swellings, located on or near the gum, are included clinically under the heading of epulis. Pathologically, however, the term applies to outgrowths from the alveolar processes of the jaws.

Types
A. *False or Cranulomatous Epulis.*—This is a heaped-up mass of granulation tissue in relation to infected gum or carious tooth, or at the site of irritation by a false tooth.

B. *True Epulis:*

   1. Benign   : (a) Fibrous or fibroid.
                         (b) Giant-cell or myeloid.
                         (c) Melanotic.
   2. Malignant   : (a) Fibrosarcomatous.
                         (b) Carcinomatous (rare).

Fibrous or Fibroid Epulis.—This is the commonest variety of epulis and if arises from either the periodontal membrane or the periosteum of the jaw. The site is on the edge of the gum at the neck of the teeth—the incisors or the premolars.

Microscopically, it consists of massive amount of fibrous tissue, loosely arranged spindle cells, and variable amount of blood vessels.

It is slow-growing, painless, has a smooth surface, and is covered by normal mucous membrane. Characteristically, it is pedunculated and has a firm feel. Sometimes it grows between the teeth and loosen them.

X-ray shows no changes.

Giant-cell or Myeloid Epulis.—This is much less frequent than the fibrous type. There are two views about its origin:
a. It is an osteoclastoma arising in the peripheral part of the jaw and therefore presenting under the gum.
b. It is a granuloma of inflammatory origin, which begins in the interior of the alveolus and projects beneath the gum. It quickly extends into the body of the bone, where it produces a cyst-like structure, surrounded by a shell of bone and thus gives the appearance of an osteoclastoma, which actually it is not.

Whatever be the origin, *microscopically* the tumour consists of fibrous tissue with abundant vascularity and giant cells of foreign body type.

It is more rapidly-growing than the fibrous type but is also painless and has a smooth surface. The overlying mucosa is dark-red or purple in colour, and ulceration and haemorrhages may occur. Characteristically, it is sessile and soft in feel.

X-ray shows bone destruction with ridging of the walls (pseudo-trabeculation).

Melanotic Epulis.—This is a rare tumour found in children and is commoner in the maxilla than the mandible.

Microscopically there are spindle cells laden with melanin. It is a benign tumour but with tendency to local recurrence.

Fibrosarcomatous Epulis.—This occurs as a result of malignant change in a fibrous epulis. The features of malignancy are as follows:

a. Rapid growth.
b. Pain.
c. Ill-defined margins with infiltration into the gum.
d. A soft feel and the tumour often bleeding to touch.
e. Regional nodes may be significant.
f. X-ray may show rarefaction of the jaw bone.

Carcinomatous Epulis.—This is actually an epithelioma of the gum, arising around a tooth or its socket. It presents all the features of an epithelioma.

Treatment of Epulis

1. *False or Granulomatous Epulis.*—Extraction of the carious tooth, treatment for the infected gum, and removal of any ill-fitting denture. The granuloma is scraped out and a biopsy of the material advised.
2. *Fibrous Epulis.*—Simple excision of the tumour is often associated with recurrence. Hence, the following structures have to be removed:
   a. The tumour with surrounding healthy gum.
   b. The tooth or teeth in relation to which the tumour is located; this removes the periodontal membrane.
   c. The margins of the alveoli of the extracted teeth (i.e. a wedge of bone); this removes the local alveolar mucosa.
3. *Giant-cell Epulis:*
   a. If the tumour is small.—Curettage.
   b. If the tumour is big.—Resection of the bone. This means maxillectomy or partial resection of mandible.
4. *Melanotic Equlis.*—The treatment is same as for fibrous epulis.
5. *Malignant Epulis.*—The treatment consists of:
   a. Adequate resection of the jaw—maxillectomy or partial resection of mandible.
   b. Block dissection of neck nodes, if necessary.
   c. Postoperative radiotherapy.

ODONTOMES

Odontomes are tumours made of constituents of dental tissue in varying proportions and different degrees of maturity, derived from one or more of the embryological components of a tooth in the process of development. The pathological character of a particular tumour depends on the stage of development of the embryonic dental element from which it originated.

Classification of Odontomes.—Of the different types available, the *Bland-Sutton's* classification appears to be the best:

A. Odontomes arising from Enamel Organs:
  1. Dental cyst.
  2. Adamantinoma.

B. Odentomes arising from Dental Sac:
  1. Dentigerous cyst (follicular odontome).
  2. Fibrous odontome.
  3. Cementome.
  4. Compound follicular odontome.

C. Odontomes arising from Dental Papilla:
  Radicular odontome.

D. Odontomes arising from the whole Tooth Germ:
  Composite odontome.

Dental Cyst (Radiculo-dental Cyst).—A dental cyst is found in relation to a normally erupted but pulpless carious tooth. The association of such a tooth in relation to a localised swelling in a jaw gives the diagnosis of the cyst. Most commonly it develops in relation to the incisors or canines of the maxilla. When it attains large size, it often extends into the maxillary air sinus and causes bulging of the cheek. Usually it occurs in adult life and is painless.

The cyst is unilocular and usually has an epithelial lining. This lining may be partially destroyed and replaced by fibrous tissue. The contents are fluid, usually crystal clear and containing cholesterol crystals.

Origin.—It is believed that a dental cyst arises from the paradental epithelial debris which are stimulated to proliferation by the infection in the neighbouring tooth.

Dentigerous Cyst (Follicular Odontome, Odontocele).—In these cases there is a localised swelling in the jaw and the characteristic feature is that one permanent tooth is missing. This tooth had neither been extracted nor fallen off. The tumour may occur in either jaw, more commonly in relation to the molars and premolars. It usually occurs in the adults immediately after the second dentition is over, and is painless.

The cyst is unilocular and usually has an epithelial lining which may be partially replaced by fibrous tissue. The content is a gelatinous white fluid and typically there is a whole tooth located inside the cyst. The roots of the tooth are often truncated in the wall of the cyst and the crown, usually fully developed, lies in the cavity. This is the missing tooth.

Origin.—There are different views:
a. It is a cyst formed by cystic degeneration of the Nasmyth's membrane.
b. It is formed by distension of the dental sac.
c. A dentigerous cyst is actually a dental cyst in relation to a milk tooth, which, during the process of development, had incorporated a neighbouring developing permanent tooth within itself.

Treatment of Dental and Dentigerous Cysts.—Before surgery is undertaken oral hygiene must be properly established. An intraoral approach is usually made, the incision being placed on the gum directly over the swelling (for large mandibular cysts, however, an external approach has to be undertaken). As the incision is deepened, the mucoperiosteum on the outer surface of the jaw, over the swelling, is incised, and it is elevated with a periosteum elevator. The outer cortex of the jaw (which is often thinned by the expanding cyst) is chiselled out. The cyst wall is now seen. If possible, the cyst is removed intact. If this is not possible, the cyst wall is removed piecemeal, care being taken not to leave behind any part of it (to prevent recurrence). This is ascertained by cauterising the wall of the cavity with carbolic acid. The excess of carbolic acid is removed by swabbing with alcohol. If the cavity is big it may be partially filled by the small pieces of bone which had been chiselled out from the outer cortex. The cavity is plugged with gauge. Subsequently, healing occurs by granulation.

Adamantinoma (Multilocular Cystic Tumour, Enameloblastoma).—This tumour is almost exclusively found in the lower jaw, only very rarely in the maxilla.
It is a locally malignant tumour. This means that simple curettage of the tumour, from inside the jaw, is usually followed by recurrence. The tumour never shows distant metastasis.

Pathology.—Macroscopically, it is a soft fleshy tumour, having a maroon colour because of haemorrhages. There are often areas of cystic degeneration (hence called multilocular cystic tumour). As the tumour grows inside the jaw, it causes an expansion and thinning of the cortex (more so of the outer cortex) and this may cause egg-shell crackling of the bone (this, however, should not be tried to be demonstrated). Also, the growth causes destruction of the jaw bone, leaving behind some of the bony trabeculae intact.

Microscopically, the cells are of basal cell type. Over some areas, the cells swell up and then liquefy, thus forming the cysts.

Clinical Features.—The tumour usually occurs in the third decade, nearly always at the angle of the mandible, in relation to the molars. It is more prominent from the skin than from inside the mouth because it causes more expansion of the outer cortex of the mandible. The teeth on the swelling are irregularly set up, often loosened, and some of them fall out.

X-ray shows an expansion and thinning of the cortex, with no new bone formation. The presence of bony trabeculae, left behind, gives a characteristic *soap-bubble appearance*. Thus there is a similarity in appearance to an osteoclastoma. However, in adamantinoma there is also an associated fine honey-comb appearance, which differentiates it from an osteoclastoma. Osteoclastoma in the jaw is also much less frequent. However, a wrong diagnosis between osteoclastoma and adamantinoma in the jaw is not much dangerous because both the tumours are locally malignant and the treatment for both is the same, i.e. partial resection of mandible.

Origin.—There are several views, but it is certain that the tumour is of epithelial origin:
1. Some pathologists believe that the tumour arises from the paradental epithelial debris.

2. Others think that it arises from the cells of the primitive enamel organ (enamel-forming cells), i.e. ameloblasts. Hence it is also known as enamel-oblastoma or ameloblastoma.

3. Another belief is that it arises from the primitive ectodermal epithelium of the stomodeum. In favour of this view is the fact that the tumour histologically looks and pathologically behaves like a basal cell carcinoma.

Treatment.—Simple curettage from inside the bone is almost invariably followed by recurrence, so this should not be done. The treatment is partial resection of the mandible, including the tumour and healthy bone on its either side.

BENIGN TUMOURS OF THE JAW BONES

A. Solid Tumours:

1. Ossifying fibroma.
2. Fibrous osteoma.
3. Fibrous dysplasias.—Either monostotic in the jaw or a local manifestation of generalized polyostotic fibrous dysplasia.
4. Osteoma:
   a. Localised.—Ivory osteoma.
   b. Diffuse.—Leontiasis ossea.
5. Paget's disease.—Either as a part of generalized Paget's disease or confined only to the jaw.

B. Cystic Tumours:

1. Solitary cyst.
2. Osteoclastoma—much rare than adamantinoma.
3. Giant cell reparative granuloma. This may be mistaken for osteoclastoma or adamantinoma. It is a painless swelling, occurring between 10 and 25 years of age, and more common in the mandible. There is a round or oval radio-translucent area, which expands but never breaks the cortex. Treatments is by curettage, approach being from the skin, without opening into the mouth.
4. Multiple cysts of hyperparathyroidism.
5. Myxoma.

MALIGNANT TUMOURS OF THE JAW BONES

A. Tumours of the Maxilla:

1. Carcinoma.—This is the commonest maxillary tumour. It may originate as follows:
   a. Primarily arising from the mucosa of maxillary antrum—columnar-cell carcinoma.
   b. Secondarily involving the maxilla from the epithelium overlying the hard palate, nostril, tooth-socket, or gum—squamous-cell carcinoma.
2. Sarcoma:
   a. Osteogenic sarcoma.
   b. Lymphoepithelioma.
3. Burkitt tumour (African lymphoma).

Maxillary carcinoma, though locally very invasive, causes distal and node metastases only late. Thus, maxillectomy (with pre- and postoperative radiation) and, if required, block dissection of neck nodes often provide good results. Three months after the operation, an obturator (bearing teeth) may be fitted.

B. Tumours of the Mandible:

1. Carcinoma.—This is virtually the only malignant tumour of the mandible but is considerably frequent. The carcinoma is always an extension of a cancer from elsewhere:
   a. By direct extension from: (i) Floor of the mouth, (ii) Tongue, (iii) Gum.
   b. Through the mental foramen—from lip.
   c. From a secondary node (facial node) attached to the bone.
2. Burkitt tumour (African lymphoma).

In cases of carcinoma, whenever possible, partial resection of the mandible is undertaken, together with excision of the original carcinoma and a block dissection of the nodes. Radiation is hazardous as it causes necrosis of the mandible.

26

Cleft Lip and Cleft Palate

Embryology. At about the sixth week of intrauterine life, the stomodeal depression develops at the cephalic end of the foetus (Fig. 26.1A). Around this depression there are five elevated processes, viz.

An upper central called frontonasal process.

Two upper lateral called maxillary processes.

Two lower lateral called mandibular processes.

The two mandibular processes fuse in the midline and form the lower lip and the lower jaw.

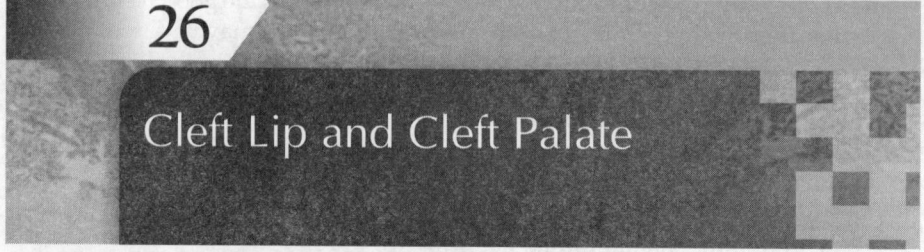

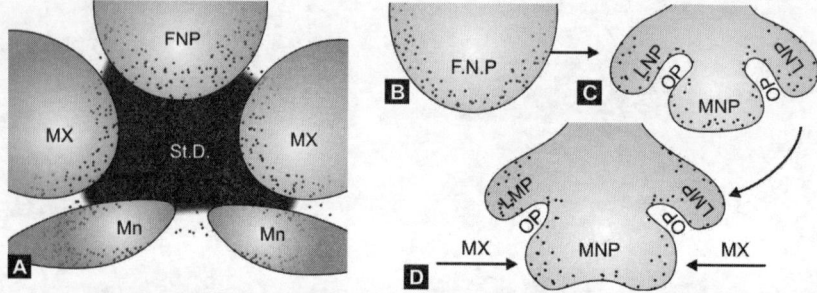

Fig. 26.1: Schematic representation of the development of the lips (A) St.D. represents the stomodeal depression around which five elevations are seen: FNP—Frontonasal process; Mx—Maxillary processes (two); Mn—Mandibular processes (two), (B, C, D)—The frontonasal process and its development. OP represents the two olfactory pits which divide the FNP into MNP and two LNPs. Note that the LNPs move up, allowing the maxillary process, on each side, to fuse with the MNP.

The frontonasal process (FNP) undergoes changes (Fig. 26.1B, C and D). On its either side a depression develops and, since this depression is destined to form the nostril, it is called the *olfactory pit*. The two olfactory pits divide the FNP into three parts a central part called the median nasal process (MNP), and two lateral parts called the lateral nasal processes (LNP) (Thus, each nose is developed from the MNP and the LNP).

The LNP moves up and, on either side, the MNP fuses with maxillary process (hence there is no midline fusion in the upper lip).

The upper lip is thus formed centrally from the superficial part of MNP (this part of the upper lip is called the philtrum) and laterally, on each side, from the maxillary process.

While the superficial part of the MNP forms the philtrum of the upper lip, its deeper part develops into the anterior central part of the palate, called the pre-maxilla (this is the area of the palate that bears the incisor teeth).

The palate develops from three components:
   i. Pre-maxilla.
  ii. Two palatine processes of maxilla one on either side.

CLEFT LIP

Developmental error in the lower lip is exceedingly rare. If it occurs at all, there will be a cleft in the midline.

Developmental error in the upper lip, however, is common. Since there is no midline fusion in the upper lip, the old term *hare-lip* is a misnomer and it should be called cleft lip; the gap is always situated laterally. This cleft is due to failure of fusion between the MNP and the maxillary process.

Classification

A. Cleft lip may be:
   1. Unilateral (common).
   2. Bilateral (occasional).
B. Cleft lip may be:
   1. Incomplete. The upper part of the lip has fused.
   2. Complete. In these cases the cleft extends to the floor of the nose. Since the same developmental elements take part in the formation of the nose, an associated deformity of the nose is always present. This is characterized by flattening and widening of the nostril on the affected side, and the deformity increases as age advances. A complete cleft lip is often complicated (vide below).
C. Cleft lip may be:
   1. Uncomplicated.
   2. Complicated, i.e. associated with:
      a. Cleft alveolus, or
      b. Cleft alveolus and cleft palate.

Difficulties of the Patient

1. Cosmesis.
2. Deformed nostril.
3. Teeth come out through the gap and dental irregularity results.

Operation. Various operations are practised to repair the cleft (a popular operation is that of Mirauit-Blair), but the principles underlying the different operations are the same, as follows:
1. It must be remembered that there is no loss of tissue, which are only developmentally misplaced. Hence, adjustment of the tissues should be so made that the repaired lip is of normal height and thickness, without any depression.
2. The gap on the floor of the nostril must be repaired. Correction of the deformity of the nostril, as well, should always be done.
3. Associated alveolar cleft, if any, cannot and need not be repaired. If the orbicularis oris is effectively reconstructed, the alveolar gap obliterates spontaneously.
4. Adequate mobilisation of the flap must be made from the underlying maxilla on each side; otherwise the sutures tend to give way under tension.
5. The margins must be made raw *(paring)*, so that they can unite.

6. The vermilion border of the lip must be made regular.
7. Sutures must include the orbicularis oris muscle, since this is the mainstay. Hence, there should be three layers of sutures, viz. mucous membrane, muscle, and skin. Alternatively, suturing may be done in two layers, viz. mucous membrane with the deeper part of the muscle in one layer, and skin with the superficial part of the muscle in another.

Postoperative Care

1. Infection must be prevented. Cleanliness is maintained and antibiotics administered.
2. Tension on the suture line is avoided by some surgeons with the help of *Logan's bow*. However, if adequate mobilisation has been done, this is seldom necessary.

Optimum Age for Operation

1. Ideally, it should be done within 48 hours of birth, when the child has still in it, the immunity of the birth-trauma and the maternal antibodies.
2. If this is not possible, one has to wait till the child is about 12 lbs of weight (about 6 months), when it can stand anaesthesia and surgical shock. Beyond this age, teeth start coming out and dental irregularity results.
3. However, even if the patient comes late, the operation has to be undertaken, though the final results may not be so satisfactory. The protruding tooth and any other tooth, that is likely to cause pressure on the suture line, has to be extracted.

CLEFT PALATE

The palate develops from 3 components, viz. the premaxilia (bearing the incisor teeth) and the two palatine processes (vide embryology).

The line of fusion is in the form of Y and fusion starts from the angle between the limbs of Y.

Classification

A. Cleft palate may be:
   1. Tripartite. Y
   2. Bipartite. Y
   3. Intermaxillary. The intermaxillary type may be:
      a. Complete.
      b. Incomplete. In these cases the cleft is situated posteriorly in the palate because fusion starts from the front. Hence the commonest type of an incomplete cleft palate is bifid uvula.
B. Cleft palate may be:
   1. Uncomplicated.
   2. Complicated with cleft lip.

Girls suffer much more frequently from cleft palate, though the incidence of cleft lip is equal in both the sexes.

Difficulties of the Patient

1. Inability to suck. Effective negative pressure cannot be produced inside the mouth because of the gap. Therefore, either the child has to be spoon-fed or the holes in the rubber teat of the feeding bottle have to be enlarged.
2. Regurgitation of food into the nose.

3. Dental crippling because of the associated maldevelopment of the maxilla.
4. Nasal intonation. This occurs because a part of the air comes out through the nose while talking. This is because:
   a. There is a free gap between the mouth and the nose.
   b. The palate in these cases is short in length, so that complete closure of the nasopharyngeal isthmus, which normally occurs during speech by the backward movement of the soft palate, is impossible in these cases.
5. Deafness. About 50 per cent of the patients suffer from deafness. This is because of the blockage of the orifice of the Eustachian tube by inflammatory oedema, resulting from the regurgitated food into the nasopharynx.
6. Cosmesis (though not so much as with cleft lip).

Operation
1. *The 2-flap Operation (Langenbeck's).*—In older days, the 2-flap operation was practised. The mucoperiosteum of the hard palate is mobilised from the underlying bone with the help of release incisions. Two such release incisions are made, one on either side, on the lateral aspect of the palate, just medial to the alveolar border. The release must be adequate so that the suture at the midline, between the flaps, is without tension. The medial margins of the flaps are made raw before suturing *(paring)*

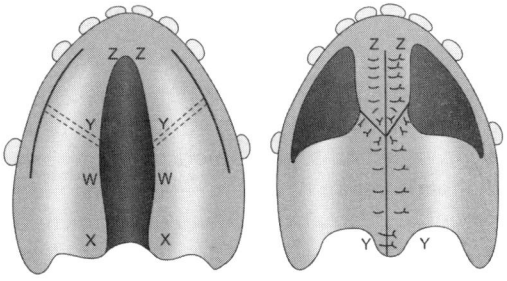

Fig. 26.2: The 4-flap (Wardill's) operation for cleft palate. The figure on the left side shows how the flaps are made. The lateral release incisions on the mucoperiosteum, on the two sides, are seen. Note how each mucoperiosteal flap is divided into two, making four flaps. The figure on the right side shows how the flaps are sutured. Note that the posterior flaps are swung towards the midline, so that, after suturing, the points W, X and Y lie apposed to each other at about the midline.

2. *The 4-flap Operation (Wardill's).*—The difficulties of the 2-flap operation are:
   i. Suture without any tension is a near impossibility, and even the slightest tension would mean failure of union and necrosis of the mucoperiosteal flaps, due to loss of vascularity.
   ii. The length of the palate remains as short as it was prior to the operation, and so nasal intonation persists.
   Hence the 2-flap operation has been abandoned and the 4-flap operation is now universally accepted. Its modifications over the 2-flap operation are:
   a. In order to overcome the tension on the mucoperiosteal flaps and on the suture line, the hamulus process, on either side, is broken. This relaxes the tensor palati muscle.
   b. Each of the 2 flaps are divided obliquely (as in Fig. 26.2) so that 4 flaps are now available. The posterior flaps from the two sides are sutured in the

midline, swinging them backwards as well as medially, as far as practicable; thereafter, the anterior flaps are apposed (the points V, W, X, Y and Z of one side are sutured to the corresponding points of the opposite side after the point X on either side is mobilised to the midline; hence the points W, X and Y now lie apposed to each other at about the midline). This causes some increase in the length of the palate (an increase of about the length of WX), which can now efficiently go back to close the nasopharyngeal isthmus during speech.

c. An operation of *pharyngoplasty* may be added, in which the nasopharynx is made narrower and the *ridge of Passavant,* on the posterior pharyngeal wall, is made more prominent.

A combination of the procedures (b) and (c), or sometimes (b) alone, makes adequate closure of the nasopharyngeal isthmus possible during speech, preventing nasal intonation.

d. The repair of the palate is made in two layers the mobilised nasal mucosa first (with catgut) and the mucoperiosteal flaps on the oral side thereafter (with silk).

Optimum Age for Operation. This operation, requiring a prolonged anaesthesia and causing considerable bleeding and surgical shock, cannot be done very early in the child s life (c.f. cleft lip). The earliest age when the child can stand the operation is when it is about 14 lbs of weight (more than 6 months). This is the age that the British surgeons prefer.

In any case, the operation should not be delayed till the child begins to speak, since, once the nasal intonation develops, it can hardly be cured. Hence the operation must be done by 18 months, and American surgeons prefer this age.

It has been found that early repair of a cleft palate often increases the already existing underdevelopment of the maxilla (due to detachment of the periosteum at operation). Hence, some surgeons advocate repair of the cleft in the soft palate only before the child begins to speak, and put an obturator to occlude the gap in the hard palate. After the age of 18 years, when maxillary growth ceases, the gap in the hard palate is repaired.

After any operation for a cleft palate, the child must have a course of *speech-training.*

27

The Salivary Glands

Surgical Anatomy.—The **parotid gland** one on each side, fits into the space behind the mandible and in front of the mastoid process, below the external ear. Its anterior border overlies the masseter. The lower pole of the gland extends into the neck below and behind the mandible, sometimes as much as 5 cm, and a swelling in relation to this part may cause diagnostic perplexity.

The gland is arbitrarily divided into two lobes, the *superficial* and the *deep,* by the facial nerve which may be looked upon as the meat in a parotid sandwich. The superficial lobe is much bigger.

The *facial nerve,* after emerging from the stylomastoid foramen, enters the posterior part of the gland a little below its middle. Inside the gland the nerve divides into its two main subdivisions, viz. the temporo-facial and the cervico-facial, and from these the terminal branches arise. All the branches of the nerve lie in one plane, which is designated as the faciovenous plane since it is in this plane that the posterior facial vein also lies (in this plane the gland may be split sagitally into two parts without damaging the facial nerve, as is done in superficial parotidectomy).

The parotid duct (*Stensen's duct*) emerges from the anterior border of the gland and passes transversely across the masseter. It makes a right-angle turn round the anterior border of the masseter and pierces the buccinator to open on the mucous membrane of the cheek, opposite the crown of the upper second molar tooth.

Many lymph glands are closely related to the parotid gland. Some of them (*the juxtaparotid lymph glands)* are located deep to the parotid fascia, either on the surface or within the substance of the parotid gland. Others (the *pre-auricular glands*) lie superficial to the parotid fascia.

The **submandibular gland**, one on each side, is situated partly below the mandible and partly deep to it. The free posterior border of the mylohyoid muscle is insinuated into the medial border of the gland, dividing the gland arbitrarily into two parts, the *superficial* and the *deep.* The superficial part is covered only by the platysma and the deep fascia. The deep part is deep to the mylohyoid, between this muscle and the hyoglossus (i.e. on the floor of the mouth, between the mandible and the tongue). Between the deep part and the hyoglossus muscle there are two important nerves—the lingual and the hypoglossal. The submandibular lymph glands are closely related to the surface of the submandibular salivary gland.

The submandibular duct (*Wharton's duct),* emerging from the medial aspect of the deep part of the gland, opens into the mouth on the sublingual papilla, at the side of the frenum linguae.

The **sublingual gland**, one on each side, lies below the termination of the submandibular duct. Of its fifteen or so ducts, half open into the submandibular duct and the remainder separately on the sublingual papillae.

Ectopic salivary glands are dotted here and there in the bucco-pharyngeal cavity, e.g. palate, cheek, tongue, lip, floor of the mouth, maxillary antrum, etc. the commonest site being the hard palate. The importance of these ectopic glands is that they may give origin to tumours which may cause diagnostic perplexity.

Special Investigations

1. *Straight X-ray.*—A stone in the submandibular duct or gland usually casts a clear shadow. A parotid calculus is usually too small or too radiotranslucent to cast a diagnostic shadow.
2. *Sialography.*—This is particularly useful for the parotid. A fine ureteric catheter or a lacrimal duct canula is gently passed into the duct, through its opening. 1 or 2 ml of an watery (and not oily) solution of lipiodol is injected with light pressure and X-ray taken. A good radiograph of the parotid tree may be obtained by this method.

Common Diseases of the Salivary Glands

1. Inflammation:
   a. Acute.—Almost always in the parotid.
   b. Recurrent Subacute and Chronic.—Common in both parotid and submandibular glands.
2. Fistula.—Almost always in relation to the parotid.
3. Stones.—Much more frequent in the submandibular.
4. Tumours.—Much the commoner in the parotid. Only 7 per cent of the tumours occur in the submandibular and 10 per cent in the ectopic salivary glands.

ACUTE PAROTITIS

Types.—There are two distinct varieties:

1. Acute epidemic parotitis, i.e. mumps. This is of viral origin, it is of a little surgical importance.
2. Acute suppurative parotitis and parotid abscess. This is of surgical importance and is discussed below.

Etiology.—Almost always the infecting organism is *Staphylococcus aureus* and the bacteria reach the gland by retrograde infection from the mouth.

The most important *predisposing factors* are:

1. Dryness and lack of cleanliness of the mouth.
2. Diminished output of secretion from the gland which may be due to:
   a. Lack of normal stimuli to secretion, e.g. fasting.
   b. Lack of pumping action on the gland, i.e. stopping mastication.
   c. Dehydration.
   d. Obstruction in the Stensen's duct, e.g. parotid calculus or (rarely) a foreign body.

A combination of many of the above factors is found in a post-operative abdominal case. The patient is fasting, not masticating, and is often dehydrated. An old and uraemic patient is particularly a sufferer. Debilitating medical diseases, especially typhoid fever and cholera, are often complicated with acute parotitis.

Pathology.—In contrast to mumps, the infection may be confined to one parotid. Often, however, both the glands are involved, either simultaneously or in succession.

Infection in the parotid is associated with early necrosis and abscess formation. This is due to two factors:

a. The necrotoxic action of the *Staphylococcus aureus*, the commonest organism.

b. The inflammatory products kept under tension within the dense parotid fascia.

For a long time the pus is kept confined within the parotid fascia. Later, it may burst through the fascia and rupture either into the external auditory meatus, or on the surface of the gland usually below the angle of the mandible.

Clinical Features.—Very often the patient is a post-operative abdominal case, ideally an elderly, dehydrated, pre-uraemic patient. The characteristic presenting features are as follows:

1. Pain over the parotid.
2. Trismus, i.e. difficulty in opening the mouth, due to spasm of the muscles of mastication.
3. Brawny edematous swelling over the parotid region with all signs of inflammation. Fluctuation, however, is late to appear because of the dense parotid fascia.
4. Pus can often be expressed from the Stensen's duct.
5. Constitutional symptoms are often severe—high fever, headache, malaise, and sometimes rigor.
6. The abscess may burst on the surface or into the external auditory meatus.

Treatment

A. *Prophylactic.*—These are of particular value in post-operative cases and debilitating medical diseases:
1. Prevention of dehydration.
2. Special nursing care to maintain oral hygiene.

B. *Treatment in Established Cases*:
1. Maintenance of oral hygiene and correction of dehydration.
2. Antibiotics.—The organisms are usually penicillin-resistant, so broad spectrum antibiotics are advised; erythromycin is often useful. If pus can be expressed from the Stensen's duct, it is sent for culture. The antibiotic is then chosen according to the drug-sensitivity of the organism.
3. Incision and Drainage.—When response is not seen within 48 hours and particularly when the condition is bilateral, incision is essential. This should not be delayed for fluctuation to appear, which is masked by the dense parotid fascia. This is because a delayed incision predisposes to the development of a parotid fistula.

A vertical incision is made through the *skin only* in the pre-auricular crease. When the surface of the gland is exposed, the *parotid fascia* is incised transversely, i.e. along the line of the branches of the facial nerve, thus avoiding injury to these branches.

Complications of Incision.—A delayed or badly placed incision, or sometimes even a proper incision, may be associated with complications in some cases. These complications may be as follows:

1. Facial palsy.
2. Auriculo-temporal syndrome (Frey's syndrome).
3. Parotid fistula.

Auriculo-temporal Syndrome (Frey's Syndrome).—This peculiar syndrome usually follows injury to the fibres of the auriculo-temporal nerve during incision of a parotid abscess. The syndrome is characterized by the following features:

1. The cheek is red, hot and painful, and there is sweating over the parotid area during consumption of meals.
2. There is a cutaneous hyperaesthesia in front and above the ear, particularly noticed during shaving.

Treatment.—Usually the patient is advised to ignore the symptoms and he often agrees.

The only effective treatment is avulsion of the auriculo-temporal nerve (*see* Chapter 15).

PAROTID FISTULA

Fistula develops only rarely in relation to the submandibular gland and even if it does, the condition may be easily treated by excision of the gland.

For practical purposes, a salivary fistula means a parotid fistula. Such a fistula may be internal or external, but the internal fistula does not produce any symptoms.

Thus, it is only an external parotid fistula that deserves consideration.

Causes

1. Following a parotid abscess which has either been allowed to rupture spontaneously, or has been incised late or incised with a badly placed incision.
2. A penetrating injury into the parotid (e.g. glass splinter).
3. Following partial parotidectomy (this is rare and the fistula, usually short-lasting, heals spontaneously).

Types.—While the external opening of the fistula is over the parotid area and usually no bigger than a pinpoint, the internal communication may be:

1. With a ductule, i.e. *gland fistula.*
2. With the main duct, i.e. *duct fistula.*

Symptoms.—There is discharge of saliva from the external opening, particularly during consumption of meals. The amount of discharge varies with the type of the fistula. A gland fistula causes only some moisture on the face when the patient eats. On the other hand, a duct fistula causes considerable and distressing output of saliva on the cheek when the patient consumes a meal or even smells food or thinks of food. Moreover, the salivary enzymes cause excoriation of the neighbouring skin.

Sialography.—This is of great value. It indicates the site and type of the fistula, i.e. whether the internal communication is with a ductule or with the main duct, and this decides the course of treatment.

Treatment

A. GLAND FISTULA.—A fistula communicating with a ductule causes little inconvenience and may be advised to be ignored. Such a fistula often heals spontaneously and this may be aided by probanthine, 50 mg every six hours, for a week (atropin-like effect).

B. DUCT FISTULA.—This is really a surgical problem and ordinary conservative methods of treatment often prove to be unsuccessful. The different types of treatment, conservative and radical, are as follows:

1. *Auriculo-temporal Avulsion.*—This procedure had been practised for many years but usually proves to be of little effect. The idea behind the treatment was to cut off the secretomotor nerve supply to the gland (*see* Chapter 15).

2. *Radiation* over the parotid, in order to diminish its secretion, also commonly proves to be futile.

3. *Reconstructive Operation (Newman and Seabrook's Operation).*—This consists of repair of the duct at the site of the injury. The site of injury is identified by passing two probes, one through the orifice of the Stensen's duct and the other through the external opening of the fistula. The repair is done with fine catgut stitches over a fine polythene catheter, passed through the duct from the mouth. The repair is successful at least in some cases.

4. *Flap Supplement.*—If the distal part of the duct has been destroyed or if it is stenosed, the distal part of the duct is made with a mucosal flap. A rectangular pedicle flap of mucosa is raised from the inner side of the cheek and is rolled into a tube. To this tube is anastomosed the proximal end of the duct.

5. *Complete Parotidectomy.*—This is the radical form of treatment and is particularly advisable when a reconstructive operation fails.

RECURRENT SUBACUTE AND CHRONIC INFECTION OF THE SALIVARY GLANDS (SIALANGIECTASIS)

Recurrent subacute and chronic inflammations may occur either in the parotid or in the submandibular salivary gland. One or a combination of the following factors is responsible:

1. Ascending infection from the mouth.
2. Dilatation of ductules in the gland, i.e. *sialangiectatis*. Rarely the main duct may also be dilated. The condition is particularly seen in the parotid. Such dilatation may be:
   a. Primary, i.e. without any obvious cause of obstruction in the main duct. The condition is often congenital (congenital sialangiectasis). This is the commoner type.
   b. Secondary, i.e. associated with an obstruction near the mouth of the main duct, e.g. stenosis.
3. Stone in the salivary duct; particularly in case of the submandibular gland.

Special Investigations
1. Straight X-ray, for evidence of stones.
2. Sialogram distinctly shows the pattern of dilatation.

Treatment
1. Maintenance of oral hygiene.
2. Removal of stone from the duct, if any, or dilatation of a stenosed orifice.
3. Gentle massaging of the gland after meals, and administration of sialogogues to prevent stasis.

4. Catheterisation of the duct with a fine ureteric catheter and injecting a weak antiseptic solution through it (in case of parotid).
5. Some cases may even require excision of the gland.

MIKULICZ DISEASE

This disease is characterized by a triad of features:
1. Symmetrical enlargement of all the salivary glands.
2. Narrowing of the palpebral fissures due to enlargement of lachrymal glands.
3. Parchment-like dryness of the mouth due to lack of salivary secretion. When there is an associated generalised arthritis, the condition is known as *Sjogren's syndrome.*

Pathology.—The salivary and lachrymal tissues are progressively replaced by lymphoid tissue. There are two views about the etiology:
1. It is a process of chronic inflammation.
2. It is an auto-immense disease like Hashimoto's disease of the thyroid. However, the pathology is self-limiting.

Treatment.—Radiotherapy is the only available treatment to check the progress of the disease.

SALIVARY CALCULUS (SIALOLITHIASIS)

Stones are 40 to 50 times commoner in the submandibular than the parotid glands. This is because of three factors:
a. The secretion of the submandibular gland is much more viscid.
b. The secretion of the submandibular gland is rich in salts.
c. There is an upward trend of the termination of the Wharton's duct and this leads to easy stagnation in the gland.
   Chemically, the stone resembles dental tartar. The stone may be located either in the main duct or in the ductules (gland substance), and may be multiple.

Clinical Features of Submandibular Salivary Calculus
1. There is swelling of the gland, characteristically aggravated during meals.
2. Sometimes there is a salivary colic, typically at the commencement of a meal. The pain is often like toothache and is sometimes referred to the tongue (due to irritation of the lingual nerve which hooks round the Wharton's duct).
3. The swelling may be reproduced during clinical examination by giving the patient a few drops of lemon juice. The orifice of the ducts are also watched. While saliva freely ejects from the non-affected side, it is scarce on the affected side.
4. If the stone is situated in the Wharton's duct, it can always be palpated by bi-digital examination, and can often be seen.

X-ray.—A submandibular calculus is usually easily seen on the straight X-ray.

Treatment
1. STONE IN THE MAIN DUCT.—This can easily be removed from inside the mouth. Local anaesthesia is sufficient. The stone is steadied by grasping the duct behind the stone since it has a notorious tendency to slip back into the gland substance. An incision is made along the length of the duct just over the stone, which is easily removed. The wound is left unsutured.

2. STONE IN THE GLAND SUBSTANCE.—This requires excision of the submandibular salivary gland. A curved incision is made over the gland, in the line of the skin crease, below and behind the lower border of the mandible. If the incision does not extend to within 2 cm of the angle of the mandible, the cervical branch of the facial nerve is not injured. The gland is usually easily dissected out. The facial artery and the veins in the location require ligation. While the gland with its duct is dissected from its bed, care is taken to avoid injury to the hypoglossal and lingual nerves in this situation. The duct and the deeper part of the gland are dissected out by retracting the mylohyoid muscle anteriorly.

TUMOURS OF THE SALIVARY GLANDS

75 per cent of salivary tumours arise in the parotid glands and 15 per cent in the submandibular glands. 10 per cent of tumours arise in the ectopic salivary glands and these may cause diagnostic problems. The salivary tumours may be classified as follows:

I. EPITHELIAL TUMOURS
   A. *Benign,* i.e. adenoma:
      1. Pleomorphic adenoma.
      2. Monomorphic adenoma:
         a. Adenolymphoma or Warthin's tumour.
         b. Oxyphilic adenoma or oncocytoma—rare.
         c. Other rare types of adenoma.
   B. *Intermediate Types,* i.e. low grade malignancy:
      1. Mucoepidermoid tumour.
      2. Acinic cell tumour.
   C. *Malignant,* i.e. carcinoma:
      1. Adenocarcinoma.
      2. Malignant change in pleomorphic adenoma.
      3. Adenoid cystic carcinoma.
      4. Epidermoid carcinoma.
      5. Anaplastic carcinoma.

II. NON-EPITHELIAL TUMOURS: These are connective tissue tumours and are rare. They may be benign or malignant, e.g. fibroma, neurofibroma, sarcoma, etc.

PLEOMORPHIC ADENOMA

This is the commonest tumour of the parotid, constituting about 60 per cent of the cases.

Histology.—The tumour is so named because it shows different pattern of cells (c.f., monomorphic adenoma, e.g. Warthin's tumour where a single type of cell is seen). There are two main groups of cells, widely varying from each other:
1. One group comprises well-differentiated epithelial cells. These may be columnar, squamous or basal, and may be arranged in acini, cords, tubules, sheets, etc.
2. The other group consists of sheets of spindle-shaped or stellate cells and these are probably of myoepithelial origin.
   There is an abundance of intercellular mucoid material. This material separates

the cells and gives a myxomatous appearance which closely resembles cartilage tissue (the so called *pseudo-cartilage*)

In the past, the tumour was popularly called *mixed parotid tumour* because the second element looked like cartilage (connective tissue) which was found in association with the epithelial cells (i.e. mixture of epithelial tissue and connective tissue).

Macroscopic Features.—The tumour is usually bulky, with a nodular outline. It has a firm-to-hard feel and usually cuts with a gritty sensation (the pseudo-cartilage). The tumour may be solid homogenous or there may be areas of cystic degeneration.

Recurrence and Malignant Change.—This tumour is essentially benign in nature. However, it has a great tendency to recur after local excision. Also, at least a small percentage (the exact figure is highly debated) tends to turn malignant, though usually after many years.

As for the recurrence of the tumour after simple enucleation and even after extracapsular excision, there are two views:

1. The tumour capsule, which may be well-formed over much of its surface, is rarely complete. There are often areas where the tumour tissue comes out from lobulated surface of the main mass through the gaps in the capsule. It is from these elements that recurrence is believed to occur.
2. The tumour is of multicentric origin, the left-out undetected tumours producing the so-called recurrences in future.

Clinical Features

1. The tumour usually appears in early adult life and the incidence is equal in both the sexes.
2. The history is usually for many years and the only complaint is the swelling.
3. For some obscure reason, it is the lower part of the parotid in relation to which the tumour is usually seen, and it commences in that part of the parotid gland which overlies the jaw.
4. The swelling is firm-to-hard, lobulated, and painless. It is free from the skin and the underlying masseter.
5. There is no involvement of the facial nerve.

Signs of Malignant Change in the Tumour

1. It starts growing rapidly.
2. It becomes painful.
3. The feel becomes stony hard.
4. Fixity with the surrounding structures sets in, i.e. the skin superficially (ultimately fungation may occur), and the masseter and the mandible in the depth.
5. Movements of the jaw may be restricted (due to infiltration of the masseter and the pterygoids).
6. The most important suggestive feature is facial nerve palsy.
7. The cervical nodes may show significant enlargement.

Treatment.—Superficial parotidectomy is the standard method of treatment. The different surgical procedures adopted for mixed tumours are as follows:

1. *Extracapsular Excision.*—This is indicated only for a small superficial tumour. There is considerable chance of recurrence for reasons already described. On no account should an enucleation of the tumour be done (leaving behind the capsule) since such a procedure is almost always likely to cause a recurrence. Some surgeons advocate post-operative radiotherapy after local excision.

2. *Superficial Parotidectomy* (Superficial Parotidectomy).—This is advised for most of the tumours. The whole of the superficial lobe of the gland is removed, particular care being taken to preserve the facial nerve and its branches. The incision begins at the level of the zygomatic arch and is carried down vertically immediately in front of the pinna, thereafter curving round the root of the lobule, and extending up to the base of the mastoid process; from here it is extended downwards along the anterior border of the sternomastoid for a short distance. The incision leaves a rather inconspicuous scar but, by raising the flaps, the whole of the superficial lobe of the gland is exposed. The dissection of the gland is commenced from its posteroinferior border and the plane of dissection is kept at the facio-venous plane in order to save the facial nerve. Since the part of the parotid gland superficial to the facial nerve is excised the operation is also designated as *superficial* parotidectomy (Fig. 27.1).

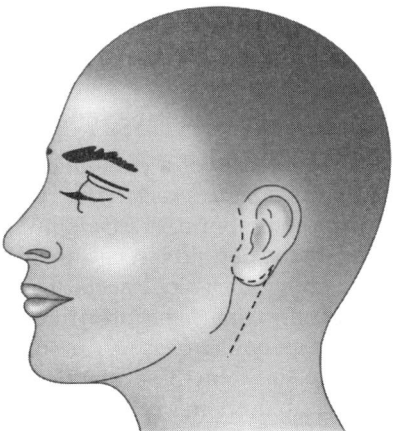

Fig. 27.1: Incision for parotidectomy

3. *Complete (Total) Conservative Parotidectomy.*—This is indicated under the following circumstances:
   a. A tumour situated in the deep part of the gland.
   b. A tumour which has broken its confines and has commenced to enlarge comparatively rapidly, i.e. suspicion of malignant change.
   c. A tumour that has recurred after local excision.

   All attempts are made to preserve the facial nerve but it is often difficult to save all its branches. The operation is called conservative because the facial nerve is preserved (c.f. radical parotidectomy for carcinoma).

WARTHIN'S TUMOUR (ADENOLYMPHOMA)

This tumour is much less frequent than pleomorphic adenoma but is not uncommon.

Clinical Features.—The tumour resembles the pleomorphic adenoma in its size, rate of growth, painlessness, and clear delination.

The points of difference from a mixed tumour are as follows:

1. The patient is almost always over forty.
2. Males are more often affected than females (5 : 1).
3. The tumour occurs much more frequently in the white races.
4. Though, like a pleomorphic adenoma, the site is the lower part of the parotid, at least some part of the swelling is situated in the neck, below the angle of the mandible.
5. The tumour is never hard, and in many cases it is sufficiently cystic for fluctuation to be elicited.
6. Sometimes the tumour is bilateral.
7. It is easily removed and seldom recurs.
8. While other tumours present as 'cold' spots in a $^{99}Tc^m$ Pertechnetate *scan*, this tumour presents as a 'hot' spot.

Macroscopic Appearance.—The tumour is essentially benign. It is either solid or partly cystic. It has a complete and well-defined capsule.

Histology.—There are two characteristic tissues:

1. Papillary columnar cells with a greater or lesser degree of cyst formation. These cells are often termed *oncocytes*.
2. Lymphoid stroma of varying amount, with or without germ centres.

Histogenesis.—As the tumour consists of a combination of adenomatous and lymphoid element, it is termed *adenolymphoma*. The presence of the lymphoid stroma strongly suggests that the tumour arises from juxtaparotid lymph nodes. These nodes are situated deep to the parotid fascia, either on the surface or within the substance of the parotid gland. Embryological studies have shown that ductal structures from the developing primary parotid bud often grow into these developing lymph nodes. These encompassed ductules ultimately loose all connections with the parotid tree. It is from these ductules that an adenolymphoma arises. In other words, an adenolymphoma is an epithelial tumour arising in a juxtaparotid lymph node.

Treatment.—As the tumour is well-limited within a fully developed capsule, extracapsular excision is sufficient. Recurrence is extremely rare.

Oncocytoma.—This resembles a Warthin's tumour, but differs from it in that it consists only of the oncocytes and no lymphoid stroma.

CARCINOMA

Types.—*See* classification of salivary tumours.

Adenoid cystic carcinoma deserves special mention. The tumour arises from the myoepithelial cells and the cells of duct epithelium. There are sheets, strands or cords of cells within which a basophilic material accumulates, giving a cystic appearance. However, it is hard and fixed. The tumour is slow-growing, compared to the other types of carcinoma. However, it has a special tendency to spread along perineural tissues of adjacent nerves for long distances and also to spread to medullary bone.

Clinical Features.—These are described under pleomorphic adenoma (signs of malignant change).

Treatment

1. *For Operable Cases.*—Complete parotidectomy with post-operative radiation is the treatment. Block dissection of the cervical nodes is not undertaken unless there are significant nodes. Adequate removal of a malignant parotid, i.e. *radical parotidectomy*, cannot be accomplished without injury to the facial nerve (c.f. conservative total parotidectomy for mixed parotid tumours).
2. *For Inoperable Cases.*—Palliative radiation is the treatment of choice.

MUCO-EPIDERMOID TUMOUR

These tumours are of low-grade malignancy and usually very slow-growing. According to some pathologists, they are of two types:

a. Low malignancy
b. High malignancys

The tumour is partly solid and partly cystic. It is so named because histologically it consists of the following elements:

i. Sheets of epidermoid cells,
ii. Cystic spaces lined by mucus-secreting cells.

The *treatment* is total parotidectomy.

ACINIC CELL TUMOUR

This rare tumour is also of low-grade malignancy and is usually slow-growing. It is soft and often cystic. It is composed of cells resembling those of serous acini.

The *treatment* is total parotidectomy.

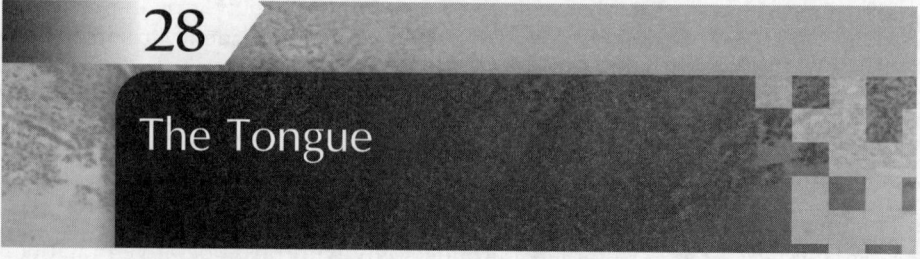

28

The Tongue

Surgical Anatomy

DEVELOPMENT AND NERVE SUPPLY

A. *The Mucosa, the Glands, and the Lymphoid Tissue* develop from the first and third branchial arches:

1. From the first (mandibular) arch three buds arise and fuse together to form the anterior two-thirds of the tongue. These are the centrally placed *tuberculum impar* and a pair of *lateral rudiments* or *lingual swellings*. The nerve supply of this part of the mucosa is, therefore, mainly from the nerve of the first arch (trigeminal)—the lingual branch of the mandibular. In addition, the pretrematic branch of the nerve of the second arch, i.e. the chorda tympani branch of the facial nerve also supplies this part. The lingual nerve mediates common sensations and the chorda tympani mediates taste.

2. From the third arch a swelling develops *(the cupola of His* or *hypobranchial eminence)* and part of this forms the posterior third of the tongue. The nerve supply of this part is, therefore, derived from the nerve of the third arch, i.e. the glossopharyngeal nerve. It mediates both common sensations and taste.

B. *The Musculature* has an extraordinary origin. Three or four occipital myotomes contribute the musculature. The musculature is thus innervated by the hypoglossal nerve which is brought down with these occipital myotomes. The only exception is the palatoglossus muscle, coming from the sixth arch myotome and therefore supplied by the cranial root of the accessory nerve.

PARTS.—For purpose of description, the tongue is divided into an anterior two-thirds and a posterior third. The circumvallate papillae, about a dozen in number and arranged in the form of a V with the apex backwards, is the anterior boundary of the posterior third of the tongue. The sulcus terminalis, which is a shallow groove behind the circumvallate papillae, is incorrectly stated to be the line of union of the two embryological components; it is a part of the posterior third.

MUSCLES OF THE TONGUE

A. *Intrinsic Muscles.*—They cause alteration in the shape of the tongue:
1. Longitudinal (superior and inferior).
2. Transverse.
3. Vertical.

B. *Extrinsic Muscles.*—They cause movements of the tongue:
1. Genio-glossus (from the superior genial tubercle of the mandible).
2. Hyo-glossus (from the hyoid bone).
3. Palato-glossus (from the palate).
4. Stylo-glossus (from the styloid process).

LYMPHATIC DRAINAGE.—The tongue is drained by four main sets of lymph vessels:
1. *Apical Vessels.*—From the tip of the tongue these vessels drain bilaterally into the submental nodes, from where efferents go to the deep cervical nodes. Some of these vessels, however, may directly drain into the jugulo-omohyoid nodes.
2. *Marginal Vessels.*—From the lateral borders of the anterior two-thirds of the tongue these vessels drain homolaterally to the submandibular nodes, from where efferents run to the deep cervical, i.e. jugulo-digastric and jugulo-omohyoid nodes.
3. *Central Vessels.*—From the central area of the anterior two-thirds of the tongue, on either side of the median raphe, these vessels drain bilaterally to the deep cervical nodes.
4. *Basal Vessels.*—From the posterior third of the tongue these vessels drain bilaterally to the deep cervical nodes.

It is important to note that many of the apical and marginal vessels run along the periosteum of the mandible on their way to the submental and submandibular nodes.

GLOSSITIS

Types

1. ACUTE:
   a. *Acute Superficial Glossitis.*—This follows scalds and superficial injuries. Herpes of the tongue may be included in this group.
   b. *Acute Parenchymatous Glossitis.*—This rare condition may occur as a sequela to deep wounds in the tongue.
2. CHRONIC: Chronic superficial glossitis.

CHRONIC SUPERFICIAL GLOSSITIS (LEUKOPLAKIA)

This is an intractable form of hyperplasia involving the superficial tissues of the tongue and showing a tendency towards cancerous change. A similar condition is also common in the buccal mucous membrane.

Etiological Factors.—The following factors, singly or, in combinations, are believed to play some role as causative agents:
1. Sharp tooth (or ill-fitting denture), i.e. trauma.
2. Smoking, spirit, spices, i.e. irritation.
3. Sepsis (chronic), i.e. infection.
4. Syphilis—a common cause in older days; now rare.
5. Susceptibility of some persons.
6. Deficiency of vitamin A, which is known to impair the nutrition of epithelial tissues.
7. Chronic intestinal disorders, especially in this country.
8. Candidiasis—long-standing infection with *Candida albicans*.

Microscopic Pathology.—Changes are seen both in the epidermis and the dermis.
A. *Epidermis.*—All the layers show changes in the form of more rapid proliferation than normal, particularly the middle layer:

1. The superficial layer (a) is increased in depth, (b) shows extensive kerati-nisation, and (c) shows cornification of the superficial cells (this causes the patchy whiteness, i.e. *leukoplakia*).

2. The middle layer shows swelling and vacuolation of the cells (sometimes resembling the Paget's cells of the breast). There is extensive proliferation of the cells.

3. The basal layer also shows proliferative changes (in some cases approximating malignancy).

As a result of the rapid proliferation of the epidermis, particularly in its middle layer, not only does the epidermis increase in its thickness but also the interpapillary processes become broader and longer (projecting more deeply into the corium).

B. *Dermis.*—It is congested, oedematous, and shows round cell infiltration.

Clinical Features (and Macroscopic Appearance).—The disease may be localised in some area of the tongue or may be diffuse. Sometimes there is simultaneous involvement of the buccal mucosa.

The presenting features may be described in stages:

I. The patient first presents with a white patch on the tongue (*leukoplakia* = white plaque), together with hypertrophy of the lingual papillae. The white patch passes through 3 stages:

1. In the first stage there is a thin milky patch over a wide area of the tongue.

2. In the next stage the patch becomes smaller in size but gets thicker, as if the tongue is covered with a smooth paint.

3. In the last stage the patch is still smaller but the surface becomes irregular and cracked, resembling wrinkled paint.

II. Subsequently, some portions of the leukoplakic patch falls off (desquamation) and this area of the tongue gets a raw beefy appearance. Such patches are often called *smoker's patches.*

III. Till later, the tongue develops:

1. Multiple cracks and fissures.

2. Little warty projections.

This is definitely a *precancerous* state.

IV. Finally, carcinoma develops at least in some of the cases. This may occur either in the depth of the cracks or in the warty projections.

Treatment

A. In the Early Stages:

1. All precautions to remove the irritating factors.

2. Maintenance of oral hygiene to prevent sepsis, and application of 2 to 4 per cent mercurochrome.

3. Supplements of vitamins A, B-complex, and C.

4. Correction of intestinal disorders.

5. Treatment of syphilis, if present.

B. In those cases

1. where a localised patch does not recede with conservative treatment, or

2. where there is a suspicion of malignancy (warty projections or chronic fissures).

—the patch must be excised and biopsy performed to exclude malignancy.

C. In cases where the affected area is larger, can be excised, biopsy is performed to exclude malignancy, and the patient is kept on a check-up every three months.

D. Radiotherapy should not be advocated. The appearance of the lesion improves but chances of malignancy are increased and, such a malignant lesion is often radioresistant.

TUMOURS OF THE TONGUE

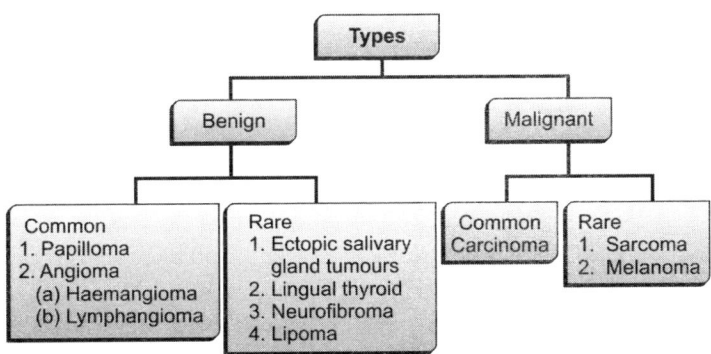

Papilloma.—This is the commonest benign tumour of the tongue. The tumour is either pedunculated or sessile. A pedunculated papilloma is easily diagnosed. A sessile papilloma may sometimes be difficult to be diagnosed from carcinoma; differentiation is done by the absence of induration at the base. A papilloma may undergo secondary malignancy.

Treatment consists in excision together with a small wedge of normal tissue round the base, followed by biopsy.

Haemangioma.—This is a fairly common tumour of the tongue and is usually of the cavernous type. The tumour is usually localised. Rarely a large haemangioma may be found and sometimes an arteriovenous aneurysm; these varieties cause *macroglossia.*

Treatment consists in excision, preferably with a diathermy. As a preliminary step, to reduce haemorrhage and prevent recurrence, sclerosing agents may be injected pre-operatively. The external carotid artery may require ligation.

CARCINOMA OF THE TONGUE

Predisposing Factors
1. Leukoplakia.
2. Papilloma.
3. Chronic irritation by sharp tooth or ill-fitting denture.
4. Syphilis—nowadays rare.

Distribution

1. Lateral margin of the anterior two-thirds   47%
2. Posterior third   20%
3. Tip   12%
4. Undersurface and frenum   9%
5. Dorsum   6%
6. Other parts   5%

Macroscopic Types

A. *Centrifugal growths,* i.e. those with tendency to expand outwards:

1. Ulcerative
2. Proliferative. } much the commoner.

B. *Centripetal growths,* i.e. those with tendency to infiltrate inwards:

1. Fissure
2. Plaque } most commonly following leukoplakia.
3. Indurated submucous nodule.
4. Diffuse scirrhous growth with extensive infiltration through the substance of the tongue, making the tongue shrunken, cracked, and fixed. This is called *woody tongue.*

Microscopic Types

1. In the *anterior two-thirds* of the tongue, where the epithelium is thick, stratified and cornified, the growth is a squamous cell carcinoma with well-formed cell nests. The degree of differentiation, i.e. the grade of the tumour, however, varies.
2. In the *posterior third* where the epithelium lacks cornification and where there are abundant racemose glands and collection of lymphocytes, the growth may be one of the following types :
   a. Lympho-epithelioma.
   b. Transitional cell carcinoma.
   c. Basal cell carcinoma.
   d. Adenocarcinoma.

Spread

A. DIRECT SPREAD

1. *By Continuity.*—The carcinoma spreads along the substance of the tongue and this is helped by the rich lymphatic plexus in the tongue. In cases of growth in the anterior two-thirds, the median raphe usually delays a spread across the midline. An anterior two-thirds growth seldom encroaches on the posterior third and vice versa.
2. *By Contiguity :*
   a. From the anterior two-thirds.—To the floor of the mouth, alveolar processes and mandible, and the cheek.
   b. From the posterior third.—To the tonsils, epiglottis, and the soft palate.

B. LYMPHATIC SPREAD.—*See* surgical anatomy of lymphatic drainage of the tongue.

It should be noted that, on an average, lymphatic metastases from growths on the margins of the anterior two-thirds are homolateral, while those from growths on the posterior third and the tip are bilateral.

C. VENOUS SPREAD.—Distant spread by venous route is rare and occurs almost exclusively with posterior third growths. The lungs, bones, or liver may be involved.

Clinical Features

A. *Distribution*
   1. The patient is usually above 50.
   2. Males suffer much more commonly than females.
B. *Presentation*
   1. For a growth in the anterior two-thirds, the patient sees the growth and seeks advice for it, though often after a long neglect.
   2. A growth in the posterior third is never seen by the patient, and an ordinary examination by the clinician often fails to detect it. For such a growth, the patient often presents late and with the following features:
      a. A cervical swelling due to metastatic nodes.
      b. Hoarseness of voice.
      A laryngoscopic examination detects the growth.
C. *Symptoms*
   1. Pain:
      a. Local, in the tongue.
      b. Referred, often to the ear, by way of the auriculo-temporal nerve which is a branch of the mandibular, of which the lingual nerve is another branch.
   2. Profuse salivation.
   3. *Ankyloglossia.*—In the early stage, as the patient is asked to protrude the tongue, the tip is found to be deviated to the side of the lesion. This is caused by the pull of the fibrous tissue in the growth. Thereafter, movements of the tongue are gradually restricted because of infiltration, i.e. the tongue gets fixed.
   4. Difficulty in articulation.—This occurs as a result of a combination of ankyloglossia, salivation, and pain.
   5. Dysphagia.—More pronounced with growths in the posterior third.
   6. Foetor.—Accumulation of profuse saliva and failure to maintain oral hygiene lead to secondary bacterial stomatitis and bad smell.

Causes of Death

1. Inanition and malignant cachexia.
2. Inhalation bronchopneumonia (from oral sepsis).
3. Secondary haemorrhage :
   a. From the primary growth.
   b. From a big vessel in the neck, eroded by a malignant node which is also ulcerated on the surface.
4. Asphyxia :
   a. Pressure on the larynx and trachea by metastatic nodes.
   b. Oedema glottis occurring in growths of the posterior third.

Special Investigations

1. Indirect laryngoscopy to visualize growths of the posterior third.
2. X-ray:
   a. Chest
   b. Mandible, to exclude its involvement.

3. Biopsy:
   a. From a primary growth.
   b. From a neck node in cases where the primary growth is undetected.

Treatment.—This may be discussed under three headings :
   I. Management of the primary growth.
   II. Management of the neck nodes.
   III. Management for advanced cases.

I. Management of the Primary Growth

A. PRELIMINARY MEASURES.—Oral hygiene must be properly maintained. This includes:
   1. Regular mouthwash with antiseptic lotions.
   2. Antibiotic treatment, the antibiotic preferably chosen on the basis of the sensitivity test of the predominant organism in the mouth, detected by culture.
   3. Treatment for carious teeth and infected gums.

B. RADIOTHERAPY.—Unless there is a contraindication, all patients should get the benefit of radiotherapy because the growths are usually radio-sensitive and a mutilating operation on the tongue can be avoided. The *contra-indications* to radiotherapy are:
   1. A growth very close (within 2 cm) to the mandible (because the radium needles, lying in close contact with the bone, cause severe bone necrosis).
   2. A growth involving the mandible (any form of radiation causes bone necrosis).
   3. Presence of gross sepsis in the mouth of jaw (as bone necrosis invariably occurs).

Radiation may be achieved in two ways:
   1. *Interstitial radiation* (i.e. direct radiation).—This is done for growths in the anterior two-thirds, i.e. the site accessible for implantation of caesium$_{137}$ needles, or iridium$_{192}$ wires. A single layer of needles are used (i.e in one plane), 1 cm apart.
   2. *Teletherapy.*—This is usually done with cobalt$_{60}$ unit. This is an indirect form of radiation, i.e. by rays from outside. This is indicated for:
      a. Growths in the posterior third, i.e. the part inaccessible for implantation of needles.
      b. Growths too big to be radiated by a single layer of needle implantations, i.e. more than 2 cm in diameter or 1 cm in depth.

C. SURGERY is indicated:
   1. Where the growth is small (i.e. less than 1 cm) and is situated in the anterior two-thirds. Here surgery is preferred to interstitial radiation because of more definite results and easy surgery.
   2. Where a growth fails to disappear within 2 months of completion of radiotherapy or recurs after radiotherapy.
   3. Where the growth is within 2 cm of the mandible or has involved the mandible.

The types of surgery are as follows (Fig. 28.1):
   1. *Excision.*—When a lesion is of doubtful malignancy or when a malignant lesion is less than 1 cm in diameter. Excision should always be followed by

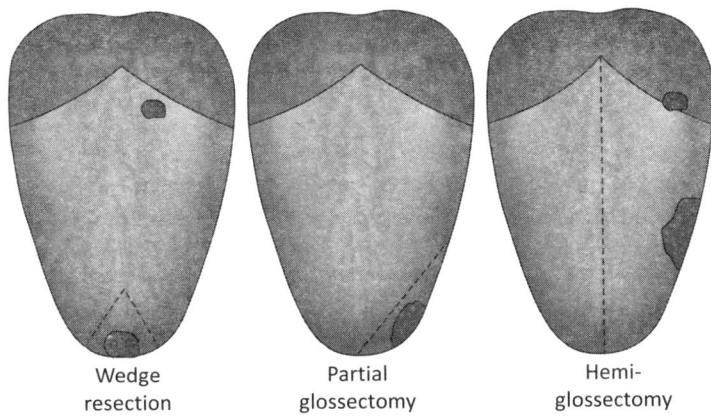

| Wedge | Partial | Hemi- |
| resection | glossectomy | glossectomy |

Fig. 28.1: Different types of resections of the tongue

biopsy. A wide margin of mucosa, not less than 1 cm round the growth, should be removed.

2. *Wedge Resection.*—For small growths near the tip.
3. *Partial Glossectomy.*—For growths on the lateral margin, close to the tip.
4. *Hemiglossectomy.*—This means excision of half of the anterior two-thirds of the tongue. This is done for growths on the lateral margin.
5. *Subtotal Glossectomy.*—i.e. excision of the whole of the anterior two-thirds, and *total glossectomy*, i.e. excision of the whole tongue are rarely done for extensive lesions. The lower lip and the mandible are bissected and the incision is prolonged down to the hyoid. The muscles are cut and the tongue is removed. The floor of the mouth is sutured.
6. *Hemimandibulectomy* has to be added to glossectomy if growth involves, or reaches to within 2 cm of the mandible.
7. *Commando Operation.*—This means glossectomy and hemimandibulectomy together with block dissection of the cervical nodes. The operation is so named because of its extensive nature.

II. Management of the Neck Nodes.—Four groups of patients may be encountered:
1. Patients with no palpable neck nodes.—In these cases, after the treatment for the primary growth, the patient is kept on a periodic check-up.
2. Patients with palpable significant (i.e. metastatic) nodes which are still mobile.—Block dissection of the cervical nodes is required (*see* below).
3. Patients with significant fixed nodes.—Only palliative treatment is advised (*see* below).
4. Patients with palpable nodes and it cannot be ascertained clinically whether the nodes are metastatic or inflammatory (because the primary growth is often grossly infected).—This is the problem group. In these cases one of the two following procedures may be adopted:
   a. With the treatment for the primary growth, a 3 to 4 weeks' antibiotic treatment is instituted. If the nodes regress, they are possibly infective and the patients are treated as in group (1). On the other hand, if they persist or progress, they are taken as malignant and a block dissection is advised.

b. Biopsy of a node is done to decide the nature of enlargement, and treatment done accordingly.

Block Dissection of the Cervical Nodes

1. If the nodes are involved on one side, unilateral block dissection is done; for bilateral involvement, bilateral block dissection is required.
2. If only the upper group of cervical nodes are involved, *suprahyoid block dissection* is advocated by many surgeons. In this operation, nodes above the level of the hyoid, on both the sides, are resected.
3. For better results, instead of ordinary block dissection, *radical neck dissection (Crile's block dissection)* may be done. This means block dissection of the nodes together with excision of the structures to which these nodes are intimately related, viz. part of the internal jugular vein (ligating it above and below), deeper fibres of the sternomastoid and, if required, parts of the omohyoid and digastric. In case a bilateral radical neck dissection is required, the internal jugular vein on one side has to be spared in order to avoid an obstructed cerebral venous flow (this idea is debatable).

(*See* Chapter 18 for details of these operations).

III. Palliation for Advanced Cases

1. *Radiotherapy.*—This is often helpful for large primary growths even if there are unresectable nodes. Radiotherapy is of a little or no value for the nodes.
2. *Chemotherapy:*
   a. Regional intra-arterial injection of amethopterin (50 mg daily for 5 days) may be used either for palliation or as an adjunct, before, during, and after excision of a growth.
   b. Systemic chemotherapy.
3. *Cryosurgery.*—This is a technique in which the tissues are exposed to extreme cold (less than –20°C) to cause irreversible cell damage.

Prognosis.—All groups of cases taken together, the 5-year survival is 25 percent.

ULCERS OF THE TONGUE

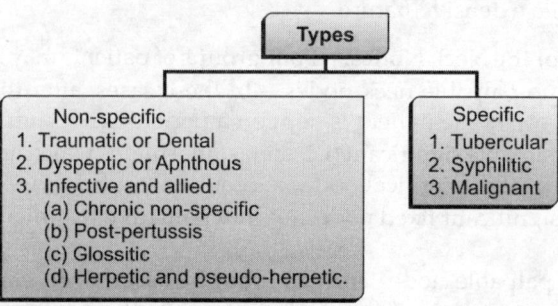

Dental Ulcer.—These result from trauma of the mucosa by sharp tooth or denture. They are always located on the margin of the tongue. The ulcer starts as a longitudinal erosion of the mucosa, which then gets infected. Left untreated, it gets chronic, and the fibrosis at its base causes induration that may lead to a wrong diagnosis of malignancy. Moreover, chronic irritation may actually turn the ulcer malignant.

Treatment
1. The irritating tooth or denture is removed.
2. Oral hygiene is maintained by regular mouthwash and application of 4 per cent of mercurochrome on the ulcer.
3. Vitamins A, B-complex, and C.
4. If the ulcer persists, it is excised and sent for biopsy.

Aphthous Ulcer.—These ulcers, common at the tip of the tongue, are often multiple. They are found on the tongue, as well as the lips and mouth, in persons suffering from intestinal disorders. They start as small blisters, which burst and produce painful superficial ulcers, surrounded by a hyperaemic zone. They tend to heal by themselves with correction of the intestinal disorder.

Chronic Non-specific Ulcer.—These ulcers often cause diagnostic difficulties. The ulcer, usually situated at the margin of the tongue, is painless and chronic. It has no attributable cause for its occurrence. Because of the induration at the base it may be mistaken for malignancy. Some of the ulcers may actually turn malignant. *Treatment* is in the same line as for dental ulcers.

Post-pertussis Ulcer.—This is found in children on the frenum linguae only, following whooping-cough.

Glossitic Ulcer.—This means the 'smoker's patch', found in chrome superficial glossitis.

Herpetic Ulcers.—There are two varieties:
1. *True herpetic ulcer* is due to a herpetic affection of the lingual nerve. Acute neuralgic pain, strictly unilateral, is followed a few hours later by the appearance of a vesicle, which bursts to form a very painful superficial ulcer.
2. *Pseudo-herpetic ulcer* has no relation to herpes and occurs in children as multiple blisters, rupturing to produce superficial ulcers.

Tubercular Ulcers.—Though rare, these occur as secondary ulcers in patients suffering from pulmonary tuberculosis expectorating out tubercle bacilli in the sputum. The ulcers are multiple and painful. Like tubercular ulcers elsewhere, they are shallow, with thin, bluish, overhanging-margins. The floor is covered by whitish granulation tissue and there is no induration at the base. X-ray shows the pulmonary lesion.
Systemic antitubercular treatment cures the ulcers.

Syphilitic Ulcers.—Syphilis may involve the tongue in all its stages.

A. Primary stage.—Extragenital chancre, occurring at the tip of the tongue. Submental nodes are enlarged but not tender. *Treponema pallidum* is seen in the scrapings from the floor of the ulcer by dark-field illumination.

B. Secondary stage
1. Multiple 'Snail track' Ulcers.—Shallow painless ulcers found on the margins and under-surface of the tongue.
2. *Mucous Patches.*—Greyish-white in colour.
3. *Hutchinson's Wart.*—This is really a condyloma and has the appearance of a papillary growth, located strictly on the midline of the dorsum of the tongue.

C. Tertiary stage
1. Chronic Superficial Glossitis (Leukoplakia).—Syphilis is nowadays only a rare cause for this condition.
2. Gummatous Ulcer.—This occurs always on the dorsum.

The ulcer has a typical appearance—clear punched-out margins, wash-leather slough on the floor, and no induration at the base.

Malignant Ulcers.—This means ulcerative type of carcinoma. As elsewhere, the ulcer is raised from the surface, with rolled-out everted margins, and induration at the base. Significant neck nodes may be present.

For treatment *see* carcinoma of the tongue.

MEDIAN RHOMBOID GLOSSITIS

This is a developmental anomaly of the tongue, believed to be due to inadequate covering of the tuberculum impar in the development of the tongue (*see* Embryology).

There is a rhomboid-shaped area on the dorsum, in the midline, just in front of the circumvallate papillae, with its long axis along the long axis of the tongue. The area is red in colour and is devoid of lingual papillae.

The condition, though chronic, produces no symptoms and requires no treatment. Its only importance is that the patient is afraid of a cancer and the clinician may also sometimes make a wrong diagnosis of cancer or smoker's patch.

FURRED TONGUE (FISSURED TONGUE)

Sometimes a patient presents with multiple fissures in the tongue. Such fissures may be of the following types:
1. Congenital.—The fissures are usually transverse. No treatment is necessary.
2. Acquired:
    a. Syphilitic.—Mainly disposed longitudinally.
    b. In association with chronic superficial glossitis.

MACROGLOSSIA

This means chronic painless enlargement of the tongue, often making it voluminous, so that it is protruded out of the mouth. This may be caused by the following anomalies when they are extensive:
1. Angioma:
    a. Lymphangioma.
    b. Haemangioma, including arteriovenous fistula.
2. Neurofibromatosis.
3. Muscular hypertrophy in idiots and cretins.
4. Amyloidosis.

29

Development of the Neck and Some Important Congenital Anomalies

BRANCHIAL ARCHES

In early intrauterine life, six transverse ridges appear on each side of the neck, opposite that part of the foregut which is destined to form the mouth and the pharynx. These are known as branchial arches. Each arch fuses ventrally in the midline with its counterpart of the other side. Each branchial arch is a mesodermal condensation, covered on the outer side by ectoderm and on the inner side by entoderm. The successive arches are separated from each other by depressions both internally (i.e. towards the pharynx) and externally. The external depressions, lined by ectoderm, are called *branchial clefts*. The internal depressions are known as *pharyngeal pouches*. The fifth branchial arch is very rudimentary and disappears so that the fourth and the fifth pharyngeal pouches become one, and open into the pharynx by a common channel.

The thin wall between a pharyngeal pouch and the corresponding branchial cleft is known as the *cleft membrane*. This membrane never disappears in man (in contrast to fishes) because a little mesoderm always lies between the ectoderm and the entoderm.

The mesoderm within each arch forms a central bar of cartilage (which later usually forms bone) and a muscle mass. Each arch has a nerve to supply its derivatives. The artery to each arch is called an *aortic arch*. The six aortic arches are the channels of communication between the ventral and the dorsal aorta.

Derivatives of the Arches

First arch (mandibular arch)

A. *Cartilage* (Meckel's Cartilage) → Bone:
   The major part disappears and the remnants form:
   1. The lingula and mental ossicles of the mandible (the remaining major part of the mandible is developed by ossification in membrane that develops in place of the cartilage).
   2. Malleus.
   3. Incus.
B. *Ligaments:*
   The fibrous perichondrium of the cartilage, which remains after disappearance of the Meckel's cartilage, forms:
   1. Sphenomandibular ligament.
   2. Anterior ligament of malleus.
C. *Muscles:*
   1. Muscles of mastication—masseter, temporal, pterygoids.
   2. Mylohyoid.

3. Anterior belly of digastric.

4. Two tensor muscles—tensor palati, tensor tympani.

D. *Nerve:*

Mandibular nerve (branch of 5th cranial).

E. *Artery:*

Maxillary (remnant of the first aortic arch).

SECOND ARCH (HYOID ARCH)

A. *Cartilage* (Reichert's Cartilage) → Bone:

1. Stapes.

2. Styloid process.

3. Lesser cornu and upper part of the body of hyoid bone.

B. *Ligaments:*

The fibrous perichondrium of the cartilage, that remains after disappearances of its central part, forms:

Stylohyoid ligament.

C. *Muscles:*

1. Muscles of facial expression, including buccinator.

2. Muscles of the scalp.

3. Platysma.

4. Posterior belly of digastric.

5. Stylohyoid.

D. *Nerve:*

Facial nerve (7th cranial)

E. *Artery:*

Stapedial artery (remnant of the second aortic arch).

THIRD ARCH (THYROHYOID ARCH)

A. *Cartilage* → Bone:

Greater cornu and lower part of the body of hyoid bone.

B. *Muscles:*

Stylopharyngeus

C. *Nerve:*

Glossopharyngeal nerve (9th cranial).

D. *Artery:*

Internal carotid artery (third aortic arch).

FOURTH ARCH

A. *Cartilage:*

Thyroid cartilage.

B. *Muscles:*

1. Cricothyroid.

2. Inferior constrictor of pharynx.

C. *Nerve:*

External laryngeal nerve (branch of 10th cranial).

D. *Artery:*

1. On the right side.—First part of the subclavian artery.

2. On the left side.—Main part of the arch of aorta.

FIFTH ARCH

Disappears.

SIXTH ARCH

A. *Cartilage:*
1. Cricoid cartilage.
2. Rings of trachea and bronchi.

B. *Muscles:*
1. Intrinsic muscles of larynx, excepting cricothyroid.
2. All muscles of the pharynx, excepting stylopharyngeus.
3. All muscles of the palate, excepting tensor palati.

C. *Nerve:*
Recurrent laryngeal nerve (branch of 10th cranial), but carrying fibres of the cranial accessory.

D. *Artery:*
1. Ventrally.—Main part of the pulmonary artery.
2. Dorsally.—The artery disappears. On the left side it persists as the ductus arteriosus.

It is easier to remember the nerve supply of the local muscles as follows:

1. All the muscles of the face are supplied by the facial nerve excepting one, i.e. masseter (supplied by the mandibular nerve).
2. All the muscles of the tongue are supplied by the hypoglossal nerve excepting one, i.e. palato-glossus (supplied by the cranial accessory nerve).
3. All the muscles of the larynx are supplied by the recurrent laryngeal nerve excepting one, i.e. cricothyroid (supplied by the external laryngeal nerve).
4. All the muscles of the soft palate are supplied by the cranial accessory nerve via the pharyngeal plexus excepting one, i.e. tensor palati (supplied by the mandibular nerve).
5. All the muscles of the pharynx are supplied by the cranial accessory nerve via the pharyngeal plexus excepting one, i.e. stylopharyngeus (supplied by the glossopharyngeal nerve).

The first and second branchial arches grow much more rapidly than the others. For the first arch, this growth is well seen as the development of the mandible. The rapid growth of the second arch, downwards, occurs superficial to the other arches (overhanging). Thus, in between the developing second arch and the lower arches, there is a space lined by ectoderm (squamous epithelium). This space, with its opening downwards, is called the *cervical sinus*. Ultimately, the overgrown second arch fuses with the sixth arch, and the cervical sinus turns into a closed space, lined by ectoderm. This space normally disappears entirely. Should this space persist, it results in a branchial cyst. Persistence of the whole of the lower part of the cervical sinus results in a branchial fistula.

BRANCHIAL CYST

Origin.—This results from non-obliteration of the closed space between the overhanging second branchial arch and the lower branchial arches (vide above). The cyst is lined by ectoderm (squamous epithelium) of the arches. The secretions of this ectoderm forms the fluid in the cyst, which is turbid, often looking like pus. However, the fluid is very rich in cholesterol crystals which can easily be identified if a drop is examined under the microscope—the crystal looks rectangular, with a notch at one corner.

Clinical Features

1. In spite of its congenital origin, the cyst makes its appearance usually between 20 and 25 years.
2. The patient complains of a gradually enlarging swelling, which is painless. Infection may sometimes occur, resulting in pain.
3. The location of the cyst is typical—it protrudes forwards from beneath the upper third of the sternomastoid.
4. Since cold abscess, originating in the cervical nodes in this situation, is very common, a branchial cyst, particularly when associated with pain, may be wrongly diagnosed as a cold abscess. Absence of palpable characteristic matted nodes underneath the swelling usually confirms the diagnosis. In cases of doubt, aspiration, followed by microscopic examination of the fluid confirms the diagnosis (demonstrating typical cholesterol crystals in cases of branchial cyst).
5. As the swelling is deep to the deep fascia, unlike other simple cysts, it can be moved transversely but not vertically.

Treatment.—Excision of the cyst has to be performed. This is done with a transverse incision placed over the cyst. As the anterior wall of the cyst is exposed, some of its contents is aspirated. The cyst can now be grasped with a suitable forceps. This procedure definitely helps in dissecting out the cyst. Sometimes a fibrous band, attached to the deeper aspect of the cyst, passes inwards, towards the pharyngeal wall, like a branchial fistula. If this is present, this has to be dissected out like a branchial fistula (*see* below).

BRANCHIAL FISTULA

Origin.—This results from persistence of the whole length or the lower part of the cervical sinus (vide development). Since the cervical sinus never communicates with the pharyngeal lumen, a branchial fistula can never have any communication with the lumen of the pharynx. When complete, it can, at the most be attached to the lateral pharyngeal wall. The cases, in which a branchial fistula at operation has been shown to communicate with the pharynx, are those where the cleft membrane has been forcibly punctured by the probe that was introduced into the fistula to define its track. Thus, in true sense, the condition is not a fistula but a sinus.

Clinical Features

1. The condition is bilateral in about 30 per cent of cases. The position is fairly constant—at the anterior border of the sternomastoid in its lower third.
2. There is a sticky mucoid discharge—the secretion of the lining ciliated epithelium. This may form a crust at the mouth of the fistula.
3. The opening of the fistula is usually found to be covered, from above, by an overhanging fold of skin. This is because of the inability of the fistula to grow in pace with the growing neck. Sometimes this skin contains fibrocartilage, and this is known as a *cervical auricle*.

Special Investigation.—Injection of a little radio-opaque medium (diodone or hypaque) into the tract demonstrates its course, and extent (*see* below).

Pre-operative Preparations.—For better definition of the tract at operation, one of the following procedures may be adopted pre-operatively:

a. A little amount of a radio-opaque dye is introduced into the tract and then the opening is closed by a purse-string suture on the skin round it. While X-ray shows the track, the dye, with the pent up secretions, produces a thickening of the wall of the fistula, and this helps in its identification and makes dissection easier.

b. Alternatively, just before operation, a small amount of methylene blue is introduced into the tract as above. The dye helps identification of the length of the tract.

Operation.—A transverse incision, split to encircle the external opening, is made through the skin, subcutaneous tissue, and the platysma. The tract has a subcutaneous course up to the level of the upper border of the thyroid cartilage. Here it pierces the deep fascia. The deep fascia at the anterior border of the sternomastoid is incised longitudinally at this level and the sternomastoid is retracted laterally. The tract is found to pass upwards and medially through the gap between the internal carotid and the external carotid arteries. The internal carotid artery develops from the third arch artery and the cranial part of the dorsal aorta. The external carotid artery is not developmentally a primary artery but is an outgrowth from the internal carotid artery and passes cranially, parallel to the dorsal aorta, towards the second arch. This is why the tract passes between these two arteries. In fact, the tract lies deep to all the structures developing from the second arch in this situation, and superficial to the derivatives of the third arch (as per the course of cervical sinus).

The tract is traced up to its upper end which, if the tract is complete, will be found attached to the pharyngeal wall just behind the tonsillar fossa, but not opening in the pharynx (as discussed above).

In carrying out dissection of the upper part of the tract, another incision at a higher level, is usually necessary. This is a transverse incision, parallel to the first. The dissected tract is brought out through this second incision. This method is popularly known as the *step-ladder* pattern of dissection.

Other Derivatives of Branchial Arches and Cervical Sinus.—Apart from the important conditions of branchial cyst and branchial fistula, these may be:

1. Branchial cartilage.—A small cartilage, covered by skin, in the lower part of the anterior border of sternomastoid.
2. Cervical auricle (vide branchial fistula).
3. Branchiogenic carcinoma.
*4. Lateral variety of sublingual dermoid.
*5. Plunging ranula.
*6. Pharyngeal pouch.
*7. Laryngocele.
      (*According to some authorities only).

DEVELOPMENT OF THE THYROID

The entoderm over the floor of the mouth, behind the tuberculum impar, is invaginated. This forms into and persists as the foramen caecum of the tongue. This entodermal invagination (which is a derivative of the first bronchial arch) grows caudally, lying ventral to the second, third, fourth, fifth, and sixth branchial arches, as far back as the commencement of the trachea. This is known as the *median thyroid diverticulum* or *thyroglossal duct*. Its caudal extremity expands and forms the bilobed thyroid with its isthmus. A portion of the distal end of this duct is represented in the pyramidal lobe of the thyroid. Except for the proximal depression (persisting as the foramen caecum of the tongue) and the distal part (represented by the pyramidal lobe), the long central part of the thyroglossal duct normally disappears.

The thyroglossal duct, as it passes ventral to (i.e. in front of) the second and third arches, should pass in front of the hyoid bone that develops from these arches. Often, however, the duct, after passing in front of the hyoid bone, curves round its lower border and runs a little upwards behind the bone and then courses down. Occasionally, the duct passes through the substance of the hyoid bone. This last variety can be explained by the fact that the hyoid bone partially develops from the second arch and partially from the third, and it is probable that the thyroglossal duct is included in between these two parts when they fuse together.

Persistence of a part of the thyroglossal duct, with pent-up secretions in it, results in a *thyroglossal cyst*.

THYROGLOSSAL CYST

Origin.—This is a cyst developing in an unobliterated thyroglossal duct (*see* above).

Sites.—A cyst may occur at any point in the course of the thyroglossal duct—from the foramen caecum to the suprasternal notch. However, remnants of the duct above the hyoid and below the thyroid are rare, so cysts in these situations are also rare. The location of the cyst may be:
1. In the substance of the tongue, below the foramen caecum.
2. In the floor of the mouth.
3. Suprahyoid.
4. Subhyoid.
5. On the thyroid cartilage.
6. At the level of the cricoid cartilage.
7. In front of the upper tracheal rings.
In order of frequency, the sites are:
1. Subhyoid.
2. On the thyroid cartilage.
3. Suprahyoid.

Clinical Features
1. Swelling in the midline of the neck, in any of the above situations. For swellings below the hyoid, the swelling is invariably displaced a little to one side, by the midline prominence of the larynx.
2. The swelling moves up and down with deglutition.
3. The swelling moves up with protrusion of the tongue (due to pull from foramen caecum).
4. Sometimes the patient first presents with an abscess in the cyst, resulting from infection.

Treatment.—The cyst, together with the whole length of the thyroglossal duct, has to be excised. Since the tract has a very intimate but indefinite and unidentifiable relationship with the central part of the hyoid bone, this part of the hyoid bone is included in the resection (*Sistrunk's operation*). This is done with a transverse incision placed over the cyst, and then dissecting out of the cyst, together with the thyroglossal duct, upwards. As the hyoid is reached, its central part is excised and included in the dissection. Above the hyoid, the tract is usually indefinite. Therefore, removal of the central core of the muscles in the floor of the mouth, together with diathermy of the central core of the tongue below the foramen caecum, is performed. The cyst is tense and thin-walled, and contains clear or mucoid fluid.

THYROGLOSSAL FISTULA

In contrast to branchial fistula, thyroglossal fistula is never congenital. It follows rupture or incision of an infected thyroglossal cyst. It may also result from incomplete excision of the thyroglossal duct while operating for a thyroglossal cyst.

The sites are the same as for thyroglossal cyst. There is often a hood of skin on the fistula (like branchial fistula), due to unequal rate of growth of the tract and the neck as a whole.

Infection of thyroglossal cyst is common because its wall contains lymphatic tissue which communicates with the cervical lymph nodes.

Treatment.—*Sistrunk's operation,* as for thyroglossal cyst. The transverse incision on the skin splits to encircle the opening.

ECTOPIC THYROID

These may be found anywhere along the course of the thyroglossal tract, from the foramen caecum above (lingual thyroid) to the front of the trachea below. Occasionally, they may be found retrosternal or in the posterior mediastinum.

The importances of an ectopic thyroid are:
1. It may present itself as an abnormal swelling.
2. It may be the only thyroid tissue so that its removal will make the patient devoid of thyroid.
3. It may be the site of a goitre.
4. A lingual thyroid may cause dysphagia, dyspnoea, or impairment of speech.

CYSTIC HYGROMA

This is a cavernous lymphangioma, most commonly found in the neck (90 per cent). The cheek and axilla are next common sites, but far less frequent. A combination of a cystic hygroma in the neck and a cavernous lymphangioma of the tongue (causing macroglossia) is occasionally found. Groin, mediastinum, and viscera are rare sites.

Clinical Features
1. The patient is usually an infant or a child. Rarely the condition is congenital and may cause obstructed labour.
2. Typically, cystic hygroma in the neck is found in the posterior triangle, increasing upwards, from the supraclavicular fossa to the ear.
3. As the swelling consists of many intercommunicating compartments, containing fluid, it shows partial reducibility on pressure.
4. It shows an increase in size when the child coughs or cries.
5. Fluctuation can be elicited.
6. It is brilliantly transilluminant.

Pathology.—The swelling consists of innumerable intercommunicating cysts, containing lymph. The deeper cysts, smaller in size, infiltrate widely into the muscles—macroscopically and microscopically.

Complications

1. Respiratory obstruction by rapidly-growing swelling (demands emergency aspiration as a life-saving measure).
2. Recurrent infection. While infection is dangerous, it may sometimes be followed by spontaneous regression.

Treatment.—Excision of the whole mass of cysts.

Preliminary injections of boiling water into the cyst, 3 to 6 injections at weekly intervals, may be beneficial since they:

a. Check the growth of the swelling.
b. Make the walls of the cysts fibrous, tough, and identifiable, thereby making dissection relatively easier.

The difficulties of the operation are:

1. Recurrence.—Even with all precautions and skill, microscopic cysts are very likely to be left behind in the muscle planes. However, many of the cases do not recur.
2. Profuse leakage of lymph from the wound in the post-operative period may cause dangerous dehydration in the child.
3. There is a high risk of surgical and anaesthetic mortality.

Origin.—Cystic hygroma results from failure of communications developing between the primitive lymph sacs in the neck and the general lymphatic system. There are two such major sacs in the developing neck, one on either side. They are located between the internal jugular vein and the subclavian vein. They are known as jugular lymph sacs and they represent the lymph hearts of the lower animals. Sequestration of a portion of a jugular lymph sac from the lymphatic system results in the formation of cystic hygroma.

STERNOMASTOID TUMOUR AND CONGENITAL TORTICOLLIS

Etiology.—There are several views:

1. This is a condition of ischemic contracture of the sternomastoid, comparable to Volkmann's ischemic contracture. It results from infarction of the central part of the muscle at the time of birth.
2. This is a fibrosis in the sternomastoid, resulting from partial rupture of the muscle, due to an injury sustained at birth.
3. This is due to a congenital aplasia.

Clinical Features

1. At birth, there is a circumscribed firm swelling in the substance of the sternomastoid. Often the swelling is seen a few weeks after birth.
2. Subsequently, a typical contracture of the sternomastoid develops, involving both the sternal and the clavicular heads of the muscle. The result is that the head is flexed, bent towards the affected side, and rotated towards the opposite side, i.e. as if the affected sternomastoid was contracting. There is gradually increasing restriction of movements of rotation and elevation of the head.

Secondary Effects
1. There is restriction of growth of all soft tissues in the affected part of the neck, including deep fascia, big vessels and scalene muscles.
2. There is asymmetry of face and skull. On the affected side the face is small and the frontal prominence flatter, while on the opposite side the occiput is more prominent. As the sternomastoid muscle is very short, the mastoid process may become abnormally large and even an exostosis may develop in it.
3. A compensatory cervical scoliosis often develops.

Treatment
1. If detected immediately after birth, the infant's head is manipulated daily through full range of movements.
2. If the condition is detected only after torticollis has developed, and this happens more commonly:
   a. Corrective brace (torticollis harness) may be tried, but usually fails.
   b. Division of the sternomastoid muscle has usually to be performed. The muscle is divided either at its distal end or at both the ends, care being taken of the spinal accessory naive at the proximal end. Postoperatively, a torticollis harness has to be worn.

CERVICAL RIB AND SCALENE SYNDROME

Morphology
1. The anterior part of the transverse process of a cervical vertebra is known as the *costal element* because it is homologus with the thoracic ribs. Sometimes the costal element of the seventh cervical may develop abnormally big and this is known as cervical rib. Rarely the sixth cervical may also have this anomaly.
2. The brachial plexus is formed by the lower four (C5, 6, 7, 8) cervical nerves and the first thoracic nerve. These nerves are relatively large during development and it is probable that the pressure of the big nerve trunks prevent the growth of the costal elements of the cervical vertebrae. Anomalies may occur in the formation of the brachial plexus as follows:
   a. When there is only a minute contribution from T1, the costal element of the seventh cervical vertebra can grow without impediment. This condition (in which the brachial plexus is shifted headwords) is known as *prefixed* brachial plexus, and in this condition, therefore, cervical rib is common.
   b. When the brachial plexus receives a big contribution from both T1 and T2, it is called *post-fixed*. In this condition, the first rib may be underdeveloped.

Types.—Cervical ribs may be of the following types:
1. *Complete*, articulating anteriorly with:
   a. Either, the manubrium sterni (rare),
   b. Or, the first rib, usually near its scalene tubercle.
2. *Incomplete:*
   a. A blunt swelling of the costal element of C7, its free, end expanding into a big bony mass.

b. A small rib with a tapering anterior end, from where a fibrous band extends to the scalene tubercle. This band passes either in the substance of the scalenus medius or closely applied to the muscle.

c. There is no rib. Instead, there is a fibrous band—extending from the costal element of C7 to the scalene tubercle—in the substance of, or closely applied to, the scalenus medius (this variety is not demonstrated on X-ray).

In a little less than half of the cases, cervical *ribs are bilateral.*

Anatomy and Pathology.—As the brachial plexus and the subclavian artery run from the neck to the arm, they pass through a narrow triangular area. The arms of this triangle are—anteriorly the scalenus anterior, posteriorly the scalenus medius, and at the base (below) the first rib. The subclavian vein is in front of the scalenus anterior.

When there is a cervical rib, the base of the triangle is raised up by the height of one vertebra, being formed by the cervical rib itself. This causes an abnormal angulation of the structures passing above it—particularly the subclavian artery and the lower trunk of the brachial plexus. This abnormal angulation causes the main difficulties in cases of cervical rib (Fig. 29.1).

Clinical Types

A. CERVICAL RIB WITH NO SYMPTOMS.—Many people show evidence of cervical rib on X-ray but have no complaints. Experience says that well-formed ribs, as seen on the X-ray, produce symptoms much less frequently than rudimentary (incomplete) ribs. It is believed that the fibrous band attached to an incomplete rib is notorious in causing symptoms.

B. CERVICAL RIB WITH LOCAL SYMPTOMS.—The patient may complain of:
a. A bony lump in the locality.

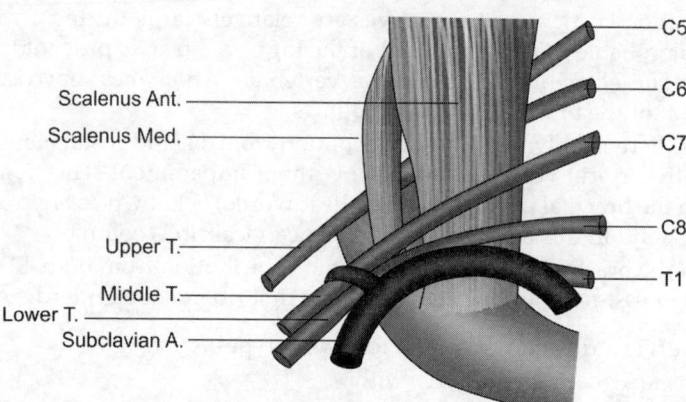

Fig. 29.1: Showing the positions of the subclavian artery and the lower trunk of brachial plexus in relation to the first rib and the scalenus muscles. In case of cervical rib there is further angulation of the artery and the nerve. The rationality of scalenotomy to relieve the pressure is obvious.

b. Tenderness in the supraclavicular fossa. In these cases the rib is usually of type 2(a).

C. CERVICAL RIB WITH VASCULAR SYMPTOMS.—The theories put forward as to the cause of the vascular symptoms are:

a. Stretching or irritation of the periarterial sympathetic fibres around the subclavian artery, causing vasoconstriction.

b. Intermittent mechanical occlusion of the artery in the triangle described above.

c. Arterial embolism, resulting from thrombosis, occurring in that part of the subclavian artery which is just distal to the site of constriction of the artery in the triangle. This part of the artery is dilated and this is called *poststenotic dilatation.* Thrombi are very likely to form here and these are carried down as emboli, which cause vascular occlusion. This is the generally accepted theory.

The vascular symptoms consist of all or some of the following features:

1. *Pain.*—This is a common complaint for all the patients. The pain is comparable to intermittent claudication in the leg. It is experienced in the forearm during exercises and is relieved on rest. The pain is maximum when the arm works in an elevated position.

2. *Vasomotor inefficiency:*
   a. Temperature.—The hand on the affected side may be colder.
   b. Colour Changes.—The hand is unduly pale when elevated and unduly blue when dependent for some time.

3. *Trophic Changes:*
   a. Numbness in the fingers, followed by—
   b. Ulceration or even gangrene in the fingers.

4. *Pulsation:*
   a. The radial pulse may become weaker when the arm is elevated.
   b. *Adson's Test* may be positive,—The radial pulse is felt with the patient sitting erect. The patient is asked to take deep breath, hold it, and then turn the chin up and to the affected side. There is diminution or obliteration of the radial pulse.
   c. A systolic bruit may be heard, on ausculation, over the distal part of the subclavian artery which feels prominent and pulsates visibly in the neck.
   d. In cases associated with trophic changes, the radial pulse, and sometimes the brachial, may be absent.

D. CERVICAL RIB WITH NERVE-PRESSURE SYMPTOMS.—The patient may present with features of compression of the lower trunk of the brachial plexus, associated with segmental sensory loss and wasting of small muscles of the hand. There may be two types of muscular wasting:

1. *Median Nerve Type* (commoner).—Opponens pollicis, abductor pollicis and flexor pollicis brevis.

2. *Ulnar Nerve Type.*—The other small muscles, particularly the interossei and the adductor pollicis.

   It should be remembered that:
   a. Nerve-pressure symptoms in case of cervical rib are of very infrequent occurrence, much less frequent than the vascular symptoms.
   b. The cases presenting with nerve-pressure are often associated with cervical spondylosis, carpal tunnel syndrome, etc. In these cases the nerve-pressure

is usually due to these conditions, and the presence of a cervical rib is just incidental.

Special Investigations

1. X-ray.—The important points to remember are:
   a. Mere presence of cervical rib does not always cause symptoms.
   b. When there are symptoms characteristic of cervical rib but X-ray fails to show a rib, the possibility is a fibrous band (Type 2c). It is a common experience that these cases produce maximum symptoms. It is to this group of cases that the term *scalene syndrome,* as opposed to cervical rib, is applied.
   c. When a patient of cervical rib presents, mainly with nerve-pressure symptoms, care must be taken to exclude other causes of nerve pressure, especially cervical spondylosis.
2. Arteriography.—This may show variable degrees of occlusion of the brachial artery and its tributaries, in patients with vascular symptoms.

Treatment

1. *Conservative Treatment.*—This is indicated in mild cases, not associated with vascular symptoms, and consists of:
   a. Use of a sling.
   b. Exercises aiming at strengthening the muscles of the shoulder girdle (because drooping of the shoulder aggravates the pressure symptoms).
2. *Operative Treatment.*—This is advisable for:
   a. Mild cases not responding to conservative treatment.
   b. Patients with vascular symptoms.
   c. Patients with nerve-pressure symptoms, provided other causes of nerve-pressure have been excluded.

Type of Operation

1. *If there is a Cervical Rib.*—Excision of the whole length of the rib, including any fibrous band that may extend from the tip of an incomplete rib to the scalene tubercle. In approaching the rib, the scalenus anterior has to be divided close to its insertion at the scalene tubercle, i.e. a *scalenotomy* has always to be done. The periosteum of the cervical rib must be removed, otherwise the rib may regenerate.
2. *In those cases where there is No Cervical Rib.*—Only scalenotomy is performed. A careful search is made for the presence of any fibrous band in the substance or neighborhood of scalenus medius, and if there be any, it is excised.

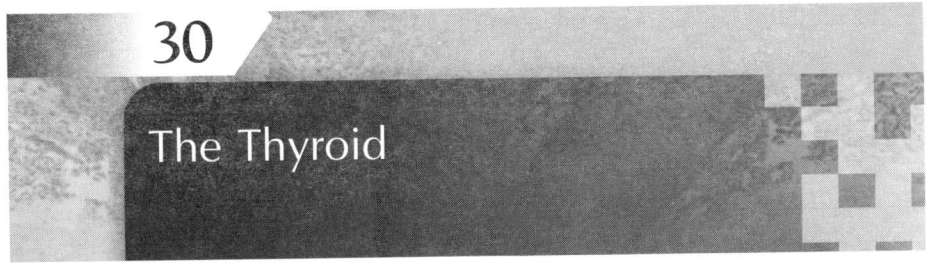

30

The Thyroid

Embryology.—*See* Chapter 29.

SURGICAL ANATOMY

Parts.—The thyroid consists of:
1. Two lateral lobes, which are symmetrical each on one side of the midline, extending above to the lamina of the thyroid cartilage and below to the sixth tracheal ring.
2. The isthmus, connecting the two lateral lobes, lies in front of and closely attached to the second, third, and fourth rings of trachea.
3. The pyramidal lobe, which is an additional lobe and not always present, projects upwards from the isthmus.

Coverings
1. True fibrous capsule or fascia propria, which envelops the gland closely and sends numerous fibrous septa into it.
2. Fascial sheath, derived from the pretracheal layer of the deep cervical fascia. This layer, as it reaches the lateral border of the thyroid on either side, splits into an anterior and a posterior lamina, in between which the thyroid gland is enveloped. On the postero-medial aspect of each lobe, this sheath is thickened and these thickenings are called (lateral) *ligaments of Berry*. These ligaments extend from the postero-medial border of the thyroid lobes to the border of the cricoid cartilage.

Movements of the Thyroid with Deglutition.—During deglutition, the larynx is pulled up by the three muscles, viz. the stylopharyngeus, the salpingo-pharyngeus, and the palatopharyngeus, which are all attached to the ala of the thyroid cartilage. The thyroid is closely attached to the larynx and trachea, therefore the gland moves up with deglutition. These attachments are as follows:
1. The posterior lamina of the pretracheal fascia, which is closely adherent to the rings of the trachea on the back and the isthmus of the thyroid in front.
2. The ligament of Berry on either side.
3. If a pyramidal lobe is present, a fibromuscular slip extends from this lobe to the inferior border of the hyoid bone. This is termed the *levator glandulae thyroidae*.

Close Relations
1. The medial surface of each lobe is closely applied to the trachea and larynx in front, and the oesophagus and pharynx behind.
2. In the interval between the oesophagus and the trachea (tracheo-oesophageal cleft) lies the recurrent laryngeal nerve. The nerve is, however, located *behind*

the posterior lamina of the pretracheal fascia, and if this fascia is kept intact, the nerve is not likely to be injured during thyroidectomy.

3. The two parathyroids, on each side, lie behind the lateral lobe, on or within the thyroid gland, *inside the pretracheal fascia.*
4. Postero-laterally, the thyroid is in contact with the carotid sheath.

Blood Supply.— On either side, there are two arteries and three veins—the superior and inferior thyroid arteries, and the superior, middle, and inferior thyroid veins. The middle thyroid vein has no accompanying artery. There is an indefinite *artery* coming up to the isthmus, called the *arteria thyroideaima;* this artery may sometimes be of considerable calibre and occasionally it comes from the arch of the aorta. The superior thyroid artery is a branch of the external carotid while the inferior thyroid artery springs from the thyrocervical trunk, a branch of the subclavian. The inferior thyroid artery runs behind the carotid sheath to reach the middle of the back of the lateral lobe. The superior and the middle thyroid veins end in the internal jugular. The inferior thyroid veins are often multiple and they drain downwards, usually into the innominate vein. Multiple unnamed vessels also feed the thyroid from the oesophagus and the trachea.

Ligature of the Vessels the Thyroidectomy.—The superior thyroid artery and vein run together to the upper pole of each lateral lobe. They can, therefore, be ligated together during thyroidectomy. As the external laryngeal nerve is located just a little away from the upper pole in this situation, these vessels are preferably ligated in the substance of the thyroid in order to avoid injury to this nerve. The inferior thyroid artery and veins do not run together, and they have, therefore, to be ligated separately. The inferior thyroid artery should be ligated as far away from the gland as possible because:

a. The recurrent laryngeal nerve is in close relation to the thyroid and if the artery is ligated close to the gland, the nerve may be injured.
b. The artery often divides into two branches before entering the gland and, if an attempt is made to put the ligature close to tile gland, only of the branches may be ligated the other escaping.

In thyroidectomy, it is usually the practice to ligate superior thyroid vessels and divide them, while the inferior thyroid artery is simply ligated in continuity (i.e. it is not cut).

When all the arteries are ligated, the thyroid (or its remaining parts) still gets a good blood supply from the many small vessels which enter the gland from the trachea and the oesophagus.

Lymphatic Drainage.—The lateral lobe and the lateral part of the isthmus, on either side, drain into the jugulo-digastric and the jugula-omohyoid nodes of the corresponding side. The central part of the isthmus drains into the prelaryngeal and pretracheal nodes; these nodes lie behind the isthmus, in front of the larynx and trachea, and are also known as *juxtathyroid nodes.* According to some authors, the major part of the lymphatics from the lateral lobes also drain primarily into the juxtathyroid nodes and then to the deep cervical nodes.

Microscopic Anatomy.— The unit of the thyroid gland is an acinus or vesicle. Thousands of acini are aggregate together in the gland, supported by connective tissue that contains numerous blood vessels, lymphatics, and aggregation of lymphocytes. This interstitial tissue also contains groups of special cells known as *parafollicular* or C-cells, which are believed to be derived from the ultimo-branchial body (which arises as diverticulum from the fourth pharyngeal pouch, on each side, and amalgamates with the lateral lobe of the thyroid).

The acini have no basement membrane and their lining cells are, therefore, in direct contact with the connective tissue stroma. The lining of the acini consists of a single layer of epithelium and the lumen of the acini contains the secretion of the thyroid in a conjugated form popularly known as the colloid material (see physiology below). This colloid stains bright-pink with eosin. It may be mentioned that thyroid is the only endocrine gland which has the capacity of storing its own secretion.

Even in a normally functioning thyroid, two types of acini may be found according to their physiological state of work:

1. *The Resting Acini.*—The cells are cuboidal, their protoplasm and nuclei stain faintly and show a few granules. The major part of the acini are filled with colloid material which stains deep with eosin and there are only a few vacuoles.
2. *The Working Acini.*—The cells are columnar, their protoplasm and nuclei stain bright and show many granules. The lumen contains much less colloid and many vacuoles, and the colloid is also only faintly stained with eosin.

While these two types of acini are found in the normal thyroid, a deviation from either of the two, to a pathological state, may be reached. This results in what is called a metabolic goitre. Such deviation may be:

a. Either, an exaggeration of the resting phase—the cells are flat, and the acini are distended with very deeply staining colloid with no evidence of vacuoles (as seen in diffuse colloid goitre).
b. Or, an exaggeration of the working phase—the cells are tall columnar, and the acini contain only a little or no colloid that stains very faint and there are many vacuoles in them (as seen in hyperplastic goitres).

In a multinodular goitre all the above four types of acini are seen.

PHYSIOLOGY OF THE THYROID

Synthesis of Thyroxin

1. *Trapping.*—The thyroid has the special capacity of abstracting iodide from the circulating blood; This iodide is mainly derived from drinking water.
2. *Oxidation.*—The iodide is converted into iodine by a peroxidase enzyme.
3. *Binding.*—Iodine combines with the essential amino-acid tyrosine to form:
   a. Mono-iodotyrosine,
   b. Di-iodotyrosine.
4. *Coupling:*
   a. Mono-iodotyrosine + di-iodotyrosine = tri-iodothyroxine (T_3);
   b. Di-iodotyrosine + di-iodotyrosine = thyroxin (T_4).
   Thyroxin is formed far in excess to T_3.
5. *Reversible Conjugation.*—Thyroxin and T_3 immediately get attached to thyroglobulin, which is a specific protein also secreted by the thyroid cells. This conjugated material is popularly called the 'colloid substance' and it is in this

form that thyroxin (and T_3) is stored in the acini. When required in the system, the conjugation breaks, and thyroxin (and a little amount of T_3) is liberated into the circulation.

Circulation of Thyroxin

1. Immediately on release into the circulation, both T_4 arid T_3 get bound to the serum proteins. There are two such proteins :
   a. Thyroid-binding globulin (TBG).
   b. Thyroid-binding pre-albumen (TBPA).
   The normal range of this 'protein bound iodine (PBI) is 3.5 to 8.0 µg per 100 ml.
2. However, a small proportion of T_4 and T_3 circulate *free* in the serum. In practice, the PBI level is considered to be a direct measure of the thyroid activity.

Utilisation in the Tissues.—Thyroxin is essential for tissue metabolism. As thyroxin enters into the tissues, it is broken up into T_3 + one atom of iodine. It is the T_3 form which is quick-acting (works in a few hours). Thyroxin, as such, can work in the tissues, but slowly (4 to 14 days). T_3, which enters the tissues, works as such.

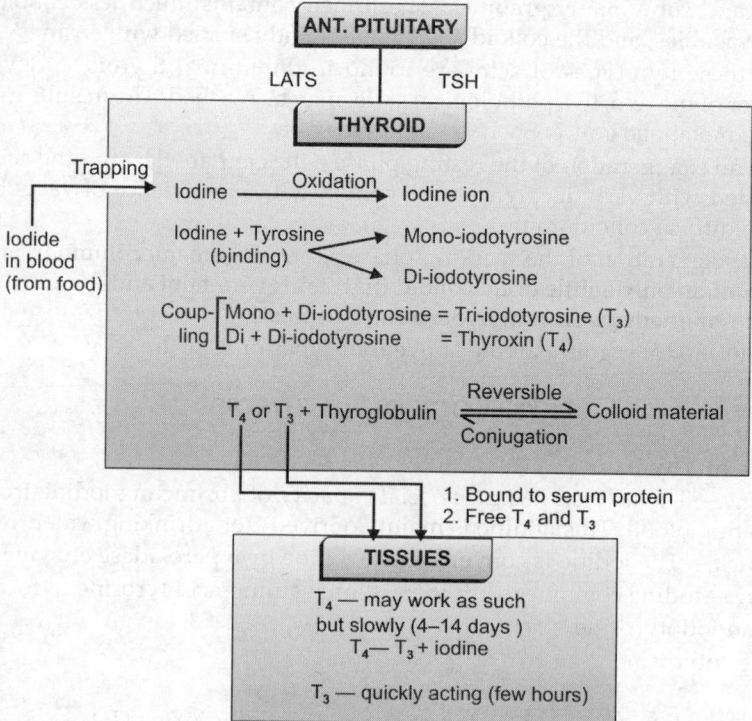

Control of Thyroid Function

A. The Thyroid-Stimulating Hormone (TSH)
   1. Synthesis and liberation of hormones from the thyroid is under direct control of TSH (thyrotropin), a hormone of the anterior pituitary.
   2. Again, there is a reciprocal relationship between the level of the circulating thyroxin and the secretion of TSH. In hyperthyroidism, when the level of

circulating thyroxin is high, the TSH production is suppressed; in hypothyroidism, the TSH production is stimulated. This reciprocal relationship is popularly termed the *feedback mechanism.*

3. The secretion of TSH is, in turn, controlled by a releasing hormone of the hypothalamus (thyrotropin-releasing hormone or TRH). There is probably also a release-inhibitory hormone of the hypothalamus.
4. TSH is quick-acting on the thyroid, its maximum effect occurs in 1½ to 3 hours.

B. LONG-ACTING THYROID STIMULATOR (LATS).—This is another substance which controls synthesis and liberation of thyroxin in patients of hyperthyroidism. It differs from TSH in the following respects:

1. It is a gamma-globulin (it is believed to be an auto-antibody to a thyroid antigen).
2. Its duration of action on the thyroid is much more prolonged—maximum effect produced in 16 to 24 hours.
3. Whether LATS works in normal persons or only in patients of hyperthyroidism is yet to be established.

Thyroid Auto-antibodies—It has recently been established that various auto-antibodies circulate in the serum of patients suffering from different types of goitre:

a. As has already been mentioned, LATS is an auto-antibody (to a thyroid antigen) and this is found in the serum of 85 per cent of patients of hyperthyroidism.
b. In Hashimoto's disease, an auto-antibody circulates in the serum and this is believed to be formed by the leakage of thyroglobulin from inside the thyroid acini into the circulation.
c. More and more evidences are now being put forward to suggest that, in all forms of goitre, there is an auto-antibody circulating in the patient's serum.

Effects of Excess of Thyroxin in the System, i.e. Thyrotoxicosis or Hyperthyroidism

A. METABOLISM.—There is an increased metabolism:

1. Increased (sometimes voracious) appetite but loss of weight.
2. Above-normal temperature.
3. High BMR.
4. Hyperglycaemia and glycosuria in some cases. These may be due to:
   a. Higher rate of glucose absorption from the gut.
   b. Excess of glycogenolysis in the liver and muscles.
   c. Excess of neoglucogenesis.
5. Creatinuria, due to direct breakdown of muscle proteins.

B. CARDIOVASCULAR SYSTEM.—Thyroxin produces its ill-effect on the heart in two ways:

a. The increased metabolism calls for more blood supply to the tissues, and the heart, having to work hard, gradually gets damaged.
b. Thyroxin is directly toxic to cardiac musculature.

The effects on the cardiovascular system are as follows:

1. Tachycardia, even when the patient is sleeping.
2. Irregularity of the pulse.
3. High systolic pressure with a little rise in the diastolic pressure. The resulting raised pulse pressure is demonstrated as *water-hammer pulse.*

4. ECG shows various types of cardiac irregularities, i.e. extrasystoles, paroxysmal auricular tachycardia, auricular fibrillation (paroxysmal or persistent), and ultimately heart failure (the heart stops at systole).
5. The patient's complaints are palpitation and dyspnoea on exertion.

C. NERVOUS SYSTEM.—There is irritation of both central and autonomic nervous systems:
  1. Central Nervous System:
    a. Insomnia and irritability.
    b. Exaggerated jerks.
    c. Fine tremors, best seen on extended fanned-out fingers and protruded tongue.
  2. Autonomic Nervous System:
    a. Flushed fades.
    b. Excess of perspiration.
    c. Dysentery and diarrhoea (the gut autonomic).

D. SKELETAL MUSCLES:
  1. Wasting of muscles (breakdown of muscle proteins), particularly frontalis, platysma, and quadriceps femoris.
  2. Weakness of the proximal limb-muscles is commonly seen; only rarely severe muscular weakness (*thyrotoxic myopathy*), resembling myasthenia gravis, occurs.

Exophthalmos and Eye Signs in Thyrotoxicosis.—Exophthalmos (which means protrusion of the eyeball) and opthalmoplegia (paralysis of the ocular muscles) are often seen in cases of primary toxic goitre. That these are not due to excess of thyroxin, i.e. hyperthyroidism, is proved by the following facts:
1. They are virtually never seen in secondary toxic goitre.
2. Following treatment (medical or surgical) for primary toxic goitre, while all other features of toxicity improve or disappear, the exophthalmos not only persists but often progresses.

The second point suggests that the exaggerated exophthalmos must be due to stimulation of the pituitary caused by the lowered thyroxin level following the treatment. So the cause of the exophthalmos lies in the pituitary and there are two possibilities:
a. It is due to TSH.
b. It is due to a special hormone liberated from the anterior pituitary and termed the *exophthalmos-producing hormone* or *substance* (EPH or EPS).

That it is not due to the TSH is proved by the fact that there is no evidence that exophthalmos can be produced by administration of TSH. The role of EPH in causing the exophthalmos is substantiated further by the fact that partial relief is obtained by pituitary ablation or stalk section.

A. EXOPHTHALMOS.—The degree of exophthalmos varies—it may be mild, moderate, or severe, and can be exactly measured by 'exophthalmometry'.

The exophthalmos, seen clinically, is partially apparent and partially true:
1. *Apparent.*— This is due to spasm and retraction of the upper eyelids. This spasm occurs because the levator palpebrae superiors is partly innervated by sympathetic fibres.

2. *True.*—The explanations put forward for this true protrusion of the eyeball are as follows:—

  a. The milder degrees of exophthalmos are due to sustained contraction of the *Muller's muscle* (unstriped muscle fibres within the orbit)—the reverse of what is seen in enophthalmos occurring after division of the cervical sympathetic trunk.

  b. The severe and progressive cases of exophthalmos are due to fatty deposits and oedema in the retrobulbar connective tissues and orbital muscles, increasing their volume. The oedema may be due to lymphatic or venous obstruction. In some cases there may be an actual enlargement of the globe.

B. THE EYE SIGNS.—These are due to:

  1. Spasm and retraction of the upper eyelid.
  2. Paralysis of the external ocular muscles.

3. Fatty deposits and oedematous infiltration the muscles inside the orbit; restricting the movements of the eyeball, particularly in an upward direction.

  Various eye signs are described, of which the following are commonly searched for:

  a. *Dalrymple's sign.*—Visibility of the upper sclera. This is due to retraction of the upper eyelids (normally the upper sclera is not visible).

  b. *von Graefe's sign.*—The upper eyelids lags behind the eyeball as the patient is asked to look downwards suddenly.

  c. *Joffroy's sign.*—Absence of wrinkling on the forehead when the patient looks-upwards with the head fixed.

  d. *Stellwag's sign.*—Infrequency of normal blinking, i.e. a staring look.

  e. *Moebius' sign.*—Lack of convergence of the eyeballs.

Signs of Hypothyroidism in association with Thyrotoxicosis.— In some cases of primary toxic goitre, signs of thyroid insufficiency may be curiously mixed with hyperthyroid features. These signs are:

1. *Pretibial Myxoedema.*—Thickening of the pretibial skin by a mucin-like deposit, often bilateral and symmetrical in distribution.
2. Thinning of the hair.
3. There may be clubbing of the fingers and toes *(thyroid acropathy).*

  These features are attributed to anterior pituitary overaction.

SPECIAL INVESTIGATIONS IN THYROID CASES

1. SLEEPING PULSE RATE—This is particularly important:

  a. In differentiating mild thyrotoxic goitres from non-toxic goitres associated with anxiety neurosis. The anxiety factor is cut off when the patient is sleeping and the actual pulse rate obtained.

  b. In determining the degree of toxicity. Here also, the factors of apprehension and anxiety are cut off and the actual degree of toxicity is indicated by the pulse rate, e.g.:

Below 90	Mild
90 to 110	Moderate
Above 110	Severe

2. TEMPERATURE.—The body temperature is always above normal in cases of hyperthyroidism (temperature is the index of metabolism).

3. ESTIMATION OF BMR.—High in cases of hyperthyroidism, low in hypothyroidism. This test is only rarely done now because of inaccuracies in the result and the time involved. However, when performed with meticulous care, it is of great value.

4. EXAMINATION OF URINE.—In cases of hyperthyroidism:
   a. Presence of sugar.
   b. Creatinuria, i.e. presence of creatine (coming from direct break-down of muscle protein).

5. BLOOD BIOCHEMISTRY
   a. Estimation of blood sugar—hyperglycaemia in cases of toxicity;
   b. Estimation of serum creatinine—a raised lever in hyperthyroidism.
   c. Estimation of serum cholesterol—a raised level in hypothyroid conditions; a lowered level in hyperthyroidism.

6. ECG.—May show cardiac arrhythmias in thyrotoxicosis.

7. X-RAY.—An anteroposterior view of the neck may show tracheal deviation or compression. A lateral view of the chest may confirm the presence of a retro-sternal goitre.

8. ESTIMATION OF THYROID HORMONES IN THE SERUM—The major part (95%) of thyroxin (T_4) and T_3 are carried in the plasma bound to the serum proteins— thyroxin binding globulin and thyroxin binding prealbumin. However, a small amount (5%) circulates free in the serum. On the basis of this knowledge, the following measurements are needful:
   a. *Serum Protein Bound Iodine* (PBI).—In practice this is considered to be a direct measurement of the thyroid activity. The normal range is 3.5 to 8.5 µg (microgram) per 100 ml of serum.
   Accepting the PBI as an absolute indication of thyroid activity is faced with difficulties since false high and false low results may be obtained under many conditions. To overcome these falacies, more accurate estimations are called for.
   b. *Total Serum Thyroxin*.—The normal range is 3.0 to 7.5 µg per 100 ml. This test is now freely available.
   c. *Total serum T_3*— Radioimmune assay has to be done. The normal range is 1.3 to 3.5 nmol/litre. This test is also freely available and is useful because there are a few cases of hyperthyroidism (T_3-toxicosis) where the thyroxin level is normal but the T_3 is raised.
   d. *Free Serum Thyroxin*.—This is also estimated by radio-immune assay. Though this is the best index of thyroid activity its estimation is difficult and the test is not generally available.

9. RADIOACTIVE IODINE TESTS (I_{131}-TESTS).—These tests are valuable since I_{131} is treated in the same way by the thyroid as is inorganic iodine (I_{127}) while it can be easily *traced in* the body, after administration, because of its radioactivity.

The *tracer dose,* which is usually 5 microcurie (one µc is millionth part of a curie), is given to the patient as a drink. As it is absorbed from the gut into the blood, there are two organs which compete for it—the thyroid and the kidneys. In hyperthyroidism the uptake by the thyroid is high and so a correspondingly less amount is excreted in the urine. In hypothyroidism the reverse occurs. I_{131} is utilised by the thyroid in making thyroxin, which comes back to the circulation and can be estimated as PBI_{131}.

The tests may, therefore, be as follows:

a. I_{131} *uptake by the Thyroid*—This again can be estimated by two methods:

    i. Direct Method.—The amount of I_{131} picked up by the thyroid can be directly read from a Geiger-Muller counter, placed on the neck after 4 hours. In the present days, this test has further been improved in the process of **thyroid scanning.** Special types of counters indicate the actual amount of I_{131} taken up by the individual nodules as well as the rest of the thyroid. Accordingly, three types of nodules are described—hot, cold, and neutral. A *hot nodule* is one which has a high I_{131}-uptake, and is likely to be toxic. A *cold nodule* is one with low I_{131}-uptake, and it is more likely to turn malignant or is actually malignant. A *neutral nodule* picks up the same proportion of iodine as does the remaining thyroid tissue, i.e. it possesses the same degree of activity as the rest of the gland.

    ii. Indirect Method.—The amount of I_{131}, excreted in the urine, is measured. When this is deducted from the total dose administered to the patient, the quantity of I_{131} picked up by the thyroid is known.

The normal iodine-uptake of the thyroid is 30 per cent. In hyperthyroidism this is raised to variable degrees according to the activity of the gland (to as high 90 per cent); in hypothyroid conditions it is correspondingly diminished.

b. *Estimation of PBI_{131}.*—This provides a very correct index of the thyroid function. The normal level should be 0.1 to 0.4 per cent of the given dose per litre of serum, 48 hours after administration of the tracer dose. In hyperthyroidism the level is raised and in hypothyroidism it is lowered.

c. *I_{131}-clearance from the Blood*—The rate of I_{131} pick-up by the thyroid is also indicative of thyroid function. In hyperthyroidism there is a very quick uptake by the thyroid.

10. I_{132}-TESTS.—I_{132} has a very short half-life, i.e. only 2.3 hours (compared to 8 days of I_{131}. It can, therefore, be used with benefit in children and in pregnant women.

11. NEEDLE OR DRILL BIOPSY.—This could have been of help in diagnosing malignant nodules but false negative results are fairly common because the needle may miss the target. It may, however, differentiate a solid from a cystic nodule.

12. ULTRASOUND.—This may be used to differentiate solid from cystic nodules. Also, it may demonstrate clinically impalpable nodule so that what appears to be a clinically solitary nodule may be ascertained as a multinodular goitre.

13. SELENIUM SCAN.—This may help differentiating between a benign and a malignant cold nodule. A highly cellular tumour, i.e. a malignant nodule, manifests itself very prominent on the scan.

GOITRE

Definition.—In the past, non-inflammatory, non-neoplastic swellings of the thyroid were called goitre. In the present days, any swelling of the thyroid is termed goitre (Latin, *guttur* = throat).

Classification of Goitres

I. Metabolic Goitres

A. SIMPLE (NON-TOXIC):

    1. Hyperplastic (physiological), 2. Diffuse colloid, 3. Nodular

B. Toxic:

    1. Primary

    2. Secondary

II. Neoplastic Goitres

A. BENIGN:

1. Adenoma 2. Rarely other tumours

B. MALIGNANT:

1. Carcinoma 2. Rarely other malignant tumours

III. Inflammatory Goitres and Allied Groups (Thyroiditis)

A. INFLAMMATORY:

1. Bacterial 2. Viral

B. AUTO-IMMUNE THYROIDITIS

Hashimoto's disease is the commonest and most important.

C. RIEDEL'S THYROIDITIS

D. RADIATION THYROIDITIS

METABOLIC GOITRES

Simple Goitres

The two cardinal features of simple goitres are:

1. There is a generalised enlargement of the thyroid
2. There is no increase in the functional activity of the gland (in some cases mild hypothyroidism may be present).

The essential prerequisite for a simple goitre is a persistently low level of circulating thyroxin. This causes an increase in the output of TSH from the anterior pituitary. The increased TSH level causes stimulation of the thyroid that results in its hyperplasia, i.e. a simple goitre.

Three types of simple goitre are described, but actually they represent various stages of the same process, i.e. hyperplasia-involution cycle of the thyroid, of which the cause of hyperplasia has already been stated:

1. **Hyperplastic or Physiological Goitre.**—The thyroid is enlarged but not greatly so, and the enlargement is uniform in nature. It is called hyperplastic because the follicles are increased in number, their lining cells are columnar, they contain a little or no colloid, whose iodine content is greatly reduced. This means that the gland is actively working.

The goitre is also called 'physiological' because it occurs during physiological stress-periods, e.g. puberty, pregnancy, lactation, etc., and because the goitre sometimes regresses spontaneously after the period of stress is over. It is believed that, during these periods, due to increased metabolism, there is an excess need of thyroxin. So, there is a relatively low level of circulating thyroxin and this causes an increase of output of TSH. The thyroid undergoes hyperplasia and enlargement. Such goitres most commonly occur at puberty and hence they are popularly known as *puberty goitres.*

A puberty goitre may have two fates:

a. It may completely involute, i.e. regress after puberty is over, if the TSH stimulation ceases.

b. It may persist and become permanent, changing its nature to a diffuse colloid goitre (*see* below).

Treatment.— No surgery should be advocated till puberty is over (21 to 22 years) since there is a chance of spontaneous regression. During this period small doses of 1-thyroxin and potassium iodide may be helpful.

2. **Diffuse Colloid Goitre**—The goitre is so named because the thyroid is uniformly (diffusely) enlarged and there is an excessive storage of colloid in the acini. The

cut surface has a fine honeycomb appearance, the spaces containing the glistening colloid material—amber-coloured or clear. Microscopically, the acini are widely dilated, contain very brightly staining colloid material with practically no vacuoles in them, and their lining cells are flattened.

A diffuse colloid goitre is believed to be a sequela to a hyperplastic goitre which has involuted beyond the normal limits when the TSH stimulation had fallen off. The excessive accumulation of the colloid material is difficult to explain. It is believed that the colloid is deficient in some respect and therefore it cannot be utilised by the body. Some pathologists ascribe it to an excessive intake of calcium and phosphorus in proportion to iodine.

Clinically, the thyroid is uniformly enlarged and has a soft consistency. The thyroid function tests usually show that the gland is hypo-functioning; however, clinical evidence of myxoedema is seldom present. Occasionally a large goitre may cause pressure symptoms.

Treatment.—This is a problem in view of the fact that partial thyroidectomy, which has to be undertaken for cosmetic reasons, makes the patient further hypothyroid by removing part of whatever normally functioning thyroid is present. Medical treatment with 1-thyroxin and iodides are of no avail. Partial thyroidectomy has to be done and some of the patients may require supplements of 1-thyroxin tablets for the future life.

3. **Nodular Goitre.**—There are multiple nodules in the thyroid, which is enlarged. Hence these goitres are popularly termed *multinodular goitre.* Occasionally, however, there may be a single palpable nodule, but even then microscopic changes are present throughout the gland. This differentiates it from the other form and the more common type of solitary nodule — adenoma of the thyroid (i.e. a neoplastic goitre). In other words, a clinically solitary nodule is more likely to be an adenoma than a part of a metabolic goitre.

While the thyroid, as a whole, is enlarged the number and size of the nodules vary greatly. On examination, it is usually found that the nodules are circumscribed areas of colloid-filled vesicles, while the intervening thyroid tissues are either normal or hyperplastic. Microscopically four types of acini are encountered in these thyroids—the two physiological types (resting and working) and the two pathological types (colloid and hyperplastic).

A multinodular goitre probably originates from irregular involution subsequent to hyperplasia in the thyroid—some parts remain in the state of hyperplasia, some involute to the normal state, while others undergo excessive involution. However, the sum total thyroxin secretion is more or less normal and hence the goitre is non-toxic. Anytime in the course of the disease, the hyperplastic tissue in the thyroid may proliferate and thus produce excess of thyroxin; the goitre then turns toxic. This is how a secondary toxic goitre forms. Hence, a secondary toxic goitre is secondary to the hyperplasia-involution changes in the thyroid.

Complications of Multinodular Goitre

1. Secondary toxicity.
2. Malignancy, i.e. carcinoma.
3. Pressure effects on the trachea (dyspnoea) and oesophagus (dysphagia).
4. Haemorrhage in a nodule—rapid increase in size with dyspnoea.

   Treatment—Partial thyroidectomy has to be undertaken:

   a. For cosmetic reasons.
   b. For prevention of complications.

TOXIC GOITRES

There are two distinct types of toxic goitres:
I. Primary toxic goitre.   II. Secondary toxic goitre.

The pathogenesis, pathology, clinical features, and also the treatment of the two types vary widely.

Primary Toxic Goitre

Nomenclature.—The cause of a primary toxic goitre is not definitely known. It is believed to be due to abnormal thyroid stimulators which are thyroid-stimulating auto-antibodies, of which LATS has been definitely detected in the serum of many patients. The enlargement of the thyroid and the features of hyperthyroidism appear simultaneously and this is why .the toxic goitre is called *primary* (which means that the toxic features have developed in a healthy thyroid). The goitre is often associated with exophthalmos and so it is called *exophthalmic goitre*. The thyroid shows a diffuse enlargement and so the condition is termed *'diffuse toxic goitre'*. According to its inventor, it goes by the name of *Graves disease*.

Pathology

MACROSCOPIC FEATURES:

1. The thyroid undergoes a diffuse enlargement but the enlargement is never great. On an average, it is 4 to 5 times its normal size. Occasionally the enlargement is not visible as the gland insinuates itself in the tracheo-oesophageal cleft (these are called *latent toxic goitre*).
2. The gland is highly vascular.
3. The cut surface is granular and friable. It lacks the normal glistening appearance because of great diminution in its colloid content.

MICROSCOPIC FEATURES

1. There is great proliferation of the epithelial cells lining the acini, so that they are arranged in several layers in the walls of the acini, often forming papillary projections into the acinar lumen. There is often an infolding of the acinar walls, so that the acini lose their normal shape.
2. The epithelial cells themselves are enlarged and are definitely columnar.
3. The colloid inside the acini is scanty, more fluid, and stains poorly with eosin. There are plenty of vacuoles.
4. The interstitial tissue shows extensive lymphocytic infiltration (sometimes with follicle formation). The capillaries are always dilated and, often, there are inter-stitial haemorrhages.

The pathological characters of the gland are greatly modified following iodine or thiouracil treatment. The hyperplasia of the epithelium may disappear over wide areas, the colloid content may increase, and the vascularity may diminish.

Clinical Features.—Primary toxic goitres occur most often in young subjects. Females preponderate in the ratio of 8:1. There may be a history of goitre in the family. Subjects of emotional temperament are more susceptible, and a history of nervous strain, sudden or protracted, may precede the onset. Some of the cases may show periodicity, i.e. phases of remission and relapse.

The three cardinal features of a primary toxic goitre are—enlargement of the thyroid, features of hyperthyroidism, and exophthalmos:

1. Enlargement of the Thyroid.—The enlargement is slight to moderate but is always diffuse, conforming to the normal shape of the gland. There may be

some cases without visible enlargement of the gland (latent toxic goitre). The gland has an elastic firm feel. It may be pulsatile and a thrill may be felt which, on auscultation, reveals a systolic bruite; these features are due to capillary dilatation, sometimes associated with arteriovenous shunts.

2 Features of hyperthyroidism, i.e. the ill-effects caused by excess of thyroxin in the body (see under physiology).

3. Exophthalmos and Eye Signs (*see* under physiology).

Secondary Toxic Goitre

Pathogenesis.—Here the features of hyperthyroidism occur in a thyroid which is already nodular. Thus, there is a non-toxic nodular goitre to start with; there is proliferation of the hyperplastic element in it, the thyroxin secretion increases, and toxicity sets in. The condition is, therefore, secondary to the hyperplasia-involution cycle in the thyroid. Also, the features of toxicity appear at a variable interval from the appearance of the thyroid swelling (hence called secondary toxic goitre).

Pathology.—There are two distinct types of secondary toxic goitre:

1. There is a multinodular goitre. Thyroid scanning with I_{131} shows that the nodules themselves show a little activity (cold nodules) while the rest of the gland is over-active. The thyroid, when examined macroscopically, also shows that the nodules are filled up with colloid material. Microscopical examination reveals that the acini at the site of the nodules show exaggeration of the resting phase, while those in between the nodules are hyperplastic.

2. There is a solitary nodule, and scanning with I_{131} shows that the nodule itself is over-active (hot nodule), while the rest of the thyroid is relatively silent. Here the nodule is a true tumour (i.e. a neoplastic goitre—an adenoma), secreting thyroxin autonomously and not subject to the control either of TSH or of LATS. This is, therefore, termed *autonomous toxic nodule.*

It is important to make a differentiation between these two types because, in the second variety, the toxicity will be cured by simple removal (i.e. excision) of the adenoma, while for the first condition, a subtotal thyroidectomy will be necessary.

Clinical Features

1. Secondary toxic goitres generally develop in older subjects—usually above thirty-five years of age, often much later in life. However, as with primary toxic goitre, females preponderate in the ratio of 8 to 1.

2. The goitre may precede toxic features for years. It is always nodular. In case of a multinodular toxic goitre; the thyroid swelling may be considerable.

3. The onset of toxicity is usually gradual, and toxicity is seldom as severe as in the primary type. The nervous manifestations (nervousness, insomnia, tremor, sweating, diarrhoea, etc.) are rather unusual. On the other hand, cardiovascular manifestations are usually more severe than is found in the primary variety.

4. Exophthalmos and eye signs are virtually never seen (only an apparent exophthalmos due to spasm and retraction of the upper eyelid may be occasionally encounted).

Differences between Primary and Secondary Toxic Goitre

PRIMARY	SECONDARY
1. The goitre and the toxic symptoms appear simultaneously—hence, called primary.	1. The toxic symptoms appear after a variable interval from the appearance of the goitre—hence, called secondary.

2. The patient is usually young.

2. Occurs in elderly subjects, rarely before the age of 35.

3. The toxicity starts suddenly and is seldom mild. Nervous manifestations are more predominant.

3. The onset of toxicity is gradual and toxicity is seldom severe. Cardiovascular manifestations are more predominant.

4. Exophthalmos and eye signs are common.

4. Virtually never seen.

5. The goitre is small to moderate in size, uniform, and firm.

5. The goitre is often big, always nodular.

Special Investigations for Toxic Goitres.—These have been described in details under physiology of the thyroid.

Treatment of Toxic Goitres.—Three forms of treatment are available:

A. Medical treatment

B. Surgical treatment

C. Radio-active iodine (I_{131}) treatment

A. MEDICAL TREATMENT.—This is done with tranquilisers and anti-thyroid drugs. Various anti-thyroid drugs are available, all of them having the effect of bringing down the level of thyroxin. However, the different drugs work at different sites in the chain of thyroxin-formation and its liberation from the gland. Thiouracil, which was popular in the past, is only rarely used now. Potassium perchlorate is sometimes used. The most widely used drug is Carbimazole (Neomercazole) because it is most effective and has least side-effects. The usual dose is 10 mg TDS, followed by a maintenance dose of 5 mg TDS.

Advantage.—Surgery and use of radioactive materials are avoided.

Disadvantages:

1. The treatment is time-consuming (at least two years) and is costly.
2. The final result is unpredictable—the failure rate is at least 50 per cent. The failure rate is more with secondary toxic goitres, for which condition, therefore, medical treatment is only rarely advised.
3. Some patients may not tolerate the drugs, i.e. idiosyncratic. Rarely, dangerous drug-reactions may occur, e.g. agranulocytosis, aplastic anaemia.
4. The anti-thyroid drugs, while diminishing the toxicity, cause an increase in the size and vascularity of the thyroid This is because, with the fall in the thyroxin level, the pituitary is stimulated to produce more TSH (feedback mechanism). This causes not only an increase in the thyroxin secretion (which is counteracted by the antithyroid drug) but also an increase in the size and vascularity of the thyroid. This has a two-fold ill-effect:
   a. The increase in size may cause pressure-symptoms which the patient did not have previously.
   b. If operation is contemplated, it becomes more difficult.

In this respect, iodine is the best antithyroid drug. This is because it has the additional capacity of directly depressing the TSH (and thus preventing the increase in size and vascularity of the gland). Unfortunately, however, the effect of iodine therapy is short-lasting and so iodine cannot be used as a long-term antithyroid drug. Its use is limited only to preparation of the toxic patients for surgery.

(It is important to note that even simultaneous administration of thyroxin and the antithyroid drugs cannot prevent the enlargement and increased vascularity of the thyroid).

B. SURGICAL TREATMENT

Nature of Surgery:
1. For a primary toxic goitre.—Subtotal thyroidectomy.
2. For a multinodular secondary toxic goitre.—Subtotal thyroidectomy.
3. For an autonomous toxic nodule.—Excision of the nodule (the suppressed normal thyroid tissue, left behind, starts functioning again).

Advantages
1. Cure rate is highest among all the forms of treatment available.
2. Cure is rapid.

Disadvantages
1. There is some risk of morality (this can, however, be minimised by proper preoperative preparation).
2. There may be some post-operative complications (*see* below).
3. The amount of thyroid to be excised is a matter of great judgement—either a recurrence or a myxoedema may occur if too little or too much is resected.

C. RADIOACTIVE IODINE (I_{131}) TREATMENT.—While the penetrating gamma rays of I_{131} are utilised as tracer substance in estimating thyroid functions, its non-penetrating β-rays are very effective in killing the thyroid cells, thereby diminishing the secretion of thyroxin.

Dosage.—This is difficult to estimate but the suggested usual dose is 160 μc. (microcurie) per 1 Gm of thyroid tissue. However, the actual weight of a particular gland, *in vivo*, is very difficult to be determined.

In general, considerable improvement is expected to start in 8 to 12 weeks' time. If, after this period, improvement is not remarkable, the first dose was inadequate and a second dose (and rarely another) has to be administered.

Advantage.—Surgery and prolonged (and indefinite) medical treatment are avoided.

Disadvantages
1. The dosage is difficult to determine and the services of an experienced radio-therapist are essential.
2. The patients are likely to become hypothyroid gradually. This is because radiation reduces the power of reproduction of those cells which survive but undergo sublethal damage, and they fail to replace the dead cells. This occurs in about 80 per cent of the cases.
3. In about 20 years, the patient is likely to develop a carcinoma in the body. Hence this method of treatment cannot be advocated before the age of 45.
4. It crosses the placental barrier and damages the foetus—hence it cannot be advised during pregnancy.
5. It may cause a genetic damage.
6. Much higher doses are necessary and the results are much less satisfactory in cases of secondary toxic goitre as compared to primary toxic goitre.

Indications for I_{131} Treatment— Radio-iodine treatment is, therefore, indicated in the following conditions, considered singly or in combinations:
1. Patients above 45.
2. Recurrence after surgery, particularly when one recurrent laryngeal nerve has been damaged at surgery (damage to the other, at the second operation, may be hazardous to the patient).
3. Patients unwilling to undergo surgery and refractory or hypersensitive to antithyroid drugs.
4. Patients with gross cardiac impairment, where surgery is contraindicated.

General Choice of Treatment in Toxic Goitres

GROUP A: UNTREATED CASES

1. Primary Toxic Goitre:
    a. Over 45 years.—Radio-iodine treatment
    b. Below 45 years:
        i. If the goitre is small.—Antithyroid drugs.
        ii. If the goitre is large.—Surgery (subtotal thyroidectomy).
2. Secondary Toxic Goitre:
    a. Multinodular Goitre.—Surgery (subtotal thyroidectomy).
    b. Autonomous Toxic Nodule.—Surgery (excision of the nodule).

GROUP B: TREATED CASES

1. Recurrence after adequate surgery:
    a. Over 45 years.—Radio-iodine treatment
    b. Below 45 years.—Anti-thyroid drugs.
2. Failure with anti-thyroid drugs.—Surgery.
3. Failure with radio-iodine treatment—Surgery.

Preparation of Toxic Patients for Surgery.—While patients of non-toxic goitre may be readily subjected to surgery, toxic patients cannot be dealt with as such because of chances of *thyroid crisis* developing in the post-operative period. They have to be prepared with the aim of bringing down the toxicity and making them *euthyroid* or near-euthyroid (i.e. normal state of function) at operation. The principles of preparation are as follows:

1. Cases of secondary toxicosis (which are usually mild) and cases of mild primary thyrotoxicosis.—In these patients, a 14-day iodine treatment just before operation is usually sufficient (the peak effect of iodine is reached by that time). For this purpose, Lugol's iodine (iodine in potassium iodide) is given 15 minims thrice daily.

2. Cases of moderate or severe primary thyrotoxicosis.—A long-term preparation with antithyroid drugs is necessary. Neomercazole (5 to 10 mg thrice daily) has to be administered till the patient reaches the euthyroid state—usually a matter of 8 to 12 weeks. With this treatment, however, the size and vascularity of the goitre increases, making operation further difficult. Some surgeons, therefore, stop or reduce the dose of the anti-thyroid drug 14 days prior to the operation and, for these 14 days, they administer iodine with the idea that iodine will cause diminution in the size and vascularity of the thyroid. While this is true, others do not favour the use of iodine since it causes an increased friability of the gland which proves troublesome at operation.

Post-operatively, all toxic patients must get a course of Lugol's iodine as a preventive measure against thyroid crisis.

NEOPLASTIC GOITRES (TUMOURS OF THE THYROID)

Adenoma (Thyroadenoma)

This presents as a solitary nodule in the thyroid—the rest of the thyroid is impalpable. Scanning studies with I_{131} show that the adenoma may have:

a. Normal I_{131}-uptake as the rest of the gland (neutral nodule).

b. Low I_{131}-uptake (cold nodule)—these adenomas are very likely to turn malignant or they are malignant, i.e. carcinoma.

c. High I_{131}-uptake (hot nodule)—these adenomas often produce excess of thyroxin and the patients present with features of secondary toxic goitre; they are termed *autonomous-toxic nodule* (already discussed).

Very often carcinoma of the thyroid also starts as a nodule in the thyroid. Similarly, some of the cancers may be secondary on a pre-existing adenoma. The differentiation between an adenoma and a carcinoma is often difficult, but the following points are helpful in making a differential diagnosis:

ADENOMA	CARCINOMA
1. May occur at any age.	1. Usually above 40, but quite common at earlier ages, even before puberty.
2. Duration usually long, with, slow rate of growth.	2. Short duration with rapid growth.
3. Usually painless.	3. May be associated with pain, Very often the patient has, at least, some sense of discomfort in the neck.
4. Pressure symptoms are usually absent. On rare occasions, when an adenoma is located in the postero-medial part of a lobe, dyspnoea or dysphagia may occur.	4. Pressure symptoms may be evident, e.g. dyspnoea, dysphagia.
5. Features of infiltration are never noticed.	5. Features of infiltration may be noticed: a. Recurrent laryngeal nerve— hoarseness of voice. b. Carotid sheath—obliteration of carotid pulsation.
6. No fixity to superficial or deep structures.	6. The growth may be fixed.
7. Firm in consistency.	7. Usually a hard consistency.
8. Cervical nodes are not involved.	8. Cervical nodes may be involved, particularly in papillary carcinoma.
9. No evidence of any distant metastasis.	9. Distant metastases may be present, particularly with follicular or ana-plastic carcinoma.

Treatment of Adenoma

1. Ordinarily, excision of the adenoma (i.e. removal with the capsule) is sufficient. The tumour must be sent for biopsy in order to exclude malignancy.
2. The toxicity in cases of toxic adenoma lies in the adenoma itself. Therefore, in cases of toxic adenoma, excision of the adenoma is the treatment. Following removal of the toxic nodule, the rest of thyroid tissue, whose function had been kept suppressed so long, resumes normal activity.
3. If there is any doubt as to whether the nodule is an adenoma or a carcinoma, a hemithyroidectomy (i.e. resection of the whole lobe of the thyroid in which the nodule lies) should be preferred to simple excision of the nodule. This is because, if the biopsy report proves to be a carcinoma, removal of the other half of the thyroid (with a view to perform a total thyroidectomy) remains an easy job (in cases of papillary carcinoma, even this may not be necessary because a hemithyroidectomy is often sufficient for this type of cancer). On the other hand, if a simple excision would have been done, a total thyroidectomy would mean

exploration of the same side again, to remove the rest of the hemithyroid, which might prove difficult.

4. For the same reason, hemithyroidectomy should be the treatment of choice for all patients above 45.

Carcinoma of the Thyroid

Very often, carcinoma starts as a solitary nodule in the thyroid; a diffuse swelling is rather rare except for the anaplastic type. This is why diagnosis may be difficult from an adenoma in the early stages of the disease (see adenoma).

While carcinoma may start *de novo* in a healthy gland, it may also occur in a thyroid, altered by disease, e.g.:

1. In an adenoma, i.e. what is called 'adenoma with infiltration'.
2. In a multinodular goitre.

Classification.—Histologically, cancers of the thyroid may be broadly classified as follows:

1. Differentiated types, i.e. Adenocarcinoma:
   a. Papillary carcinoma.
   b. Follicular carcinoma.
   c. Mixture of papillary and follicular carcinoma—these behave just like papillary carcinoma.
2. Undifferentiated Type.—Anaplastic carcinoma.

Other Malignant Tumours of the Thyroid.—Some uncommon malignant growths are encountered in the thyroid:

1. Squamous cell carcinoma.
2. Medullary carcinoma (discussed later).
3. Malignant lymphoma—arising from the interstitial lymphoid tissue.
4. Secondary carcinoma, i.e. metastatic lesion from other sites (very rare).

Papillary Carcinoma.—This is the commonest type of thyroid cancers, accounting for more than 60 per cent of the cases. It usually occurs in a healthy thyroid, i.e. a *de novo* cancer.

The cells in the acini, undergoing malignancy, spread in branching papillary processes into the lumen of the acini—hence the tumour is called papillary.

This variety of cancer has a special tendency to spread by lymphatics into the regional nodes, viz. the juxtathyroid (pretracheal and paratracheal) lymph nodes as well as the deep cervical nodes.

The tumour usually affects only one lobe of the thyroid; only in 20 per cent of cases both the lobes are involved. However, almost always there are multiple foci, i.e. the growth is *multifocal*. This is possibly due to spread in the intraglandular lymphatics.

The tumour is almost always TSH dependent.

Papillary carcinoma bears the best prognosis amongst all thyroid cancers, if properly treated, even when node metastasis has occurred.

Follicular Carcinoma.—Such a cancer may originate in a healthy thyroid or in a thyroid already, altered by disease, e.g.:

a. Adenoma, i.e. adenoma with infiltration.
b. Multinodular goitre.

Microscopically, the tumour presents an acinar arrangement, the cells being cubical or low columnar. It is, therefore, known as *alveolar carcinoma* as well.

This variety has a special tendency to spread by the veins.

Macroscopically, the tumour appears to be encapsulated but microscopical examination usually shows invasion of the capsule by tumour cells. Those tumours, in which such invasion is minimal, are called *'non-invasive'* while the others are termed *'invasive'*. The non-invasive type has a prognosis comparable to that of papillary carcinoma while the invasive variety bears a worse prognosis because of chances of local recurrence after surgery, and lung and bone metastases.

The tumour is usually unifocal and involves only one lobe of the thyroid.

Anaplastic Carcinoma.—The cells lose thyroid character, hence called anaplastic. The tumour is highly invasive, so that it involves not only the greater part of the thyroid but frequently the surrounding structures as well. Spread by lymphatics and veins is also frequent.

Medullary Carcinoma.—This tumour deserves special mention because of the following points:
1. It originates in the parafollicular or C-cells in the interstitial tissue of the thyroid (these cells are derived from the ultimo-branchial body).
2. The tumour is slow-growing, though microscopically it represents and undifferentiated character. It consists of sheets of round cells and, histologically, often resembles carcinoid tumour of the gut.
3. Characteristically, the tumour contains an amyloid material, whose presence is detectable both macroscopically and microscopically (hence the name 'medullary').
4. The disease may be familial and may be associated with multiple neuromas on the mucous membranes or with pheochromocytoma.
5. The tumour may secrete a number of hormones:
   a. Calcitonin.—This hormone, which lowers the level of blood calcium, may cause bone pains and parathyroid enlargement.
   b. 5-hydroxytryptamine (5-HT).—This hormone may cause severe diarrhoea (carcinoid syndrome).
   c. A substance like ACTH. —This may cause Cushing's syndrome.
6. The tumour may involve the whole of the thyroid gland and has a tendency to spread by lymphatics. Its treatment is, therefore, total thyroidectomy with clearance of involved lymph nodes.
7. The prognosis is midway between a follicular adenocarcinoma and an anaplastic carcinoma.

Spread of Thyroid Cancers
1. *Direct Spread.*—Almost always starting as a nodule in the thyroid, the growth spreads to the surrounding thyroid tissue. Coming out of the thyroid, the tumour may infiltrate into the overlying muscles (infrahyoid muscles and sterno-mastoid), larynx and trachea oesophagus, recurrent laryngeal nerve, and carotid sheath. Anaplastic carcinoma has the tendency for extensive direct spread while papillary carcinoma the least; follicular carcinoma lies in between.
2. *Lymphatic Spread.*—While all the varieties may spread by lymphatics, papillary carcinoma has special predilection for this route. The nodes involved are the deep cervical nodes (jugulo-digastric and jugulo-omohyoid) and, particularly with the papillary carcinoma, the lymph node metastasis is almost always homolateral. The prelaryngeal and pretracheal nodes (juxtathyroid nodes) are often involved in papillary carcinoma.
3. *Venous Spread.*— Follicular carcinoma has special tendency to spread by veins.

Analplastic carcinoma also, often shows venous spread. Venous embolism as well as permeation may occur. Lungs and bones are especially involved. Thyroid is an important primary site for skull metastasis.

Special Features of Thyroid Metastasis

1. Whatever be the histological type of the primary lesion, the metastatic tumours often show a remarkable degree of differentiation, so that they may closely resemble normal thyroid tissue. It is because of this resemblance that such metastatic lesions in older days were called *'benign metastasizing goitre'*. Such metastatic tumours are even capable of producing thyroxin.
2. Papillary carcinoma often spreads early to the deep cervical nodes and, even when the primary growth is clinically unrecognisable, metastatic nodes may appear. The histological character of a metastatic node may be that of normal thyroid tissue. Such nodes were wrongly termed *lateral aberrant thyroid* in the past. In other words, they used to regarded as developmentally aberrant thyroid tissue on the lateral side of the neck. Actually, they are secondary tumours in the cervical lymph nodes from small, unrecognised, and slowly-growing papillary carcinoma in the thyroid.

Hormone-Dependence of Thyroid Cancers.—Thyroid cancers are often hormone-dependent, depending on TSH stimulation. This is because the activity of the thyroid gland is regulated by TSH papillary carcinoma, in particular, and follicular carcinoma, to certain extent, are dependent on TSH stimulation. Anaplastic carcinoma (which has lost thyroid character) is, however, independent of TSH.

It is, therefore, very useful to administer thyroxin in all cases of thyroid cancers (irrespective of the histology and the type of resection performed). Thyroxin depresses the TSH secretion of the pituitary and so the stimulus to tumour growth (i.e. recurrence) is curtailed.

Iodine-Uptake by Thyroid Cancers

1. Follicular carcinoma shows a good iodine-uptake as is demonstrable by I_{131} tests. Papillary and anaplastic cancers show a little or no uptake.
2. Metastatic lesions from any type of thyroid cancer usually shows good iodine-uptake. This is because the metastatic lesions often show normal thyroid structure.

Clinical Features of Thyroid Cancers.—While cancers of the thyroid usually occur above the age of 40, papillary carcinoma, in particular, may occur in younger age groups, even in children. Females suffer three times more commonly than males. The cases may be divided into three categories:

  I. The clinically doubtful group.
 II. The clinically certain group.
III. The metastatic group.

THE CLINICALLY DOUBTFUL GROUP.—The patient presents with a solitary nodule, and it is very difficult to differentiate it from an adenoma. The points that may be helpful in differentiation have been discussed under adenoma of the thyroid. Papillary and follicular carcinoma usually belong to this group.

In many cases, differentiation is impossible and only histology reveals the correct diagnosis.. This is the reason why, in any doubtful case of a thyroid nodule, hemithyroidectomy is preferred to simple excision of the tumour. If the report is a papillary carcinoma, no further surgery is usually necessary since the growth is limited usually to one lobe. If the report is a follicular carcinoma, a total thyroidectomy can now be done just by removing the remaining half of the thyroid without opening up the already handled counter-half of the neck.

THE CLINICALLY CERTAIN GROUP.—This group may present with either of the following features:
1. A hard, irregular, infiltrating lump, involving the whole of the thyroid, i.e. an anaplastic carcinoma.
2. A suspiciously firm or hard, irregular nodule, associated with:
    a. Discomfort in the neck or pain, often referred to the ear.
    b. Pressure symptoms—dyspnoea, dysphagia.
    c. Features of infiltration—recurrent laryngeal palsy (hoarseness of voice), obliteration of carotid pulsation.
    d. Metastatic deep cervical nodes.
    e. Distant metastases—lung, bones

THE METASTATIC GROUP.—The patient has no complaint about the thyroid but presents with features of metastasis:
1. Significant deep cervical nodes.
2. Pain chest, haemoptysis, cough, dyspnoea, fever (lung metastasis).
3. Pathological fracture or a pulsating bone tumour (bone metastasis).

Special Investigations
1. I_{131}-uptake usually reveals a 'cold nodule'. Follicular carcinoma, however, may show a 'neutral' nodule. A 'hot' nodule is very unlikely to be a cancer, i.e. cancer and thyrotoxicosis only rarely co-exist. Metastatic lesions often show a good I_{131}-uptake.
2. Biopsy:
    a. Excisional biopsy is the usual procedure for a resectable nodule and, for this purpose, a hemithyroidectomy is preferable to simple excision.
    b. Incisional biopsy is always avoided in cases of resectable nodules for fear of seeding of malignant cells and local recurrence. However, incisional or needle biopsy may be indicated in cases of anaplastic carcinoma or irremovable growths (anaplastic carcinoma may be difficult to be differentiated clinically from Riedel's thyroiditis and Hashimoto's disease).
3. X-ray of the chest
4. X-ray of a suspicious bone metastasis.

Treatment.—The available forms of treatment are:
1. Surgery.
2. Irradiation.
3. Radioactive iodine (I_{131}) treatment
4. Hormone treatment.

SURGERY
1. As the patient usually presents with a resectable nodule, hemithyroidectomy is the treatment of choice. If the nodule extends into the isthmus, the isthmus should be included in the resection. When the nodule occupies only the isthmus, isthmusectomy is sufficient.

The biopsy report is of great importance for the subsequent treatment:
    a. If the report is a papillary carcinoma, a total thyroidectomy should be undertaken because the tumour is multifocal and both the lobes may be involved. Since, however, the chances of involvement of the other lobe is only 1 in 5, some surgeons do not advocate any further surgery after hemithyroidectomy and leave the cases to be treated by thyroxin (see below).
    b. If the report is a follicular carcinoma, no further surgery after hemithyroidectomy is necessary because these tumours are unifocal and involve only one lobe. Some surgeons, however, prefer a total thyroidectomy.

2. If simple excision of a nodule has been performed and biopsy reveals a carcinoma, the subsequent procedure is as follows:
   a. For a Papillary Carcinoma—Total thyroidectomy.
   b. For a Follicular Carcinoma—Removal of the rest of the hemithyroid on the affected side (because the follicular cancers are unifocal and usually limited to one lobe). Some surgeons, however, advocate total thyroidectomy.
3. Anaplastic carcinoma, still limited within the capsule, can best be treated by total thyroidectomy, followed by irradiation.
4. Medullary carcinoma are treated by total thyroidectomy.
5. During operation for any thyroid tumour, the deep cervical nodes should be carefully examined (these are well exposed at operation). If there are no enlarged nodes, no treatment is necessary. If, however, there is involvement of nodes, the procedure should be:
   a. Individual excision of the nodes.
   b. Block dissection only if the nodes are grossly involved.

IRRADIATION.—This is always a palliative measure and is indicated for:
1. Anaplastic carcinoma (papillary and follicular cancers are radio resistant).
2. Solitary bone metastasis.

RADIO-IODINE TREATMENT.—This is also a palliative measure and is used for:
1. Non-resectable primary growths, particularly of the follicular variety (papillary and anaplastic cancers have low iodine-uptake).
2. Metastatic lesions—pulmonary or multiple bone metastases.

HORMONE TREATMENT.—As has already described, thyroxin, in good quantity, should be an adjunct to all forms of treatment, irrespective of the type of cancer. A maximum dose of 0.3 mg to 0.4 of 1-thyroxin, per day, is recommended for complete suppression of TSH production. Papillary carcinoma responds most because the tumour is usually TSH dependent.

Summary of Treatment
1. For all resectable growths.—Surgery.
2. For non-resectable growths:
   a. Anaplastic carcinoma.—Irradiation.
   b. Follicular carcinoma.—I_{131}-treatment.
   c. Papillary carcinoma.—Thyroxin (papillary cancers are radioresistant and also have a poor iodine uptake capacity; moreover, they are almost always TSH dependent).
3. For metastasis:
   a. Nodes.—Surgery.
   b. Solitary bone metastasis.—Irradiation.
   c. Pulmonary or multiple bone metastases.—I_{131}-treatment.
4. Thyroxin should be an adjunctive treatment in all cases.

THYROIDITIS

Inflammatory Goitres
These are rare and may be of three types:
1. Acute Thyroiditis.—Bacterial.
2. Chronic Thyroiditis.—Tubercular or syphilitic.
3. Subacute Thyroiditis.—This is of viral origin and is also known as *granulomatous thyroiditis* or *de Quervain's thyroiditis*. There is a painful swelling of the thyroid,

associated with fever. There may be pressure on the trachea. The condition lasts usually for a few weeks and gradual recovery occurs. Prednisone, 10 to 20 mg daily to start with, and then in reduced dosage for a month, is the treatment.

Hashimoto's Disease

Etiology.—It is an auto-immune disease and hence known as *auto-immune thyroiditis*. The patient's serum contains an antibody to the patient's own thyroglobulin and thus an antigen–antibody reaction takes place. The site of such reaction is the thyroid gland itself and the gland shows characteristic pathological changes. The antibody in the serum is demonstrable by serological precipitation tests.

Why such an antibody should develop in the patient's serum is a matter of controversy. The normal rule is that the body develops an immunological tolerance to its own proteins. This should also have happened with thyroglobulin, but this protein, because it is confined within the thyroid acini, does not come in contact with the serum and does not therefore, give a chance for such tolerance to develop. It is believed that in Hashimoto's disease, a leakage of thyroglobulin occurs into the circulation and this brings about the antibody response.

The condition is not infrequently associated with other auto-immune diseases, e.g. auto-immune gastritis, pernicious anaemia, myasthenia gravis, etc.

Pathology.— Usually the disease runs in two stages:
1. At first there is a moderate and uniform enlargement of the thyroid; the gland has a firm feel.
2. Thereafter, usually it turns hard and nodular.

Histologically, there is widespread lymphocyte infiltration inside the thyroid and often germ follicles (as found in lymph nodes) are seen. These replace the thyroid tissue gradually. This is why the condition is also known as *lymphadenoid goitre* (i.e. resembling lymph gland) *and struma lymphomatosa* (struma is the name of a river in Bulgaria, along the banks of which goitres are found in endemic form; hence many thyroid swellings go by the name Struma).

Gradually, a diffuse fibrosis sets in and, depending on the degree of fibrosis, the gland becomes hard and nodular.

The thyroid function is always low, as evidenced by low I_{131}-uptake; in some cases features of myxoedema may be present. This is because of replacement of thyroid tissue by lymphoid and fibrous elements.

Clinical Features
1. For some unknown reason, the disease occurs almost exclusively in the females (95 per cent), and usually above the age of 45.
2. The goitre is usually of moderate size. It may be firm and uniform, or hard and nodular (depending on the degree of fibrosis).
3. Sometimes there may be pressure symptoms (dyspnoea or dysphagia) and a sense of discomfort in the neck.
4. In some cases the deep cervical nodes may be enlarged.
5. Features of myxoedema are seen in 20 per cent of cases.

The age of the patient, the hard nodular feel of the thyroid, occurrence of pressure symptoms and discomfort in the neck, involvement of the cervical nodes, and a low I_{131}-uptake may lead to a wrong diagnosis of carcinoma of the thyroid.

Special Investigations
1. Radio-iodine uptake—invariably shows a low level

2. Serological tests (precipitin), for thyroglobulin-antibody, provide some accurate means of diagnosis.

Treatment

1. MEDICAL.—In those cases where the diagnosis is certain and there are no pressure symptoms or discomfort due to a large goitre, medical treatment with 1-thyroxin is ideal. Thyroxin is necessary because:
   a. The patient is always hypothyroid.
   b. The early cases may show regression of the goitre.
2. SURGICAL:
   a. If diagnosis from a carcinoma is not certain, a total thyroidectomy (followed by biopsy).
   b. If the diagnosis is certain but there are pressure symptoms or discomfort due to a large goitre—subtotal thyroidectomy.

Riedel's Thyroiditis

This is a rare condition, in which the thyroid tissue is gradually replaced by fibrous tissue. Hence, it is also known as *struma fibrosa*. The fibrosis extends beyond the limits of the gland, into the adjacent muscles, trachea, and the carotid sheaths. The cause is not definitely known but it is believed to be a collagen disease; it may be associated with mediastinal and retroperitoneal fibrosis. Hashimoto's disease *never* leads to this condition.

However, the thyroid function is not diminished, as is shown by I_{131}-uptake and PBI estimation. This is because normal thyroid tissue is usually present at the periphery.

The importance of the condition lies in the facts that:
1. It may strangle the trachea.
2. It may be mistaken for an anaplastic carcinoma.

A wedge resection of the isthmus is the *treatment* because it releases the trachea and also provides an excellent material for biopsy, in order to make a differential diagnosis from carcinoma.

OPERATIONS ON THE THYROID

Types

1. Excision of a nodule, e.g. adenoma.
2. Hemithyroidectomy, i.e. resection of one lobe of the thyroid. This is done for:
   a. Some cases of adenoma, e.g. where there is a suspicion of malignancy.
   b. Papillary carcinoma.
3. Hemithyroidectomy with isthmusectomy, i.e. resection of one lobe together with the isthmus. This is done where a suspicious nodule or a papillary carcinoma occupies partially a lobe and partially the isthmus.
4. Isthmusectomy, i.e. excision of the isthmus. This is done for a nodule occupying only the isthmus.
5. Partial thyroidectomy.—This is done in cases of non-toxic metabolic goitres, i.e.
   a. Diffuse colloid goitre.
   b. Multinodular goitre.
   Thyroid tissue, amounting to a normal-size thyroid, is left behind and the excess is resected. In practice, the whole of the isthmus and parts of each lateral lobe from the surface is removed, flush with the tracheal surface, so that there is no undue prominence at the front and sides of the neck.
6. Subtotal thyroidectomy.—This is done for cases of toxic goitre, primary or secondary. Almost the whole of the thyroid is removed, leaving behind only a

small strip on either side, in the tracheo-oesophageal cleft. It is safe to keep this part intact because it is the part which lies in close relationship to the important structures like the recurrent laryngeal nerve, parathyroids, etc. As the thyroid tissue is hyperfunctioning, these small strips, left behind, are sufficient to produce the required quantity of thyroxin.

7. Total thyroidectomy, i.e. removal of the whole of the thyroid. This is done for:
   a. Anaplastic carcinoma of the thyroid, still limited within the capsule of the gland.
   b. Papillary carcinoma.
   c. Cases of Hashimoto's disease, where diagnosis from an anaplastic carcinoma cannot be made clinically.
   All cares must be taken to preserve:
   i. Both recurrent laryngeal nerves.
   ii. Both external laryngeal nerves.
   iii. All the parathyroids with their blood supply intact. It is of particular importance to see that at least two parathyroids (with their blood supply intact) are preserved in order to avoid post-operative tetany and hypoparathyroidism. A little thyroid tissue may have to be left to protect the parathyroid arterial supply. Hence the operation should preferably be called *near-total thyroidectomy*.

Steps of Operation.—The incision is a cosmetic one, that is a *collar incision* along the lowest natural crease of the neck which runs transversely about one inch above the suprasteraal notch. The incision must extend from the posterior border of one sternomastoid to the posterior border of the other. This is because the carotid sheaths, in whose relation the blood vessels of the thyroid run, have to be exposed and for this purpose the sternomastoid have to be retracted backwards (and so the sternomastoids have to be exposed). In the operation of excision of a nodule or of hemithyroidectomy, however, the incision need not be so long but then again it must be adequate enough to allow palpation of the rest of the thyroid to exclude presence of other nodules.

The skin, subcutaneous tissue, and platysma are cut It is better that the platysma is cut at a different level from the skin because this procedure minimises the scar. The skin flaps are mobilised up and down, as far as is necessary, for proper exposure. Thereafter, the ensheathing layer of the deep cervical fascia is cut in the line of the incision.

The infrahyoid (strap) muscles are split in the midline and retracted on either side. If the goitre is big and a wider exposure is necessary, the muscles may be cut transversely instead of being split. If this is done, the muscles should be cut through their upper part since their nerve supply comes from below.

The anterior layer of the pretracheal fascia, covering the thyroid, is carefully incised and the thyroid is exposed.

The vessels are now to be dealt with, one side first and then the other. The middle thyroid veins is cut between ligatures, so that the thyroid lobe can be pulled anteromedially and the other vessels can be dissected (vide ligature of vessels in thyroidectomies—discussed under surgical anatomy).

After the vessels have been ligated, resection of the thyroid is done as is required, i.e. partial, subtotal or total.

The cut surface of the remaining thyroid tissue (which often bleeds considerably, particularly in toxic goitres, even after all the named vessels have been ligated) is sutured with mattress stitches to achieve haemostasis which must be perfect.

A drain of corrugated rubber sheet is put on each side of the trachea and the wound is closed in layers. The platysma must be sutured, and this suturing should be made separately from the skin to avoid an ugly scar.

POSTOPERATIVE COMPLICATIONS

A. IMMEDIATE COMPLICATIONS

1. Haemorrhage.
2. Infection.
3. Recurrent laryngeal nerve palsy.
4. Respiratory obstruction.
5. Thyroid crisis.
6. Parathyroid insufficiency.
7. Mediastinal emphysema.

B. LATE COMPLICATIONS

1. Recurrence.
2. Hypothyroidism.
3. Progressive exophthalmos.
4. Keloid scar.

Haemorrhage.—This is a reactionary haemorrhage. The bleeding may occur from:

1. A main vessel, most commonly the superior thyroid, from where the ligature has supplied.
2. Cut surface of the thyroid.

Either there is a soakage of the bandage or the patient develops sudden dyspnoea because of pressure on the trachea by blood clots.

If there is dyspnoea, the wound should be opened up *immediately* (in the ward). All the stitches should be cut and the trachea should be exposed to relieve the pressure, exerted on it, by the accumulated blood clots. Thereafter, proper exploration should be made in the theatre, haemostasis achieved, and the wound closed with adequate drainage.

Infection.— This is commoner if there has been post-operative haemorrhage. The abscess should be drained properly.

Recurrent Laryngeal Nerve Palsy.—A temporary hoarseness of voice, immediately after the operation, is of common occurrence after operation on big goitres because of slight oedema of the glottis and pressure on the recurrent laryngeal nerves by the exudates.

Injury or inclusion of the nerve in ligature may, however, occur and this may be unilateral or bilateral. Damage to the nerve may be prevented by adopting the following measures:

1. Careful identification of the nerve while ligating the inferior thyroid artery.
2. Ligating the inferior thyroid artery as far away from the thyroid as is possible, thus keeping well away from the course of the nerve.
3. Keeping the posterior lamina of the pretracheal fascia intact—the nerve lies behind the fascia.

Since the recurrent laryngeal nerve supplies all the muscles of the larynx excepting the cricothyroid, which is the strongest adductor of the larynx (this muscle is supplied by the superior laryngeal nerve), injury of this nerve will cause abduction palsy of the vocal cord:

1. In *unilateral* nerve injury, the vocal cord of the affected side is adducted, i.e. it is drawn to the midline, by the unparalysed cricothyroid. The opposite vocal cord is normal in position and normally functioning. The patient's difficulties are:
   a. Hoarseness of voice.   b. Cough.
   c. Tendency of liquids to go down the larynx during deglutition.

In the majority of cases, accommodation occurs and the difficulties pass off in a few months.

2. *Bilateral* nerve injury is very dangerous. Both the vocal cords are adducted, i.e. they are apposed to each other in the midline causing complete closure of the glottis. Immediate asphyxia may develop as soon as the endotracheal tube is withdrawn by the anaesthetist.

Immediate tracheostomy is a life-saving measure in these cases.

Injury to the superior (external) laryngeal nerve is seldom associated with any symptoms since the other abductors of the larynx, supplied by the recurrent laryngeal nerve, are functioning. However, if the superior and the recurrent laryngeal nerves are both injured, the vocal cord assumes a position midway between abduction and adduction, and hangs without tension, as seen in the dead (*cadaveric position* of the cord). Such injuries are, however, extremely rare (this is more commonly seen in vagal palsy; both these nerves are branches of the vagus).

Respiratory Obstruction.—This may be due to:
1. Pressure on the trachea by blood clots.
2. Bilateral recurrent laryngeal nerve injury.
3. Laryngeal oedema caused by trauma to the larynx by endotracheal intubation.

Thyroid Crisis.—This is also known as *thyrotoxic crisis* (which is a better name) or *thyroid storm*. There is acute exacerbation of thyrotoxic features.

CAUSE.—This complication occurs after operation for toxic goitres, particularly when the patient has not been properly made euthyroid prior to operation. The condition results from sudden entry of a huge quantity of thyroxin into the circulation, and this may be due to:

a. Pumping out thyroxin from the gland during manipulation at operation.

b. Absorption of thyroxin from the raw cut surface of the thyroid.

CLINICAL MANIFESTATIONS

1. Hyperpyrexia.—The temperature may be as high 108 °F.
2. Cardiovascular Features.—Severe tachycardia (e.g. 180 per minute), gross cardiac irregularities extrasystoles, auricular fibrillation, and ultimately heart failure (in systole).
3. Nervous Features:
   a. CNS—Delirium, coma, convulsions.   b. Autonomic.—Severe diarrhoea.

TREATMENT

1. *Symptomatic Treatment:*
   a. Sedation.—Morphine or pethidine.
   b. Control of hyperpyrexia by all possible means.—Ice bag, ice-sponging, rectal ice-irrigation, air-conditioning of the room. Severe cases demand 'controlled hypothermia'.
   c. For cardiac control.— Digitalis may be necessary.
2. *Specific Treatment:*
   a. β-adrenergic blocking drugs are most useful for immediate control of the condition—Propranolol, 20 mg every 6 hours, is administered.
   b. Cortisone is often life-saving and may have to be combined with ACTH.
   c. Lugol's iodine by all possible routes. To start with, it is administered 2 ml IV and then 2 ml IM every 6 hours. Thereafter, it is given orally, 60 minims every 8 hours for 48 hours, and then the dose is gradually reduced.

Hypoparathyroidism.—Hypoparathyroidism, causing tetany, may occur as a result of:

a. Removal of the parathyroids with the thyroid.
b. Impairment of blood supply to the parathyroids (the arteries to the parathyroids are end-arteries).

If two of the four parathyroids are intact, tetany does not develop.

TREATMENT

A. *Prophylactic:*
1. During dissection and ligature of the vessels at thyroidectomy, the parathyroids and their blood supply must be carefully preserved.
2. After the thyroid is removed, the specimen should be carefully examined for inclusion of the parathyroids. If more than two parathyroids are present in the specimen, they should be taken and implanted into a sternomastoid muscle. The glands do not live permanently but they are likely to tide the patient over in the immediate post-operative period.

B. Curative:
1. Immediate.—Calcium is to be administered by all possible routes:
   a. Calcium gluconate (10 per cent), 10 to 20 ml is given IV.
   b. Thereafter, a similar dose is given IM for a prolonged effect
   c. In severe cases, the IM dose is repeated till the spasms are controlled
   d. Soluble calcium aspirin is given orally in doses of 1 gm daily when the patient can swallow.
2. Long Term
   a. Calcium.—A diet rich in calcium. In severe cases, calcium lactate or soluble calcium aspirin.
   b. In addition to calcium, one of the following drugs has to be administered:
      i. Parathormone.—It is expensive, has to be administered intramuscularly, and loses effect when given for long periods.
      ii. Calciferol (vitamin D_2), 10 mg twice daily, orally.
      iii. Dihydrotachysterol or irradiated ergosterol in those cases which prove refractory to calciferol.

Mediastinal Emphysema.—This rare complication occurs if air gains entry into the mediastinum along pretracheal space.

Recurrence

1. Recurrence of toxicity.—This is more likely to occur if considerable amount of thyroid tissue has been left behind. However, it may also occur after adequate surgery.
2. Recurrence of malignancy.

Hypothyroidism.—This is rather easy to treat with 1-thyroxin.

Progressive (Malignant) Exophthalmos.—As has been stated, after treatment for hyperthyroidism, while the thyrotoxic features regress, the exophthalmos may increase (*see* physiology).

Keloid Scar.—This is more likely to occur:

a. If there is infection.
b. If the scar overlies the sternum.

RETROSTERNAL GOITRE

Only rarely a goitre arises from ectopic thyroid tissue in the superior mediastinum, i.e. a *true retrosternal goitre*.

The common form of retrosternal goitre is an extension downwards of a nodule from the lower pole of the thyroid. Such an extension is likely to occur if:

a. The goitre is big.
b. The neck is short.
c. The pretracheal muscles are so strong that they prevent much of forward expansion of the gland and thus forces it to grow downwards.

Once the nodule enters into the mediastinum, the negative intrathoracic pressure sucks it further downwards.

According to the degree of descent, 3 types are described:

1. **Substernal.**—The lower pole of the nodule is palpable during the act of swallowing.
2. **Plunging.**—The lower pole is occasionally forced up into the neck when there is a raised intrathoracic pressure.
3. **Intrathoracic.**—The lower pole never comes up to the neck.

Clinical Features

A. GOITRE
   1. In the majority of cases, the cervical part of the goitre is visible and a clinical examination suggests a downward prolongation.
   2. In some cases, no goitre is visible. In these patients, history of a previous cervical goitre, which subsequently disappeared, is often present.
   3. When a retrosternal goitre arises from intrathoracic ectopic thyroid tissue, no goitre is visible, neither a suggestive history is elicited.

B. SYMPTOMS
   1. Many of the retrosternal goitres are symptomless.
   2. Toxicity.—Clinical diagnosis may be very difficult in cases of intrathoracic toxic goitres.
   3. Pressure Symptoms:
      a. Dyspnoea and stridor (harsh sound during inspiration).
      b. Cough, particularly when the patient lies down. Many patients get the cough only when they lie on one side, very commonly the right side.
      c. Dysphagia—rare
      d. Hoarseness of voice—rare
      e. Prominent neck veins (and sometimes the veins on the chest wall) due to pressure on the big thoracic veins.

Special Investigations

1. X-ray of the Chest:
   a. Lateral view of the chest may be very helpful. A shadow in the superior mediastinum may be due to other conditions as well, e.g. persistent thymus, thymic tumours, mediastinal tumours, etc. However, if calcification is present, diagnosis of a goitre is almost certain.
   b. Anteroposterior view may show deviation and compression of the trachea.
2. I_{31}-uptake test may be valuable but it is of a little value if iodine affinity of the goitre is poor.

Treatment.—This is always surgical. Treatment with anti-thyroid drugs or radio-iodine may prove dangerous as the goitre may increase in size and cause severe obstructive features.

As the blood supply of a retrosternal goitre comes from the neck, the operation is usually not very difficult. It can well be done from the neck by digital manipulation and delivery of the retrosternal part, after ligation of the blood vessels at the neck. If, however, adhesions inside the mediastinum or the big size of the goitre makes its delivery difficult, one of the following two procedures may be adopted:

1. The impacted goitre is broken up and removed piecemeal. Before doing this, the possibility of a carcinoma has, however, to be excluded.
2. A sternal split, i.e. splitting the sternum in the midline, to expose the mediastinum, is performed.

31

The Parathyroid Glands

Surgical Anatomy.—These endocrine glands, usually two pairs—superior and inferior, develop from the pharyngeal pouches. The superior parathyroid, on each side, develops from the fourth pouch (hence called parathyroid IV). Paradoxically, the inferior parathyroids develop from the third pharyngeal pouch (parathyroid III). The inferior parathyroids develop together with the thymus and, since the thymus descends low down, the glands come down to a lower level than their counterparts developing from the fourth pouch. For the same reason, the inferior parathyroids may be situated in the superior or posterior mediastinum instead of their usual anatomical position.

The glands are oval in shape, about the size of small peas, the inferior glands being larger than the superiors. Their colour varies from red or pink to yellow depending on the amount of fat deposition as age advances. They have, however, a distinctly different colour from the thyroid and this factor is of great help in their identification either at thyroidectomy or at parathyroidectomy. Though they vary greatly in their position (particularly the inferior parathyroids), the usual disposition is that the superior one is situated on the posterior surface of the lateral lobe at about its middle, and the inferior is located on the posteromedial aspect of the lateral lobe where the inferior thyroid artery enters the thyroid. The inferior parathyroid may be located either above or below the inferior thyroid artery.

It is generally agreed that the parathyroids are located between the true fibrous capsule (fascia propria) of the thyroid and fascial sheath of the thyroid derived from the pretracheal fascia. However, in some cases, the glands may lie outside the fascial sheath of the thyroid or inside the true capsule of the thyroid.

The *blood supply* to all the parathyroids is mainly derived from the inferior thyroid artery, by way of an anastomotic channel connecting the superior and the inferior thyroid artery on each side.

Microscopically, the parathyroids contain three types of cells:
1. Basophilic or chief cells.
2. Eosinophilic cells (their number increases as age advances).
3. Water-clear cells.

Surgical Physiology.—The hormone of the parathyroid is *parathormone,* which is polypeptide. It regulates the calcium and phosphorous metabolism of the body, maintaining a balanced ratio between the two. The normal level of serum clacium is 9 to 11 mg per 100 ml and that of serum phosphorus is 3 to 4.5 mg per 100 ml (4.5 to 5.5 and 1.8 to 2.7 mEq. per litre respectively). The product between calcium and phosphorus in mg, i.e. Ca × P is about 40 in a normal subject.

The control on the calcium and the phosphorus metabolism is maintained by the effect of parathormone on two organs, viz. bone and kidney. As to the exact mode of control, there are two views:

1. Parathormone stimulates osteoclasts to bone destruction; thus mobilising calcium and phosphate from bone to blood. This theory fails to explain why the serum phosphorus level should be low when the calcium level rises in hyper-parathyroidism.
2. Parathormone controls reabsorption of phosphates by the renal tubules. Since there is a reciprocal relationship between phosphorus and calcium, any change in the serum phosphate level brings in a compensatory change in the calcium level by mobilisation from the bone. This view is more commonly accepted.

One important point about the serum calcium is as to how it is held in solution in the blood plasma. From this point of view, the calcium may be divided into three parts:

a. About one-third is held adsorbed on plasma proteins; this is non-ionised and is physiologically inactive.
b. A small part is in close attachment with organic acids; this also is non-ionised and, hence, physiologically inactive.
c. The remainder is held in solution by parathormone. It is only this part which is ionised and is physiologically active, i.e. dynamic. The rise or fall of serum calcium, as seen in hyper- and hypo-parathyroidism respectively, is only with respect to this part.

HYPERPARATHYROIDISM

Local Pathology.—This condition, in which there is an excess of parathormone secretion, may be due to one of the following conditions:

1. *Solitary adenoma* in a parathyroid, obviously hormone-secreting— these account for 80 per cent of the cases.
2. *Hyperplasia* involving all the parathyroids—these account for about 20 per cent of the cases.
3. *Multiple adenoma* usually in one, exceptionally in two parathyroids— rare.
4. *Carcinoma* in a parathyroid—extremely rare.

Biochemical Changes

1. *Elevation of the Serum Calcium Level.*—In the majority of cases there is considerable rise in the level of serum calcium. There are two views to explain this rise:
   a. That parathormone directly mobilises calcium from the bone by stimulating the osteoclasts to bone destruction.
   b. That parathormone diminishes tubular reabsorption of phosphate in the kidney so that there is increased phosphate excretion in the urine. The serum phosphate level, therefore, falls. Since there is a reciprocal relationship between the phosphate and calcium levels in the serum, the serum calcium level is elevated.

The serum calcium level often rises to 12 to 16 mg (sometimes 20 mg) from the normal level of 9 to 11 mg per 100 ml.

As has already been stated, this elevation is only in respect to that part of the serum calcium which is held in solution by parathormone and is ionised and physiologically active, i.e. dynamic. The actual level, to which the serum calcium rises, depends on four factors:

i. Rate of mobilisation from the bones.

ii. Rate of absorption from the gut (i.e. food).

iii. Rate of excretion by the kidneys.

iv. Rate of excretion from the gut.

2. *Increased Excretion of Calcium in the Urine.*—There are two routes of excretion of calcium from the body, viz., the stool and the urine. In a normal individual most of the calcium is eliminated in the stool and only 10 to 30 per cent in the urine. In hyperparathyroidism this ratio is reversed and the urine is supersaturated with calcium. This calcium is excreted:

a. As calcium phosphate, if the urine is alkaline;

b. As calcium oxalate, if the urine is acid

3. *Increased Excretion of Phosphorus in the Urine.*—As has been stated, this is the prime factor in the biochemical disturbances. However, when gross renal damage sets in, in the late stage of the disease (see below), the phosphorus excretion may fall.

4. *Diminished Level of Serum Phosphorus.*—As phosphorus is excreted in high quantities in the urine, its level in the serum falls (normal 3 to 4.5 mg/100 ml).

5. *Elevation of Serum Alkaline Phosphatase Level.*—As in all bone dystrophies, there is an elevation in the level of serum alkaline phosphatase (normal 3 to 13 KA units/100 ml).

Distant Pathological Changes and Clinical Features

A. THE BONE LESIONS.—Lesion in bones, i.e. *parathyroid osteodystrophy*, is the most well-recognised manifestation of hyperparathyroidism but it is not invariable. In at least some cases, the bones may be spared by increased utilisation of dietary calcium. The changes may involve the entire skeleton and are as follows:

1. Generalised demineralization with subperiosteal bone resorption (*von Recklinghausen's disease of bone*).

2. In some areas there may be complete replacement of osseous structure by fibrous tissue (i.e. *osteitis fibrosa*) in which there is an abundance of osteoclast giant cells (the so-called *brown tumour of hyperparathyroidism*). Such areas of fibrous replacement may become cystic (*osteitis fibrosa cystica*). Some bones are commonly affected, viz. the metaphysis of long bones, mandible, maxilla, and phalanges.

3. Softening of bones may lead to deformities.

4. Pathological fractures may occur through the cystic areas.

B. THE KIDNEY LESIONS.—The increased urinary output of calcium may lead to the following changes:

1. Formation of urinary calculi (hyperparathyroidism should be excluded especially in cases of multiple and recurrent calculi).

2. *Nephrocalcinosis.*—Radiologically seen as streaks of calcification in the line of renal tubules. Calcific foci block the renal tubules and cause fibrosis and obliteration of the corresponding nephrons.

3. Widespread obliteration of nephrons, resulting in renal damage, may cause polyuria, hypertension, and renal failure. Renal failure is often the *cause of death* in these cases.

C. THE ABDOMINAL LESIONS:
1. Anorexia, nausea and vomiting may be the presenting features.
2. Peptic ulcer may occur in 15 per cent of cases. The pain is worsened by alkalis. Recurrent bleeding may occur. The ulcer may not be demonstrable radiologically.
3. Acute, subacute, or chronic pancreatitis may occur in some cases.

Special Investigations

A. BIOCHEMISTRY
1. Elevation of serum calcium.
2. Increased urinary excretion of calcium.
3. Increased urinary excretion of phosphorus.
4. Diminished serum phosphorus.
5. Elevation of serum alkaline phosphatase.
6. Elevation of serum parathormone (upper limit of normal is 0.5 microgram per litre of serum). The hormone is always detectable in hyperparathyroidism patients while it may be undetectable in many normal subjects.
7. *Sulkowitch Test.*—The patient is given a diet containing 125 mg of calcium daily, for three successive days. In hyperparathyroidism more than 200 mg of calcium is excreted in the urine daily (in a normal subject this level will be less than 100 mg).

B. X-RAY OF BONES
1. Generalised decalcification, often with cyst formation.
2. Subperiosteal resorption, best seen in the middle phalanges. There is often an associated reabsorption of the tufts of the terminal phalanges.
3. Pathological fractures.
4. The skull may have a 'ground glass' appearance due to decreased density.

C. X-RAY OF THE KIDNEYS may show stones or nephrocalcinosis.

D. METASTATIC CALCIFICATION in soft tissues may be occasionally seen.

Treatment.—Surgery is the only method of treatment. The actual type of surgery depends on the pathology, and may be as follows:
1. If there is a parathyroid adenoma, it should be excised. However, after excising the tumour, all the other three parathyroids are to be explored and examined. This is because multiple adenoma may occur, involving more than one parathyroid. The operation is performed with a collar incision, as for subtotal thyroidectomy. While the parathyroids may be found in their normal positions behind the thyroid lobes, they may be located in abnormal situations as well, e.g.
   a. Embedded in the substance of the thyroid,
   b. In the tracheo-oesophageal groove.
2. If no adenoma is detectable and all or several parathyroids are found to be larger than normal, parathyroid hyperplasia is the diagnosis (had there been a hidden adenoma, the parathyroids would be smaller in size due to disuse atrophy). In such cases, three or three and a half of the parathyroid glands are removed.
3. When the parathyroids appear normal or smaller in size, adenoma in an ectopic parathyroid is the likely pathology. In these cases, after careful search of the

thyroid lobes and the tracheo-oesophageal grooves, the mediastinum has to be explored. For this purpose, a sternal split is done. An ectopic parathyroid may be located:

a. retrosternal

b. on the pericardium

c. in relation to the thymus (a thymectomy may have to be done).

4. If some of the parathyroids (particularly the inferior glands) are not traceable in the neck, the mediastinum has to be explored, as above, in order to find out the glands.

HYPOPARATHYROIDISM

Causes

1. POST-OPERATIVE.—These account for the majority of the cases. They occur after thyroidectomies, but only in about one per cent of the cases. The features appear in one to five days after the operation but, if the symptoms are mild, the condition may remain unrecognised for weeks (*see* complications of thyroidectomy, Chapter 30).

2. INSIDIOUS.—These occur spontaneously in some people. The condition is characterised by weakness, opacity of the lenses, brittleness of the nails, loss of dental enamel, loss of hair, and a low serum calcium level.

3. IDIOPATHIC.—This occurs in children, usually in the active stages of rickets.

4. SECONDARY.—These cases occur secondary to alkalosis and may be found in:

a. Long-continued vomiting.—Pyloric stenosis, high intestinal obstruction.

b. Prolonged administration of alkalis.—Peptic ulcer.

Clinical Features.—The features of tetany set in when the blood calcium level comes down to the *'tetany level'* which is usually below 6 mg per 100 ml of serum. It takes a few days for this level to be reached, so post-operative tetany (the commonest form) takes about 2 to 5 days to appear. The milder forms may be missed clinically for longer periods. The earlier the features appear, the delayed is the recovery.

The clinical features are all motor, resulting from muscular irritability:

1. Widespread fibrillation of the muscle fibres may give the patient a sensation of tingling and numbness of the lips, nose, and extremities; there may be a typical circumoral pallor.

2. The muscles of the forearms and legs go into spasm, resulting in what is called the 'carpopedal spasm'. The characteristic features are:

a. The foot assumes an equinus position (i.e. plantar-flexion).

b. The hand assumes the *'obstetrical position'*—the fingers are extended except at the metacarpophalangeal joints (which are flexed), and the thumb is adducted.

3. In latent cases, muscle spasms which are not ordinarily seen, may be induced as follows:

a. *Trousseau's Sign.*—A sphygmomanometer cuff is applied round the arm and the pressure is raised to above the systolic level—the hand assumes the 'obstetrical position'.

    b. *Chvostek's Sign.*—Tapping the facial nerve, just in front of the ear, with a percussion hammer, provokes twitching of the facial muscles.

4. In severe cases, the spasms may be more pronounced, e.g.
   a. Generalised fits.
   b. Spasm of the muscles of respiration—dyspnoea.
   c. Spasm of intra-ocular muscles—blurring of vision.
5. The insidious cases may present with weakness, cataracts, brittle nails, lack of dental enamel, and loss of hair.

Special Investigations

1. *Estimation of Serum Calcium.*—This is always low, usually below 6 mg per 100 ml, in frank cases of tetany.
2. *Erb's Sign.*—A hyperexcitability of the muscles can be seen on galvanic stimulation.

Treatment.—*See* Chapter 30, under 'post-thyroidectomy complications'.

32

The Adrenal Glands

The adrenal gland, one on each side, is enclosed, together with the kidney, within the renal fascia but a lamina of fibroareolar tissue separates the two structures, so that they occupy separate compartments. The right adrenal is triangular in shape and the left is semilunar.

Each gland has usually three arteries but a single vein. The arteries are:

1. The superior adrenal artery, branch of inferior phrenic.
2. The middle adrenal artery, branch of abdominal aorta direct.
3. The inferior adrenal artery, branch of renal.

The veins on the two sides differ from each other:

a. The right adrenal vein is very short and drains directly into the inferior vena cava, distal to the hepatic vein. The vein is so short that the gland actually sits on the inferior vena cava.
b. The left adrenal vein is longer and it drains into the left renal vein. Anatomical communications exist between the renal vein and the azygos vein, so that the venous blood from the left adrenal has direct access into the vertebral, intercostal, and internal mammary veins of the left side.

These differences in the veins of the two sides are important in two ways:

1. Adrenalectomy is a little more difficult on the right side because the vein is so short that it may tear even with mild traction on the gland, and, as the tear is practically on the inferior vena cava, the bleeding may prove very difficult to be controlled.
2. Metastatic lesions from malignant tumours of the adrenal (e.g. neuroblastoma) may show differences in their distribution. With growths on the right side, hepatic metastasis is commoner; with tumours on the left side, bone metastasis is commoner (especially the skull, by way of vertebral veins).

The adrenal gland (like the pituitary) consists of two different tissues—the cortex and the medulla. Except for the fact that these two parts are in so intimate anatomical relationship as to deserve description together, there is every reason to consider the two parts separately, because developmentally, structurally, as well as functionally, the two behave as separate endocrine organs.

THE ADRENAL MEDULLA

Embryology.—The adrenal medulla is ectodermal in origin. It is developed, together with the sympathetic nervous system, from the neuroectoderm. Hence, it is in close functional relationship with the sympathetic nerves, its secretions acting on the sympathetic nerve endings.

Histology.—The adrenal medulla consists of:

1. Mainly chromaffin tissue, an aggregation of chromaffin cells. These are large polyhedral cells and are so named because they contain granules which stain yellow with chromic acid. These granules are actually the secretions of the adrenal medulla and they are found, as such, inside the small radicles of the adrenal vein.

2. Some nerve cells of the sympathetic nervous system.

Functions.—The secretion of the adrenal medulla consists of different catecholamines, of which only two are important:

1. Adrenaline.

2. Noradrenaline.—This is the unmethylated precursor of adrenaline.

In health, 80 per cent of the medullary secretion is adrenaline and only 20 per cent noradrenaline.

Adrenaline causes peripheral vasoconstriction but muscular vasodilatation. Noradrenaline causes an overall vasoconstriction. However, the action of noradrenaline is short lived. These effects are produced by the action of adrenaline and noradrenaline on the sympathetic nerve-endings. In conditions like fear, anger, and pain (i.e. when the body is subjected to noxious stimuli), the adrenal medulla is stimulated by way of the splanchnic nerves and it quickly liberates its hormones in the blood to make a rapid response. Adrenaline has an additional effect of glycogenolysis.

TUMOURS OF THE ADRENAL MEDULLA

There are three common tumours—pheochromocytoma, ganglioneuroma, and neuroblastoma.

Classification

A. ACCORDING TO ORIGIN

1. Those arising from the chromaffin cells.—Pheochromocytoma.
2. Those arising from the nerve cells (mature or immature) of the sympathetic nervous system:
    a. Arising from and reproducing nerve cells of very immature type.—Neuroblastoma.
    b. Arising from and reproducing ganglion nerve cells of adult type.—Ganglioneuroma.

B. ACCORDING TO AGE INCIDENCE

1. Those occurring at any age.—Ganglioneuroma.
2. Those occurring in children.—Neuroblastoma.
3. Those occurring usually in adults.—Pheochromocytoma.

C. ACCORDING TO PATHOLOGY

1. *Benign*
    a. Ganglioneuroma.
    b. Pheochromocytoma (90 per cent).
2. Malignant
    a. Neuroblastoma
    b. Pheochromocytoma (10 per cent).

PHEOCHROMOCYTOMA

Origin.—These tumours originate in the chromaffin cells of the adrenal medulla. Rarely a tumour may originate from extra-adrenal chromaffin tissue (i.e. at ectopic sites), e.g.:

a. Retroperitoneal tissues—along the aorta, at the base of the mesentery, etc.

b. Sympathetic ganglia.

c. Mediastinum.

Pathology

1. The tumour is usually benign, but may be malignant (10 per cent). Metastasis may occur from a malignant growth.
2. In about 15 per cent of cases the tumour is bilateral. Sometimes there are multiple tumours.
3. The tumour is usually small (less than 5 cm). It has a thin but definite capsule. It is soft and is brownish in colour.
4. *Microscopically,* it consists of phaeochromocytes in large numbers. These are large, well-differentiated round cells, which characteristically stain black with chromium salts.
5. Occasionally the condition may be associated with neurofibromatosis or with medullary cancer of the thyroid.

Pathological Effects.—This tumour is important because it secretes the adrenal medullary hormones in excess—both adrenaline and noradrenaline. The proportion between the two differs from case to case, but in a vast majority it is the noradrenaline which preponderates. The normal ratio of adrenaline to noradrenaline (80:20) may just be reversed. A tumour in an ectopic site and one in a child is more likely to produce noradrenaline. These hormones, released into the blood stream, cause hypertension. In all the cases, to start with, the hypertension is paroxysmal, the systolic blood pressure rising to alarmingly high levels during the attacks. In at least 50 per cent of the cases the hypertension becomes persistent, though paroxysms may be superadded even on such cases. As the hypertension becomes persistent all its complications may set in.

A similar type of paroxysmal hypertension may occur in the rare condition of hyperplasia of the adrenal medulla, in which both the adrenals share.

Clinical Features.—Almost always the patient is an adult, both the sexes being equally affected. The presenting features are:

1. Paroxysms of hypertension, associated with some symptoms, which, in order of frequency, are—headache, palpitation, vomiting, sweating, dyspnoea, weakness, and pallor. The systolic blood pressure is raised enormously during the attacks.
2. Persistent hypertension in about 50 per cent of cases. Even in these cases, attacks of paroxysmal increase may occur from time to time. Cardiovascular changes may set in, and hypertensive retinopathy may occur.
3. 10 per cent of cashes develop diabetes mellitus.
4. A pheochromocytoma may originate or may be switched into activity during pregnancy.

Special Investigations

A. RADIOGRAPHY

1. A straight X-ray may very occasionally show a soft tissue shadow in the adrenal region. Usually, however, the tumour is too small to cast such a shadow.

2. IVP may show displacement of the pelvicalyceal system at the upper pole of the kidney. This may sometimes be mistaken for a renal tumour.

3. *Paracoccygeal air insufflation* into the retroperitoneal tissues.—A lumbar puncture needle is passed in and 500 ml of air is introduced with the help of a pneumothorax apparatus. The air moves upwards to the perirenal areas and an adrenal swelling may be made out by contrast. The contrast may be made stronger, and diagnosis from a renal neoplasm easier, by adding one of the following procedures:

    a. IVP.

    b. Aortography.—As the tumours are usually vascular, the increased vascularity may be well-demonstrated.

    c. Retrograde venous catheterisation and injection of a contrast medium.

4. CAT scan may be of great help in the diagnosis.

B. HORMONE TESTS

1. *Urine tests:*

    a. Estimation of VMA (vanillyl mandelic acid), which is a metabolite of the catecholamines, i.e. nor-adrenaline and adrenaline. A colorimetric examination is done. The normal output is 2< to 8 µg in 24 hours. In phacochromocytoma this level is significantly raised.

    b. Direct estimation of catecholamines in the urine by fluorimetric method. This may be done as an alternative to (a).

    c. Animal Test.—Extracts from the patient's urine, containing the catecholamines, are injected into a cat to find if there is a rise in blood pressure.

2. *Blood Examination.*—A retrograde venous catheterisation is done, and blood from the inferior vena cava is directly drawn for estimation of nor-adrenaline.

3. *Pharmacological Tests.*—These are done by administration of drugs, which either provoke or diminish the hypertension, and their effects are studied:

    a. *Drugs provoking hypertension.*—Histamine or mecholyl is injected intravenously and an attack of hypertension is provoked for confirmation of diagnosis. The procedure is dangerous for the patient, and is therefore condemned.

    b. *Drugs diminishing hypertension.*—Adrenaline-antagonist drugs are administered and the blood pressure is reduced; this confirms the diagnosis. This procedure is safe and therefore standard. Piperoxane or dibenamine may be used, but the most commonly used drug is Rogitine (phentolamine), 5 mg given intravenously.

Treatment.—The only available treatment is removal of the adrenal gland on the affected side. If the side is certain, an extra-peritoneal approach by the lumbar route (as for the kidney) is done. The twelfth (sometimes also the eleventh) rib is excised to expose the adrenal. If the side of the tumour is uncertain, a transperitoneal approach has to be made, so that both the adrenals can be examined.

Special Precautions at Operation.—During anaesthesia and while manipulating the adrenal, there is every possibility of rise of blood pressure to serious levels. After removal of the adrenal, with the tumour, there is again the possibility of a sudden fall of blood pressure. These may be combated by the following procedures:

1. Rogitine, 20 to 40 mg thrice daily, is given orally for a few days prior to the date of operation.
2. Before induction of anaesthesia, Rogitine 5 mg is administered intravenously.
3. While manipulating the adrenal, Rogitine 5 mg is again given intravenously, and repeated if required.
4. As soon as the adrenal gland is removed (or the vein ligated), noradrenaline is given intravenously to combat hypotension. A nor-adrenaline drip may have to be continued for the first forty-eight hours and then the drug is gradually tailed off over a week.

NEUROBLASTOMA

Origin.—This tumour arises from immature nerve cells of the sympathetic nervous system (neuroblasts), contained in the adrenal medulla. Occasionally it may arise from neuroblasts located at extra-adrenal sites, e.g. retroperitoneal tissues, mediastinum, and along the sympathetic chain.

Pathology

Microscopic Features.—The tumour consists of small round cells which are often arranged in *rosette-forms*. The cells have a special affinity for silver salts and are, therefore, known as *argentophil cells.* The cells are of highly immature and undifferentiated type.

Macroscopic Features.—The tumour is usually of massive size, like Wilms' tumour of the kidney. Characteristically, the surface is *nodular.* It has a maroon colour and there are big areas of necrosis and haemorrhage.

Spread

1. *Direct Spread.*—A very quickly growing tumour, it attains very large size and comes out of the confines of the adrenal gland to involve neighbouring structures, viz. the liver and the spleen, the adrenal vein, the renal vein, and the inferior vena cava. Peculiarly, the kidney is often spared.
2. *Lymphatic Spread.*—Para-aortic nodes may be involved.
3. *Venous Spread.*—This is a very important channel of spread. Spread occurs to the bones and the liver. There is a special tendency for the right-sided growths to metastasize into the liver and the left-sided ones to disseminate into the bones. This is explained by the difference in the venous drainage of the two adrenals; the right adrenal vein drains into the inferior vena cava just distal to the hepatic vein while the left adrenal vein drains into the left renal vein which communicates, through the azygos vein, with the vertebral, intercostal and internal mammary veins of the left side. Skull is a very favourite site for osseous metastasis and it is believed that the malignant cells reach there by way of the vertebral veins.

Clinical Features

1. This is a tumour of the children, more than 80 per cent occurring below the age of 5 years. Sometimes an infant may be born with a neuroblastoma. Both the sexes are equally affected.

2. The child is presented with an abdominal lump. The lump starts in the loin but very quickly spreads to the major part of the abdomen. The age of the patient and the quick growth closely resembles a Wilms' tumour, from which it is clinically differentiated by two points:

   a. Neuroblastoma has characteristically a nodular surface, while Wilm's tumour is smooth.

   b. Haematuria, which sometimes occurs in Wilms' tumour, is very rare with neuroblastoma.

3. In all the cases there is pallor, with loss of appetite and weight.

4. Many of the children show evidence of bone metastases, especially in the skull. The liver is the next common site of metastasis. Symptoms due to involvement of the lung and soft tissues may occur.

5. Occasionally the tumour shows evidence of hormone production—there is flushing, sweating, hypertension.

6. In some cases the child may have *coeliac syndrome*, characterised by diarrhoea, weight-loss, and abdominal enlargement.

Types of Neuroblastoma.—It is customary to describe two types:

Pepper type

1. The growth is in the right adrenal.
2. Occurs very early in life.
3. Liver metastasis is characteristic.
4. Histologically, the cells are very immature.
5. Prognosis is grave.

Hutchinson type

1. The growth is in the left adrenal.
2. Occurs in older children.
3. Bone metastasis is characteristic.
4. Histologically, the cells are relatively mature.
5. Prognosis is relatively better.

Special Investigations

1. Hormone Assay.—Estimation of vanillyl mandelic acid (VML) in the urine may show a high level (see pheochromocytoma).

2. Aspiration of bone marrow may show malignant cells.

3. Bone-scanning may detect deposits even before metastases are evident on the X-ray.

4. Straight X-ray shows a huge soft tissue shadow in the kidney region, sometimes with areas of calcification.

5. IVP shows a displacement of the pelvi-calyceal system (c.f. Wilms' tumour, where there is distortion and disappearance of the calyces involved).

6. Paracoccygeal air insufflation into the retroperitoneal tissues may be helpful to show the tumour by contrast. The contrast is made further strong by adding:

   a. IVP.

   b. Aortography (renal angiogram).

   c. Retrograde venogram.

   (*see* phaeochromocytoma).

7. X-ray of the bones:

   a. The skull is often involved, particularly in the region of the orbit. There is often an evidence of new bone formation in the form of *'pins and needles'*.

b. The metastases in the long bones have characteristically the appearance of *Ewing's tumour*. This is the reason why, in older days, Ewing's tumour was believed to be a secondary deposit from neuroblastoma unrecognised.

Treatment

1. Excision, followed by radiotherapy, is the usual method of treatment. Sometimes a course of pre-operative radiation is helpful, as it brings down the size and vascularity of the tumour, making resection a little easier. One characteristic feature of the tumour is that, even when it cannot be excised radically, the tumour shows a regression in the post-operative period (even if radiotherapy is omitted). Further, the secondary lesions, also, often show tendency for spontaneous regression.

2. In this respect, high doses of vitamin B_{12} often achieve miracles. The explanation often put forward is that such cases are borderline between ganglioneuroma (benign) and neuroblastoma (malignant), and a high dose of folic acid converts the tumour into a ganglioneuroma, thus improving the prognosis.

3. Radiation of the bone metastases.

4. Chemotherapy in advanced cases.

GANGLIONEUROMA

Only 15 per cent of ganglioneuromas occur in the adrenal medulla, the remaining occurring along the sympathetic chain in the paravertebral recess of the abdomen or thorax.

The tumour is of developmental origin, sometimes associated with developmental defects in the ribs or vertebrae. It originates from the mature nerve cells of the sympathetic nervous system and reproduces ganglion cells of adult type, i.e. it is benign. This feature is of importance because normally ganglion cells are incapable of division. The bulk of the tumour, however, is not made of these cells but of collagenous fibrous matrix, as in neurofibroma.

The patient may be of any age, and the presenting feature is an abdominal lump. The tumour is incapable of producing any hormone.

Removal of the tumour usually brings a cure.

THE ADRENAL CORTEX

Embryology.—Unlike the medulla, which is of ectodermal origin, the cortex of the adrenal is mesodermal in origin. It arises in a ridge, which appears just by the side of the mesonephros (Wolffian body).

Structure.—The adrenal cortex is composed of large polyhedral cells, rich in lipoids, and the cells are arranged in three different layers, which from outside inwards, are named:

1. Zona glomerulosa.
2. Zona fasciculata.
3. Zona reticularis.

Adrenal Cortical Hormones.—The hormones of the adrenal cortex are all esters of cholesterol; the polycyclic nucleus of cholesterol is modified by the addition of O_2, OH, or other complex groups, by the action of different enzymes. More than fifty such compounds have been isolated. The more important of these are divided into three groups:

1. Glucocorticoids.
2. Mineralocorticoids or salt-regulating hormones.
3. Sex hormones.

GLUCOCORTICOIDS.—These hormones are so named because they favour neoglucogenesis. They are concerned in the metabolism of protein and carbohydrate, favouring formation of glucose from non-carbohydrate sources. *Hydrocortisone* (cortisol) is the chief of these hormones. It is so called because it possesses a hydroxyl (OH) group at the 11-position—it thus belongs to the class of 11-oxysteroids. It is essential for life because it has an overall effect on general metabolism and also some effect on water and electrolyte balance. *Cortisone* is a synthetic preparation and is converted into hydrocortisone in the body, exerting same effects.

Hydrocortisone, after metabolism, is excreted in the urine chiefly as 17-hydroxycorticoids.

Hyperplasia or tumours of those cells which produce glucocorticoids, results in what is known as *Cushing's syndrome.* The glucocorticoids are chiefly produced in zona fasciculata and zona reticularis.

MINERALOCORTICOIDS.—These are concerned in the maintenance of water and electrolyte balance. *Aldosterone* is the most important of these hormones. It is also known as 11-desoxycorticoid because it possesses neither an oxygen atom nor a hydroxyl group at the 11-position (c.f. hydrocortisone). The control on water and electrolyte balance is effected mainly by the agency of the cells in the renal tubules. Excess of the hormones causes increased tubular reabsorption of sodium and chloride, which are retained along with water in the blood (oedema, hypertension); there is loss of potassium in the urine resulting in hypopotassaemia. Conversely, a deficiency of the hormones results in loss of sodium in the urine and retention of potassium. The excess loss of sodium causes a fall in the osmotic tension of plasma and extracellular fluid; water now leaks into the cells and a dehydration (extracellular) results.

The synthetic mineralocorticoid is *desoxycorticosterone* (DOCA) and it has the same effects as aldosterone.

Hyperplasia or neoplasm of those cells, which produce aldosterone, results in what is known as *Conn's syndrome (primary aldosteronism).* Aldosterone is produced in the zona glomerulosa.

SEX HORMONES.— Both androgenic and oestrogenic hormones are produced in the adrenal cortex. The sex hormones are known as 17-ketosteroids or 17-oxosteroids because they possess an oxygen atom at the 17-position.

The male (androgenic) hormone is androsterone.

The female (oestrogenic) hormones are oestrone, oestriol, and oestradiol-17β.

Excess of the androgenic hormones may cause virilism in the females. Excess of the oestrogens may (very rarely) cause effeminancy in the males.

Control of Cortical Function.— The adrenal cortex is under control of the anterior pituitary through the agency of ACTH, i.e. adrenocorticotrophic hormone (corticotrophin), which stimulates the adrenal cortex. Conversely hydrocortisone of the adrenal cortex inhibits the secretion of ACTH (feedback mechanism).

Role of Adrenal Cortex in 'Stress'— The adrenal cortex quickly responds to all types of stress (trauma, haemorrhage, burn, acute infection, acute perforations, etc.), and this is well-demonstrated by the microscopical appearance of the gland. The cells of the adrenal cortex are normally laden with lipid materials, which represent the storehouse of the hormones of the gland. Under conditions of stress, there is a depletion of this lipid storage (as the hormones are discharged into circulation). Thereafter, there is a phase of cellular overgrowth, associated with re-accumulation of the lipid materials (suggesting return to normalcy).

Tests for Adrenal Cortical Function

A. By measuring the blood level of the hormones directly:
1. Plasma cortisol (hydrocortisone) level.—Normally 8 to 28 micrograms per 100 ml.
2. Other cortical hormones.—Using radio-activation techniques, it is now possible to estimate the levels of the other cortical hormones individually.

B. By measuring the urinary output (24 hours) of the metabolites of individual cortical hormones or of the hormones themselves:
1. 17-hydroxycorticoid (for hydrocortisone).
2. 17-oxosteroid, i.e. 17-ketosteroid (for androgens and oestrogens).
3. Aldosterone itself.
4. The three oestrogens themselves.
   (1 and 2 are usually measured for testing cortical function).

C. Similar estimations made after stimulating the adrenal cortex by administering ACTH (ACTH stimulation tests):
These are done with the idea that patients with adrenal hyperplasia respond much more than persons with normal cortical function.

The urinary output of the 17-hydroxycorticoid and 17-ketosteroid in 24 hours are measured first. Thereafter, the cortex is stimulated by ACTH gel (40 units given intramuscularly twice, in a span of 24 hours). The urinary output of the two metabolites are measured in the urine of the next 24 hours.

D. Similar estimations made after suppressing the adrenals by inhibiting ACTH.

ACTH suppression is usually done by injecting hydrocortisone or, more commonly, dexamethasone (which suppresses the pituitary by the same feedback mechanism as hydrocortisone). The urinary excretion of 17-hydroxy corticoid and 17-ketosteroid in 24 hours prior and after the injection is measured. It is found that there is a far more severe depression in the excretion of the metabolites in patients with adrenal hyperplasia than in normal subjects. Curiously, however, in patients of adrenal tumours with overactivity, this depression is not noticed. This is explained by the fact that the secretion of the cortical hormones from adrenal tumours is autonomous, i.e. not under control of ACTH. Thus the ACTH suppression test is valuable not only in diagnosing cortical overactivity but also making a differential diagnosis between adrenal hyperplasia and neoplasm.

Therapeutic Uses of Hydrocortisone (and Cortisone)

1. In Endocrine (adrenocortical) Deficiency:
   a. After bilateral adrenalectomy.
   b. Adrenocortical insufficiency, i.e. hypocorticism—acute or chronic (Addison's disease).

2. In Non-endocrine Conditions:
   1. Allergic conditions.
   2. Blood dyscrasias.
   3. Collagenoses.
   4. Granulomatous disorders.
   5. Rheumatoid arthritis.
   6. Different skin and eye conditions, acting as an anti-allergic agent (applied locally).

CUSHING'S SYNDROME

This is the commonest form of hypercriticism and is due to an excessive production of the glucocorticoids, chiefly hydrocortisone. It occurs in the adults and is, therefore, also known as postpubertal or adult hypercriticisms.

The other types of hypercorticism are:
1. Infantile.
2. Pre-pubertal.
3. Post-menopausal.

Pathology.—The excessive production of the hydrocortisone (cortisol) may be brought about by one of the following conditions:

A. Bilateral Adrenal Hyperplasia (60 per cent):
   1. Primary or idiopathic.
   2. Secondary, i.e. due to stimulation by excess of ACTH from:
      a. Basophil adenoma or invasive carcinoma of the anterior pituitary.
      b. Ulcerogenic islet-cell tumour of the pancreas, producing ACTH (rare).
      c. Bronchial carcinoma (rare).
B. Adrenal Tumours (35 per cent):
   1. Benign (adenoma).
   2. Malignant (carcinoma).
C. No Structural Alteration in the Adrenal Cortex (5 per cent):
   In some of these cases there may be a tumour of the thymus or of the pineal glands (located between the posterior parts of the thalamus of the two sides).
D. Drug-induced:
   Cushing's syndrome is seen in its most typical form in persons treated with cortisone over long periods for non-endocrine conditions, particularly rheumatoid arthritis.

Clinical Features.—Females suffer more commonly than males (3 : 1). A typical patient is a female between 15 and 30 years of age (excepting the cases where the condition is drug-induced).

The clinical features may be divided into 5 broad groups:
A. Those due to metabolic disorders.
B. Those due to fluid and electrolyte disturbances.
C. Sexual disorders.
D. Mental changes.
E. Other features.

A. THOSE DUE TO METABOLIC DISTURBANCES.—These disturbances are related to fat, protein, sugar, and calcium metabolism:

1. Obesity.—There is excessive deposits of fat over some particular parts, resulting in:
   a. Protuberant abdomen.
   b. Buffalo hump (fatty pads over the scapulae).
   c. Moon face with pursed lips.
   d. Obliteration of supraclavicular fossae.
   e. Increased body weight.

2. Protein breakdown:
   a. Thinning of the arms and legs due to muscle breakdown (the swollen abdomen with the thinned-out legs may be compared to 'a lemon on the match-sticks').
   b. Increasing muscular weakness.

3. Atrophy of the dermis and inhibitory effect on fibrous tissue:
   a. Skin gets inelastic and assumes a tissue-paper consistency; on the abdomen this gives the same pattern as striae gravidarum.
   b. There is a high-coloured complexion due to transparency of the skin.
   c. Purpura and bruising to minimal trauma (due to atrophy of capillary walls).

4. Diabetes, due to increased neoglucogenesis.

5. Negative calcium balance causing gross osteoporosis and, sometimes, pathological fractures (particularly of the vertebrae).

B. THOSE DUE TO FLUID AND ELECTROLYTE IMBALANCE.—These occur because, hydrocortisone has a weak aldosterone effect. There is retention of sodium and water with excessive loss of potassium. This results in:

1. Hypertension, which may lead to cardiac hypertrophy, myocardial ischaemia, cerebrovascular accidents, and congestive heart failure.

2. Hypokalaemic alkalosis.

C. SEXUAL DISORDERS:

1. Common types:
   a. Sterility and impotency in the males.
   b. Sterility and menstrual disorders in the females (oligomenorrhoea, amenorrhoea, or menorrhagia).

2. Uncommon types, i.e. *Adreno-genital Syndrome:*
   These are the cases where the sexual disorders are more predominant than the metabolic disorders:
   a. Most commonly it occurs in females due to excessive secretion of androsterone. The condition usually starts at about the age of 20. There is oligomenorrhoea, atrophy of the breasts, enlargement of the clitoris, deepening of the voice, and a change of body structure to a manly build.
   b. Very rarely it may occur in young males due to excessive secretion of oestrogens. There is gynaecomastia, atrophy of the testes, change in voice, etc.

D. MENTAL CHANGES.—Various types of psychosis may set in (more than half of the cases).

E. OTHER FEATURES
1. Increased growth of lanugo hairs, sometimes frank hirsutism.
2. Acne and skin infections (due to suppressed inflammatory reaction).
3. Recurrent intercurrent infections (due to same reason).
4. Excessive pigmentation of the skin (this is not due to excess of hydrocortisone but because of increased ACTH).

Special Investigations

1. *Blood Count.*—Polycythaemia and leucocytosis (with lymphopenia and eosinopaenia).
2. *Urine Examination:*
   a. Glycosuria.
   b. Hypercalciuria.
3. *Blood Biochemistry:*
   a. Hyperglycaemia.
   b. Hypercholesterolaemia.
4. *BMR—Low.*
5. *X-ray:*
   a. Skeleton.—There may be gross osteoporosis, particularly in the vertebrae and pelvis.
   b. Pituitary fossa (sella turcica).—An enlargement may sometimes be seen if the condition is due to a pituitary tumour.
   c. Lungs.—Rarely presence of a bronchial carcinoma.
   d. Kidneys.—Rarely presence of stones or nephrocalcinosis.
   e. X-rays to demonstrate adrenal tumours (*see* under phaeochromocytoma).
6. *Hormone Assays:*
   a. Estimation of plasma cortisol level.
   b. Estimation of urinary 17-hydroxycorticoid and 17-ketosteroid.
   c. ACTH stimulation test.
   d. ACTH suppression test.
   (*see* tests for adrenal cortical function).

Treatment

1. *When the pathology is primarily in the adrenal:*
   a. In cases of adrenal hyperplasia (which is bilateral).—Total adrenalectomy on one side and resection of seven-eighth of the adrenal gland on the other side.
   b. In cases of adrenal neoplasm (adenoma or carcinoma).—Excision of the adrenal gland that contains the tumour.
   If the diagnosis is a tumour and the side is ascertained, an extraperitoneal approach by the lumbar route (as for the kidney) is done; the twelfth rib (sometimes also the eleventh) is excised to expose the adrenal. In other cases, a transperitoneal approach has to be made, so that both the adrenals can be examined.
2. *When the adrenal condition is secondary to a pituitary tumour:* Two forms of treatment are available:
   a. Surgical removal of the pituitary (hypophysectomy).

b. Radiation-ablation of the pituitary by implanting Yttrium-90 pellets into the gland.

Cortisone Replacement in Adrenalectomy.—The daily output of hydrocortisone from the adrenals, in a normal subject, is about 25 mg. After bilateral adrenalectomy, this amount has to be supplied from outside, throughout the lifetime of the patient. Following subtotal adrenalectomy, however, the remnant of the adrenal tissue gradually picks up function and the external supply may be withdrawn after sometime. Similarly, even after bilateral adrenalectomy, the adrenal cortical rests in the body may be geared into action in some cases and the external supply may be discontinued.

Again, the stress of the operation and anaesthesia, for adrenalectomy, requires a high supplement during and after the operation. It is desirable that the higher supplement is instituted from one or two days prior to the date of operation. The following is a tentative routine of cortisone replacement in cases of adrenalectomy:

A. *Before Operation:*
   For 1 or 2 days.—Cortisone acetate, intramuscularly, 100 mg daily.

B. *On the Day of Operation:*
   1. 1 to 2 hours before operation.—Cortisone acetate, intramuscularly, 100 mg.
   2. During operation.—Hydrocortisone hemisuccinate, 100 mg in the intravenous drip. Alternatively, the hydrocortisone is pushed directly intravenous just after extirpation of the adrenals.
   3. After operation.—Cortisone acetate, intramuscularly, every 6 hours.

C. *Until 5th Post-operative Day:*
   Cortisone acetate, 100 mg, intramuscularly or orally, according to the patient's condition.

D. *After 5th Day:*
   Cortisone acetate is given, but the dose is gradually reduced to 25 to 50 mg in cases of total adrenalectomy, and to nil in subtotal adrenalectomy (the remaining adrenal tissue picks up function).

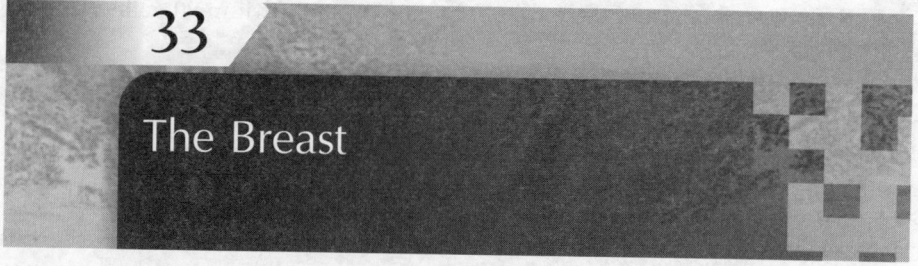

33

The Breast

Embryology.—The glandular element of the breast is derived from the surface ectoderm and is actually a collection of highly modified sebaceous glands. The connective tissue element of the breast, i.e. fat and fibrous tissue, develops from mesoderm.

Towards the end of the second month of the intrauterine life, an ectodermal thickening appears on each side of the embryo, along a line, which extends obliquely from the axilla to the corresponding groin. This ectodermal proliferation is known as the *milk ridge* or *milk line*. In both the sexes, the major length of this line quickly disappears, leaving behind only that part which overlies the pectoral region. Persistence of the milk ridge at other sites, along its length, results in supernumerary breasts or nipples.

In the fourth month of the foetal life, this pectoral plaque of ectodermal proliferation grows towards the depth, into the underlying mesoderm, in the form of 15 to 20 solid pencils. These are the precursors of the main lactiferous ducts. The growing end of each pencil divides and subdivides to form the precursors of the ductules and the acini.

Towards the end of the foetal life, the ectodermal plaque over the pectoral region breaks down on its surface and forms what is known as the *mammary pit*. The process of breakdown is also continued into the depth, and the hitherto solid lactiferous ducts, ductules, and acini are canalised. The mesoderm, into which the ectodermal infiltration occurs, develops into the connective tissue of the breast. Just before birth, a process of differential growth occurs in the region of the mammary pit, and what actually was a pit is converted into an elevation, forming the nipple. Failure of this differential growth to occur results in an *inverted* or *crater nipple*.

In the males and also in the females up to puberty, the gland does not develop appreciably. In the females, at puberty, there is proliferation of the epithelial element to some extent and the connective tissue (fat) to a great extent. Thus the breast takes its typical feminine appearance.

Surgical Anatomy.—The base of the breast extends from the second rib to the sixth costal cartilage, and from the lateral border of the sternum to the anterior axillary fold. Actually, in addition to this, a thinned out breast tissue spreads all round from this boundary to extend to the clavicle above, eighth costal cartilage below, midline medially, and posterior axillary fold laterally (hence, in radical mastectomy, the subcutaneous tissue over this wide part is excised). From the superolateral part of the breast, the *axillary tail (of Spence)* extends upwards and laterally towards the axilla, under cover of the pectoralis major and closely applied to the pectoral group of lymph nodes there. The breast is, therefore, superimposed on:

a. The pectoralis major with its fascia.—Two-thirds of the breast lies on this muscle. Deep to this muscle is the pectoralis minor with its fascia, and the clavipectoral fascia.
b. The serratus anterior.—The lower lateral third of the breast lies on this muscle.
c. The upper fourth of the anterior rectus sheath.—The inner lowermost part of the breast lies on it.
d. The external intercostal muscles, which lie under cover of (a).

In addition, the lymph vessels draining the breast are closely applied to:

e. The subscapularis muscle.
f. The latissimus dorsi muscle.

This is the reason why the pectoralis major (excepting its clavicular head) and pectoralis minor, together with their covering fasciae, as well as the fasciae covering, and some superficial fibres of the other muscles, mentioned above, are included in the resection of radical mastectomy.

The shape of the breast is given by the fat in which the breast tissue is accommodated.

The support to the breast is provided by the multiple *ligaments of Cooper.* These are hollow cones, made of fibrous tissue. The base of the cones is attached to the underlying deep fascia and the apex to the overlying skin of the breast. As they run through the breast substance, the hollow in the cones is filled up by breast tissue.

Each breast drains by 15 to 20 main lactiferous ducts, which open at the summit of the nipple. To each lactiferous duct is attached, and drains into it, a lobe of the breast. Each lobe consists of hundreds of lobules. The unit structure of the breast is a lobule, which consists of a ductule and an acinus. Both of these are lined by a single layer of epithelium, lined by a basement membrane. The fibrous tissue in the breast consists of two distinct components. There is a layer of fibrous tissue immediately outside the acini and ductules, and limited within the elastic lamina that wraps the ductules. This is known as the *periductal* and *periacinar fibrous tissue.* This fibrous tissue undergoes the same types of hyperplasia and involution as does the glandular element of the breast, during the whole lifetime of a female. The other component of the fibrous tissue, lying outside the internal elastic lamina, possesses no such character.

Lymphatic Drainage of the Breast.—This has to be considered under three headings:
 I. The lymph nodes concerned in the drainage.
 II. The lymph vessels and their course.
 III. The special points of importance in the lymphatic drainage, particularly in relation to spread of breast cancers.

I. The Lymph Nodes.—There are three sets of nodes into which the breast drains:
A. The Axillary Nodes.
B. The Internal Mammary Nodes.
C. The Supraclavicular Nodes.
A. THE AXILLARY NODES.—There are five groups of nodes:
 1. *Anterior* or *Pectoral Group.*—Located behind the pectoralis muscles, in close relation to the axillary tail of Spence.

2. *Posterior* or *Subscapular Group.*—Lying in front of the subscapularis muscle.

3. *Lateral* or *Humeral Group.*—Lying on the axillary vessels.

4. *Central Group.*—Located at the base of the axilla, just under cover of the axillary fascia.

5. *Apical Group.*—*Lying* at the apex of the axilla, just below the clavicle (infraclavicular group).

(The axilla is a pyramidal space and the nodes are located on the three walls, the base, and the apex of the pyramid.)

Of the above groups of nodes, the anterior, posterior, central, and apical groups are concerned in the lymphatic drainage of the breast. The apical and the central groups of nodes receive the lymphatics either directly or via the anterior and posterior nodes.

In addition, the following nodes, located in the vicinity of the axilla, also drain the breast tissue:

a. A few nodes along the upper part of the cephalic vein, in the delto-pectoral groove.

b. A few nodes lying between the pectoralis major and the pectoralis minor (*Rotter's nodes*).

The efferent lymphatics from the axillary nodes drain into the supra clavicular nodes.

B. THE INTERNAL MAMMARY NODES.—These nodes are situated in the anterior mediastinum, on the internal mammary vessels, closely applied to the parietal pleura. Usually they lie between the second, third, fourth, and fifth costal cartilages and the intervening intercostal vessels.

C. THE SUPRACLAVICULAR NODES.—These are located in the supraclavicular fossa. There are three groups—medial, intermediate, and lateral.

II. The Lymph Vessels.—The lymph vessels draining the breast may be divided into two broad groups:

A. Those draining the skin overlying the breast, excluding the areola and the nipple.

B. Those draining the breast parenchyma, together with the areola and the nipple.

A. LYMPHATICS OF THE SKIN.—These lymphatics run radially and, therefore:

1. Those from the lateral part drain into the axillary nodes.

2. Those from the upper part drain into the supraclavicular nodes.

3. Those from the medial side drain into the internal mammary nodes and also communicate with the lymphatics of the opposite breast, across the midline.

B. LYMPHATICS FROM THE PARENCHYMA

1. The lymphatics from the superficial part of the parenchyma, together with those draining the areola and nipple (and these constitute about 75 per cent of the lymphatics), run along the substance of the axillary tail of Spence to enter the axilla and drain into the axillary nodes.

2. The lymphatics from the deeper part of the parenchyma pierce the underlying muscles:

a. On the lateral side they pierce the pectoral muscles, to drain into the axillary nodes.

b. On the medial side they pierce the pectorals and the intercostal muscles, to drain into the internal mammary nodes.

c. On the lower inner side they pierce the rectus sheath, to reach the extraperitoneal space. Here they may have free communications with the subperitoneal plexus of lymphatics. Cancer cells entering these lymphatics may, therefore, pass into the subperitoneal plexus. A secondary growth in this plexus may erupt on the inner surface of the peritoneum and this may be a route of peritoneal dissemination.

III. The Special Points of Importance

1. Though, for the purpose of description, a segmental lymphatic drainage of the breast has been described above; lymphatics from any part of the breast may drain into any set of nodes. Any group of nodes may, therefore, be involved from cancers in any quadrant of the breast.

2. There is a free communication between the lymphatics of the two breasts, so carcinoma from one breast may spread to the other.

3. In older days, it was believed that all the lymphatics of the breast primarily drain into the *subareolar plexus of Sappey* (a collection of large lymph vessels located under the areola) and many of them would have communications with the *deep fascia plexus* (a network of lymph vessels on the deep fascia under the breast). This idea has now been abandoned. Though such plexuses do exist, it is not .necessarily that all the lymph should primarily drain into them.

4. The supraclavicular nodes may be involved in breast cancers by different ways:

a. By efferents from the axillary nodes (which occurs late).

b. Directly, by lymphatics from the skin overlying the upper part of breast (which may occur early).

CONGENITAL ANOMALIES OF THE BREAST

1. **Amazia.**—Congenital absence of one or (rarely) both breasts. The condition is commoner in males.

2. **Polymazia.**—Accessory breasts may be present anywhere along the line of the milk ridge, the commonest site being the axilla. They may produce milk. *Treatment* consists in excision of the accessory breast.

3. **Athelia.**—Congenital absence of the nipple.

4. **Polythelia.**—Accessory nipples.

5. **Congenitally Retracted Nipple** *(Crater nipple).*—*See* embryology.

BREAST ABSCESS

Classification

A. Breast abscesses, according to their clinical behaviour, may be:

1. Acute.

2. Subacute.

3. Chronic.

B. Breast abscesses, according to their position, may be:

1. Premammary (including subareolar).

2. Intramammary.

3. Retromammary.

Of all the types, acute intramammary abscess is much the commoner and about 85 per cent of breast abscesses belong to this category.

Intramammary Abscess

About 85 per cent of breast abscesses, if not more, are located within the breast tissue, i.e. they are intramammary.

Etiology.—In more than 90 per cent cases, the disease occurs in a lactating breast. However, it may occur in non-lactating breasts and even in the breast of nulliparous women. Most commonly it occurs during the *first lactation*.

The infecting organism is usually Staphylococcus (often penicillin-resistant), which enters the breast from the infant's throat, either along a milk duct or through a crack in the nipple. The organism enters the infant's throat from the hospital wards, so breast abscess may sometimes be *endemic*.

The abscess occurs frequently during the first month of lactation. Another common period of occurrence is when the child is more than six months old and is developing teeth. The teeth cause trauma to the nipple and make the portal of entry for the organisms.

Formation of an abscess is favoured by milk stagnation and, therefore, it is more likely to occur in women having difficult suckling (e.g. retracted nipple). This is because the stagnated milk is a good nidus for bacterial growth. Also, Staphylococci cause milk coagulation and this may cause obstruction to the flow of milk.

Pathology and Clinical Features

1. STAGE OF CELLULITIS.—The whole of the breast is swollen, congested, and painful. There are associated constitutional symptoms, including fever. This stage is more prominent in a lactating breast.
2. STAGE OF LOCALISATION AND ABSCESS FORMATION.—The inflammation now localises to one part of the breast. However, the Staphylococcal necrotoxin causes much tissue-sloughing, so that the abscess quickly spreads to the adjacent lobes. Commonly, therefore, a *multilocular* abscess cavity is formed, traversed by fibrous bands. Left untreated, the abscess may destroy a wide part of the breast. Since the abscess is located inside the breast tissue, fluctuation is late to appear (and should not be waited for before incision is made). However, the overlying skin shows an oedema, and an area of tense induration may be made out in the breast, after the breast has been evacuated of milk. These two clinical points indicate that localisation has occurred. In general, localisation usually occurs by 48 hours.

Treatment

A. STAGE OF CELLULITIS.—The treatment is strictly conservative, and consists of:
   1. Good support to the breast.
   2. Antibiotics.—The organism is usually a penicillin-resistant staphylococcus, and erythromycin works well.
   3. Examination of the urine for sugar.
B. STAGE OF LOCALISATION.—Immediate incision has to be made, notwithstanding whether fluctuation is present (see clinical features). The incision should be made *under general anaesthesia* because:

a. The abscess is very painful.

b. Considerable manipulation has to be made during drainage:

One of the following *incisions may* be employed:

i. *Radial Incision.*—This avoids injury to the main milk ducts. It may, however, leave an ugly scar.

ii. *Para-areolar Incision.*—This is a cosmetic incision as the scar merges with the coloured areola. It is made along the cutaneoareolar margin, over the abscess; keeping parallel to the areolar margin. Its disadvantage is that it may cause injury to a main milk duct (Fig. 33.1).

As the pus comes out, a finger is put into the abscess cavity and all fibrous strands are broken, to make the multilocular cavity into one.

For better drainage, *a counter incision* should always be made at the most dependent part of the breast.

The cavity is *tightly* packed with roller gauge. This is essential to control haemorrhage that may be considerable because a lactating breast is highly vascular. A tight bandage is also applied.

Postoperative Management

1. Antibiotics should be continued as long as there is evidence of pus formation. A sensitivity test of the organism should preferably be done.
2. Regular change of dressings. From the first postoperative dressing, onwards, the cavity should be packed only *lightly,* since continued tight plugging may make the abscess chronic.
3. Suckling:
   a. The infant is allowed to suck the opposite breast:
   b. The milk from the affected breast is pumped either with a breast pump or manually, boiled for five minutes, and then given to the'infant.
   c. Weaning, i.e. stopping milk formation, is usually unnecessary. It has however to be done if:
      i. The abscess fails to heal, or there is formation of a milk fistula due to injury to a main milk duct.
      ii. Expression of the milk is very painful for the mother.
      iii. The child has been breastfed too long.
   Stilboestrol tablets, 10 mg thrice daily, usually serve the purpose.

Premammary and Subareolar Abscesses

These abscesses are located in front of the breast tissue. They may be due to:
1. Furuncle in the skin overlying the breast.
2. Inflammation of *glands of Montgomery* (these are sebaceous glands located in the areolar skin).

Being close to the surface, the abscess quickly points. Constitutional symptoms are also minimum. There is a little or no damage to the breast tissue itself.

Incision is easy and cures the condition.

Retromammary Abscess

These abscesses have usually no relation with the breast proper and are located in the tissue planes behind the breast. Occasionally, however, an abscess may be collar stud, with a small pocket in the breast substance and a large pocket in the retromammary tissues.

Causes

1. Infected haematoma in the pectoral muscles.
2. Cold abscess from:
   a. Caries spine.
   b. Tubercular rib (rare).
3. Osteomyelitic abscess from rib.
4. Empyema *necessitatis* (the abscess shows an expansile impulse on coughing).

Treatment.—This depends on the cause. When an incision is necessary, it is best done with a *Galliard Thomas' (submammary) incision.* The incision is made in the submammary sulcus, between the chest wall and the overhanging inferolateral quadrant of the breast (Fig. 33.1). Thus there is a direct approach behind the breast and the scar is cosmetic, hidden by the breast itself.

Chronic Breast Abscess

This usually results from faulty management of an acute intramammary abscess, e.g.

1. Administering antibiotics without incising the abscess. The abscess wall becomes fibrous (lined inside by granulation tissue), and the pus within turns sterile. This condition is popularly known as *antibioma.*
2. Undue delay in draining the abscess.
3. Continuing tight packing of the abscess cavity for a long period after incision.

The first type may sometimes be mistaken for a carcinoma because of its consistency and because the overlying skin is attached to it and often shows a peau d'orange appearance.

Treatment

1. Excision of the abscess cavity is the best treatment.
2. Alternatively, incision with curettage of the wall, to remove all fibrous and granulation tissues on the wall, may be done.
3. Sometimes a simple mastectomy has to be performed (if the diagnosis is doubtful or if the abscess occupies almost the whole of the breast).

FIBROADENOSIS

Synonyms

1. Cystic lobular hyperplasia.
2. Fibrocystic dysplasia of the breast.
3. Chronic mastitis.
4. Cystic mastitis.
5. Involution disease of the breast.

This multiplicity of nomenclature points to the complicated morphology, obscure etiology, and varying pathology of the disease.

Pathology.—The disease occurs in *two distinct forms,* in two different age groups:

1. In the commoner type, occurring in young women, the condition is usually bilateral, and there are multiple ill-defined lumps. The lumps have no capsule and are white in colour (cf carcinoma, which has a greyish colour). A lump can be easily cut (cf the gritting sensation while cutting through a carcinoma), and the cut surface keeps flat (cf the concavity assumed by the cut surface of a carcinoma).

2. In the less common type, occurring in older women nearing menopause, the condition is usually unilateral, and also affects only one segment of the breast. In this group, it is usually one lobe of the breast that is affected and its whole duct system—from the nipple to the periphery—undergoes dilatation, forming one or more cysts. In older days, the condition of multiple cysts was known as *'fibrocystic disease'*. Sometimes there may be a solitary big cyst—the *'blue-domed cyst of Bloodgood'*.

Microscopic Appearance.—Microscopically, the following features are noticed:

1. EPITHELIAL PROLIFERATION.—The lobular epithelium (i.e. epithelium lining the ductules and acini) shows evidence of varying degrees of hyperplasia (hence called 'lobular hyperplasia'). The hyperplasia may be of two types:

   a. *Adenosis.*—The number of lobules over the affected part of the breast increases considerably. Thus the proliferation conforms to the physiological pattern, comparable to that seen in pregnancy.

   b. *Epitheliosis.*—The epithelial cells, lining the lobules, show proliferation, and the proliferating cells encroach into the glandular lumen. This may either be in the form of simple overgrowth of the epithelial lining or there may be papillary projections into the ductules and acini.

      Adenosis and epitheliosis may occur separately or they may be found in the same breast. The unit of proliferation in adenosis is the lobule itself, while that in epitheliosis is the epithelial cell lining the lobule. Since adenosis conforms to a physiological pattern of proliferation, it never leads to carcinoma, while epitheliosis, being an atypical proliferation, may be regarded as precancerous, at least in some percentage of cases.

2. FIBROUS TISSUE HYPERPLASIA.—The periductal and periacinar fibrous tissue, lying just outside the basement membrane of the lobules, also shows different degrees of proliferation.

3. CYST FORMATION.—These cysts represent the dilated duct system, mainly the ductules. The cause of the dilatation may be:

   a. Failure of involution to occur in a ductule that had dilated during the phase of hyperplasia.

   b. Obstruction in the distal part of the duct system due to epithelial proliferation.

      This cyst formation, as has been described above, is more marked in the elderly subjects.

4. LYMPHOCYTIC INFILTRATION (sometimes plasma cells as well) is a common accompaniment, and it was for this finding that the condition was believed to be a chronic inflammation and termed 'chronic mastitis' in the past.

5. APOCRINE EPITHELIUM (found in the axilla) may replace the breast epithelium in some places.

Clinical Features

1. The patient is either a young lady or an elderly nearing menopause. The disease is commoner in those breasts which had been denied their usual function, i.e. nulliparous women and women who did not suckle their children.
2. The younger patients usually complain of multiple swellings in both breasts. The lumps in one or both the breasts usually become painful and extremely tender (and sometimes enlarge) just before menstruation. The elderly patients usually present with solitary lump in one breast, which is symptomless.
3. On examination, the lumps, as presented by the younger group, are multiple and ill defined. They may be made out when examined between the fingers and the thumb, but not when palpated by the flat of the palm against the chest wall. The lump, in case of the elderly patients, is usually well-felt but never so easily as a fibroadenoma or a carcinoma. In any case, the lumps are adherent neither to the skin nor to the pectorals.
4. There is no retraction of the nipple but there may be a serous or dark-green *discharge* from the nipple.

Etiology.—The etiology of the disease is disputed. One point is, however, certain that the process is not an inflammatory one. The term 'chronic mastitis' is a misnomer and the lymphocytic infiltration, found under the microscope, is a reactive phenomenon. It is also argued that all the cases are not due to the same cause. Thus:

1. The nodular breast in the younger women is a form of dysplasia, resulting from an endocrine imbalance (possibly due to an excess of oestrogen). This means that there is an aberration in the hyperplasia-involution cycle of the breast. That the nodules become enlarged and painful during the premenstrual period, and that many of the sufferers also complain of menstrual irregularities, strongly support this view.
2. The lobar type that occurs in the elderly group is possibly more related to defective drainage. According to many pathologists, the primary factor in these cases is fibrosis around a main duct that causes partial obstruction to the duct with some dilatation. The associated retention of secretions causes irritation of the lining epithelium of the whole ductular and acinar tree attached to the duct, and leads to epithelial hyperplasia The proliferated epithelium causes further obstruction and the dilatation progresses to cyst formation. A vicious cycle is thus established and the pathology progresses.

Relationship to Cancer

1. Adenosis never leads to cancer; epitheliosis, however, may progress to a cancer, though possibly only in a small percentage of cases.
2. The nodular breast of the younger women usually shows adenosis, and at least in some cases a fibroadenoma results. The lobar type of the elderly women often shows epitheliosis but only a few of these lead to carcinoma.

Treatment

A. CONSERVATIVE TREATMENT.—Ideally, the management of the patient is on conservative lines and consists of the following:
   1. Reassurance to the patient that the condition is not a cancer and is not likely to lead to a cancer.

2. Good support to the breast—this minimises pain.
3. Systemic injections of non-specific proteins, e.g. milk with iodine.
4. Correction of menstrual disorders.

B. OPERATIVE TREATMENT.—Surgery is indicated only in a few cases:
 1. If there is real doubt whether the lump is a cancer.
 2. If the patient cannot tolerate the pain.
 3. If the patient cannot be reassured and suffers from persistent anxiety.
 4. If the condition turns into a very well-localised solitary lump. This means
    that the pathology has turned into either a fibroadenoma (in the young) or a
    solitary cyst (in the elderly).

The type of surgery, in all these cases, is excision followed by biopsy. Facility of freeze-section is of immense help.

Flowchart 33.1: Tumours of the breast

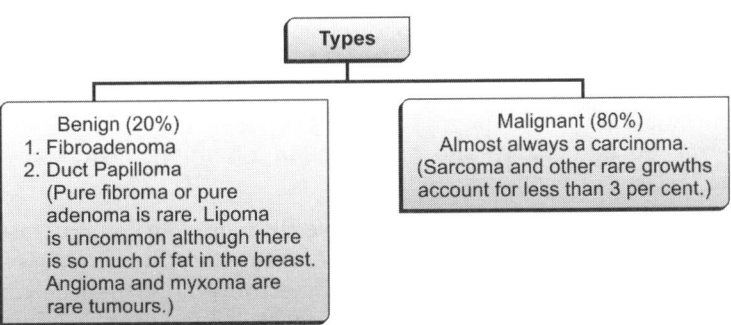

FIBROADENOMA

Pathology.—It has been stated earlier that the fibrous tissue of the breast possesses the character of undergoing hyperplasia and involution as does the glandular element. It is possibly for this reason that pure adenoma or pure fibroma is rare in the breast and fibroadenoma is of common occurrence.

It has been seen that the fibrous tissue of the breast has two distinct components, separated by the elastic lamina that wraps the ductules. Depending on which of these two components shares in the proliferative process, with the glandular element, two types of fibroadenoma may be found:

1. *Pericanalicular Fibroadenoma.*—The fibrous tissue, outside the elastic lamina, undergoes proliferation.
2. *Intracanalicular Fibroadenoma.*—The fibrous tissue, lying within the elastic lamina (i.e. the periductal and periacinar fibrous tissue), undergoes proliferation. This hyperplastic fibrous tissue projects into the lumen of the ductules, invaginating the overlying epithelium, hence the tumour is called 'intracanalicular'.

Macroscopically, both varieties present as solid, white, usually solitary tumours that are characteristically well-localised and well-encapsulated. When the capsule is incised and opened, the tumour may be enucleated as easily as a 'pea from a pod'.

Both the types are usually of a firm feel, though the intracanalicular type has sometimes a tendency to be a little soft (as the fibrous tissue often becomes delicate and takes a myxomatous appearance). Thus, from the clinical point of view, fibroadenoma may be of two types:

Pericanalicular = Hard fibroadenoma

Interclavicular = Soft fibroadenoma.

The interclavicular type has usually a more rapid rate of growth so that the tumour may occasionally be of massive size *(cystosarcoma phylloides)*. It has also more a tendency to undergo malignancy (carcinoma or, rarely, adenosarcorna).

Clinical Features

1. The patient may be of any age, the hard fibroadenoma usually occurring in the age group of 20 to 30, and the soft usually in that of 30 to 50.
2. The patient characteristically presents with a painless, slowly growing lump in the breast. In some cases of hard fibroadenoma, there is a past history of pain, and this suggests that the fibroadenoma is a sequela to fibroadenosis.
3. Usually there is a solitary lump, but sometimes there may be more than one lump or both the breasts may contain a tumour.
4. Typically, the lump is freely mobile and it moves so freely that it is often termed a 'breast mouse'.
5. There is no skin change and no change in the nipple, neither any discharge from it. The axillary nodes are free.

Treatment.—Excision of the tumour, followed by biopsy. In doubtful cases, facilities of a freeze-section are of immense help; if unfortunately the tumour is found to be a carcinoma, an immediate radical mastectomy may then be undertaken. Enucleation should not be performed as the left-behind capsule is susceptible to form a recurrent tumour and that may prove malignant.

One of the following incisions may be used for the purpose of excision (Fig. 33.1):

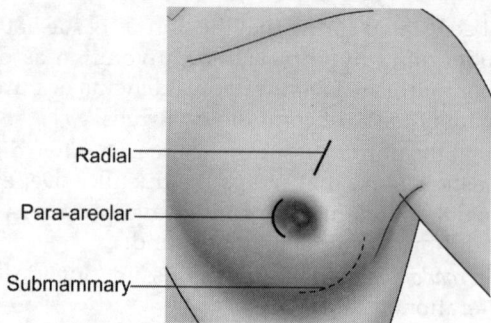

Radial

Para-areolar

Submammary

Fig. 33.1: Incisions on the breast

1. *Para-areolar Incision.*—This is a cosmetic incision as the scar merges with the coloured areolar skin. It is made along the cutaneo-areolar margin. Majority of the tumours may be removed by this incision, as they are highly mobile and can be drawn to the areola.
2. *Galliard Thomas Incision.*—This incision is indicated for tumours located in the lower outer quadrant of the breast. The breast is lifted up and the incision is

placed along the submammary sulcus, between the chest wall and the overhanging inferolateral aspect of the breast. The breast tissue is approached from behind and the tumour is excised. The scar is hidden by the breast itself and thus the incision has a cosmetic value.

3. *Radial Incision.*—This incision is usually not preferred as it leaves behind an ugly scar. However, this has to be made in cases where the tumour is located too far away from the areola and cannot be mobilised towards it, or is too big to be removed by a para-areolar incision.

CYSTOSARCOMA PHYLLOIDES

This is really a massive soft fibroadenoma and is not a malignant condition. In older days, all fleshy tumours were called sarcoma and this tumour looks fleshy on cut section. Due to rapid growth, degeneration and cyst formation are characteristic (*serocystic disease of Brodie*). The cut surface has the appearance of leaves arranged side by side, hence the term 'phylloides' (Greek *phylloid* = leaf-like). Thus the name of the tumour is explained.

However, massive a size the tumour may attain, it shows no evidence of malignancy, e.g.

1. No rapid growth.
2. No pain.
3. No fixity to the skin and no skin changes, as seen in cancer. With big tumours, the skin is stretched, thin, tense and glistening, with prominent veins on it. Ultimately the tumour may fungate through the skin (*cystosarcoma fungoides*).
4. No elevation of the breast, no retraction of the nipple, and no discharge from the nipple.
5. No fixity to deeper structures.
6. No involvement of axillary nodes, neither any distant metastasis.

Treatment.—Simple mastectomy is all that is necessary. Even in the recent past, some surgeons would prefer a radical mastectomy thinking that the tumour is never as benign as it is described to be. In any case, simple excision of the tumour should not be done, even if the tumour is not massive. This is because recurrence is very common in the left-out breast tissue.

DUCT PAPILLOMA

Pathology.—This is a benign tumour, arising from the epithelial lining of one of the *main* lactiferous ducts. The tumour is usually of a small size (3 to 4 mm) but as it projects into the lumen of the duct, the duct is dilated and may even become cystic.

As to the nature of the tumour, there is great diversity of opinion:

a. It is not precancerous.
b. At least some of the tumours are precancerous and may turn into duct carcinoma.
c. It is, by itself, an evidence of malignancy, and should be regarded and treated as such.

Clinical Features

1. The commonest age group is 35 to 50.

2. The commonest and earliest symptom is a discharge from the nipple—most commonly bright red blood, sometimes dark blood-stained fluid, rarely serous fluid (not blood-stained).

3. A rounded mass of any size (sometimes as big as an egg), often cystic in feel, may sometimes be felt close to the nipple. Pressure on the swelling often brings out a discharge on the nipple, from the affected duct.

4. The nipple may be unduly prominent or (rarely) retracted.

Treatment

1. *Microdochectomy.*—The duct, containing the papilloma, together with a little of healthy tissue on all sides, is excised. The affected duct is identified by noticing the discharge. A straight blunted sewing needle is passed into it to act as a probe. The duct, with the probe inside it, is removed as a whole, together with a little healthy tissue around it.

2. *Simple Mastectomy* is advocated by some surgeons.

CARCINOMA OF THE BREAST

Incidence

1. This is the commonest cancer in the females—one female child out of 25 is destined to develop a breast cancer in future.

2. If there is cancer in one breast, the other breast is five times more likely to develop a cancer than a normal breast.

3. Carcinoma may occur in a male breast, but the incidence is less than 1 per cent. However, in the males the prognosis is worse because the tumour, as it occurs in a breast of small dimensions, easily transgresses the limits of the breast tissue and involves the pectorals, chest wall, skin, and lymph nodes.

Etiological Factors

1. The disease is commoner in certain countries (the western countries), and it is presumed that diet and environment have some role to play.

2. Heredity is also believed to play a role—there are evidences of frequency of the cancer in some families.

3. There is definite evidence that suckling reduces the incidence of breast cancer—unmarried and less fertile women develop the cancer more frequently than the multipara.

4. Obstruction to the flow of milk from the breast is believed to be a predisposing factor—women with history of difficult suckling are common sufferers.

5. *Bittner's milk factor*, which is a filterable virus, passing with the milk from the mother to the offspring, definitely makes it susceptible to breast cancer in the mice. Whether such a factor also works in the human beings has not yet been established.

6. Hormonal factors:
   a. In the past, excess of oestrogen was believed to be an important etiological factor. It has since then been established that many of the breast cancers are either oestrogen-stimulated or dual hormone stimulated (i.e. oestrogen and mammotrophin working together), and this is the basis for hormone treatment in advanced breast cancers.

b. It is more or less established that adrenocortical hormones have some role to play in the development of breast cancers as well as in deciding their behaviour and prognosis. There are two hormones of particular importance:
   i. Aetio-cholanolone (an androgen derivative), which is excreted in lower quantities, and
   ii. 17-Hydroxycorticosteroid, which is excreted in higher quantities, in the urine of patients with breast cancer. Also, those women who excrete the latter hormone in higher quantities in the urine are found to be more prone to subsequent development of breast cancers, i.e. they belong to the *'higher risk' group*.
7. Certain existing pathology in the breast may secondarily lead to cancer:
   a. Fibroadenoma, particularly the soft fibroadenoma. When a fibroadenoma turns malignant, it usually develops into a carcinoma and only rarely into an adenosarcoma.
   b. Fibroadenosis.—While adenosis never leads to a cancer, epitheliosis, in certain cases, is believed to be precancerous.
   c. Duct papilloma may change into duct carcinoma.

Types of Breast Carcinoma.—Majority of the breast cancers originate in the cells lining the terminal ductules, presumably because these are the cells on which the hormones, concerned in the normal development of the breast, have their maximum influence. An unqualified term of breast carcinoma, therefore, means a growth originating in the ductules. Far more rarely, cancers originate in the cells lining the acini but the pattern and behaviour of these cancers are the same as those originating in the ductules.

Carcinoma may originate in the main lactiferous ducts and then they are called 'duct carcinoma'. In addition, there is a slow-growing cancer in relation to the nipple and the areola, and this is known as 'Paget's disease'.

Gross variations, however, exist in the histology and behaviour of the cancers arising in the ductules. To start with, the epithelial cells, lining the ductules, proliferate entirely within the lumen of the ductules, limited by the basement membrane of the ductular wall. As long as they remain in this state they are called the 'non-infiltrating cancers'. Sooner or later, they infiltrate outside the basement membrane, into the neighbouring breast tissue, and become 'infiltrating cancers'. On assuming infiltration however, the nature of invasion, the histological picture, and the degree of malignancy show wide variations. Only in some cases the cells still show a glandular arrangement and these growths are termed 'adenocarcinoma'. In the vast majority of cases, the cells, which were originally cylindrical, now assume a spheroidal shape. They no longer show any regular glandular pattern and grow in the form of solid processes, into the surrounding tissues. They are now designated as 'spheroidal-cell carcinoma'. The nature of these spheroidal-cell cancers again vary widely, depending on the functional activity of the affected breast. In an atrophic breast, with scanty blood supply and poor lymphatic drainage, the malignant cells grow slowly but induce an extensive proliferation of fibrous tissue, resulting in what is known as 'schirrhous carcinoma', the commonest cancer of the breast. On the other hand, when a growth occurs in a well-developed breast with abundant blood supply and perfect lymphatic drainage, the malignant cells grow in large solid masses while the fibrous tissue proliferation is much less marked. This is known as the 'encephaloid' or 'medullary' carcinoma. The term 'mastitis carcinomatosa' or 'acute cancer' is applied to a rapidly growing tumour, usually found in pregnancy and lactation. In some cases the growth may show large areas of mucoid degeneration, and then it is known as 'colloid carcinoma'.

Classification.—From what has been detailed above, cancers of the breast may be broadly classified as follows:

I. Cancers arising in the ductules (and acini)

A. Non-infiltrating (2 per cent):
   1. Papillary type, including intracystic papilliferous carcinoma
   2. Comedo type.

B. Infiltrating:
   1. Adenocarcinoma (1 percent)
   2. Scirrhous carcinoma (65 per cent)
   3. Atrophic scirrhous carcinoma (5 per cent)
   4. Medullary or encephaloid carcinoma (15 per cent)
   5. Mastitis carcinomatosa (2 per cent)
   6. Colloid carcinoma (1 per cent)

 II. Cancers arising in a main lactiferous duct
   Duct carcinoma (8 per cent)

III. Cancers closely related to the areola and nipple
   Paget's disease (1 per cent)

Non-infiltrating Carcinoma.—The ductular epithelium has turned malignant. It has proliferated, but entirely within the lumen of the ductules, limited by the basement membrane lining the ductules. This is the *pre-invasive state,* i.e. *carcinoma in situ* or *intraductular carcinoma.* The proliferation of the cells may be of two types:

1. PAPILLARY TYPE.—The cells proliferate into the ductules in finger-like projections. In some cases, the ductules undergo a cystic dilatation and the condition is then known as *intracystic papilliferous carcinoma.*

2. COMEDO TYPE.—The cells proliferate rapidly from all round the circumference of the ductule, and fill up its lumen. The central mass of cells undergoes necrosis, because of lack of blood supply, and turns into a semi-solid mass, which can be ejected out of the ductules like toothpaste, on application of pressure (hence the name *comedo).*

Adenocarcinoma.—In this variety, the tumour is invasive but it still shows a glandular arrangement of its cells. There are tubules lined by several layers of hyperplastic epithelial cells. The tumour is often well-localised and is of low-grade malignancy. It thus offers a good prognosis.

Scirrhous Carcinoma.—This is the *commonest type* of breast cancer. The malignant cells are spheroidal and are arranged in small groups, separated by wide masses of fibrous tissue.

The tumour has a typical hard feel (*skiros* = hard) and, when it is cut through, there is a typical gritty sensation. The cut surface becomes slightly concave because of pull by the preponderent fibrous tissue; it has a typical greyish appearance with white specks in it, comparable to the cut surface of an unripe pear. The tumour is usually of small size but having no capsule, invades the breast in all directions.

As has already been said, this type of tumour occurs in atrophic breasts, where the blood supply is poor and the lymphatic drainage is scanty. The tumour is slow-growing but highly infiltrating.

Atrophic Scirrhous Carcinoma.—This is a variant form of an ordinary scirrhous carcinoma. It occurs in the grossly atrophic breasts of very elderly women. Having all the characters of a scirrhous carcinoma, the tumour histologically shows much more abundance of fibrous tissue with relatively scanty spheroidal cancer-cell masses.

Medullary Carcinoma.—This type is much less common than scirrhous cancers. It usually occurs in well-developed breasts, which possess good blood supply and free lymphatic drainage. The spheroidal cells grow in big solid masses, separated only by small areas of fibrous tissue. The tumour is less hard than the scirrhous type, nevertheless, it is hard in feel. Though it grows rapidly, it has less power of infiltration. On the other hand, it possesses the power of quick lymphatic and venous spread. The cut surface has the appearance of brain tissue, hence the name *encephaloid carcinoma.*

Mastitis Carcinomatosa.—This rare type of cancer, unlike other cancers of the breast, has an acute onset, associated with pain, resembling acute lactational mastitis (hence called *acute lactational cancer)*. It usually occurs during pregnancy and lactation, thus making diagnosis further difficult. A highly malignant type, this tumour grows rapidly to a large size and ends fatally in a few months. The breast is swollen, painful, and hot (because of vascularity). The overlying skin is reddened and oedematous (due to blockage of subdermal lymphatics by the cancer cells), and there are dilated veins on the surface. The axillary nodes are always enlarged. The points of difference from an acute lactational mastitis are:

a. Absence of temperature.

b. Widespread oedema.

c. Absence of leucocytosis.

d. Failure of response to antibiotics.

Colloid Carcinoma.—This results from widespread mucoid (gelatinous) degeneration, usually in a medullary carcinoma. The tumour is bulky and soft. The progress varies from case to case.

Duct Carcinoma.—This occurs in a main lactiferous duct. These cancers may arise *de novo* or by malignant change in a duct papilloma. The lymphatic spread of the cancer is slow, hence the prognosis is a little better. Usually the only complaint .of the patient is painless bleeding (fresh blood) from the nipple and, because of the alarming symptom, the patient often reports early, making another point for better prognosis. In some cases, a small lump may be made out, as in duct papilloma. The condition is often difficult to be diagnosed from a duct papilloma.

Paget's Disease.—This condition starts as a small erosion on the nipple and then the areola. The erosion turns into ulceration. The ulcer slowly progresses peripherally. In about 2 years time (often much later), a tumour appears in the breast tissue proper, usually close to the nipple but sometimes well away from it.

Microscopically, the characteristic features are as follows:

a. Thickening and widening of the epidermal papillae in the dermis, together with thickening of the surface epidermis.

b. Presence of vacuolated cells (called *Paget's cells*) in the depths of the epidermis, especially in the prickle cell layer.

c. Infiltration of the dermis with lymphocytes and plasma cells.

d. Epithelial hyperplasia with dilatation of the ducts in the underlying breast. These proliferative changes are very slow.

It is believed that the lesion starts in the main lactiferous ducts, close to the nipple. The lining epithelial cells proliferate and invade the epidermis, causing the ulcerative lesion. Simultaneously, but much more slowly, they grow intra-ductally, to invade the proximal parts of the duct system and ultimately come out of the duct wall, forming a scirrhous carcinoma.

Spread of Breast Carcinoma

1. INTRA-DUCT SPREAD, occurring along the lumen of the ductules and ducts. The best example of this form of spread is seen in Paget's disease.

2. DIRECT SPREAD.—Most commonly the tumour starts in the upper outer quadrant of the breast, presumably because this is the largest quadrant. It then spreads peripherally, along the breast tissue. Though all breast cancers are notorious for infiltration, the scirrhous and atrophic scirrhous varieties are the worst in this respect. Gradually, the tumour comes out of the breast tissue and infiltrates into the surrounding structures:

   a. Overlying skin. In very advanced stages, the growth may fungate through the skin.

   b. Underlying muscles, usually the pectoralis major and then the pectoralis minor. Growths located laterally may infiltrate into the serratus anterior and those located in the lower inner quadrant into the upper part of the anterior rectus sheath.

   c. The chest wall, i.e. intercostal muscles, ribs and costal cartilages, may be infiltrated in more advanced cases.

   While infiltration occurs through the breast tissue, two components therein deserve special mention:

   i. Infiltration into the ligaments of Cooper causes shortening in the height of these conical ligaments, resulting in dimpling of the skin overlying the tumour. Hence, fixity to the skin may be of early occurrence (the area of skin adherence is, however, limited within the limits of the boundary of the tumour).

   ii. Infiltration into the wall of the main milk ducts causes shortening in their length, resulting in retraction of the nipple (this retraction is of quick onset; hence called *recent retraction,* as opposed to long-standing congenital retraction).

3. LYMPHATIC SPREAD:

   a. The lymphatic drainage of the breast, together with special points of importance in the spread of cancers, has been fully discussed earlier in this chapter.

   b. Lymphatic spread from breast cancers may occur in two ways:

   i. *By embolism.*—Detached cancer cells are swept along the lymph channels.

   ii. *By permeation.*—Solid columns of cancer cells grow along the lumen of the lymph vessels, keeping continuity with the parent tumour. This is corroborated by the fact that groups of radiating nodules may be found on the skin over the breast, around the main tumour mass, with gaps of healthy skin between one group and another.

c. Secondary to the blockage of the lymph nodes by the malignant cells and the lymphatic stasis thereupon, oedema of the skin, overlying the breast, ensues. This oedematous skin has characteristically the appearance of the peel of an orange *(peau d'orange) or pig-skin*. The multiple pin-point depressions (pits) in the oedematous skin represent the sites of attachment of the hair follicles. These hair follicles are more firmly fixed to the subcutaneous tissue than the rest of the skin and, as they maintain their height through the swollen skin, their surface attachments are retracted beneath the level of the surrounding skin, thus causing the pits.

4. VENOUS SPREAD—This may cause metastases to:
   a. Lungs.
   b. Liver (the liver may also be involved via lymphatics piercing the rectus sheath and via the falciform ligament).
   c. Bones.—The bones of the thoracic cage (ribs, sternum, and thoracic vertebrae), the head of the humerus, the bones of the pelvis (pelvic bones and lumbar vertebrae), the head of the femur, and the skull are favourite sites. The lesions are almost always of *osteolytic* nature.
   d. Brain and central nervous system.
   e. Adrenals.

5. TRANSPERITONEAL SPREAD.—Cancer cells may gain entrance into the peritoneal cavity by way of the lymphatics piercing the rectus. These lymphatics, on reaching the extraperitoneal space, communicate with the sub-peritoneal plexus of lymphatics. Cancer cells thus reach the subperitoneal plexus. A secondary growth in the plexus may erupt on the inner surface of peritoneum. Considerable peritoneal dissemination may occur, including Krukenberg's tumour in the ovaries, i.e. secondary deposits on the ovaries.

Clinical Presentation of Breast Cancers.—The incidence is highest between the age of 40 and 50 years, but no age after menarche is immune. The presenting features may be as follows:

1. Typically, the patient presents with a painless lump in the breast, most commonly in the upper outer quadrant. Unless there are other alarming features, the patient seldom reports before 6 months of the onset of the tumour.
2. Pain may sometimes occur and it is always present in the advanced stages.
3. A discharge from the nipple, of varying nature, is sometimes complained of. Discharge of fresh blood is usually the only complaint in case of a duct carcinoma.
4. Recent retraction of the nipple may be complained of by an intelligent patient.
5. Ulceration may sometimes be the first presenting feature and may be due to:
   a. Paget's disease.—The ulceration starts on the nipple and spreads peripherally, often associated with itching.
   b. Fungation in a late case.
6. Sometimes the patient is ignorant about the breast tumour and presents with features due to metastases, e.g.
   a. Axillary or supraclavicular swelling due to metastatic nodes.
   b. Pain chest, cough, haemoptysis, dyspnoea, and fever due to lung metastasis.

c. Jaundice and ascites, caused by liver metastasis.

d. Bone pain, referred pain, and pathological fractures due to bone metastases.

Examination of the Patient

I. Simultaneous inspection of both the breasts, with patient either sitting erect or standing, is essential in order to compare:

1. Size of the two breasts.
2. Level of the two breasts.
3. Level of the two areola and nipples.
4. Axis of the two areola and nipples.

The affected breast shows an enlargement due to the lump. In the commonest scirrhous variety, the affected breast, together with its areola and nipple, is elevated to a higher level and there may be a deviation of the normal axis of the nipple and areola because of pull by the fibrous tissue contained in the tumour.

II. Palpation of the normal breast first.

III. Palpation of the affected breast with a complete examination of the lump:

A. Shape, size, position and extent.

B. Consistency and tenderness.

C. Fixity to the underlying muscles, particularly the pectorals.

D. Fixity to the chest wall.

E. Fixity to the skin, and other skin changes, if any, e.g.:

1. Dimpling of the skin, caused by infiltration of the ligaments of Cooper.
2. Fixity to the skin.—It should be carefully ascertained whether the area of skin fixity extends beyond the periphery of the tumour (this suggests an advanced growth).
3. Peau d'orange appearance.
4. Fungation of the growth through the skin.
5. Multiple skin nodules radiating from the main mass (due to lymphatic permeation).
6. *Cancerous pachydermia.*—This occurs rarely in the advanced stages, due to direct invasion of the skin and the dermal lymphatics by malignant cells. Progressively larger areas of skin, over the thorax, gets infiltrated with scirrhous cancer, so that the chest is enclosed in a semi-rigid case, likened to a coat of armour *(cancer en cuirasse).*

IV. Examination of the nipple for:

a. Retraction.
b. Discharge.
c. Ulceration (Paget's disease).

V. Palpation of the lymph nodes in *both* the axillae.

VI. Palpation of the supraclavicular nodes.

VII. Clinical examination of the chest, for evidence of metastasis.

VIII. Examination of the abdomen for malignant liver and ascites.

IX. Vaginal examination for evidence of pelvic metastasis.

Special Investigations

1. Biopsy in doubtful cases, which approximate to 25 per cent, even with the expert clinicians. Biopsy is not required where the diagnosis is clinically certain. An incisional biopsy (i.e. cutting out a part of the tumour for the purpose of examination) should never be performed as it invariably causes dissemination. The types of biopsy advocated are:

   a. *Aspiration Biopsy.*—This is safest but may provide false negative results if the needle misses the malignant area. Moreover, the amount of material may be so small that a proper histological examination is impossible. *Drill biopsy*, with a wide-bore vibrating needle, overcomes these difficulties to a great extent and is being recently practised.

   b. *Excision Biopsy.*—The whole mass, together with a margin of apparently healthy tissue, is removed. This is done for small and superficial growths.

   c. *Simple Mastectomy.*—This is advocated if the growth is not small enough or superficial enough for an excision.
   If facilities for *freeze-section* are available, the patient is kept prepared for a radical mastectomy while undertaking an excision biopsy or a simple mastectomy. If the report (which is immediately available) is positive, radical mastectomy is performed immediately. If such facilities are not available, radical mastectomy should be undertaken as soon as a positive histological report is received.

2. Discharge from the nipple is subjected to cytology.
3. X-ray of the chest in all cases.
4. X-ray of any suspected bony lesion.
5. In the recent days, various investigations are advised to detect very early lesions, even when there is no palpable lump. These include:

   a. Mammography—Straight X-rays of the breast are taken (two views). A characteristic soft-tissue shadow with calcification suggests malignancy.

   b. Thermography.—Rise of temperature in the breast containing a carcinoma.

   c. Xero-radiography

6. Assay of urinary steroids.—Aetio-cholanolone and 17-hydroxy-corti-costeroids predict the clinical behaviour and overall prognosis of the growth. A low level of the former and a high level of the later (in the urine) indicate a bad prognosis.

Clinical Assessments.—There are two popular methods:

A. CLINICAL STAGING (MANCHESTER).—The patients may be grouped into four stages:

Stage I: The tumour is confined within the limits of the breast tissue (an area of adherence to the skin, limited within the boundaries of the tumour, which is only due to involvement of the ligaments of Cooper, does not affect staging).

Stage II: The tumour is limited within the breast tissue locally but there are significant axillary nodes, the nodes being mobile.

Stage III: The tumour has extended beyond the limits of the breast tissue locally, i.e. either infiltrated into the pectorals or involved wider areas of skin. The axillary nodes may or may not be involved, but if they are involved, they are still mobile.

1. Tumour fungating through the skin.
2. Tumour fixed to the chest wall.
3. Fixed axillary nodes.
4. Significant supraclavicular nodes.
5. Distant metastases.
6. Spread to the opposite breast.

B. TNM CLASSIFICATION.—T denotes the tumour, N the draining (axillary or supraclavicular) nodes, M the distant metastases. Points are attached to each of these, e.g. $T_2N_1M_0$, $T_2N_1M_1$, etc. The total score gives an idea about the extent of the malignant process (*see* Chapter 22).

Operative, Pathological, and Histological Grading.—The clinical staging may prove wrong at operation, e.g. axillary nodes, not detected clinically, may be found enlarged at operation.

The operative findings, again, may prove wrong at the pathological examination, e.g. the removed nodes may not be metastatic.

The histological grading gives a comprehensive idea about the degree of malignancy. In this respect, *Broder's classification* is valuable, the grading depending upon the percentage of undifferentiated cells in the tumour:

Grade I: Up to 25 per cent cells undifferentiated.

Grade II: 25 to 50 per cent cells undifferentiated.

Grade III: 50 to 75 per cent cells undifferentiated.

Grade IV: More than 75 per cent cells undifferentiated.

Outline of Treatment for Breast Cancers.—In general, Stage I and Stage II cases are believed to be curable, and curative surgery, followed by radiotherapy, is the treatment of choice (in selected cases, some surgeons advocate a course of pre-operative radiation as well). Stage III and Stage IV cases are believed to be too advanced for any radical treatment, and different types of palliative treatment are advocated.

It should, however, be noted that there is a big fallacy left in such discrimination, since the all-important internal mammary group of nodes are never taken into account while judging the stage in these cases, simply because these nodes are not available for clinical examination.

However, the above outline has been time-old and is still recognised very widely. For purpose of description here, the Stage I and Stage II cases will be called *early cases* and Stage III and Stage IV *late cases*.

Management of Early Cases.—The usual management is curative surgery, followed by radiotherapy. The area of radiation includes the area of the breast, the axilla, the supraclavicular region, and the internal mammary nodes.

Other adjunctive treatment, sometimes advocated in these cases, includes:

a. Androgen treatment.

b. Oopherectomy.

Their value, as prophylactic measure in the early cases, is greatly debated and is yet to be proved.

A. THE STANDARD SURGERY that is most widely advocated is *radical mastectomy*, which means *en bloc* removal of the following structures:

1. The whole of the breast with the tumour.
2. An elliptical flap of skin, the centre of the ellipse corresponding to the centre of the tumour, but always including the areola and the nipple.
3. The subcutaneous fat, extending above to the clavicle, below to the upper fourth of the rectus sheath, medially to the midline, and laterally to the posterior axillary fold.
4. The pectoralis major with its fascia (the clavicular head of the muscle is spared).
5. The pectoralis minor with its fascia.
6. The clavipectoral fascia.
7. The covering fascia together with some of the superficial fibres of the following muscles, on which the breast and its lymphatics are located:
   a. External intercostal.
   b. Serratus anterior.
   c. Subscapularis.
   d. Latissimus dorsi.
   e. Upper fourth of rectus abdominis.
8. All fat, fasciae, and lymph nodes in the axilla.

The following structures are to be carefully preserved:

i. Nerve to serratus anterior.
ii. Nerve to latissimus dorsi.
iii. Axillary vein.
iv. Cephalic vein.

The veins require to be preserved in order to avoid the occurrence of postoperative oedema of the arm.

The incision on the skin is an elliptical one, as mentioned above; from its upper end it is prolonged along the anterior axillary fold to the upper fourth of the arm, and from its lower end it is prolonged to the upper fourth of the rectus abdominis.

When the wound is closed, the scar mark has a gentle 'S' curve. The skin sutures must be without tension and, if this is not ordinarily possible, release incision should be applied to the flaps. The gaps created at the areas of release should be covered with split-skin graft. This is a better procedure than putting split-skin grafts over the breast-area itself, because this area has to undergo early radiation, and radiation may damage the grafts. In no case, split-skin grafts should be applied over the axilla.

Radiotherapy should be instituted as soon as the wound heals. Therefore, all attempts should be made to see that there is a primary healing of the wound.

B. MORE EXTENSIVE SURGERY

1. Biopsy of the internal mammary node in the second intercostal space is sometimes added to radical mastectomy. This, however, only gives a clue to the prognosis.
2. *Ultra-radical Mastectomy (Urban).*—Block dissection of the internal mammary nodes of the affected side *en masse*, with radical mastectomy, is done. The second, third, and fourth costal cartilages, together with the corresponding

part of the lateral margin of the sternum, are to be excised in order to gain access to the internal mammary nodes. These nodes are removed together with the underlying part of the parietal pleura and the internal mammary vessels, to which they are closely related.

3. *Extended Radical Mastectomy (Dahl-Iverson).*—This is a more radical surgery, in which, in addition to what is done in the ultra-radical mastectomy, the supraclavicular nodes are resected. In order to perform this, the central part of the clavicle has to be excised.

C. LESS RADICAL SURGERY

1. *Simple Mastectomy,* as advocated by Mc. Whirter, followed by radiation of the muscles as well as all sets of nodes (axillary, internal mammary, and supraclavicular), is practised in some centres. The logic put forward by Mc. Whirter in support of this procedure is that, if the internal mammary nodes may be left behind after radical mastectomy (to be treated by radiation), the other nodes and lymphatics may also be left behind and treated as such. The contour of the chest wall is then preserved and a massive excision is avoided. The practical point against Mc. Whirter's view is that, for some obscure reasons, the axillary nodes are not as radiosensitive as the internal mammary nodes.

2. *Modified Radical Mastectomy (Patey).*—In this operation, the pectoralis major is left intact. It is retracted upwards and medially, making the pectoralis minor available for excision. The pectoralis minor is excised from its insertion and this gives access to the axilla for its clearance. The advantages of this operation, over standard radical mastectomy, are:

a. The shape of the chest and the anterior axillary fold is maintained.

b. The pectoralis major offers an ideal bed for split-skin grafts, if these are necessary.

c. The arm is kept stronger.

3. *Segmental Mastectomy.*—This means excision of the tumour with adequate margin of healthy tissue. This is followed by extensive radiation.

Till date, radical mastectomy is the most favourite type of curative surgery.

Management of Advanced Cases.—The aim of treatment is palliation, and the following methods of treatment are used either singly or in different combinations:

A. Surgery.

B. Radiotherapy.

C. Chemotherapy

D. Endocrine Treatment.

A. Surgery.—This may be as follows:

1. For an ugly-looking, foul-smelling, fungated mass, much relief is offered to the patient by performing a simple mastectomy. This is called *toilet mastectomy.*

2. For solitary local recurrence.—Excision may be done.

3. For solitary distant metastasis.—Excision may be performed.

4. For pathological fracture in a metastatic bone.—Internal fixation gives good results.

B. Radiotherapy.—This is possibly the commonest and the best form of palliative treatment.

C. Chemotherapy.—Cytotoxic drugs and antimetabolites; used with precision, may prolong the patient's life and bring her comfort.

D. Endocrine Treatment.—The basis of this form of treatment is that about 50 per cent of the. cases of breast cancer are *hormone dependent.* This means that the progress and spread of these tumours depend on the circulation of certain hormones in the body, to be more specific, the hormones that are concerned in the normal mammogenesis. These hormones are oestrogen (derived from the ovary and the adrenals) and mammotrophin (derived from the anterior pituitary). The remaining tumours are *autonomous,* i.e. independent of any hormone stimulation. The real difficulty is to ascertain whether the cancer is hormone-dependent. Recently methods of searching for oestrogen-receptors in the tumour-cells or of examining the direct effect of the different hormones on the tumour-cell cultures are being tried.

From the point of view of endocrine treatment, the hormone-dependent cases may be divided into two broad groups:

Group I: Patients who have crossed menopause more than 5 years back.

Group II: Patients who are pre-menopausal or who have crossed menopause but less than 5 years back.

Group I Cases: It is found that, in these patients, oestrogen in high dosage causes regression of the tumour or arrests its progress. The reason for this paradox is not known. However, the dose of oestrogen must be high, because small .doses often cause an increase in the rate of growth. Stilboestrol, 25 to 50 mg per day, or (better) ethinyloestradiol, 0.5 mg daily, should be administered.

Group II Cases: The tumours in this group are of two types:

1. Oestrogen-stimulated tumours.—This is the main group.
2. Dual-hormone stimulated tumours.—This is a small group in which the tumour depends on the combination of two hormones, viz. oestrogen and mammotrophin.

ENDOCRINE TREATMENT FOR THE OESTROGEN-STIMULATED TUMOURS.— *Anti-oestrogenic* line of treatment has to be instituted in these cases and this may consist of the following measures:

1. *Androgen Therapy.*—Injections of male hormones, like testosterone, are often effective, but their masculinising side-effects are disturbing. In this respect Durabolin (25 mg intramuscularly bi-weekly) is better. Long-acting androgens of this form, e.g. Decadurabolin, are also popularly used.
2. *Oopherectomy.*—Bilateral oopherectomy removes the main source of oestrogen in the pre-menopausal age. Radiation-ablation of the ovaries is a substitute to this, but is less definite.
3. *Adrenalectomy.*—After oopherectomy, the adrenals are the source of oestrogen. Hence, if the patient is benefited with oopherectomy, bilateral adrenalectomy should be considered.
   As an alternative, long-term cortisone treatment, with a view to depress the adrenals, has not proved to be much effective.
4. *Hypophysectomy.*—After adrenalectomy, the small but multiple adrenal rests in the body are stimulated to growth and they produce oestrogen. As these rests cannot be detected separately and removed, the only way to overcome their activity is to remove the pituitary, i.e. hypophysectomy. As an alternative to hypophysectomy, radiation-ablation of the pituitary, by implanting pellets of Yttrium-90 into the pituitary fossa, by the transnasal route, may be undertaken.

TREATMENT FOR THE DUAL-HORMONE STIMULATED TUMOURS.—Since one of the two hormones is mammotrophin from the anterior pituitary, hypophysectomy or radiation-ablation of the pituitary is the only answer to the problem.

Complications following Radical Mastectomy

A. IMMEDIATE COMPLICATIONS
1. Injury to nerves (nerve to serratus anterior or latissimus dorsi) or veins (cephalic or axillary).
2. Sloughing of skin, which may be due to:
   a. Suturing under tension.
   b. Very thin skin flaps, developing ischaemia.
   c. Tension caused by collections.
   d. Infection, particularly if there are collections.

B. LATE COMPLICATIONS
1. Local recurrence:
   a. Skin nodules,
   b. Cancer-en-cuirasse.
2. Axillary recurrence.
3. Distant metastases, including involvement of opposite breast or axilla.
4. Limitation of shoulder movements (this can always be avoided by proper exercises, started early after the operation).
5. Oedema of the arm.—This may be of two types:
   a. *Pitting Oedema.*—This usually occurs in early postoperative days, rarely late. It is generally caused by inflammation of the lymphatics, i.e. lymphangitis, and tends to pass off with conservative management.
   b. *Solid Oedema* or *Brawny Arm.*—This occurs months or years after the operation and is due to a permanent defective fluid drainage from the limb. It usually occurs if the veins have been blocked either by inflammation or by injury. This is because the other channel of drainage, namely the lymphatics, are always obliterated after gland extirpation. Sometimes, axillary recurrences are the causes of such oedema.

CYSTS IN THE BREAST

Classification

A. CYSTS RELATED TO MAMMARY DYSPLASIA
1. Usually multiple.
2. Occasionally solitary (Blue-domed cyst of Bloodgood).

B. RETENTION CYSTS
Galactocele (*see* below).

C. CYSTS IN RELATION TO TUMOURS
1. Benign:
   a. Cystosarcoma phylloides.
   b. Papillary cystadenoma.
2. Malignant:

2. Lymphatic cyst (localised lymphangioma).
3. Dermoid cyst.
4. Hydatid cyst.

Treatment

A. *If there are Multiple Cysts.*—Simple mastectomy, preferably with a Galliard Thomas incision.

B. *If there is a Solitary Cyst:*
1. For cysts in relation to tumours.—Treatment for the tumour itself (i.e. excision, simple mastectomy, or radical mastectomy).
2. For a galactocele.—Excision.
3. For other cysts or where the cause of the cyst is unknown, two procedures may be adopted:
   a. Excision, followed by macroscopic examination and biopsy. If required, further treatment according to necessity.
   b. Aspiration.

USES OF ASPIRATION
1. To know the nature of the cyst by examination of the aspirate.
2. Repeated aspirations (followed by pressure bandaging) may cure an ordinary cyst.

DISADVANTAGES AND CONTRAINDICATION OF ASPIRATION.—A false negative result may be dangerous, i.e. an intracystic neoplasm may be missed. Aspiration is contraindicated if:

a. The cyst refills.
b. The fluid withdrawn is blood-stained.
c. There is a residual lump following aspiration.

In any of the above circumstances, an excision should be advocated, followed by biopsy.

Galactocele or Milk Cyst.—This is a rare variety of solitary cyst in relation to a main lactiferous duct. It is a form of retention cyst, caused by obstruction to the flow of milk from a milk duct. It develops during or immediately after lactation, and presents as a painless and localised swelling situated close to the nipple. To start with, it is tense-cystic and mobile, but later the consistency may be softer and the mobility restricted (due to development of fibrous adhesions). Sometimes a little milky discharge may be expressed from the nipple. The history is usually suggestive of the diagnosis but sometimes an aspiration is necessary for confirmation. The cyst contains milk—liquid or inspissated. The lining epithelium is gradually lost and the wall becomes fibrous and thick, sometimes calcified (demonstrated in a mammogram).

Treatment.—Excision of the cyst with a para-areolar incision.

DISCHARGE FROM THE NIPPLE

Diagnosis.—The following points require consideration:

A. Nature

4. Blackish.—Old blood from duct papilloma or duct carcinoma.

5. Purulent.—Mammillary fistula (resulting from a chronic and recurrent subareolar abscess in relation to a milk duct).

6. Milky.—Galactocele.

7. Creamy.—Duct ectasia.

B. Quantity.

C. Association of any lump in the breast.

D. If the discharge is from one particular duct or it cannot be localised to one duct.

E. Age of the patient.

F. Duration.—Sometimes the discharge stops spontaneously.

G. Onset, e.g.

1. Galactocele starts during or shortly after lactation.

2. Painful start, followed by recurrent abscesses, suggests mammillary fistula.

Treatment

A. WHENEVER A DISCHARGE IS ASSOCIATED WITH A LUMP IN THE BREAST.—The lump is removed and biopsy done. If necessary, a simple mastectomy is performed instead. When the discharge is definitely due to a carcinoma, a radical mastectomy has to be undertaken.

B. WHEN THE DISCHARGE IS FOUND TO BE RELATED TO ONE DUCT.:

1. If it is a blood-stained discharge, the condition is a duct papilloma or duct carcinoma. A microdochectomy is done, i.e. the duct probed with a blunted sewing needle and is excised intact, with the needle still inside it. The excised mass should contain about an inch of breast tissue, centered by the duct. If the report is a duct carcinoma, radical mastectomy is undertaken. Facilities of freeze-section biopsy are of great help.

2. Even when the discharge is not blood-stained, a microdochectomy is done and biopsy performed. Further treatment depends on the biopsy findings.

C. WHEN THE DISCHARGE CANNOT BE LOCATED TO ONE DUCT.—Two points are of importance:

1. Whether it contains blood (frank or occult).

2. The age of the patient.

Treatment depends on these two points is as follows:

a. If the discharge does not contain blood, whatever be the age of the patient, no active treatment is advised. The patient is kept on a periodic check-up and, on each occasion, the discharge is tested for occult blood. If, at any time, blood is detected, treatment is in the same line as for the following group.

b. If the discharge contains blood:

i. If the patient is above 40 years.—Simple mastectomy followed by careful biopsy.

ii. If the patient is below 40 years.—The patient is kept under careful observation; if at any time a lump appears, it has to be removed.

D. SOMETIMES A DISCHARGE CANNOT BE LOCALISED TO ONE DUCT TO START WITH, BUT SUBSEQUENTLY THE DISCHARGING DUCT CAN BE IDENTIFIED—A microdochectomy is performed in such cases, on identification of the offending duct.

TRAUMATIC FAT NECROSIS

This is an aseptic saponification of neutral fat, occurring in the fat of the breast. It is, in no way, related to the glandular element of the breast but the clinical appearance has close resemblance to, and may be mistaken for, a breast cancer. There is a lump, which is of stony hard consistency. It is often adherent to the underlying pectorals and/or the overlying skin. Occasionally, a peau d'orange appearance of the skin is seen, and sometimes the nipple is retracted. However, the lump is well-circumscribed and the patient is always obese.

The condition results from trauma, known or unrecognised:

1. *Known trauma:*
   a. A blow on the breast.
   b. Subcutaneous administration of saline solution.
2. *Unrecognised trauma:*
   a. Pressure of tight brassieres.
   b. Drag by a heavy pendulous breast.

The pathology, as has been said, is an aseptic saponification of the neutral fat and this excites a slow foreign body reaction in the form of fibrous tissue formation. Thus, there is a central area which contains chalk-like material (i.e. the saponified fat, resembling that seen in acute pancreatitis), surrounding which there is a layer of tough fibrous tissue. The facts that the condition is very well-circumscribed, that there is no evidence of infiltration, and that there is absence of the characteristic greyish spots (due to epithelial debris) seen in carcinoma, differentiate the condition from carcinoma of the breast.

Treatment.—Usually the diagnosis is doubtful in these cases and an excision is performed for the purpose of biopsy. The naked-eye appearance of the lump immediately tells the diagnosis, which is confirmed by histology.

GYNAECOMASTIA (GYNAECOMAZIA)

This is a condition in which the breast of a male looks like that of a female. The breast is enlarged to varying degrees, while the areola and the nipple assume a feminine appearance.

The condition may be unilateral or bilateral. Usually it is painless but sometimes there may be a little pain, particularly in the elderly patients.

Histological examination shows that there is actually no increase in the glandular element; it is only the fibrofatty tissue of the breast that proliferates.

A. IDIOPATHIC.—This is the commonest group and the patient is usually a boy, just crossed puberty. Some of the patients, however, may be between the ages of 20 and 30. There is no apparent cause for the condition and the probable explanation is some hormonal imbalance.

B. SECONDARY.—There is an attributable cause, resulting in a rise in the oestrogen level or a fall in the androgen level in the system:

1. *Hormonal Group:*
   a. Prolonged oestrogen therapy in patients of carcinoma of the prostate.
   b Testicular tumours, e.g. chorionepithelioma and some other varieties of teratoma.

   c. Bilateral ill-developed testes or atrophy of the testes (e.g. following mumps).

   d. Following castration.

   e. Some adrenal and pituitary tumours.

   f. *Klinefelter's syndrome.*—A sexual anomaly, producing a chromatin-positive male.

2. In patients of leprosy, possibly because of bilateral testicular atrophy.

3. In advanced portal cirrhosis, possibly because of the failure on the part of the liver to break down oestrogen.

4. Rarely, in cases of carcinoma of the bronchus.

Treatment.—It is usually the idiopathic group that comes for treatment of the gynaecomastia because of psychological reasons. The treatment is a simple mastectomy. The areola and the hippie are preserved, and the breast tissue is scraped from within. If the breast is small, this can be done with a para-areolar incision, but for a big breast, a Galliard Thomas incision is required.

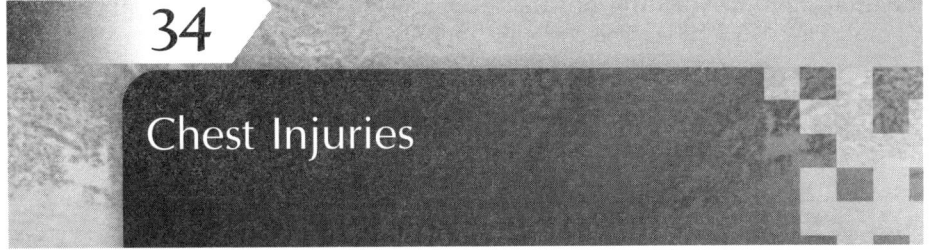

34

Chest Injuries

FRACTURE OF THE RIBS

Incidence.—Fracture of the ribs is less frequent in children, in whom the ribs are malleable. The first and second ribs, protected by the clavicle, are seldom fractured. Again, the eleventh and twelfth ribs being floatable, seldom fracture.

Trauma
1. *Direct Trauma.*—By a hard object. This generally results in fracture of a single rib, usually at the site of the trauma.
2. *Indirect Trauma.*—By severe crushed injuries, often automobile accidents. Several ribs are usually fractured. The fracture occurs at the site of maximum curvature and stress, i.e. at the anterior and/or posterior angles of the ribs.
3. *Insignificant Trauma.*—In very elderly people, in whom the ribs are rigid, a violent paroxysm of cough may cause fracture of a rib.

Uncomplicated Rib Fractures.—This condition is painful but rarely disturbing. The presenting features are:
1. Local pain, exaggerated by deep respirations, coughing, sneezing, etc.
2. Respirations are shallower and painful.
3. Tenderness at the fracture site, elicited by :
   a. Direct pressure.
   b. *'Springing ribs'.*—On pressing the chest, with one hand in front and another behind, the patient experiences pain at the fracture site.

X-RAY.—The fracture is usually seen. Occasionally, however, it may be difficult to be demonstrated radiologically.

TREATMENT.—Irrespective of the nature of treatment, the fracture heals by itself. The only aim of treatment is to relieve the pain:
1. Systemic analgesics.—Orally or, better, by injections, e.g. Novalgin, every 8 hours, for the first 2 or 3 days
2. Injection of 2% Novocaine:
   a. at the fracture site, and
   b. intercostal nerve block.
3. Immobilisation of the fracture by *strapping* the chest with adhesive plaster had been in practice since long and is still advised by many surgeons as it definitely relieves pain. Strapping, to be effective, must cross the midline both anteriorly

Strapping is discouraged in many centres because of the following disadvantages:—
a. It diminishes the respiratory movements and this may be harmful particularly in the elderly people, in whom all attempts must be made to establish full respirations.
b. Occasionally, the strapping may force the broken rib-ends inwards, causing damage to the underlying structures.

Complications of Fractures of Ribs.—Complications usually occur only in cases of multiple rib fractures. The complications are caused:
a. either, by the trauma that had caused the fracture:
b. or, by the fractured rib-ends.

The different complications may be enumerated as follows:
  1. Shock.
  2. Surgical emphysema. .
  3. Pneumothorax (traumatic).
  4. Haemothorax (traumatic).
  5. Stove-in chest and flail chest.
  6. Contusion and laceration of the lung, and wet-lung.
  7. Injury to the heart and hemopericardium (cardiac tamponade).
  8. Traumatic asphyxia.
  9. Injury to subdiaphragmatic organs—liver, spleen, kidneys, stomach, colon.
  10. Injury to the diaphragm and occurrence of diaphragmatic hernia.

Surgical Emphysema.—This is a condition in which air infiltrates into the subcutaneous tissue (hence also called *subcutaneous emphysema*).

MECHANISM.—The compressing force, that causes the fracture, forces inwards the sharp fracture-end and this stabs into the underlying lung. Air escapes into the chest wall, around the fractured rib and this makes the subcutaneous emphysema.

This phase of escape of air from the lung is momentary and air is injected into the subcutaneous tissues without allowing entrance into the pleural cavity, the rent in the lung being sealed off.

There may be variations to the above procedure:
a. In some cases, the rent in the lung persists and this results in:
  i. an associated pneumothorax,
  ii. a spreading subcutaneous emphysema, which extends widely along the chest wall encroaches the neck and in an advanced case, may even go up to the face and the limbs.
b. Rarely, air escapes from a ruptured bronchus and collects in peribronchial space, resulting in *mediastinal emphysema*. The emphysema is first evident over the suprasternal notch and then rapidly spreads into the neck, face, chest wall, abdominal parieties and scrotum. Often the tension is sufficient to cause cardiac embarrassment and pressure on great veins.

CLINICAL FEATURES
1. On inspection, the area involved (which may extend to the neck, face, and sometimes the limbs) looks bloated up with the air.
2. On palpation, there is a typical crepitus.
3. Percussion elicits a resonant node, which may be due to:
  a. the emphysema.
  b. associated pneumothorax, if any.

4. Auscultation reveals:
   a. the crepitus of the emphysema;
   b. absence of breath sounds due to associated pneumothorax.

X-RAY
   1. Gas in the soft tissues.
   2. Fractured ribs.
   3. Associated pneumothorax, if present

MANAGEMENT
1. In an uncomplicated case, no treatment is required; the air in the subcutaneous tissue is gradually absorbed. Some surgeons advocate multiple incisions along Langer's lines, through the skin, down to the subcutaneous tissues, to allow the air to escape. This is better avoided since it invites infection.
2. In localised emphysema associated with pneumothorax, an intercostal needle drain through the second space, connected to a water-seal bottle, is established.
3. In progressively increasing emphysema (mediastinal emphysema), associated with ruptured bronchus:
   a. Intercostal needle drain.
   b. Tracheostomy.
   c. If required, exploratory thoracotomy and repair of the bronchus.

OTHER CAUSES OF SUBCUTANEOUS EMPHYSEMA
1. Localised emphysema around abdominal or thoracic incisions.
2. In the neck, following ruptured oesophagus.
3. In the loin, following extraperitoneal injuries of ascending or descending colon, or of rectum.
4. On the face, following fractures of nasal bones and paranasal sinuses.

Traumatic Pneumothorax.—This means air in the pleural cavity, following trauma. In the majority of cases, there is blood as well in the pleural cavity, so that the condition is more often a *haemopneumothorax*.

In cases of fractured ribs, a pneumothorax may be as follows:
1. Air leaks from the lung that has been damaged by the fractured rib-ends.
2. If the lacerated lung communicates with a branch of the bronchial tree, it allows air to enter the pleural cavity from the lung during inspiration but does not permit its escape during expiration, i.e. the leak is *valvular*. Air quickly accumulates within the pleural cavity, causing total collapse of the lung. This is called *tension pneumothorax*. There is mediastinal displacement towards the opposite side.
3. In penetrating injuries of the chest (seldom associated with fractured ribs), air enters the pleural cavity through the wound, i.e. it is sucked in. This is called *sucking wound*. This also produces a tension pneumothorax if the air cannot simultaneously escape through the wound.

TREATMENT
1. A small pneumothorax, without much symptoms, requires no active treatment
2. A sucking wound is an emergency. This should be *immediately* covered up by occlusive pad and then surgical repair arranged.
3. A tension pneumothorax is also an emergency.—As an emergency procedure, an aspirating needle (unmounted) is plunged into the pleural cavity; this allows

cannula, a narrow soft catheter is introduced into the pleural chamber and is connected to a water-seal bottle.

Traumatic Haemothorax.—This is a common complication of fractured ribs and other chest injuries. The source of the blood may be:

1. Intercostal vessels
2. Injured lung
3. Big vessels and heart.

TREATMENT

1. In massive haemorrhage, blood transfusion and treatment for the associated shock. In many cases, other associated chest injuries (e.g. a stove in chest) require active treatment
2. Ordinarily, the haemothorax *requires repeated aspiration.* The first aspiration is performed after 24 hours, allowing the bleeding vessel to seal (in massive haemorrhages, however, earlier aspiration has to be instituted). Subsequently, aspiration has to be repeated, to start with daily and then at increasing intervals. At the close of each aspiration 10 lac units of penicillin is pushed into the pleural chamber through the aspiration needle, in an attempt to prevent secondary infection. Aspiration has to be continued till:
   a. No further material comes out, the lung shows clinical evidence of expansion, and X-ray shows full lung expansion and no further pleural collection.
   b. When the blood is so clotted that aspiration fails. In these cases a *decortication* operation has to be undertaken—the blood clots from the pleural cavity and the surface of the lung have to be removed.
3. In many cases, the haemothorax changes into an empyema and the treatment is in the same lines as for subacute empyema, i.e. repeated aspirations with local antibiotic instillation or, subsequently, a decortication.
4. If the haemothorax is progressive, *exploratory thoracotomy* has to be undertaken and the bleeding vessel secured. Any contused segment of lung may have to be resected. In many such cases, the offending vessel is an intercostal artery.

Stove-in Chest and Flail Chest.—A *stove-in chest* is one in which-there is a permanent indentation (i.e. depression) of the chest wall, resulting from fracture of several consecutive ribs, each fractured either at one site or more than one, due to crushing force.

A *flail chest* is an extreme degree of stove-in chest, in which a part of the chest wall, having lost its support, becomes so flail (i.e. unstable or floating) as to exhibit paradoxical respirations. This means that this segment of the chest wall is sucked inwards during inspirations and pushed out at expirations (the reverse of the usual chest movements). This may occur under two conditions:

1. Several consecutive ribs are fractured at two or more places, so that the segment of chest wall, made up by these fragments, becomes flail or floating. An associated fracture of the clavicle, if present, enhances the condition.
2. A sudden backward displacement of the sternum (as in steering-wheel injury) produces fractures—superiorly across the sternum, laterally across the ribs or costal cartilage on both the sides, and sometimes interiorly across, the sternum as well. This results in an unstable floating section of the anterior chest wall.

1. With a depressed segment (stove-in chest), there is considerable reduction in the size of the hemithorax and the function of the underlying lung may be grossly reduced, i.e. there is *reduction in the ventilatory lung surface.*
2. With a flail chest, a *paradoxical* respiration occurs in the flaccid unstable segment of the chest wall. Ordinarily, during inspiration, the diaphgram moves down and the chest wall expands (the drawing in of the chest wall, by the negative intrapleural pressure, is prevented by the rigidity of the wall). During expiration, the diaphragm moves up and the chest wall is also forced in (its outward bulging by the high pressure is also prevented by its rigidity). When a flail chest occurs, the unsupported part possesses no more that rigidity which can stand the effects of the intrapleural pressure. So, during inspiration, as there is an intrapleural negative pressure, this part is sucked in. Similarly, during expiration, with rise of pressure, it is forced out. Thus, it shows just the reverse of the movements of the normal chest, hence called paradoxical.
3. The paradoxical respiration causes:
   a. Imperfect ventilation, because the lungs are not allowed to inflate and deflate normally.
   b. Pendulum movement of air from one lung to the other. This is particularly likely to occur when the upper respiratory passages are blocked, e.g. accumulated secretion. The expired air from one bronchus is sucked into the opposite bronchus and vice-versa, and this process is continuously repeated, so that only de-oxygenated air is entering the lungs.
   c. Movement of the mediastinal structures, during each phase of respiration, i.e. *'mediastinal flutter'*. This causes shock as well as imperfect ventilation.
4. There is *accumulation of the bronchopulmonary secretions* because:
   a. The patient does not cough for fear of pain.
   b. There is relative immobility of the underlying lung. The results of such accumulation are:
      i. Imperfect air entry.
      ii. Pendulum movement of air from one lung to the other,
      iii. *Wet-lung,* i.e. the lung accumulates its own secretions.

The above factors, together, lead to hypoxia and carbon dioxide accumulation, and these may cause rapid death.

TREATMENT
1. Tracheostomy is urgently required and often produces dramatic improvement The advantages of tracheostomy are:
   a. It decreases the *dead space of* the respiratory tract (i.e. from nose and mouth to the trachea, the area which is not concerned in ventilation).
   b. It keeps the airway patent and provides a ready route for tracheobronchial suction.
   c. It provides relief from exhausting cough.
   d. It often corrects the paradoxical respiration.
   e. It minimises the breathing resistance and makes the work of the respiratory muscle easier.
2. If facilities for immediate tracheostomy are not available, an endo-tracheal intubation is done and ventilation carried out with an anaesthetic machine. This is replaced by a tracheostomy at the earliest.

3. Wherever facilities are available, the tracheostomy tube is connected to a respirator (ventilator), and a well-managed positive-pressure respiration with the ventilators is all that is needed in these cases. Care must be taken to see that the expanding lung is not lacerated by the fractured rib-ends.

4. *External stabilisation of the flail segment may* have to be done if, in spite of tracheostomy, the paradoxical respiration persists. This may be done by the following, methods:
   a. For minor degrees.—By simple pad and strapping.
   b. In severe cases.—By elevating the depressed chest wall with towel clips placed round the ribs *(external fixation).* Traction is applied on these towel clips.
   c. If the deformity tends to recur after (b), the ribs are exposed and the fractures fixed with nails or wires *(internal fixation).* If the clavicle is fractured as well, it must be controlled with a plate or pin.

5. Any associated traumatic pneumothorax or haemothorax (which is often present) has to be promptly treated.

6. Antibiotics to combat infection.

7. Breathing exercises, after tracheostomy has been established.

Contusion and Laceration of the Lung.—These may be minor, moderate, or severe. The results in the different cases are:

1. Surgical emphysema.
2. Traumatic pneumothorax, sometimes valvular.
3. Traumatic haemothorax or haemopneumothorax.
4. Haemoptysis.
5. Consolidation, following contusion, usually resolving spontaneously.
6. Persistent collapse of a grossly lacerated segment.
7. Secondary infection of the damaged lung.

Only occasionally there is the necessity for a thoracotomy and repair or resection of the affected segment.

Wet-Lung.—Inability of the patient to cough out the secretions and relative immobility of the underlying lung in cases of fractured ribs, result in accumulation of the secretions in the lung. This condition is called 'wet-lung'. Secondary infection is very likely to set in. A tracheostomy, breathing exercises, encouraging cough, and administration of antibiotics, overcome this difficulty.

Injury to the Heart and Hemopericardium.— Injury to the heart, resulting in quick accumulation of blood in the small pericardial space, causes what is called *'cardiac tamponade'*. There is gross interference with the functions of the heart. There are three classical signs:

1. Silent heart, i.e. diminution of heart sounds.
2. Increased area of cardiac dullness.
3. Rapid fall in the arterial pressure with concomitant rise in the venous pressure.

As a life-saving measure, immediate aspiration of the pericardial chamber has to be undertaken. This is done through the left costoxiphoid angle.

Traumatic Asphyxia.—This is a rare complication that may follow compression of the chest. The compressing force (causing the rib fracture), momentarily raises the intrathoracic pressure. Blood, from the intrathoracic big veins, is forced back into the veins of the head, neck, upper part of the chest, and arms. The pressure is transmitted to the smaller veins and venules, resulting in intense venous congestion and petechial haemorrhages:

1. There is a dusky appearance of the head, neck, upper chest, and sometimes arms, due to venous congestion and extravasation. Petechial haemorrhages may be seen.
2. X-ray of the lungs, taken later, may suggest a picture of miliary deposits.

   No special treatment is required for this condition, excepting a propped up position for easy venous drainage.

MANAGEMENT OF CHEST INJURIES

Types of Injury.— Injuries of the chest may be:
1. Closed Injuries, i.e. crushed injuries with fractured ribs.
2. Open Injuries:
   a. Penetrating, e.g. stab wounds.
   b. Perforating, i.e. through and through injuries, e.g. gun-shot wounds.
   To these may be added—
3. Thoraco-abdominal Injuries.

Crashed Injuries.—These are the cases of multiple rib fractures with different complications, as described above. The principles of treatment may be .summarised as follows.

A. IMMEDIATE EMERGENCY MANAGEMENT IN SOME CASES
1. If there is tension pneumothorax.—Immediate plunging of an aspiration needle into the second intercostal space.
2. If there is stove-in chest or flail chest —Tracheostomy or endotracheal intubation, and ventilation with an aneasthesia machine.
3. If there is 'cardiac tamponade'—Percardial aspiration through the left cos-toxiphoid angle.

B. USUAL MANAGEMENT
1. Treatment in propped-up position.
2. Relief of pain :
   a. Systemic sedatives and analgesics.
   b. Intercostal nerve block.
3. Adequate oxygen therapy.
4. Treatment of shock, including blood transfusion, if necessary.
5. Maintaining air-entry and adequate ventilation:
   a. Suction of tracheobronchial secretions, including bronchoscopic aspiration.
   b. Tracheostomy:
      i. If profuse secretions persist.
      ii. In cases of flail chest and stove-in chest.
      iii. In mediastinal emphysema.
   c. The tracheostomy tube is connected to a ventilator (where available), if required.
6. Removal of pleural blood and air:
   a. Continuous aspiration of air with water-seal arrangement.
   b. Repeated aspiration of blood.
   c. Thoracotomy for arrest of haemorrhage, if there is rapid accumulation of blood.

7. Stabilisation of the chest wall:
   a. Simple strapping for minor cases.
   b. External stabilisation with towel clips for stove-in chest.
   c. Internal fixation with nails or wires for flail chest or severe cases of stove-in chest.
   d. Tracheostomy in ease of stove-in or flail chest.
8. Exploratory thoracotomy, when indicated (e.g. ruptured bronchus or quickly accumulating haemothorax).
9. Exploratory laparotomy of the abdomen for injuries of subdiaphragmatic organs, e.g. liver, spleen, kidneys, etc.

The above points have been discussed in details under complications of fractures of ribs.

Open Injuries.—These are penetrating or perforating (through and through) wounds. Such wounds may be:
1. Simple.
2. Complicated with serious damage to underlying viscera, viz. pleura, lung, heart, and abdominal organs (liver, spleen, kidneys, stomach, colon).

The management of open injuries of the chest may be summarised as follows:

A. EMERGENCY MANAGEMENT IN SOME CASES
1. If there is a sucking wound, it should be immediately covered up with occlusive pad, pending surgical repair.
2. If there is uncontrollable external or internal haemorrhage, immediate thoracotomy has to be undertaken.
3. If there is severe respiratory difficulty, tracheostomy often improves the condition.

B. FOR SIMPLE WOUNDS
Provided gross injury to the lung and bronchi, injury to the heart or big vessels, and injury to abdominal viscera or diaphragm have been excluded, the management is conservative. Usually, it consists of one of the following:
1. No active treatment.
2. Continuous pleural aspiration for pneumothorax.
3. Repeated aspiration for haemothorax.

C. FOR WOUNDS COMPLICATED WITH UNDERLYING VISCERAL DAMAGE
1. Exploratory thoracotomy has to be undertaken *after* the patient has been resuscitated.
2. *Immediate* exploratory thoracotomy has to be considered only in presence of uncontrollable internal or external bleeding.

Thoraco-abdominal Injuries.—Since there is an abdominal component of the injury, it is obligatory that these wounds are explored. The exploration is better done with a thoracic approach because:
   a. It permits correction of thoracic injuries.
   b. It gives easy and adequate exposure of the upper abdomen through the diaphragm.

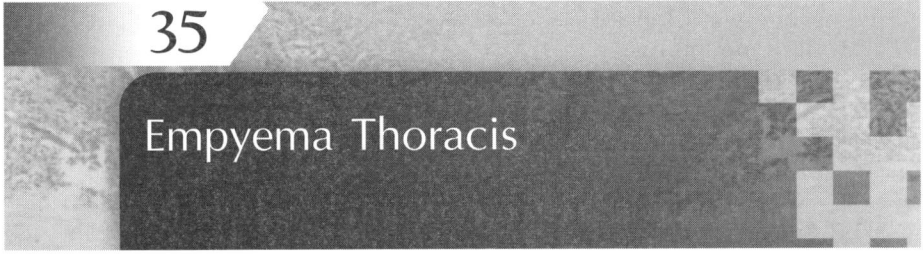

35

Empyema Thoracis

Definition—If the term is applied rigidly, empyema thoracis means a pleural abscess, i.e. collection of thick pus, usually localised, in the pleural cavity. However, the term is usually used in a much broader sense, and often, a generalised pleural effusion with a little turbidity, due to infection, goes by the name of empyema. This latter condition should better be termed *'diffuse suppurative pleurisy'*. It may be said that the difference between an empyema and diffuse suppurative pleurisy is more or less the same as that between an abscess and diffuse cellulitis, in other parts of the body.

Causes—An empyema is never primary. The source of infection may be the underlying lung. However, there may be other sources as well, and the causes of empyema may be detailed as follows:

1. FROM OUTSIDE
   a. Penetrating injuries of chest
   b. Haemothorax secondarily infected during the process of repeated aspirations.
   c. Following thoracotomy, i.e. post-operative.

2. FROM THE CHEST WALL
   a. Osteomyelitis of rib.
   b. Parietal abscess.

3. FROM THE UNDERLYING LUNG
   a. Pneumococcal pneumonia.
   b. Streptococcal bronchopneumonia.
   c. Lung abscess, often staphylococcal.
   d. Tuberculosis.
   e. Bronchiectasis.
   f. Malignant growth.
   g. Actinomycosis.

4. FROM THE OESOPHAGUS
   a. Rupture.
   b. Carcinoma.

5. FROM BELOW THE DIAPHRAGM
   Subphrenic abscess (by way of lymphatics).
   Of the above sources, those in groups 1 and 3 are the commonest causes of empyema.

Pathology.

I. ACUTE EMPYEMA—In the older days, when empyema was believed to be almost always due to a secondary infection of the pleura from the underlying lung, there were two distinct types of empyema to be recognised—synpneumonic and metapneumonic. The *synpneumonic empyema* was seen in cases of streptococcal bronchopneumonia and, because the empyema occurred synchronously with the bronchopneumonia, it was called synpneumonic. The *metapneumonic empyema* was seen in cases of pneumococcal lobar pneumonia and, because the process of empyema usually started after the resolution of pneumonia, it would be called metapneumonic. In general the streptococcal synpneumonic empyema was of the nature of a diffuse suppurative pleurisy while the pneumococcal metapneumonic empyema was usually of a localised abscess type.

In the present days, availability of antibiotics and better management have reduced the incidence of either of the above types of empyema. Nevertheless, empyema is still common nowadays, though the sources of infection may have changed.

In almost all the cases, the pathology starts as a diffuse suppurative pleurisy. In the majority, however, the process of infection in the pleural chamber gets localised. This process of localisation is primarily achieved by deposits of fibrin, which cause adhesions to develop between the visceral and parietal pleurae, around the site of localisation. Certain types of infection, e.g. pneumococcal favour the formation of such adhesions, while in others, e.g. streptococcal infection (because of streptokinase, liberated by the bacteria), adhesion formation may be much delayed.

In the next phase, fibrous tissue is deposited on the inner surface of the parietal pleura and the outer surface of the visceral pleura, i.e. around the empyema cavity. Gradually this fibrous tissue is changed into vascular granulation tissue and, in the meantime, the fluid inside turns into thick pus. This is actually the stage of empyema.

This process of localisation is usually towards the parieties, i.e. peripheral. Occasionally, localisation may occur at other places in the pleural cavity. Accordingly, empyema may be.—
1. Peripheral (commonest).
2. Mediastinal.
3. Apical.
4. Basal.
5. Interlobar.

II. CHRONIC EMPYEMA—If, at this stage of acute empyema proper drainage is not established, the empyema turns into chronicity—the fibrous tissue in the wall gradually gets thicker. The secondary effects of this thick fibrous tissue may be as follows:
a. No antibiotic reaches the empyema cavity.
b. The underlying lung cannot expand, so it does not work.
c. The overlying chest wall gets rigid and immobile and may be drawn inwards. The ribs are drawn close together and may overlie one another.
d. There may be mediastinal shift towards the affected side, caused by the pull of fibrous tissue.
e. When the diaphragmatic pleura is affected, the diaphragm is usually fixed in an elevated position.
f. When the pericardial pleura is involved, the resulting adhesions may embarrass the action of the heart (pleuropericardial adhesion).

It may be mentioned that the fibrous tissue deposit on the parietal pleura is much thicker than that on the visceral pleura. It is often three or more centimeters in thickness, oedematous, and bleeds exceedingly freely. In older cases it is absolutely unyielding, often, like leather. There is usually a plane of cleavage between the fibrous tissue and the visceral pleura (and its advantage is taken of in the operation of decortication).

Clinical Types

I. ACUTE FULMINATING EMPYEMA.—This is rather uncommon and occurs only if the empyema follows oesophageal rupture or lung abscess. The patient is severely toxic and, unless quick drainage is established, death occurs.

II. ACUTE EMPYEMA.—Though called acute, the course of the empyema is actually subacute, so it should better be termed *subacute empyema.* This is much the commoner variety. The onset is generally insidious because of early administration of antibiotics for the primary condition. The presence of such an empyema is elicited by the following features:

1. A continuing, often low grade temperature.
2. Some amount of dyspnoea and, sometimes, cough. In synpneumonic empyema the dyspnoea may be considerable because of the underlying generalised lung pathology (bronchopneumonia) and the patient may have a little cyanosis as well— hence called *blue dyspnoea.*
3. A little pain or discomfort in the chest.
4. Clinical signs of fluid in the pleural cavity:
   a. Diminished chest movements on the affected side.
   b. Mediastinal displacement to the opposite side.
   c. Stony dullness on percussion.
   d. Diminished breath sounds.
5. Diagnosis is usually confirmed by :
   a. Straight X-ray.
   b. Aspiration of pleural cavity.

III. CHRONIC EMPYEMA

A. *Close Type.*—This may occur if an acute empyema has not been drained. The walls become covered with thick fibrous tissue and may even be calcified The pus inside may be small in quantity, thick, and often sterile.

B. *Open Type:*
   1. Either, a *bronchopleural fistula,* i.e. empyema cavity communicates with a bronchus, into which it discharges from time to time.
   2. Or, a parietal fistula *(pleuroparietal fistula),* when there is a persistent discharging sinus on the chest wall following open drainage for acute empyema (see below).

Treatment of Acute Empyema.—The principles, underlying the treatment, are:

A. Control of infection.
B. Elimination of the dead space of the cavity.

A. CONTROL OF INFECTION
   1. Systemic Antibiotics.—The specific antibiotic is preferably chosen on the basis of culture and sensitivity test of the aspirate.
   2. Local instillation of penicillin (10 lacs) and streptomycin (1 gm) into the empyema cavity, through the aspiration needle, at each aspiration.

B. Elimination of dead space
1. *Drainage of the empyema cavity.*—There are two forms of drainage:
    a. *Close Drainage*, i.e.. repeated aspiration.
    b. *Open Drainage*—either by rib resection or by intercostal drainage.
In all cases, to start with, drainage by aspiration is the routine. Particularly when the stage is one of diffuse suppurative pleurisy, open drainage is dangerous since pleural adhesions have not yet developed and the patient may die of a mediastinal shift.

Repeated aspirations are performed, usually on alternate days. On each occasion, as much pus as possible is removed, and antibiotics are introduced locally through the aspiration needle. Aspiration is usually easy, provided a correct site is chosen. A careful clinical and radiological examination usually provides proper information. At the end of the first aspiration, radio-opaque iodised oil may be injected into the cavity, so that at subsequent X-ray, the lower limit of the space is easily outlined.

Open drainage has to be thought of, to replace aspiration, when :
    i. The pus has turned too thick to come out even through a widebore needle.
    ii. Aspirations fail to produce expansion of the lung.

Open drainage of an empyema may be achieved either by *rib resection* or by *intercostal drainage*. Majority of surgeons prefer rib resection and keep intercostal drainage reserved for children and for absolutely feeble patients. This is because they believe that the tube of an intercostal drainage is likely to be pressed between the ribs at each respiration and so the drainage is unsatisfactory. Many surgeons, however, advocate intercostal drainage for all the cases because of the simplicity of the procedure and because they believe that this provides an adequate drainage (rib resection and intercostal drainage are described below).

After rib resection or intercostal drainage, the drainage tube is connected to a *water-seal bottle*, i.e. a closed drainage is maintained. This is continued till the daily output of pus is less than two ounces. When this state is reached, the cavity has become small, and now the tube may be allowed to have an open drainage into the dressings.

Only when the cavity has been completely obliterated (which it usually takes about 6 to 8 weeks), that the tube should be withdrawn.
2. Well-guided and vigorous *breathing exercises* must be undertaken routinely so that the underlying lung can re-expand and obliterate the cavity. They also overcome residual deformity and limitation of movements.

Rib Resection.—The most suitable rib for resection and the part of it to be resected, in a particular case, are chosen on the basis of:
a. the findings of diagnostic aspirations,
b. X-ray findings.

For efficient drainage, the rib, corresponding to the lowermost part of the empyema cavity, should always be resected. Since, in the majority of cases, the pus has a tendency to collect in the lowermost part of the pleural chamber, a lower rib should generally be resected. Since, however, the diaphragm moves up and down with every respiration and causes a hindrance to drainage, the lowermost ribs are unsuitable for resection. Making a compromise between these two factors, the 8th or 9th rib is the ideal to be resected.

As the patient will lie recumbent after the drainage, the most dependent part in that position is the paravertebral region and it is this part of the rib that should be resected. So it stands that for an ordinary empyema, the 8th or 9th rib in the posterior axillary line is the ideal to be resected.

The operation is done with local infiltration anaesthesia, and, to start with, the integument, upto the intercostal muscles, are infiltrated. The patient preferably sits on a stool with the arms and head supported on a table. If he is unable to do so, he lies on his sound side.

The incision is commonly a transverse one, along the rib to be resected. If, however, it is not very sure whether a lower rib has to be resected, a vertical incision is preferred as it provides an easy approach to the lower rib, if required.

All tissues, down to the outer periosteum of the rib, are incised and the periosteum from both the surfaces of the rib are elevated (see Doyen's raspatory— Chapter on instruments). At this stage, a further infiltration of the local anaesthetic is made subperiosteally on the outer surface of the rib and also just deep to its lower border to block the intercostal nerve.

About 3 inches of the rib is resected with a rib shear, after having ligated the intercostal vessels at either end (see Doyen's raspatory).

The inner periosteum, with the parietal pleura attached to it, is carefully infiltrated with local anaesthetic for prevention of *pleural shock.* The empyema cavity is opened by thrusting a sinus forceps through these structures and then opening its blades. At this stage, the patient usually gets a bout of cough. The cavity is explored with a finger and all fibrous loculi are broken. A self-retaining catheter is then introduced into the cavity. The excess of the opening is sutured by the side of the tube. The muscles and the skin are sutured.

Intercostal Drainage.—The choice of site is in the same principles as for rib resection (8th intercostal space in the posterior axillary line). The skin and muscles, and the parietal pleura are infiltrated with a local anaesthetic. A small transverse skin incision is made, just enough to admit the tip of a trocar for puncture. A two-way trocar and canula is now made to puncture all soft tissues, down to the pleural cavity. After the puncture is made, the trocar is withdrawn. A self-retaining catheter, with its introducer, is passed through the canula into the empyema cavity. The introducer and the canula are withdrawn together, keeping the tip of the catheter inside the empyema cavity.

CHRONIC EMPYEMA

Types.—As has already been discussed, there are two types:

A. Close Type.

B. Open Type:
 1. Bronchopleural fistula
 2. Pleuroparietal fistula, following open drainage.

Pathology

CLOSE TYPE.—This occurs if an acute empyema has not been drained. The walls become covered with thick fibrous tissue and may even be calcified. The pus inside is small in quantity, thick, and often sterile.

OPEN TYPE.—These are the cases where the cavity communicates with the exterior:—

1. *Bronchopleural Fistula*, i.e. the pleural empyema cavity is communicating with a bronchus, into which it is discharging from time to time. This may occur:
   a. If the empyema cavity ruptures into a bronchus.
   b. If a lung abscess ruptures into the pleural cavity on one side, and into a bronchus on the other.
2. *Parietal Fistula (pleuroparietal fistula)*, when there is a persistent discharging sinus on the chest wall following open drainage for an empyema. This is described below in details.

Causes of Persistent Discharging Sinus

1. *Defective Drainage Operation :*
   a. Drainage done too late so that the wall of the cavity is grossly thickened and fibrous and the cavity does not obliterate.
   b. Drainage done too high:
      i. The lower part of the cavity could not drain itself,
      ii. The scapula presses on the drainage tube.
   c. Drainage done too low.—The diaphragm hinders drainage.
2. *Defective Post-operative Management:*
   a. Early omission of antibiotics or use of antibiotics to which the organisms are insensitive.
   b. Omission of breathing exercises.
   c. Withdrawal of the drainage tube before the cavity has obliterated completely.
   d. Leaving behind a foreign body or part of the drainage tube, inside the cavity.
   e. Osteomyelitis of the cut rib ends.
3. *Repeated Re-infection from an Underlying Lung Pathology :*
   a. Bronchopleural fistula.
   b. Tuberculosis.
   c. Lung abscess.
   d. Bronchiectasis.
   e. Malignancy.
   f. Actinomycosis.

Special Investigations

1. Probe examination of the sinus to know its length and direction.
2. X-ray of the chest, to demonstrate:
   a. The location of the cavity.
   b. Any gross lung pathology.
   c. Osteomyelitis of a resected rib end.
   d. Foreign body in the cavity.
3. *Sinugraphy*—A radio-opaque dye (lipiodol) is introduced into the sinus and X-ray taken. This may suggest the position and extent of the cavity.
   In those cases, where there is a bronchopleural fistula, this dye may enter the bronchial system and the same examination produces an *ascending bronchogram*. In such a case, addition of colours like Sudan III to the lipiodol and expectoration of the colour by the patient, confirms the diagnosis of a bronchopleural fistula.
4. All investigations for the underlying lung.

Management of Chronic Empyema

A. SIMPLER CASES.—These are the cases where:

1. The drainage has been imperfect.
2. The post-operative management has been faulty.
3. There is a foreign body in the cavity or there is osteomyelitis of the rib ends.

In those cases where the rib resection was not done at a proper level, a fresh rib resection is performed at a suitable place.

Any foreign body is removed or osteomyelitic rib ends are resected.

Culture of the discharge and sensitivity test of the organisms are done, and a suitable antibiotic administered.

Vigorous breathing exercises are advocated in all the cases.

B. MORE DIFFICULT CASES.—In these cases there may be:

1. Extensive deposit of fibrous and granulation tissues on the wall of the empyema cavity.
2. A gross pathology in the underlying lung, causing repeated reinfection.
3. A combination of the above two factors.

In the first group of cases, the operation of *decortication* has to be undertaken. In this operation, all fibrous tissue from the wall of the empyema cavity is dissected out. On the inner side such dissection is rather easy since there is usually a plane of cleavage between the visceral pleura and the fibrous tissue. As the fibrous tissue is removed, together with the abscess cavity, the underlying lung gets elastic again and re-expands, causing obliteration of the space.

In the second and third groups of cases, in addition to decortication, an appropriate operation for the lung pathology has to be undertaken, e.g. segmental resection, lobectomy, pneumonectomy.

C. MOST DIFFICULT CASES.—These are the cases where, even after decortication and lung resections, the cavity persists. They pose some of the most serious problems in surgery. Thoracoplasty and various types *of flap operations* have been advocated. The idea behind all these operations is to make the chest wall soft and mobile, and to press it down into the empyema cavity, with the idea of obliterating the cavity.

36

Surgical Treatment of Pulmonary Tuberculosis

PRINCIPLES OF TREATMENT IN PULMONARY TUBERCULOSIS

I. ENCOURAGEMENT OF ACTIVE RESISTANCE by dietetic and other general measures.

II. CHEMOTHERAPY.—To start with, three anti-tubercular drugs are used (triple drug therapy). There are two popular combinations:
1. Streptomycin, ethambutol and INH (isoniazid).
2. Rifampicin, ethambutol and INH

Rifampicin, INH and streptomycin are bactericidal while ethambutol is bacteriostatic.

When streptomycin, INH and ethambutol are used, streptomycin is given intramuscularly, 1 gm daily, usually up to a maximum of 90 gm. In the later stages the drug may have to be used on alternate days if the patient cannot tolerate daily administration. INH is given 300 mg daily as a single dose. Ethambutol is administered 20 mg/kg body weight, i.e. 800 to 1200 mg per day in single dose. While streptomycin is omitted after administration of 90 gm, INH and ethambutol have to be continued for at least 18 months or till clinical cure occurs, whichever is later.

Rifampicin, INH and ethambutol is a better combination because rifampicin is much more bactericidal than streptomycin. However, it is costlier. It is particularly indicated for elderly patients who cannot tolerate streptomycin because of vestibular damage. The advantage of rifampicin is that, when it is used, INH and ethambutol can usually be discontinued after 9 months therapy. Rifampicin is administered 450 to 600 mg orally daily (commonly in single dosage) usually for a period of three months.

III. RELAXATION.—This means diminution or abolition of expansion of the lung and permitting its natural elasticity to induce an artificial collapse, not only of the cavities but also of the bronchi draining them. The collapse and the resultant rest to the part (i.e. 'functional stenosis') provide great help to the healing of tuberculosis. Healing occurs by fibrosis. This fibrous tissue causes contraction of the diseased area and obliteration of the destroyed areas and cavities (i.e. 'organic stenosis').

There are two types of relaxation:
A. *Passive Relaxation.*—This is achieved by rest in bed. The patient's oxygen requirement is lessened, the inspiratory excursion of the chest is diminished, and the pull on the bronchial walls and the lung tissue around them is reduced. This provides relaxation.
B. *Active Relaxation.*—This is the main aim of surgical treatment in pulmonary tuberculosis. The methods may be divided into two groups:

1. Minor Procedures:
    a. Artificial pneumothorax.
    b. Phrenic paralysis.
    c. Intrapleural pneumolysis.
    d. Pneumoperitoneum.
2. Major Procedures:
    a. Thoracoplasty.
    b. Extrapleural pneumolysis.

These operations are described below in detail.

IV. EXCISION OF THE DISEASED LUNG—With the introduction of the efficient antitubercular drugs, resection of the diseased segment of the lung has almost totally replaced the major procedures of collapse therapy, e.g. thoracoplasty. The *advantages* of resection, over collapse therapy, are:

a. It removes the major foci of the disease, leaving only very little of the residual disease to be dealt with by the body.
b. It leaves no external deformity and disturbs the respiratory functions very little.
c. It is a surer method.

This is why resection is presently the treatment of choice in nearly 90 per cent of cases requiring surgical aid Before undertaking resection :

a. *Tomography* and *bronchography* should be undertaken to know whether the lung and bronchi, to be left behind, are free from the disease.
b. *Bronchoscopy* should be done to exclude active tuberculous bronchitis. If this is present the operation should be deferred till the bronchitis is controlled by chemotherapy.

At operation, it is necessary to remove all obvious tubercular lesions. Accordingly, segmental resection, lobectomy, or pneumonectomy is undertaken. Over-distension of the remaining lung tissue may cause reactivation of the dormant foci, and this must be prevented by either of the following procedures: —

  i. A temporary phrenic paralysis.
 ii. A small apical thoracoplasty.

V. OPERATIONS FOR TUBERCULOUS EMPYEMA.—Open drainage should be avoided for the risk of secondary infection.

1. Decortication, combined if possible, with complete excision of the cavity, is the treatment of choice.
2. If active disease is present in the lung, the affected part may be removed together with the thickened pleura *(pleuro-pneumonectomy or pleuro-lobectomy)*.

THE DIFFERENT OPERATIONS

Thoracoplasty.—In the present days, lung resection has widely replaced thoracoplasty, which had been a standard surgical procedure for pulmonary tuberculosis even few years back. Thoracoplasty is preferred to lung resection only under the following circumstances:

1. Cavities in the upper lobe with a persistently positive sputum and resistant organisms.
2. Where the risks of resection are unduly high because of extensive disease.

In the first group of cases, only the upper 4 or 5 ribs (sometimes the first three) are resected subperiosteally so that the collapse is confined to the upper lobe *(selective thoracoplasty)*. In the second group, an *extensive* or *complete thoracoplasty* has to be undertaken.

After thoracoplasty, the chest wall falls inwards, achieving a lateral relaxation. Apical and mediastinal relaxation may be simultaneously achieved by separating the lung from the apex and the mediastinum *(apicolysis)*.

Artificial Pneumothorax.—This aims at abolition of the negative pressure in the pleural cavity, by injection of air into it. Refilling at intervals are required to maintain efficient collapse for two years or longer. Its advantage is its simplicity. Its disadvantage is that active disease might persist or even progress in the collapsed lung.

Phrenic Paralysis.—This may be made:
a. *Temporary*—by crushing the nerve.
b. *Permanent*— by avulsing the nerve.

The idea is to produce hemiparesis of the diaphragm. This reduces the capacity of the hemithorax and thus promotes collapse. The results are uncertain.

Intrapleural Pneumolysis.—This is usually employed as an adjunct to pneumothorax. With a thoracoscope, introduced through an intercostal space, adhesions, which prevent the lung from collapsing, are divided.

Extrapleural Pneumolysis.—This method was previously employed for upper lobe cavities but is no longer used because of risks of infection. It consists of separating the parietal pleura in the apical region from the surrounding structures, thus creating an extrapleural artificial space:
1. This space may be filled up with air, which depresses the apex together with the pleura, thus causing collapse— *extra-pleural pneumothorax.*
2. As an alternative to air, the apex may be kept depressed by some form of *plombage*—fat, muscle, or paraffin (used in older days), or solid balls of polytheline.

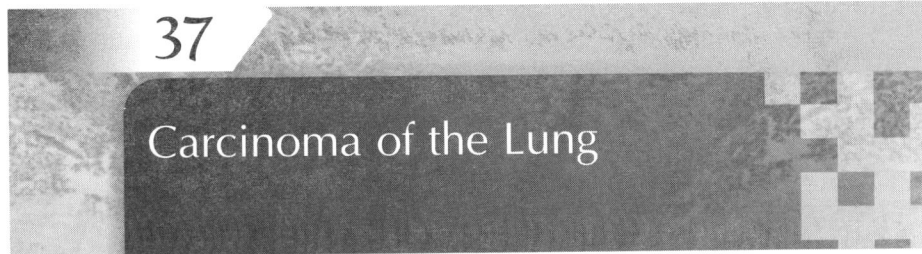

37

Carcinoma of the Lung

Lung cancers may be primary or secondary, the latter much the commoner.

SECONDARY CANCERS

The Primary Lesion.—While the primary disease may be located in almost any organ or tissue of the body, cancers which notoriously metastatise to the lungs are those of the kidney, breast, prostate, thyroid, testis and uterus.

Routes of Spread.—These cancers may reach the lung by one of the following routes.:

1. *By bloodstream.*—When the primary growth is situated in the area of systemic circulation, the cancer cells in the blood stream meet the first set of capillaries in the lungs, where they can rest and proliferate to form the secondary tumours, This is why lung secondaries are so common. Where the primary growth is situated in the drainage area of the portal circulation, the first set of capillaries that the cancer cells encounter is in the liver, so that liver is the usual site of first metastasis in these cases.

2. *By the lymphatics.*

Types.—The secondary deposits in the lungs may be of two types:

1. Multiple, peripheral and often bilateral deposits— the usual type.
2. A solitary central deposit, known as *'cannon-ball' metastasis* sometimes occurs, particularly from hypernephroma.

Tumours which metastatise in the lungs are:

1. Carcinoma.
3. Sarcoma.
2. Melanoma.
4. Chorionepithelioma.

PRIMARY CANCERS (BRONCHIAL CARCINOMA)

Etiological Aspects

1. This is the commonest cancer in the males now. The incidence is much lesser in the females (1:8).
2. Usually it occurs above the age of 40, but younger people may suffer and then, often, from the more malignant types.
3. During recent years, there has been a steady increase in the rate of bronchial cancers. The important factors, held responsible for this, are:
   a. Cigarette smoking.
   b. Atmospheric pollution, including smoke.
   c. Industrial hazards—dusts, fumes, dyes, etc.

Origin

1. From a main bronchus, close to the hilium— commonest.
2. From a small bronchiole, close under the pleura.
3. Midway between the above two.

Microscopic Types.—The lining epithelium of the bronchus, from which the cancer originates, is ciliated columnar. The histological types of the carcinoma may be:

1. Squamous-cell type (due to metaplasia)—60%
2. Adenocarcinoma—10%
3. Anaplastic, i.e. differentiated—30%

There is a special variety, included under the anaplastic group, which is known as the 'oat cell' type. These account for about 5 per cent of the cases and are the most malignant of all. The tumour consists of small cells with large nuclei.

Squamous cell cancers are the least malignant.

Spread

1. *Intrabronchial Spread.*—Along the wall of the bronchus there may be considerable spread through the submucosa. A main bronchus tumour may thus reach the trachea or even the opposite bronchus.
2. *Direct Spread:*
   a. Commonly to the overlying pleura or mediastinum.
   b. Sometimes to the chest wall or pericardium.
3. *Lymphatic Spread:*
   a. Primarily to the hilar nodes.
   b. Then to the subcarinal nodes (below the bifurcation of trachea) and paratracheal chain.
   c. From the paratracheal chain, the supraclavicular nodes (including the scalene nodes) may be involved
4. *Blood Spread*—To the liver, brain, other lung, and bones (particularly the ribs, vertebrae, and pelvis).

Clinical Features

1. Due to presence of the irritating lesion in the bronchus:
   a. Cough with expectoration.
   b. Haemoptysis.
2. Due to pleural irritation.—Pain in the chest.
3. Due to secondary pathological changes in the lungs:
   a. Complete bronchial obstruction.—Atelectasis.
   b. Partial bronchial obstruction.—Bronchiectasis, emphysema.
   c. Secondary infection.—Bronchopneumonia, pneumonia, lung abscess.
   Features of any or many of the above may be present, particularly dyspnoea and rise of temperature.
4. Due to pressure effects:
   a. Oesophagus.—Dysphagia.
   b. Trachea.—Stridor.
   c. Recurrent laryngeal nerve.—Hoarseness of voice.
   d. Superior vena caval obstruction.
5. Due to the malignant process.—Anorexia, loss of weight.

Pancoast Tumour.—This cancer, originally designated by Pancoast as 'superior pulmonary sulcus tumour' was believed by him to arise from the fifth branchial pouch.

It has now been established that this is actually a peripheral bronchial carcinoma, arising at the apex of the lung. It invades the neighbouring structures, viz. the brachial plexus, sympathetic chain, upper ribs and adjacent vertebrae, and this produces what is known as the 'Pancoast syndrome':

   a. Lower brachial plexus palsy.
   b. Horner's syndrome.
   c. Shadow of the growth at the apex of the lung, on the X-ray.
   d. Erosion of rib, seen on the X-ray.

The tumour is distressing because of the intractable pain that it causes. Also, the tumour is slow-growing and the patient has to live for a long period with this intractable pain.

Special Investigations for Primary Lung Cancers

1. X-ray chest.—This usually gives the most valuable informations.
2. Bronchoscopy.—This is an important diagnostic procedure. Centrally located tumours are seen and biopsy can be done. Operability of the growth may also be assessed—involvement of the trachea, paralysis of vocal cord and widening of the carina indicate inoperability. However, peripherally placed tumours may not be seen by a bronchoscope.
3. Laryngoscopy, to show evidence of paralysis of vocal cord (involvement of recurrent laryngeal nerve).
4. Tomography:
   a. Detecting and delimiting the tumour.
   b. Detecting enlarged mediastinal nodes.
5. Bronchography.—This may provide valuable information in cases of doubtful diagnosis.
6. Barium Swallow of the Oesophagus.—This may suggest extension of the growth into the mediastinum or enlargement of mediastinal nodes.
7. Cytological examination for cancer cells in:
   a. The sputum.   b. The pleural aspirate.
8. Scalene node biopsy.—If positive, radical surgery is contra-indicated.
9. Thoracoscopy, to demonstrate pleural metastasis.
10. Mediastinoscopy, to reveal involvement of paratracheal nodes.
11. CAT whole body scanning is being done in many centres for detection of distant metastases.

Treatment

I. RADICAL RESECTION —This is the method of choice, wherever practicable. It includes adequate removal of the primary tumour and the regional paratracheal, subcarinal and para-aortic nodes, preserving as much healthy lung tissue as possible. Thus, it may be:

1. Pneumonectomy—for main bronchial lesions.
2. Lobectomy—for peripheral lesions.
3. Lobectomy with '*sleeve resection*' of the main bronchus, for the intermediate growths. The affected lobe with a cylinder (inner layers) of the main bronchus is resected.

II. PALLIATIVE RESECTION.—Even when the growth cannot be radically removed, the affected lung tissue may be resected as this gives a good palliation.

III. RADIOTHERAPY

A. *Interstitial Radiation* with radio-active gold (Au_{198}):
   1. At thoracotomy, when the growth is found irremovable or is only incompletely removed, i.e. after palliative resection.
   2. Bronchoscopic insertion.

B. *External Radiation,* with super-voltage machines. The results are good as far as palliation is concerned.

IV CHEMOTHERAPY.—The results are not encouraging.

Staging of the Growths.—Lung cancers are divided into 4 stages:

Stage I. — The growth is limited within the lung.

Stage II. — Involvement of the broncho-pulmonary nodes at the hilum.

Stage III. — Involvement of the mediastinal (tracheo-bronchial) nodes.

Stage IV. — Distant metastasis.

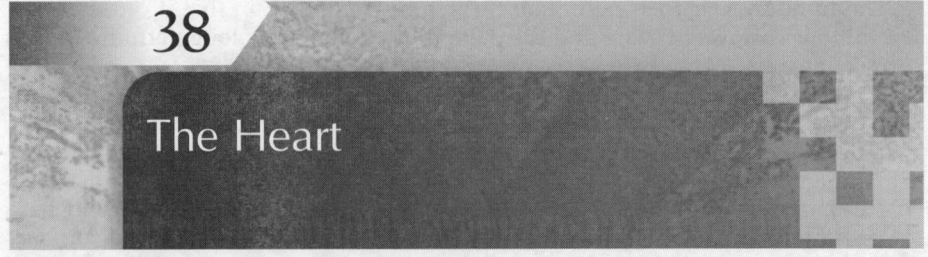

38

The Heart

SPECIAL INVESTIGATIONS

Remarkable advancement in the field of cardiac surgery in the recent years has been possible not only because of introduction of modern appliances (especially the heart-lung bypass machines) but also for introduction of excellent methods of investigations that provide accurate assessment of the patient and the pathology. The important available methods of investigations are described below:

1. **Electrocardiography (ECG).**—This is still the most commonly practised investigation and provides great details about the functions of the heart.
2. **Radiological Investigations.**—
   a. PLAIN X-RAY.—X-ray of the heart as well as the lungs are important:
      1. The shape and size of the heart can be made out
      2. In many pathological conditions of the heart there are gross changes in the pulmonary circulation and these may be demonstrated in the lung X-rays.
   b. FLUOROSCOPY.—Cardiac borders are better observed in postero-anterior (PA), right anterior oblique (RAO), left anterior oblique (LAO) and right lateral positions.
   c. TOMOGRAPHY, i.e. body section radiography, is not as useful for the heart as for the lungs but is helpful in determining certain conditions, e.g. coarctation of aorta, calcified valves, etc.
3. **Angiocardiography:**
   a. ORDINARY ANGIOCARDIOGRAPHY.—Sufficient quantity of a radio-opaque solution (Hypaque 85% or Urograffin) is introduced rapidly into the venous circulation and its consecutive passage through the right heart, pulmonary circulation, left heart, aorta and major arteries is recorded by serial X-rays taken at frequent intervals.
   b. BIPLANE ANGIOCARDIOGRAPHY.—The best X-ray machines for the purpose of angiocardiography are fitted with two roll-film changers at right angle to each other and allowing 12 exposures per second in both frontal and lateral planes. Bi-dimensional anatomical details of all the above structures are obtained.
   c. CINEANGIOCARDIOGRAPHY OR CINEFLUOROGRAPHY.—This is done by focussing a movie camera so as to illustrate the dynamic pattern of blood flow through the heart. The presence of a shunt or of obstruction or incompetence of a valve is recorded nicely.
   d. SELECTIVE ANGIOCARDIOGRAPHY.—This is a method in which the radio-opaque substance is introduced directly into the right ventricle. As the right atrium is bypassed. In this method, overlapping shadows are avoided.
   e. RADIO-ISOTOPIC ANGIOCARDIOGRAPHY.—This provides better sensitivity, safety and accuracy than ordinary contrast medium studies 99-Tc labelled albumin

or RBC is usually used. The course of the intravenously injected material is depicted as it passes through the chambers of the heart, the lungs and the great vessels.

4. **Cardiac Catheterisation:**

   a. RIGHT HEART CATHETERISATION.—A fine radio-opaque nylon catheter, 100 to 125 cm long (several calibres available) is passed from the medial cubital vein of the *right side* (entry into the heart is easier from this side than from the left arm vein). The catheter passes into the superior vena cava, then the right atrium, the right ventricle and, if desired, into the pulmonary artery. The passage of the catheter can be followed by fluoroscopy. Blood pressure is recorded at different levels as the catheter is connected to an electromanometer. Blood samples may be drawn from different sites, especially to know the oxygen saturation.

   b. LEFT HEART CATHETERISATION.—If there is atrial or ventricular septal defect, a catheter from right heart may be passed through the defect into the left heart. Alternatively, left heart catheterisation is done by the arterial route. The brachial artery is exposed in the cubital fossa and the catheter passed retrograde through the axillary and subclavian artery into the aorta. It is then pushed through the aortic valve into the left ventricle.

The normal pressure in the different chambers of the heart and the oxygen saturation of blood in these chambers are as follows:

Chamber	Pressure S/D	O$_2$-saturation%
Right atrium	+2/–2	60
Right ventricle	30/1	60
Left atrium	3/0	95
Left ventricle	120/0	95

5. **Coronary Arteriography.**—A soft tappered-tipped woven-dacron catheter is used. As for left heart catheterisation, the catheter is passed by the arterial route and as it enters the aorta, its tip is manipulated into the coronary orifices. It is much easier to enter the right coronary orifice than the left. A dye is injected and X-rays are taken. The state of the coronary arteries may be noted and the results of coronary bypass anticipated.

6. **Left Ventriculography**—After the catheter has been passed into the left ventricle, a dye is injected and X-rays are taken.

7. **Cardiac Ultrasound or Echocardiography.**—Beams of high speed ultrasound waves are directed through the heart. For a routine examination the transducer is usually placed in the left 4th intercostal space, close to the sternal margin. The beam is usually passed in three directions, one after another.

Position 1: The beam is directed medially and upwards. The anterior heart wall, the root of the aorta, the cusps of the aortic valve and the cavity of the left atrium are demonstrated.

Position 2: The beam is now angulated a little laterally and downwards. The right ventricle, the interventricular septum, the anterior and posterior leaflets of the mitral valve and the posterior wall of the left ventricle are shown.

Position 3: The beam is angulated into the cavity of the left ventricle. The interventricular septum and the posterior wall of the left ventricle are better demonstrated.

An ECG is simultaneously recorded with all ultrasound examinations.

CARDIAC ARREST

Factors to be Considered Together

1. Two conditions, viz. cardiac arrest (asystole) and ventricular fibrillation, should be considered together because either of them causes immediate cessation of effective circulation:

   a. ASYSTOLE.—This is due to. severe myocardial depression. The cause is very often either massive coronary thrombosis or severe anoxia. The contractions of the heart become feeble and slow, and the heart finally stops.

   b. VENTRICULAR FIBRILLATION.—This usually occurs in a heart which has been made irritable by drugs or manipulation or trauma (including cardiac catheterisation and cardiac operations). The ventricular myocardium contracts irregularly and feebly so that the cardiac output is practically nil. While on one hand the myocardium is less depressed than it is in asystole, so that cardiac activity is more likely to return to normal, on the other hand, unless promptly treated, asystole quickly supervenes. Considered from another point, when an asystolic heart is being resuscitated, it may pass through the phase of ventricular fibrillation before returning to normalcy.

2. While considering the dreadful condition of cardiac arrest, the work of the heart and that of the lung should be considered together. To start with there may be cessation of function of only one of these two, but very quickly the other stops functioning. Thus, cardiac arrest very quickly brings in respiratory failure while respiratory failure is the commonest cause of cardiac arrest.

Common Causes of Cardiac Arrest

1. ANOXIA.—Myocardial anoxia is the commonest cause. The anoxia may be due to:
   a. Respiratory obstruction or depression.
   b. Severe hypotension (usually from haemorrhage).
   c. Coronary thrombosis.

2. DRUGS:
   a. Drugs directly depressing the myocardium, e.g. digitalis.
   b. Drugs depressing the heart indirectly by way of circulation— vasodilators.

3. MANIPULATION.—Operations on the heart, including cardiac catheterisation and angiocardiography.

4. SERUM POTASSIUM.—Both hyper- and hypo-potassaemia, especially the former.

5. ANAESTHESIA.—Almost all anaesthetic agents, when used in excessive amounts, depress the myocardium. A combination of inadequate ventilation of the lungs and injudicious use of anaesthetic agents is the cause of cardiac arrest, in many cases.

6. REFLEX MECHANISMS.—Vagal stimulation, e.g. endotracheal suctioning, insertion of Ryle's tube, etc. particularly in the presence of diseased myocardium, may reflexly cause cardiac arrest.

7. DISEASED MYOCARDIUM.—A healthy myocardium can stand the distress of any of the aforesaid factors better than a diseased myocardium, which therefore is more vulnerable to arrest.

Diagnosis.—Cessation of circulation produces significant and often irreversible brain damage in 3 to 4 minutes. Hence diagnosis has to be made almost immediately so that the major part of these valuable few minutes are utilised for resuscitation.

The four cardinal features for diagnosis are:
1. Abrupt disappearance of peripheral pulses, best confirmed by palpating the carotids.
2. Absent respiration or gasping.
3. Dilated pupils.
4. Loss of consciousness.
No time should be wasted on complex diagnosis procedures since every second counts.

ECG is of *no value* in diagnosing cardiac arrest. ECG can only make possible a differentiation between cardiac asystole and ventricular fibrillation and this is of no importance as regards the starting of resuscitative measures, which are the same for both the conditions. The real value of ECG is to find the presence or absence of ventricular fibrillation after resuscitation measures have been instituted, in order to decide whether defibrillation should be incorporated in the treatment.

Treatment—Just to remember what to do in such a serious condition, when everyone is apt to be puzzled, the following formula is popularly advised:

A—To maintain the Airway. B—To breathe for the patient.
C—Cardiac massage.   D—Drugs.
E—ECG.   F—defibrillation, if necessary.

The first three of these are carried out as *emergency measures* by the person or persons present on the spot. The other three are employed in *subsequent management* as and when expert help and appropriate drugs and equipments arrive.

I. EMERGENCY MEASURES.—Maintenance of the airway and breathing for the patient are considered together as *ventilation*. This should go hand in hand with cardiac massage. To start with, ventilation is most readily accomplished by mouth to mouth insufflation of the lungs. This should be started instantaneously and has to be continued till less laborious methods can be arranged. A laryngoscope, an endotracheal tube and a ventilator should be waited for and when these arrive an endotracheal intubation is done and the tube connected to a ventilator. No attempt should be made for a tracheostomy which may be difficult under such conditions, wasting a valuable part of the available short time for resuscitation.

Cardiac massage and ventilation can both be performed by one person but are more efficient and less exhausting if two persons are available. This is a *closed chest cardiac massage* and is done at the rate of 60 per minute, a very exhausting procedure for the operator. The heart is compressed between the sternum and the vertebral column (the intact pericardium prevents lateral slipping of the heart). The heel of one hand is placed on the lower third of the sternum while the other hand is put on this hand to press the sternum for 3 to 4 cm intermittently. The compression should be brisk to depress the sternum sharply and should be released immediately to allow filling of the heart. The procedure should be continued uninterrupted till a heart beat or spontaneous respiration returns. There is no definite time limit after which cardiac massage is abandoned for death but the majority of successful resuscitations are accomplished within a few minutes.

Open cardiac massage, performed through an incision along the left 5th intercostal space, is only rarely employed:

1. It is usually done when the chest has already been opened for an operation.
2. It is preferred to closed massage by some surgeons if the patient is already on the operation table.
3. It is a must when there is cardiac tamponade or massive intrathoracic haemorrhage.

II. SUBSEQUENT MANAGEMENT:

1. *ECG* is done, preferably with a monitor, to determine the type of arrest, viz. asystole or fibrillation and to know how the heart is progressing to recovery.
2. *Defibrillation* should be arranged if ventricular fibrillation is detected. A defibrillator is used for the purpose. 100 to 400 watt-second are used on the close chest and 10 to 40 watt-second, if the stimulation is put directly on the open heart. There is a standstill of the heart, followed by normal rhythm.
3. *Drugs:*
   a. *To stimulate the heart:*
      i. If fibrillation persists even after external defibrillation has been attempted, calcium chloride (a powerful cardiac stimulant) is injected. 5 to 10 ml of a 10 per cent solution is used. Lignocaine 100 mg or procaine amide 250 mg may also be administered. These drugs are used either intravenously or by direct intracardiac injection.
      ii. If asystole persists, 10 ml of adrenaline (1 in 10,000 solution) or 0.01 mg of isoprenaline is injected directly into the heart. This usually converts asystole into fibrillation and then treatment for fibrillation is continued.
   b. *To correct metabolic acidosis.*—Cessation of circulation and the resultant continued tissue anoxia produce a state of metabolic acidosis and, unless this is corrected quickly, the heart may not recover, 60 ml of a 8.4 per cent of sodium bicarbonate is given intravenously and further additions are made, as necessary, to restore the normal pH of blood.
   c. *To correct hypovolaemia.*—Many cases of cardiac arrest are due to hypovolaemia. This has to be corrected quickly and an amount upto 1 litre or even more may have to be administered in jet by the intravenous route.

APPROACH TO CARDIAC SURGERY

A. Closed Heart Surgery.—The heart is allowed to work while it is operated upon. Access inside the heart is obtained by making a rent in the atrial or ventricular wall. The operation is done blindly (like Freyer's prostatectomy) either by finger alone or by finger and some instrument, controlled by touch. The heart continues to work during the operative procedure so that blood supply to the tissues is not interfered with. Majority of the cardiac conditions for which surgery is undertaken cannot be corrected by the blind method and with the heart moving continuously. Mitral valvotomy is possibly the only operation done nowadays by this closed technique.

B. Open Heart Surgery—Every surgeon would like to operate on the heart under direct vision (i.e. opening it) and also having it motionless. If the heart is made motionless, blood supply to the tissues will be stopped and, as in the cases of cardiac arrest, irreversible tissue damage (especially the brain) will set in within 3 to 4 minutes. No open heart surgery is possible within this short period. Devices have, therefore, been introduced to overcome this difficulty and these are as follows:

1. HYPOTHERMIA.—If the body temperature is cooled down to 28–30°C, the basic metabolism of the vital organs is so reduced that they can survive total deprivation of oxygen for a period of 10 minutes. This time is sufficient for correction of some conditions of the heart, e.g. atrial septal defect, pulmonary stenosis, etc. Such hypothermia may be achieved in two ways :
   a. Surface cooling.—The whole body is cooled either by immersion in cold water or by application of cooled blankets.
   b. Veno-venous cooling.—Only the blood is cooled. The superior and inferior vena cava are cannulated. Blood is drawn from the superior vena cava, passed through a cooling chamber, and returned to the inferior vena cava.
2. DEEP HYPOTHERMIA.—The body temperature is reduced to as low as 15° C. This is done by cannulating each side of the heart separately and taking the blood to separate cooling chambers. As the heart starts fibrillating at about 25°C, it becomes unable to pump out this cold blood when returned to it. A pump is, therefore, incorporated in each circuit. The patient's lungs, however, do the oxygenation of the blood. At a low temperature like this, the tissues can tolerate oxygen deprivation for as long as 45 to 60 minutes. This technique is very useful for correction of congenital heart diseases in the infants.
3. HEART-LUNG BYPASS.—This is achieved by heart-lung machines, which are basically pump-oxygenators. The pump works for the heart and the oxygenator for the lungs, so that an *extracorporeal circulation* is established. This puts the patient's heart and lungs at rest during the operation while maintaining blood supply to the tissues. The surgeon gets a safe period of several hours by which time complicated abnormalities like ventricular septal defect, valvar anomalies, Fallot's tetralogy, etc. can be corrected.

Any heart-lung machine basically consists of four parts:
1. Canulae and tubing which connect the patient to the machine.
2. An oxygenator.
3. A pump.
4. A heat exchanger to control the temperature of the blood.

Venous blood is withdrawn from the terminal parts of the two venae cavae, passed through the oxygenator, and then the pump returns it to the ascending aorta. At some point in the circuit, the blood passes through the heat exchanger.

The two vanae cavae are separately cannulated, approaching through the right atrium. The ascending aorta is cannulated through a purse-string suture.

Just before connection is established between the patient's circulation and the machine, the patient is heparinised (3 to 4.5 mg/kg body weight). At the completion of operation, the heparin is counteracted with protamine (6 mg/kg body weight). The extra-corporal circulation has a capacity of about 2.5 litres and the machine is filled with this amount of Ringer's solution just before it starts working.

4. OTHER FORMS OF BYPASS:
   a. *Left Heart Bypass*.—This is of great help in operation on the thoracic aorta. The left atrium is cannulated and blood drawn from it is pumped into the femoral artery (i.e. atrio-femoral bypass). With this procedure the aorta can be cross-clamped. The left ventricle pumps blood into the upper part of the body while the blood thrust into the femoral artery with the bypass supplies the lower part.

b. *Femoro-femoral Bypass*—The femoral artery and the femoral vein are each cannulated. Blood is drawn from the vein, passed through the oxygenator, and returned to the body through the artery. Indications for such bypass are the same as for the left heart bypass and this is done where the left atrium is not easily accessible.

c. *Regional Bypass.*—Blood may be withdrawn from the left subclavian artery and returned to the femoral artery while operating for aortic aneurysm or coarctation.

COMMON CONDITIONS WHERE SURGERY IS UNDERTAKEN

I. Acquired Heart Diseases:

A. DISEASES OF THE HEART VALVES.—In order of frequency these are:
1. Mitral valve disease—stenosis or regurgitation.
2. Aortic valve disease—stenosis or regurgitation.
3. Tricuspid valve disease—rare.
4. Pulmonary valve disease—very rare.

B. CORONARY HEART DISEASE, i.e. arteriosclerotic narrowing of the coronary arteries.

II. Congenital Heart Diseases:

A. DISEASES NOT ASSOCIATED WITH CYANOSIS:
1. Atrial septal defect (ASD).
2. Ventricular septal defect (VSD).
3. Congenital anomaly of the valves—stenosis and/or regurgitation. Stenosis of the pulmonary and the aortic valves are the commoner of these anomalies.

B. DISEASES ASSOCIATED WITH CYANOSIS:
1. Fallot's tetralogy.
2. Transposition of the great vessels—the aorta arises from the right ventricle and the pulmonary artery from the left ventricle.

III. Congenital Disorders of the Great Vessels:

1. Patent ductus arteriosus.
2. Coarctation of the aorta.

Shunts in Congenital Heart Diseases.—The main effect of a defect in either the atrial or the ventricular septum is an abnormal passage (shunt) of blood from the left side of the heart to the right (L-R shunt). This is because of the higher pressure in the left heart than the right. For the same reason, blood is shunted from the aorta to the pulmonary artery in cases of patent ductus arteriosus.

On the other hand, the shunt may be from the right side of the heart to the left (R-L shunt), if there is a septal defect *plus* an obstructive lesion at the exit of the right heart (i.e. pulmonary stenosis) or in the pulmonary vasculature. This latter lesion raises the pressure in the right heart to such a great extent that it surpasses the pressure in the left. Such a shunt adds venous blood of the right heart to the systemic circulation and causes cyanosis (cyanotic group of congenital heart diseases). The commonest example of this defect is Fallot's tetralogy.

While R-L shunts cause cyanosis, L-R shunts increase the volume of blood-flow through the pulmonary circulation because of the added blood from the left heart via the defect. This results in pulmonary hypertension (hilar dance) and dilatation of pulmonary vessels (pulmonary plethora). However, there is no cyanosis (acyanotic group of congenital heart diseases).

Mitral Valve Surgery

I. MITRAL STENOSIS.—The different operations available are:
1. Closed mitral valvotomy
2. Open mitral valvotomy.
3. Valve replacement.

1. *Closed Valvotomy.*—This is one of the oldest operations practised on the heart with good results. The heart is approached through a left anterolateral thoracotomy incision. The leaflets of the stenosed valve may be split apart with the right index finger inserted into the left atrium through its appendage. A better splitting is done by a valvotome (expanding dilator) inserted through a stab in the apex of the left ventricle and controlled by the right index finger inserted through the left atrium, as above.

Closed valvotomy can effect good results only when the valve is mobile and the leaflets are not thickened or calcified.

The ill-effects of the operation are :
 i. Re-stenosis.—50 per cent of the patients who had a valvotomy done more than 10 years back develop re-stenosis.
 ii. Incompetence.—This occurs if a valve leaflet is torn during splitting.
 iii. Systemic embolism.—The risk may be minimised if the appendage of the atrium (which harbours the emboli) is excised at the end of the operation.

2. *Open Valvotomy.*—This is done with the aid of heart–lung machines. The defects in the valve are carefully noted and dealt with as necessary. The fused leaflets are accurately incised and the fused chordae tendinae are carefully separated. The irregularities and tears in the leaflets are corrected.

3. *Valve Replacement.* —If the valve is grossly deformed or calcified it has to be replaced. The valve is excised and is replaced by a prosthesis. Three types of prosthesis are available,
 i. Ball valve,
 ii. Disc or hinge valve,
 iii. Tissue valve—usually procine graft is used.

II. MITRAL INCOMPETENCE.—Open heart surgery has to be undertaken with the help of a heart–lung bypass:
1. Usually the choice of operation is valve replacement.
2. If the valve leaflets are still pliable, some form of valvuloplasty may be done.

Aortic Valve Surgery—There may be stenosis, regurgitation or both. The cause may be congenital, rheumatic or degenerative. The cases of rheumatic origin are often associated with mitral valve disease.

The surgery is almost always an *aortic valve* replacement because, by the time symptoms appear and surgery is contemplated, the architecture of the valve is so damaged that any form of valvuloplasty is impossible. The types of valve replacement are the same as described under mitral valve replacement. Some surgeons, however, use homografts—taking human mitral valve and placing it upside down to replace the aortic valve.

Surgery for Coronary (Ischaemic) Heart Diseases.—The chief aim of surgery is to relieve the anginal pain (claudication). The principal group of patients for whom surgery is contemplated is those with angina of a degree that alters the life pattern of the patient and remains unresponsive to drug therapy.

All the cases should be primarily investigated by :

1. Coronary arteriography.—This will demonstrate the site and the length of the obstructive segments. Obviously, those having central obstructions with good distal lumens will benefit with the bypass operation. Bypass will be of little avail in the cases with extensive peripheral occlusions.

2. Left ventriculography.—If there is a diffusely dyskinetic (i.e. poorly contracting) left ventricle, the patient is bad-risk for any operation and the results of the operation are also poor. On the other hand, if there is a localised area of poor contraction or ventricular aneurysm, surgery is definitely indicated since excision of this area of the aneurysm will surely improve ventricular function.

The patient's saphenous vein is used for the purpose of grafting (*autogenous vein graft*). There are three main coronary vessels and some or all of these may require grafting. Proximally the graft is attached to the ascending aorta and distally to the affected coronary artery beyond obstruction.

Surgery for Atrial Septal Defect.—The defect is closed under direct vision, using heart-lung bypass. A small defect (less than 2 cm) can be repaired by direct sutures. For larger defects a dacron or terylene patch is used to cover the hole. Alternatively, pericardium may be used as a patch.

Surgery for Ventricular Septal Defect.—The gap is closed under direct vision with the help of heart-lung bypass. A dacron or terylene patch, or a piece of pericardium is used to cover the rent. The chief *hazard* of the operation is heart block because the Bundle of His, which runs along the lower border of the gap, is sometimes caught by the stitches.

Surgery for Fallot's Tetralogy.—In Fallot's tetralogy there are three primary defects and one secondary feature.

1. Stenosis of the pulmonary tract.—Causing arise of pressure in the right ventricle.
2. Ventricular septal defect.—Allowing deoxygenated blood from the right ventricle to pass to the left ventricle (the shunt is R-L and not L-R because of the rise of pressure in the right ventricle, as mentioned under (1) above).
3. Root of the aorta is displaced to the right so that it overrides the septum and therefore receives blood from both the ventricles (much of the blood is therefore deoxygenated and the body is cyanosed).
4. Gross hypertrophy of the right ventricle as a result of increased workload— this is the secondary feature.

Surgery for this condition may be considered under two headings:

1. COMPLETE CORRECTION.—Patient who have only a moderate degree of pulmonary stenosis and minimal cyanosis can be made to wait till they are sufficiently grown upto stand complete correction of the defects which is a major surgical procedure. The operation is usually undertaken between 5 and 10 years of age. It is done with the help of heart–lung bypass. The VSD is closed with a dacron or terylene patch. The pulmonary stenosis is cut and relieved.

2. TEMPORISING PROCEDURES.—These operations are relatively simple and aim at improving the blood flow to the lungs by creating an anastomosis between the aorta or one of its main branches and pulmonary artery. This allows the child to

live and grow so that he becomes fit to stand the operation of complete correction:

a. *Blalock's Operation.*—This is the most popular operation. The left subclavian artery (which arises from the arch of the aorta) is mobilised from its origin upto the first rib. Here it is divided and the cut proximal end is anastomosed end-to-side with an opening made on the left pulmonary artery. If this operation cannot be performed for technical reasons, one of the following anastomoses may be done.

b. Ascending aorta—right pulmonary artery (Waterson–Cooley).

c. Descending aorta—left pulmonary artery (Pott's).

Surgery for Patent Ductus Arteriosus.—The ductus connects the main pulmonary artery (at its bifurcation) with the aorta just distal to the origin of the left subclavian artery. It is less than 1 cm in length and usually less than 1 cm in diameter. The shunt is L-R because of the higher pressure in the aorta than in the pulmonary artery.

Results of surgery are very gratifying with practically no risk of mortality. Ligation of the ductus is the standard procedure, chances of recanalisation being very rare. Non-absorbable sutures are used—one at either end of the ductus and a central transfixion suture.

Surgery for Coarctation of the Aorta.—This is a stenosis of the aorta which is nearly always located just distal to the origin of the left subclavian artery. The constriction is close to the insertion of the ductus arteriosus or its ligamentous remnant—either above it (pre-ductal type) or below it (post-ductal type). The obstruction in the aorta results in hypertension above and hypotension below the constriction. An enormous collateral circulation develops in an attempt to supply the lower part of the body—branches of the subclavian (internal mammary, scapular) anastomosing with the intercostal arteries arising from the aorta below the block.

Surgery aims at excising the constricted segment and restoring continuity. In the majority of cases direct end-to-end anastomosis can be done because the excised constricted segment is short. In the cases where a long segment has to be excised, grafting is necessary to bridge the gap. Aortic homografts, which were originally used, tend to calcify. Teflon or dacron grafts are, therefore, preferred. When operation with grafting is necessary in a child, every effort must be made to leave some of the circumference of the aorta intact so that the reconstructed segment can grow with the child.

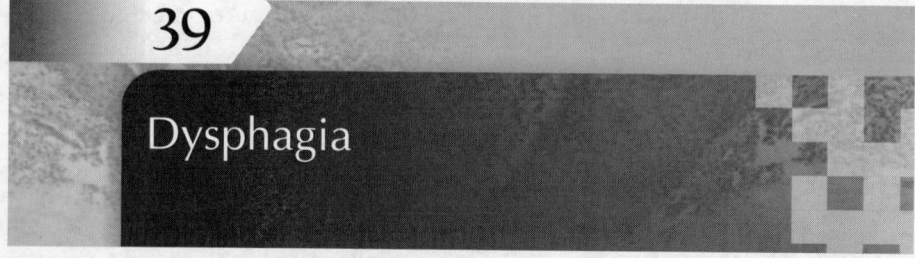

39

Dysphagia

This means difficulty in swallowing. The causes of dysphagia may be listed as follows:

I. Local Causes in the Alimentary Canal

A. ACUTE AND PAINFUL
1. Acute inflammation in the floor of mouth.
2. Cancer of the posterior third of the tongue, tubercular ulcers of the tongue.
3. Acute tonsillitis, quinsy, acute laryngitis, acute pharyngitis, retropharyngeal abscess.
4. Acute oesophagitis, reflux oesophagitis, peptic ulcers of the oesophagus.
5. Corrosion.
6. Foreign bodies.—Impaction, effect of transit, effect of removal.

B. CHRONIC AND USUALLY PAINLESS
1. Laryngeal tuberculosis, laryngeal carcinoma.
2. Pharyngeal pouch (third stage), pharyngeal carcinoma.
3. Oesophageal causes:
   a. Localised muscular spasm:
      i. Cardiospasm (achalasia of oesophagus).
      ii. Plummer-Vinson syndrome (glossitis, anaemia, dysphagia, brittle spoon-shaped nails; occurring exclusively in women of about 40).
      iii. Multiple ring contractions of oesophagus.
   b. Congenital stricture.
   c. Simple strictures:
      i. Following corrosion by swallowed poisons.
      ii. Secondary to reflux oesophagitis and peptic ulcer.
      iii. Secondary to Plummer-Vinson syndrome (oesophageal web).
      iv. Schatzki's ring (mucosal stenosis just above the cardia).
      v. Hypertrophic stenosis of oesophagus (muscular hypertrophy).
      vi. Scleroderma strictures.
   d. Tubercular strictures.
   e. Carcinoma of oesophagus.

II. Local Causes Outside the Alimentary Canal

A. ACUTE AND PAINFUL
1. Acute submandibular sialoadenitis.
2. Acute cervical lymphadenitis.
3. Acute cellulitis of neck, including Ludwig's angina.

4. Acute thyroiditis.

5. Acute suppurative pericarditis.

6. Acute mediastinitis.

B. CHRONIC AND USUALLY PAINLESS

1. Carcinoma of thyroid, big goitres and retrosternal goitres.

2. Malignant cervical lymph nodes.

3. Aortic aneurysm, abnormal arteries (dysphagia lusoria), pericardial effusion, dilatation of heart.

4. Mediastinal tumours or abscesses, malignant deposits in mediastinal nodes.

III. Distant Causes

1. Paralysis of palate, pharynx and vagus nerves :
   a. Diphtheria in children.
   b. Bulbar paralysis or lead paralysis in adults.

2. Hysteric spasm.

3. Hydrophobia.

4. Tetanus.

5. Myasthenia gravis.

6. Polio-encephalitis.

CARDIOSPASM

This condition, also known as *achalasia of the oesophagus,* is characterised by dilatation and hypertrophy of the oesophagus, without any demonstrable obstructive lesion.

Pathological Changes

1. The oesophagus is dilated, often grossly, the dilatation being most obvious in its distal two-thirds. Also, it is lengthened, sometimes by more than an inch, so that it also becomes tortuous.

2. There is considerable muscular hypertrophy.

3. The mucous membrane is stretched and thinned, and usually shows features of inflammation and, sometimes, ulceration.

4. The most characteristic changes are seen at the lower end of the oesophagus. As the dilatation is traced downwards, it narrows in a funnel-shaped manner, but a short distance above the cardia, the oesophagus attains normal dimensions. The musculature and the mucosa in the last inch of the oesophagus are normal.

Etiology.—The cause of the disease is still obscure and the various theories put forward are as follows:

1. It is due to spasm of the cardiac sphincter (hence called cardiospasm). However, there is nothing like a sphincter, anatomically, at this point.

2. It is a functional obstruction due to achalasia, i.e. failure of relaxation, which normally precedes a peristaltic wave. There are various views about this achalasia again, and the most popular belief, now, is that the condition is due to an autonomic nerve imbalance. It consists essentially of a failure of integration of the parasympathetic impulses (the vagus nerves supply the whole length of the oesophagus). The result is an irregular peristalsis in the oesophagus as well as failure of relaxation of the cardia, which together amount to *a functional obstruction.* The Auerbach's plexus (connected to the vagus), located between

the longitudinal and circular muscle fibres, are present but defective (c.f. Hirschprung's disease, where they are absent).

3. It is essentially a mega-oesophagus, the result of a congenital abnormality. It is actually due to a failure of propulsive effort rather than an obstruction, comparable to paralytic ileus.

4. Occasionally an epidemic variety occurs, associated with vitamin B_1 deficiency and trypanosomiasis *(Chaga's disease)*.

Clinical Features

1. The patient is more often a female, usually above 40.
2. The chief complaint is long-standing and progressive dysphagia characterised by :
   a. Insidious onset.
   b. Intermittent symptoms.
   c. More marked with liquids and less so with solids (weight of the food helps its passage).
3. The patient complains of 'vomiting' but actually it is a regurgitation, often several hours after the meal *(oesophageal pseudo-vomiting)*. In addition, abundance of froth and mucus are brought up. There is a foetid flatulence.
4. There may be a retrosternal or interscapular discomfort.
5. An aspiration pneumonitis and, occasionally, a toxic rheumatoid arthritis may occur.

Special Investigations

1. BARIUM MEAL EXAMINATION:
   a. Enormous dilatation of the oesophagus, with smooth termination of the barium meal. There is a smooth pencil-shaped narrowing of the lower segment (c.f. carcinoma, where the lower end of the oesophageal shadow is irregular and there is not much dilatation above).
   b. Absence of gas bubble in the stomach.
   c. An incoordinated peristalsis in the oesophagus; the incoordination is more evident if carbachol is injected.
2. OESOPHAGOSCOPY:
   a. There is a grossly dilated lower oesophagus, containing dirty water, moving to and fro with respirations.
   b. After the fluid has been sucked out, the cardiac orifice is difficult to be seen because of its contracted state.

Treatment.—The *principle* behind any treatment is disrupting the constricting fibres at the cardia.

A. CONSERVATIVE TREATMENT.—Here the constricting fibres are disrupted from within. There are two methods to achieve this:

1. Intermittent dilatation with oesophageal bougies. Dilatation must be done regularly.
2. Continuous dilatation with *Plummer's hydrostatic bag.* This often succeeds where dilatation fails, because the bag (balloon) can be distended to a transverse diameter of 5 cm. The bag consists of a tube, at the end of which a balloon is attached (comparable to Foley's catheter).

B. OPERATIVE TREATMENT.—This is required in about 20 per cent of cases, where:

   a. There is failure with conservative treatment.
   b. There are secondary organic changes in the oesophagus.

The universally accepted operation is *Heller's operation* (oesophagocardio-myotomy), comparable to Ramstedt's operation for congenital hypertrophic pyloric stenosis. The approach may be:

i. *Abdominal.*—A midline or left upper paramedian incision is made. The left lobe of the liver is mobilised after cutting the triangular ligament, and the cardiac end of the oesophagus is exposed.

ii. *Thoracic.*—After the lower end of the oesophagus is mobilised, a longitudinal incision is made through the constricted segment, and extending 3 cm proximally and 5 cm distally. The incision is deepened upto the submucous coat only, taking care not to cut through the mucosa, which bulges out through the gap.

CARCINOMA OF THE OESOPHAGUS

Microscopic Types
1. Squamous-cell carcinoma.—Majority of the cases.
2. Adenocarcinoma:
   a. Carcinoma arising from the lowest inch of oesophagus, which is lined by columnar epithelium.
   b. An extension upwards of a gastric cancer.
   c. Rarely, in the upper oesophagus. —A carcinoma occurring in heterotopic gastric epithelium in the oesophagus or at a site where there is columnar cell metaplasia.

Macroscopic Types
1. Annular stenosing type.—Scirrhous in nature, usually found at the cardia.
2. Ulcerative type.—A typical malignant ulcer.
3. Proliferative type.—A friable cauliflower mass, medullary in nature.

Sites—Cancer is said to be commoner at the sites of anatomical narrowing of the oesophagus:
1. At the level of the cricoid (15 cm from incisor teeth).
2. At the level of the aortic arch and, a little below, at the level where the left bronchus crosses the oesophagus (25 cm from incisor teeth).
3. At the level of the diaphragm and, a little below, at the cardia (40 cm from incisor teeth).

Spread
I. DIRECT SPREAD.—This is the main method of spread:
   1. *By Continuity.*—The growth spreads by direct extension in the wall, encircling it and causing narrowing of the lumen (more prominent with the annular type). There is also an extension longitudinally, for a variable distance. Submucous spread may extend far beyond the visible and palpable limits of the growth.
   2. *By Contiguity.*—Eroding through the muscular wall, the growth infiltrates into contiguous tissues:
      a. In the neck to:
         i. Recurrent laryngeal nerve,
         ii. Thyroid,
         iii. Trachea, sometimes causing tracheo-oesophageal fistula.
      b. In the mediastinum to:
         i. Mediastinum (mediastinitis and subcutaneous emphysema).
         ii. Recurrent laryngeal nerve (the left nerve is longer, hence more likely to be involved).

   iii. Trachea or left bronchus (fistula or fatal bronchopneumonia).
   iv. Lung (lung abscess).
   v. Pleura (empyema).
   vi. Aorta (sometimes with fatal haemorrhage).
   vii. Pericardium (suppurative pericarditis).
  c. In the abdomen to:
   i. Diaphragm.
   ii. Adrenals.

II. Lymphatic spread.—The lymphatic spread tends to be:
  a. in a downward direction, and
  b. initially to the nodes located actually on the surface of the oesophagus.
The nodes involved are as follows:
  i. In the Neck.—Lower deep cervical and supraclavicular nodes.
  ii. In the Thorax.—Para-oesophageal and tracheo-bronchial nodes, from where downward extension to subdiaphragmatic nodes may occur.
  iii. In the Abdomen.—Nodes along the upper part of the lesser curvature, viz. the upper coronary and paracardial nodes, from where efferents run to the coeliac group.

III. Venous spread.—It is exceptional for oesophageal cancers to spread by the blood stream. Only the cancers at the lower end may metastatise to the liver, by way of the left gastric vein (oesophageal tributaries). Rarely, the lungs may be involved.

Clinical Features

1. The disease is much commoner in men. Persons between 45 and 70 are the usual sufferers.
2. The leading and often the only symptom is progressive dysphagia— first with solids, and then with liquids as well. The patient often suggests the level where the food is held.
3. Regurgitation (*oesophagus pseudo-vomiting*) of food, mixed with froth and saliva, often streaked with blood, and alkaline in nature.
4. Discomfort—retrosternal, interscapular, or epigastric. Pain is usually absent till late in the course of the disease.

Special Investigations

1. Barium swallow examination shows a persistent irregular filling defect or a persistently stenotic segment. In cancers of the lower part of the oesophagus, the irregular narrowing is typically described as a '*rat-tail deformity*. A retrograde radiography, i.e. with the patient in the Trendelenburg position, may indicate the longitudinal extent of the growth.
2. Oesophagoscopy is the surest way to reach the diagnosis. A biopsy must be done while doing the oesophagoscopy.
3. Bronchoscopy should be done to exclude involvement of, or fistula formation with, the bronchus, in patients presenting with cough and purulent expectoration.
4. Exfoliative cytology.—The finding of cancer cells in the fluid obtained by oesophageal lavage may provide a very early diagnosis.

Causes of Death

1. Starvation, dehydration, and malignant cachexia.
2. Bronchopneumonia, resulting from fistula with the bronchial tree.
3. Mediastinitis and extensive subcutaneous emphysema, due to perforation into the posterior mediastinum.
4. Sudden haemorrhage due to erosion of the aorta (rare).

Treatment.—The aims of the treatment are:
I. *To Relieve Dysphagia.*—This may be done by radical resection, by palliative methods (conservative or operative), or by radiotherapy.
II. *To Treat the Cancer.*—Either by radical excision or by radiotherapy. Thus, the available methods of treatment may be considered under three headings:
   A. Radical resection.
   B. Radiotherapy.
   C. Palliative procedures.

Radical Resection or Radiotherapy—While both these methods are regarded as definitive treatment for oesophageal cancers, the choice between the two has to be based on the following points:
1. Almost all the growths in the upper and middle thirds of the oesophagus are squamous-cell carcinoma, while those in the lower third are either adeno-carcinoma or squamous-cell carcinoma.
2. Squamous-cell cancers of the oesophagus are fairly radiosensitive while adenocarcinoma seldom responds to radiation.
3. Radical excision, for growths in the upper and middle thirds of the oesophagus till remains a formidable procedure, carrying a high mortality, in spite of all improvements achieved in the exposure of the oesophagus, surgical techniques, and perfection of anastomosis.
    Judged from the above points, the usual trend of opinion is—radical excision for growths in the lower third and radiotherapy for growths in the upper two-thirds.

Radical Resection.—A radical resection implies resection of the tumour-bearing area together with the *entire oesophagus below this level.* Thus, the higher the situation of the growth, the more extensive is the operation. The upper limit of resection and the type of anastomosis depends on the situation and extent of the growth : —
1. For growths at the gastro-oesophageal junction:
   a. Some surgeons advocate excision of the lower oesophagus and the cardia of the stomach. Continuity is restored by anatomosing the upper oesophagus to the cut end of the stomach, the latter being made in the form of a tube and drawn up into the thorax.
   b. Others advocate excision of the lower oesophagus with total gastrectomy (together with spleen and tail of pancreas). An oesophagojejunal anastomosis is done by Roux-Y method.
2. For growths in the lower third, not involving the cardia.—The lower oesophagus is excised. The upper oesophagus is anastomosed to the stomach, drawn up into the thorax.
3. For growths in the middle third, if surgery is undertaken, the technique is the same as in (2) but much more difficult.
4. For growths in the upper third.—Surgery is only rarely undertaken. The whole length of the oesophagus is excised. The gap is bridged by an isolated loop of jejunum or transverse colon or by a polyethylene prosthesis, which is anasto-mosed at the upper end to the pharynx and at the lower end to the stomach. The jejunal or colonic loop is usually placed in a subcutaneous tunnel in front of the sternum *(ante-sternal),* so that it is not compressed by recurrence of the tumour. Also, if there is any leakage from the anastomic line, it is not in the mediastinum.

Radiotherapy.—Almost all cases of upper-third growths are treated by radiation. Majority of the growths in the middle third are also similarly treated. Introduction of cobalt-60, which has a high penetrating but surface-sparing power, and the institution of rotational device, have substantially improved the effects of radiation. Ability to swallow is usually restored.

Palliative Procedures

I. WHEN IMPROBABILITY IS DECIDED STRAIGHTWAY (CLINICALLY):

1. In the present days, introduction of a tube in the oesophagus is, more or less, the universally accepted procedure. It keeps the passage open, allows the patient to eat and drink as long as he lives, and also prevents aspiration pneumonia (none of these can be achieved by gastrostomy). There are two types of tubes :

   a. *Celestins Tube*—This is made of flexible polyethylene and carries, at its upper end, an oval barrel-shaped funnel of the size of a bolus. The tube passes through the carcinomatous segment and the funnel keeps at the upper end of the growth. For the purpose of introduction, the tube is threaded to a pilot bougie, which is passed under direct vision with an oesophagoscope. A gastrotomy is done to remove the bougie and to cut the excess of the tube. The stomach wound is closed.

   b. *Souttar's Tube.*—This is made of German silver and may be pushed blindly or with an oesophagoscope. It is less effective than Celestin's tube and is reserved only for the terminal cases with severe dysphagia.

2. *Gastrostomy.*—It is seldom done except when there is complete obstruction and intubation is impossible.

II. WHEN INOPERABILITY IS DECIDED AFTER THORACOTOMY.—The growth may be by-passed as follows:

1. *For growths in the lower third*—By oesophago-jejunostomy; the oesophagus is transacted above the growth, its lower end closed, and the cut upper end anastomosed, Roux-Y, with the jejunum.

2. *For growths in the middle third.*—By oesophago-gastrostomy; as above, the anastomosis is done with the stomach mobilised up.

3. *For growths in the upper third.*—By isolated jejunal or colonic loops placed ante-sternal, i.e. subcutaneously.

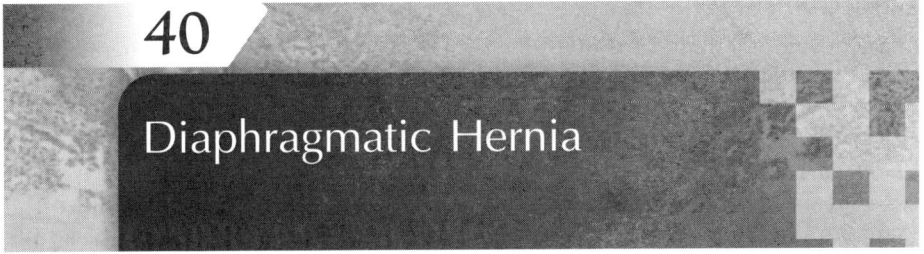

40

Diaphragmatic Hernia

Displacement of abdominal viscera into the thorax, through a gap in the diaphragm makes a diaphragmatic hernia. The fixation of the thoracic contents prevents prolapse in the reverse direction.

98 per cent of diaphragmatic herniae occur through the oesophageal hiatus, i.e. oesophageal hiatus hernia.

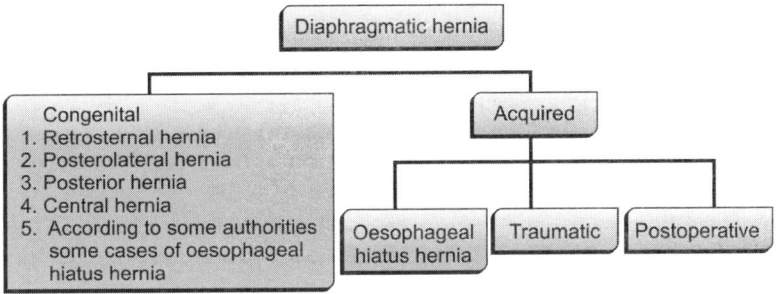

CONGENITAL DIAPHRAGMATIC HERNIA

Development of the Diaphragm.—Developmentally, the diaphragm is a composite structure and the septum transversum plays a major role in its formation. This septum is derived from the caudal wall of the pericardium. The septum, the pericardium and the heart are formed in the neck and obtain their innervation there (C 3, 4, 5). They migrate caudally to their ultimate destinations, carrying their nerve supply with them.

Developmentally, the diaphragm has five parts:

1. The *ventral part* is developed from the septum transversum. It is attached to the xiphisternum and forms:
   a. The central tendon.
   b. The central part of the muscle of the diaphragm, as far back as the oesophageal hiatus (including the venacaval opening).
2. The *two dorsal parts*, which form:
   a. The crura.
   b. The part of the diaphragm from the vertebrae posteriorly to as far forwards as the oesophageal hiatus (including the aortic opening)
3. The *two ventrolateral parts*, which form that part of the diaphragm which is attached to the ribs.

Types of Congenital Diaphragmatic Herniae.—These herniae result from errors in the development and fusion of the different embryological components of the diaphragm. Congenital diaphragmatic herniae are rare in that they constitute only two per cent of *all* diaphragmatic herniae. The different types of these rare herniae are as follows:

1. *Retrosternal Hernia* (through the Foramen of Morgagni).—This foramen exists between the ventral (xisphisternal) and lateral (costal) slips or origin of the diaphragm, i.e. between (1) and (3) of the embryonal components. In the adults the superior epigastric vessels pass through this foramen. This hernia is commoner on the right side.

2. *Posterolateral Hernia* (through the Foramen of Bochdalek, i.e. the Pleuroperitoneal Hiatus).—This results from failure of fusion between the dorsal and ventrolateral parts of the developing diaphragm, i.e. between (2) and (3) of the embryonal components. So, the hernia is located between the lumbar and costal parts of the muscle. It is commoner on the left side. Almost always there is no hernial sac, and the abdominal organs, usually consisting of small intestines and colon, move freely in the chest.

3. *Posterior Hernia* (Hernia Diaphragmatica Transversa).—This results from failure of development of the dorsal parts of the diaphragm, i.e. (2) of the embryonal components. There is a wide gap and there is no sac.

4. *Central Hernia* (through the Dome of the Diaphragm).—This is believed to result from an intra-uterine rupture of the central membranous part of the developing diaphragm. It is usually left-sided. There is no sac.

Some Important Points

1. *Eventration.*—Eventration of the diaphragm is not a true hernia because the gut lies below the diaphragm. It is due to absence of muscle in the left half of the diaphragm; which is replaced by fibrous tissue covered with pleura and peritoneum. There are usually no symptoms and the condition is noticed during routine X-rays. It may result from:
   a. Congenital defect.
   b. Paralysis of phrenic nerve.
   c. Anterior poliomyelitis.

2. *Congenital Oesophageal Hiatus Hernia.*—According to many authorities, all oesophageal hiatus herniae are acquired. Others believed that:
   a. The 'rollin' type of hiatus hernia is congenital.
   b. There is an entity known as *congenital short oesophagus* and this accounts for at least some cases of congenital 'sliding' type of hiatus hernia.

ACQUIRED DIAPHRAGMATIC HERNIA

1. *(Oesophageal) Hiatus Hernia.*—This is the commonest type of diaphragmatic hernia and is discussed below in details.

2. *Traumatic Diaphagmatic Hernia.*—This may occur after gun-shot injuries or crushed injuries, causing severe lower thoracic or upper abdominal compression. It may occur:
   a. At the time of the injury.
   b. More commonly, in course of time, as the scar gradually stretches.

3. *Post-operative Diaphragmatic Hernia.*—This may follow thoraco-abdominal operations.

(OESOPHAGEAL) HIATUS HERNIA

These account for 98 per cent of all diaphragmatic herniae. According to many authorities, all hiatus herniae are acquired. According to others:
a. The 'rolling' type is congenital.
b. A small percentage of the 'sliding' type is also congenital, resulting from congenital short oesophagus.

Types.—There are three types:
  I. Sliding of oesophago-gastric — 85%
  II. Rolling or para-oesophageal — 10%
  III. Mixed or transitional   — 5%

Sliding Hernia

Anatomy.—The oesophago-gastric junction, in these cases, passes upwards through the oesophageal hiatus into the posterior mediastinum; also, it comes to lie at or near the highest point of the stomach. There is a small peritoneal sac, drawn along with the left side of the stomach. Thus, the pathology is precisely similar to that of sliding inguinal hernia.

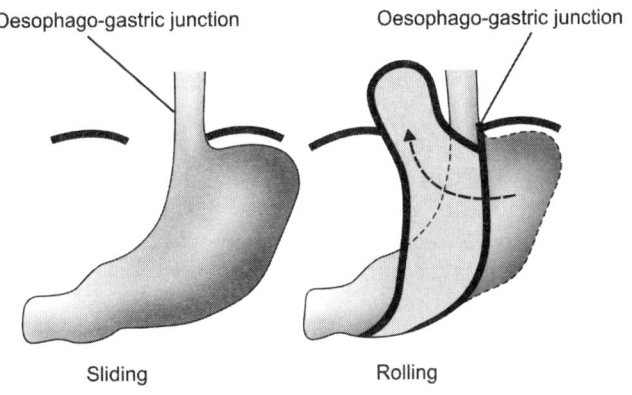

Figure 40.1: Two types of hiatus hernia

Etiology

A. According to some authorities, at least some of these cases are congenital, resulting from a congenital short oesophagus, which draws up the cardia and the upper part of the stomach. They believe that 5 per cent of sliding herniae belong to this group. Others discard this view and believe that all the cases are acquired since, at operation, there is usually no difficulty in restoring the gullet to its normal length. They think that the shortening is more often due to, or is exaggerated by, spasm of the oesophagus.

B. There are several factors in the development of the hernia:
1. Enlargement of the hiatus.—This is believed to be the primary factor and may be caused by:
   a. Muscular degeneration and relaxation (advanced age).
   b. Increasing adiposity (obese women).
   c. Aplasia of the right crus or decreased elasticity of the crus (obese women).
2. Laxity of the tissues which normally bind the cardiac end of the stomach and oesophagus. These tissues are:
   a. Perivascular tissues around the left gastric artery.
   b. Gastrophrenic ligament.
   c. Phreno-oesophageal ligament. This is a fascial layer connecting the fascia on the undersurface of the diaphragm to the fascia surrounding the terminal oesophagus.
C. Once the hernia starts, it is aggravated by:
1. Oesophageal spasm and, later, fibrosis resulting from reflux oesophagitis (*see* below).
2. Recurring negative intrathoracic pressure during respirations.
3. Increased intra-abdominal pressure, e.g. ovarian cysts, pregnancy, etc.

Pathology.—The real danger of a sliding hernia is the development of reflux oesophagitis. This results from postural regurgitation of acid gastric contents into the squamous-cell lined oesophagus. The factors, which normally prevent regurgitation of the gastric contents into the oesophagus, are:
1. The sling, i.e. the right crus of the diaphragm, which exerts a pinch-cock action (the left crus does not contribute to the formation of the hiatus).
2. The intrinsic cardio-oesophageal mechanism:
   a. The valvular effect of the oesophago-gastric angle due to the oblique entry of the oesophagus into the cardia.
   b. Interlacement of oesophageal and gastric musculatures.
3. Presence of a length (4 cm) of abdominal oesophagus.
4. The 'rossette-like' folds of gastric mucosa at the cardia.
5. Presence of the phreno-oesophageal ligament.

In cases of sliding hernia, as the cardiac orifice and a part of the stomach adjacent to it move up into the posterior mediastinum, all the above factors are disturbed. There may be a reflux of acid gastric contents into the oesophagus.

Reflux of acid does not occur in all cases of sliding hernia nor does oesophagitis occur in all cases with reflux of acid. It is likely to occur where the acid level is high or where the intragastric tension is released. So, it is commoner in patients with associated duodenal ulcer, pylorospasm, or pyloric obstruction. Gall stones, diverticulosis of colon, and hiatus hernia sometimes co-exist (*Saint's triad*).

The characteristic features of reflux esophagitis are as follows:
1. It is restricted to a narrow zone of terminal oesophagus.
2. The squamous-cell mucosa becomes inflamed, oedematous, and shows superficial erosions. These erosions tend to bleed insidiously so that there may be a gross secondary anaemia. Rarely, haematemesis and malaena may occur.

3. There is a spasm of the circular fibres at the end of the oesophagus. Later, a stricture may actually form due to fibrosis at the site of the erosion. These factors lead to dysphagia and impaired nutrition.
4. Still later, the inflammatory process extends through the wall of the oesophagus, resulting in *peri-oesophagitis,* so that:
   a. the hernia becomes fixed in the intrathoracic position;
   b. there is a shortening of the oesophagus, which exaggerates the hernia.

Clinical Features

A. Many cases of hiatus hernia are symptomless, i.e. silent.
B. Some cases (according to some authorities about 20 per cent) may occur in children under 10 years. It may even occur in infants soon after birth and they present with effortless vomiting, small in amount, often blood-tinged.
C. In some cases, regurgitation of gastric contents into the oesophagus may occur in absence of a sliding hernia. In these cases the hiatus is patulous (normally the hiatus admits the tip of two fingers).
D. The usual group of patients present with features of reflux esophagitis, viz.
   1. Pain.—Usually retrosternal. It may radiate to the interscapular region, to either arm, or to the neck. The pain occurs more commonly when the patient lies down, and does not allow him to sleep. It is relieved on sitting.
   2. Dysphagia.—At first because of oedema and spasm, later due to stricture.
   3. Heart burn is a common symptom.

Special Investigations

1. *Blood Examination.*—Secondary anaemia.
2. *Stool Examination* shows occult blood in almost all the cases.
3. *Oesophagoscopy* shows the following:
   a. Inflammation, oedema, erosions and, occasionally, ulcers in the terminal oesophagus.
   b. Reflux of gastric juice through the cardia (this is the surest sign).
   c. The cardia opens on inspiration (normally it closes).
4. *Barium Meal Examination* has to be done with the patient turned into a semi-prone position on the right side and the table tilted to 20° Trendelenburg position. The meal regurgitates into the hernia from the stomach automatically, in cases of true hiatus hernia.

Treatment

A. Simple radiological finding of a hiatus hernia in a patient who has no symptom of the hernia, requires *no treatment.* In these cases, the patient should not be told that he has a hiatus hernia, for psychological reasons.
B. In all cases with symptoms, a course of rigid *medical treatment* must be advised. The essentials of the treatment are as follows:
   1. Sleeping in a semirecumbent position (propped-up), with the foot end of the bed raised by about 18 inches.
   2. Avoiding heavy work, excessive bending, and weight lifting.
   3. Diet every 3 to 4 hours, moderate in quantity.
   4. Maintaining an upright position after the meals.

5. Reducing the body weight if the patient is obese.
6. Antacids.

C. *Indications for Surgery:*
1. Patients not improving with medical treatment.
2. Symptoms interfering with the patient's occupation or if the patient's occupation demands heavy work, weight lifting, or excessive bending.
3. Onset of complications—stenosis, haemorrhage.
4. When an abdominal operation has to be undertaken, e.g. for gall stones, peptic ulcer, etc. the hernia should be repaired.

Operative Treatment

PRINCIPLES

a. To ensure a length of at least 4 cm of abdominal oesophagus.
b. To prevent this segment from returning to the chest.

OPERATION

a. *Trans-abdominal Approach:*
   i. After reducing the hernia, the hiatus in the right crus is narrowed by two or three stitches, which approximate the muscle fibres *behind* the oesophagus (in order to restore its normal angulation at this level).
   ii. *Fundo-plication.*—The mobilised fundus of the stomach is wrapped round the terminal oesophagus and sutured anteriorly by four stitches. This prevents the reflux as well as recurrence of the hernia,
   iii. Operation for any other associated abdominal pathology.

b. *Trans-thoracic Approach.*—This is done through the bed of the 8th rib on the left side:
   i. After reduction, the stretched phrenooesophageal ligament is sutured to the undersurface of the diaphragm.
   ii. The hiatus in the right crus is narrowed, as described above.

Para-oesophageal (Rolling) Hernia

This is a true hernia and is believed to be due to the presence of a preformed sac in the posterior mediastinum. According to many authorities, this sac is congenital.

The oesophagus is normal in length and position, and the cardia lies at a normal level below the diaphragm. The mechanism of the cardia is normal so that there is no acid reflux and no oesophagitis.

The hiatus is enlarged, particularly in the forward direction. Through this gap the fundus of the stomach rotates anti-clockwise, alongside the terminal oesophagus, into the mediastinum and towards the right side of the chest. Thus, there is a rolling upwards of the anterior wall of the stomach.

Symptoms, therefore, occur only when the hernia is large. The presenting features may be:
1. Intermittent dysphagia.
2. Cardiac symptoms due to pressure on the heart.
3. Bouts of hiccough due to irritation of the phrenic nerve. Operative repair has to be undertaken when there are symptoms. Usually the approach is intra-abdominal.

Mixed or Transitional Hernia

In these cases, there is a combination of sliding and para-oesophageal hernia. Operative repair has always to be undertaken.

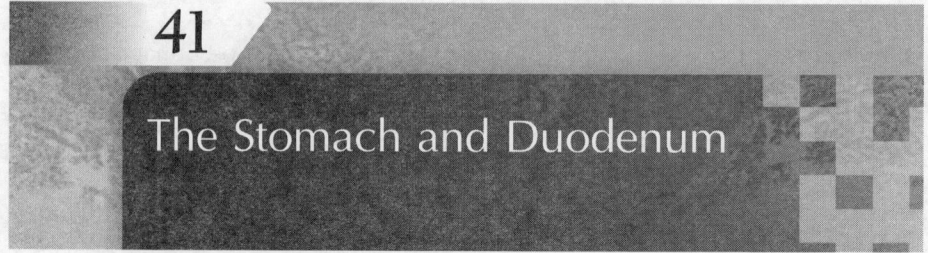

41

The Stomach and Duodenum

SURGICAL PHYSIOLOGY

Some Aspects of Gastric Secretion

1. THE CELLS.—The cells that secrete the acid are the parietal or oxyntic cells, lying in the fundus and body of the stomach. Strangely, the secretion of the antrum is alkaline.

2. MAXIMAL ACID SECRETION.—Each oxyntic cell has a uniform acid output and consequently the maximum acid secretion in a particular person depends on the number of parietal cells, i.e. the *oxyntic cell population*. The oxyntic cell population, in a normal subject, is one billion and in patients with duodenal ulcer it is 1.75 billion. Kay's augmented histamine test may be used as a method of assessing the cell population, i.e. maximal acid secretion (*see* under special investigations for peptic ulcer). In duodenal ulcer patients this is always high

3. BASAL SECRETION.—This is the secretion collected for one hour, from a fasting stomach, in the morning. In duodenal ulcer patients this is often high. It is very high in Zollinger-Ellison syndrome, i.e. non-insulin-secreting alpha-cell tumours of the pancreas.

4. VARIATION IN GASTRIC ACIDITY.—As seen on gastric analysis, the variation depends on:
   a. The proportion of oxyntic cell population that is working at the time of observation (dependent on nervous and hormonal stimulation).
   b. Neutralising factors.—Saliva, food, mucus, and alkaline pyloric and duodenal secretions.

5. CONTROL OF ACID PRODUCTION.—The acid secretion depends on two mechanisms:
   a. *Nervous Mechanism.*—Vagal stimulation is an important factor. The vagus carries parasympathetic stimuli from the hypothalamus to the ganglionic cells in the stomach wall. The impulses are transmitted across the synapase, through the agency of acetylcholine, and thence to the parietal cells. The importances of vagal stimulation are:
      i. It conditions the oxyntic cells to gastrin.
      ii. It controls the release of gastrin from the antrum.
      The nervous phase of secretion occurs before the food has come in contact with the stomach, e.g. looking at food, smelling food, thinking of food, chewing food, etc. It has been established that acid secretion, in this phase, is very high in the duodenal ulcer patients.
   b. *Hormonal Mechanism.*—This occurs when food enters the stomach. It is due to the hormone *'gastrin'*, elaborated in the wall of the pyloric antrum. The

hormone is probably released from the modified ganglion cells in the antral mucosa. The gastrin secretion is caused by:

   i. Contact of food with the antral mucosa, and

   ii. Distension of the antrum.

It is now believed that the vagal effect and the gastrin effect are not two distinct and separate mechanisms but are closely inter-related. Vagal stimulation controls the release of gastrin from the antrum. The practical importance of this point is that vagotomy not only abrogates the nervous phase of secretion but also may reduce its hormonal phase.

6. RELATIVE SECRETION IN THE TWO PHASES.—It is believed that, in some people, the vagal element predominates and, in others, the gastrin element. An approximate indication of their relative proportion, in a particular person, may be obtained by the *medical vagotomy test*. A Kay's augmented histamine test is done to assess the maximal acid secretion. On the next day, the same test is performed but, on this occasion, the vagal stimuli are blocked by a ganglion blockade agent. The amount of secretion due to gastrin mechanism now shows itself.

7. ACTUAL STIMULATION OF THE PARIETAL CELLS.—It was formerly believed that both nervous and hormonal stimuli exert their effect through the agency of histamine, which works on the parietal cells. Recently, this view has been antagonised. It has been shown that all the effects of histamine on acid secretion can be produced by a synthetic pentapeptide, *pentagastrone* (*see* under special investigations for peptic ulcer). This substance has a chemical structure like that of gastrin, and it is therefore probable that this is the final effector agent.

8. INHIBITION OF ACID SECRETION.—This is caused by:

   a. *The Antrum.*—The increasing acidity of the antral contents reflexly diminishes the secretion of the parietal cells.

   b. *The Duodenum.*—When the acidity of the duodenal contents rises or when fat is present in the duodenum, the parietal cell secretion is inhibited. This is probably due to a hormone, *'enterogastrone'*.

Functions of the Stomach

1. It acts as a reservoir for food.

2. It acts as a mixing chamber for food and renders its fluid for easy passage along the intestines.

3. It makes the food:

   a. colder or warmer, to make it to the temperature of the body,

   b. sterile,

   c. isotonic,

   d. adjusted to such a physical and chemical character that it can be effectively broken down by the enzymes.

4. It passes this prepared content into the duodenum in small amounts, at regular intervals (12 ml/minute).

5. It secretes pepsin and hydrochloric acid for the first stage of protein digestion. Equally, it secretes mucus to prevent autodigestion of the stomach by the acid.

6. It produces an internal secretion, i.e. *intrinsic factor,* which is essential for the absorption of vitamin B_{12}, and is thus concerned in haematopoiesis.

PEPTIC ULCERS

These are ulcers either formed or maintained by acid-pepsin secretion of the stomach. The commonest site is the duodenum and then the stomach. Sometimes ulcers may occur at rather unusual sites, e.g.

1. The cardiac end of the oesophagus.
2. The jejunum, at the site of gastrojejunostomy (stomal ulcer).
3. A Meckel's diverticulum, due to the presence of heterotopic gastric epithelium in its mucosa.

Sites of Gastric and Duodenal Ulcers

A. ACUTE ULCERS.—These occur anywhere in the stomach but usually only in the first part of the duodenum.

B. CHRONIC ULCERS.—There are special sites where these ulcers tend to occur *(ulcer-bearing area)*:
1. *Gastric Ulcer:*
    a. Typically, they occur on the lesser curvature of the stomach (and, thereafter, encroaching on the adjacent anterior and -posterior walls), anywhere from the oesophageal opening to within 3 cm of the pylorus. This is the area in the stomach:
        i. which is non-acid secreting, and
        ii. through which the food passes *(gastric magenstrasse)*, i.e. the area maximum exposed to trauma.
    b. Some ulcers occur in the pylorus or the pre-pyloric region.
    c. Rarely, ulcers may occur on the greater curvature or even the fundus (in these cases, all care must be taken to exclude malignancy).
2. *Duodenal Ulcer.*—Typically, it occurs in the first part of the duodenum. This is the area which is continuously struck by the acid chyme ejected from the pylorus, i.e. exposed to trauma.

Rarely, a duodenal ulcer may occur in the second part, but then always above the opening of the common bile duct.

Etiology

A. ACUTE ULCERS
1. About half of the cases follow ingestion of aspirin or butazolidine.
2. Many cases occur after acute infective and toxic conditions.
3. Sometimes ulcers occur in cases of burn and then they are called *Curling's Ulcer.* They are found in the first part of the duodenum and are often multiple. They often cause haemorrhage and may sometimes perforate.

Majority of the acute ulcers heal but a small percentage may persist and form chronic peptic ulcers. The chronic ulcers, that are encountered, represent this small percentage of persisting acute ulcers.

B. CHRONIC ULCERS.—These are possibly always sequelae to acute ulceration. Since peptic ulcer occurs only in those areas to which gastric juice has access, it is certain that peptic digestion is the sole cause for its origin. Also, since autodigestion of the mucosa of the stomach or duodenum does not occur normally, it may be assumed that an ulcer may occur either if the acidity is very high or, if there is a lowered resistance of the mucosa. It is believed that the first factor is responsible for duodenal ulcer and the second for gastric ulcer.

1. DUODENAL ULCER.—The important etiological factors may be as follows:

   a. *Hyperacidity.*—The acid secretion in duodenal ulcer patients is always very high. Moreover, these patients produce an excess of acid in the empty stomach (including at night), i.e. in the neurogenic phase of secretion. Autodigestion of the duodenal mucosa by the high acid, secreted from an empty stomach, is quite likely to occur, and this results in ulceration.

   b. *Genetic and Hereditary Factors:*

      i. It is found that persons of blood group O are three times more likely to develop duodenal ulcer than those belonging to other groups. So, there must be a genetic factor. Probably the blood group modifies the oxyntic cell population.

      ii. In many instances, chronic ulcers are found to run through generations.

   c. *Susceptibility and Emotional Factors.*—There are typical vagotonic patients who suffer more from duodenal ulcer. These people are tall and thin, and are energetic, restless, and emotional.

      It is believed that the stomach is the mirror of the mind, and so anxiety and mental strain are important etiological factors. Under these circumstances, there is not only an excess of secretion in the stomach but also increased vascularity and hypermotility. These effects are probably exerted through the vagus.

   d. *Endocrine Factors.*—In addition to the neurogenic (vagal) factor, the effects of emotional and other stresses are transmitted to the stomach also by way of the pituitary-adrenocortical axis. Moreover, specific endocrine disorders have been proved to be associated with peptic ulceration. The important endocrine factors may be enumerated as follows:

      i. Excessive adrenocortical activity (including long use of cortisone and ACTH).

      ii. Zollinger-Ellison Syndrome.—Ulcers occurring in association with non-insulin-secreting alpha-cell tumours of pancreas.

      iii. Hyperparathyroidism.

      iv. Multiple adenoma syndrome, i.e. adenoma in pituitary, adrenal, parathyroid, and pancreas.

   e. *Trauma.*—Caused by continuous ejection of the acid chyme against the duodenal wall.

   f. *Dietary Factors,* including deficiency of vitamins and proteins, may be responsible.

2. GASTRIC ULCER.—In contrast to duodenal ulcer, the acidity in the gastric ulcer patients is seldom high; commonly it is either normal or below normal (possibly due to the associated chronic gastritis). Hence the cause of gastric ulcer is believed to be a lowered mucosa resistance to autodigestion, rather than hyperacidity. This lowered resistance may be due to the following factors:

   a. *Dietary Deficiencies,* particularly of vitamins and proteins. Gastric ulcer is commoner in the poorer section of people, as compared to duodenal ulcer.

   b. *Trauma and Irritation.*—Trauma by inadequately masticated, indigestible, and hot food is an important etiological factor. This is substantiated by the fact that gastric ulcer usually occurs on the gastric magenstrasse. Irritation by alcohol or excessive smoking may also be responsible.

Pathology

Acute ulcers	Chronic ulcers
1. May occur in any part of the stomach or duodenum.	1. Occur, in 90 per cent of cases, over the 'ulcer-bearing areas'.
2. Usually multiple.	2. Usually single. Kissing duodenal ulcers (that is one on anterior wall and another, opposite it, on the posterior wall), and synchronous gastric and duodenal ulcers may, however, occur.
3. Usually shallow, not more than erosion of the mucosa. When they get deeper, they diminish in dimensions at the depth progressively, so that they have a typical 'terraced' appearance. Usually, there is not much evidence of the ulcer from the peritoneal surface.	3. Usually deep, but the walls are vertical, giving it a clear punched-out appearance. There is usually complete breach of the muscle coat and the ulcer extends to the subserous layer, which is fibrous, oedematous, thickened, and often puckered.
4. The surrounding mucosa is grossly congested and oedematous, or shows more ulcers.	4. Surrounded by a smooth mucosa, which overhangs the ulcer
5. Irregular in shape	5. Duodenal ulcers are round or oval. Gastric ulcers are bigger, round to start with, sometimes getting saddle-shaped.
6. Haemorrhage is common, perforation rare, penetration usually does not occur.	6. Haemorrhage and perforation both less common in proportion to the number of ulcers. However, perforation and penetration are relatively common.
7. Microscopically, there is a striking absence of inflammatory changes and there is no fibrosis.	7 There is a central area of necrosis, surrounding which there is lymphocytic infiltration. The most characteristic feature is an abundance of fibrosis. This fibrous tissue indicates stages of healing. A chronic ulcer repeatedly heals (even spontaneously), only to re-break. This accounts for the typical periodicity encountered in the course of the disease.

Incidence.—Duodenal ulcers are much commoner than gastric ulcers (at least 4:1; usually the ratio is much higher). Males suffer much more commonly than females both from gastric and duodenal ulcers. In this country, duodenal ulcer is rare in the females; gastric ulcer is not so infrequent.

Clinical Features.—The commonest presenting feature of the peptic ulcer patients is pain, usually having definite relationship to food. Haemorrhage is rather a common complaint and sometimes there may be haemorrhage from an ulcer which never had any symptom of pain. Though there are many features in common for gastric and duodenal ulcers, there are points of difference as well:

Gastric ulcers	Duodenal ulcer
1. *Periodicity.*—Less marked.	1. *Periodicity* usually well-marked and often the symptoms occur during the periods of stress and mental anxiety.
2. *Pain.*—Burning, spasmodic, or pricking in nature and, in cases of deep ulcers, there may be a penetrating pain to the back.	2. *Pain.*—Types of pain are the same as in gastric ulcer.
a. The pain starts almost instantaneously after taking food as the ulcer is irritated by the food and acid.	a. The pain usually starts 2 to 2½ hours after taking food, i.e. the time when the acidity in the stomach reaches its peak, the pylorus opens up, acid chyme enters the duodenum and irritates the ulcer. In some patients, however, the stomach is hypermotile and the pylorus opens up very quickly. In these cases, the pain may start much earlier, even 15 to 30 minutes after taking food
b. There is no pain in empty stomach as there is no acid secretion then.	b. These patients, securing good amount of acid, even in empty stomach (neurogenic phase), have nothing to dilute the acid there. The raw acid, entering the duodenum, causes irritation of the ulcer, and pain. So, there is pain in empty stomach.
c. Food never relieves pain.	c. While the patient is getting pain in empty stomach, if he takes some food, there is dilution of the acid and he is relieved of the pain for the time being. Since food relieves pain which the patient was having in empty stomach, the pain is described as '*hunger pain*'.
d. No pain at night when the stomach is empty.	d. Nocturnal pain, awakening the patient, is common because the patient secretes in empty stomach at night.

3. *Vomiting.*—Fairly common, often after food. Vomiting relieves pain, therefore, often self-induced.

3. *Vomiting.*—Not so common, nor so typical, unless it is self-induced.

4. *Haemorrhage.*—A big haemorrhage from the ulcer is manifested usually as haematemesis. Also, because some of the blood passes down the gut, there is often malaena (altered or reduced blood, giving the stool a tarry black colour; the blood is digested and reduced as it comes down).

4. *Haemorrhage,* if it occurs, is usually manifested as malaena. Only when the haemorrhage is so massive as to force open the pylorus, that haematemesis occurs.

5. *Appetite.*—Gradually there is a loss of appetite. Primarily, this is because the patient is afraid of taking food but later because of the associated chronic gastritis

5. *Appetite* is good and the patient is usually advised to take food at regular intervals. He does it to avoid pain of empty stomach. However, he knows which foods are to be avoided.

6. *Loss of Weight.*—Hence, by the time the patient presents, there is loss of weight and anaemia

6. *Weight* is usually not lost. On the contrary, the patient often gains weight because of regular diet and a diet rich in milk.

7. *Malignancy* is sometimes a sequela to a chronic gastric ulcer, though the frequency of such malignant change is debatable.

7. *Malignancy* virtually never occurs

8. *On Examination.*—Tenderness is usually elicited to the left of the midline on the epigastrium.

8. *On Examination.*—Tenderness is elicited:
   a. At the duodenal point (in the transpyloric plane, just lateral to the lateral border of the right rectus), in some cases;
   b. Over the midline on the epigastrium, in some cases;
   c. At both the above points in the others.

Special Investigations

I. OCCULT BLOOD IN THE STOOL is detectable in all cases of active ulcer because a little oozing constantly occurs from its surface. While testing for occult blood, all iron-containing food and drugs, as well as green vegetables, must be stopped in order to avoid false positive results (occult blood means hidden blood, which cannot be seen by naked eye but is demonstrable by chemical tests, e.g. benzidine test).

II. TESTS FOR GASTRIC ACIDITY

A. THE OLDER METHODS:

1. *Fractional Test-Meal Analysis (FTM).*—A Ryle's tube is inserted in the morning, and all contents from the stomach aspirated and measured (this is *the fasting content,* normally 50 to 70 ml). The patient now drinks the test meal, which is

either gruel or 7 per cent alcohol. Thereafter, every 15 minutes, a fraction of the gastric contents, about 10 ml each time, is drawn out and collected in separate test tubes. 12 such samples are obtained over a period of 3 hours. These samples are titrated for hydrochloric acid as well as total acid (i.e. including organic acids). They are also tested for the presence of blood, bile, and mucus.

2. *Insulin Analysis.*—The procedure is same as above but instead of the test meal, crystalline insulin, 15 units, is given intravenously and samples collected as above. Insulin causes temporary hypoglycaemia that stimulates the hypothalamus→vagal centres→vagus nerves, and thus initiates a nervous phase of secretion in the stomach. Hence, this test was used to assess the neurogenic phase of secretion in the ulcer patients.

This insulin analysis (Hollander's test) is nowadays abandoned ordinarily as a preoperative investigation. Its only application, now, is to test for completeness of vagotomy in the duodenal ulcer patients. If, after vagotomy, the acid secretion in response to insulin is more than 20 m Eq. per litre above the basal level, vagotomy is believed to be incomplete.

B. THE RECENT METHODS:

1. *Kay's Augmented Histamine Test.*—The idea behind this test is to assess the oxyntic cell population. It is now confirmed that the amount of hydrochloric acid secretion is directly proportionate to the number of oxyntic cells in the stomach wall. Stimulation of the total cell population to activity may be readily achieved by injecting a *heavy dose* of histamine (4 times the usual dose) and so this test is known as *augmented* histamine test.

   To counteract the side-effects of this excess of histamine, an anti-histamine drug, mepyramine malleate, 100 mg, is given intramuscularly half an hour prior to the injection of histamine. The dose of histamine advocated is 0.04 mg/kg of body weight and this is administered subcutaneously. An alternative method is to give a continuous intravenous infusion of histamine. Alternatively, *histology* may be used.

   From a fasting stomach, the *basal secretion* is collected for one hour, with a Ryle's tube. The anti-histaminic drug and then the histamine are injected. During the subsequent one hour, the gastric secretion is drawn out by the Ryle's tube. This gives the *maximal acid secretion.*

2. *Pentagastrone (Peptavlon) Test.*—Recently, a synthetic penta-peptide, with a structure comparable to that of gastrin, is being used with the same purpose as the augmented histamine test. With this, the gastric acid secretion can be maximally stimulated without any side-effects. Peptavlon, 6 mg/kg of body weight, is given subcutaneously or intramuscularly, and subsequently the gastric secretion is drawn out every 15 minutes, for one hour.

3. *Night Secretion (Dragstedt's).*—This test aims at assessing the inter-digestive or resting (neurogenic) phase of secretion by measuring the amount of acid secretion at night, when the stomach is empty. A Ryle's tube is inserted and the gastric contents are continuously sucked out for 12 hours from 9 PM to 9 AM In a normal subject, the amount of this secretion is about 400 ml. In duodenal ulcer patients, the amount as well as the acidity are very high.

4. *Assessment of the Humoral Phase of Secretion.*—A Kay's augmented histamine test is done to know the maximal acid secretion. On the next day, the same test is performed but, on this occasion, the vagal stimuli are blocked by a ganglion blockade agent. The amount of secretion effected by the gastrin mechanism, i.e. the humoral phase, now shows itself.

III. Barium meal examination.—This is done with barium sulphate. The findings are as follows:

A. Gastric ulcer
  1. *Screen Examination:*
    a. Tenderness at the ulcer-bearing area.
    b. Folds of scar tissue converging on the ulcer site (rugal convergence).
    c. Evidence of chronic gastritis.
  2. *X-ray Plates.*—A typical *ulcer crater (niche)* is seen at the site of the ulcer (usually on the lesser curvature), where the meal projects outwards from the smooth outline of the stomach. In some cases, due to the spasm of the circular muscle fibres locally, there is evidence of a *notch* (indrawing) on the opposite curvature of the stomach.

B. Duodenal ulcer
  1. *Screen Examination:*
    a. Hypermotility of the stomach.
    b. Tenderness at the duodenal point.
    c. Rugal convergence.
  2. *X-ray Plates:*
    a. An ulcer crater may be seen.
    b. In the majority of cases, there is a deformity of the *duodenal cap*. The duodenal cap represents the normal radiological appearance of the first part of duodenum. In chronic ulcers, the extensive fibrosis causes a deformity of the normal pyramidal appearance of the cap.

IV. Gastroscopy.—If a gastroscope is available, the ulcer and the whole of the interior of the stomach may be seen. The progress with medical treatment can also be studied at intervals. Recent introduction of the flexible fiberscope has overcome the technical difficulties of introduction of the stiff gastroscope.

Treatment

A. Medical treatment.—Unless there is a strong indication for early surgery, every patient should get the benefit of a course of medical treatment. However, the treatment must be very rigid. The outlines of the treatment are as follows:—
  1. Rest as far as practicable, and tranquilizers at night.
  2. Balanced diet at two-hourly intervals. Milk is the best diet and, wherever possible, a milk-regime should be instituted. Otherwise, milk and rice should be the main diet. In cases of acute exacerbation, a transnasal intragastric milk drip with a Ryle's tube gives remarkable relief.
  3. Antacids in suitable quantities and with each feed.

4. Antispasmodics at regular intervals. Probanthine is the best. It is an anticholinergic drug that diminishes secretions, particularly at night, and relieves pain.

5. H_2-receptor antagonists are administered. The drug used is Cimetidine. The parietal cells secrete acid when histamine acts on these cells. Specifically histamine acts on the H_2 histamine receptors. Cimetidine blocks these receptors and thereby prevents acid secretion. It is given in doses of 200 mg thrice daily after each meal and 400 mg at night (to control the night secretion). The treatment is continued for 6 weeks, after which only the night dose is given for about 3 months.

How long the medical treatment should be tried before it is discarded in favour of surgery is a matter of controversy. In duodenal ulcers it is customary to try it for six months. With gastric ulcers, however, because of the possibilities of malignant change, this period is usually shorter. It is customary to review the ulcer after 6 weeks. A barium meal X-ray is usually done and this is compared with the previous films—healing, even if partial, is usually manifested. If there is no evidence of healing, a gastroscopy is done and, if possible, four-quadrant biopsy is performed to exclude malignancy, if facilities of gastroscopy are not available, surgery is undertaken.

B. INDICATIONS FOR SURGERY

1. Failure of the ulcer to heal, or recurrence, after rigid medical treatment (6 months for duodenal ulcer, 3 to 4 weeks for gastric ulcer).
2. If the patient is unwilling or unable to undergo medical treatment.
3. Intractable pain with frequent loss of work.
4. Persistence or reappearance of pain after the patient has undergone surgical repair of perforation.
5. Repeated haemorrhages.
6. Appearance of complications, e.g. pyloric stenosis.
7. Suspicion of malignancy in a gastric ulcer, and for the same reason, all gastric ulcers above the age of 45.
8. Usually, an ulcer of over 5 years' duration.

C. SURGICAL TREATMENT FOR GASTRIC ULCER.—The rational surgery is partial gastrectomy, which resects the distal 3/5th of the stomach, including the ulcer-bearing area (the ulcer is usually located here), together with the pylorus. The ulcer is removed since it may turn malignant. As the acid secretion is seldom very high in the gastric ulcer patients, a limited resection like this is usually sufficient (c.f. subtotal gastrectomy for duodenal ulcer).

If the ulcer is located high up in the stomach, resection of the stomach *below* the ulcer always results in healing of the ulcer. The operative difficulty, mortality and morbidity are greatly reduced by this procedure than a high resection of the stomach including the ulcer. However, it must be ascertained that the ulcer is benign.

Some surgeons advocate vagotomy with pyloroplasty (*see* under treatment of duodenal ulcer) for gastric ulcer. As above, it must be confirmed that the ulcer is not malignant. Results are claimed to be satisfactory.

D. SURGICAL TREATMENT FOR DUODENAL ULCER.—There are two ways of approach to the surgical treatment for duodenal ulcer:

A. *Vagotomy.*—Resection of the anterior (left) and posterior (right) vagus nerves is performed at the cardiac end of the oesophagus. The rationality of vagotomy is that the major part of the hyperacidity in duodenal ulcer is neurogenic, mediated by way of the vagus nerves.

The operation is usually performed with an upper midline incision. The stomach is pulled outwards and downwards to approach the abdominal oesophagus. The vagi, which stand up in this situation by the pull of the stomach, are easily identified by palpation. A part of each vagus is resected to prevent regeneration.

Since the vagal fibres are not only secretomotor but also motor to the stomach, gastric stasis is likely to occur after vagotomy. Hence, the stomach has to be drained. The different drainage operations, that may be added to vagotomy, are:

1. Gastrojejunostomy.

2. Pyloroplasty.—The pylorous is cut through longitudinally 6 cm, opening up its lumen, and then sutured transversely. This widens the lumen of the narrow pylorus and provides easy drainage from the stomach *(Heineke-Mikulicz Pyloroplasty)*. Alternatively, a *Finney's pyloroplasty* may be done in which the adjacent antrum and duodenum are approximated to each other and an inverted U-shaped incision made on the two is sutured to provide a wide gastroduodenal anastomosis.

3. Antrectomy.—The pyloric canal, together with the pyloric antrum, is excised. In addition to helping drainage, this procedure cuts down the chemical phase of secretion considerably.

B. *Subtotal Gastrectomy.*—This is performed with the idea of bringing down the acid secreting cell population. Since the patients of duodenal ulcer usually produce very high quantities of acid, a major part of the stomach has to be resected, i.e. the distal 7/8th. The pylorus is included in the resection. Whether the ulcer-bearing area in the duodenum shall be removed depends on the technical feasibility in the individual cases. If gross adhesions around the ulcer makes mobilisation of this part difficult, the ulcer may be left behind since it heals spontaneously as the acid secretion is cut down. Moreover, duodenal ulcers virtually never turn malignant.

The operations of gastrojejunostomy and gastrectomy have been described in details in the Chapter on instruments, under gastrointestinal clamps.

Types of Vagotomy

I. TRUNCAL VAGOTOMY.—This is the operation described above. The trunks of the anterior and posterior vagus are resected at the cardiac end of the oesophagus. Thus there is a total vagal denervation *(total abdominal vagotomy)*.

2. SELECTIVE VAGOTOMY.—One of the complications of truncal vagotomy is diarrhoea. The anterior vagus gives a hepatic branch which supplies the liver and stimulates its secretion. The posterior vagus gives a branch which passes via the coeliac plexus to supply the pancreas. If a truncal vagotomy is performed, the liver and the pancreas are denervated of their vagal supply, their secretion is diminished

and the patient may suffer from steatorrhoea and diarrhoea. In selective vagotomy the supply to the liver and the pancreas are kept intact. The anterior vagus is traced downwards and the hepatic branch is identified. The vagus is cut below this branch. Similarly, the posterior vagus is cut below the site where the coeliac branch leaves the trunk.

3. HIGHLY SELECTIVE VAGOTOMY.—This operation aims at avoiding the drainage operation obligatory for truncal vagotomy. This is done by preserving the vagal innervation of the pylorus. The anterior and the posterior nerves of Latarjet supply the pyloric antrum and the pylorus, reaching the antral wall 5 to 7 cm above the pylorus. The trunk of the anterior vagus is traced downwards and its twigs supplying the terminal oesophagus and the fundus and body of the stomach are cut, till the nerve ends as the anterior nerve of Latarjet, which is carefully preserved. The same procedure is carried out with the posterior vagus. Thus the parietal cells are denervated (*parietal cell vagotomy*). This operation has not been very popular because, though theoretically sound, there are practical difficulties in identifying the small vagal filaments supplying the stomach so that the denervation may be incomplete.

Complications of Peptic Ulcer

A. ACUTE COMPLICATIONS
   1. Perforation.
   2. Haemorrhage.—Haematemesis and/or malaena.

B. SUBACUTE COMPLICATIONS
   Residual Abscess.—This may sometimes occur after conservative treatment for perforation.

C. CHRONIC COMPLICATIONS
   1. *Penetration.*—A posteriorly situated ulcer in the stomach or duodenum does not usually perforate because the adjacent viscera get fixed to it by adhesions and the ulcer does not get a free peritoneal surface to perforate through. Thus, the ulcer, deepening out of the wall of the stomach or the duodenum, penetrates into the adjacent viscera, most commonly the pancreas, occasionally the liver, and rarely the colon (gastrocolic fistula).

   2. *Malignant change* in a gastric ulcer.—The frequency of such change is widely debated and the modern belief is that the incidence is definitely low. There is some evidence to suggest that the prepyloric ulcers carry the greatest risk. Duodenal ulcers virtually never turn malignant.

   3. *Stenosis.*—The extensive fibrosis at the base of the ulcer may be sufficient to cause obstruction to the lumen of the duodenum or even the stomach, i.e. stenosis. The types of stenosis may be as follows:
      a. Duodenal Ulcer.—The popular term applied to the obstruction is 'pyloric stenosis'. This is a misnomer since it is actually a duodenal stenosis, occurring in the first part of the duodenum.
      b. Gastric Ulcer:
         i. If the cicatrisation is in the transverse axis, the result is an *hour-glass stomach.* As the ulcer is commonly located more towards the pylorous, the upper pouch is always bigger.

ii. If the cicatrisation is in the longitudinal axis, in a lesser curvature ulcer, the result is a *tea-pot stomach.*

iii. With a pyloric ulcer, a true pyloric stenosis may occur.

PEPTIC ULCER PERFORATION

Duodenal ulcer perforation is far more common than gastric ulcer perforation. If there is perforation of a gastric ulcer, malignancy should be carefully excluded. Ulcers on the anterior wall tend to perforate while those on the posterior wall tend to penetrate into neighbouring organs, usually the pancreas. When an ulcer is located on the anterior wall of the stomach or duodenum, its perforation occurs into the greater sac of peritoneum. If an ulcer on the posterior wall of the stomach perforates, the perforation occurs in the lesser sac. In these cases, on opening the abdomen, no collection may be found in the general peritoneal cavity if the epiploic foramen is occluded, and only on exploration of the lesser sac, the collection can be detected.

Pathology

A. THE USUAL TYPE

Stage I: The contents of the stomach or duodenum enter the peritoneal cavity and cause an irritation of the peritoneum. This is the *stage of peritonism.* As the escaping contents are highly acid, there is no question of peritonitis at this stage. This is simply a chemical irritation and the peritoneal contents are sterile.

Stage II: The peritoneum reacts to this irritation by pouring in a large quantity of effusion, in an attempt to dilute the irritating fluid. This is the *stage of reaction.*

Stage III: Thus neutralised, the peritoneal fluid is now secondarily infected by bacteria, either from blood stream or from lymphatics. Now the *stage of peritonitis* sets in. This is helped by reflex inhibition of the acid secretion in the stomach, soon after perforation has occurred. In general, peritonitis does not set in before 6 hours of perforation.

B. LEAKING PERFORATION.—If a perforation is very small and if it occurs when the stomach is empty, very little fluid and more of gas escapes into the peritoneal cavity. The irritation and reaction are localised, without features of general peritoneal irritation. This is called leaking perforation.

Clinical Features.—Almost always the patient is a male. In more than 80 per cent of cases there is a history of peptic ulcer but in the remaining cases, a silent ulcer perforates.

In some cases, at least, perforation and haemorrhage occur simultaneously, and the prognosis is worse in these cases.

Clinically, also, the three pathological stages are represented:

I. STAGE OF PERITONISM.—Usually the attack occurs after a meal but a duodenal ulcer may perforate even when the stomach is empty.

The patient feels an acute agonising pain in the epigastrium and sometimes typically describes it as something having 'given way' inside the abdomen. In some cases, the patient may describe the pain as *migrating* from the epigastrium, along the right paracolic gutter, to the pelvis and then on the left side of the abdomen, i.e. the course of the irritant fluid inside the peritoneal cavity.

There is vomiting, once or twice, till the stomach gets empty.

On examination, the patient looks anxious and the tongue is a little dry. Temperature is usually normal and sometimes subnormal. The pulse rate is about 80 per minute.

Respiratory movements of the abdomen are usually absent and often the abdomen is scaphoid. There is generalised tenderness all over the abdomen. There is an extensive rigidity compared to that of *card board*. The escaping gas tends to collect under the diaphragm, so that the normal *liver dullness* is either *obliterated* or is brought down at a lower level. Irritation by the fluid causes intestinal paresis and so intestinal sounds are not heard. A rectal examination may elicit tenderness in the pelvis due to collection of the irritant fluid.

II. STAGE OF REACTION.—At this stage, the patient may feel a little better but the general look and the abdominal findings do not show any improvement. So, this is a *phase of illusion*. However, because of dilution of the irritating fluid, the tenderness and rigidity may be a little less marked.

III. STAGE OF PERITONITIS.—At this stage the patient rapidly deteriorates. Incessant vomiting starts and the temperature shoots high. There is a toxic look (peritonitic facies), a rapidly deteriorating quick pulse, rapid shallow respiration, and gradual fall of blood pressure.

The abdominal rigidity is now replaced by gross distension of the abdomen.

Special Investigations.—Diagnosis is usually made on clinical examination. In doubtful cases, a straight X-ray of the abdomen, with the patient in the sitting posture, is often helpful. In this posture, the escaping gas tends to collect under the diaphragm, so that *subdiaphragmatic gas shadow* may be seen. This shadow is often crescentic because of the fluid level below.

Treatment.—In almost all the cases, immediate exploration and repair of the perforation is the treatment. A conservative treatment is indicated only in the few cases of leaking perforation. In some cases, a definitive surgery, instead of a simple repair of the perforation, is indicated.

As soon as the patient has been admitted, diagnosis confirmed, and operation decided, the following treatment is instituted:

1. Rest and injection of pethidine or morphine (sedatives should only be administered after the diagnosis has been confirmed).
2. Stoppage of oral feeding, introduction of a Ryle's tube and institution of gastric suction.
3. Intravenous fluid drip, which has to be continued in the postoperative period. To start with, the fluid is transfused rapidly to make up for the fluid lost in the peritoneal cavity. Thereafter, it replaces the daily fluid requirement, together with the amount of loss in gastric suction, i.e. approximately 2500 ml plus the amount of suction, daily.
4. A parenteral antibiotic.

Operation.—The abdomen is opened with a right paramedian incision. A hissing sound, on nicking the peritoneum, due to escape of the free gas from the peritoneum, confirms perforation. All peritoneal collections are sucked, and the stomach is drawn out to locate the perforation. Repair of the perforation may be difficult as the sutures tend to cut through the fibrous and oedematous tissues at the base of the ulcer. This difficulty may be overcome by taking the bites of the needle a little away from the ulcer, through the neighbouring healthy wall. Before the knots are tied, a piece of omentum is placed on the surface of the ulcer, and the knots are tightened on it—this prevents the cutting through. Finally, peritoneal toileting is done. A drain is put down to the right paracolic gutter, where the fluid tends to collect. The end of the drain is brought out through a stab in the loin.

Definitive Operation of the Ulcer in Cases of Perforation.—Ordinarily, repair of a perforation has to be followed later by the definitive operation for the ulcer. In some cases, however, the definitive operation has to be performed straightway in a case of perforation, e.g.

1. Suspicion of malignancy in a perforated gastric ulcer.
2. Perforation associated with gross haemorrhage.
3. Recurrent perforation.
4. As a method of choice by some surgeons in any patient, if received within 6 hours of the perforation, i.e. before peritonitis has set in. A straight-way definitive operation, i.e. partial gastrectomy for gastric ulcer, and vagotomy with gastrojejunostomy (together with repair of the ulcer) for duodenal ulcer, saves the patient from two operations and two convalescences. In absence of peritonitis, the results are believed to be excellent.

Management of Leaking Perforation.—Provided the diagnosis is certain, a conservative treatment may be tried in these patients. This consists of the following:
1. Rest.
2. No sedative should be administered because the progress cannot be studied as the symptoms are masked.
3. Stoppage of oral feeding, introduction of a Ryle's tube and continuous gastric suction.
4. Intravenous fluid drip to replace the daily fluid requirement and the loss in the gastric suction.
5. Parenteral antibiotics.

A close watch is kept on the patient. Any sign of a spreading peritonitis is an indication for immediate exploration and repair of the perforation.

A residual abscess may sometimes occur in these cases. Should this happen, drainage of the abscess has to be undertaken.

PEPTIC ULCER HAEMORRHAGE

Haemorrhage occurs due to erosion of an artery in the wall, usually the base of an ulcer.
1. *Acute Ulcers.*—The bleeding may be considerable because of severe congestion of the surrounding mucosa and because the ulcers are often multiple.
2. *Chronic Ulcers:*
   a. In case of gastric ulcer, the bleeding is usually from a moderate size vessel, often a branch of the left gastric or right gastric artery. Only

occasionally does a main artery, e.g. left gastric, right gastric, or splenic artery bleeds, causing a massive haemorrhage.

b. In case of duodenal ulcer, the ulcer is almost always situated on the posterior wall and the bleeding occurs from a branch of the gastroduodenal artery. Sometimes the gastroduodenal artery itself bleeds and this results in massive haemorrhage.

In cases of chronic ulcer, the bleeding often continues because the eroded vessel cannot retract to effect a natural haemostasis. This failure of retraction may be due to several reasons:

a. The erosion in the artery is on its lateral wall and thus there is an incomplete injury to the vessel, which, therefore, cannot retract.

b. Extensive fibrosis at the base of the ulcer prevents retraction of the vessel situated in this fibrous bed.

c. If the patient is elderly, the vessels are often arteriosclerotic and do not retract.

The initial haemorrhage, excepting when the bleeding vessel is unusually big, is usually not fatal. The patient deteriorates or dies under the following conditions:

i. Persistent oozing of blood or recurrent haemorrhages at a few hours' or days' intervals. There is progressive anoxia, resulting in complications like renal failure, coronary thrombosis, etc.

ii. The initial small haemorrhage, being repeated at intervals, is followed by a sudden severe haemorrhage (comparable to the warning haemor-rhages preceding severe secondary haemorrhage).

iii. Rarely, on the first occasion, a very big vessel like the left gastric, gastro-duodenal, or splenic artery bleeds.

Clinical Features.—While majority of these patients have a definite history of ulcer pain, there are many in whom the haemorrhage is the first manifestation of an ulcer, i.e. the ulcer was silent. In many cases of acute ulcer, haemorrhage is the only symptom.

As soon as the haemorrhage starts, the patient has a sense of ill-being, e.g. reeling, sweating, etc., the degree of which is proportionate to the amount of bleeding. In many cases there is a definite abdominal discomfort,

In the majority of cases it is a duodenal ulcer that bleeds (because, on the whole, duodenal ulcer is much commoner than gastric ulcer) and the presenting feature is malaena. Only when the duodenal bleeding is massive or when it is a gastric ulcer that bleeds, that haematemesis occurs first; malaena follows at a variable interval.

The initial bleeding often stops and, in many cases, within a few hours or days, recurrent haemorrhages occur. One of such haemorrhages may be severe and fatal. In other cases, repeated or persistent haemorrhage leads to a continued state of anoxia that may cause renal failure or coronary thrombosis. The majority of the patients, however, improve and survive.

On examination, there are all features of haemorrhage, viz. cold skin which may be clammy if the haemorrhage is severe, progressive fall of blood pressure, increasing and gradually weakening pulse, and rapid respiration.

The abdomen, except for a little fullness, usually does not show any abnormality. In some cases there may be gross distension. In other cases rigidity may be marked, and in these cases, an associated perforation has to be carefully excluded.

Treatment.—In the majority of patients, conservative treatment arrests the haemorrhage. This consists of the following:

1. Absolute bed rest.
2. Sedation.—Morphine or pethidine.
3. Immediate fluid transfusion.
4. Blood is grouped and cross-matched, and is kept ready. Transfusion is started as soon as indicated.
5. Ryle's tube.—It is safer to put in a Ryle's tube and institute gentle gastric suction so that:
   a. The amount of haemorrhage can be assessed in cases of gastric ulcer bleeding.
   b. The strain of vomiting, which forces more blood out is avoided.
   c. Sucking the blood out of the stomach cuts short the vicious cycle, bleeding → collection of clots → gastric distension → mucosal congestion → more bleeding.
   d. Ice-cold milk drip may be started. This provides nutrition and also acts as local haemostatic.
   Some surgeons discourage introduction of Ryle's tube for fear of its tip causing trauma to the ulcer and further bleeding. Also, the suction must be gentle because a strong negative pressure causes more bleeding.
6. Oesophagogastroscopy.—If a fibre-optic endoscope is available, this provides very valuable information. If the bleeding is from oesophageal varices, the condition is detected. Otherwise, the site and nature of the bleeding ulcer can be made out.

A close watch is kept on the patient and the progress carefully recorded. In absence of the facilities for blood volume estimation, blood pressure is the best guide. If, in spite of blood transfusion, the haemorrhage is not controlled and/or the blood pressure continues to fall, surgery has to be undertaken.

Indications for Surgery

1. Patient deteriorating with conservative treatment.
2. Haemorrhage repeating in quick successions.
3. Recurrent haemorrhages, i.e. bleeding frequently at a few months' interval.
4. A patient above 45 years, particularly if there are evidences of arteriosclerosis.
5. If the possibility of an associated perforation cannot be excluded.

Operation.—At operation, the ulcer is carefully discovered. At times this may be difficult and the stomach has to be opened up to locate the bleeding ulcer. A definite surgery for the ulcer has to be done, e.g. partial gastrectomy for gastric ulcer, and subtotal gastrectomy or vagotomy with gastrojejunostomy for duodenal ulcer. At the same time, the bleeding vessel at the base of the ulcer must be carefully ligated or cauterised after the ulcer-bearing area has been dissected out.

PYLORIC STENOSIS

The common pyloric stenosis, following chronic duodenal ulcer, is a misnomer; this is actually a duodenal stenosis in the first part of the duodenum, caused by the extensive fibrosis on the wall of the ulcer. A true pyloric stenosis results from a pyloric ulcer or a pyloric cancer.

There is a typical history of duodenal ulcer, usually for a long period. When stenosis sets in, characteristic clinical features are noted as follows:

1. Periodicity is lost.
2. Pain changes its character. It becomes less intense and loses relationship to food. More distressing is a sensation of fullness in the epigastrium, which is continuous but is exaggerated after taking food.
3. Vomiting becomes a constant feature:
   a. It is projectile.
   b. It is copious.
   c. It is often self-induced.
   d. It usually contains *old food.*
4. Majority of the patients complain of a lump, moving in the upper abdomen, particularly after taking food.
5. Constipation becomes more severe.
6. There is rapid loss of weight due to inanition.

On Examination
1. A cricket ball-size lump is seen moving across the epigastrium, from left to right, at the rate of 3 to 4 per minute. It is particularly noticed after the patient is asked to drink something.
2. A *suction splash,* due to presence of large quantities of fluid together with gas in the stomach, is heard by the naked ear, on vigorously shaking the abdomen.
3. On *ausculto-percussion,* as the greater curvature is traced, it is found that the stomach is grossly dilated.

Special Investigations
1. *FTM Analysis:*
   a. Huge quantity of fasting content, often containing old food.
   b. A low hydrochloric acid level. This is due to lack of function of the oxyntic cells, resultant upon the severe chronic gastritis set up by fermentation of food from stasis.
   c. A high total acid level because of organic acids derived from fermentation.
   d. Absence of bile in all the samples.
   e. Copious amount of mucus because of chronic gastritis.
2. *Barium Meal Examination:*
   a. A grossly dilated stomach.
   b. Evidence of gross chronic gastritis.
   c. Failure of the stomach to evacuate the meal even after 6 hours (stasis of the meal may also be found in cases of pylorospasm; in these cases, however, injection of an antispasmodic evacuates the meal; this does not occur in cases of actual stenosis).
   d. Simultaneous finding of the meal in the stomach and the transverse colon.

Treatment.—The treatment is operative and consists of either a vagotomy with gastrojejunostomy or a subtotal gastrectomy, as is done for chronic duodenal ulcer. Though the acid secretion in these patients is low and the only problem is the obstruction, a simple gastrojejunostomy is not advisable. As soon as the obstruction is relieved, the fermentation stops, the chronic gastritis disappears, and the original high acidity reappears, resulting in recurrent ulceration. A simple gastrojejunostomy is only advised for elderly patients of pyloric stenosis, in whom atrophic gastritis has already set in and the acidity is not likely to go high again.

GASTRIC CARCINOMA

Predisposing Factors.—Majority of the cases are believed to occur in previously healthy stomach. Some of the predisposing factors are:

1. Gastric polyp.
2. Chronic gastric ulcer.—The incidence is debated. In general, it is now believed that only a small percentage of chronic gastric ulcers turn malignant.
3. Atrophic gastritis associated with pernicious anaemia.
4. Blood group A.

Sites

1. The pyloric region is the commonest site.
2. Lesser curvature.
3. Any part of the stomach, viz. greater curvature, fundus and cardia.

Microscopic Types

1. Almost all the cases are columnar-cell adenocarcinoma.
2. Squamous cell carcinoma, that is occasionally seen, is actually an extension from an oesophageal carcinoma.

Macroscopic Types

1. Ulcerative.—This is the commonest type. The ulcer is raised from the surface, with rolled out everted margins.
2. Proliferative or cauliflower, i.e. polypoid.
3. Infiltrating type.—Though all cancers of the stomach show infiltration, this particular type is characterised by widespread infiltration in the submucous and subserous coats (scirrhous type of growth). There are two varieties of this infiltrating type:
   a. Generalised.—The wall of the whole stomach gets grossly thickened. The stomach is greatly contracted and is rigid like a hosepipe, with gross narrowing of its lumen. When the process is extensive, the condition is called *'leather-bottle stomach'* or *'linitis plastica'*.
   b. A localised variety, limited to the pyloric region, and giving rise to a quick-onset pyloric stenosis (i.e. malignant pyloric stenosis).
4. Colloid cancer.—The submucous and subserous coats are infiltrated with a mucoid material. This is a highly malignant variety of cancer.
5. Ulcer cancer.—This means malignant change in a gastric ulcer.

Spread

I. DIRECT SPREAD
   a. *By Continuity.*—The wall of the stomach is greatly infiltrated, particularly along the submucous coat, to far beyond the visible limits of the growth. The infiltration is seen at its maximum with the infiltrating type of growths.
   b. *By Contiguity.*—The growth, infiltrating out of the wall, may spread to the omentum, pancreas, liver, colon, and rarely the spleen and small gut.

2. LYMPHATIC SPREAD.—This may occur either by embolism or by permeation. The lymphatics from the stomach drain into a wide chain of nodes around the stomach. The nodes concerned in gastric lymphatic drainage are as follows:
   i. Around the Pylorus:
      a. Suprapyloric Glands.—Just above the pylorus.
      b. Subpyloric Glands.—Below the pylorus, in the angle between the first and second parts of the duodenum, in contact with the head of the pancreas. These glands are very important since cancer of the stomach (which is commonest in the pyloric area) almost always metastatises into these nodes.

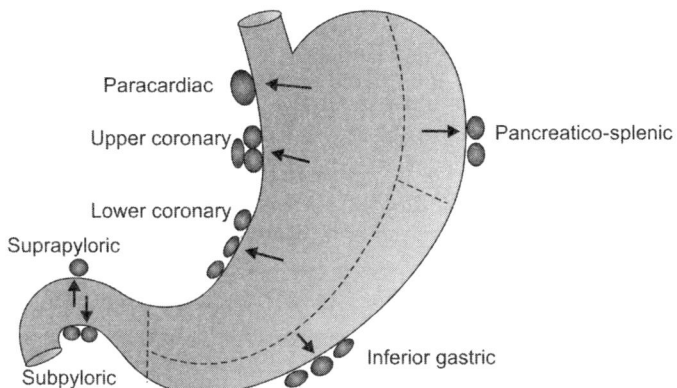

Paracardiac

Upper coronary

Lower coronary

Suprapyloric

Subpyloric

Pancreatico-splenic

Inferior gastric

Fig. 41.1: The lymphatic drainage of the stomach

   ii. Along the Lesser Curvature:
      a. Paracardiac Glands.—Around the cardia.
      b. Upper Coronary Glands.—In relation to the upper part of the left gastric artery.
      c. Lower Coronary Glands.—In relation to the lower part of the left gastric artery, i.e. along the left half of the lesser curvature of the stomach between the layers of the lesser omentum.
   iii. Along the Greater Curvature:
      a. Pancreatico-splenic Glands.—At the fundus of the stomach, near the spleen and the tail of the pancreas.
      b. Inferior Gastric Glands.—Along the lower part of the greater curvature, in relation to the right gastroepiploic artery.

The efferents from all these nodes drain into the coeliac nodes situated at the origin of the coeliac axis from the abdominal aorta.

Though cancer cells from any part of the stomach may metastatise into any group of nodes, for purpose of description of lymphatic drainage, the stomach is divided into three parts. A line is drawn along the long axis of the stomach, dividing it into an upper two-thirds and a lower third. The lower third is subdivided, by a vertical line, into a left one-third and a right two-thirds. The pylorus is taken separately for description. The corresponding lymph vessels are believed to drain into adjacent nodes as shown in Fig. 41.1.

3. Venous spread.—As the veins of the stomach drain into the portal system, metastasis to the liver is commonest. The lung and other organs may also be involved.

4. Transperitoneal spread.—Widespread metastasis may occur on the peritoneum, particularly:
   a. the omentum,
   b. the pelvic floor,
   c. the surface of one or both the ovaries (Krukenberg's tumour)—especially with colloid cancers.

Clinical Features.—The disease, a little commoner in the males, usually occurs above 45 years, but is not uncommon in the younger group. The presenting features are variable and the following groups of patients may be encountered:

Group A: New dyspepsia.—A person above the age of 45, previously healthy, suddenly developing a vague but persistent dyspepsia. The dyspepsia is caused by the associated chronic gastritis as well as atrophic gastritis (due to wide infiltration in the submucous coat), resulting in gross hypochlorhydria or achlorhydria.

Group B: Insidious group.—These patients present with:
- Anorexia.
- Asthenia.
- Anaemia.
   The anaemia is due to: (i) Chronic blood loss from the growth, (ii) Interference with gastric haemopoeitic factor.

Group C: Pain.—Vague pain or discomfort in the epigastrium, constant in nature, without periodicity, and not relieved by food. Vomiting is usually present, sometimes coffee-ground in character.

Group D: Haemorrhage.—Some patients may present with severe haematemesis and malaena.

Group E: Ulcer-cancer.—The features, which suggest that a chronic gastric ulcer has turned malignant, are:
1. Loss of periodicity.
2. The sharp burning pain of the ulcer replaced by a dull aching pain, constant in character.
3. Vomiting getting more frequent, often coffee-ground.
4. Quick loss of appetite.
5. Rapid loss of weight.

Group F: Obstruction
1. Pyloric Obstruction.—In contrast to ordinary pyloric stenosis, this is of quick onset and is rapidly fatal.
2. Dysphagia.—This occurs in cases of growths obstructing the cardiac end of the stomach.

Group G: Lump.—The palpable lump may be:
1. The growth itself. The major part of the lump is, however, made by the omentum wrapping up the growth.
2. The metastatic nodes.

3. The deposits on the omentum.
4. The dilated stomach above the growth, presenting as a soft cricket ball-size swelling moving from left to right (as in cases of pyloric stenosis).

GROUP H: METASTATIC GROUP.—The presenting features are due to metastases:
1. Liver.—Pain, jaundice, ascites.
2. Peritoneum.—Ascites.
3. Enlargement of the left supraclavicular nodes. The nodes located between the sternal and clavicular heads of the sternomastoid (Virchow's nodes) are of particular importance *(Troisier's sign)*.

Special Investigations
1. *Blood Examination:*
   a. Low haemoglobin.
   b. Low RBC count.
   c. High ESR.
2. *Occult Blood* in the stool is almost always present.
3. *Gastric Analysis:*
   a. Gross hypochlorhydria or achlorhydria. If the maximum acid output is more than 20 mEq/litre, carcinoma can usually be excluded.
   b. Blood in all the samples of FTM analysis.
   c. Excess of mucus (due to chronic gastritis).
4. *Barium Meal Examination.*—There is a persistent filling defect at the site of the growth, associated with diminished peristalsis. Early lesions, and lesions in the upper part of the stomach, may be missed.
5. *Gastroscopy* shows the growth. Multiple biopsies should be taken.
6. *Exfoliative Cytology.*—The gastric washings with a Ryle's tube are centrifuged and the sediment is examined for cancer cells. Positive results confirm the diagnosis but there may be false negative reports.
7. *Tetracycline Flourescence Test.*—Orally administered tetracyclines are quickly absorbed by the rapidly growing cancer cells and the cells are stained yellow. When these cells are seen in ultraviolet light they show their yellow flourescence. This can either be seen by gastroscopy or by examining *in vitro* the gastric washings containing such cells.
8. *Laparotomy.*—If the diagnosis is still doubtful, early exploration should always be advised.

Treatment.—Unless there is a definite clinical contraindication, all cases must get the benefit of exploration, to confirm the diagnosis and to assess operability. The clinical contraindications to exploration are:
1. Metastatic liver.
2. Gross ascites, indicating peritoneal dissemination.
3. Distant metastases, including Virchow's nodes.
   On exploration, it has to be decided whether radical surgery can be performed. The contraindications to radical surgery are:
   1. Growth fixed to the posterior abdominal wall or to the mesentery, particularly at the origin of the superior mesenteric artery.
   2. Nodes well fixed to the posterior abdominal wall.
   3. Liver metastases (a solitary metastasis in the liver may be resected).
   4. Widespread peritoneal dissemination.
   In the presence of such contraindications, only a palliative surgery is indicated.

Radical Surgery.—This is called *radical gastrectomy* which means en bloc resection of the growth-bearing area of the stomach with at least 1½ inch of healthy stomach wall at either end, together with all the nodes draining the stomach. According to the situation of the growth, radical gastrectomy may be:

1. *Lower Radical Gastrectomy.*—For growths in the lower part of the stomach.
2. *Upper Radical Gastrectomy.*—For growths in the upper part of the stomach.
3. *Total Radical Gastrectomy.*—The whole of the stomach is resected in cases of growths infiltrating widely along the wall of the organ.

Gastrectomy has been described in details in Chapter on instruments under gastrointestinal clamps.

Palliative Surgery

A. FOR INOPERABLE PYLORIC GROWTHS:
   1. *Gastrojejunostomy.*—The difficulties after a simple gastrojejunostomy are:
      a. The bleeding from the growth still continues.
      b. Loss of appetite and vomiting continues.
      c. The stoma is quickly infiltrated by the growth.
      Thus, a better procedure is:
   2. *Devine's exclusion operation.*—In this operation, the stomach is transected well above the growth and the distal cut end is closed. A gastro-jejunostomy is then performed between the proximal cut end of the stomach and the jejunum. The disadvantages of a simple gastrojejunostomy are overcome as the growth is excluded from the pathway of food. This operation is contraindicated if the pylorous is completely occluded because the secretions of the isolated chamber cannot come out.

B. FOR INOPERABLE GROWTHS IN THE UPPER PART OF THE STOMACH AND FOR LEATHER-BOTTLE STOMACH:
   1. Oesophagojejunostomy.
   2. Permanent jejunostomy for feeding.

C. FOR INOPERABLE GROWTHS AT THE CARDIAC END:
   An oesophageal tube, as used for oesophageal cancers, is passed down to the stomach through the growth, and the patient is fed through it.

CONGENITAL HYPERTROPHIC PYLORIC STENOSIS

Etiology and Pathology.—This is a congenital condition of pyloric obstruction and distinctly differs from the common post-ulcer pyloric stenosis of the adults in that there is no fibrosis in the pylorus or duodenum; instead, there is a gross hypertrophy of the pyloric musculature, so much so that its lumen is obliterated.

The factors, leading to this pyloric obstruction, are as follows:

1. Gross hypertrophy of the musculature of the pyloric antrum, particularly the circular muscle fibres, and the hypertrophic musculature encroaching into the lumen of the pylorus. Distally, the hypertrophic fibres end abruptly at the pylorus, so that the duodenum is absolutely normal. Proximally, the hypertrophy gradually fades off into normal gastric musculature.
2. A spasm of the hypertrophic musculature. Whether the spasm is primary and the hypertrophy is secondary to it, or whether the hypertrophy is congenital and the spasm is secondary, is a matter of debate. According to

many pathologists, again, the condition is due to an achalasia of the pylorus (i.e. primary failure to relax) and, in order to overcome this, the antral musculature hypertrophies.

3. Oedema of the pyloric mucous membrane. This is believed to be due to irritation by curd, resulting from stasis of milk in the stomach.

Onset.—Though the condition is called congenital, the symptoms of obstruction seldom start at birth. In the majority of cases, symptoms begin between the second and third weeks of life. This may be explained by two factors:

a. The oedema of the mucous membrane, which makes the obstruction complete, takes 2 to 3 weeks' time to develop.

b. The spasm of the pyloric musculature starts at that time.

Incidence.—There are certain interesting features as regards the incidence of the disease:

1. Males suffer much more frequently than females (9:1).
2. It is usually the first-born male child that suffers and the incidence steadily declines according to the position of the child in the stem.
3. There is often a hereditary factor—the disease appears in some families with greater frequency.

Symptoms.—As has already been stated, symptoms usually start between the second and third weeks of life. A child, who was so long healthy and gaining weight, suddenly starts deteriorating as follows:

1. Vomiting.—Forcible and projectile, and not containing bile. It occurs almost after every feed. In spite of vomiting, the appetite is good and the child wants food after each vomit.
2. Constipation.—Small, dry stools.
3. Urine output diminishes gradually, so that there is less wetting of the napkins.
4. Loss of weight.

Physical Signs

1. There are signs of dehydration, including depressed frontanalles.
2. Visible Peristalsis.—The dilated stomach, proximal to the obstruction, is seen as a ball-shaped lump, moving from left to right across the epigastrium, particularly after a meal.
3. If, by gentle palpation, the firm hypertrophic pylorus can be felt as a lump just below the right costal margin, the diagnosis is confirmed.

Special Investigations.—Diagnosis is usually made on clinical examination. In case of difficulty, a *barium-meal examination* may be done and this shows:

a. Dilated stomach.
b. Retention of the meal in the stomach even after six hours.
c. The pyloric canal shows an elongation and persistent gross narrowing—the 'string sign'.

If a barium examination is done, the remnant meal must be sucked out since, otherwise, the child may vomit and aspirate the meal.

A better procedure, to avoid the hazards of a barium examination, is to give the child a measured quantity of milk and to aspirate the stomach after 4 hours. Recovery of more than 75 per cent of the meal confirms the diagnosis.

Treatment.—In the majority of cases the treatment is surgical. Medical treatment may be tried under the following circumstances:

1. Cases of late onset, i.e. after 6 weeks of birth.
2. Cases in which the obstruction is not absolutely complete.
3. Children suffering from intercurrent infection.

Medical Treatment.—This consists of:

1. Stoppage of breastfeeding.
2. Feeding at regular 3-hourly intervals.
3. Administration of antispasmodics, of which Eumydrin is the best. This is given as drops, 15 minutes before each meal.

If the condition does not improve or deteriorates with medical treatment, surgery should be undertaken without delay.

Surgical Treatment.—The universally accepted surgical procedure is *Ramstedt's Operation.*

Before operation is undertaken, the child requires preparation, and this consists of:

1. Subcutaneous saline, 50 to 100 ml in each thigh.
2. Penicillin, by parenteral route.
3. Gastric lavage with saline, several times, finally one hour before the operation.

Ramstedt's Operation.—This may be done either under general or under local anaesthesia.

Either a right paramedian or a transverse incision is made. On opening the abdomen, the dilated stomach is brought out. The hypertrophic pylorus has a tendency to be invaginated into the adjacent duodenum like the cervix uteri into the vagina, making the so-called 'duodenal fornices' (this is due to gastric peristalsis). The pylorus is pulled out of the duodenum and is held between the fingers of the left hand. The hypertrophic musculature of the pylorus has to be cut longitudinally, so that the intact mucous membrane can bulge out through the gap made in the muscle. For this purpose, a rather avascular part of the pylorus has to be selected and this is usually its anterosuperior surface. While cutting the pyloric musculature, care must be taken that the duodenal fornix is not injured and, to do this, the pylorus should be completely drawn out of the duodenum. Hence, while cutting through the pyloric musculature, the points of importance are:

1. The pyloric mucous membrane must not be injured.
2. The duodenal fornix must not be injured.
3. The hypertrophic muscle must be cut along its whole length, otherwise the obstruction persists.

On division of the muscle, the stomach is squeezed, and if air freely enters the duodenum, division of the muscle is complete. At the same time, any hissing sound suggests mucosal injury (either in the pylorus or in the duodenal fornix), which must be carefully repaired.

The opening made in the musculature has to be left unsutured.

Post-operative Complications
1. Gastroenteritis
2. Peritonitis and burst abdomen—if there is injury to the mucosa and it has been left unrepaired.
3. Wound infection, particularly with local anaesthesia.
4. Chest complications, particularly with general anaesthesia.

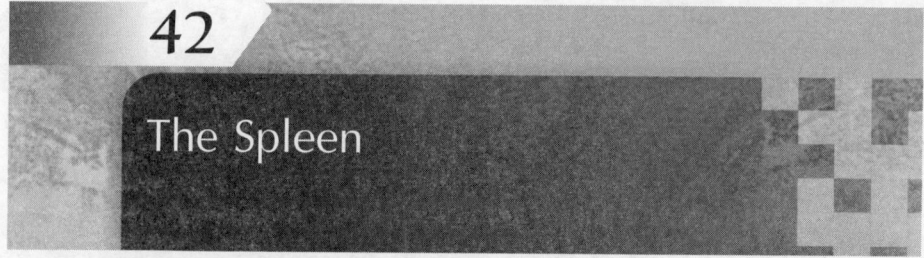

42

The Spleen

Surgical Anatomy.—The spleen develops in the dorsal mesogastrium. Hence it has two ligaments of attachment, one of these stretches between it and the stomach anteriorly, and this is called the *gastrosplenic ligament (omentum)*. This contains the short gastric and left gastroepiploic vessels. The other ligament, posteriorly situated, extends from the spleen backwards to the posterior abdominal wall, where the left kidney is located. Thus, the ligament extends from the spleen to the left kidney, hence it is called the *lienorenal ligament*. The splenic vessels, i.e. the main pedicle of the spleen, lies between the layers of the lienorenal ligament.

The splenic artery is a branch of the coeliac axis. The splenic vein joins the superior mesenteric to form the portal vein, and just before its termination it receives the inferior mesenteric vein. The artery is situated at a higher level than the vein. The pedicle of the spleen is in close relation to the pancreas, the tail of which is in the danger of being included in the ligature applied to the pedicle during splenectomy.

Functions of the Spleen.—The spleen is intimately connected with three important systems:

1. It is the most important member of the reticulo-endothelial system. It is, therefore, the principal site of destruction of blood cells of all types.
2. It takes part in the formation of blood cells, especially in the embryo.
3. It takes active share in the metabolism of blood pigment.

The functions that the spleen is definitely known or is believed to possess may be enumerated as follows:

A. HAEMATOPOIETIC FUNCTION
   1. The spleen is the site of red-cell formation in the foetus. This function is in abeyance after birth, but may sometimes be resumed during adult life if the red bone marrow is extensively destroyed by tumours, or is replaced by fibrous tissue or bone.
   2. The spleen produces lymphocytes and monocytes throughout life.

B. HAEMATOCLASTIC FUNCTION.—As the most important member of the reticulo-endothelial system, the spleen is the principal site of destruction of blood cells of all types. In health, this process is limited to the ageing or disintegrating cells. In diseases, however, the bounds of this normalcy may be exceeded and healthy cells may be destroyed.

C. RESERVOIR FUNCTION.—As a reservoir of blood, spleen is not so important in man as in the lower animals, e.g. dogs, in whom the organ can accommodate even one-fifth of the total blood volume. This is because of the relatively small size of the organ. However, a big spleen may contain a good proportion of the blood volume. The capsule and trabeculae of the spleen, rich in plain muscle fibres, can contract actively in response to certain stimuli, e.g. exercises, asphyxia, haemorrhage, etc., to meet the demand for sudden increase in the circulating blood.

D. DEFENSIVE FUNCTION
1. Phagocytic activity.—As a member of the reticulo-endothelial system, again, the spleen possesses strong phagocytic properties. Organisms, foreign materials, etc., coming in contact with the phagocytic cells of the splenic pulp, are quickly removed from the blood stream. This is favoured by the sluggish flow of blood through the splenic sinusoids, allowing these foreign materials to come into intimate contact with the phagocytic cells.
2. Protection against infection.—Spleen, having the largest aggregation of lymphoid tissue in the body, may be believed to have the capacity of offering protection against infections.

E. METABOLIC FUNCTION.—The spleen takes active share in the metabolism of blood pigments. It is closely related to the regulation of iron metabolism and iron storage.

F. HORMONE FUNCTION.—There are evidences that the spleen secretes a hormone that inhibits the production of thrombocytes and leucocytes by the bone marrow. According to some pathologists, an excess of this hormone is the cause of thrombocytopenic purpura and splenic neutropaenia.

Indications for Splenectomy

1. Rupture of the spleen, usually due to trauma, either close or penetrating. Spontaneous rupture may rarely occur in a huge spleen, e.g. kala-azar, malaria, etc.
2. Splenomegaly associated with certain blood dyscrasias, though it is difficult to ascertain whether the splenomegaly is the cause or the effect of the dyscrasia:
   a. Idiopathic thrombocytopenic purpura.
   b. Haemolytic anaemia.—Splenectomy is far more effective in continental haemolytic anaemia (acholuric jaundice or congenital spherocytosis) than in acquired haemolytic anaemia.
   c. Early cases of splenic anaemia (Banti's disease).
3. Conditions related to the spleen itself:
   a. Cysts, abscesses, tubercular infection, and tumours.
   b. Aneurysm of the splenic artery.
   c. Wandering or mobile spleen.
4. As a part of certain other operations, e.g. total gastrectomy.
5. In surgical treatment of portal hypertension, in selected cases, e.g.
   a. Splenic vein thrombosis.
   b. Persistence of a big spleen after shunt operation.
   c. When a spleno-renal anastomosis is done. This is done when a porto-caval anastomosis, which is the standard shunt operation, is not possible because of thrombosis in the portal vein. The spleen is removed and the splenic vein is anastomosed, end-to-side, with the left renal vein.

The Operation of Splenectomy.—The *incisions,* employed, may be as follows:

a. Left paramedian (extended as 'T' or 'L' by cutting the fibres of the rectus, if necessary).

b. Oblique subcostal incision (same as Kocher's incision for cholecystectomy on the right side).

c. An abdomino-thoracic approach may have to be made if the spleen is very big in size, and has too many adhesions with the diaphragm.

A hand is passed between the spleen and the diaphragm, and the adhesions, which are often vascular, are carefully dissected. As the spleen is now drawn forwards and medially, the posterior layer of the lienorenal ligament is encountered. This is carefully divided and now the spleen is well mobilised. The gastrosplenic ligament is divided in sections, between clamps, and the vessels therein properly secured. The anterior layer of the lienorenal ligaments is then cut and the splenic vessels are exposed. These are carefully ligated (see pedicle clamp and pedicle needle—Chapter on instruments) and the spleen removed.

RUPTURE OF THE SPLEEN

Rupture of the spleen usually occurs as a result of traffic or industrial accidents. The injury is often associated with fracture of the left lower ribs. Sometimes, there are associated injuries to the left kidney, the gut, or the liver.

Penetrating wounds may also injure the spleen.

Spontaneous rupture may rarely occur in huge spleens, as after kala-azar or malaria

Clinical Features.—There may be three types of cases:

A. THE USUAL TYPE.—Following the initial shock, features of an intra-abdominal catastrophe set in. The suggestive features of splenic rupture are as follows:

1. Profound shock, associated with rapidly progressing pallor, rapid fall of blood pressure, and quickly deteriorating pulse.

2. There is often a referred pain in the left shoulder *(Kehr's sign),* where sometimes a hyperaesthesia also be elicited. This is due to irritation of the left dome of diaphragm by the blood clots and is particularly noticed if the foot end of the bed is raised.

3. Tenderness and rigidity all over the abdomen but more marked over the left hypochondrium.

4. Shifting dullness on the flanks because of blood in the peritoneal cavity. Since the blood on the left side, near the spleen, is clotted, the dullness on the right side can be made to shift but that on the left is constant. This is called *Ballance's sign.*

5. Intestinal sounds are absent due to paralytic ileus, which also causes abdominal distension.

6. Rarely *Cullen's sign* may be positive—there is a black discolouration around the umbilicus.

7. Rectal examination may elicit tenderness and a soft swelling, due to blood clots in the rectovesical pouch of Douglas.

B. THE HURRICANE TYPE.—The patient never recovers from the initial shock and succumbs before any treatment can be instituted. This may happen:

i. If there is avulsion of the spleen from its pedicle.

ii. If the splenic vessels are torn.

iii. If a big vascular spleen ruptures.

C. THE DELAYED TYPE.—Following the initial shock, there is quick recovery, but after a variable interval, usually two weeks or more, suddenly the features of splenic rupture appear. This may be due to:

1. A haematoma under the capsule (subcapsular), gradually increasing in size, rupturing at a later date.

2. A small ruptured area, plugged by omentum for the time being, which later detaches.

3. A small ruptured area, sealed by blood clot temporarily, the clot thereafter being digested by ferments released from the lacerated pancreatic tail.

X-ray.—Though there is no confirmatory sign on the X-ray, the following points are suggestive:

1. Obliteration of the splenic outline.

2. Obliteration of the left psoas shadow.

3. Indentation in the normal gas shadow of the gastric fundus.

4. Fractured lower ribs on left side.

5. Elevation of the left dome of diaphragm.

Treatment

1. Immediate treatment for shock:
   a. Rest.
   b. Sedation.—Injection of morphine or pethidine.
   c. Fluid transfusion.
   d. Arrangement for blood transfusion.

2. Splenectomy has to be undertaken without delay. If blood is not readily available, *autotransfusion* of the blood, sucked out from the peritoneal cavity, may be done. The blood, sucked through sterile equipments, is mixed with citrate solution, strained through a few layers of sterile gauze, and is transfused.

43

The Liver

Blood Supply to the Liver.—The liver is the only organ to have dual blood supply— it receives blood from the portal vein as well as the hepatic artery (blood is drained from the liver by the hepatic veins). The portal vein carries about 80 per cent and the hepatic artery 20 per cent of the total blood supply to the liver. Blood from both these sources carries oxygen to the liver. The portal vein also carries the products of digestion from the gut as well as the secretions of the pancreas (insulin, glucagon).

Functions of the Liver

1. SECRETION—Bile.
2. STORAGE:
   a. Carbohydrates.
   b. Minerals.—Iron, copper.
   c. Vitamins.—A, B12 (cyanocobalamin).
3. SYNTHESIS:
   a. Glycogen from monosaccharides (e.g. dextrose).
   b. Phospholipids and cholesterol.
   c. Fatty acids from carbohydrates, and fat synthesis.
4. PRODUCTION:
   a. Albumin.
   b. Fibrinogen.
   c. Prothrombin.
5. BREAKDOWN:
   a. Glucose from glycogen (glycogenolysis).
   b. De-amination of amino-acids, with formation of urea.
6. DETOXICATION:
   a. Hormones.—Oestrogens.
   b. Removal of ammonia from portal blood.
   c. Drugs.—Barbiturates.
7. RETICULOENDOTHELIAL ACTIVITIES and destruction of the bacteria that gain entrance into the body by portal circulation, especially gram-positive cocci.
8. HEAT PRODUCTION.

Liver Function Tests.—As the liver has to perform so many functions, no single test can assess the function of the organ. Moreover, even when as much as 80 per cent of the liver is out of activity, there may be little or no effect on any individual liver function test. The best example is found in cirrhosis of the liver, where all the liver function tests may be within normal limits.

Some of the commonly practised liver function tests are mentioned below:

1. SERUM BILIRUBIN ESTIMATION.—The normal level is 0.2 to 0.8 mg per 100 ml. Higher levels indicate either biliary obstruction or hepatocellular damage. So, a rise in the bilirubin level confirms jaundice but does not indicate the type of jaundice— obstructive or hepatocellular. A steroid test, however, may be helpful. If 40 mg of cortisone is given daily, there is a significant fall in the serum bilirubin level after 4 days if the jaundice is hepatocellular but not so if the jaundice is obstructive.

2. SERUM ALKALINE PHOSPHATASE ESTIMATION.—The enzyme alkaline phosphatase is excreted in the bile by the liver cells. Its serum level, therefore, indicates hepatic function. The normal value is 3 to 13 King Armstrong (K-A) units or 1.5 to 4 Bodansky units per 100 ml of serum. Values above 30 K-A units indicate obstructive jaundice while values above normal but below 30 K-A units indicate hepatocellular jaundice. This test is, therefore, helpful in differentiating the two types of jaundice.

3. SERUM ALBUMIN ESTIMATION.—Albumin is produced in the body only by the liver. Serum albumin level is, therefore, a useful guide to liver function. A level above 3 gm per 100 ml denotes satisfactory liver function. Levels below 2 gm indicate gross liver damage. A rise in the serum globulin level is also an indication of liver damage. However, this is of less significance than serum albumin estimation since, unlike albumin, globulins are, at least in part, formed elsewhere than the liver. Also, because albumin and globulin measure different functions, the albumin–globulin ratio is rather meaningless in ascertaining liver functions. However, many authorities still believe that a reversed A/G ratio is an index of impaired liver function.

4. PLASMA PROTHOMBIN INDEX.—This is an important guide to liver function. In vitamin K deficiency also, there is a low prothombin index. If, in spite of administration of vitamin K, the prothombin index keeps low, gross hepato-cellular damage is present.

5. ESTIMATION OF SERUM TRANSAMINASES.—There are two glutamic transaminases— serum glutamic oxaloacetic transaminase (SGOT) and serum glutamic pyruvic transaminase (SGPT). These are present in the liver and the heart muscle. Increased transaminase levels in the serum (above 100 units) are found in hepatocellular jaundice but not much in obstructive jaundice (unless hepato-cellular damage has set in). These levels are, therefore, valuable in assessing liver function as well as in differentiating the two types of jaundice. SGPT estimation is of more significance because it is found in much greater concen-tration in the liver than in the cardiac muscle.

6. BROMOSULPHTHALEIN TEST.—In the absence of jaundice, this test is of great value as it indicates even mild degrees of derangement of liver function. The dye bromosulphthalein is quickly picked up from the blood by the liver cells and is excreted in the bile. The dye is injected intravenously, 5 mg/kg of body weight. Not more than 10 per cent of the dye should be present in the serum 45 minutes after the injection, if the liver is healthy. The value of the test is greatly diminished if jaundice is present.

7. TURBIDITY AND FLOCCULATION TESTS.—These tests are used to distinguish hepato-cellular from obstructive jaundice and also in differentiating the different types

of. hepatocellular derangements, i.e. different types of hepatitis. This is because they depend mainly upon the increased serum gamma-globulin concentration, as found in different liver diseases. Various tests are used, e.g. thymol turbidity and flocculation, zinc turbidity, cephalin cholesterol flocculation, etc. Of these, the first one is the most commonly practised.

8. LIVER BIOPSY.—A needle biopsy may be done in selected cases. Menghini needle or Vim-Silvermen needle may be used for the purpose. Liver biopsy should always be done by expert hands and should never be attempted if the patient has a bleeding tendency. The prothombin time should be taken into account.

9. LIVER SCANNING.—Different isotopes are available, of which Rose Bengal labelled with I_{131} is commonly used. The emitted gamma rays serve the purpose of scanning. The liver cells pick up the isotope, so that areas devoid of functioning liver cells, e.g. abscesses, cysts, tumours, etc. are seen as 'cold' areas on the photoscan.

10. ULTRASONOGRAPHY.—This gives an idea about the liver and the intrahepatic biliary channels. Tumours and abscesses in the liver may be outlined.

AMOEBIC LIVER ABSCESS

Etiology.—Amoebic collitis → amoebic hepatitis → amoebic liver abscess. The condition is always secondary to amoebic ulcers on the colonic wall. *Entamoeba histolytica,* from lesions in the colonic wall, enter into the venules and thereafter pass up along the inferior mesenteric vein → splenic vein → portal vein → liver.

Pathology.—In the liver, *Entamobae* multiply and live at the expense of the liver cells. They cause multiple foci of liquefaction necrosis in the liver substance. Coalescence of these necrotic areas forms the abscess. The characters of an amoebic liver abscess are as follows:

1. *Site.*—In 70 per cent of cases the abscess is in the right lobe and in the remainder in the left lobe. The most favourite site of an abscess is the postero-superior surface of the right lobe.
2. *Number.*—In 70 per cent of cases the abscess is solitary; in 30 per cent more than one abscess is present.
3. *Content:*
   a. Characteristically, the pus is chocolate-coloured as it results from degenerating liver substance; it is often viscid and glairy. Hence, it is popularly known as *'anchovy sauce'.*
   b. In many cases the pus is green because of its bile content.
   c. In rare instances the pus is creamy.
4. *Wall:*
   a. The wall is primarily composed of necrotic liver tissue and is usually shaggy.
   b. Later, fibrous tissue may be deposited on the wall, making, as if, a capsule.
   c. Perihepatitis develops early and the liver gets fixed, by adhesions, to the diaphragm and the abdominal wall.
   d. The wall of the abscess and the surrounding liver tissue always contain *Entamoebae* that can be demonstrated in the scrapings from the abscess wall.
5. *Microscopic Nature of the Pus:*
   a. The pus consists of broken-down liver cells and leucocytes.

b. In about half of the cases, the pus contains only *Entamoebae*.
c. In the remaining half, the pus also contains Staphylococci, Streptococci, and *B. coli*.
d. In occasional cases, the pus is sterile.

6. *Fate:*
   a. The abscess gradually enlarges, and this is usually in an upward direction. Drainage is usually called for at this stage.
   b. Untreated, the abscess reaches the surface of the liver and bursts. In order of frequency, the rupture occurs into:
      i. Right lung,
      ii. Peritoneal cavity,
      iii. Right pleural cavity,
      iv. A hollow viscus, e.g. colon,
      v. On the skin surface.
   c. Occasionally, a very small abscess may undergo complete resolution under medical treatment, instituted early.
   d. Rarely, the abscess becomes encapsulated and remains as a cyst, lying dormant for long periods.

Clinical Features.—Amoebic liver abscess is almost confined to persons living in the tropics; hence it is also known as *tropical liver abscess.*

Symptoms
1. History of dysentery.—This is usually present but there may be some cases with no previous history of dysentery.
2. Pain over the liver area, worsened by movements. Sometimes the patient supports the enlarged liver with his hand while walking. In some cases the pain may be referred to the right shoulder (as the abscess gets adherent to the diaphragm).
3. Temperature of varying range, often nocturnal, sometimes associated with chill and rigor, and often associated with profuse sweating.
4. Quick loss of weight.
5. Change of complexion.—A characteristic earthy complexion sets in.

Physical signs
1. There is a progressive anaemia.
2. Tenderness over the liver area.
3. Rigidity over the right hypochondrium may be present in some cases.
4. Enlargement of the liver is usually found on palpation. However, even with a big abscess, the enlargement may be insignificant because the abscess is usually located at the superior surface of the right lobe and the liver is fixed, by perihepatitis, to the diaphragm. A careful percussion may, however, demonstrate this upward enlargement of the liver.
5. The base of the right lung may present rales and rhonchi.

Presentation of Complications
1. When an abscess bursts into the right lung, there may be expectoration of a huge quantity of chocolate-coloured sputum (and there may be a natural cure).
2. When an abscess ruptures into the peritoneum, the patient presents with features of acute abdomen, associated with severe shock.

3. When an abscess ruptures into the right pleural cavity, there are clinical features of pleural effusion.
4. When an abscess points under the skin, it may be difficult to be differentiated from a parietal abscess.

Special Investigations
1. *Stool Examination* for presence of *Entamoebae*.
2. *Blood Examination*.
   a. Anaemia.
   b. Leucocytosis.—Often a polymorphonuclear leucocytosis with eosinophilia.
3. *Radiography:*
   a. Straight X-ray shows an irregularly elevated and fixed right dome of the diaphragm (i.e. tenting). A little pleural effusion and a basal collapse on the right side are sometimes evident. Both antero-posterior and lateral views should be taken.
   b. Outlining the abscess cavity with dye (*see* under treatment).
4. *Liver Scanning.*—This is done with substances emitting gamma-rays (e.g. Rose Bengal labelled with I_{131}). Liver cells pick up these substances while the abscess cavity, devoid of cells, appears as a defect on the photoscan. Thus, the diagnosis is confirmed and the position of the abscess ascertained. Employment of *ultrasonic techniques* may be further helpful in outlining the abscess cavity.
5. *Aspiration* may be a valuable method of diagnosis in doubtful cases.

Treatment

A. SPECIFIC TREATMENT
   1. *Emetine hydrochloride* is the drug. 60 mg is given deep intra muscularly, daily, for six consecutive days. Then there is an interval of three days, and three further injections are made on three consecutive days. The disadvantages of the drug are that it may cause myocardial damage, the injections are really painful, and unless injected deep, they may form abscess.
   Dehydroemetine is a better substitute, 60 mg injected daily for 10 consecutive days.
   2. *Chloroquin* may be used as an adjunct to *emetine* or it may be administered singly in persons in whom emetine is contraindicated (e.g. cardiac patients). The drug is given orally, 0.9 gm daily for 10 days, followed by 0.6 gm daily for 20 days (a total course of one month).
   3. *Tetracyclines* may have to be added where a secondary infection is suspected, e.g. high fever, presence of large number of pus cells in the aspirate, etc. The dose is 250 mg administered four times a day.
   4. *Metronidazole* (e.g. Flagyl) is often advocated after the course of emetine, in place of chloroquin. The drug is effective in the treatment of amoebic colitis and amoebic hepatitis, the two conditions which are always associated with (pre-exist) amoebic liver abscess. The dose is 400 mg thrice daily for 5 days.

B. ASPIRATION.—The indications for aspiration are:
   a. When presence of an abscess is radiologically confirmed.
   b. When the temperature does not come down and/or the pain persists, in spite of specific drug treatment.

The values of aspiration are three-fold:
  i. It confirms the diagnosis.
  ii. It brings out the necrotic (and often secondarily infected) material, thus improving the general condition of the patient and relieving pain.
  iii. It reduces the tension within the abscess cavity and this encourages outpour of emetine-saturated lymph from the wall.

Aspiration should be done only after the commencement of specific drug treatment. There are two types of aspiration—close and open:

1. *Close Aspiration.*—This is the method tried first, in all the cases. The aspiration must be done with a wide-bore (1–2 mm) needle because the pus is always thick. The site of puncture depends on the location of cavity:

  a. If (as in the majority of the cases) the abscess is located in the upper part of the liver (shown by 'tenting' of the diaphragm), a transpleural route is adopted. Chances of pleural contamination are remote because the two layers of the pleura usually get adherent in the neighbourhood of the abscess. The site of puncture is the 9th intercostal space, in the midaxillary line. The needle is passed to a depth of not more than 4 inches and is directed upwards, towards the superior surface of the liver. The angle is changed till the abscess cavity is reached and pus starts coming out in the aspiration syringe. Only as much of the pus as comes out easily should be withdrawn (forceful aspiration may cause haemorrhage). At each aspiration, a solution of quinine bihydrochlor (1:1000), which is lethal to the Amoebae, may be injected into the cavity before withdrawing the needle. Aspiration has to be repeated at gradually increasing intervals, till the cavity is dry. After aspiration, either air or lipiodol is injected into the cavity to make it visible on X-ray. By this method shrinkage of the cavity may be ascertained. Also, if the cavity eludes the aspiration needle in future aspirations, help of X-ray may be taken.

  b. If the abscess is located in the lower part of the liver (the liver is then enlarged downwards considerably), the aspiration needle is introduced below the costal margin.

2. *Open Aspiration.*—This means aspiration after laparotomy. This is required when the abscess cavity eludes the aspiration needle even with the best of efforts. The abdomen is opened, packs are placed around the liver, and the abscess is aspirated under direct vision, with a needle and syringe. The abdomen is closed without a drain. Once the location of the cavity is known, future aspirations, if required, may be carried out blindly.

TUMOURS OF THE LIVER

Benign Tumours.—Haemangioma is the commonest benign tumour. Next to skin, liver is the commonest site of haemangioma. The haemangioma is of cavernous type.

Hepatoadenoma arises from, and consists of, hepatic cells. Cholangioadenoma arises from intrahepatic bile ducts. Hepatocholangioadenoma originates from both hepatic cells and bile ducts.

Primary Malignant Tumours

1. HEPATOCARCINOMA.—This is the commonest type of primary malignant tumour of the liver. The tumour may originate in a healthy liver, but is commoner in cirrhotic livers. In cirrhosis, there is great regeneration of liver cells and if this regeneration crosses the physiological limits, a hepatocarcinoma originates. In such cases, therefore, the tumour is often multicentric. The degree of malignancy varies greatly—the tumour may be relatively benign or highly malignant. In the latter case, there is a large mass of soft solid tissue that may show metastases in the hilar nodes, in the liver itself, or even at distant sites (chest and supraclavicular nodes). *Microscopically,* the tumour consists of masses of liver cells that show evidences of malignancy.

2. CHOLANGIOCARCINOMA.—This tumour originates in the intrahepatic bile ducts. It is a columnar-cell adenocarcinoma. It is much less common than hepatocarcinoma.

3. HEPATOBLASTOMA.—This tumour is also known as *embryonic malignant hepatoma.* It occurs in children below four years of age. The tumour shows very rapid growth as well as early metastases (liver, lung, nodes). There are two *histological types:*
   a. Simple liver cell carcinoma, consisting of immature liver cells only.
   b. Mixed tumour, in which, in addition to the immature liver cells, there are mesodermal (sarcomatous) elements, e.g. spindle cells, muscle, cartilage, bone.

Secondary Carcinoma of the Liver.—Liver is the commonest organ in the body to develop secondary tumours. Also, secondary tumours are very much more common than primary tumours in the liver.

In the majority of cases, the primary lesion is located within the portal area. Of these again, the stomach with the lower part of the oesophagus, and the colon account for more than half of the cases.

In many cases, however, organs outside the portal area are the sites of primary lesion. Of these, the lung, breast and kidney are more important.

As a rule, secondary growths are multiple, scattered all over the liver. Occasionally, however, there may be a solitary deposit. In many cases one lobe is more involved than the other. A solitary deposit is amenable to excision, which is advisable if the primary growth is resectable.

The multiple nodules of secondary deposit cause an enlargement of the liver, which is hard in feel. Because of their size and consistency, these nodules are often palpable clinically. The central part of the nodules, deprived of blood supply, undergoes degeneration and softening, so that the big nodules are usually *'umbilicated'.*

Other Secondary Malignant Tumours.—Melanoma metastasises to the liver frequently, particularly when the primary growth is in the eye. Both melanoma and chorionepithelioma reproduce their histological characters in the metastases. Sarcoma, sometimes, and carcinoid tumours, rarely, metastatise into the liver.

From what has been discussed above, the tumours of the liver may be summarised in the flow chart given on the next page.

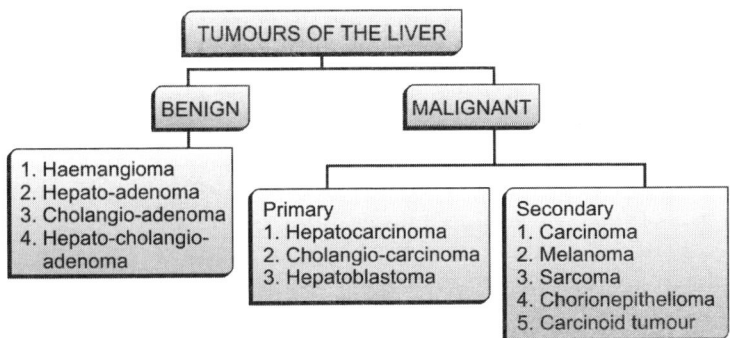

Of all the tumours, secondary carcinoma is the commonest.

PORTAL HYPERTENSION

The blood pressure within the portal vein, in a normal person at rest, is between 6 and 12 cm of water; in no case it exceeds 25 cm in a healthy subject. Any rise in the portal venous pressure, above this level, indicates portal hypertension.

Causes.—In the majority of the cases, the cause of obstruction is within the liver, i.e. intrahepatic. Sometimes, however, the obstruction is below the liver, i.e. pre-hepatic, and rarely above the liver, i.e. post-hepatic.

1. INTRAHEPATIC LESIONS.—These account for 80 per cent of the cases. The obstruction is due to fibrotic changes in the liver that strangle the branches of the portal vein within that organ. The fibrosis is almost always due to cirrhosis of the liver but may be rarely due to other causes, e.g. hepatosplenic fibrosis (Banti's) or a sequela to acute virus hepatitis.

2. PRE-HEPATIC LESIONS.—These account for 20 per cent of the cases. As the cause is usually congenital, the condition is most commonly encountered in the children and the adolescents. The occlusion is either in the main portal vein or in the splenic vein, i.e. before the portal vein has entered the liver. Such obstruction may be due to:
   a. Congenital malformation of the vein, the vein being represented only by cavernous spaces in the mesenchyme; rarely, the vein may be congenitally absent.
   b. Thrombosis of the portal vein, usually as a result of extension upwards of the normal process of obliteration of the umbilical vein in the neonates. Such extension of thrombosis is usually the result of umbilical sepsis. Rarely, thrombosis of the portal vein may be post-traumatic, occurring in the adults.

3. POST-HEPATIC LESIONS.—These are extremely rare. The obstruction is in the hepatic vein or still above, i.e. above the liver, e.g.
   a. Occlusion of the hepatic vein by malignant metastases or by thrombosis *(Budd-Chiari syndrome)*.
   b. Constrictive pericarditis.

Cirrhosis of the Liver and Portal Hypertension.—As has already been said, 80 per cent of cases of portal hypertension are due to cirrhosis of liver. The rise in the portal venous pressure has been attributed to several causes:

1. *Mechanical obstruction,* i.e. pressure by:
   a. Fibrosis.
   b. Regenerated mass of liver tissue in the compensated cases.
2. *Arterio-venous fistulae.*—Multiple minute intrahepatic arterio-venous fistulae develop between the smaller branches of the hepatic artery and those of the portal vein. These are believed to develop as a result of deformity in the liver architecture in portal cirrhosis. The result is that the pressure of the hepatic arterial system is transmitted to the portal venous system.

Pathological Changes

A. OPENING UP OF COLLATERAL CIRCULATION.—As the blood in the portal circulation finds an obstruction, it tries to reach the heart by way of the systemic circulation. The naturally existing collateral channels between the portal and the systemic circulations open up. The sites of portasystemic anastomosis are as follows:
   1. At the lower end of the oesophagus.—Oesophageal branches of the left gastric vein (portal), and lower oesophageal veins (systemic).
   2. Around the umbilicus.—Para-umbilical veins accompanying the round ligament of the liver (portal), and superficial veins of the anterior abdominal wall (systemic).
   3. At the Hilton's line in the anal canal.—Superior haemorrhoidal vein (portal), and middle and inferior haemorrhoidal veins (systemic).
   4. In the retroperitoneal tissues and extraperitoneal surfaces of the abdominal organs, including the bare area of the liver.—Tributaries of the superior and inferior mesenteric veins (portal), and retroperitoneal and subdiaphragmatic veins (systemic).

   The effect of the first is the occurrence of *oesophageal varices.* Though called oesophageal, the varices extend well down into the stomach. There may be severe haemorrhage from rupture of the varices. About 25 per cent of the cases die because of the first haemorrhage from the oesophageal varices. The actual site of bleeding usually lies within a few centimetres of the lower end of the oesophagus.

   The effect of the second is the formation of what is known as *caput medusae,* i.e. a network of dilated veins around the umbilicus.

   The effect of the third should have been occurrence of haemorrhoids but this is extremely rare.

   The effect of the fourth is not clinically manifested.

B. ENLARGEMENT OF THE SPLEEN.—This is believed to be the result of venous stasis.

C. BLOOD CHANGES:
   1. Anaemia.
   2. Leukopenia.
   3. Thrombocytopenia.
   The blood changes are believed to be due to hypersplenism.

D. ASCITES.—There are several factors to account for the ascites:
   1. Portal hypertension.—There is transudation of fluid due to raised venous pressure.

2. Reduction in plasma proteins, particularly albumin (which is synthesised only in the liver and the liver is damaged). This causes ascites in two ways:
   a. Low osmotic pressure of blood.
   b. Impairment of nutrition of the capillary endothelium, raising their permeability.
3. Excess of mineralo-corticoids because of failure on the part of the damaged liver to inactivate them.

Clinical Features

1. Bleeding from oesophageal varices, usually recurrent and often massive, manifested as haematemesis. About 25 per cent of the cases die of the first haemorrhage. Sometimes it is difficult to differentiate the haemorrhage from the bleeding of peptic ulcer. Also, hepatic cirrhosis and peptic ulcer may co-exist in some cases. In some cases, again, oesophageal varices may exist without causing haemorrhage (portal hypertension *au Froid*).
2. Ascites, sometimes associated with oedema of the legs (caused by pressure of the abdominal fluid on the inferior vena cava).
3. Splenic enlargement, usually marked.
4. Presence of caput medusae around the umbilicus.
5. Anaemia.

Special Investigations

1. *Blood Examination.*—Anaemia (microcytic hypochromic), leukopenia, and thrombocytopenia.
2. *Liver Function Tests.*—Poor liver function (*see* above).
3. *Barium Swallow Examination* of the oesophagus demonstrates the oesophageal varices as filling defects, particularly noticed in the lower few centimetres of the oesophagus.
4. *Oesophagoscopy* is the surest method of demonstrating the varicose veins, but great care must be taken in doing this, since even a minor trauma may cause severe bleeding. The findings are:
   a. Submucous veins, following a longitudinal course, raising the mucosa in three parallel ridges (like the piles).
   b. Subepithelial dilated veins, running a zig-zag course.
5. *Measurement of Intrasplenic Pressure.*—Under local infiltration anaesthesia, a fine lumbar puncture needle is passed upwards and backwards, through the 9th intercostal space in the left midaxillary line. As the needle enters the spleen, free respiratory movements are seen on the needle. The stylet of the needle is removed (blood comes out) and the intrasplenic pressure is recorded. The importance of this test lies in that the intrasplenic pressure is closely related to the portal venous pressure. It thus confirms the diagnosis of portal hypertension and also indicates its severity.
6. *Transplenic Portal Venography.*—The preliminary steps are the same as for measurement of intrasplenic pressure. When the needle is inside the splenic substance, 40 ml of 70 per cent *Diodone* is injected quickly, and a series of X-rays are taken at short intervals. The dye enters the portal tree via the splenic vein. When the portal circulation is normal, the dye reaches the liver within 2 to 3 seconds, and the splenic and portal veins are filled but no other vessels are outlined. In portal cirrhosis the venogram varies widely from patient to patient.

In some cases it may be completely normal. However, the commoner findings are as follows:

a. The intrahepatic radicles of the portal vein are distorted ('tree in winter' appearance) and there is a delay in their filling.

b. There may be evidence of filling of large number of porta-systemic collateral vessels, of which the oesophageal varices are the most constant.

c. If there is any block in the portal vein (i.e. pre-hepatic obstruction), it may be demonstrated.

   Before doing the splenic needling, the prothombin time and the platelet count must be ascertained to avoid the risk of haemorrhage.

7. *Measurement of Wedged Hepatic Venous Pressure* (WHVP).— This is an indirect method of ascertaining portal hypertension and is of particular value in those cases where the intra-splenic pressure cannot be measured because of previous splenectomy. A cardiac catheter is passed from the antecubital vein to the right atrium, and then along the inferior vena cava into a hepatic vein. The catheter is pushed further till it reaches the periphery of the liver and its progress is resisted. The pressure, now recorded, is the WHVP. Normally it is about 10 mm of Hg. In portal hypertension there is a considerable rise in this pressure.

Management of Portal Hypertension.—This may be considered under three headings:

I. Medical treatment.

II. Emergency management of massive haemorrhage from oesophageal varices.

III. Surgical treatment.

I. Medical Treatment

1. Diet.—In chronic cases, a high carbohydrate, low protein (but containing essential aminoacids), low fat, high vitamin diet is advocated. Vitamins K and B-complex must be supplemented adequately.

   In acute cases, all dietary proteins are withheld. At least 1600 calories must be given daily as glucose drinks. If necessary, this has to be given by an intragastric drip or even by an intravenous drip. Vitamins K and B-complex are given parenterally.

2. Bowel evacuation must be regular. Purgatives and enema may be necessary to evacuate the bowels, which is effective in bringing down the blood ammonia level, minimising the incidence of hepatic coma.

3. Antibiotics.—*Neomycin* is the drug of choice, though it is expensive. In acute cases, the dose is 6 gm daily, in divided doses. Thereafter, it has to be continued for a long period in a dose of 4 gm daily.

4. Blood transfusions are necessary in the majority of the cases to combat the anaemia.

II. Emergency Management of Massive Haemorrhage from Oesophageal Varices

A. Conservative treatment

1. Rest and sedatives. Morphine is contraindicated; barbiturates are used.

2. Pitressin (pituitrin), which lowers the portal venous pressure by constricting the splanchnic arterioles, should be used with caution. It allows thrombosis of the bleeding vessels by lowering the portal pressure but its prolong use

may induce substantial liver damage because of reduction in hepatic blood flow. 20 units of *pitressin*, diluted in 200 ml of normal saline, is given as a slow intravenous drip.

3. Blood transfusion for replacement.

4. Vitamin K by parenteral route, to make up for the prothombin deficiency.

5. Evacuation of blood from the alimentary tract.—As soon as possible, the blood has to be evacuated because of the risk of encephalopathy due to absorption of protein metabolites. Bowel washes are given for the purpose.

B. TAMPONADE.—This is required when conservative methods fail to control the haemorrhage. The *Sengstaken tube* is used for the purpose. This is designed to occlude the varicose veins by direct pressure. There is a cylindrical balloon for the lower oesophagus and a spherical balloon for the stomach, to press upon the veins (the varicose veins extend into the upper gastric wall). The tube must not be kept in position for more than 72 hours, otherwise ulceration and rupture of the oesophagus may occur from pressure-necrosis. After the balloons are deflated there is the risk of renewed haemorrhage. Therefore, 24 hours after the introduction of the tube, the balloons are deflated but the tube is kept in position for few more hours. If bleeding recommences, the balloons are inflated again and emergency operation is arranged.

C. EMERGENCY OPERATIONS.—When bleeding recommences after deflation of the balloons of the Sengstaken tube, emergency operation has to be undertaken to save the patient. The operation aims at interruption of the oesophageal varices. Since the operation interrupts the communications between the portal (left gastric vein) and azygos (oesophageal veins) systems, it is also known as *porto-azygos disconnection*. Three types of operation are practised:

1. *Ligation of the Varices (Crile's).*—The oesophagus is isolated and is clamped at the cardia. It is opened up longitudinally and the margins are held apart. The columns of varices, usually three in number (like the piles), are under-run with catgut sutures. The rent in the oesophagus is carefully closed.

2. *Oesophageal Transection (Milnes Walker's).*—This operation aims at complete interruption of the submucosal and subepithelial varices. The oesophageal musculature is incised longitudinally and the mucosa and submucosa are isolated as a tube. They are now divided across completely. Thereafter, a repair of the tube is done by a continuous catgut suture and this, by itself, obliterates all the varicose veins. The musculature is repaired separately.

3. *Sub-cardiac Gastric Transection (Tanner's).*—The stomach is completely transected, 2 inches below the cardia. All the vessels here are divided and ligated. The stomach is then resutured. The aim is the same as for the oesophageal transection, which is an easier procedure and is, therefore, preferred.

III. Surgical Treatment

A. Decompression Operations.

B. Splenectomy.

A. DECOMPRESSION OPERATIONS.—Every patient of portal hypertension, who has bled from oesophageal varices, must have the benefit of a portal decompression.

Otherwise, 95 per cent of these patients are destined to die within 5 years. These operations cannot cause any improvement in the liver function but they definitely prevent further haemorrhage. Decompression is achieved by shunting the blood from the portal circulation to the systemic circulation, thus by-passing the liver, where the obstruction exists. However, a shunt operation can be undertaken only when a reasonable level of liver function can be attained, i.e. the serum albumin should be at least 3 gm and the serum bilirubin 10 mg per 100 ml.

Three types of shunt operation are available:

1. *Porta-caval Anastomosis.*—This is the operation of choice. The portal vein is anastomosed to the inferior vena cava. A side-to-side anastomosis between the two veins may be done. Alternatively the portal vein is divided, the upper cut end closed, and the lower cut end anastomosed end-to-side with the inferior vena cava.

2. *Spleno-renal Anastomosis.*—This has to be undertaken when the portal vein is occluded by thrombosis and cannot be utilised for anastomosis. The operation is also of value where the spleen is grossly enlarged and is hyperactive, so that it requires removal. It is contraindicated if the splenic vein is less than 1 cm in diameter. The spleen is removed and the cut end of the splenic vein is implanted into the left renal vein, end-to-side.

3. *Superior Mesenterico-caval Anastomosis.*—This means anastomosis between the superior mesenteric vein and the inferior vena cava. This operation is only rarely performed. It is indicated when the portal vein is thrombosed, and the splenic vein is less than 1 cm in diameter or the spleen has been removed earlier. The inferior vena cava is divided just above its lower end. The lower cut end is closed, while the upper cut end is implanted end-to-side on the superior mesenteric vein, at the root of the mesentery.

B. SPLENECTOMY.—This has no place in the treatment of portal hypertension but it may have to be undertaken under the following circumstances:

a. As a preliminary step for spleno-renal anastomosis.

b. If there is splenic vein thrombosis.

c. Where a big spleen persists after a porta-caval anastomosis and causes symptoms.

Complications of Shunt Operation

A. IMMEDIATE:

1. Haemorrhage from the suture line.

2. Hepatic coma, i.e. liver-failure.

3. Occlusion of the anastomosis by thrombosis, making the shunt operation ineffective. Occlusion is more likely to occur if veins of narrow calibre are used for anastomosis, e.g. spleno-renal or superior mesenterico-caval anastomosis.

B. DELAYED:

Portal-systemic Encephalopathy.—This due to the toxic effects of the products of protein breakdown (of which ammonia is the chief) on the brain and spinal cord. Normally, the ammonia-laden portal blood enters the liver, where it is detoxicated. After a shunt operation, the ammonia-rich blood enters the systemic circulation directly and ammonia exerts its ill-effects on the nervous system, i.e. there is *ammonia intoxication*. The symptoms usually appear suddenly, most commonly 2 to 3 days after the shunt operation. There is disorientation, cogwheel rigidity of the limbs, flapping of the outstretched hands and, ultimately, deep coma.

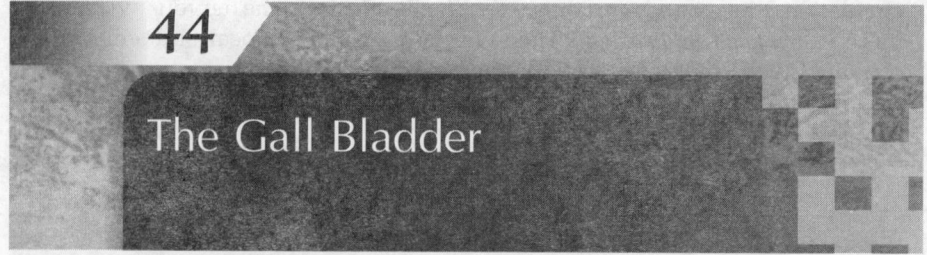

44

The Gall Bladder

Surgical Anatomy
1. The capacity of the gall bladder is about 50 ml.
2. The parts of the gall bladder are:
   a. *The Fundus.*—This is the part which can be palpated when the gall bladder is distended.
   b. *The Body.*—This is attached to the under-surface of the liver by the peritoneum covering it.
   c. *The Neck.*—The somewhat angulated distal part of the neck often makes a pouch, when stones harbour in it. This is called the *'Hartmann's pouch'*. The neck ends in the cystic duct and the Hartmann's pouch overlies the cystic duct.
3. The cystic duct and the cystic artery are not parallel to each other; they make an angle between themselves. Hence they should not be included in the same ligature while performing cholecystectomy (the ligature may slip through the angle). The cystic artery is shorter in length than the cystic duct and so the duct is curled. During cholecystectomy, the artery should be cut first so that the curling of the duct is undone, the duct can be stretched, and ligature can be placed on it right at its junction with the common bile duct. The cystic artery, the cystic duct, and the common hepatic duct make the three arms of an arbitrary triangle, at the neck of the gall bladder—the *Callot's triangle*.
4. The gall bladder has no submucous coat.

Surgical Physiology.—The functions of the gall bladder may be summarised as follows:
1. Storage and Concentration of Bile.—Since the capacity of the gall bladder is only 50 ml, bile is kept in the gall bladder in a concentrated form for efficient storage. This is possible because the gall bladder mucosa has the capacity of absorbing water. It also possesses the property of selective absorption of bile pigments, as well as sodium, chloride, and bicarbonate (liver bile is alkaline, gall bladder bile is acid).
2. Expulsion of Bile.—When needed (as after a fatty meal), the gall bladder musculature can contract actively in order to expert bile into the duodenum. Contraction of the gall bladder requires simultaneous relaxation of the sphincter of Oddi. These two functions occur synchronously and is brought about by a hormone, called *cholecystokinin*, which is liberated in the duodenal mucosa in response to fatty meals.
3. Secretion of Mucus.
4. Relation to Cholesterol Metabolism.—Some authorities believe that cholesterol is excreted (from blood) into bile by the gall bladder mucosa while others believe

that cholesterol is absorbed by the gall bladder mucosa and conserved (in blood). Possibly both the views are correct, the direction of the passage of cholesterol depending on the serum cholesterol level.

Special Investigations in Gall Bladder Cases.—The investigations may be grouped under four headings:

GROUP A: Investigations for confirmation of the diagnosis.

GROUP B: Investigations for jaundice.—Even if jaundice is not present clinically, there may be a sub-clinical (latent) jaundice. If there is jaundice, its nature and severity should be assessed.

GROUP C: Liver-function tests.—Patients suffering from chronic cholecystitis often have impaired liver function. The liver function is grossly damaged in cases of obstructive jaundice.

GROUP D: Other investigations.

GROUP A: INVESTIGATIONS FOR CONFIRMATION OF DIAGNOSIS

1. *Straight X-ray of the Abdomen:*
   a. Shadow of gall stones. Majority (90 per cent) of gall stones are radio-translucent, i.e. not seen in straight X-rays. Only some mixed stones are radio-opaque. They have a typical appearance—regular outline with a signet-ring appearance, i.e. a central dark zone with a white rim at the periphery. Such shadows are often multiple (multiple stones).
   b. Rarely, the gall bladder wall is calcified and this casts a shadow on straight X-ray.
2. *Oral Cholecystography.*—This is done with the idea of assessing two important functions of the gall bladder, viz. concentration of bile and expulsion of bile in response to fatty meal.
   An iodine-containing radio-opaque dye, sodium tetra-iodo-phenolpthalein *(telepaque)* is given orally, as six tablets. This dye, passing down the gut, is absorbed by the portal circulation and is taken to the liver. The liver cells excrete the dye into bile. The dye-containing bile comes down along the biliary passages and part of its enters into the gall bladder by way of the cystic duct. If the gall bladder possesses the normal power of concentration, the dye is concentrated along with the bile, and the concentrated dye casts the shadow of the gall bladder, its container, on X-ray. The whole process (absorption from the gut, excretion by the liver, entry and concentration in the gall bladder) takes about 14 hours' time. It is, therefore, customary to give the six tablets of the dye at 9 PM and to take the X-ray at 11 AM on the following day. This is done when the gall bladder is at rest (i.e. not actively contracting), and for the purpose, the patient is kept on an absolutely fat-free diet throughout the day on which he takes the dye.
   When the gall bladder has been visualised, the patient is given a fatty meal and another X-ray is taken after about an hour. If the size of the gall bladder shadow is now considerably reduced, the second function of the gall bladder (viz. expulsion of bile in response to fat) is present and the gall bladder is declared to be fully functioning. On the other hand, if the gall bladder fails to contract in response to fatty meal, it is said to be *dyskinetic* (kinesia = to move).
   If the gall bladder shadow is not visualised, the gall bladder is declared to be "non-functioning". There are possibilities of so many lapses in the procedure (*see* below) that, before declaring a gall bladder as non-functioning, the patient

is given a 'double dose' of the dye in the next evening to have another trial. If, even with the double dose, the gall bladder is not visualised, it is called non-functioning.

If the gall bladder shadow is not seen, the possibilities are as follows:

- The gall bladder is non-functioning.
- There is obstruction in the cystic duct (the dye could not enter the gall bladder).
- The liver is grossly damaged (its cells could not excrete the dye). This is one reason why oral cholecystography is contraindicated in presence of jaundice.
- The dye has been vomited out or has not been taken.
- The dye has not been absorbed because of diarrhoea and quick excretion (this may be prevented by giving tinct. opii, 15 drops, with the dye).

An oral cholecystography, therefore, shows both the anatomy and the physiology of the gall bladder. It only occasionally visualises the ducts, which are shown by different types of cholangiography (*see* below).

3. *Ultrasonography.*—Stones in the gall bladder and the bile ducts can be detected in an ultrasonogram. The size of the gall bladder as well as the ducts can also be made out. Even presence of biliary mud can be detected. This investigation is of particular value when oral cholecystography cannot be done because of presence of jaundice.

4. *Barium Meal Examination.*—If a patient presents with obstructive jaundice, a barium meal examination, in order to demonstrate the C-loop of duodenum (to exclude carcinoma of the head of the pancreas), is very useful.

GROUP B: INVESTIGATIONS FOR JAUNDICE

1. *Estimation of Serum Bilirubin.*—This is raised in any case of jaundice, the level being directly proportional to the severity of jaundice.

2. *Icteric Index.*—Same as with serum bilirubin.

3. *van den Bergh Test.*—The report may be negative, indirect positive, or direct positive (immediate or delayed). A positive van den Bergh reaction is obtained in presence of jaundice, while an immediate direct positive result indicates obstructive jaundice.

4. *Urine Examination.*—Bile pigments and bile salts are present in all types of jaundice. Continued absence of urobilinogen suggests total obstruction of the common bile duct.

5. *Stool Examination.*—Pale-white bulky stool is found in cases of obstructive jaundice.

GROUP C: LIVER FUNCTION TESTS

1. *Estimation of Serum Alkaline Phosphatase.*—The normal value is 3 to 13 King Armstrong units. In liver damage, the level is proportionately elevated.

2. *Estimation of Serum Albumin.*—Since liver is the only site of its production, the albumin level in the serum is a good index of liver function. A level below 2 G per 100 ml indicates very poor liver function. Levels above 3 G per 100 ml are satisfactory.

3. *Estimation of Serum Transaminases.*—High levels (above 100 units) of SGOT and SGPT indicate liver damage.

GROUP D: OTHER TESTS
1. *Estimation of Serum Cholesterol.*—The level is often raised in gall bladder diseases.
2. *ECG.*—Gall bladder patients occasionally suffer from decreased coronary blood flow, arrhythrnia or heart block (cholecystic heart), because of vagal reflexes from a diseased gall bladder.
3. *Cholangiography* of different types (*see* below).

Different types of Cholangiography.—A cholangiogram means an X-ray of the biliary passages, shown by radio-opaque (iodine-containing) dyes. According to the nature of administration of the dye, the cholangiographies are named as follows:
1. Intravenous cholangiography.
2. T-tube cholangiography (surgical cholangiography).
3. Percutaneous transhepatic cholangiography.

INTRAVENOUS CHOLANGIOGRAPHY.—The dye used is Biligrafin (20 ml) and it is given intravenously. Some patients may have idiosyncracy to iodine and, for them, the procedure is dangerous. To exclude any complication, the patient is given a test dose (supplied in a separate small ampoule with the main vial) and watched for any reaction. If he is idiosyncratic, the cholangiography should be abandoned.

Intravenous cholangiography has the advantage of demonstrating the bile ducts (intra- and extra-hepatic) but, for the gall bladder, it is inferior to oral cholecystography. Its main indications are:
a. To demonstrate any stone or obstruction in the bile ducts in patients suffering from post-cholecystectomy syndrome.
b. In cases where early confirmation or exclusion of acute cholecystitis is urgently required for the purpose of differential diagnosis.

T-TUBE CHOLANGIOGRAPHY.—This is so called because it is done with the help of a T-tube, introduced into the common bile duct. As the procedure entails an operation, it is also known as *'surgical cholangiography'*. The dye (Hypaque) is introduced through the T-tube. There are two-types of T-tube Cholangiography:
a. *Pre-operative.*—The cholangiography is done during operation.
b. *Post-operative.*—The cholangiography is done after the operation, usually before the T-tube is withdrawn. Absence of any filling defect (due to stones) and a normal flow of the dye into the duodenum suggest that the T-tube may be removed.

PERCUTANEOUS TRANSHEPATIC CHOLANGIOGRAPHY.—The dye is injected directly into the liver, along a needle, passed through the overlying skin and integuments. The procedure is unsafe and unreliable, but it is of great help in differentiating between intrahepatic and extrahepatic causes of obstructive jaundice.

Endoscopic Retrograde Cholangio-pancreatography (ERCP).—This is a highly specialised type of investigation. A side-viewing fibre-optic duodenoscope is passed and the ampulla of Vater is seen. A canula is made to pass through the ampulla (through the duodenoscope) and 65% Angiografin is injected through the canula. The entire biliary duct system as well as the pancreatic duct are outlined. Stones (as negative shadows) dilatations, strictures or growths in the biliary ducts can be made out.

CHOLESTEROSIS

This is a condition in which cholesterol crystals are deposited in the mucous membrane of the gall bladder. As has been mentioned (under surgical physiology), cholesterol passes through the mucosa of the gall bladder, either from blood to the bile or from bile to the blood.

Pathology.—From outside, the gall bladder looks normal. When cut open, the mucous membrane shows small yellowish elevated specks, like the seeds of a ripe strawberry—*'strawberry'* or *'fish-scale'* gall bladder. These specks contain the cholesterol crystals. Sometimes the cholesterol deposits may be excessive so that they are found hanging from the mucous membrane— *cholesterol polypi.* Occasionally a polyp may get detached and lie loose in the lumen, and it is believed that this makes the starting point of a cholesterol stone.

Clinical Features.—Cholesterosis, as such, should not produce any symptom. If symptoms are present, they must be due to some other pathology, e.g. associated gall stone or cholecystitis, pancreatitis, peptic ulcer, appendicitis, etc.

Treatment.—Cholecystectomy should *never* be performed for simple cholesterosis. The patient is advised fat free diet and cholagogues.

GALL STONES

TYPES

Metabolic
1. Cholesterol stones
2. Pigment stones

Infective
mixed stones

Metabolic Stones.—These stones are believed to be of aseptic origin, resulting from derangement in metabolism, either of cholesterol or of bile pigments. Accordingly, there are two types, viz., cholesterol stones and pigment stones. There is no infection in the gall bladder, at least to start with.

1. CHOLESTEROL STONES (8 per cent).—Cholesterol is normally present in bile in large quantities and so it has to be held in a colloidal solution, by the process of adsorption, on the surface of bile salts. The normal ratio of bile salts to cholesterol is 25:1. If the level of bile salts declines or that of cholesterol elevates to make the proportion less than 13:1, cholesterol gets precipitated and stones start forming. Sometimes a cholesterol stone starts in a detached cholesterol polyp in a cholesterotic gall bladder.

   These stones are usually solitary (*'cholesterol solitaire'*), accommodated in the Hartmann's pouch. They are big, round, white (or light yellow), soapy to touch, and lighter than water. The cut surface shows a typical radiating appearance. Since there is no calcium, the stone does not cast a shadow on straight X-ray.

2. PIGMENT STONES (12 per cent).—These stones are made either of pure bilirubin or of calcium bilirubinate. They may form either in the gall bladder or in the bile ducts (*primary ductal stones*). They occur particularly under those circumstances in which there is excess of pigment in the bile, e.g. haemolytic jaundice.

These stones are always multiple, small, dark green, and they are either hard or soft putty-like masses. Because of their small size and very little calcium content, they do not cast any shadow on straight X-ray.

Infective Stones or Mixed Stones (80 per cent).—These stones are always preceded by infection- in the gall bladder. The evidence of this infection may lie in the centre (nucleus) of the stone, which is formed by dead bacteria, pus cells, RBC, or epithelial debris. On this nucleus, alternate layers of calcium bilirubinate (sometimes calcium carbonate) and cholesterol are deposited. Since these stones are mixtures of cholesterol and bile pigments, they are called mixed stones.

The stones are usually multiple, moderate to large in size, and are faceted (by mutual pressure or friction against each other). The surface is either white or green in colour, depending on whether the outermost layer consists of cholesterol or of bilirubin. However, the cut surface typically shows the alternate layers.

These stones sometimes cast shadow on the straight X-ray (10 per cent). They have a regular outline and typically a *'signet ring'* appearance (the central black area in the signet-ring contains cholesterol and the white area at the periphery contains calcium bilirubinate or calcium carbonate).

Causative Factors.—It is believed that there are three principal factors which predispose to gall stone formation, viz.
1. Infection in the gall bladder.
2. Stasis of bile.
3. Increase in the cholesterol content of blood.

Pathological Changes due to Stones

A. In the gall bladder:
1. Chronic cholecystitis.
2. Acute cholecystitis:
    a. Mucocele.
    b. Empyema.
    c. Gangrene and perforation.
    d. Penetration and fistula formation.
3. Calcification.—Rare.
4. Carcinoma.—The carcinoma is often of the epidermoid type since chronic irritation by the stone may change the columnar cell lining of the gall bladder to squamous cell, by the process of metaplasia.

B. In the common bile duct, due to impaction:
1. Obstructive jaundice.—White bile and hydro-hepatosis, followed by liver failure.
2. Cholangitis.

C. In the pancreas:
1. Acute pancreatitis.
2. Chronic relapsing pancreatitis.

D. In the small intestine:
Gall stone ileus.—This may occur if a stone gains entry into the small intestine. The stone is too small to cause intestinal obstruction but, as it comes down the gut,

faecal deposits occur on its surface. The stone now gets bigger in size, sufficient to cause obstruction. Impaction of the stone most commonly occurs in the terminal part of the ileum, which is the narrowest segment of the gut.

Clinical Features.—8 to 10 per cent cases have *silent stones,* which do not produce symptoms and are detected only incidentally at X-ray, operation, or post-mortem. The patients, having symptoms, do not present with same types of features and, according to their presenting symptoms, they may be grouped as follows:

1. Presenting with features of chronic cholecystitis:
   a. Pain in the right hypochondrium, sometimes with radiation (*see* chronic cholecystitis).
   b. Biliary dyspepsia, i.e. dyspepsia for fatty food and flatulent dyspepsia.
   c. Acidity and heartburn.
2. Presenting with features of acute cholecystitis, including mucocele and empyema.
3. Presenting with biliary colic.—This occurs when a stone tries to pass down a narrow duct, typically when a stone from the gall bladder tries to come down the cystic duct. The colic continues till the stone gives up its attempts to come down or till it is successful in coming down to the common bile duct.

   There is an acute agonising spasmodic pain, which often doubles the patient up. The pain is located in the right hypochondrium and sometimes radiates to the inferior angle of the right scapula (vide chronic cholecystitis). As with any colic, pain is intermittent in character, continuing for varying periods, and thereafter passing off as suddenly as it came.

   There is an associated vomiting and retching. The pulse and respiration are hurried and the tongue is dry. Abdominal examination at this stage elicits only severe rigidity.

   After the colic passes off, jaundice sets in, in about 20 per cent of cases. This may be:
   a. Obstructive jaundice, the stone having come down to the common bile duct, or
   b. Inflammatory jaundice due to cholangitis.
      A definite tenderness and rigidity can now be elicited over the gall bladder area and there may be a positive Murphy's sign. Sometimes the gall bladder is palpable.
4. Presenting with features of obstructive jaundice.—This is due to impaction of a stone in the common bile duct.
5. Presenting rarely as acute or relapsing pancreatitis, and still rarely as gall stone ileus.

Special Investigations.—Vide above (special investigations in gall bladder cases).

Treatment
1. For stones in the gall bladder.—Cholecystectomy.
2. For stones in common bile duct.—Choledocholithotomy with cholecystectomy (the gall bladder has to be removed because, almost always, a diseased gall

bladder is the source of the stone). If there is jaundice, the patient has to be primarily treated conservatively and, when the jaundice disappears, choledocholithotomy is undertaken. If, with conservative treatment, the jaundice does not abate, operation has to be undertaken even in the presence of jaundice, though with a risk (for details, see stones in the common bile duct, described below).

STONES IN THE COMMON BILE DUCT

Origin
1. Majority of the stones originate in the gall bladder and come down to the duct, usually via the cystic duct, rarely through a fistula formed between the gall bladder and the common bile duct. These are, therefore, *secondary* duct stones.
2. Rarely stones form in the duct itself, i.e. *primary* duct stones. Such stones are:
   a. usually pigment stones;
   b. rarely mixed stones, formed as a result of infection and biliary stasis due to obstruction in the common bile duct.

Progress.—The bile ducts, in contrast to the gall bladder, have no muscle in their wall that can effectively contract to expel a stone through the sphincter of Oddi. When the gall bladder is pathological and fibrotic (as is usually the case) or the gall bladder has been already removed, the flushing action on the common bile duct (normally brought about by a healthy gall bladder) is absent. Thus, a stone in the duct has only remote chances to be expelled by natural process, unless it is very small in size.

Behaviour
1. Many duct stones do not cause any symptom and are discovered only during routine palpation of the common bile duct at cholecystectomy.
2. A stone may move inside the duct and form a kind of ball-valve, and this gives rise to intermittent obstructive jaundice. The obstruction is believed to be due to oedema of the adjacent duct wall, caused by the stone.
3. Sometimes the stone becomes fixed, i.e. impacted, in some part of the duct, the commonest site being just above the sphincter of Oddi.

Pathological Effects of an Impacted Stone
1. Obstructive jaundice.
2. Gradual hepatic failure.
3. White bile.
4. Hydro-hepatosis (rare).
5. Acute pancreatitis (rare).

WHITE BILE.—This is the name given to the contents of the bile ducts in cases of complete obstruction of the common bile duct. The term is a misnomer since the content is neither bile nor it is white in colour (it is opalescent). Bile secretion by the liver cells ceases when the pressure in the common bile duct rises above 300 mm of water. The ducts then contain a secretion, mainly of mucus, secreted by the mucous glands in the wall of the ducts. This is what is called white bile *(surgical bile)*.

Hydro-hepatosis.—This term denotes gross dilatation of the intra-hepatic biliary canaliculi, which are filled .up with white fluid (the liver cells having stopped secreting bile against enormous pressure), in cases of long-continued complete obstruction of the common bile duct. The condition is rather uncommon in cases of impacted stones where the ducts fail to dilate much because of fibrosis in their wall, resulting from recurrent cholangitis, associated with the obstruction (c.f. obstruction due to carcinoma of the pancreatic head, where hydro-hepatosis is commoner).

Clinical Features of Duct Stones

1. As has already been said, some of the stones in the duct may be symptomless.
2. Stones producing ball-valve obstruction at intervals (due to oedema of the duct wall) typically produce *'Charcot's triad'*, characterised by:
   a. recurrent pain (biliary colic),
   b. fluctuating jaundice,
   c. intermittent fever with rigor (due to ascending cholangitis).
3. Stones impacted anywhere in the common bile duct cause:
   a. Severe biliary colic.
   b. Progressive jaundice.

Courvoisier's Law.—According to this law, which applies to patients of obstructive jaundice, if the gall bladder is palpable, the cause of obstruction is not an impacted duct stone, and is usually a carcinoma of the head of the pancreas. There are two explanations for this:

a. The stone in the duct is usually the product of diseased gall bladder and such a gall bladder is fibrotic and inelastic, incapable of dilatation against raised pressure in the duct system. On the other hand, in pancreatic carcinoma, the gall bladder wall is usually healthy and the gall bladder dilates under pressure of obstruction.
b. In pancreatic carcinoma, the biliary pressure rises unrelentingly, whereas in cases of duct stones, the rise of pressure is intermittent.

Special Investigations.—*See* special investigations in gall bladder cases (discussed earlier in this chapter).

Treatment

1. When the stone is detected during a cholecystectomy.—Choledocholithotomy is done to remove the stone.
2. When the patient presents with obstructive jaundice.—The treatment is discussed below in details.

Management of Obstructive Jaundice due to Stone Impacted in the Common Bile Duct.—Immediate surgery, to perform choledocholithotomy with cholecystectomy, is contraindicated as the patient is one of poor risk because of the following factors:

1. Obstruction in the duct causes back pressure in the liver and so the liver function deteriorates quickly. Moreover, stagnation of bile in the dilated bile radicles is associated with cholangitis. Altered metabolism following surgery and anaesthesia, and toxic effects of the anaesthetic drugs (including the muscle

relaxants) are likely to cause further damage to the liver and this may prove fatal.

2. There is considerable risk of haemorrhage at and after operation due to diminished coagulability of blood. This results from failure of absorption of vitamin K from the gut in the absence of bile salts.

3. The patients of obstructive jaundice are very prone to infections due to lowered resistance.

These patients are, therefore, subjected to conservative treatment as follows:—

A. *Support to the liver by:*
   1. High calorie, high carbohydrate, low protein and no fat diet, rich in vitamins and containing essential aminoacids.
   2. Administration of glucose—to start with intravenously (25% glucose solution 100 ml BD), and thereafter orally.
   3. Administration of vitamin B-complex and vitamin C—to start with IV with the glucose, and thereafter orally.

B. *Overcoming risks of haemorrhage by:*
   1. Supplementing vitamin K by IV or IM injections.
   2. Blood transfusion, preferably fresh blood, in serious cases.

C. *Combating infection* in the biliary system as well as providing prophylaxis against intercurrent infections.—Broad spectrum antibiotics, to start with parenterally and thereafter orally. Biliary antiseptics like hexamine (IV with glucose) or calomel may be administered.

Results with the above conservative treatment may be as follows:

1. In the majority of cases the jaundice gradually abates. After complete disappearance of the jaundice the patient is subjected to a cholecystography for confirmation of diagnosis and, on confirmation, a cholecystectomy with choledocholithotomy is performed as a planned operation.

2. In some cases the jaundice either persists or progresses, even with a careful conservative treatment. The patients cannot be allowed to continue as such for a long period because of the grave risks of hepatic coma and suppurative cholangitis setting in. In these cases, operation has to be undertaken, even against odd risks, after preparing the patient with glucose, and vitamins B-complex, C and K. Provision for fresh blood transfusion, in adequate quantities, has always to be kept. The exact type of operation, performed, varies:

   a. The safer procedure consists of minimum manipulations and simply aims at relieving the obstructive jaundice. This is done by performing a *choledochostomy* and providing a T-tube drainage from the proximal dilated part of the duct. Only when a stone is freely available in the duct that it should be removed. Drainage of bile along the T-tube, for a few days, makes the jaundice disappear, together with its ill-effects. Thereafter, the final operation of cholecystectomy with choledocholithotomy may be safely undertaken.

   b. With vast improvement in modern anaesthesia and with the availability of broad spectrum antibiotics, a *first stage choledocholithotomy with cholecystectomy* is often undertaken in these jaundiced patients in the present days. The little increased mortality is well balanced by making two postoperative convalescences into one, and by avoiding a second exploration, which is always made difficult by gross adhesions developing after the primary choledochostomy.

CHOLECYSTITIS

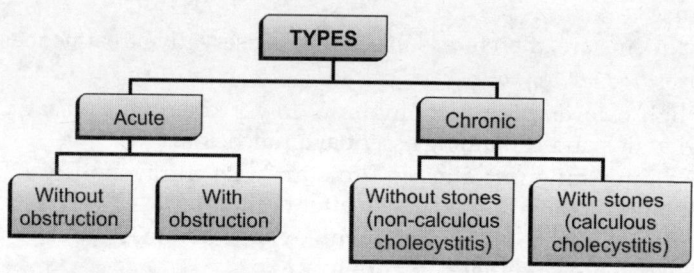

Bacteriology of Cholecystitis.—The infecting organisms are *B. coli*, Streptococci, Salmonella, Staphylococci, and rarely, *Cl. welchii*. Actinomyces can sometimes be isolated from gall stones.

Route of Infection.—There are two views:

1. The infection reaches the wall of the gall bladder by way of the blood stream or via lymphatics. The fact that organisms are often absent from the bile in a diseased gall bladder while they are present in the wall, supports this view.
2. The infection reaches the gall bladder by way of the bile. The types of the infecting organisms (those common in the gut) supports this view.

ACUTE CHOLECYSTITIS

Types

1. *Without Obstruction.*—Where bile has free entry into and exit from the inflamed gall bladder.
2. *With Obstruction.*—Where, together with the inflammation, there is an obstruction to the flow of bile in and out of the gall bladder. The obstruction may be caused by:
   a. a stone in the cystic duct, or
   b. a stone impacted in the Hartmann's pouch and causing pressure on the cystic duct from outside.

Fate of Acute Non-obstructive Cholecystitis.—Depending on the virulence of the infecting organisms and the resistance of the patient (including the treatment received), this may be:

1. Acute catarrhal cholecystitis.
2. Acute suppurative cholecystitis.
3. Acute gangrenous cholecystitis.—This is rare (as compared to appendicitis) because of the ample blood supply to the gall bladder.

Fate of Acute Obstructive Cholecystitis.—This depends on 3 factors, viz:

   a. The condition of the gall bladder wall at the time of the present infection. There are two possibilities. Either the gall bladder wall is healthy, capable of doing normal functions, or the wall has already lost its functions because of previous inflammations.

b. The virulence of the organisms.

c. The resistance of the patient, including the treatment received.

Depending on these three factors, the outcome in acute obstructive cholecystitis may be as follows:

1. *If the gall bladder is healthy to start with:*
   a. When the virulence of the organisms is low and the patient's resistance high, the obstruction is the sole feature. The stagnated bile is worked upon by the still healthy gall bladder mucosa. Water and bile pigments are absorbed from it and mucus is poured in. The bile, therefore, changes into a colourless mucoid fluid. The gall bladder, distended with this fluid, is called *'hydrops'* or *'mucocele'*.
   b. When the virulence of the organisms is high and the resistance low, the gall bladder wall does not get time to work on the stagnated bile, which is quickly changed into pus. The gall bladder, distended with pus, is termed *'empyema'*.

2. *If the gall bladder wall is already non-functioning,* because of previous inflammations, whatever be the virulence of the organisms or the resistance, the bile changes into pus, resulting in an empyema.

Fate of Mucocele

1. Surgically removed.
2. May get secondary infection and change into an empyema.
3. With certain degree of distension of the gall bladder, the wall tends to be lifted away from the sides of the stone, i.e. a disimpaction occurs. The stone slips back into the lumen of the gall bladder, allowing it to drain itself into the common bile duct.

Fate of Empyema

1. With efficient antibiotic treatment, the inflammation is localised and the pus inside, gets sterile. Such a sterile empyema is later removed surgically.
2. If infection is uncontrolled, the tension in the gall bladder mounts, and the wall undergoes gangrenous changes because of obliteration of blood supply. The usual sites of gangrene are:
   a. At the fundus, which is most distal from the supply of the cystic artery.
   b. At the Hartmann's pouch, where there is pressure-necrosis of the wall by the impacted stone.

Such a gangrenous change results in perforation of the gall bladder. When perforation occurs, the result may be:

i. Generalised peritonitis.

ii. Localised abscess, limited by adhesions.

iii. Fistula formation with common bile duct, duodenum, colon or stomach (in that order of frequency).

Mucocele and Empyema.—A myelocele has a thin healthy wall, without congestion and without much adhesions with the surrounding structures.

In empyema, the gall bladder wall is grossly thickened, congested, oedematous, and shows considerable adhesions with the surrounding structures.

Symptoms in Acute Cholecystitis

1. *History.*—In many cases there is a history suggestive of chronic cholecystitis or previous acute cholecystitis.
2. *Pain.*—The pain is more sudden with the obstructive type, less so in the non-obstructive cases. It is either spasmodic or aching in nature, the former being commoner with the obstructive type. The pain starts in the right hypochondrium and occasionally in the epigastrium. Very often the pain is radiated to the inferior angle of the right scapula, an area which has the same segmental (T_7) nerve supply as the gall bladder itself. Occasionally the pain radiates to the tip of the right shoulder because of irritation of the diaphragm by the fundus of an enlarged gall bladder (this is by way of the phrenic nerve, the C_4 component of which also supplies the tip of the shoulder).
3. *Nausea and Vomiting.*—This is reflex and, therefore, occurs only till the stomach is empty. If the attack starts in an empty stomach, there may be only nausea.
4. *Temperature.*—Variable, high and hectic in cases of empyema. There may be associated rigors.
5. *Jaundice.*—Occurs only in a few cases and is due to an associated cholangitis.

Physical Signs

1. The patient is anxious in pain and there is a variable amount of toxicity. The tongue is dry, temperature raised, the pulse and the respiration rapid.
2. There is rigidity in the right upper abdomen, sometimes more extensive.
3. There is acute tenderness over the right hypochondrium, maximum at the gall bladder point (tip of the right 9th costal cartilage). *Murphy's sign* is usually positive. This means there is a catch in the breath at the height of inspiration, when pressure is put over the gall bladder point and the patient is asked to take deep respiration. This catch in breath is nature's attempt to prevent a hurt to the inflamed gall bladder by the examining fingers (in cases where the liver is small, the patient may have to be seated to elicit the Murphy's sign—the liver with the gall bladder coming down with gravity).
4. *Boas's sign* is positive in some cases, particularly with the obstructive type. There is an area of hyperaesthesia between the 9th and 11th ribs, *posteriorly,* on the right side.
5. In case of mucocele or empyema, the enlarged gall bladder is usually palpable.
6. *Leake's Oedema Test.*—Oedema may be demonstrated in the skin and subcutaneous tissues overlying the gall bladder point.
7. There may be an associated abdominal distension with diminished intestinal sounds.

Management of Acute Cholecystitis.—In contrast to acute appendicitis, the management of acute cholecystitis is usually conservative. This is because of the following points:

1. Cholecystectomy, in presence of acute inflammation, is really difficult since the important structures at the neck of the gall bladder are grossly oedematous, friable, non-identifiable, and liable to injury, which is not the case with appendicectomy.
2. There are no weak spots in the musculature of the gall bladder and there is an abundant blood supply. Hence, chances of perforation and spreading peritonitis are remote, as compared to acute appendicitis.

Unless, therefore, there is a gross contraindication, the management of acute cholecystitis is immediate conservative treatment, followed by interval cholecystectomy.

CONSERVATIVE TREATMENT

1. Rest in bed.
2. Rest to the gall bladder by:
   a. Stopping oral feeding.
   b. Introducing a Ryle's tube and instituting gastric suction.
3. Intravenous fluid in drip to supply the daily fluid requirement, 2 to 2.5 litres a day.
4. Antibiotics, broad spectrum, administered parenterally to start with and thereafter orally.
5. Antispasmodics to relieve pain. Analgesics and sedatives may be given if the pain is severe. Morphine is avoided because it causes spasm of the sphincter of Oddi, thus increasing tension and pain.
6. A close watch is kept on the patient to assess the progress:
   a. If the condition improves (which is usually the case), oral feeding is gradually started and antibiotics withdrawn. When the patient is more or less normal, investigations are undertaken to confirm the diagnosis (in doubtful cases). With the diagnosis confirmed, cholecystectomy is performed *(interval cholecystectomy)*.
   b. If the temperature does not come down and the toxicity increases even after 48 hours of rigid conservative treatment, the case is one of empyema, not responding to antibiotics and likely to perforate if kept as such. In these cases conservative treatment has to be abandoned in favour of immediate surgery.

INDICATIONS FOR IMMEDIATE SURGERY

1. When the diagnosis is doubtful, e.g. from peptic perforation or acute appendicitis.
2. Empyema, not responding to 48 hours' rigid conservative treatment.
3. Perforation of the gall bladder.

NATURE OF IMMEDIATE SURGERY

1. Majority of the surgeons, in the present days, prefer *Cholecystectomy*.
2. If, however, the structures at the neck of the gall bladder are very oedematous and friable, so much so, as to make, cholecystectomy dangerous, *cholecystostomy* is done for the time being to drain the gall bladder and release the tension. Cholecystectomy is undertaken at a later date.

CHRONIC CHOLECYSTITIS

Types

1. Usually the condition is associated with gall stones *(calculous cholecystitis)*.
2. Sometimes stones are not associated *(non-calculous cholecystitis)*.

Pathology

1. The gall bladder is contracted and small
2. The wall is thickened with fibrous tissue.

3. The colour of the gall bladder becomes white because of:
   a. Presence of fibrous tissue in the wall.
   b. Subserous deposits of fat.
4. There is variable amount of adhesions with the surrounding structures, e.g. omentum, common bile duct, duodenum, colon, stomach; etc. Sometimes, there is fistula formation with the stomach or duodenum, or with the common bile duct.
5. The mucous membrane is thickened, oedematous, and often shows cholesterosis.
6. Stones are usually present.

Presenting Features.—Typically, the patient is described as a *fat, fair, fertile female* above *forty* but any exception is common. The patients may present with a variety of features and these may be grouped as follows:

GROUP I: Chronic pain in the right hypochondrium or epigastrium, often radiating to the back and rarely to the tip of the right shoulder (*see* acute cholecystitis);

GROUP II: Biliary dyspepsia, characterised by:
             a.   Qualitative dyspepsia for fatty food.
             b.   Flatulent dyspepsia.

GROUP III: Acidity and heartburn, due to reflex gastric irritation and pylorospasm. Sometimes this may cause pain, typical of peptic ulcer.

GROUP IV: Acute cholecystitis.

GROUP V: Biliary colic.

GROUP VI: Obstructive jaundice, due to a stone coming down to the common bile duct.

GROUP VII: Acute pancreatitis or chronic relapsing pancreatitis.

GROUP VIII: Cardiac complaints, like angina pectoris, may rarely occur. It is believed that the gall bladder is sometimes the *trigger point* for cardiac pains.

Special Investigation.—These have been discussed in details earlier in this chapter.

Treatment.—Whatever be the function of the gall bladder (usually these gall bladders are non-functioning), if stones are detected on X-ray, cholecystectomy has to be undertaken. Conversely, even if no stones are seen on the X-ray but the gall bladder is non-functioning, cholecystectomy is obligatory.

Operations.—The operations of cholecystectomy and choledocholithotomy are described in details in the chapter on instruments, under cholecystectomy forceps and choledocholithotomy forceps, respectively.

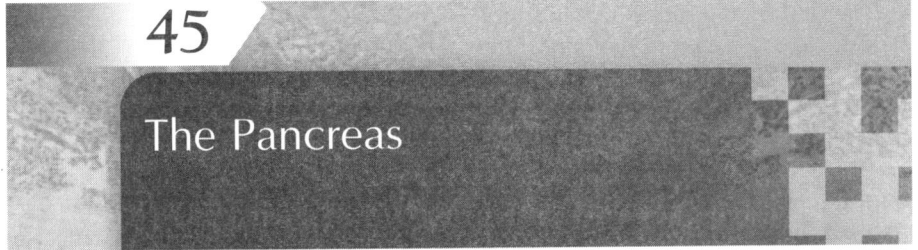

45
The Pancreas

SURGICAL ANATOMY

Parts.—The pancreas consists of the following parts:

1. THE HEAD.—It is surrounded on its upper, right and lower aspects by the duodenum. The lower part of the common bile duct lies between the head and the second part of the duodenum.

2. THE NECK AND UNCINATE PROCESS.—The neck marks the junction of the head and the body. From the lower and left part of the head projects the uncinate process. The superior mesenteric vessels run in front of the uncinate process. These vessels make a deep groove on the posterior surface of the lower part of the neck. The upper part of the posterior surface is grooved by the portal vein, formed here by the junction of the superior mesenteric and the splenic veins.

3. THE BODY.—The splenic vessels are closely related to the body of the pancreas along its whole length. The artery runs along its upper border and the vein along its posterior surface.

4. THE TAIL.—It rests on the splenic hilum and care should be taken not to injure it during splenectomy.

Ducts.—The pancreas has two ducts:

1. THE MAIN DUCT OF WIRSUNG.—This runs along the whole length of the pancreas, towards the head. Thereafter, it joins the ampulla of Vater, which is the dilatation formed by the junction of this duct with the common bile duct. The ampulla opens at the summit of the duodenal papilla, located on the posteromedial aspect of the second part of the duodenum. The papilla is surrounded by the sphincter of Oddi. This arrangement is believed to have considerable importance in the pathogenesis of pancreatitis.

2. THE ACCESSORY DUCT OF SANTORINI.—This drains a part of the head and opens into the duodenum, about half an inch above the main duct. In about 10 per cent of cases, this becomes the main secretory duct of the pancreas. Developmentally, this is the major duct of the pancreas, as this is the duct of the dorsal bud of the pancreas (*see* below).

Embryology.—The pancreas develops as two buds, a dorsal and a ventral, growing in the dorsal and ventral mesoduodenum respectively. The dorsal bud forms the body, tail, and ventral part of the head, i.e. the major part of the pancreas. Its duct is the duct of Santorini, which, however, becomes the accessory duct in future.

The ventral bud forms only the dorsal part of the head and the uncinate process. Its duct forms the proximal part of the main pancreatic duct (Wirsung). This bud is intimately attached to the developing choledochus and the duodenum. Its duct maintains this close attachment and this is why the common bile duct, the main pancreatic duct, and the duodenum are so closely related.

The ventral bud swings to the right and then dorsally, and fuses with the dorsal bud, to complete the head of the pancreas. In this attempt, a ring of pancreatic tissue may encircle the second part of the duodenum. This is what is called an annular pancreas.

An *annular pancreas* is often symptomless. However, it may cause obstruction:
1. To the Duodenum.—Acute or chronic obstruction—at birth, in early childhood, or in the adult life.
2. To the Common Bile Duct.—Rarely the common bile duct may pass through this ring of pancreatic tissue and may be compressed, causing obstructive jaundice.

The treatment for an annular pancreas, producing duodenal obstruction, is as follows:
1. In the Children.—Duodenojejunostomy. Simple division of the anterior part of the ring does not provide satisfactory results.
2. In the Adults.—Gastroduodenectomy, i.e. resection of lower part of the stomach and the upper part of the duodenum to just above the ring, followed by a poly A gastrojejunostomy.

PHYSIOLOGY

Cells.—Broadly, there are two types of cells:
1. ACINAR CELLS, which line the acini and are responsible for the external secretion of the pancreas that is ejected through the pancreatic ducts.
2. ISLET CELLS, which are arranged in islets or clumps, and are responsible for the internal secretion. There are three types:
   a. *Alpha Cells,* secreting glucagon, which has a hyperglycaemic (i.e. anti-insulin) action.
   b. *Beta Cells,* secreting insulin.
   c. *Non-beta Cells,* believed to produce a substance pharmacologically identical with gastrin. A tumour arising in these cells causes fulminating peptic ulceration *(Zollinger-Ellision Syndrome).*

External Secretion.—The normal adult secretes about one litre of pancreatic juice daily. The juice, which is highly alkaline because of high sodium bicarbonate content, contains digestive enzymes, which act on starch, fat, and protein:
a. Amylase (diastase), for carbohydrate digestion.
b. Lipase, for fat digestion.
c. Trypsinogen, for protein digestion. Trypsinogen, as such, is inactive; it has to be activated into *trypsin* and normally this is done by the succus entericus. It is believed that trypsinogen may be activated to trypsin also by bile, by the tissue juices, and by the products of bacterial growth. *Chymotrypsin* is another proteolytic enzyme secreted by the pancreas.

Control of Secretion.—The external secretion of the pancreas is controlled by humoral and nervous mechanisms, of which the latter is less significant:

1. HUMORAL.—This involves two hormones, both of which are liberated in the mucosa of the duodenum and upper jejunum, chiefly by the action of acid and also by food. They are carried by blood to the pancreas. The hormones are:
   a. *Secretin.*—This produces large amounts of secretion, rich in sodium and bicarbonate but poor in enzymes.
   b. *Pancreozymin.*—It produces small amounts of secretion, viscid and rich in enzymes.
2. NERVOUS.—Initiated by vagal stimulation. The secretion is small, viscid, and rich in enzymes.

PANCREATITIS

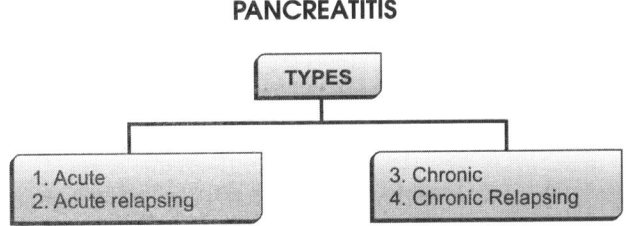

In acute and acute relapsing pancreatitis:
a. There is necrosis of the pancreas (of different degrees).
b. The clinical picture is acute.
c. If the patient survives, the attack subsides, without leaving behind any structural or functional deficit in the gland. The pancreas returns to normal. In no case an acute pancreatitis leads to a chronic pancreatitis. In the acute relapsing type there are repeated attacks of acute pancreatitis (usually not very severe).

In *chronic and chronic relapsing pancreatitis:*
a. There is a slow and progressive destruction of the pancreatic tissue.
b. The areas of destruction are replaced by fibrous tissue. The fibrosis gradually increases, with corresponding functional failure.

As regards etiological similarity between the acute and chronic forms, two factors are found to play important roles in both the conditions:
   i. Gall stones and/or infected biliary tract.
   ii. Chronic alcoholism.
   In both the conditions, naturally, the liver function is depressed.

ACUTE PANCREATITIS

Etiology.—There are various theories as to the cause of acute pancreatitis, as described below. However, the first, i.e. autodigestion, is more or less the established one:
   I. Autodigestion
   II. Infection
   III. Trauma
   IV. Embolism of pancreatic arteries.

AUTODIGESTION.—It is now generally accepted that the condition is essentially an acute necrosis of the pancreas, resulting from autodigestion of the gland by its own proteolytic enzyme, trypsin. Normally trypsin is secreted by the pancreas in an inert form, i.e. trypsinogen, and it is activated in the duodenum by the enzyme enterokinase. Therefore, the cause of this autodigestion is a condition in which trypsinogen is activated into trypsin while it is still within the pancreas. The different views about this cause are as follows:

A. *Regurgitation of Bile.*—It has been established that regurgitation of bile, especially if infected, into the pancreas, causes pancreatitis. For regurgitation to occur, there must be two factors:
   a. The common bile duct and the pancreatic duct must open by a common channel, i.e. ampulla, into the duodenum (while this is the usual anatomy, many people have separate openings for the two).
   b. There must be an obstruction to the outflow of bile into the duodenum through this channel.

While the first factor depends on the anatomical arrangement in the particular subject, the second factor may be brought about by either of the following:
   1. Stone impacted at the sphincter of Oddi.
   2. Spasm of the sphincter of Oddi, caused by:
      a. Gall bladder diseases.
      b. Digestive disturbances.

The common association of acute pancreatitis and gall bladder diseases substantiates this view.

B. *Duct Distension.*—Pancreatitis may be produced by injecting even sterile water into the pancreatic duct, causing a duct distension. It is therefore believed by many pathologists that the cause of acute pancreatitis lies in simple distension of the duct by its own secretion. This causes mechanical rupture of the pancreatic acini and the resultant products of tissue destruction activate trypsinogen into trypsin. Such duct distension may be caused by:
   1. Stone impacted at the sphincter of Oddi.
   2. Spasm of the sphincter of Oddi.
   3. Squamous metaplasia of the lining epithelium of the smaller ducts, causing heaping in the wall that obstructs the lumen.
   4. Sudden stimulation of the pancreas to secrete in excess, as in alcoholics or after a heavy meal.

II. INFECTION
1. Blood-borne infection may rarely be the cause of acute pancreatitis, as is occasionally seen in the course of typhoid fever, mumps, and other diseases.
2. Lymphatic infection from the gall bladder.
3. Direct spread of infection from the lesser sac.

III. TRAUMA.—This may rarely be the cause, e.g.
1. Blow on the epigastrium or automobile injury.
2. Crush fracture of the vertebrae behind.
3. Surgical trauma, e.g. at gastrectomy.

IV. EMBOLISM OF PANCREATIC ARTERIES
1. By thrombus.
2. By fat emboli.

Nomenclature.—Depending on the degree of necrosis, the damaging effect of the pancreatic enzymes, and the rapidity of the process of necrosis, different nomenclatures have been in use to qualify acute pancreatitis:

A. ACCORDING TO THE CLINICAL COURSE

1. *Acute Fulminating Pancreatitis or Fulminating Pancreatic Necrosis.* — The disease originates with dramatic intensity and kills the patient within 2 to 3 days.
2. *Subacute Pancreatitis* or *Subacute Pancreatic Necrosis.*—The disease proceeds less urgently and recovery is usual. Acute relapsing cases usually belong to this group.

B. ACCORDING TO THE PATHOLOGICAL CHANGES

1. *Acute Oedematous Pancreatitis.*—There is a generalised oedema of the gland. This is the mildest form.
2. *Acute Haemorrhagic Pancreatitis.*—There are wide areas of necrosis, with gross haemorrhages within and outside the gland. This is the most severe form.
3. *Acute Suppurative Pancreatitis.*—There are isolated areas of necrosis, wherein secondary suppuration occurs. This is intermediate in severity between the above two types.

Pathology

1. THE PANCREAS.—In the mildest form, the pancreas shows a generalised (rarely localised) oedema. In severe forms it is grossly haemorrhagic and necrotic. Suppuration may follow subsequently.

2. HAEMORRHAGE.—The haemorrhage, which occurs in the gland itself, usually spreads to the vicinity. The peritoneal cavity, especially the lesser sac, contains a blood-stained fluid. Occasionally, there may be haemorrhages at distal sites, e.g. the abdominal wall. The haemorrhages are believed to occur as a result of degenerative changes, brought about in the walls of blood vessels, by the liberated pancreatic enzymes.

3. FAT NECROSIS.—This is caused by the lipase escaping from the pancreas. The lipase splits fat into glycerol and fatty acids. The fatty acids combine with calcium to form soaps. This soap is represented in the areas of fat necrosis, which are dull, opaque, yellowish white, raised areas, suggestive of drops of wax. The sites of these deposits are as follows:
   a. Most abundantly in the neighbourhood of the pancreas.
   b. In the fat, especially of the greater omentum, and also that of the mesentery, transverse mesocolon, extraperitoneal tissues or anterior abdominal wall. This occurs by the permeation of the lipase along lymph vessels.
   c. At distant sites occasionally, e.g. in the bone marrow, under the pleura and pericardium, or in subsynovial fat of the knee joint. This occurs possibly as a result of excessive amounts of lipase being carried in the blood stream.

4. BILIARY TRACT.—Gall stones, infected bile, and chronic cholecystitis are commonly associated. The liver function is often depressed.

Clinical Features

A. INCIDENCE

1. Both sexes are equally affected, there is no special predilection for obese people, and often the patient is between fifty and sixty.
2. The attack often follows a heavy meal or alcohol consumption.

B. Symptoms

1. Pain.—Epigastric, often radiating to the back; the pain gradually increases in intensity and usually becomes unbearable.
2. Vomiting.—Constant and repeated. To start with, it is due to reflex gastric irritation (due to tension in the pancreatic capsule as well as compression of the adjacent coeliac plexus), but thereafter, it is obstructive.
3. Constipation.

C. General signs

1. Profound shock and features of collapse are often found. These are due to the vasodepressor activity of:
   a. The circulating 'kinins', produced by the action of trypsin on the plasma proteins.
   b. The circulating products of protein breakdown, absorbed from the autodigested pancreas.
2. Cyanosis is present in some of the cases. The same factors, which produce shock, cause the cyanosis because of generalised capillary paralysis.
3. Jaundice.—A faint jaundice may sometimes be seen, usually after 24 hours. This is because of the oedema of the pancreatic head, obstructing the common bile duct.
4. Temperature.—Subnormal at first, rises with the onset of peritonitis.
5. Pulse rate may often be abnormally slow.

D. Local signs

1. *Rigidity.*—Generalised all over the abdomen, but not so marked as in peptic perforation.
2. *Tenderness.*—Over the whole abdomen and sometimes at the left renal angle (the tail is nearer that surface).
3. *Ante-mortem Lividity.*—Ecchymosis and pigmentation of the skin may be seen in some cases, 48 hours after the attack. This is due to spread of blood and pancreatic ferments from the retroperitoneal tissues to the subcutaneous fat and skin. Typically, there are two sites:
   a. On the back, spreading forwards from the back to the loin. This is caused by simple gravitation into the dilated capillaries of the dependent skin of the back.
   b. Round the umbilicus. This is known as *Grey Turner's* sign, comparable to Cullen's sign, as described in ruptured ectopic gestation. The retroperitoneal blood and ferments may reach this area either directly or via the round ligament of the liver.
4. Paralytic ileus sets in early.

E. Later features

1. Signs of peritonitis may set in.
2. A tender palpable lump may appear in the epigastrium. This may be due to:
   a. Pseudopancreatic cyst, if it appears towards the end of the second week.
   b. Peri-pancreatic abscess, if it appears later than the third week.

Causes of Death.—Death often follows the fulminating type of acute pancreatitis and may be due to:

1. Peripheral circulatory failure (soon after the onset).

2. Toxaemia caused by the products of protein breakdown (few hours after the onset).
3. Peritonitis (after a few days).

Special Investigations

A. BLOOD COUNT.—A high leucocytosis is found.

B. BLOOD BIOCHEMISTRY:
1. *Serum Calcium.*—Usually shows a low level, because calcium is utilised for the formation of soap. The fall is generally delayed (about a week). A level below 7 mg/100 ml indicates a grave prognosis (normal 10 mg/100 ml).
2. *Serum Bilirubin.*—Raised, even if jaundice is not clinically detected.
3. *Blood Sugar.*—May be elevated in some cases.
4. *Serum Fibrinogen.*—This is raised at the end of the first week. This is of prognostic value.
5. Presence of *methaemalbumen* in blood indicates a bad prognosis as it suggests haemorrhagic necrosis.

C. ENZYME STUDIES
1. *Serum Amylase.*—The normal level is 80 to 150 Somogyi units. Levels higher than 500 units are suspicious but levels above 1000 units are highly suggestive. The highest level is reached within one hour of the onset and a gradual fall occurs during the next few days. Thus, this test is valuable only in the earlier phase of the disease.
2. *Urinary Diastase (i.e. amylase).*—Normally the diastatic index is below 50 units. It starts rising after 12 hours and remains elevated for a few days. Thus, this test is of value in the late stages. Levels above 100 units are suggestive but considerably higher levels may be reached.

D. X-RAY.—A straight X-ray of the abdomen may be helpful:
1. *'Cut-off' Sign.*—There is an isolated gas-filled solitary loop, consisting of the duodenum and proximal jejunum.
2. Gall stones may be seen.
3. Absence of subdiaphragmatic gas shadow excludes peptic perforation, from which condition the disease is sometimes really difficult to be diagnosed.

E. ECG.—This is mainly helpful in making a differential diagnosis from myocardial infarction. Insignificant ECG changes, which are sometimes seen in pancreatitis, disappear as the patient recovers.

Treatment

I. WHEN THERE IS NO DOUBT ABOUT THE DIAGNOSIS.—The treatment is always *conservative* and consists of the following:

A. *Relief of Pain:*
1. Morphine *should not be used* as it causes spasm of the sphincter of Oddi. Pethidine also causes some spasm but may be used in conjunction with other drugs as mentioned below.
2. Instead of doping the patient with sedatives, relief may be provided by dorso-lumbar paravertebral block with 1 per cent lignocaine. There is interruption of the afferent pain fibres of the sympathetic splanchnics.
3. Suppression of pancreatic activity will greatly relieve pain (*see* below).

B. *Suppression of Pancreatic Activity:*
1. Gastroduodenal suction with Ryle's tube subdues the humoral secretion (i.e. caused by secretin and pancreozymin).
2. Inj. Atropin 1/100 gr, every 6 hours, abolishes the nervous (i.e. vagal) phase of secretion. Inj. Baralgan may be used instead, as it overcomes the spasm of the sphincter of Oddi and also acts as a pain reliever.
3. Anti-trypsin drugs, e.g. Trasylol, administered IV or intraperitoneally, are recommended by some authorities to inhibit the destroying effect of trypsin.

C. *Treatment for Shock:*
1. Relief of pain (discussed).
2. Suppression of pancreatic secretions (discussed).
3. Fluid and electrolyte replacement:
    a. The profound shock often demands blood and/or plasma transfusion.
    b. If plasma is not available, low-molecular dextran may be used with advantage.
    c. Glucose and glucose-saline.
    d. Calcium gluconate, 10 ml of a 10 per cent solution IV, should be administered daily, to make for the low serum calcium level.
    e. Hydrocortisone 100 mg IV, repeated as necessary, in cases of persistent hypotension.

D. *Prevention of Secondary Infection:*
Tetracyclines should be administered parenterally, 250 mg every 6 hours.

II. WHEN THE DIAGNOSIS is DOUBTFUL.—There should not be any hesitation in performing an exploratory laparotomy in cases of doubtful diagnosis (e.g. perforated peptic ulcer). If, on exploration, acute pancreatitis is detected:
1. Any drastic handling should be avoided; no attempt should be made to manipulate anywhere near the ampulla of Vater.
2. Some surgeons advocate drainage of the gall bladder (cholecystostomy) to release the tension in the biliary tract.
3. The abdomen should always be closed with *non-absorbable* sutures because the trypsin activity may result in a burst abdomen.

III. DELAYED SURGERY.—This may be as follows:
1. Drainage of a pancreatic abscess in or after the third week.
2. Operation for a pseudopancreatic cyst, when it localises.
3. Cholecystectomy, choledocholithotomy and sphincterotomy in cases of gall stones, when the patient's condition permits.

CHRONIC AND CHRONIC RELAPSING PANCREATITIS

Pathology.—The pancreas undergoes gradual but progressive and permanent loss of structure and function. The acini and/or the islet cells undergo progressive destruction. The destroyed areas are replaced by fibrous tissue, in which there are multiple foci of calcification. The calcification, however, is almost always intraductal and not interstitial, i.e. presenting as *pancreatic stones.* The duct system shows irregular segments of constriction, with proximal dilatation.

Etiology.—As has already been said, the condition is never a sequela to acute pancreatitis. The two common associations of the condition are:

1. Gall stones, particularly those impacted in the common bile duct.
2. Chronic alcoholism.
   Both these conditions are associated with depressed liver function.

Presenting Features.—The patients may present with different features, which may be grouped as follows:

1. Pain, characteristically pancreatic.—Located centrally in the epigastrium, often radiating to the back.
2. Gastrointestinal upsets.—Anorexia, nausea, vomiting.
3. Jaundice.—Obstructive.
4. Malabsorption symptoms, e.g. steatorrhoea, loss of weight. These are due to failure of external secretions.
5. Diabetes.—Due to failure of internal secretion.
6. X-ray.—Pancreatic calcification (pancreatic calculi).
7. ERCP (*see* carcinoma of the pancreas, later in this Chapter).— Strictures (usually .multiple) with proximal dilatations (sacculations) and stones may be demonstrated. There may be a *'chain of lakes'* appearance due to alternating strictures and sacculation along the duct.
8. Operating Pancreatography.—If an ERCP has not been done, 60% Hypaque solution is injected into the pancreatic duct through the duodenum at operation and X-ray taken. The state of the duct system is demonstrated.
9. At laparotomy.—The pancreas feels indurated, with nodularity and restricted mobility (this is the feel of the *'banting pancreas'* that develops in laboratory animals when the pancreatic duct is ligated). The condition may be difficult to be diagnosed from a carcinoma.

The difference between chronic and chronic relapsing pancreatitis is mainly clinical. The chronic variety presents as persistent upper abdominal pain, while the relapsing type manifests itself by recurrent acute upper abdominal pain with minor residual symptoms in between the acute attacks.

Treatment.

I. Conservative.—Unless the symptoms are intolerable, the only treatments advisable is conservative (medical) treatment:

1. Low fat, high protein, high calorie, high vitamin diet. Iron should be supplemented if there is anaemia.
2. Absolute stoppage of alcohol consumption.
3. Pancreatic enzyme, e.g. pancreatin, 5 mg tablet, with each meal.
4. Control of diabetes.

II. Surgery

A. For gall stones:

If there is evidence of gall stones or cholecystitis, the patient must undergo an operation—cholecystectomy with choledochostomy. Some surgeons advocate simultaneous sphincterotomy.

B. For the pancreas:

1. *Sphincterotomy.*—To give a free drainage to both the common bile duct and the pancreatic duct. The results are not satisfactory.

2. *Pancreato-jejunostomy.*—The pancreatic duct is opened with a longitudinal incision and to this the first loop of jejunum is anastomosed side-to-side. All stones, encountered in the duct, are removed prior to the anastomosis.

3. *Partial Amputation of the Pancreas (Distal Pancreatectomy).*—The portion of the pancreas towards the tail is amputated when the disease is more manifested in this part of the gland. The cut end may either be closed with non-absorbable sutures or a loop of jejunum may be anastomosed to it, i.e. *retrograde pancreato-jejunostomy.* With simple closure of the stump there is a high risk of pancreatic fistula.

4. *Pancreato-duodenectomy.*—Excision of the head of the pancreas and the duodenum (as done for carcinoma of the head of the pancreas) may be done when the disease is manifested at its maximum at the head of the gland.

C. For intractable pain:

Splanchnicectomy, i.e. resection of a part of the right greater splanchnic nerve.

PANCREATIC CYSTS

```
                          ┌──────────┐
                          │  TYPES   │
                          └──────────┘
              ┌───────────────┴────────────────────┐
        ┌───────────┐                    ┌─────────────────────┐
        │ True—20%  │                    │     False—80%       │
        └───────────┘                    │ (Pseudopancreatic   │
                                         │       cyst)         │
                                         └─────────────────────┘
    ┌──────────┴─────────────┐
```

| Congenital
1. Dermoid cyst
2. Congenital cystic disease
3. Fibrocystic disease (mucoviscidosis)
4. Lymphangiomatous cyst | Acquired
1. Degeneration cyst
  (a) Cystadenoma
  (b) Cystadenocarcinoma
2. Retention cyst (secondary to
    duct obstruction in chronic pancreatitis)
3. Haemorrhagic cyst
4. Hydatid cyst |

PSEUDOPANCREATIC CYST

Definition.—False, i.e. pseudopancreatic cysts, largely outnumber true cysts of the pancreas (4:1). The cyst is called false because it does not originate in the substance of the pancreas but is located in close proximity to it and attached to it. The relationship between the cyst and the pancreas is so intimate that, on exploration, it is almost impossible to decide whether the cyst is in the gland or outside it, and it is equally impossible to dissect the cyst from the pancreas.

Origin.—A pseudocyst is actually a collection of fluid in the parapancreatic cellular tissues or the lesser sac, the collection having been so encapsulated as to give it the shape of a cyst. Such collection of fluid, with subsequent encapsulation, may result under the following circumstances:

1. Injury to the pancreas, together with laceration of the posterior wall of the lesser sac (that covers the pancreas). Blood and pancreatic secretions accumulate in the parapancreatic cellular tissues and the lesser sac. The epiploic foramen is sealed and so the collections get localised. The cyst increases in size by the

drawing in of fluid into the cyst because of the high osmotic tension of its contents. The surrounding peritoneum (i.e. the peritoneum of the lesser sac) becomes so condensed as to make a capsule for the cyst.
2. Acute haemorrhagic pancreatitis may be followed by the formation of a pseudocyst because of the outpour of blood and pancreatic ferments around the pancreas and into the lesser sac.
3. Perforation of a posterior wall ulcer of the stomach, the epiploic foramen having been previously sealed. The gastric contents escape only into the lesser sac and may form a cyst there.
4. Healed tubercular peritonitis, localised in the lesser sac.

Sites of Presentation.—There being the tough posterior abdominal wall on the back, the cyst projects anteriorly and, in order of frequency, this may be as follows:
1. Between the stomach and the transverse colon.
2. Between the liver and the stomach.
3. Between the layers of the transverse mesocolon, with the colon stretched on the surface of the cyst.

Clinical Features.— Pseudopancreatic cysts are not of common occurrence. Their importance lies in that they have to be taken into consideration while making the differential diagnosis of an upper abdominal swelling. The main features of presentation are as follows:
1. There is either a history of trauma or an acute abdominal pain (suggestive of pancreatitis, rarely of peptic perforation) in the majority of the cases.
2. At a variable interval, usually about two weeks, a swelling appears in the epigastrium. The swelling gradually increases in size.
3. To start with, there is pain, but this is usually replaced by an epigastric discomfort, often associated with severe anorexia, nausea and vomiting (due to pressure on the stomach). Because of inanition, the patient often loses weight quickly.
4. The swelling is localised and its surface is smooth (c.f. retroperitoneal sarcoma, which is nodular).
5. The swelling cannot be moved (c.f. mesenteric cyst, ovarian cyst, cyst of greater omentum). It does not move with respiration (c.f. liver, gall bladder, spleen, kidney) and it is not ballotable (c.f. hydronephrosis).
6. As the cyst is usually tense, it has often a firm rather than a cystic feel, and fluctuation is often absent.
7. There is often a transmitted pulsation of the abdominal aorta (c.f. aneurysm of the abdominal aorta, where the pulsation is expansile, much diminished in the knee-elbow position, and there is the presence of a bruit on auscultation).

Special Investigations
1. A Barium-meal X-ray is done and the lateral views are more important. The stomach is pushed anteriorly, i.e. the vertebro-gastric interval is increased.
2. An IVP may be necessary to exclude the possibility of a hydronephrosis.

Complications
1. Infection (commonest).
2. Haemorrhage.
3. Rupture.

Treatment.—Operation is the only available treatment and this should be done early.

Excision of the cyst is impracticable because of the intimate relationship of the cyst wall to the stomach, colon, mesocolon, pancreas, and liver, from which structures it cannot be separated. The available operations are as follows:

1. INTERNAL DRAINAGE.—This means anastomosing the cyst to the stomach (*cysto-gastrostomy*) or to the jejunum (*cysto-jejunostomy*). Cysto-gastrostomy is the most commonly practised procedure. The stomach is opened through an incision on its anterior wall. The posterior wall of the stomach and the anterior wall of the cyst, which are closely adherent to each other, are now incised together for about 5 cm. The contents of the cyst are sucked out. Several interrupted stitches are applied between the anterior cyst wall and the posterior gastric wall, around the stoma. The opening made on the anterior gastric wall is closed. Fortunately, the drainage is always from the cyst into the stomach and food never enters into the cyst. This operation is highly favoured because the convalescence is short and the patient has no discomfort.

2. EXTERNAL DRAINAGE.—This is also known as *marsupialisation*. The cyst is exposed, part of its wall is removed, the cut edges of the wall are sutured to the skin, and the cyst is packed. The track usually closes in about a month's time, but there may be considerable delay because of skin digestion by the pancreatic enzymes (which may be disastrous) and because of secondary infection. Also, a permanent fistula may develop. These are the reasons why this operation is seldom practised now.

TUMOURS OF THE PANCREAS

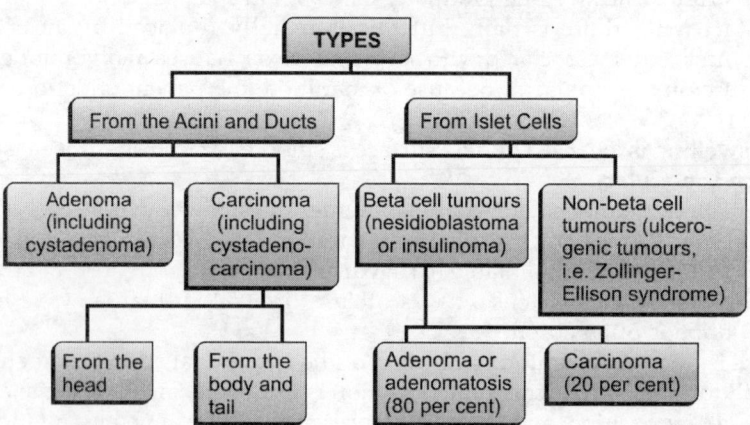

Beta-cell Tumours or Nesidioblastoma.—These tumours, which originate from the beta-cells, produce an excess of insulin, hence they are also known as *insulinoma*.

In a typical case, the patient present with *Whipple's triad*, characterised by a complex of three symptoms, viz.

1. Attacks of nervous of gastro-intestinal disturbance, coming on in a fasting state (e.g. in the morning) or after an exercise, when
2. The fasting blood sugar is less than 50 mg per cent and
3. The attack is relieved immediately by the ingestion of glucose.

Pathologically, the tumours may be:
1. Benign.—Adenoma or adenomatosis (i.e. multiple adenoma)—80 per cent.
2. Carcinoma—20 per cent.

CARCINOMA OF THE PANCREAS

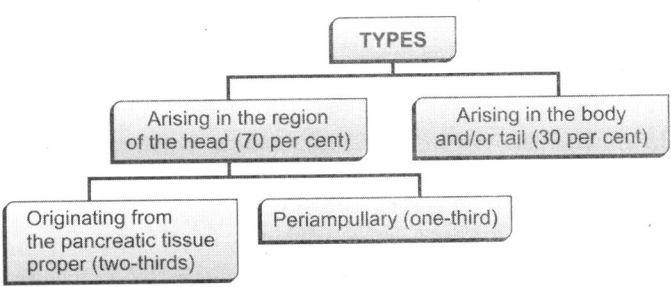

Pathology

I. CARCINOMA OF THE HEAD PROPER.— The tumour arises from the glandular epithelium of the head. It is a spheroidal-cell carcinoma. The tumour is characterised by:

   a. Scirrhous (i.e. hard) nature.
   b. Rapid growth and early metastasis.
   c. Rapidly-progressing obstructive jaundice, leading to death from cholaemia, because of compression of the common bile duct.

II. PERIAMPULLARY CARCINOMA.—Cancers may arise in the:

   a. Termination of the common bile duct or pancreatic duct.
   b. Common ampulla of Vater.
   c. Duodenal papilla or the duodenal mucosa adjacent to the papilla.

On exploration, it is usually impossible to decide in which of the above structures the tumour had originated. This is why these tumours are collectively termed periampullary cancers, i.e. cancers around the ampulla of Vater. The tumours are closely related to the head of the pancreas and so they are considered together with cancers of the pancreatic head. These tumours are of columnar-cell type. They are characterised by:

   a. Encephaloid (i.e. softer) nature, thus more likely to undergo central degeneration.
   b. Slow growth and late metastasis.
   c. Early jaundice which progresses at a lesser speed than that associated with cancer of the head proper.
   d. Anaemia due to slow bleeding from the tumour into the duodenum.

III. CARCINOMA OF THE BODY AND/OR TAIL.—When the tumour arises from the glandular epithelium, it is of the spheroidal-cell type. When it arises from the cells lining the excretory duct, it is of columnar-cell type. These tumours usually differ from the above types in the following points:

   a. Bigger size.
   b. More widespread metastases (death is due to liver metastasis).
   c. Often painful.

Spread

1. DIRECT SPREAD.—Cancers arising in the pancreatic tissue proper tend to spread more quickly than the periampullary cancers. Again, cancers of the body and tail spread quicker than those of the head. Coming out of the pancreatic tissue, the growth may spread to the bile ducts, duodenum or pyloric antrum. Growths of the body and tail may infiltrate into the stomach wall, transverse mesocolon or coeliac plexus (causing pain).

2. LYMPHATIC SPREAD
   a. *From the Head.*—To the nodes in the capsule of the head, and then to the nodes on the bile ducts and those at the porta hepatis. Portal metastasis is relatively late.
   b. *From the Body and Tail.*—To the nodes along the upper border of the pancreas, and then to the coeliac and splenic nodes.

3. VENOUS SPREAD.—These are commoner with cancers of the body and tail. Spread occurs to the liver by way of the portal vein. Usually the metastases are multiple and small. Rarely there may be lung metastasis.

4. TRANSCOELOMIC SPREAD.—Peritoneal dissemination may occur in some cases.

Symptoms

1. *Obstructive jaundice* is the most important presenting feature of cancers of the head, because of obstruction to the common bile duct. The jaundice is progressive and the patient may turn green in colour. In some cases of periampullary carcinoma, the jaundice may show periodical waxing and waning. This is because of a periodic necrosis, occurring in some part of the growth (since it is soft in nature), allowing the pent-up bile to be excreted into the duodenum. During these periods, the stools may get coloured.

2. *Itching.*—This is often distressing and is due to the circulating bile salts.

3. *Pain.*—Though the characteristic presentation of head cancers is stated to be a painless jaundice, many of the patients get pain sometime or other. The pain may be of variable nature and intensity, and may precede or follow the jaundice. Cancers of the body and tail are usually painful because of:
   a. Early involvement of coeliac plexus.
   b. Spread along nerve trunks.

4. *Gastroduodenal Symptoms.*—Anorexia is fairly common; vomiting is a late symptom.

5. *Diarrhoea* may occur in some cases and may be due to:
   a. Pancreatic insufficiency in cases of head cancers due to obstruction of the pancreatic duct (steatorrhoea).
   b. Involvement of the transverse colon by growths of the body and tail.

6. *Diabetes.*—There is a reciprocal relationship between diabetes and pancreatic cancers:
   a. Diabetes is commoner in patients with cancers of the pancreas.
   b. Pancreatic cancers are about 10 times more frequent in the diabetics than the normal people.

7. *Malaena* may occur, especially in periampullary cancers that erode into the duodenum.

8. *Loss of Weight* is a constant feature.

9. *Anaemia.*—More severe in cases of periampullary cancers because of oozing into the duodenum (occult blood in stool).

10. *Thrombophlebitis Migrans.*—There is often a fleeting thrombophlebitis in the different superficial veins, one after the other *(Trousseau's sign)*. This is commoner with cancers of the body and tail.

PHYSICAL SIGNS

1. The gall bladder is often palpable in accordance with *Courvoisier's law* (*see* stone in the common bile duct, Chapter 44).

2. The liver is nearly always palpable and this may be due to:
   a. Biliary obstruction, resulting in dilatation of biliary channels, sometimes amounting to hydrohepatosis (*see* Chapter 44). The palpable liver is smooth, i.e. *cholestatic liver* (on exploration, the liver looks green).
   b. Metastasis.—Hard and nodular liver.

3. The tumour itself is seldom palpable, excepting very rarely, e.g. a large growth in the body or tail.

4. Ascites is a common feature, particularly in a late case. This may be due to:
   a. Compression or invasion of the portal vein by the growth.
   b. Portal obstruction within the liver, when hepatic metastases occur.
   c. Peritoneal dissemination.

Differences between Cancers of the Head Proper and Periampullary Cancers.—Differentiation is usually impossible but the following points may be helpful:

1. JAUNDICE:
   a. After the appearance of the jaundice, the duration of life is usually longer, and the health better maintained, in periampullary cancers.
   b. The jaundice may show waxing and waning in cases of periampullary cancers, and may occasionally disappear completely for some period (already explained).

2. PAIN.—Less common and less severe in periampullary cancers.

3. MALAENA.—Commoner with periampullary cancers because they tend to ulcerate into the duodenum.

4. GALL BLADDER.—More often palpable in periampullary cancers.

Special Investigations

A. TESTS FOR JAUNDICE.—Features of obstructive jaundice are universally found in cancers of the head of any type:
   1. *Blood:*
      a. Serum bilirubin is raised.
      b. Icterix index is high.
      c. There is an immediate direct positive van den Bergh reaction.
   2. Urine:
      a. Urobilinogen is grossly diminished.
      b. Conjugated bilirubin is present in excess.
   3. *Stool:* Stercobilinogen content is grossly lowered (less than 10 mg per cent).

B. TESTS FOR DUODENAL BLEEDING.—This is commoner with periampullary cancers:
   1. Blood may be present in the duodenal aspirate.
   2. Occult blood in the stool is a valuable finding.

C. TESTS FOR PANCREATIC INSUFFICIENCY.—This is due to occlusion of the duct of Wirsung:
1. The stools are bulky, with increased fat content.
2. The duodenal aspirate may show lack of pancreatic secretion. This lack is more significant if it persists even after stimulation by injection of secretin and pancreozymin *(secretin-pancreozymin test).*

A double-lumen radio-opaque *Dreiling tube* is passed and is so placed that one lumen aspirates the stomach and the other aspirates the duodenum (in this way the aspirated duodenal contents are not allowed to be contaminated by the gastric contents). After the duodenum is made empty by suction, secretin 100 units is injected intravenously. The duodenal contents are sucked out every 10 minutes for 30 minutes. Pancreozymin, 1 unit/kg body weight, is now injected intravenously and the duodenal contents aspirated similarly for 30 minutes. Comparison is now made with normal data—in carcinoma lack of secretion is conspicuous.

D. *Exfoliative Cytology.*—The duodenal contents, as aspirated above by stimulation with secretin and pancreozymin, are centrifuged and the deposit is subjected to examination for cancer cells. A positive finding is almost confirmatory.

E. LIVER FUNCTION TESTS:
1. Estimation of serum alkaline phosphatase.
2. Estimation of serum albumin.
3. Estimation of serum transaminases.
(*see* under investigations for gall bladder—Chapter 44).

F. BARIUM-MEAL EXAMINATION.—This is helpful only in relatively advanced cases:
a. In cancers of the head proper there is a positive 'pad sign', i.e. the duodenal C-loop is widened (as if padded), by the growth in the pancreatic head.
b. In periampullary cancers, a persistent filling defect may be detected on the medial wall of the second part of the duodenum. In a typical case this takes the form of a 'reversed 3' i.e. ε
c. *Hypotonic Duodenography.*—A Dreiling tube is passed in 4 mg of Antrenyl (antispasmodic) is injected intravenously to make the gut atonic. 20 to 40 ml of barium solution is run through the tube into the duodenum and then air is injected through the tube to distend the duodenum. This gives a clear outline of the duodenum (by contrast of air and barium). In headproper carcinoma a *'rose-thorn' appearance* of the medial border of the duodenum is seen. Periampullary carcinoma shows a filling defect.
[With the Dreiling tube, therefore, a *'triple test'* can be done:
i. Test for pancreatic secretion,
ii. Exfoliative cytology,
iii. Hypotonic duodenography.]

G. EXPLORATORY LAPAROTOMY AND BIOPSY
1. Many surgeons advocate exploration whenever there is suspicion of a pancreatic cancer and the diagnosis cannot be substantiated otherwise.
2. On exploration, if a growth is suspected, many surgeons prefer a freeze-section biopsy prior to resection of the pancreas. This is because cancers of the pancreas are often very difficult to be diagnosed from chronic pancreatitis by simple palpation of the pancreas. For the purpose of biopsy:

a. Some take a specimen from the pancreas itself.
b. Others consider pancreatic biopsy to be hazardous and select a neighbouring suspicious node for the purpose

Treatment for Causes of the Pancreatic Head

1. *Radical Surgery,* i.e. *Pancreato-duodenectomy.*—This is possible if the growth is not fixed to important structures (e.g. the portal vein), if the nodes at the porta hepatis are free, and if liver secondaries are absent, provided the patient's general condition permits this formidable procedure. The resection, consists of:
   a. The head of the pancreas.
   b. The duodenum, including the pylorus and the duodenojejunal flexure.
   c. The terminal part of the common bile duct.
   After resection, continuity is established as follows:
   i. The end of the common bile duct is anastomosed to the cut upper end of the jejunum. This end-to-end anastomosis is possible because the common bile duct is grossly dilated;
   ii. The cut pancreatic duct is anastomosed, end-to-side, to the jejunum.
   iii. The next loop of jejunum is anastomosed, side-to-end, to the cut end of the stomach.

2. *Palliative Surgery,* i.e. *Cholecystojejunostomy.*—If radical resection is impossible, attempts are made to relieve the patient of the obstructive jaundice and impending liver failure. This can well be achieved by anastomosing the fundus of the gall bladder to a loop of jejunum. To obviate the risk of the jejunal contents entering the gall bladder, a side-to-side anastomosis, between the two limbs of the jejunal loop (used for the anastomosis), is performed.

The high mortality rate of pancreato-duodenectomy makes this palliative procedure an operation of choice to many surgeons, particularly for growths of the head proper, where the patient often dies early of metastasis.

Treatment for Cancers of the Body or the Tail.—*Distal pancreatectomy,* i.e. partial amputation of the pancreas is performed (described under chronic pancreatitis).

46

The Appendix

Anatomical Considerations

1. The appendix is a narrow blind tube, its only open end communicating with the caecum:
   a. One of the most important factors in appendicitis is obstruction to the drainage of the appendix. This is because the appendix has a narrow lumen and it is closed at one end. In infancy the lumen of the appendix is relatively wide; as age advances it gradually undergoes narrowing. This is one of the reasons why appendicitis is rather uncommon in infancy *but* common after first few years of life. In old age the appendix atrophies and, consequently, appendicitis is again relatively rare.
   b. By virtue of its communication with the caecum, this blind tube is likely to lodge substances which may occlude its lumen, e.g. ingested foreign bodies, faecoliths, undigested elements of food, worms, etc.
2. The *submucous coat* of the appendix is very rich in lymphoid tissue. This may be a good barrier against infection but once the lymphoid tissue itself catches the infection, it cannot be eradicated unless the appendix is removed. Because of its lymphoid tissue content, the appendix is called the *abdominal tonsil*.
3. *Musculature:*
   a. Through developmentally the appendix is a part of the large intestine, its musculature resembles that of the small intestine in that the longitudinal coat is continuous, i.e. there are no *Taenia coli.*
   b. There are gaps in the musculature, called *hiatus muscularis:*
      i. Through these gaps, infection from the submucous coat directly comes down to the peritoneum, so that appendicitis virtually means a regional peritonitis, and spreading peritonitis is so common from appendicitis.
      ii. Through these weak spots the appendix may easily perforate when there is a rise of tension inside the organ. This is one of the reasons why appendicular perforation is so common.
4. *Blood Supply:*
   a. The appendicular artery, which is a branch of the inferior division of the ileocolic artery and runs along the free margin of the mesoappendix, i; shorter in length than the appendix itself. This is why the appendix is curved like a comma.
   b. The appendicular artery is end-artery. Inflammatory thrombosis of the artery, which sometimes occurs in acute appendicitis, may, therefore, lead to gangrenous changes in the distal part of the appendix, which has no other source of blood supply. This is another reason why appendicular perforation (following gangrene) is so common.

c. The artery does not reach the tip of the appendix, which has to live on lymphatics only and is, therefore, very prone to gangrenous changes.

d. The additional supply to the base of the appendix, by way of the posterior caecal artery, is of no importance.

5. *Anatomical Positions of the Appendix:*

a. Retrocaecal and retrocolic — 74%

b. Pelvic — 21%

c. Splenic: (i) Pre-ileal (ii) Post-ileal

d. Para-caecal — 5%

e. Subcaecal

f. Subhepatic (maldescended) .

APPENDICITIS

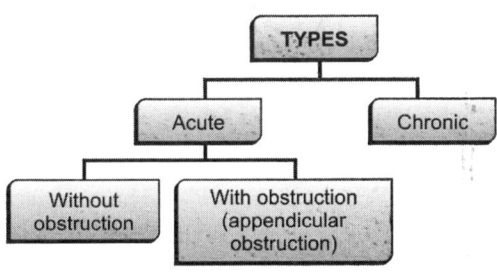

CHRONIC APPENDICITIS

Types.—There are 3 types:

1. Chrome Recurrent Appendicitis.—There are recurrent attacks of acute appendicitis.

2. Chronic Simple Appendicitis.—There is a chronic vague pain in the right iliac fossa, which may be difficult to be diagnosed from amoebic colitis.

3. Appendicular Dyspepsia.—A patient of chronic appendicitis may present with features of duodenal ulcer. In these cases there is no tenderness at the duodenal point but pressure on the Mc. Burney's point causes pain over the epigastrium.

The treatment for any form of chronic appendicitis is appendicectomy (appendectomy).

ACUTE APPENDICITIS

1. WITHOUT OBSTRUCTION *(non-obstructive appendicitis).*—Where the entire length of the lumen can drain into the caecum.

2. WITH OBSTRUCTION *(obstructive appendicitis* or *appendicular obstruction).*—Where there is an obstruction to the flow of the contents into the caecum:

a. *In the lumen.*—Foreign body, undigested bolus of food, faecolith, roundworms, plug of threadworms, etc.

b. *In the wall.*—Stricture (fibrosis resulting from earlier inflammations) or tumour (not very common; the commonest tumour of the appendix is *carcinoid tumour'* which is a locally malignant tumour).

c. *Outside the wall.*—Kinks, adhesions, folds, etc.; the appendix may rarely be a component of an obstructed hernia.

Fates of Acute Appendicitis

1. Surgical removal.
2. *Appendicular Lump.*—This is nature's attempt to localise the infection, which would otherwise lead to a spreading peritonitis. The structures, forming the lump, are the inflamed appendix with the adjacent caecum and colon, the greater omentum (the policeman of the abdomen, which attempts to wrap up any pathological organ to localise the pathology), and the surrounding coils of terminal ileum. These structures are bound together by the plastic inflammatory exudate and this is made possible by a temporary paralytic ileus, set up by the bacterial exotoxins. The usual fate of the lump is a gradual resolution, but it may turn into an abscess or lead to a spreading peritonitis.
3. *Appendicular Abscess.*—When there is a considerable quantity of pus in an appendicular lump.
4. *Spreading Peritonitis*—The process of inflammation is not localised, and a generalised peritonitis supervenes.
5. *Gangrene, Perforation,* and *Faecal Peritonitis.*—The reasons for the rather frequent occurrence of gangrene and perforation of the appendix have been discussed under anatomical considerations.
6. *Mucocele of the Appendix.*—When the virulence of the organisms is low, an obstructed appendix may be distended with a mucopurulent fluid and the condition is known as mucocele. This leads to a chronic form of appendicitis.
7. *Fibrosis.*
8. *Resolution.*—This is most fortunate but least common.

Clinical Features.—These may be discussed under three headings:

Group I: Features common for all the cases.

Group II: Features modified according to the anatomical position of the appendix.

Group III: Differentiating features between non-obstructive and obstructive appendicitis.

Group I: Features of Common for All the Cases

A. Symptoms.—Typically, there is pain, vomiting and temperature, and commonly in that sequence, when it is termed *Murphy's triad.* Often the attack starts in the early morning hours.

1. *Pain.*—The pain, in almost all the cases, is spasmodic to start with; this is due to a rise of tension in the organ because of collection of inflammatory exudates in the wall. Subsequently, however, the pain often becomes dull aching and this is due to the regional peritonitis. In appendicular obstruction, the spasm is more severe because of excessive rise of tension in the organ, and the pain is spasmodic throughout the course of the disease. As for the location of the pain, there may be four types:

a. In the majority, the pain starts around the umbilicus (this area having the same segmental nerve supply as the appendix itself, i.e. T10), and after a few hours it shifts to the right iliac fossa (when regional peritonitis has set in). The initial pain is felt in the midline because, developmentally, the appendix is a diverticulum of the primitive midgut and the primitive midgut is a midline structure.

b. The pain starts over the epigastrium and then shifts to the right iliac fossa.

c. The pain is in the right iliac fossa from the beginning.

d. To start with, there is a vague pain, all over the abdomen but, subsequently. there is localisation at the right iliac fossa.

2. *Vomiting.*—This is reflex because of an associated pylorospasm and, therefore occurs only once or twice, till the stomach is empty. In case an attack starts in empty stomach. there may be only nausea and no vomiting.

3. *Temperature.*—This is rarely high, usually 99 to 100 °F.

4. *Constipation.*

B. PHYSICAL SIGNS

1. The patient looks anxious in pain the tongue is dry, the pulse and respiration rates are high.

2 *Rigidity* over the right iliac fossa.

3. *Tenderness* over the right iliac fossa, maximum at the McBurney's point.

4. *Hyperaesthesia* is sometimes found over the *Sherren's triangle* (the angles of the triangle are the anterior superior iliac spine, the symphysis pubis and the umbilicus).

5. A *rebound tenderness* may sometimes be elicited and is due to the associated parietal peritonitis at the right iliac fossa.

6. *Rovsing's sign* is often positive, i.e pressure on the left iliac fossa causes pain over the appendicular region. There two explanations for this:

a. Retrograde displacement of the colonic gas, striking the base of the inflamed appendix.

b. Displacement of the iliac loops to the right side of the abdomen, irritating the inflamed appendix.

7. The intestinal sounds may be absent because of the paralytic ileus.

Group II Clinical Features Modified according to the Anatomical Position of the Appendix.

A. RETROCAECAL APPENDIX

1. In this position, the inflamed appendix is buffered in front by the caecal gas, so that tenderness and rigidity at the right iliac fossa may be minimum.

2. The patient may have pain in the back, near the loin. Deep tenderness may be present in the loin.

3. The inflamed appendix, lying in contact with the psoas major, causes spasm of this muscle. The patient prefers to keep the right hip flexed, and may attempt to extend the hip causes pain over the appendicular area—this is called *Cope's psoas test.*

B. PELVIC APPENDIX

1. The tip of the inflamed appendix may irritate the urinary bladder, causing frequency of micturition.
2. Rarely the tip may be in contact with the rectum, causing tenesmus and diarrhoea.
3. The appendix, hidden under the pelvic bones, may not cause abdominal tenderness or rigidity, but an internal examination (rectal or vaginal) definitely elicits tenderness in the right side of the pelvis.
4. The inflamed appendix, if it lies on the psoas major, may cause a positive 'Cope's psoas test'.
5. Alternatively, if it lies on the obturator internus, there may be a positive *Cope's obturator test*—attempts to flex and internally rotate the hip causes abdominal pain.

C. SPLENIC APPENDIX

1. The inflamed appendix may either cause pressure on the ileum (preileal appendix) or irritate the ileum (preileal or postileal appendix), resulting in absolute constipation and diarrhoea, respectively.
2. Continued irritation of the ileum may cause incessant vomiting. This factor, together with the above, may lead to a wrong diagnosis of intestinal obstruction.
3. Tenderness, instead of being located at the McBurney's point, may be maximum by the side of the umbilicus.

D. SUBHEPATIC APPENDIX

The pain and tenderness may be in the subhepatic region, leading to a wrong diagnosis of acute cholecystitis or leaking peptic ulcer.

Group III : Differentiating Features between Non-obstructive Appendicitis and Appendicular Obstruction.—The features of the obstructive type are as follows:

1. The pain is spasmodic although.
2. Vomiting is often persistent.
3. Temperature may not be elevated.
4. The extensive spasms may cause diarrhoea.
5. The patient looks more anxious and more toxic.
6. The pulse is out of proportion to the temperature.
7. Hyperaesthesia at the Sherren's triangle is very common.
8. The intestinal sounds may suggest hyperperistalsis.
9. Rebound tenderness is more often elicited.

Management of Acute Appendicitis.—Unless there is a contraindication (*see* below), the only treatment advisable is *immediate appendectomy* because:

1. Spreading peritonitis is a common sequela to acute appendicitis,
2. Perforation of the appendix is fairly common.
3. The operation is rather easy, even in presence of acute inflammation.

The only *contraindication* to immediate appendectomy is the presence of an appendicular lump. This usually takes about 48 hours, time to form. Time, however, is not the criterion and the decision is taken only on the basis of clinical examination as to whether a lump is palpable. Immediate appendectomy is inadvisable in presence of a lump because:

1. The infection, that has been localised by nature, will be disseminated by the surgeon's knife.
2. The operation is technically difficult.
3. The tissues become so friable that intestinal injury is likely to occur during the process of dissection, and faecal fistula may form.

Treatment for Appendicular Lump.—This consists of *an immediate conservative treatment* followed by an *interval appendectomy*, i.e. after the lump has undergone resolution. The lines of conservative treatment are the same as for acute cholecystitis (see Chapter 44), excepting that no sedatives are given to the patient (because the symptoms and physical signs may be masked and a deterioration in the patient's condition may be overlooked).

Under usual circumstances, the lump takes about 3 to 4 weeks' time to resolute, after which appendectomy is undertaken (interval appendectomy).

A close watch is kept on the patient while he undergoes the conservative treatment, and any deterioration during this period calls for abandoning the conservative treatment in favour of an immediate appendectomy. The indications or deterioration are:

a. A rising pulse rate.
b. Vomiting or copious gastric suction.
c. Spreading abdominal pain, suggesting spreading peritonitis (one of the earliest features of spreading peritonitis is pain and tenderness over the left iliac fossa).
d. Diarrhoea or passage of mucus in the stools during the later stages of treatment (these suggest pelvic abscess formation)

Particular Indications for Immediate Appendectomy.—Whatever time has elapsed after the onset of pain, immediate appendectomy is particularly indicated under the following circumstances:

1. If the diagnosis is doubtful (e.g. ruptured ectopic, peptic perforation, etc.).
2. If the patient is a child. The greater omentum is too short in the children to reach and wrap the inflamed appendix efficiently.
3. If the patient is very old. These patients have very low resistance, so spreading peritonitis is fairly common. Further, the onset of peritonitis often goes unrecognised and the patient quickly passes to irreversible uraemia.
4. If the patient has taken a purgative (perforation may easily occur).
5. Any evidence of deterioration during conservative treatment for a lump (*see* above).

Treatment of Appendicular Abscess.—Immediate drainage, under antibiotic cover, is the treatment. Even if the appendix is readily found at drainage, appendectomy should not be done for fear of a faecal fistula. Appendectomy is postponed till the abscess dries up. If, however, the appendix has perforated, its removal is obligatory. The routes of drainage are as follows:

1. If it is a retrocaecal abscess, the drainage is made extraperitoneal, through a Rutherford Morison's incision (see Chapter 53). The peritoneum is not opened but is pushed medially and forwards. From behind the caecum, the abscess is drained extra-peritoneally.

2. In other types, e.g. pre- or post-ileal abscess, intraperitoneal drainage has to be undertaken with a Rutherford Morison's incision.
3. A pelvic abscess may be drained in the females into the vagina and in the males into the rectum.

Differential Diagnosis of Acute Appendicitis

GROUP A.—PELVIC CAUSES:
1. Ruptured ectopic gestation.
2. Ruptured Graffian follicle.
3. Acute salpingitis.

GROUP B.—ABDOMINAL CAUSES:
1. Amoebic colitis.
2. Intestinal obstruction (late cases of acute appendicitis and pre-ileal appendix).
3. Meckel's diverticulum.
4. Acute form of Crohn's disease.
5. Non-specific mesenteric lymphadenitis.
6. Peptic ulcer perforation.
7. Acute cholecystitis.

GROUP C.—RETROPERITONEAL CAUSES:
1. Pyelitis.
2. Ureteric stone.
3. Torsion of undescended testis.
4. Vertebral lesions, e.g. caries spine, metastatic deposits, etc.

GROUP D.—THORACIC CAUSES:
Basal pleurisy, etc.

The Operation of Appendicectomy.—This is described in the Chapter on instruments under mosquito forceps.

47

Anomalies of the Vitello-Intestinal Duct

The vitello-intestinal duct starts from the antimesenteric border of the midgut, passes through the umbilicus, and communicates with the yolk sac. After birth, no remnant of the duct is usually to be found because the duct, together with its lumen, undergoes complete obliteration. Anomalies may, however, occur in this obliteration and produce different pathological conditions which are as follows (Fig. 47.1):

1. The whole length of the duct may persist, resulting in an umbilical fistula. This is called *vitello-intestinal fistula.* Such a fistula usually brings out mucus and, only rarely, stool.

   The *treatment* of a vitello-intestinal fistula is excision of the whole tract, together with the umbilicus, and repair of the rent in the ileum.

   [The other cause of congenital umbilical fistula is a *patent urachus.* The lower end of the urachus communicates with the fundus of the bladder. During the act of micturition, it is the fundus of the bladder that contracts first, occluding the opening of the urachus, situated here. Hence, no leakage of urine occurs through the umbilicus, even in the presence of the fistula. Only when there is an obstruction to the natural flow of urine (e.g. enlarged prostate, stricture urethra, etc.), that such leakage is likely to occur. Hence, though the pathology is congenital, symptoms usually start only late in life. The treatment for a patent urachus is excision of the whole tract and closure of the bladder opening.]

2. The distal part of the tract may remain unobliterated while the proximal part (i.e. towards the intestine) obliterates. This results in an *umbilical sinus.* The epithelial lining of the sinus usually becomes everted and prolapses through the umbilicus in the form of a (false) tumour. This is called *umbilical polyp* or *raspberry tumour* or *enteroieratoma,* all of which are misnomers.

   Treatment consists of excision of the tumour with the umbilicus and the whole length of the tract.

3. Both the proximal and the distal ends of the duct may be obliterated, keeping only the central part patent. This part, with its secretion in the closed space, forms an intraperitoneal cyst, often called *enterocystoma.*

   Treatment is excision of the cyst.

4. The proximal part of the duct may remain unobliterated while the distal part obliterates. This results in a *Meckel's diverticulum* (*see* below).

5. The lumen of the vitello-intestinal duct may be obliterated but the duct itself may persist in the form of a cord. This is called *vitello-intestinal cord.* This may be of the following types:

   a. One end of the cord is attached to the antimesenteric border of the ileum and the other to the umbilicus. This forms an intraperitoneal band. Coils of small intestine may pass under or over this band, or may be twisted around it, causing intestinal obstruction.

b. The umbilical end of the cord may remain free and the cord may move like a free whip inside the peritoneum. It may strangle a loop of gut, causing obstruction.

c. The intestinal end of the cord may not be attached to the ileum but to the tip of a Meckel's diverticulum. In such a case, if there is an umbilical hernia, the cord may pull the Meckel's diverticulum into the hernial sac.

d. The cord may start from the end of an umbilical sinus and extend either to the ileum or to the tip of a Meckel's diverticulum.

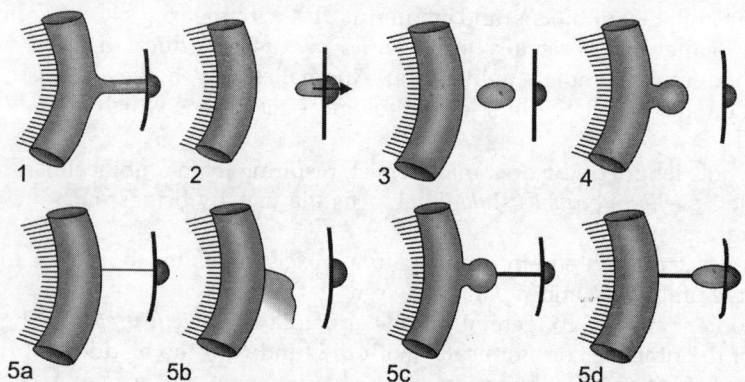

Fig.47.1: Anomalies of the vitello-intestinal duct

6. Occasionally, a cord-like structure stretches from the umbilicus, across the ileum, to end in the mesentery. This is not a vitello-intestinal cord but an obliterated vitelline artery.

MECKEL'S DIVERTICULUM

Incidence.—This represents the unobliterated proximal end of the vitello-intestinal duct.

It is found in 2 per cent of the population (but detected only in a few who produce complications or in whom it is seen at operation or at post-mortem). Usually it is 2 inches in length and located at about 2 feet above the ileo-caecal junction. The incidence is equal in both the sexes but, as complications are commoner in the males, leading to detection of the condition, there is an apparent frequency in the males.

The diverticulum is typically located at the antimesenteric border of the ileum. Since it is a congenital diverticulum, it is thick-walled, possessing all the coats of the small gut, to which it is attached. Typically, therefore, the mucosa is that of the small intestine. However, in about 20 per cent of cases there is presence of heterotopic epithelium, e.g. gastric, colonic, pancreatic, etc. Usually such heterotopic element presents in the form of a swollen mucosa that is commonly found at the base of the diverticulum, encroaching onto the adjacent small intestine.

Complications.—While majority of these diverticula are *silent,* complications often occur, producing symptoms. In order of frequency, these complications are as follows:

1. Haemorrhage.—This occurs from a peptic ulcer that may form in the diverticulum because of acid-pepsin secretion by the heterotopic gastric epithelium that may be present in its wall. Typically, the patient is a young boy and the blood is passed per rectum. As the source of the blood is the midgut, it is neither bright red nor tarry black.

2. Intestinal obstruction.—This may be caused in different ways:
   a. *Intussusception:* The invagination usually starts at the base and not at the apex of the diverticulum. This means that the apex of the intussusception is the base of the diverticulum, where a swollen mucosa is possibly the cause.
   b. Obstruction by a vitello-intestinal cord, which stretches from the tip of the diverticulum to the umbilicus. Loops of small intestine may pass over or below this band or be twisted around the band *(volvulus).*

3. Meckelian diverticulitis (inflammation).—This is usually caused by foreign bodies, and may be with or without perforation of the diverticulum. The clinical features of a diverticulitis without perforation are similar to those of acute appendicitis. The features of a diverticulitis with perforation are usually like those of peptic ulcer perforation. In either case, the correct diagnosis is reached only at operation.

4. Chronic peptic ulcer.—The ulcer is usually found at the base of the diverticulum. The pain is related to meals like a duodenal ulcer but is felt around the umbilicus.

Special Investigations.—A careful barium meal examination may show the diverticulum. Usually, however, a diverticulum is detected only at operation, either when the patient comes with complications related to it or during routine exploration of the abdomen at some other operation.

Treatment

Group A: When the patient comes with a complication related to the diverticulum, excision has to be done. A part of the small intestine attached to the base of the diverticulum should be included in the excision, since pathological areas are usually located here. The opening in the gut is closed in two layers. Alternatively, a portion of the ileum, together with the diverticulum, is resected.

Group B: When a diverticulum is detected at routine exploration of the abdomen at some other operation, unless there is an extra risk on the patient, it should be excised in order to avoid complications in future.

48

Intestinal Tuberculosis and Crohn's Disease

INTESTINAL TUBERCULOSIS

Types

1. Ulcerative tuberculosis.
2. Hyperplastic ileo-caecal tuberculosis. (Miliary tuberculosis is not considered here.)

ULCERATIVE TUBERCULOSIS	HYPERPLASTIC ILEO-CAECAL TUBERCULOSIS
1. Secondary to pulmonary tuberculosis and caused by ingestion of the bacilli in the sputum.	1. Primary, there is usually no pulmonary lesion.
2. Occurs in people with low resistance against tubercle bacilli; so there is caseation and breakdown of tissues, resulting in ulceration.	2. Occurs in people who have acquired high immunity against tuberculosis and they respond by excess of fibrous tissue formation, hence called hyperplastic.
3. The site is the terminal part of the ileum.	3. Occurs in the ileo-caecal region (the terminal inch or two of the ileum and the caecum are affected).
4. Due to human type of bacillus.	4. May be caused by both bovine and human types, and the infection is due to a small number of bacilli of an avirulent strain.

ULCERATIVE TUBERCULOSIS

Pathology.—The distal part of the ileum is the usual site because this is the most actively absorptive part of the gut and is rich in lymphoid tissue (Peyer's patches).

The ulcers start on the Peyer's patches and extend along the transverse axis of the gut, i.e. the direction of the lymphatic vessels along which the bacilli pass. They have all the characters of tubercular ulcers. As the ulcers are usually shallow, they perforate only rarely. Their importance lies in the fact that, during healing, they may cause extensive fibrosis and lead to strictures, single or multiple. As the small-gut contents are liquid, obstructive features, however, are late to set in—at first chronic and then acute.

Clinical Features

1. The patient is usually a known person of pulmonary tuberculosis.
2. Diarrhoea is the main symptom, stools often containing pus.
3. Quick loss of weight.
4. Constitutional symptoms of tuberculosis.

Special Investigations
1. Stool Examination.—Pus and occult blood are present.
2. X-ray chest and ESR.
3. Barium meal examination may fail to show the terminal ileum (and sometimes the proximal colon) since the meal passes very quickly through the ulcer-bearing irritable loop.

Treatment.—Conservative (anti-tubercular) treatment is the rule. Surgery may have to be undertaken for:
1. Strictures causing obstruction.
2. Perforation (rare).

HYPERPLASTIC ILEO-CAECAL TUBERCULOSIS

Pathology.—The terminal inch or two of the ileum and the caecum are affected. The affected gut shows gross thickening of its wall, resulting from chronic inflammation. The thickening is partly due to tubercular granulation tissue and oedema, but is mostly due to deposits of excess of fibrous tissue, which is maximum in the submucous and subserous planes. Unlike other tubercular lesions, there is no ulceration and no breakdown of tissues. Also, unlike Crohn's disease, abscess and fistula formation are rare. Microscopically, tubercular lesions, as usual, are noted but areas of caseation are neither numerous nor extensive.

The regional mesentery is usually thickened and oedematous. The mesenteric nodes are involved in the tubercular process but these nodes, again, rarely soften.

The effect of the excess of fibrous tissue in the wall is an intestinal obstruction. This is due to:
a. Encroachment on the lumen by the thickened wall.
b. Contraction of the fibrous tissue.

Clinical Features
1. As the patients have good resistance against tuberculosis, constitutional features are often minimum (only a vague ill-health).
2. These patients usually present with features of chronic intestinal obstruction, characterised by *alternate constipation and diarrhoea,* associated with attacks of *abdominal pain.* Often the patient presents with *blind-loop syndrome* because of stasis, resulting from obstruction. The stasis causes an abnormal bacterial flora and the resultant infection leads to anaemia (due to vitamin B_{12}-deficiency), steatorrhoea, and loss of weight, i.e. 'blind-loop syndrome'.
3. Often the patients present with lump in the right iliac fossa.
4. Some patients may first present with acute intestinal obstruction.

Special Investigations
1. Stool examination shows presence of blood and mucus.
2. ESR may not be high.
3. X-ray chest is usually negative.
4. Barium Enema Examination.—A barium meal usually gives a better picture of the ileo-caecal region than a barium enema but should be avoided lest it precipitates an acute intestinal obstruction. The findings in case of hyperplastic ileo-caecal tuberculosis are as follows:

a. Persistent irregular narrowing of the lumen of the terminal ileum, caecum and ascending colon.
b. Widening of the ileo-caecal angle, caused by the pull of the fibrous tissue. This angle, which is normally 90 degrees, may become as wide as 180 degrees, so that the terminal ileum lies vertically in line with the caecum and the ascending colon.
c. The caecum is pulled up and may become subhepatic.

Treatment
A. If there is no intestinal obstruction, conservative (antitubercular) treatment is advised.
B. Majority of the patients present with chronic obstruction. They should undergo surgery, under cover of anti-tubercular treatment. There is, however, a diversity of opinion as regards the nature of the surgery:
1. Some surgeons advocate radical surgery, i.e. right hemicolectomy.
2. Since the main problem in these cases is the obstruction and not the tuberculosis, many surgeons advocate a conservative surgery and this means ileo-transverse anastomosis. If the patient's symptoms still persist or if the features of 'blind-loop syndrome' set in, hemicolectomy may be undertaken at a second stage.
C. Patients presenting with acute intestinal obstruction should be treated by ileo-transverse anastomosis.

CROHN'S DISEASE

This disease, in the majority of cases, occurs in the terminal part of the ileum, and hence it is popularly known as *regional ileitis*. However, it may occur in any part of the gut, and hence it is better called *regional enteritis*.

Etiology.—The cause is not understood, but the process is undoubtedly one of non-specific inflammation. There are different views as to the cause:
1. It is due to Streptococci, *B. coli*, or dysenteric organisms.
2. It is due to an acid-fast bacillus (no such organism has, however, been demonstrated in the lesion).
3. It is a type of sarcoidosis.
4. It is due to lymphatic blockage.
5. It is a foreign body reaction to silica (in ingested toothpastes) or other chronic irritants. This is the most popular view.

Pathology.—The disease typically occurs in the terminal ileum, involving a limited segment, usually twelve inches (but this may vary). Distally the pathology stops sharply at the ileo-caecal valve. Proximal to the lesion there is healthy gut, but still proximal to it there is usually a small lesion, i.e. a *skip lesion*. It is believed that further skip lesions, often microscopical, do exist, and are the causes of recurrence which is so frequent even after resection of the affected loop (50 to 60 per cent of the cases recur).

There are two forms of the disease:
a. Acute—5 per cent.
b. Chronic—95 per cent.

ACUTE FORM.—The affected loop is grossly congested and somewhat oedematous. The adjacent mesentery is congested and contains enlarged soft nodes. There is no evidence of caseation anywhere.

CHRONIC FORM

1. There is gross thickening of the wall due to granulomatous and fibrous tissue deposits, particularly in the submucous and subserous coats. The hypertrophic wall makes the lumen irregularly narrow and the gut becomes stiff, like a hose-pipe, with loss of capacity to contract. The granulomatous tissue does not show any caseation but there is a giant cell system. The mucous membrane shows patchy ulcerations.
2. The adjacent mesentery is grossly thickened and oedematous. It contains enlarged and fleshy lymph nodes, which, however, neither caseate nor calcify (c.f. tuberculosis).
3. Subsequently, multiple strictures develop in the gut.
4. Still later, dense adhesions, abscesses, and fistulous tracts are likely to develop (*see* clinical features).

Clinical Features

ACUTE FORM.—The presenting features are very similar to acute appendicitis, excepting that, instead of constipation, diarrhoea usually occurs.

CHRONIC FORM.—The disease runs in 3 stages:

Stage I: The patient presents with features of ulceration, characterised by long-continued irregular diarrhoea and dysentery, abdominal pain, mild pyrexia, constitutional symptoms, loss of weight, and a secondary anaemia. An ill-defined lump is often felt in the right iliac fossa.

Stage II: There are features of chronic intestinal obstruction, characterised by alternate constipation and diarrhoea. The lump becomes more definite. Sometimes an acute obstruction may set in.

Stage III: Dense adhesions develop with surrounding structures. Localised peritoneal abscesses may form. Fistulae may develop:

1. *Internal fistula,* e.g. with pelvic colon, bladder, etc.
2. *External fistula*—if there is a recent abdominal scar (e.g. appendectomy), a fistula may occur through it. Spontaneous perianal fistulae may occur.

Special investigations

1. Stool examination.—Blood, mucus, and often steatorrhoea.
2. Barium enema usually provides the diagnosis:
   a. *In the non-stenosing stage,* the affected loop shows:
      i. Lack of segmentation with loss of peristalsis,
      ii. Straightening of valvulae conniventes.
      iii. The oedematous mucosa, in between the ulcers, produce multiple filling defects (*cobblestone appearance*), seen after evacuation of the meal.
   b. *When stenosis sets in,* there is gross irregular narrowing of lumen, which in its extreme stage, shows the barium as narrow as a string—*string sign of Kantor.*

Treatment

A. ACUTE CASES.—These require no special treatment and, in the majority of cases, the acute process subsides. In the great majority, there is no recurrence. If the abdomen is explored on a wrong diagnosis of acute appendicitis, the one thing *not to do* is appendectomy since a faecal fistula may easily form through the scar.

B. CHRONIC CASES

1. *Medical Treatment* for the early cases:
   a. High calorie, high protein, high vitamin, low carbohydrate diet.
   b. Sulphathalidine or other antibiotics.
   c. Cortisone, ACTH, and salazopyrine are better avoided as they usually fail to produce long-lasting effects.
   d. Azathioprine, in small doses, is under trial.

2. *Surgical Treatment.*—This is indicated under the following conditions:
   a. Failure with medical treatment.
   b. Presence of intestinal obstruction.
   c. Fistula formation.

   There is a diversity of opinion as to the nature of surgery:
   i. Some surgeons advocate radical operation, i.e. right hemicolectomy with resection of the affected loop of ileum.
   ii. Since, even after such extensive resections, recurrence is fairly common (evidently due to unrecognised skip-lesions), many surgeons advocate a 'defunctioning ileo-transverse anastomosis'. In this operation, the ileum is bisected proximal to the lesion and the distal cut end is closed; the proximal cut end is taken for an ileo-transverse anastomosis, end-to-side. Should toxicity or other complications (e.g. blind-loop syndrome) occur in future, a hemicolectomy may still be undertaken.
   iii. If, however, fistulae have formed, resection is obligatory.

49

Disease of the Colon

MEGACOLON

This is a condition of dilatation and hypertrophy of a part or whole of the colon, occurring in the absence of any demonstrable obstructive lesion. Two distinct types are recognised:

1. Hirschprung's Disease or Congenital Megacolon.
2. Idiopathic Megacolon.

HIRSCHPRUNG'S DISEASE

Pathogenesis.—This is a congenital malformation (hence called congenital megacolon). There is a defect in the intrinsic innervation of the gut, which results in defective propulsion of its contents, i.e. a functional obstruction. Such obstructions are not visible to the naked eye but their effects are manifested as dilatation and hypertrophy of the gut proximal to the site of obstruction.

This functional obstruction is caused by the absence of ganglion cells in the submucous and intermuscular myenteric plexuses, their place being taken by clusters of unmedullated nerve fibres. Normally this plexus transmits the parasympathetic stimulation from the nerve roots to the motor end-organs. In the absence of the ganglion cells of the plexus, the transmission mechanism is lost, resulting in loss of the normal peristaltic movement of the affected part of the gut. This is the functional obstruction. As the aganglionic segment is the cause of the obstruction, the disease is also known as *aganglionosis* or *congenital aganglionic megacolon*.

Characteristically, the aganglionic segment commences at the lower end of the rectum and extends proximally for a variable distance. In 80 per cent of cases it does not extend beyond the sigmoid colon. These are known as *short segment aganglionosis*. In the remaining, it extends proximally; to involve variable lengths of the colon and may even involve the terminal ileum. These are the rare cases of *long segment aganglionosis*. There are some cases where aganglionosis occurs in 'skip areas'; these are known as *segmental aganglionosis*. Because of these variations, the disease is more correctly termed *congenital intestinal aganglionosis*

Just proximal to the aganglionic segment, there is an area of transitional zone, usually 1 to 5 cm in length. Here ganglion cells are present, but fewer than normal. Above the transitional zone the distribution of ganglion cells, in the plexuses, are normal.

Pathology

1. The aganglionic segment, which is the cause of the disease, looks normal to the naked eye (this should be carefully remembered—Fig. 49.1).

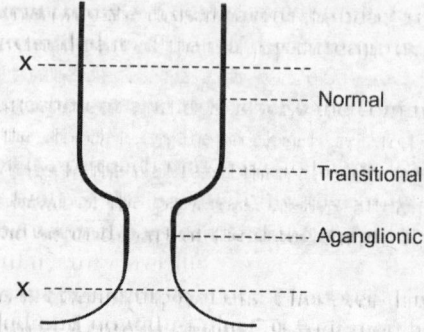

Fig. 49.1: Hirschprung's disease. The two lines marked 'X' denote the levels of resection

2. The transitional zone also looks normal macroscopically.
3. The proximal gut, which is almost always the colon, undergoes gross dilatation and hypertrophy. This is most marked in the sigmoid colon, which lies just proximal to the obstruction. The dilated gut is partly filled up by gas and partly by faecal matter, which is hard, pultaceous, and offensive-smelling. The hypertrophy is mostly marked in the circular muscle fibres. The mucous membrane undergoes secondary inflammation and often develops stercoral ulcers. The pelvic mesocolon is elongated and its vessels are elongated, dilated and tortuous.

Clinical Features.—The disease is at least 5 times commoner in the males. In some instances it has been found to run in families, suggesting a genetic bearing. The patient usually comes in infancy, sometimes in early childhood, and occasionally in the adult life.

A. INFANTS.—The patient usually presents within 3 days of birth and the presenting features are as follows:
1. *Onset:*
   a. No passage of meconium. After insertion of the little finger into the rectum, meconium is passed. Thereafter, stools are passed like *toothpaste,* only on great straining and in inadequate quantities.
   b. Abdominal distension sets in within 3 days. There are visible peristalsis and loud borborygmi.
   c. Vomiting starts within a few days of birth. The vomitus contains bile.
2. *Progress.*—There may be two types of cases, of which the first one is commoner:
   a. Acute-on-chronic obstruction sets in, anytime from within a few days of birth. The obstructions are usually recurrent, till the patient undergoes colostomy or till death occurs. The earlier attacks of acute obstruction are often relieved by insertion of examining fingers or by small enemas, and sometimes spontaneously.
   b. Chronic obstruction, characterised by chronic constipation alternated by episodes of diarrhoea, associated with passage of large amount of foul-smelling gas.

B. CHILDREN.—Those infants who survive the odds of infancy may present during childhood. The child presents with:

1. Constipation, dating from birth. The stools are hard and likened to 'goat-pellet'.
2. Malnutrition.—Wasted limbs with wrinkled skin; small face with sunken eyes and hollowed-out cheeks.
3. Abdominal distension.—The abdomen has a characteristic appearance. Its muscles become thin from stretching, and there are prominent veins on it. The costal angle is widened and its margins are everted.
4. Rectal examination reveals that the anal sphincter is normal and the rectum is empty. Faecal impaction may be felt above it, by the tip of the examining finger.

C. ADULTS
1. Only occasionally the symptoms become severe as late as in the adult life, when the patient seeks advice.
2. Some of the adult cases present with a colostomy, performed in infancy or childhood.

Causes of Death.—50 per cent of the untreated cases die during the first year of life. The causes of death, in Hirschprung's disease, are:
1. Acute intestinal obstruction that may result in:
   a. Electrolytic imbalance and dehydration.
   b. Strangulation.
   c. Perforation of the colon;
2. Malnutrition, anaemia, and toxaemia ('toxic megacolon', characterised by bloody diarrhoea, persistent anorexia, loss of weight, fever and leucocytosis, comparable to ulcerative colitis).
3. Enterocolitis.
4. Chest infections.

Special Investigations
1. BARIUM ENEMA EXAMINATION.—This should be done in an unprepared bowel, i.e. without administering the preliminary colonic washouts, as is done in other cases. This is because a preliminary washout often minimises the dilatation of the gut above the obstruction. The barium enema should be prepared with normal saline and not with water because the megacolon absorbs water much more rapidly than normal colon and this may result in 'water intoxication' with disturbance of electrolyte balance, especially of sodium.
   a. *In infants.*—The most distinctive feature in the infants is retention of the barium for 24 hours or more. In the infants the proximal colon has not yet become permanently dilated, so that a change in the calibre from it, to the aganglionic segment, is not well defined. Thus, in case of the infants, delayed films after 24 hours are obligatory.
   b. *In Children.*—The characteristic radiological finding is a narrow aganglionic segment, the funnel-shaped transitional zone, and the increasingly dilated proximal colon. Most important of these is the visualisation of the narrow segment because this gives the diagnosis and also provides an idea about the length of the aganglionic segment. However, it may be difficult to be demonstrated in many cases, particularly if it is short in length, because it is overlapped by the dilated over-filled proximal colon. Therefore, a frontal as well as a lateral view must be taken.

2. RECTAL BIOPSY.—Demonstration of the absence of ganglion cells in the submucous and intramural myenteric plexuses, and presence of clusters of unmedullated nerve fibres in their place is confirmatory of Hirschprung's disease. The biopsy must be taken at least 2 cm from above the mucocutaneous junction. A block of full-thickness rectal wall, measuring 5 mm × 10 mm, must be taken for biopsy. Only superficial biopsy provides no confirmatory evidence since the intermuscular plexus has to be seen. The defect made in the muscle and mucosa has to be carefully repaired.

3. EXPLORATORY LAPAROTOMY.—This has to be undertaken:
   a. As an emergency procedure, when the patient presents with an acute-on-chronic obstruction.
   b. As a cold operation, when diagnosis cannot be established by barium enema examination and rectal biopsy.

Treatment

AIM.—The only curative treatment is surgery. The aim of the surgery is to excise the whole length of the aganglionic segment (which is the cause of the functional obstruction) and to restore continuity by a method which will retain the normal sphincteric control at the anus. In other words, the upper limit of resection must include the transitional zone and a little of the healthy (dilated) colon above it, while the lower limit should be so designed as to preserve the anal canal with its sphincters.

ONE-STAGE OR TWO-STAGE?

A formidable procedure like this, compared to the age of the patient, is possible only when the patient is moderately healthy. The majority of the patients are neonates or infants, presenting either seriously ill or in a state of acute intestinal obstruction. In such cases an emergency colostomy is required to save the life of the patient and the definitive operation of resection has to be postponed to a later date, i.e. two-stage operation. One-stage surgery (primary resection) is limited only to the patients who present after the age of 18 months in a moderately fair health.

Colostomy.—As to the siting of the colostomy, there are two views:
1. Some surgeons prefer a transverse colostomy.
2. Others prefer a colostomy placed just above the transitional zone.

The advantages of the latter procedure is that the loop of colostomy may be resected together with the aganglionic segment, so that the whole operation can be completed in two stages, viz. colostomy and resection. The advantages of a transverse colostomy is that it leaves a clean operative field for the resection and it protects the anastomosis after resection by defunctioning it, because the colostomy still works. Its only disadvantage is that it requires a third operation, viz. closure of the colostomy.

During the operation of colostomy, it is always advisable to put a marker with black silk at the lowermost limit of the dilated ganglionic segment, i.e. just above the transitional zone. This is of great help during the operation of resection. After a colostomy has been done, the distended gut usually collapses to the calibre of normal colon and, during resection, it may be very difficult to demarcate it from the aganglionic segment. A previously placed marker helps a great deal.

The definitive operation is postponed until the child attains a normal weight for its age. It is usually advised after the age of one year.

Definitive Operation.—Three types of operation are practised:

1. Swenson's operation or its modification.
2. Duhamel's operation.
3. Soave's operation.

SWENSON'S OPERATION.—The operation requires a combined abdominal and anal approach. The inferior mesenteric artery is divided between ligatures, and the sigmoid colon and the rectum are mobilised to as far down as possible. from the abdomen. During mobilisation, dissection is done as close to the wall of the gut as possible, in order to avoid injury to the pelvic nerves and thereby to avoid interference with the bladder and ejaculatory functions. The line of junction between the ganglionic and the aganglionic segments is now made out. The identification of this level may be helped if a marker had been placed during the earlier operation of colostomy. Confirmatory evidence may be obtained if freeze-section biopsy from the gut wall possible at operation. The gut is divided through the lower part of the ganglionic segment. The distal cut end is closed in the form of a stump. A long artery forceps is now introduced per anum and the stump is hold with the tip of the forceps. As the artery forceps is withdrawn from the anus, the distal loop of gut, containing the aganglionic segment and the normally innervated anal canal, is everted (i.e. mucosa outside), A transverse incision is made on the anterior wall of this everted loop, 2 cm from (now below) the anus, i.e. on the anal canal. Through this opening the long forceps is reintroduced and the proximal divided end of the colon is pulled through it (since a loop of gut is pulled through another loop, the operation is known as *pull-through operation*). The anal canal is completely divided along the same line in which it was incised on its anterior wall. Thus the whole length of the aganglionic segment is resected. To the cut end of the anal canal is anastomosed the cut end of the pulled through colon. The resection of the gut and the anastomosis are, therefore, done outside the anal canal. The anastomosis is done in two layers and the suture line, together with the anal canal, is pushed back, i.e. inverted, through the anus.

MODIFIED SWENSON'S OPERATION.—In the original Swenson's operation, the patient often complains of a tightness of the sphincter, resulting in difficulty in defaecation: This difficulty may be overcome by bisecting the anal canal obliquely, instead of transversely, so that 2 cm of the anal canal remains anteriorly and only 1 cm posteriorly. The resection thus includes a substantial portion of the internal sphincter and thereby overcomes the tightness (this is the modification).

DUHAMEL'S OPERATION.—One difficulty of Swenson's operation (or its modification) is that the normal rectal sensation is lost in the absence of the rectum, so that the defaecation reflex is disturbed. This difficulty is overcome in the Duhamel procedure. In this operation, only the aganglionic segment of the colon is excised per abdomen and the rectum is preserved. The cut end of the rectum is closed. The upper cut end of the colon is brought down behind the rectum (in front of the sacrum). It is then made to traverse through the posterior wall of the anal canal, between the fibres of the internal sphincter, so that it finally emerges at the anus posteriorly but in the submucous plane (i.e. not in the anal lumen). After an interval of 3 weeks, an enterotribe (crusher) is used to crush the partition between the two lumens. As the extrinsic nerve supply of the rectum is left undisturbed, the normal rectal sensation and the defaecation reflex are preserved.

SOAVE'S OPERATION.—This operation, like the Duhamel procedure, retains the rectum, excising only the aganglionic part of the colon from the abdomen. The rectum is denuded of its mucous membrane. Thereafter, the proximal colon is pulled through the lumen of the rectum and anal canal, and is sutured to the anus. Thus, it preserves the rectal sensation as in Duhamel's operation but avoids the blind rectal loop of that operation.

IDIOPATHIC MEGACOLON

This type of megacolon is now regarded as a distinct entity from congenital megacolon, i.e. Hirschprung's disease, from which it differs in two respects:

i. It occurs in older children or in adults.

ii. The dilatation of the gut extends up to the anus, which means that the rectum is also dilated.

As to its *pathogenesis*, there are two views:

1. It is a variant form of Hirschprung's disease, in which the aganglionic segment is so short as to avoid detection, even on careful and repeated biopsies.

2. It is an acquired condition, resulting from either or a combination of the following causes: .

   a. There is a long dilated loop of the pelvic colon, which provides a large surface for water absorption, so that the stools are unduly hard, too hard to be evacuated normally. In other words, there is a habitual constipation.

   b. Faulty bowel habits (commoner in females).

   c. Spasticity of the anal sphincters.

Inability to detect any aganglionic segment, even on careful biopsies, and failure to cure by resection of the rectum, discard the first view; the second view is more commonly accepted.

Rectal examination reveals that the anal sphincter is tight and the rectum is loaded with hard stool (c f Hirschprung's disease).

When medical treatment (regularisation of bowel habits, use of laxatives and analgesic ointments) fails, a left hemicolectomy may be required to cure the condition. The absorptive surface of the colon is thus minimised and the stools are made softer, to be easily evacuated.

ULCERATIVE COLITIS

Definition.—This is a condition of severe non-specific inflammation of the colon, associated with various degrees of ulceration.

Pathology

ONSET AND PROGRESS.—Almost always the disease starts in the rectum and extends proximally. In most of the cases, sooner or later, the whole of the colon is involved. If the ileo-caecal valve is incompetent, retrograde extension into the terminal ileum (usually involving the last one foot), i.e. ileitis, is apt to occur. In some cases 'skip lesions' occur in the colon, i.e. in between the affected areas there are lengths of healthy colon. In any case, the distal part of the colon nearly always shows the pathology at its maximum. Rarely, the proximal colon escapes completely.

MACROSCOPIC APPEARANCE

1. To start with, there is swelling, oedema, and intense congestion of the mucous membrane, associated with minute ulcers. The ulcers may be few and far between, or there may be a 'sea of ulceration'. The ulcers are shallow and irregular, with sloughs adherent to their floor. Pin-point abscesses are often visible in the depth of the mucous membrane.

2. As the disease progresses and extends along the length of the colon, the severity of the ulceration and the underlying pathology also increase. The mucous membrane becomes bright red or purple in colour, associated with purpuric haemorrhages. The small ulcers coalesce to form big ulcerations, chiefly because the crypts of Lieberkuhn become distended with pus and burst into the bowel. These big ulcers may be round or linear, but usually they are irregular in shape with undermined irregular margins. The mucous membrane, in between the ulcers, is usually swollen and oedematous. In many cases, mucosal tags, having the pattern of polyps, are found to be hanging. These are called *'pseudopolyps'* and are caused by epithelial thickening, resulting from attempts at healing. In very advanced cases the ulcers are so numerous and extensive that wide areas of colon appear to be completely denuded of mucosa.

As the ulcers get deeper and extend into the submucosa, they cause reflex muscular spasm, giving the appearance of strictures. In long-standing cases actual fibrosis occurs in the wall of the colon. The colon now becomes thick-walled and rigid. It loses its normal sacculations and becomes smaller than normal, both in calibre and in length.

The lymph nodes in the mesocolon are enlarged but the mesocolon remains thin, devoid of fat.

Etiology.—The exact cause of the disease is still unknown. Infection has some part to play in its genesis. Organisms of the dysenteric group, *B. coli*, enterococci and haemolytic streptococci are sometimes found but their mere presence does not prove that the disease is entirely due to them. There must be a constitutional factor, unknown at present, which is the root cause. There are different views as to this *unknown constitutional factor.*

1. *Allergy.*—It is believed by many people that the disease is an allergic manifestation to an allergen in the food. Milk has been incriminated most, because a high titre of antibodies to milk proteins has been found and because relief has often been obtained by switching to a milk-free diet.

2. *Autoimmune Disease.*—Some pathologists regard the disease as an autoimmune disorder. This view is supported by the common association of arthropathy, hepatitis, iridocyclitis, etc. The fact that no specific antibody has been identified, goes against this view.

3. *Lack of Lysozyme.*—This is a mucolytic ferment and is found in lowest concentration during an acute attack of the disease.

4. *Psychosomatic Disorder.*—According to many, the disease is a psychosomatic disorder linked with emotional stresses.

5. *Genetic Factor.*—There may be a genetic basis as the condition has been reported in twins.
6. *Crohn's Disease.*—According to some workers, ulcerative colitis is a form of Crohn's disease, affecting only the large intestine. That in some cases 'skip lesions' occur and that in some patients the disease spreads to the terminal ileum, are taken as positive points in support of this view.

Complications

I. LOCAL COMPLICATIONS

A. *Acute Complications:*
1. Perforation.
2. Diffuse peritonitis (unassociated with perforation).
3. Massive haemorrhage.
4. Acute dilatation of the colon.—This is also known as *'toxic megacolon'* and is caused by damage to the muscle cells in the wall of the gut, so much so, that they lose their power of contraction (it is not caused by damage to the myenteric plexus). The characteristic feature is that the patient, who was having diarrhoea, suddenly develops features of intestinal obstruction, associated with visible peristalsis. -

B. *Chronic Complications:*
1. Pseudopolyposis.—This occurs in about 15 percent of the cases. It must be distinguished from true polyps, which are real pedunculated tumours of the colon.
2. Carcinoma.—The overall incidence is 5 per cent. A colon of ulcerative colitis is five to ten times more likely to develop cancer than a normal colon. Incidence of carcinoma of the colon is 20 years earlier in the patients suffering from ulcerative colitis than in the normal population. The risk of carcinoma increases with the duration of the disease, and cancers are more apt to occur when ulcerative colitis starts early in life. Again, its incidence is more where the whole of the colon is involved in the colitis. The colon develops cancer much more frequently than the rectum, though the inflammation usually starts in the rectum.
3. Fibrous stricture.—The commonest site is the rectosigmoid junction but there may be multiple strictures.
4. Paracolic infection and abscess formation.
5. Internal fistulae.—Colovesical, rectovaginal, etc.

II. GENERAL COMPLICATIONS AND SYSTEMIC CHANGES

A. *Acute Cases:*
1. Dehydration, mineral loss, and depletion of protein (may be more than 50 gm per day).
2. Portal bacteraemia.
3. Liver damage, as a consequence of the above two factors.

B. *Chronic Cases:*
1. Malnutrition from protein loss.
2. Anaemia from recurrent bleeding.
3. Liver changes, e.g. cirrhosis, as a result of massive protein loss.
4. Vitamin deficiencies, e.g. stomatitis.

5. Skin lesions, e.g. pyodermia, erythema nodosum.
6. Eye conditions, e.g. iridocyclitis.
7. Arthritis and ankylosing spondylitis.

Clinical Features.—The onset of the disease is in the third, fourth and second decades of life, in that order of frequency. It is uncommon after 60 years, but then the prognosis is bad.

The disease starts suddenly. A person, who so long had a normal bowel habit, suddenly gets an attack of diarrhoea, occurring day and night. The stools are watery but are blood-stained. There is a rectal discharge, commonly mucoid, sometimes purulent. Pain is usually absent.

Two clinical types are encountered:

1. *Acute Fulminating Type.*—Fortunately, these account for only 5 per cent of the cases. There is incessant diarrhoea, the stools containing blood, mucus and pus. There may be an abdominal distension due to acute dilatation of the colon. The patient is highly toxic and runs temperature (102° to 103° F). With the onset of colonic dilatation, diarrhoea may give way to features of intestinal obstruction.

2. *Chronic and Chronic Relapsing Types.*—These account for 95 per cent of the cases. The initial attack is of moderate severity. Thereafter, at variable intervals, the patient gets bouts of attacks of diarrhoea. The intervals vary from days to months, but gradually the attacks become more frequent. During the attacks, stools are passed ten to twenty times in 24 hours. There is an associated tenesmus. The number of stools and the days of suffering depend on the length of the colon involved. With every episode, the patient gets emaciated and anaemic, and develops different complications, as mentioned above.

Prognosis.—A bad prognosis is associated with the following conditions:

1. Acute fulminating onset.
2. Advanced age, especially after 60.
3. Involvement of the whole length of colon.

Special Investigations

1. *Barium Enema Examination:*
   a. The earliest sign is the loss of normal colonic haustrations. This, again, is to be seen earliest in the distal colon.
   b. The colon is narrow and contracted (*pipe-stem colon*).
   c. Pseudopolyposis, characterised by small filling defects, may be well demonstrated in some cases.
   d. When the ulcers penetrate the muscularis mucosae, to involve the musculature, the barium enema reveals the telltale collar stud projections from the lumen.
2. *Sigmoidoscopy.*—Except for the acute fulminating cases, sigmoidoscopy should always be performed for the purpose of diagnosis:
   a. The earliest finding is a proctitis. The mucous membrane of the rectum is congested, bleeds to touch, and may show a mucoid or purulent discharge.
   b. Later, small pin-point ulcers are seen in the rectum as well as the sigmoid colon.

c. Still later, these ulcers coalesce to form large ulcers. In between the ulcers, the mucous membrane is congested, oedematous, and inflamed (c.f. amoebic ulcers, where the ulcers are large and deep from the beginning, and the intervening mucosa is healthy).

3. *Rectal Biopsy.*—This is important not only in establishing the diagnosis but also in assessing the effect of medical treatment.

4. *Straight X-ray* is of value in acute cases where barium enema is contraindicated. It is of particular help in suggesting whether the muscularis mucosae has been penetrated and the muscular coat involved. When this occurs islands of intervening mucosa of sufficient size are visualised as soft tissue shadows (berry-like in shape) against the relative radio-translucency of the gas in the lumen of the colon.

Treatment.—From the view point of treatment, ulcerative colitis closely resembles duodenal ulcer in many respects:

1. Two methods of treatment are available—medical and surgical.
2. All cases, acute or chronic, deserve a course of rigid medical treatment, unless there is specific contraindication to it.
3. Surgery is reserved for those cases which fail to respond to medical treatment or where complications set in.

Medical Treatment.—The general principles of medical treatment are as follows:

1. Adequate nutrition with high protein, high carbohydrate and high vitamin but low fat diet. A minimum of 3000 calories per day must be provided. Replacement of protein is the most important factor since it is lost in large quantities from the ulcerated bowel.
2. Maintenance of fluid and electrolyte balance, particularly during the periods of acute exacerbation and in the acute fulminating cases.
3. Anaemia should be corrected, if necessary with blood transfusions.
4. Tranquilizers and antispasmodics are very useful.
5. *Chemotherapy.*—Salazopyrine is believed to be the specific drug. This is an non-absorbable sulphonamide, exerting local effect possibly because of its salicylic acid component, which has an anti-inflammatory property. The drug is particularly useful for distal disease, confined to rectum and sigmoid colon. Proctosigmoiditis responds better to salazopyrine than to steroids (*see* below). The drug is given *orally*, 4 to 6 gm daily, in 4 to 6 divided doses, for 7 days. Thereafter, the dose is reduced to 2 gm per day and may have to be continued up to 6 months, according to the response, in order to prevent relapses.
   Salazopyrine, administered as *retention enema,* often gives encouraging results.
6. *Steroid Therapy.*—Hydrocortisone, administered *as retention enema,* often works miraculously. It is given as prednisolone phosphate, 20 mg in 100 ml daily, for 7 days. Such enema is sometimes advocated simultaneously with oral salazopyrine and sometimes after a 7 day course of salazopyrine.

Prednisolone may have to be given *orally* in those cases which do not respond to salazopyrine therapy and prednisolone enema. It is given 20 mg daily, for 2 to 3 weeks. Oral prednisolone is of particular value in acute fulminating cases. It is also of value in chronic cases, either during acute episodes or in improving the general condition of the patient to an extent when radical surgery becomes a relatively safe procedure.

Should prednisolone fail, a switch-over to ACTH may be effective.

While response to oral cortisone is almost certain, its use, particularly if prolonged, is associated with the following disadvantages:

a. There is increased risks of haemorrhage and perforation.

b. It makes the patient more susceptible to secondary pyogenic infections.

c. If the patient does not respond to cortisone, the colonic wall becomes extremely friable, sometimes degenerated, its place being taken by the wall of adjacent organs, often the small intestine. Surgery in such a case is extremely difficult.

7. *Immunodepressive Therapy.* — This is of particular value in acute fulminating cases. Drugs, such as azathiopurine, have been used with success in some cases.

Indications for Surgery

A. IN CHRONIC CASES

1. Progressive disability in spite of conservative treatment:
   a. When persistent diarrhoea limits the ability to work and participations in the enjoyment of life.
   b. Exacerbations recur at increasing frequency so that time is lost from work.
2. Chronic invalidism, resulting from malnutrition, anaemia and liver damage.
3. When the whole length of the colon is involved.
4. Advent of complications:
   a. Local.—Stricture, abscess, fistula.
   b. Systemic.—Eye complications, arthritis, skin lesions.
5. Risk of neoplastic change.—Pseudopolyposis;
6. Suspicion of malignancy.—It is, however, very difficult to detect when malignancy has set in. This is one strong reason why cases of long standing should be advised surgery.
7. When the onset is in the childhood.

B. IN ACUTE CASES

1. If remission is not achieved within 3 weeks of conservative treatment, particularly when oral cortisone has also failed;
2. Advent of complications—Massive haemorrhage, perforation, acute dilatation of the colon.
3. When straight X-ray suggests that the muscularis mucosae has been penetrated. Here surgery should replace conservative treatment because:
   a The stage is set for disintegration, so that acute dilatation, perforation, and portal bacteraemia are highly probable.
   b. Irreversible damage has occurred to the colonic wall and, even if the acute phase is tided over, operation will be necessary on grounds of disability and complications.

Surgical Treatment.—The choice lies between two procedures:

1. Total excision of the large intestine, including the rectum, i.e. *total procto-colectomy.* This causes a complete cure but necessitates an artificial stoma, i.e. permanent ileostomy. The cut end of the ileum is brought out on the abdominal wall.
2. Excision of the colon alone, i.e. *total colectomy,* preserving the rectum, and establishing continuity of the gut by ileo-rectal anastomosis.

This second operation is thought of in those cases where the rectum appears to be free. Its advantage is that the patient has not to bear an abdominal anus, i.e. ileostomy permanently.

However, total procto-colectomy with permanent ileostomy is the procedure favoured by the majority of surgeons for the following reasons:

a. The rectum is usually involved to a greater or lesser extent, and the patient may continue to suffer from intractable diarrhoea; hence little benefitted by the operation.

b. The risk of development of cancer and other complications is left behind.

c. The pathological changes, if present in the rectum, interfere with its normal functions, including the all important reservoir action.

d. Though apparently normal at the time of the operation, the rectum may develop the ulcerative lesions in future.

e. The patients of ileo-rectal anastomosis may, at best, have two loose motions a day, commonly four, sometimes more. Associated with this, pre-cipitancy, i.e. urgency (because of factor 'c' above) may be further distressing. In some cases the ileal contents, coming direct to the rectum, may cause perineal excoriation. It is much easier to manage an ileostomy, with an ileostomy bag fitted to it, than this perineal distress.

The only point to be careful is that the ileostomy must have an efficient stoma and it must be fitted with a correctly fitting ileostomy bag. In other words, it has to be so made that repeated operations are not necessary to correct the functioning of the ileostomy itself.

The ileostomy is placed in the right iliac fossa, through a small incision, separate from the main wound of procto-colectomy. It is best placed at a point which is equidistant from the umbilicus, the anterior superior iliac spine and the inguinal fold. A circular skin flap, 2 cm in diameter, is excised and the ileum emerges through it.

The operation of total procto-colectomy or total colectomy was formerly carried out in two or more stages, i.e. part by part excision, and this may still be the procedure in bad-risk cases. Multiple operations like this are associated with increased risk of complications and additional problems of wound infection. It is now the trend to perform one-stage operation in selected cases and after suitable preparation of the patient with medical treatment.

CARCINOMA OF THE COLON

(The benign tumours of the colon are described with those of the rectum—
see Chapter 50).

Pre-cancerous Conditions

1. Familial Adenomatous Polyposis.—Malignancy is to be apprehended practically in all of these cases.
2. Adenoma and Villous Papilloma (Non-familial Neoplastic Polyps).— The risk of malignant change is much less than that with familial polypi, but the rate is significant.
3. Ulcerative Colitis.—About 5 per cent of the cases turn into carcinoma.

Sites.—The distal part of the colon, viz. the pelvic colon and the pelvirectal junction, is the commonest site; more than half of the cases occur here. Next in order of frequency are the caecum and ascending colon transverse colon, descending colon; and the flexures.

Microscopic Types

1. Almost always it is a columnar-cell adenocarcinoma.
2. Sometimes a colloid cancer, i.e. a colloid degeneration in a massive adenocarcinoma, is seen.
3. Anaplastic cancers are rare.

Macroscopic Types

A. *Non-stenosing Varieties:*
1. Proliferative or cauliflower.
2. Ulcerative.—A typical malignant ulcer.
B. *Stenosing Varieties,* i.e. the gut is stenosed:
1. Annular.—The stenosed segment is short in length (like a ring).
2. Tubular.—The stenosed segment is rather long.

Spread

1. DIRECT SPREAD
   a. *By Continuity.*—The carcinoma, starting in the mucous membrane, spreads in all directions. The submucosa and the muscle coats are infiltrated. Spread occurs in transverse as well as longitudinal directions, in the gut wall, but it is always more rapid in the transverse axis. The best examples of rapid transverse-axial spread are the stenosing varieties of cancers.
   b. *By Contiguity.*—Coming out on the peritoneal surface, the carcinoma infiltrates into the surrounding structures, viz. i.e. retroperitoneal tissues including muscles, liver, pancreas and small intestine. When a hollow viscus is infiltrated, an internal fistula results.

2. LYMPHATIC SPREAD.—The lymphatics pierce the gut wall and drain successively into four sets of nodes:
   a. *Epicolic.*—On the wall of the colon.
   b. *Paracolic.*—By the (mesenteric) side of the colon.
   c. *Intermediate.*—By the side of the main vessels which supply the colon, viz. ileo-colic, right colic, middle colic, left colic, and the sigmoid arteries.
   d. *Main.*—These are .the preaortic nodes, situated at the origin of the superior and the inferior mesenteric arteries.
   The normal absorptive function of the proximal colon demands an abundant lymphatic drainage as compared to the distal colon. Thus, a large number of nodes are related to the proximal colon and fewer in relation to the distal. However, in colonic cancers, at any site, the nodes are rapidly involved.

3. VENOUS SPREAD.—Located in the area of the portal circulation, colonic cancers usually involve the liver and rarely more distal sites, e.g. lungs.

4. TRANSPERITONEAL SPREAD.—Peritoneal dissemination may occur, particularly the pelvic peritoneum. *Krukenberg's tumours* may be formed on the ovaries.

5. IMPLANTATION OF FREE CELLS.—During operation, cancer cells may be liberated into the lumen of the colon and may get implanted at the anastomotic suture lines, unless special care is taken. This may be a common cause of recurrence after operation.

Clinical Features.—As the colon is a long loop of gut and as the cancers may be of different types, the presenting features vary widely in the different groups of patients. These may be summarised as follows:

1. Passage of blood and mucus; sometimes only mucus, with stool.
2. Change in the bowel habit:
   a. In the non-stenosing lesions frequent attacks of dysentery and diarrhoea are common.
   b. In the stenosing lesions chronic obstruction, characterised by alternate constipation and diarrhoea, often occur. The constipation is progressive. The diarrhoea is due to two factors. One is excessive use of purgatives to overcome the constipation. The other is irritation by the accumulated scybala that cause excessive mucus secretion; sometimes 'stercoral ulcers' are formed in the proximal colon.
3. Some patients may present with acute intestinal obstruction. Both acute and chronic obstructions are commoner with left-sided colonic cancers because:
   a. Stenosing lesions are commoner on the left side of the colon.
   b. The left colon has anatomically a narrower lumen than the right.
   c. The stool in the left colon is more solid.
4. There may be a lump, and this may be due to:
   a. The growth itself (only occasionally).
   b. The affected puckered omentum.
   c. The nodes.
   d. Faecoliths, accumulated in the proximal gut (very common).
   e. Metastatic liver.
5. Pain.—To start with, colonic cancers are usually painless. In stenosing lesions, colicky pains are common. In any type, when the cancer is advanced, pain may be severe.
6. Metastatic features:
   a. Liver.—Jaundice and ascites.
   b. Peritoneum.—Ascites.
7. Features characteristic of particular locations:
   a. *Pelvic Colon:*
      i. Tenesmus.
      ii. Colicky pains.
   b. *Transverse Colon:*
      Reflex gastric symptoms, e.g. acidity and heartburn, nausea and vomiting.
   c. *Caecum and Ascending Colon:*
      i. Some cases may present as appendicular lump that fails to resolve.
      ii. Persistent or progressive anaemia.
      iii. A proliferative growth may start an intussusception.

Special Investigations

1. *Stool Examination.*—Presence of blood and mucus.
2. *Sigmoidoscopy.*—This is an important examination because majority of cases occur in the sigmoid colon and the pelvirectal junction, and because early growths, missed radiologically, are often diagnosed. If a growth is visualised, a biopsy may well be done to confirm the diagnosis.

3. *Barium Enema.*—This shows a persistent irregular filling defect, but an early growth may be missed. For the right side of the colon, a barium meal examination gives a better picture but this should be avoided if there is any evidence of chronic obstruction, since an acute obstruction may be precipitated by the meal.

4. *Contrast Enema.*—This is very useful for early cases, which are often missed by ordinary barium enema examination. The usual barium enema examination is done and, then some amount of the barium is allowed to be evacuated. Air is then injected, per rectum, into the colon and further films taken. The white shadow of the barium on the wall of the colon is very clearly seen against the black background of the air, and even very early cases, which have just produced irregularity of the mucosa, may be diagnosed.

5. *Exfoliative Cytology.*—Repeated enemas are given till the return fluid is clear. A bowel wash is now made and the return fluid (kept for 5 to 10 minutes) is collected. This is centrifuged, and the residue is examined for cancer cells. A positive result confirms the diagnosis but there may be false negative results.

6. *X-ray Chest.*

Treatment

A. *Radical Surgery* is the ideal. The contraindications to radical surgery are:
1. Growth extensively fixed to the posterior abdominal wall.
2. Nodes fixed to the posterior abdominal wall or to important vessels.
3. Liver metastasis.
4. General peritoneal dissemination.

According to the site of the growth, the radical resection may be:
1. Right hemicolectomy
2. Left hemicolectomy
3. Wedge resection of the transverse colon with mesocolon.
4. Resection of the pelvic colon with mesocolon.

B. *Palliative Surgery for non-resectable growths:*
1. For right-sided growths.—Ileo-transverse anastomosis.
2. For left-sided growths.—Permanent colostomy, proximal to the growth.

(All the above operations are described in details in the Chapter on instruments, under gastrointestinal clamps).

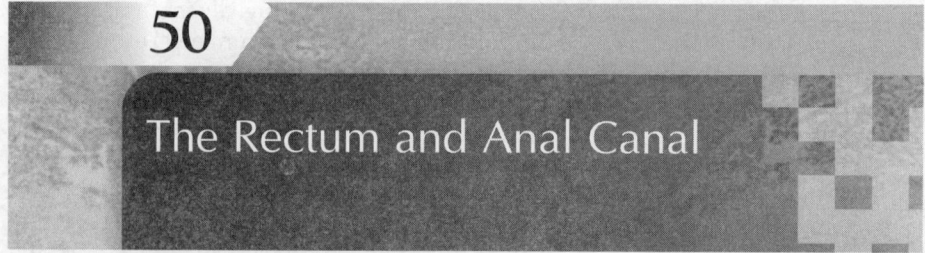

50

The Rectum and Anal Canal

MALFORMATIONS OF RECTUM AND ANAL CANAL

Embryology.—In the fifth week of intrauterine life, the hindgut opens into the cloaca above the opening of the Wolffian ducts, i.e. in the future bladder. The rectum develops as an offshoot from the hindgut. This offshoot grows, behind the cloaca, till it reaches the proctodeum. The proctodeum is a depression occurring in the surface ectoderm at the site of the future anus. The hind gut opens into the proctodeum and thus the gut opens at the anus. The rectal offshoot from the hindgut develops a temporary communication with the cloaca at the level of the opening of the Wolffian ducts, i.e. in the prostratic urethra. This communication develops in the sixth week and closes by the eighth week, i.e. when the rectal offshoot opens into the proctodeum. The rectal offshoot passes in the midline through the pelvic floor, i.e. the developing levator ani muscle, a part of which becomes the puborectal sling, which is strongest anorectal sphincter.

Anorectal Anomalies.—These may be divided into two broad groups:

1. HIGH ANOMALIES.—The rectum ends above the pelvic floor, i.e. *supralevator anomaly*. As the rectum has not passed through the pelvirectal sling, there is no sphincter mechanism to work on it. Incidence of associated urological and sacral anomalies are high.

2. LOW ANOMALIES.—The gut has developed to a point below the pelvic floor, i.e. *infralevator anomaly*. This is much less serious. As the rectum has passed through the pelvirectal sling, there is an effective sphincter mechanism. Associated urological or sacral anomalies are rare.

High Anomalies

A. IN THE MALE INFANTS.—The commonest of all anorectal anomalies is a high anomaly in a male infant:

1. When the rectal offshoot from the hindgut does not develop at all, the rectum does not develop, i.e. *total rectal agenesis.* In such cases the communication with the cloaca is very likely to persist, so that there is an associated recto-vesical fistula.

2. The rectal offshoot starts developing but has a stunted growth, its caudal migration ceasing somewhere above the level of the future pelvic diaphragm. There is *subtotal rectal agenesis.* The opening into the prostatic urethra usually persists, resulting in recto-urethral, i.e. recto-prostatic fistula.

3. There may be a complete or partial rectal agenesis without any fistulous communication, either with the bladder or with the urethra. This is *blind rectal agenesis,* the rarest of all anomalies.

There is absence of the normal sphincter mechanism in all these cases.

B. IN THE FEMALE INFANTS.—High anomalies in the female infants are much rare than in the males:

1. The rectal offshoot has a stunted growth and opens into the top of the vagina— *subtotal rectal agenesis with recto-vaginal fistula.*
2. There is no development of the rectal offshoot and the embryonic cloaca persists as a common rectogenitourinary canal. This is called *cloacal type of anomaly.*

Low Anomalies.—These anomalies are rather minor developmental errors, in which the rectal offshoot has developed fully. *The sphincter mechanism is normal in all the cases.* The defect lies with the opening. Such defects may be as follows:

A. The opening is located at the right place but is unusually *narrow:*

1. *Anal stenosis,* i.e. a narrow opening, which may look normal. The child is presented usually when it is few months old because of increasing constipation and dyschezia (difficulty in passing stools).
2. *Microscopic anus.*—This is an extreme variety of the above. The opening is so small that it has to be identified with a magnifying glass. The condition is suspected when just a speck of meconium is noticed on what appears to be an intact perineum.

B. The opening migrates unusually forwards and opens at an *ectopic* site, and it is often narrow, i.e. stenotic:

1. *Ectopic anus in the females.*—This is the commonest of all anorectal anomalies in the females. There may be two types:
   a. *Vulval ectopic anus.*—The anus and vagina open close together, without any intervening skin.
   b. *Vaginal ectopic anus.*—The anus opens just within the vagina and may be easily seen, and there is complete sphincteric control (c f the rare high anomaly of subtotal rectal agenesis with recto-vaginal fistula, where the anus opens at the top of the vagina, cannot be seen easily, and has no sphincteric control).
2. *Ectopic anus in the males.*—This is rarer than in females. The anus is located under the scrotum, in the perineoscrotal junction.

C. The anus is located normally but is covered by a thin layer of skin, i.e. *covered anus.* A blue line of meconium can be seen, extending as a sinus, under the translucent skin, from the site of normal anus to a small hole behind scrotum. The explanation for this anomaly is an excessive fusion of the genital folds, extending backwards to cover the anus.

Summary of Anorectal Anomalies

I. HIGH (SUPRALEVATOR) ANOMALIES

A. *In the Males:*
1. Total rectal agenesis with recto-vesical fistula.
2. Subtotal rectal agenesis with recto-urethral fistula.
3. Blind rectal agenesis.

B. *In the Females:*
1. Subtotal rectal agenesis with recto-vaginal fistula.
2. Cloacal type of anomaly.

II. Low (INFRALEVATOR) ANOMALIES
A. *Narrow Orifice:*
1. Anal stenosis.
2. Microscopic anus.
B. *Ectopic Orifice:*
1. In the females:
a. Vulval ectopic anus.
b. Vaginal ectopic anus.
2. In the males.—At the perineoscrotal junction.
C. *Covered anus* in the males.

Complications of Anorectal Anomalies

A. Low ANOMALIES are not associated with any serious complication. Anal stenosis, microscopic anus, and covered anus may have some degree of intestinal obstruction.
B. HIGH ANOMALIES
1. *Acute Intestinal Obstruction:*
a. In blind rectal agenesis this must occur.
b. In total or subtotal rectal agenesis with recto-vesical or recto-urethral fistula in the males, the fistulous opening is usually extremely narrow and may be blocked. Intestinal obstruction, though not complete, may be acute.
c. In similar conditions in the females, associated with recto-vaginal fistula, the fistulous opening is usually wide. Acute intestinal obstruction does not occur.
2. *Urinary Tract Infection:*
a. In the males the fistulous opening is very likely to cause ascending urinary infection, particularly because the sphincter mechanism is ineffective. In only 10 per cent of cases there is a blind rectal agenesis, whereas in the remaining 90 per cent there is a fistula. Hence, chances of urinary infection are very high. Presence of a fistula is diagnosed by passage of gas or meconium per urethra (a speck of meconium on the tip of the penis may be the first sign of the fistula).
b. In the females the risk of urinary infection is much less.

Clinical Diagnosis

A. Low ANOMALIES
1. Anal stenosis, microscopic anus, and covered anus should be easily diagnosed by close inspection, if necessary with a magnifying glass. The patient may have some degree of intestinal obstruction.
2. Ectopic anus in the males is easily identified. Ectopic anus in the females should also be diagnosed if the condition is kept in mind. The opening is easily seen in the vulva or vagina, and has sphincteric control. There is no intestinal obstruction.

B. HIGH ANOMALIES, i.e. RECTAL AGENESIS
Except on rare occasions, the patient is male infant. There is acute intestinal obstruction. In the majority of cases gas or meconium is passed per urethra, or there is a speck of meconium on the tip of the penis. In 10 per cent of cases, where there is a blind agenesis, no gas or meconium comes out of urethra.

The only difficulty in diagnosis may be with female infants having rectal agenesis with recto-vaginal fistula. Such cases have to be carefully diagnosed from ectopic vaginal anus (already discussed).

X-ray Examination

1. *Straight X-ray with the Child Inverted* (Invertogram).—The idea behind this examination is to establish the diagnosis of rectal agenesis, i.e. high anomaly, and to find out the distance of the blind end from the surface of the perineum. A metal object (e.g. a coin) is fixed to the skin by adhesive plaster at a site, where the normal anus should lie. The child is kept inverted about 5 minutes so that the sticky meconium falls down and gas moves upwards to the blind loop. Frontal and lateral views are taken to show the end of the gas shadow and its distance from the metal marker. Instead of using the metal marker, some authorities advocate simple X-ray, finding out the relationship of the gas shadow with bony landmarks. The puborectalis sling is located just below the pubococcygeal line and the levator ani muscle is situated just below the junction of the body and tail of the comma-shaped ischium.

Straight X-ray is of a little value since diagnosis should be made clinically. Moreover, the infant must be at least 12 hours old, if enough gas is to penetrate the meconium. Further, the level of the gas shadow varies considerably in the same patient, depending on the contractions of the perineal and pelvic muscles. Much valuable time is also lost in arranging the X-ray, while each hour is precious for a neonate with acute intestinal obstruction.

The chief value of straight X-ray lies in:
   a. Detection of any accompanying sacral defect (the information can well be had from simple ventral and lateral views).
   b. Presence of gas in the urinary tract to suggest a fistula.

2. *Intravenous Pyelogram* may be done when urological involvement is suspected. However, it is difficult to be performed in a neonate.

3. *Cystogram* may show a recto-vesical fistula.

   In general, X-rays are not much important in deciding the type of anomaly and the immediate treatment.

Treatment.—As has already been stated, treatment is easy and results very satisfactory in cases of low anomalies, particularly because there is an effective sphincter mechanism. In cases of high anomalies treatment is really difficult. It is not of much importance where the rectum opens; of far more importance is the point whether an effective sphincter mechanism is present.

Treatment for Low Anomalies

1. ANAL STENOSIS.—Regular dilatations. This is started with a rubber catheter, then changing to a bougie. Thereafter, digital dilatation is done, first with the little finger and then with the index finger. This is continued for about six months, by which time usually the tendency to contract passes off.

2. MICROSCOPIC ANUS.—To start with, an incision is made to enlarge the opening. Thereafter, dilatations are done as for anal stenosis.

3. VULVAL ECTOPIC ANUS.—No treatment, except dilatation of the anal orifice, if it appears to be stenosed. Any attempt to shift the anus backwards only causes

more deformity, more stricture, and more disability. Often the patient is unaware of the condition. Sexual activities and child bearing are normal.

4. VAGINAL ECTOPIC ANUS.—Two types of operation are advised:

a. *Cutback Operation.*—One blade of a scissors is passed through the ectopic anus, into the bowel, and the other blade is on the perineal] skin at the site of normal anus. The intervening tissues are cut as the blades are forcefully apposed. No suturing is done. The opening is kept fully patent with a metal dilator till, in a few months' time, the raw area gets covered with skin. Thus, a vulval anus is created. The operation is done rather easily.

b. The vaginal end of the fistulous tract is dissected, from the vagina. This end is brought down to the site of normal anus, where it is sutured. An intact bridge of skin, making the perineum, is thus left between the new anus and the vulva, as it is in a normal female. The vaginal defect is repaired. The operation is really difficult.

5. ECTOPIC (SUBSCROTAL) ANUS IN THE MALE.—The orifice is usually stenosed. The opening is enlarged a little by a backward incision, and regular dilatation is done.

6. COVERED ANUS IN THE MALE.—The skin, overlying the anus and the sinus, is excised. The anal opening, if stenosed, is dilated.

Treatment for High Anomalies.—In the vast majority of cases it is a male infant and there is acute intestinal obstruction, in addition to the malformation. Two courses are open for the purpose of treatment:

1. Immediate colostomy to relieve the obstruction, postponing the reconstructive operation to a later date, i.e. a two-stage procedure.

2. Immediate reconstructive operation to create the anorectal passage, and this automatically relieves the obstruction, i.e. one-stage procedure (without a colostomy). At reconstruction, the fistulous communication with the bladder or urethra is closed.

There are supporters of both the above procedures.

Points in favour of two-stage and against one-stage procedure:

a. The operation of reconstruction may prove to be too formidable to be survived by a neonate, particularly where there is an acute intestinal obstruction. Moreover, in many cases, there is coexistence of other serious congenital anomalies, e.g. cardiac anomalies, oesophageal atresia, urogenital anomaly, vertebral anomaly, etc., when such surgery becomes far more dangerous.

b. The bowel cannot be accurately placed in the puborectalis sling in a neonate. This is highly important in maintaining continence in the newly made anorectum.

Points in favour of one-stage and against two-stage procedure:

a. Just after birth, the infant has a great power to survive surgical shock and possesses the maternal immunity against infection. Thus, there is not much danger in undertaking the reconstructive operation.

b. Following reconstruction, dilatations are necessary. This is more easily performed in a neonate than in a child above one year, in whom it is more painful.

c. 'Sluggish rectum' is more likely to develop if the reconstructive operation is delayed.

d. If a colostomy is done, three operations are necessary, viz. colostomy, reconstruction, closure of colostomy. Of these, colostomy, just after birth, is not at all a simple operation free from danger—it carries considerable mortality and morbidity. The closure of colostomy, again, is not a minor procedure.

e. When reconstructive operation is undertaken, the fistula with the bladder or urethra is closed. This has the tremendous advantage of eliminating all dangers of ascending urinary infection.

IN THE FEMALES.—The female infants with high anomaly have usually large recto-vaginal fistula, so there is no acute intestinal obstruction. Therefore, the condition may be allowed to persist till the age of 5 to 6 years, after which reconstruction is undertaken. If, however, a female infant has no fistula or has a fistula too narrow to relieve obstruction, the patient should be treated exactly as in a male infant.

The Reconstructive Operation.—An *abdomino-perineal pull-through operation* is usually practised. It should be remembered that simply bringing the gut down to the perineum is of no avail unless sphincteric control is achieved. Since the anus has not developed, there are no sphincters available at the end of the gut. Whatever sphincteric activity can be achieved is by the puborectal sling. The gut must therefore be made to pass exactly between the two halves of the puborectalis muscle, which must be preserved intact to effect continence.

Through an abdominal incision, the sigmoid colon and the blind pouch are mobilised, till the fistula (with the urethra or bladder) is reached. This is carefully excised and closed.

A small incision is made on the perineum at the normal site of the anus. A forceps is pushed in, care being taken to keep exactly in the midline, between the two halves of the puborectalis muscle. Through the gap, made in the muscles, the blind bowel loop is brought down. It is opened at the lower end and the margins are sutured to the skin margins of the perineal wound to make the anus.

Summary of Treatment for High Anomaly

1. Male infants otherwise healthy.—One-stage abdomino-perineal pull-through operation.
2. Male infants who are unlikely to stand such procedure due to prematurity, illness, or other congenital anomalies.—Immediate colostomy with a delayed reconstructive operation, usually between 6 and 12 months of age. At a third operation the colostomy is closed.
3. Female infants.—One-stage abdomino-perineal pull-through operation, at the age of 5 to 6 years.
4. Female infants with cloacal anomaly.—Permanent colostomy.

BENIGN TUMOURS OF THE RECTUM (AND COLON)

Different benign tumours may occur in the rectum and the colon but the epithelial tumours are the only common varieties. These benign epithelial tumours of the rectum and the colon are collectively termed polyps. These are divided into four main groups:

I. Hamartomatous Polyps.
II. Neoplastic Polyps.

III. Inflammatory Polyps.
IV. Metaplastic Polyps.

Hamartomatous Polyps.—These are local tissue malformations, having *no malignant potential*. There are mainly two types:

1. JUVENILE POLYP.—The common *rectal polyp* of the children. There is a spherical mass, usually of the size of a pea, having a long narrow pedicle. The child presents with passage of fresh blood (sometimes with mucus) in the stool. Sometimes the fleshy mass is prolapsed through the anus during defaecation. Rarely, following such a prolapse, the pedicle may be tightly caught by the sphincter and an auto-amputation of the polyp may occur. Diagnosis is easily made by digital examination and with an anal speculum.

    As the pedicle is usually long, the tumour can well be delivered through the anus, the pedicle ligated, and the polyp excised. If the tumour is high up or if the pedicle is short, a snare may have to be used.

2. PEUTZ-JEGHERS SYNDROME.—This is rare in the rectum or colon, and is typical of the small intestine. Its characteristic features are:
    a. It is familial.
    b. There are multiple polyps, particularly in the jejunum (but malignancy never occurs, c f colonic polyposis).
    c. There is a melanosis of the oral mucosa and the lips.

Neoplastic Polyps.—These are the actual benign tumours of the large gut. There are mainly two types:
1. Adenoma.
2. Villous Papilloma.

    While an adenoma arises from the cells at the depth of the crypts of Lieberühn, a papilloma originates from the cells at the surface of the crypts.

ADENOMA.—An adenoma (or *adenomatous polyp*), as compared to the juvenile polyp, is either sessile or has a tougher stalk and, therefore, cannot be plucked off the rectal wall so easily. The patient, often an adult, presents with rectal haemorrhage. The tumour may occasionally turn malignant and should, therefore, be removed:
1. *If there is a pedicle:*
    a. For growths in the lower two-thirds of the rectum, the tumour can be delivered through the anus, the pedicle transfixed, and the growth excised.
    b. For growths higher up, a sigmoidoscope has to be used and the tumour removed with a snare.
2. *If there is no pedicle, i.e. sessile adenoma:*
    The tumour has to be fulgurated with a stiff insulated electrode, passed through a sigmoidoscope.

VILLOUS PAPILLOMA.—The surface of this tumour has fine finger-like projections, i.e. villi. Hence it is called villous papilloma. Like papilloma elsewhere, it has a central connective tissue stroma, on which columnar epithelium is laid down. The tumour may sometimes attain a considerable size.

    While papillomas may remain benign throughout, some of them do turn malignant; the chances of malignancy are a little more than with adenomas.

The patient presents with passage of profuse mucus (which may occasionally be as high as 2 to 3 litres a day), and a little blood per rectum. Diagnosis is made by digital examination and by proctoscopy.

For smaller growth, either excision or diathermy-coagulation of the tumour is the treatment. For large growths, excision of the rectum has to be undertaken.

Inflammatory Polyps.—These are also called pseudo-polyps because they are not actually tumours and consist of granulation tissue, covered with mucosa. They may be found in cases of ulcerative colitis, amoebic colitis and Crohn's disease. They are usually multiple (pseudo-polyposis).

Metaplastic Polyps.—These are only sesile mucosal excrescences.

Familial Polyposis of the Colon and Rectum.—This is a hereditary condition, transmitted from both the sexes to both the sexes, characterised by multiple (hundreds) adenomas, scattered over the colon, particularly the sigmoid, and often the rectum as well.

If the rectum is free, a total colectomy is done and the ileum is anastomosed to the rectum. If the rectum is involved as well, a proctocolectomy is undertaken and a permanent terminal ileostomy has to be done.

CARCINOMA OF THE RECTUM

Precancerous Conditions
1. Familial adenomatous polyposis.
2. Adenoma and villous papilloma (non-familial neoplastic polyps).

Sites
1. The commonest site is the pelvirectal junction. The growth may be either at or just below the peritoneal reflection.
2. The next common site is the ampulla of the rectum.
3. The anorectal junction.

Microscopic Types
1. Almost always it is a columnar-cell adenocarcinoma.
2. Sometimes a colloid cancer, i.e. colloidal degeneration in massive adeno-carcinoma, is encountered.
3. Anaplastic carcinoma is rare.
4. If there is a squamous-cell carcinoma, the tumour must have arisen from the anal canal and extended up to the rectum.

Macroscopic Types.—Same as colonic cancers (see Chapter 49). As with the colonic cancers, the stenosing types (i.e. *annular or tubular)* have a tendency to occur in the relatively narrow parts of the rectum, viz. the pelvirectal junction and the anorectal junction, while the non-stenosing types (i.e. *proliferative or ulcerative)* tend to occur in the spacious ampulla.

Spread

1. DIRECT SPREAD.—The tumour, starting as an irregularity in the mucosa, spreads in all directions. As a rule, spread in the longitudinal direction is restricted to a maximum of 2 to 3 cm. Spread occurs more rapidly in the transverse axis and, on

an average, the growth takes six months to cover up one-fourth of the circumference and 1½ to 2 years to completely encircle the rectum. Starting from the mucous membrane, infiltration occurs into the depth. The muscles are penetrated first, and then the fat and areolar tissues around the rectum. Beyond this, extension of the growth is restricted for a considerable period by the fascia propria. However, once this fascia is infiltrated, rapid spread occurs as follows:

Anteriorly.—The prostate, seminal vesicles, and bladder in the males. The uterus and vagina in the females.

Laterally.—The ureter (this may cause secondary hydronephrosis).

Posteriorly.—The sacrum and the sacral plexus (causing severe pain).

2. LYMPHATIC SPREAD.—Unlike colon, there are no nodes on the wall of the rectum, i.e. similar to the epicolic nodes. The nodes concerned in the lymphatic drainage of the rectum are:
 a. The *pararectal nodes of Gerota* (like paracolic nodes).
 b. The *intermediate nodes* (like colon), along the lower part of the superior haemorrhoidal artery and its terminal branches.
 c. The *main nodes* (like colon) at the origin of the inferior mesenteric artery.

Except for the main nodes (which are only rarely involved), the glands are situated within the fascial sheath of the rectum and, when the rectum is removed with its sheath, the nodes are automatically included in the resection.

The lymphatic drainage of the rectum, as considered from the point of view of spread of cancer, may be summarised as follows:
 A. The majority of the lymphatics of the rectum have an upward course. The lymphatics from above the level of the peritoneal reflection primarily drain into the intermediate and then into the main nodes.
 B. The lymphatics from below the level of the peritoneal reflection to a level of 2 cm above the anal orifice drain as follows:
  i. Majority run upward as in A, but the first halting station is the pararectal nodes of Gerota.
  ii. Some of the lymphatics drain laterally on the pelvic floor, along the middle haemorrhoidal vein. These drain that part of the rectum which is between 4 cm and 8 cm of the anal orifice.
 C. Virtually none of the lymphatics of the rectum drain downwards. It is only when a growth has encroached on the anal canal or the upper lymphatics have been completely blocked by the malignant process, that downward spread to the inguinal nodes may occur.

3. VENOUS SPREAD.—This is usually late except with the anaplastic variety. The liver is the commonest site for metastasis, and then the lungs.

4. TRANSPERITONEAL SPREAD.—This occurs only with growths that are located as high as the level of the peritoneal reflection.

Stages of Progress (Duke's Classification).—There are 3 stages:
Stage A: The growth is still limited to the rectal wall (15 per cent).
Stage B: The growth has extended beyond the rectal wall but there is no involvement of lymph nodes (35 per cent).

Stage C: The growth has extended beyond the rectal wall and there is also lymph node involvement (50 per cent). These cases are sub-divided into two groups:

C_1—Where only the pararectal nodes are involved.

C_2—Where more distal nodes are involved.

Symptoms

1. Passage of blood per rectum, often with mucus, is the most constant and the earliest symptom. This may be little or considerable, bright red or a little black, painful or painless, and either at defaecation or unrelated to it. Very often the nature of bleeding is just as what is found with internal haemorrhoids, and these cases are often overlooked and treated as piles.
2. Sense of incomplete defaecation because of the presence of the growth as well as blood and mucus in the rectum. This is likely to occur especially with the proliferative growths. The patient visits the toilets frequently (*Spurious diarrhoea* = false diarrhoea) and, instead of stool, passes blood and mucus (*bloody slime*).
3. Alteration in the bowel habits. A patient with a stenosing type of lesion suffers from increasing constipation and requires gradually increasing doses of purgatives. Conversely, a patient with a proliferative or ulcerative growth has to wake up gradually earlier in the morning to evacuate the bowels (*early morning diarrhoea*).
4. Pain is usually absent in the early stages but, with a stenosing lesion, there may be colicky pains. When infiltration into neighbouring structures occurs, pain is severe, particularly so when the sacral plexus is involved.
5. An abdominal lump is occasionally present and may be due to:
   a. Solid stool, accumulated proximal to a stenosing lesion.
   b. Metastatic liver.
6. Acute intestinal obstruction may be the first presenting feature in some cases of stenosing growths.
7. Metastatic group, i.e. patients presenting with jaundice and ascites, and a hard nodular liver.

Physical Signs

1. *Abdominal Examination* may elicit:
   a. Distended colon.
   b. Metastatic liver.
   c. Ascites.
2. *Digital Examination.*—In the majority of cases the growth can be palpated by the examining digit, and its characters may be ascertained. Sometimes a growth may be located just a little higher up than the reach of the tip of examining finger, and is missed. Such a growth may be palpable by a bimanual examination, i.e. with a digit in the rectum and the other hand on the abdomen. With a bimanual examination, the details of the growth are better known as well. In the females with growth on the anterior rectal wall, one finger in the rectum and another in the vagina give a good idea about the degree of infiltration.
3. *Proctoscopy.*—Usually shows the growth.

Special Investigations

1. *Sigmoidoscopy* may be required for high-up growths.
2. *Biopsy.*—This must be done in every case. It is done either with a proctoscope or with a sigmoidoscope.

3. *Barium enema examination* is usually not required unless sigmoidoscopy fails to show the growth.

Treatment.—Fortunately, majority of the cases give a chance for radical resection. This means *en masse* excision of:

1. The rectum with its sheath (almost all the nodes are located within the sheath).
2. The anal canal with its sphincters.
3. Lowest part of the sigmoid colon.
4. Part of the pelvic floor musculature (on which the lateral lymphatics run).
5. All the nodes draining the rectum.

This will require ligation of the superior haemorrhoidal artery high up. The most radical measure would be a *'flush ligation'*, i.e. ligature of the inferior mesenteric artery just at its origin from the aorta. Only by doing this, removal of the 'main' node is possible, and this makes the operation most radical, as far as the lymphatic spread is concerned. Such high-up ligature may, however, endanger the vascularity of the sigmoid colon at the site of colostomy (see below), and so some surgeons prefer ligating the artery a little low down, i.e. below the origin of one or two branches *(critical point of Sudek)*.

As the anal canal is removed with its sphincters, there is no good in bringing down the cut end of the sigmoid colon to the perineum; there will be incontinence. The patient, therefore, has to live with a permanent colostomy.

The operations for carcinoma of the rectum may be grouped as follows:—
A. Standard Operation.
B. Less Extensive Operations.
C. More Extensive Operations.

A. Standard Operation.—This is the radical resection, as mentioned above, and requires approach both from the abdomen and from the perineum. Depending on how the dissection progresses, the operation may be:—

1. ABDOMINO-PERINEAL RESECTION (APR).—The abdominal part of the operation is done first and the dissected mass is pushed down into the pelvis. Above this, the pelvic floor is repaired by apposing the peritoneal margins. Thereafter, the perineal dissection is done and the whole mass is removed from the perineum.

2. PERINEO-ABDOMINAL RESECTION.—The perineal dissection is done first and the dissected mass is pushed up to the abdomen, above the pelvic floor. The pelvic floor is repaired below it. The abdominal dissection is done next and the whole mass is removed per abdomen. However, the abdomen has to be opened first to assess resectability.

3. COMBINED SYNCHRONOUS ABDOMINAL AND PERINEAL RESECTION.— This is the type of operation most commonly done in the present days. Two surgeons operate simultaneously, one doing the abdominal dissection and the other the perineal, and the two meet at the pelvic floor. This gives the advantages and overcomes the disadvantages of the above-mentioned two operations, and also reduces the operating time considerably.

B. Less Extensive Operations

1. SPHINCTER-CONSERVING RESECTION (ANTERIOR RESECTION OR ABDOMINAL RADICAL RESTORATIVE RESECTION).—This may be done in a patient who is too feeble to stand

the shock of the perineal dissection, provided the growth is situated high-up in the rectum. The anal canal is preserved and so its sphincters. The pelvic colon is anastomosed to the anal canal. The operation avoids a permanent colostomy as well.

2. ABDOMINAL EXCISION ALONE (HARTMANN'S OPERATION).—This is also done for the above group of patients. By an abdominal approach, the pelvic colon and rectum are mobilised to a level as far below the growth as possible. The rectum is bisected here and the distal stump is carefully closed. The pelvic colon is bisected at a suitable level and the portion of the gut, in between, bearing the growth, is removed. A permanent colostomy is done with the proximal cut end of the pelvic colon.

3. PALLIATIVE COLOSTOMY.—This is done if:
   a. The growth is inoperable.
   b. The patient comes with acute intestinal obstruction.
   c. The patient is very feeble and cannot stand any major surgery.
   d. There is gross infection in the growth.

C. More Extensive Operations
1. In the females, if the vagina or the uterus is infiltrated, these organs may be resected with the standard operation.
2. In the males, if there is anterior infiltration into the bladder, *pelvic evisceration (Brunschwig's operation)* may be done. This removes all the pelvic organs and the nodes. The cut ureters are transplanted on the pelvic colon, with which the permanent colostomy is done (this is called *'wet colostomy'* since it brings out urine as well as stool).

SURGICAL ANATOMY OF THE RECTUM AND ANAL CANAL

The rectum is 5 inches in length, and the anal canal one and a half inches. From the pelvirectal junction the rectum is directed backwards, but a little down, it changes direction to curve anteriorly. From the anorectal junction, the anal canal is again directed backwards. There are three lateral flexures in the rectum and, corresponding to each flexure, there is a horizontal fold of mucous membrane with circular muscle coat, projecting into its lumen *(Houston's valves)*. The flexures are convex to right, left, and again right. The lower part of the rectum is dilated and this is called the *ampulla*.

The Mucous Membrane.—The pink columnar epithelium of the rectal mucosa changes into the red cubical epithelium in the anal canal. Traced further downwards, the anal canal mucosa is plum coloured. The mucous membrane of the anal canal is very loosely attached to the underlying musculature by means of lax submucosa. The mucosa is thrown into 8 to 12 folds, called the *anal columns*. These folds are joined at their lower ends by crescentic folds, known as *anal valves*. The level of the anal valves is marked by a white line, called the *pectinate* or *denate line (Hilton's)*. This pectinate line clearly divides the anal canal into an upper and a lower segment, which differ from each other as follows:

Upper	Lower
1. Developed from the post-allantoic gut.	1. Developed from the proctodeum.
2. Lined by plum coloured cubical epithelium, representing the mucous membrane.	2. Lined by white squamous epithelium, representing the anoderm, which is continued downwards as the pigmented perianal skin.
3. Supplied by autonomic nervous system and is non-sensitive.	3. Supplied by spinal nerves (somatic) and is highly sensitive.
4. Drains into portal venous system.	4. Drains into systemic venous system.

The submucosa of the anal canal is lax. It contains the veins, which, therefore, practically lie unsupported here. This lacks of support of the veins, together with their direct upward drainage against gravity, account for the frequency of these veins getting varicose, i.e. resulting in haemorrhoids.

The Musculature.—This is in three layers and, from inside outwards, these are as follows:

1. *Circular Muscle Coat.*—This is the continuation downwards of the circular muscle of the colon. At its lower end it expands to form the internal sphincter. This sphincter is typically white in colour, about an inch in height, and about 3 mm in thickness.
2. *Conjoined Longitudinal Muscle.*—This is so named because its fibres are derived from the longitudinal muscle coat of the large gut, as well as from the puborectalis part of levator ani muscle. It has a wide fan-shaped insertion:
   a. The innermost fibres pass through the internal sphincter, to be inserted into the anoderm.
   b. The central fibres are directly inserted into the perianal skin.
   c. The outer fibres pass through the external sphincter, to be attached to the perianal skin.
   [Fibres (b) and (c) constitute the *corrugator cutis ani*.]
3. *External Sphincter.*—In the past, this was described as having three components, viz., subcutaneous, superficial and deep. In the present days, it is considered as a single sphincter.

Anal Glands.—In the region of the anal valves, closely related to many of these, lie the opening of the anal glands. The duct of each anal gland, traced retrograde from its opening, passes through the submucosa and the internal sphincter, to reach the space between the internal sphincter and the conjoined longitudinal muscle. This space is known as the intermuscular space. In this space, the duct bifurcates. The upper branch is straight. The lower branch dilates in an ampulla, from where subbranches arise.

Infection is fairly common in the anal glands. The resulting inflammatory exudate, if it collects in the upper branch, can easily drain out, helped by gravity. On the other hand, exudates collecting in the lower branch, accumulate in the ampulla and its subbranches, and therefore cannot drain out properly, particularly against gravity.

Due to these factors, abscess formation in the intermuscular space is common and such abscesses are more likely to occur in the lower part of this space than in the upper part.

ANO-RECTAL ABSCESSES

These are abscesses around the anal canal and the rectum.

Types

1. Low Intermuscular Abscess	80%
2. High Intermuscular Abscess	10%
3. Ischiorectal Abscess	6%
4. Subcutaneous, Subanodermal, and Submucous Abscess	3%
5. Pelvirectal Abscess	1%

Intermuscular Abscess

ORIGIN.—These abscesses result from the acute inflammation in anal glands. The pus collects in the space between the internal sphincter and the conjoined longitudinal muscle. Low intermuscular abscess is much more common than high intermuscular abscess (see surgical anatomy of anal gland).

CLINICAL FEATURES.—The patient complains of throbbing pain inside the anal canal, aggravated after defaecation, and associated with fever and constitutional disturbances.

On examination, nothing is evident from outside. A digital examination elicits swelling and acute tenderness in the wall of the anal canal, low or high, depending on the type of the abscess.

SPREAD.—Untreated, the abscess may spread as follows:
1. Rupture into the anal canal or rectum, by penetrating through the internal sphincter and the mucous membrane.
2. Rupture into the ischiorectal fossa, by penetrating through the external sphincter, and thus presenting as an ischiorectal abscess.
3. Spread all round the intermuscular space.

TREATMENT.—Early incision, under antibiotic cover, is the treatment. A delayed, inadequate, or otherwise defective incision, or else, a spontaneous rupture of the abscess invariably leads to an anal fistula. (The abscesses demanding early incision are perianal abscess, parotid abscess, breast abscess and hand infections).

The incision is placed on the perianal skin and, in order to be adequate, always under general anaesthesia. A sinus forceps is thrust into the inter-muscular space and the abscess is drained. A digital exploration is done to break all loculi. The internal sphincter is separated from the underlying mucosa and is cut through (i.e. a sphincterotomy is done). This is of great value in preventing fistula formation. The cavity is packed and allowed to heal by granulation.

Ischiorectal Abscess

ORIGIN.—Located in the ischiorectal fossa, the abscess may arise by:
1. Direct infection, either by blood or by lymphatics.
2. Extension outwards of a low intermuscular abscess.
3. Extension downwards of a pelvirectal abscess (*see* below).

The second type of origin is very common. That is why ischiorectal abscesses are so frequent (it should be noted that the incidence of a true ischiorectal abscess, i.e. originating in the fossa itself, is only 6%).

CLINICAL FEATURES.—Apart from fever and constitutional symptoms, there is acute pain in the ischiorectal fossa, particularly during defaecation and on attempts to sit on the buttock.

TREATMENT.—Early incision under general anaesthesia. As the fossa is deep and as the overlying skin is considerably thick, fluctuation is elicited only very late, and incision should never be delayed to that date.

A large crucial incision is made on the ischiorectal fossa. As the abscess drains, a digital exploration is made:

a. To break all fibrous loculi.
b. To find out if the abscess is an extension outwards of an inter-muscular abscess or (as is rarely) extension downwards of a pelvirectal abscess. If it is so, an internal sphincterotomy should be performed.

The corners of the skin may be cut away so that the opening is circular and represents the entire floor of the abscess. The cavity is packed and is allowed to heal by granulation.

Subcutaneous, Subanodermal and Submucous Abscesses.—These abscesses are superficial, lying just deep to the skin, anoderm, or mucous membrane, respectively. A small incision, on the overlying skin, anoderm, or mucosa provides easy drainage.

Pelvirectal Abscess.—These abscesses, fortunately rare, are located very deep and high up, between the rectum and the levator ani. They usually result from pelvic cellulitis. The abscess may either burst into the rectum or penetrate downwards, through the levator ani, to present as an ischiorectal abscess. In the latter case, incision is made as for an ischiorectal abscess, and then the opening in the levator ani is enlarged to provide adequate drainage.

FISTULA-IN-ANO

This is the commonest type of external fistula. It is lined by unhealthy granulation tissue and fibrous tissue, and has one end communicating with the perianal skin and the other end with the anal canal or with the rectum.

Origin.—Usually, it is a sequela to a perianal abscess, which has either been allowed to rupture spontaneously, or has been incised late or in an inadequate or incorrect manner. Occasionally, however, a fistula may be:

a. Tubercular.
b. In association with Crohn's disease.
c. A complication of carcinoma of the rectum.

Classification and Nomenclature
A. The fistula may be classified as:
1. *Extra-sphincteric*, where the track lies immediately deep to the skin and mucous membrane.
2. *Trans-sphincteric*, where the track traverses through the fibres of the external and internal sphincters (commonest).
3. *Subsphincteric*, where the track passes entirely deep to both the sphincters (rare).
4. *Pararectal (high-level)*, where the track passes deep to both the sphincters and then through the levator ani, to enter the rectum. This type, fortunately uncommon, is a sequela to a pelvirectal abscess.

B. The fistula may be:
   1. *Complete.*
   2. *Incomplete.*—Here the track ends blindly (this should be called a sinus). However, a minute internal opening should always be searched for.
C. The fistula may be:
   1. *Single.*
   2. *Multiple.*—There is more than one external opening. In these cases there may be one or more internal openings. If there are multiple external fistulous openings, the condition is often termed *"water-can perineum'.*
D. The fistula is called:
   1. *Anterior,* or
   2. *Posterior,*
   according to the position of the external opening. This is important in view of the *Goodsall's Rule.* According to this rule, if the external opening of the fistula is in relation to the anterior half of the anal opening, the fistula is straight, running radially into the anal canal. If, however, the external opening is in relation with the posterior half of the anal opening, the fistula is a curved one, opening internally in the midline posteriorly, and often this is a *horseshoe fistula.*

Clinical Features.—There is a typical history of a perianal abscess, which, following rupture or incision, fails to heal and leaves behind a discharging opening. If this is neglected, there are recurrent attacks of perianal abscess formation. The new abscesses burst out either through the old opening or make fresh external openings. This is how multiple fistulae are formed.

Treatment.—*Excision* of the fistula is the only treatment.
1. For the commoner varieties of fistula (which are either extra-sphincteric or trans-sphincteric), the excision is fairly simple. A probe is passed in and, guided on it, a director. The track is now opened on the director. Thereafter:
   a. either the unhealthy granulation tissue on the wall is fully scraped with a Volkmann's spoon.
   b. or, the whole track, with its fibrous tissue lining, is excised.
   The cavity is packed to heal subsequently by granulation.
2. For the subsphincteric variety (which is relatively less frequent) the above type of operation may lead to anal incontinence because the whole thickness of the sphincteric mechanism is cut through. In order to make a compromise between total excision of the track and maintenance of sphincteric activity, either of the following procedures may be adopted:
   a. The lower part of the track, together with the superficial sphincteric fibres, is excised as above. A stout silk, threaded on the eye of a malleable probe, is now passed through the deeper part of the track, round the intact fibres of the sphincter and the anal canal mucosa, and is tied loosely. After about two weeks, at a second stage, the remaining part of the track, incorporated within the silk, is excised. Fibrosis, resulting from the previous operation, prevents retraction of the freshly cut sphincteric fibres, which later unite and again make up the sphincter (*Gabriel's two-stage operation*).
   b. Instead of passing the silk as above, a stainless steel wire is passed round the deeper part of the track. Starting from after two weeks, the knot on this wire is gradually tightened during subsequent dressings. The wire gradually cuts

through the remaining part of the track, thus opening it up. Since the sphincters are, in the meantime, being cut through gradually, parts of it, cut earlier, heal up by the time the remaining parts are being cut.

3. For the rare variety of pararectal fistula, the treatment is unsatisfactory since it cannot be completely opened up or completely excised. The only way is to excise the part up to the levator ani (to as high a level as possible), and the remnant is left to nature to heal. A temporary defunctioning colostomy may help obliteration of the deeper part of the track.

FISSURE-IN-ANO

This is a crack in the extremely sensitive mucous membrane of the anal canal. The condition is very painful and this pain causes spasm of the underlying internal sphincter. As long as this spasm remains, the crack in the overlying mucosa does not heal. Thus a vicious cycle is set up. Hence, a fissure, which to start with is acute, becomes chronic.

Fissures are commonest in the midline posteriorly: In males 90% occur posteriorly and 10% anteriorly, in the midline. In females, the incidence is 60% and 40% respectively. The relative frequency of the anterior fissures in the females may be explained by the trauma caused by the foetal head on the anterior anorectal wall. The overall frequency of the posterior fissures can be explained by the natural curvature of the anal canal, which takes a sharp forward bend from the rectum. A hard stool, coming down the rectum, strikes hard on the posterior wall of the anal canal. Constipation, therefore, is a common etiological factor.

Description.—To start with, a fissure is a superficial ulcer. As it gets chronic, it becomes converted into a canoe-shaped ulcer. At its upper end there is frequently a hypertrophic anal papilla. At its lower end a tag of hypertrophic skin hangs. This is called the *sentinel pile* (sentinel = sentry), and this is found only with long-standing fissures. A constant feature is a severe spasm of the internal sphincter, felt by digital examination. Frequently, a small subcutaneous fistula underlies the sentinel pile.

Types

1. Acute.—Superficial crack with thin margins.
2. Chronic.—A deeper ulcer, sometimes exposing the internal sphincter at its base. The margins are thick and oedematous. Usually there is an associated sentinel pile.

Clinical Features.—Typically, the patient presents with severe pain, during and after defaecation, often associated with a few drops of fresh blood with the stool. A history of constipation is very common.

Treatment

A. IN ACUTE CASES.—A *conservative treatment* is often successful:
1. Use of laxatives and application of a local analgesic ointment.
2. If this does not work, injection of a local anaesthetic agent in an *oily base* (for prolonged effect) into the tissues around the fissure (to relieve pain) and into the internal sphincter (to allay spasm). The disappearance of the spasm lasts for two to three weeks, by which time the fissure often heals. If required, the procedure may be repeated.

3. If the injection therapy fails, forcible digital stretching of the internal sphincter, done under general anaesthesia, often succeeds in curing the condition.

B. IN CHRONIC CASES.—*Operative treatment* has to be undertaken. The different operations, practised, are as follows:

1. *Internal Sphincterotomy.*—A Sim's speculum is introduced and the anal canal is opened up to expose the fissure. At its base, the fibres of the internal sphincter are seen. These fibres are cut through, in one line, till the conjoined longitudinal muscle is seen. Sentinel pile, if there be any, is also excised.

2. *Excision of the Fissure.*—The whole length of the fissure, together with the sentinel pile and a little of perianal skin around it, is excised in the shape of an wedge. The wound is allowed to heal by granulation.

3. *Excision of the Fissure with Sphincterotomy.*—This is the most commonly practised procedure. After the fissure is excised, a sphincterotomy is also performed as described above.

HAEMORRHOIDS OR PILES

This is a varicose condition of the veins of the anorectum, which means that the veins are .congested, dilated, elongated and, therefore, tortuous.

In the beginning, a clear differentiation should be made between an *internal* piles and an *external.* In the former variety, the veins are covered by mucous membrane, and in the latter, they are covered by skin. There may be a combination, when the veins are clothed above by the mucosa and below by the skin, and this variety is called the *interno-external* piles. An interno-external piles just represents an advanced stage of an internal piles.

While internal piles represents a single category, external piles denotes several distinct clinical entities and these are:

1. In association with an internal piles, i.e. interno-external piles.
2. In association with an anal fissure, i.e. sentinel piles.
3. Dilatation of the veins of the anul verge, as is seen in persons of sedentary life, during straining.
4. Perianal haematoma *(acute external plexus haematoma)* which results from bursting of an anal venule during straining. There is a painful, small superficial haematoma, often termed *thrombotic pile.* The condition either resolutes by itself in about a week or requires a small incision to drain the haematoma.

The majority of cases of piles are internal, and etiologically there are two groups:

I. IDIOPATHIC OR PRIMARY.—There is no definite cause to explain the varicosity. The factors believed to play their role are:

a. *Anatomical Factors:*
   i. The veins in the anal canal lack proper support since they lie in the lax submucous coat.
   ii. The veins have no valves,
   iii. The veins have to drain against gravity,
   iv. The veins pass through muscle mass and may, therefore, be constricted by the contraction of these muscles during defaecation.

b. *Hereditary Factors:*
The condition often runs in families (congenital weakness of vein wall).

c. *Exciting Factors:*
Long-continued strain, e.g. constipation (very common), over-purgation, colitis, dysenteries, etc.

2. SYMPTOMATIC OR SECONDARY.—The haemorrhoids are secondary to pressure effects, caused by some other pathology:
   a. Carcinoma of rectum.
   b. Pregnancy, uterine tumours.
   c. Persistent straining at micturition e.g. enlarged prostate.
   d. Portal hypertension, systemic hypertension, inferior vena caval congestion, etc. (rare).

Clinical Features.—The patient typically complains of fresh blood coming out with stool (hence called *bleeding piles).* In an uncomplicated case, the condition is always painless. Almost always there is a history of constipation.

As the veins get heavier in weight due to varicosity, the overlying mucosa (being very loosely attached to the underlying musculature) tends to hang down through the anal opening, together with the varicose veins underneath. Thus, there is a partial prolapse of the rectum. Depending on this factor, piles are graded as follows:

FIRST DEGREE. —No associated mucosal prolapse.

SECOND DEGREE.—Prolapse occurring during defaecation, but getting reduced spontaneously after defaecation.

THIRD DEGREE.—Same as above, but the prolapse has to be reduced manually

FOURTH DEGREE.—The piles always keep prolapsed.

A digital examination should always be done—piles can never be felt by the digit but this examination may sometimes detect a carcinoma or a polyp.

The piles are well visualised with an anal speculum or with a proctoscope. Typically, they are seen at 3, 7, and 11 o'clock positions, since these are the sites where the anorectal veins are normally bunched together. While the piles in these situations are termed *primary* piles, anastomotic veins often develop between these sets of veins, in long-standing cases. These may get varicose, and then they are termed *secondary* piles.

Treatment

A. CONSERVATIVE TREATMENT.—This consists of regular use of laxatives and local application of astringent ointments. *Injection of sclerosing agents* into the submucous coat of the gut often works well. The idea is to cause thrombosis of the piles as well as the vessels draining them, and to create fibrosis in the submucous coat, so that the lax mucous membrane retracts. The commonly used agents are 5% phenol in almond oil or arachis oil, or 3% sodium morrhuate. The injection is made with a special syringe and needle, under direct vision with an anal speculum. There are two types of injection:

a. *High Injection.*—Made into the submucosa, just above a group of piles (usually preferred nowadays).
b. *Low Injection.*—Made directly into the centre of the piles itself (done usually where high injections fail).

Injection treatment is best indicated in all cases of first degree piles but it is effective in other cases as well, where the prolapse can be replaced, i.e. second and third degree piles.

The disadvantages of this otherwise simple procedure are:

1. The results are unpredictable and the injection may have to be repeated; often frequently.
2. It is contraindicated:
   a. Where the piles tend to remain prolapsed (fourth degree).
   b. In cases of arterial piles (i.e. piles, where an artery communicates with the venous mass; diagnosed by presence of pulsation in the piles).
   c. In presence of infection.
3. A faulty technique may lead to sloughing, which may be dangerous.

B. OPERATIVE TREATMENT

1. *Ligation of the Piles* at its pedicle, after drawing the piles down. The idea is that the veins will be thrombosed, fibrosed and obliterated. This is only rarely done.
2. *Excision of Piles.*—There are two methods:
   a. Ligation of the pedicle as above, and then excising the mass of piles, together with the overlying mucosa and perianal skin, in the form of an wedge. This method of excision is easier but the loss of mucosa (particularly when three piles are excised in this way) may lead to stricture formation.
   b. *Submucous Dissection (Park's).*—An incision is made longitudinally on the mucosa, over the mass of the piles. The mucosal flaps are raised up on either side, and the venous mass is dissected out from the underlying musculature. The pedicle of the piles is now ligated. The venous mass, together with the abundant perianal skin below it, is excised. The mucosal flaps are resutured and the mucocutaneous junction is restored. The triangular gap on the skin is left open, to heal by granulation. This is a much better and logical method of excision as it avoids the risk of stricture formation.
3. *Clamp and Cautery Operation.*—A special clamp is applied on the piles on which the excess of the piles is excised. Thereafter, the tissues held in the clamp are cauterised by special technique. This method is nowadays obsolete.

Complications of Piles

1. Profuse haemorrhage.
2. Strangulation.—The piles, prolapsed out, are gripped by the internal sphincter and get irreducible. This complication is often loosely termed 'prolapsed piles' or 'acute attack of piles'.
3. Thrombosis, occurring in strangulated piles.
4. Ulceration, occurring on strangulated and thrombosed piles.
5. Fibrosis—An after-effect of thrombosis.
6. Gangrene.—If the constriction at the internal sphincter is sufficient to cause arterial obstruction, the mass of piles gets gangrenous.
7. Suppuration, due to infection in strangulated piles.
8. Portal pyaemia (pylephlebitis)—rare.

PROLAPSE OF THE RECTUM

Types.—There are two distinct types:

1. *Partial or Mucosal Prolapse.*—The everted tissue consists of mucosa alone, which is both lax and redundant. Its characteristic features are:

a. Its length is always between half and one and a half inches.

b. Palpation of the prolapse reveals that it consists of no more than a double layer of mucosa.

2. *Complete Prolapse or Procidentia.*—The prolapse consists of the entire thickness of the rectal wall. Its characteristic features are:

a. Its length is always more than one and a half inches and may be as much as 6 inches.

b. Palpation reveals that the prolapse is bulky, consisting of a double thickness of the entire rectal wall.

c. Since the upper part of the rectum has a peritoneal covering (the posterior wall of the rectovesical or rectouterine pouch), any prolapse, which is more than 2 inches in length, contains anteriorly, between its layers, the pouch of peritoneum. This means that there is a sliding hernia occurring through the pelvic diaphragm. In case of a big prolapse, this pouch may contain coils of small intestine.

PARTIAL PROLAPSE

Etiological Factors

1. *In infants and children:*

a. Rather straight course of the rectum due to as yet undeveloped sacral curvature.

b. Faulty bowel training.

c. Straining.—Attacks of diarrhoea, whooping cough.

d. Loss of weight and subsequent diminution of pararectal fat.

2. *In adults:*

a. Prolapsing haemorrhoids, i.e. second-degree onwards.

b. Torn perineum in the females.

3. *In old age:* Atony of the sphincter mechanism,

4. *At any age:* Same factors as are responsible for complete prolapse, whose primary stage is always a partial prolapse.

Treatment

A. CONSERVATIVE

1. *In infants and children.*—Digital reposition of the prolapse regularly, attention to bowel training, avoiding straining at stools, control of diarrhoea, improving general health.

2. *In adults.*—Submucous injection of 5 per cent phenol in almond oil, as is used for the haemorrhoids. The injection is made both at the apex and the base of the prolapse, after the prolapse has been brought down. After the injection, the mucosa is replaced in position.

B. OPERATIVE

1. *Thiersch's Operation.*—This operation is suitable for patients of any age. The operation is a simple one. Its aim is to reinforce the internal sphincter with a stainless steel wire and, at the same time narrowing the anal opening. Two small midline incisions are made, one in front and another behind the anal opening, about half an inch away from it. A suitably curved round body needle is passed from the posterior wound in such a way as to pass round one half of

the circumference of the anal canal, through the substance of the internal sphincter (which is situated about half an inch deep to the mucosa), and come out through the anterior wound. One end of a stainless steel wire is threaded on the needle and the wire thus traverses the track. In the same way the needle is passed round the other half of the anal canal, and the other end of the wire, threaded on it, traverses the internal sphincter. The assistant now puts a finger through the anus (the index finger in an adult, the little finger in a child), and the surgeon tightens the knot made between the two ends of the wire emerging at the anterior wound, till the assistant feels the ring sufficiently tight. The ends of the wire are clipped short and bent back. The wounds are then closed.

The only complication of the operation is infection in the wire that results in a discharging sinus. If this happens, the wire has to be removed, but by this time there is sufficient local fibrosis that prevents recurrence of the prolapse. If required, the operation may be repeated in future, and this is a great advantage of this operation, apart from its simplicity.

2. *Excision of the prolapsed mucosa.*—When a partial prolapse involves only part of the circumference of the anal canal, the prolapsed mucosa is excised and the cut margins are sutured to each other by interrupted stitches. In cases of prolapse associated with haemorrhoids, the excess of mucosa is automatically excised with excision of the piles.

COMPLETE PROLAPSE

Etiological Factors.—Several factors have been mentioned as possible causes of complete rectal prolapse:

1. *Lax Muscles:*
   a. Muscles of the pelvic floor, the opening through which the rectum passes being widened.
   b. Anal sphincters.
2. *Lack of Rectal Fixation.*—At operation it is always found that the rectum is unduly mobile and there is lack of its fixation to the bed of the sacrum.
3. *Sliding Hernia.*—As has already been stated, complete prolapse is usually associated with a sliding hernia, consisting of the rectovesical or rectouterine pouch, on its anterior aspect. It is believed by some surgeons that the process of rectal prolapse is actually an after-effect of the sliding hernia. This means that a complete rectal prolapse is nothing but an advanced stage of a sliding hernia of the anterior rectal wall.
4. *Rectal Intussusception.*—Some workers suggest that rectal prolapse actually starts as an infolding, i.e. intussusception of the rectal wall. The process starts about 3 inches above the anus, passes through the pelvic diaphragm, and ultimately comes out of the anus. According to this view, the laxity of the pelvic floor muscles and anal sphincters, the undue mobility of the rectum, and the associated sliding hernia are all secondary effects of this chronic form of intussusception.

Treatment.—Varieties of operation have been designed for complete prolapse and the number of such operations virtually indicates that none of these is fullproof. The more commonly practised procedures are mentioned below:

1. RESECTION
   a. Recto-sigmoidectomy, i.e. amputation of the prolapse from below. The prolapse is amputated outside the anus and anastomosis made between the

two ends of the bowel, the suture line thereafter being pushed in through the anus.

b. Anterior Resection, i.e. resection of the rectum and lower sigmoid per abdomen, followed by anastomosis between the sigmoid colon and the anal canal (as is done for some cases of carcinoma of the rectum).

2. FIXATION

a. *Well's Operation.*—This operation is done from the abdomen. The rectum is separated from the sacrum and a sheet of polyvinyl alcohol sponge is inserted between the rectum and the sacrum. This material induces marked fibrosis that fixes the rectum to the sacrum.

b. *Lockhart-Mummery Operation.*—Here the fixation is done from below. A transverse incision, about 2 inches in length, is made midway between the anus and the tip of the coccyx. The incision is deepened. Thereafter, the fingers, and finally, the hand is passed in the gap between the rectum and the sacrum in order to mobilise the rectum to as high a level as possible. The resulting cavity is plugged with a roller gauge so that it heals by granulation and finally by fibrosis, that fixes the rectum to the sacrum. Alternatively, a piece of polyvinyl alcohol sponge, as is used in Wells' operation, may be used to pack the cavity.

3. PLASTIC REPAIR.—This is the popular *Roscoe-Graham's operation.* Its principles are:

a. Thorough mobilisation of the rectum and pulling it up.

b. Suturing of the pubo-rectalis muscles (in the pelvic diaphragm) in front of the rectum, so as to provide adequate support to the rectum.

c. Elimination of the deep rectouterine or rectovesical pouch to exclude the sliding hernia.

The operation is usually done by an abdominal approach (some surgeons prefer an abdominoperineal approach). The rectum is thoroughly mobilised and drawn upwards, as high as possible. In doing this, the peritoneal flap in front of the rectum has to be incised, i.e. the rectouterine or rectovesical pouch is opened up. After the rectum has been mobilised, it is pushed firmly backwards and the pubo-rectalis muscles of the two sides, lying laterally, are drawn together in front of it, with a few (3 or 4) stitches. Finally, the anterior cut flap of the rectouterine or rectovesical peritoneal pouch is sutured to the rectum at a high level, so that the depth of the pouch is obliterated.

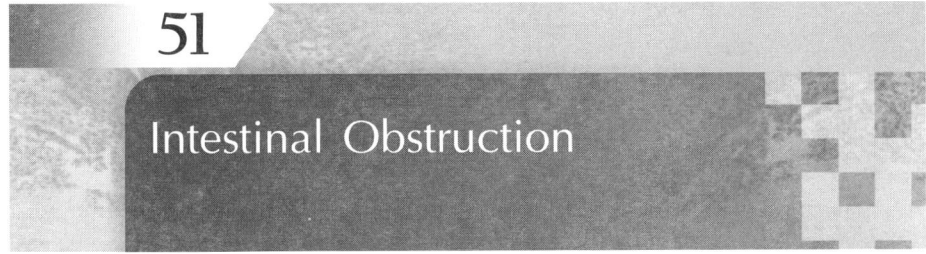

51

Intestinal Obstruction

Types

A. *Pathologically*, there are two varieties:
1. Dynamic or Mechanical.
2. Adynamic or Paralytic.

In dynamic obstruction there is a vigorous attempt on the part of the gut, proximal to the obstruction, to overcome the obstruction; hence there is hyperperistalsis.

In adynamic obstruction there is no organic block but there is a functional obstruction as the intestines fail to transmit peristaltic waves; hence there is absence of intestinal sounds *(silent abdomen)*. This is due to failure in the neuromuscular mechanism, normally conducted by the Auerbach's (myenteric) and Meissner's (submucous) plexuses. This may be due to:
a. Paralytic ileus *(see below)*.
b. Mesenteric vascular thrombosis.

B. *Clinically*, there are three varieties:
1. Acute (including acute recurrent), usually occurring in the small gut.
2. Chronic, usually occurring in the large gut.
3. Acute-on-chronic, i.e. onset of features of acute obstruction in a patient having chronic obstruction. This usually occurs in large gut obstruction that extends to the small gut if the ileo-caecal valve is open, the contents then passing up the ileum.

PARALYTIC ILEUS

Paralytic ileus may occur under several conditions, as enumerated below, of which the first two are, by far, the commoner:
1. Post-operative, following any abdominal operation.
2. Infective, i.e. associated with peritonitis.
3. Uraemia or hepatic failure.
4. Reflex, rather commonly associated with:
   a. Fracture of the spine or multiple rib fracture.
   b. Retroperitoneal haemorrhage.
   c. Tight plaster jacket.

DYNAMIC OBSTRUCTION

Causes

A. In the lumen *(intermural)*:
Foreign body, undigested bolus of food, faecolith, plug of round worms, gall stone.

B. IN THE WALL *(intra-mural):*
1. Inflammatory strictures, particularly tubercular.
2. Thickening of gut wall, e.g. Crohn's disease, hyperplastic ileocaecal tuberculosis.
3. Tumours.—Benign or, more commonly, malignant, i.e. carcinoma.

C. OUTSIDE THE WALL *(extra-mural):*
1. Hernia.—External or internal (obstructed inguinal hernia is the commonest cause of intestinal obstruction).
2. Bands and adhesions.
3. Extrinsic tumours, pressing on the gut.

D. OTHERS:
This group includes two special and rather common types of intestinal obstruction, which cannot be strictly grouped under either of the above headings, i.e.
1. Intussusception.
2. Volvulus.

Types.—Pathologically, the cases may be grouped under three headings:
1. Simple obstruction (i.e. non-strangulated).
2. Strangulation, where, in addition to obstruction, the blood supply to a loop of gut is impaired.
3. Closed loop obstruction, where a segment of gut is shut off both from above and below. This is present in almost all cases of strangulation, e.g. strangulated hernia.

Pathology and Effects of Obstruction; Causes of Death

NON-STRANGULATED OBSTRUCTION
 I. The *distal loop* (i.e. below the obstruction) looks normal for the first few hours and shows evidence of normal peristalsis. Thus, the patient may pass one or two normal stools with flatus. This is also the reason why there may be a positive result with an enema, given for the first time. However, if a second enema is given, the result is negative *(two-enema test).*
 II. The *proximal loop* shows evidence of progressive distension. The distension is due to gas and fluid:
   A. *Gas.*—There are three sources of the gas:
      1. The swallowed air.
      2. Diffusion from the blood into the lumen of the gut.
      3. Products of digestion and bacterial action.
   B. *Fluid.*—Apart from the little amount of ingested fluid, the major part is made up by the digestive juices. About 8000 ml of fluid is secreted daily into the bowel lumen:
      1. Above the Pylorus, 4000 ml.
         Saliva —1500 ml.
         Gastric secretion—2500 ml.
      2. Below the Pylorus, 4000 ml.
         Bile and pancreatic juice—1000 ml.
         Succus entericus—3000 ml.
Normally, major part of this 8000 ml is reabsorbed from the bowel lumen. In intestinal obstruction this reabsorption fails to occur because:

a. Major part of the reabsorption occurs from the colon, where the fluid is failing to reach because of the obstruction.

b. Occlusion of the veins in the walls of the distended gut which, therefore, fail to reabsorb.

III.   *Ill-effects of Distension.*—There are several effects:

1. Occlusion of the veins in the gut wall, impeding normal reabsorption.
2. The same occlusion of veins also leads to accumulation (i.e. sequestration) of fluid into the bowel wall and into its lumen. If a long .segment of gut is involved, this loss of fluid and electrolytes from the circulation may be considerable.
3. Stimulation of the afferent nerves in the bowel wall and in the mesentery of the distended loop causes not only the pain but also vomiting and, occasionally, collapse.
4. Pressure on the diaphragm causes cardiorespiratory embarrassment.

The first two factors result in considerable loss of fluid and electrolytes. There is gross deficit of chlorides and sodium, but even the relatively small loss of potassium may be equally dangerous. From what has been stated above, it is evident that distension plays a very bad role, and deflation of the distended loop, by gastrointestinal suction (preferably by a Miller-Abbott tube), is of immense value.

IV. *Causes of Death*

A. Majority of the patients die of fluid and electrolyte loss, caused by:
1. Vomiting.
2. Defective absorption.
3. Sequestration in the bowel lumen.
4. Absence of normal daily intake.

The amount of fluid and electrolyte loss, however, depends upon the level of the obstruction. If there is a high small intestinal obstruction, saliva, gastric secretion, bile and pancreatic juice, all are lost, so that gross dehydration results. On the other hand, with a low small intestinal obstruction, some reabsorption takes place, at least in the early stages, so that dehydration is less severe and late to appear. In colonic obstruction dehydration is minimum.

B. Some deaths may be caused by intestinal toxins, which have definite depressor effects. These toxins are bacterial as well as metabolic (from protein breakdown), and are elaborated either in the lumen or in the wall of the gut. As long as the obstruction is present, these are not absorbed. As soon as the obstruction is relieved, sudden and quick absorption of these toxic materials in the blood may cause death. This is believed to be an important cause of death in low small gut obstructions. .

C. Some patients may die of cardiorespiratory embarrassment, caused by the distension.

STRANGULATED OBSTRUCTION AND CLOSED LOOP OBSTRUCTION.—These two conditions are usually associated with each other, and are most commonly seen in a strangulated hernia. Here, to the effects of simple obstruction, are added those of the impaired blood supply to the loop of gut:

I. *Changes in the Strangulated Loop and Causes of Death:*
1. Distention is severe but is mostly due to gas. This, however, is only rarely the cause of death.

2. In the earlier hours of strangulation, the veins are occluded by the obstructing band while the arteries are still open. Blood reaches the gut but cannot return and, therefore, accumulates in the wall as well as in its lumen. For a short loop of gut, this may be insignificant. On the other hand, when a long loop is involved in strangulation, there may be considerable sequestration of blood in this way and this, by itself, may be a cause of death.

3. Ultimately, swelling of the strangulated loop causes obstruction of the arteries as well. Consequently, the gut wall turns gangrenous. Toxins and bacteria, from the bowel lumen, come out through the gangrenous wall, to be absorbed. Absorption is maximum if the leakage occurs into the peritoneal cavity (e.g. with internal hernia), which provides a wide field for absorption; in these cases, this is the commonest cause of death. On the other hand, absorption is slow and minimum from the scrotal tissues, so that this factor is of less importance in external herniae. (This is the reason why the fluid from the sac of a strangulated external hernia should be removed by opening the sac, before cutting the constriction band, so that entry of this toxic fluid into the peritoneal cavity is avoided).

II. *Proximal and Distal Loops.*—For a long period they keep normal. Only when retrograde thrombosis from the strangulated mesentery spreads to the mesentery of these loops that they undergo changes. Both these loops then undergo distension and paralysis.

General Clinical Features of Intestinal Obstruction

A. ACUTE OBSTRUCTION: These are usually small intestinal, and the features are:
1. Pain.—Colicky in nature.
2. Vomiting.—The higher the obstruction, the more is the vomiting.
3. Distension.—Not very evident in the early stages but appear later; the distension is centrally placed.
4. Absolute constipation.—To start with, there may be one or two stools, but then there is passage of neither faeces nor flatus, i.e. absolute constipation (*obstipation*).
5. Visible peristalsis.—This takes the typical ladder-pattern, in small intestinal obstruction. Intestinal sounds are highly exaggerated. Borborygmi may be loud enough to be heard by the naked ear.
6. Evidences of dehydration.—Dry tongue, dry skin, sunken eyes.
7. An obstructed external hernia may be evident.

B. CHRONIC OBSTRUCTION: These are commonly large intestinal, and the features are:
1. Constipation.—This appears first and, to start with, may not be absolute; gradually absolute constipation sets in.
2. Distension then appears, especially marked on the flanks.
3. Vomiting is very late to appear.
4. Dehydration is thus exceptional.

C. ACUTE-ON-CHRONIC OBSTRUCTION: This occurs when, following a large gut obstruction, the ileo-caecal valve is forced open and the contents pass up the ileum. To start with, there are features of chronic obstruction; after a few days, pain, vomiting, dehydration and central abdominal distension set in.

D. STRANGULATION: This may complicate any of the common types of mechanical obstruction, early or late, excepting carcinoma of the colon. Its presence should be suspected under the following conditions:

1. If an external hernia is tense and tender.
2. If pain is severe and comes in frequent spasms; if the pain persists for more than two hours after effective gastroduodenal suction has been instituted.
3. If there is rise of temperature and an out-of-proportion pulse rate.
4. If there is a rebound tenderness.   ..
5. If shock and toxic features are predominant.

General Management of Acute Intestinal Obstruction.—There are three principles to combat and overcome the ill-effects of acute intestinal obstruction:—

1. GASTROINTESTINAL SUCTION.—In ordinary practice, a Ryle's tube is employed and a gastroduodenal suction is effected. A better method is gastrointestinal suction with a Miller-Abbott tube. This aims at removal of fluid and gas from the stomach and upper intestines. When strangulation can be ruled out, a few hours'suction is the best form of preliminary treatment. However, even when strangulation can be excluded, not more than six hours should be spent in this form of treatment; further delay in operative interference increases the mortality considerably.

2. REPLACEMENT AND MAINTENANCE OF FLUID AND ELECTROLYTES.—The first aim is to replace what has been lost, and as much as 3.5 litres of normal saline, intravenously, may be necessary if the patient shows signs of severe dehydration. Subsequently, the daily requirement (approx. 2 litres), plus the amount drained by suction, has to be maintained by intravenous drip.

3. OPERATIVE RELIEF OF THE OBSTRUCTION.—Operation should be undertaken immediately if strangulation is evident or suspected. Otherwise, conservative treatment with gastrointestinal suction may be tried for the first few hours. If, however, the obstruction persists or the condition deteriorates even after six hours' conservative treatment, operation is imperative. Further delay simply invites strangulation in non-strangulated cases, and also increases the mortality from irreversible fluid and electrolyte imbalance.

INTUSSUSCEPTION

Definition and Nomenclatures.—Intussusception means invagination of a loop of gut into an immediately adjacent loop. Usually a proximal loop is invaginated into the distal gut (i.e. the direction of peristalsis). Rarely the distal gut may be invaginated into the proximal loop; this is called *retrograde intussusception* (e.g. jejunogastric intussusception, following gastrojejunostomy).

Occasionally, the mass of intussusception may reinvaginate into the distal gut; this is called *compound* or *double intussusception.*

Usually intussusception is single; rarely there may more than one intussusceptions, at different levels, i.e. *multiple intussusceptions.*

The condition is usually acute, but sometimes *chronic intussusception* may occur, persisting for months or even years. In rare instances, there may be *recurrent intussusception.*

Etiology.—The cases belong to two distinct categories:

GROUP A; There is a definite cause for the intussusception, e.g. polyp, submucous lipoma, carcinoma, stump of appendix, diverticulum, etc. These are the cases of *secondary intussusception*. Adults and older children are usually the victims.

GROUP B: In this type, there is no definite cause for the intussusception. Majority of the cases of intussusception belong to this group, which is known as *primary* or *idiopathic intussusception*. This type occurs, most commonly, in children between the sixth and ninth months. Various theories are put forward to explain the cause in these cases:

1. Derangement of the normal peristaltic mechanism, probably initiated by faulty diet. It is at this age that injudicious additions are made in the child's diet.
2. An inherent defect in the neuromuscular coordination in the intestines, resulting in a persistent localised contraction. This constricted segment is pushed into the immediate distal passive loop of gut by the proximal peristalsis. In the children the inhibitory nervous apparatus develops later than the motor apparatus, and are weaker than it. In other words, tonicity of the gut musculature is much greater than the capacity of relaxation.
3. Inflammatory hypertrophy of the Peyer's patches may initiate the intussusception. This view is substantiated by the fact that idiopathic intussusception most commonly occurs in the terminal part of the ileum, which is rich in Peyer's patches. A swollen Peyer's patch causes an elevation, protruding into the lumen of the gut, and this is believed to initiate the intussusceptions. As for the cause of the inflammation of the lymphoid tissue, there are two views again:
   a. Change in the intestinal flora, caused by the change in the child's diet at this age.
   b. Infection, secondary to upper respiratory tract infections, sometimes viral.
4. Structural peculiarities of that part of the intestine where intussusception commonly occurs, i.e. the terminal ileum, caecum and ascending colon, may play some role:
   a. An unusually mobile ascending colon, resulting from presence of an abnormal mesocolon.
   b. Obliquity of the opening of the ileum into the caecum.
   c. Excessive lymphoid tissue, i.e. Peyer's patches, in the terminal ileum (already discussed).

Types
1. Only Small Gut, i.e. ileo-ileal (ileum is invaginated into ileum)— 8 per cent.
2. Only Large Gut:
   a. Colo-colic (colon is invaginated into colon)—8 per cent.
   b. Caecal (the caput caeci is invaginated)—2 per cent.
3. Combination of Small and Large Guts:
   a. Ileo-caecal—46 per cent.
   b. Ileo-colic—36 per cent.

In ileo-caecal intussusception, the starting point is the ileo-caecal valve. The starting point of ileo-colic intussusception is a little proximal, i.e. the terminal ileum, so that it actually starts as an ileo-ileal intussusception that passes through the ileo-caecal valve to enter the colon.

Anatomy.—As a loop of gut passes into an immediate adjacent loop, and the two loops are continuous, the intussusception consists of three layers (Fig. 51.1). From inside outwards, these are:

1. Entering layer.
2. Returning layer.
3. Ensheathing (or receiving) layer.
   On cross section, these appear as concentric tubes.

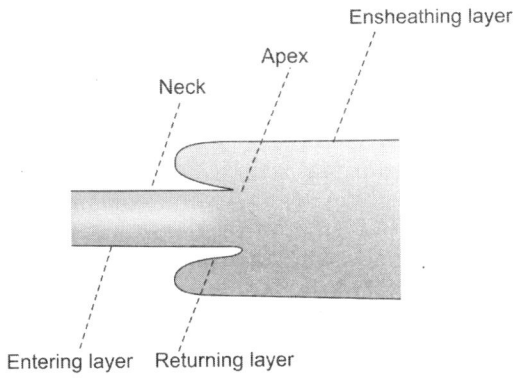

Fig. 51.1: Intussusception

The entering and the returning layers, together, make what is known as the *intussusceptum*, while the ensheathing (receiving) layer is called the *intussuscipiens*. The starting point of the intussusception is called its *apex*. It marks the junction of the entering and the returning layers, and is the most advanced part of the intussusception. It is a fixed point and so the intussusception progresses at the cost of the ensheathing layer. The site, where the returning layer and the ensheathing layer meet, is called the *neck* of the intussusception, and this point varies as the intussusception progresses.

Pathology.—Intussusception is virtually an intestinal obstruction with risk of strangulation. The course and progress of the pathology may be summarised as follows:

1. Simple telescoping of the gut does not cause total intestinal abstraction. In an attempt to overcome the obstruction, the peristalsis, behind, pushes the intussusception further along the intussuscipiens, and the intussusceptions progress.
2. The mesentery of the entering and returning layers, which is also dragged in with the gut, is crowded at the neck of the intussusception. The mass of the intussusception becomes *sausage-shaped* by the pull of the mesentery. The concavity of the sausage is towards the line of attachment of the mesentery, i.e. facing towards the umbilicus.
3. The mesentery is compressed between the entering and the returning layers, on the concave side of the sausage. For some period, the veins are occluded while the arteries are still open. This causes severe congestion and oedema in the wall of the intussusceptum, so much so, that the lumen of the gut is occluded now, causing total intestinal obstruction. The oedema and congestion in the wall of

the gut pours out into its lumen a mixture of blood and mucus, which is termed *red-currant jelly*. This is passed per rectum or is found on an examining finger after rectal examination.

4. The congestion and oedema make the apex of the intussusception so stiff that the inner tube cannot roll round and become part of the middle, i.e. returning layer. This is why the apex is always a fixed point. Elongation of the returning layer occurs at the expense of the ensheathing layer. This process of elongation continues till there is tension on the mesentery. After that, further onward movement occurs by stretching, angulation, or torsion of the mesentery. In those rare cases where the intussusceptum comes down to the rectum, it is not necessarily that the process is long-standing; it simply implies that the gut possesses a long mesentery that makes it unduly mobile.

5. Finally, pressure on the mesentery is sufficient to occlude the arteries, and gangrene sets in. The returning layer, near the apex, is the first site to become gangrenous; the ensheathing layer usually remains unaffected. As a result of gangrene, perforation and peritonitis set in.

6. In very rare instances, gross adhesions may develop at the neck, and the whole mass of intussusceptum may become necrosed and sloughed out. This results in a *natural cure.*

Clinical Features

1. *Incidence.*—Except for the secondary cases, the condition is almost, always confined to children. The commonest age is between the sixth and ninth months. Healthy, first-born, male children are common sufferers.
2. *Symptoms:*
   a. The child gets paroxysms of abdominal pain, draws up the legs, and screams. During the pain, there is often a facial pallor.
   b. Vomiting is late to appear because the obstruction is in the lower gut.
   c. There may be one or two normal stools, after which there is absolute constipation. Often, there is passage of red-currant jelly.
3. *Physical Signs:*
   a. The child is dehydrated.
   b. There is usually a little or no abdominal distension.
   c. The mass of intussusception may be made out by gentle abdominal palpation, but it may be hidden under the costal margin or in the pelvis.
   d. There may be a peculiar sensation of emptiness at the right iliac fossa, on palpation. This is called *'signe de Dance,'* and is caused by the shifting of the contents of the right iliac fossa.
4. *Rectal Examination* must be done. Usually the examining finger is smeared with red-currant jelly. Occasionally, the intussusception may be felt at the tip of the finger, like the cervix uteri in the vagina. Very rarely, the intussusceptum may hang out of the anus.

Special Investigations

1. *Straight X-ray* of the abdomen shows increased gas shadows in the small intestine, and there may be suggestion of absence of the caecal gas shadow.
2. *Barium Enema Investigation* is diagnostic in the majority of the cases. The enema is stopped as it reaches the intussusceptum, which produces a *pincer-like* or *horseshoe deformity,* caused by the cupping in of the mass of the intussusceptum.

The pressure of the barium enema may cause a spontaneous reduction of the intussusception. This was the basis of reduction of an intussusception by hydrostatic pressure in the older days (*see* below).

Treatment.—Usually the treatment is operative reduction. Some surgeons attempt reduction by hydrostatic pressure.

A. REDUCTION BY HYDROSTATIC PRESSURE.—Water is pushed under pressure, per rectum, through a catheter, from an enema can, and the returning fluid is collected. The procedure is repeated several times and the returning fluid is found to contain red-currant jelly. If, thereafter, the returning fluid contains faecal matter and flatus is passed with it, reduction has been achieved.

B. OPERATIVE REDUCTION.—In an ordinary case, this is usually not difficult. This should not be done by attempting to pull the entering layer out; instead, the intussusceptum should be squeezed out by pushing the apex towards the neck, through the intussuscipiens.

In cases of difficulty, reduction may be achieved by:
1. Dissecting the adhesions at the neck and stretching the neck gently.
2. Squeezing on the intussusceptum by fingers, in an attempt to displace the oedema from the region of the ileo-caecal valve.

C. INDICATIONS FOR RESECTION AND ANASTOMOSIS:
1. If there is gangrenous change.
2. If reduction is impossible.
3. If there is gross injury to the gut during the process of reduction.

In the usual types, i.e. ileo-caecal and ileo-colic, a right hemicolectomy has then to be performed.

VOLVULUS

Definition.—This means twisting or axial rotation of a loop of bowel, so that:
   a. both its ends are closed, and
   b. the mesenteric vessels are occluded.

Sites
1. The commonest site is the sigmoid colon (sigmoid volvulus),
2. A rather common site is the midgut in the newborn (volvulus neonatorum).
3. The small intestine (occasional).
4. The caecum and ascending colon (rare).
5. The stomach (very rare).

VOLVULUS OF THE SIGMOID COLON

Pathogenesis
1. There is a redundant loop of pelvic colon, which is chronically distended and loaded, because of constipation.
2. This hangs down into the pelvis, causing an elongation of the pelvic mesocolon. This elongation is possible as the peritoneum from the posterior abdominal wall is raised and becomes part of the mesocolon. Thus, the attachment of the pelvic mesocolon becomes narrow.

3. As a result, the two ends of the pelvic colon are approximated to each other and a twist can easily follow.
4. A horizontal attachment of the pelvic mesocolon to the posterior abdominal wall may be an additional predisposing factor.
5. A band of adhesion, stretching from the anti-mesenteric border at the summit of the pelvic colonic loop, may also be an aiding factor. The gut rotates between two fixed points.

Pathology.—To start with, the upper loop falls downwards in front of the lower, thus making half a turn. It commonly falls by gravity into the pelvis, so that the rotation is usually anti-clockwise. From this stage there may be a spontaneous de-rotation.

1. When the rotation progresses to one and a half turns, the veins in the mesocolon are occluded.
2. When the rotation is more than this, e.g. two and a half turns, arterial occlusion occurs, gangrene sets in, and peritonitis follows.

   Thus there is a closed-loop strangulated obstruction with its associated ill-effects (discussed earlier in this chapter).

Clinical Features

1. Middle-aged males are the commonest sufferers.
2. There is usually a long history of habitual constipation. In some cases there may be history of previous acute attacks of left-sided abdominal pain, caused by half-a-turn volvulus, spontaneously reduced.
3. There is severe acute colicky pain, followed by absolute constipation. This being a low-intestinal obstruction, vomiting is late to appear. However, distension of the gut causes hiccough and retching.
4. Abdominal distension is great; in no other condition there is so much of abdominal distension. At the onset the distension is mainly left-sided.
5. Features of peritonitis set in when gangrene occurs.

X-ray.—A straight film shows a huge oval gas shadow on the left side of the abdomen, with the typical appearance of a colonic distension.

Treatment

1. SIGMOIDOSCOPIC INTUBATION.—A sigmoidoscope is passed in and, when the obstruction is reached, an attempt is made to negotiate a flatus tube, through the sigmoidoscope, into the twisted gut. If this is possible, immediate deflation occurs. An emergency operation is thus avoided and the patient can be operated when he becomes fit (about two weeks later).
2. EXPLORATION.—When sigmoidoscopic intubation fails or when there is a suspicion of perforation immediate exploration should be undertaken with a left paramedian incision. De-rotation is considerably aided if a flatus tube is simultaneously passed in, through the rectum, by an assistant. The surgeon guides the tube, pass the obstruction, with his hand inside the abdomen. Once the gut is deflated, its handling and rotation become much easier. The direction of rotation is noted and the gut is rotated in the opposite direction. Usually rotation is anti-clockwise, so that the gut has to be rotated clockwise.

Simple de-rotation is not sufficient because recurrence is fairly common. Additional procedures are thus recommended:

  a. *If the gut is viable.*—Resection of the redundant loop with end-to-end anastomosis is the treatment of choice. Some surgeons advocate this to be performed at a second stage after the de-rotation operation. No form of anchoring of the pelvic colon by sutures, or of plication of the pelvic meso-colon, offers sure guarantee against recurrence.

  b. *If the gut is gangrenous.*—Exteriorisation of the affected loop, followed by resection by the Paul-Mikulicz procedure, is the treatment of choice.

In either case, redundancy of the colon and the mesocolon makes the re-section a rather simple procedure.

VOLVULUS NEONATORUM

This is due to an arrested rotation of the midgut during the second stage of intestinal rotation in foetal life. Hence, it is also called *volvulus of the midgut.*

Mechanism of Normal Rotation.—The developing midgut is concerned in this rotation. The midgut extends from the duodenal papilla at the middle of the second part of the duodenum to the neighbourhood of the left colic flexure. At the onset, the midgut is a single short loop, with its long axis along the long axis of the body. Shaped like a C, it has a fan-shaped mesentery, which suspends it from the posterior abdominal wall. This narrow pedicle of mesentery is called the duodenocolic isthmus, which corresponds above and below to the two ends of the midgut, which are thus closely apposed to each other in the midline. Along the mesentery, the artery of the midgut, i.e. the superior mesenteric artery, passes to the apex of the loop. The branches which are given to the proximal loop of the gut are called the pre-arterial branches (i.e. vasa intestinales, supplying the jejunum and the ileum), while those given to the distal loop are called the post-arterial branches (which become the ileo-colic and right colic arteries). The midgut subsequently grows voluminous, but its mesentery is attached by a very narrow pedicle, on which it may swing and rotate easily. This is the basis of rotation of the gut.

Extrusion from the coelomic cavity.—The greater part of the midgut is extruded from the coelomic cavity by the increase in size of the abdominal organs, especially the liver. It now comes to lie in the umbilical cord, i.e. a physiological hernia occurs (persistence of part or whole of the hernia results in exomphalos). The voluminous development of the midgut occurs here. The developing midgut undergoes rotation. The complicated process of rotation is described in three stages (Fig. 51.2).

First stage of rotation.—This occurs inside the physiological hernia and consists of a simple 90-degree anti-clockwise rotation of the midgut loop, whose long axis now comes to lie across the long axis of the body. The proximal end, i.e. the duodenum, is taken to the right side and the distal end to the left. Thus the base of the midgut loop lies transversely, with the duodenal papilla and the left colic flexure at almost the same level. The small intestine is now to the right of the midline and the proximal colon to the left.

Second stage of rotation.—This occurs as the midgut re-enters the abdomen. The first part to return is the smaller pre-arterial segment, i.e. the duodenum and the jejunum. The last part to enter is the bulky caecum, carrying back the superior

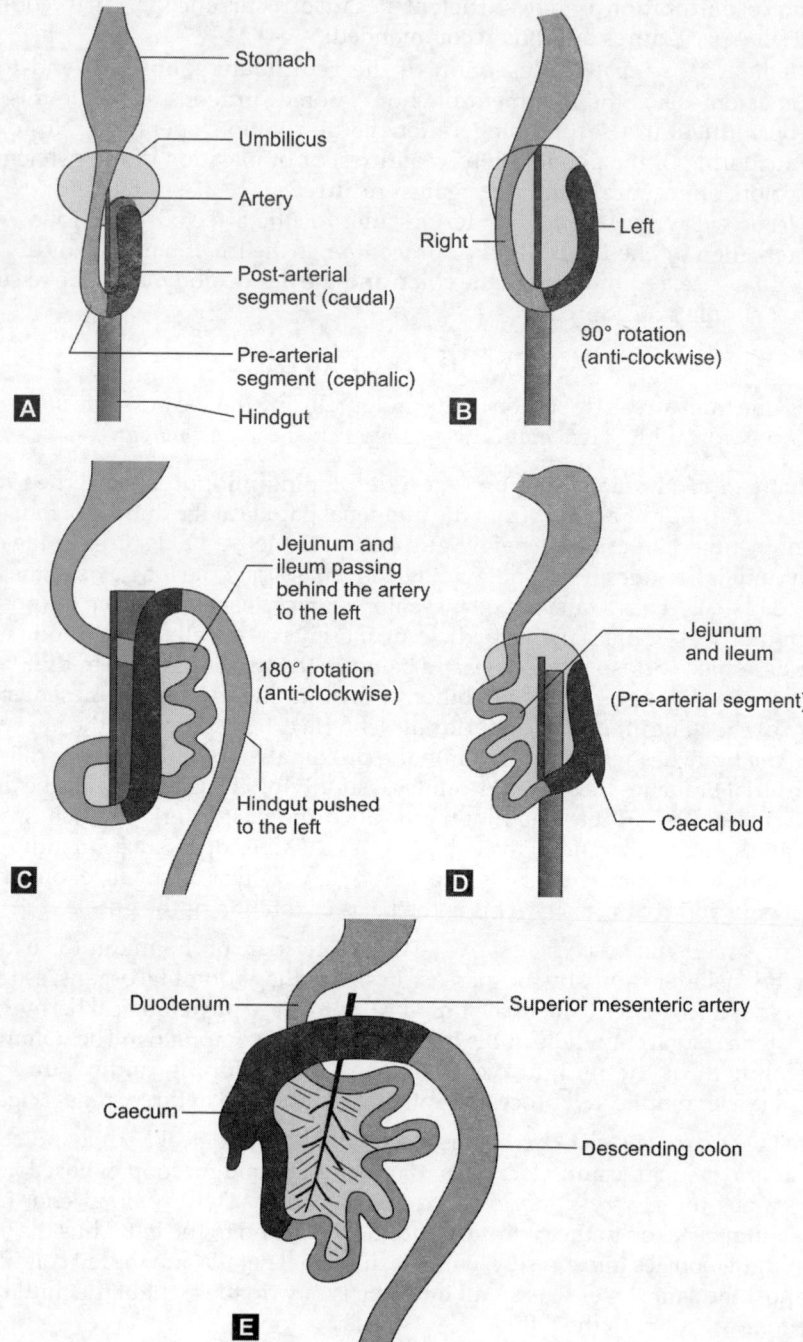

Fig. 51.2: Normal rotation of the gut

mesenteric artery with it. This fact is important because the caecum holds the superior mesenteric artery tensely forwards and this provides an axis, around which rotation of the gut is possible.

The first re-entering structure, i.e. the small intestine (pre-arterial segment), meets the unyielding bulk of liver and is thus rotated to the left side of the abdomen, below and behind the stretched superior mesenteric artery. The later-returning post-arterial segment, including the caecum, lies on the right side of the abdomen, in direct relation to the undersurface of the liver, above and in front of the artery. Thus, there is a 180-degree anti-clockwise rotation, around the artery, in this second stage.

THIRD STAGE OF ROTATION.—This is rather simple. The caecum and proximal colon descend to their adult position, and the right colon becomes fixed to the posterior abdominal wall.

Derangements of Rotation

A. FIRST STAGE: Derangements are rare.

B. SECOND STAGE:
1. Failure of re-entry into the abdomen from the umbilical cord.— Exomphalos (*see* umbilical hernia, Chapter 52).
2. Non-rotation.—Volvulus neonatorum.
3. Reversed entry and rotation.—This occurs if the post-arterial segment returns first and is pushed to the left side of the abdomen, below and behind the superior mesenteric artery. The transverse colon lies behind the artery.
4. Malrotation.—This results in anomalies, of different degrees, in the relationships of the mesenteries of the pre-arterial and post-arterial segments.

C. THIRD STAGE: The caecum fails to descend and remains subhepatic.

Pathogenesis of Volvulus Neonatorum

1. The normal 180-degree anti-clockwise rotation of the midgut (in the second stage of rotation), as it re-enters the abdomen, does not occur.
2. The whole bulk of the midgut, from the duodenum to near the left colic flexure, remains unfixed and unduly mobile. It hangs from a narrow mesenteric attachment, i.e. the duodenocolic isthmus. It may, therefore, easily undergo abnormal rotations, i.e. volvulus.
3. Such abnormal rotations do occur and usually the rotation is clockwise (c.f. adult sigmoid volvulus and normal intestinal rotation). This occurs during the first few days of life (probably initiated by feeding), and hence this is called volvulus neonatorum.

Pathology

I. THE VOLVULUS.—This differs from an adult volvulus in three respects:
   a. The whole midgut is affected but, since its lower end is less acutely twisted, the loop of gut remains collapsed.
   b. Serious occlusion of the mesenteric vessels does not occur. Hence, the typical discolouration of the adult volvulus is not seen and gangrene never supervenes.
   c. The rotation is usually clockwise.

II. THE TRANSDUODENAL BAND OF LADD.—As the caecum remains in the left hypochondrium, a peritoneal band is found, running from the caecum to the right side of the abdomen, and then across the front of the second part of the duodenum. This is called the band of Ladd and this causes *total duodenal obstruction*.

III. THE NATURE OF OBSTRUCTION.—Unlike adult volvulus, the neonatal volvulus is not a closed-loop strangulated obstruction since its lower end is open and the mesenteric vessels are not seriously occluded. However, there is an acute obstruction at the second part of the duodenum, and this is because:

a. The twist at the upper end of the volvulus is acute.

b. There is the presence of the band of Ladd.

Clinical Features

1. A young infant, previously healthy, starts bilious vomiting during the first few days of life.
2. There is abdominal distension, but limited to the upper abdomen.
3. Signs of dehydration set in.

X-ray.—The stomach and upper part of the duodenum are grossly distended with air.

Treatment.—The abdomen is explored and:

1. The gut is de-rotated (usually it has to be rotated anti-clockwise).
2. The transduodenal band of Ladd is divided.
3. The right colon is anchored to the posterior abdominal wall in order to prevent recurrence of the volvulus.

52

Hernia

INGUINAL HERNIA

Surgical Anatomy of the Inguinal Canal

POSITION AND EXTENT.—The inguinal canal is an oblique intermuscular cleft in the anterior abdominal wall, above the medial half of the inguinal ligament. It commences at the deep inguinal ring and ends at the superficial inguinal ring. In the adults, the canal is about 4 cm long, and is directed downwards and medially. In infants, the superficial and deep rings are almost superimposed and thus there is only a little obliquity of the canal.

The *deep inguinal ring* is an opening in the fascia transversalis, ½ inch above the mid-inguinal point and immediately lateral to the inferior epigastric vessels. The opening is U-shaped, incomplete above, and at its margins the fascia transversalis is condensed.

The *superficial inguinal ring* is a triangular opening in the external oblique aponeurosis. The medial and lateral margins of the opening are known as the *crura*, which are joined by criss-cross *intercrural fibres.* Normally the ring admits only the tip of the little finger.

BOUNDARIES

Anteriorly.—The external oblique aponeurosis, along the whole length of the canal. In the lateral third, in addition, are those fibres of the internal oblique muscle which arise from the intermediate part of the inguinal ligament. Superficial to these are the skin and the *two layers* of the superficial fascia; in between these two layers lie the superficial epigastric and superficial external pudendal vessels.

Posteriorly—The thickened fascia transversalis, along the whole length of the canal. In the medial half, in addition, there is the conjoint tendon (i.e. combined internal oblique and transversus).

Roof.—Formed by the lower borders of the internal oblique and transversus abdominis muscles, which arch over the canal before fusing together to form the conjoint tendon.

Floor.—The upper surface of the inguinal ligament, which forms a furrow.

CONTENTS
1. (a) In the male, the spermatic cord and the vestigial remnant of the processus vaginalis (i.e. the foetal prolongation of the peritoneum, which accompanies the testis in its descent into the scrotum).
   (b) In the female, the round ligament of the uterus.
2. Ilio-inguinal nerve (lies in the medial part of the canal).

3. Ilio-hypogastric nerve is not strictly a content of the canal but is displayed when the canal is exposed. It lies in front of the internal oblique, just above its lower border.

COVERINGS OF THE SPERMATIC CORD.—These coverings are derived as the testis descends from the abdomen into the scrotum. From inside outwards, these are:

1. The internal spermatic fascia, derived from the fascia transversalis at the deep ring.
2. The cremasteric muscle and fascia, derived from the internal oblique inside the canal.
3. The external spermatic fascia, derived from the external oblique aponeurosis at the superficial ring.

The cremasteric muscle is fairly strong in the children. The contraction of the muscular fibres can draw the testis up, from the scrotum to the superficial inguinal ring.

CONSTITUENTS OF THE SPERMATIC CORD

1. The vas deferens with its artery.
2. The testicular artery.
3. The pampiniform plexus of veins.
4. Lymph vessels.
5. Sympathetic nerve fibres.

The Mechanism of the Inguinal Canal.—Rise of intra-abdominal pressure (e.g. during defaecation, micturition, coughing, or even ordinary muscular effort) is associated with a diminution of the intra-abdominal space and there is a natural tendency for the abdominal organs to be protruded out through areas of weakness in the abdominal wall. The inguinal canal is one such weak area and an indirect inguinal hernia (the commonest of all forms of herniae) comes out through it. However, the canal possesses different defensive mechanisms, of considerable efficiency, to prevent such protrusion:

1. The canal is oblique and, therefore, to a great extent, valvular. When the intra-abdominal pressure rises, the posterior wall of the canal is pushed forwards into apposition with the anterior wall.
2. Opposite the area of greatest weakness in the posterior wall (i.e. the deep ring), is placed the strongest part of the anterior wall (where it is reinforced by the fibres of internal oblique). Similarly, at the site where the anterior wall is weakest (i.e. the superficial ring), is placed the strongest part of the posterior wall (where it is reinforced by the conjoint tendon).
3. When the intra-abdominal pressure rises, the arched fibres of the internal oblique and transversus, which form the roof of the canal, contract and straighten, so that the muscles are drawn down like a shutter, along the posterior wall of the canal, towards its floor.
4. With rise in intra-abdominal pressure, the cremasteric muscle fibres contract (because they are divided from the internal oblique) and draw the spermatic cord up into the canal, to act as a kind of plug. Simultaneously, the contracting transversus pulls the deep ring upwards and laterally, behind the muscle mass.

Hesselbach's Triangle.—This is another weak spot on the anterior abdominal wall and it is through this weak spot that a direct inguinal hernia protrudes.

The triangle is bounded medially by the lateral border of the rectus muscle, laterally by the inferior epigastric vessels, and below by the medial part of the inguinal ligament.

Classifications of Inguinal Herniae.—The two cardinal features of an uncomplicated hernia are—(i) expansile impulse on straining (e.g. coughing), and (ii) reducibility. There are different ways of classifying the inguinal herniae. These are described below in details.

A. *According to the Extent:*

1. INCOMPLETE.—Where the hernia has not at all entered the scrotum, i.e. it has not passed through the neck of the scrotum. According to some, there is a ring at the neck of the scrotum, comparable to the superficial and deep inguinal rings, and called the *third inguinal ring.* A hernia is said to be incomplete when it has not crossed this ring. The other name for an incomplete hernia is *bubonocele.*

2. COMPLETE.—Where the hernia has entered the scrotum, no matter how far down it has gone into the scrotum.

B. *According to the Site through which the Hernia comes out of the Abdomen:*

1. INDIRECT.—An indirect (i.e. oblique) inguinal hernia comes out through the deep ring and traverses the inguinal canal. The sac, i.e. the peritoneal tube, through which the abdominal contents protrude, accompanies the spermatic cord. It has, therefore, all the coverings that the spermatic cord possesses. According to many people, an indirect hernia, at whatever age it may appear, occurs into a preformed sac and this sac is a partially or completely patent processus vaginalis. Depending on the extent of this patency, indirect hernia may be of three types:

   a. Bubonocele.—The hernia does not reach the scrotum and is limited to the inguinal canal, the processus vaginalis having been obliterated at the superficial ring.

   b. Funicular.—The hernia extends only up to the top of the testis, inside the scrotum. This is because the processus vaginalis has remained patent as far as the top of the testis, being shut off from the tunica vaginalis. The testis can be felt separately below the hernia.

   c. Vaginal.—This occurs when the whole length of the processus vaginalis remains patent and the hernia descends down to the bottom of the scrotum, passing in front of the testis. The testis cannot be felt separately from the hernia.

2. DIRECT.—A direct hernia comes out through the Hesselbach's triangle, along a spot of weakness or defect in the fascia transversalis here. It passes forwards, either below the arch of the conjoint tendon or through a weak area in this tendon, and thereafter emerges through the superficial inguinal ring. It is only rarely complete, i.e. only rarely it descends down to the scrotum. It is always acquired.

The differences between an indirect and a direct inguinal hernia are many and may be enumerated as follows:

I. *Differences Found at Operation (i.e. Anatomical Differences)*

INDIRECT	DIRECT
1. The neck of the sac lies lateral to the inferior epigastric vessels.	1. The neck lies medial to these vessels.
2. The wall of the sac is intimately attached to the spermatic cord and requires skilful separation from it.	2. The wall of the sac is not attached to the cord.
3. The sac is pyriform in shape, with little or no fat on its wall.	3. The sac is often smaller than the hernial mass would indicate the protruding mass mainly consisting of extraperitoneal fat.
4. The neck of the sac is its narrowest	4. The neck of the sac is wide (this is why direct herniae only rarely strangulate).

II. *Clinical Differences*

INDIRECT	DIRECT
1. Occurs at any age.	1. Uncommon before the age of 40.
2. Much commoner in the males but not infrequent in the females.	2. Practically never occurs in the females.
3. Usually unilateral; about 30 per cent of the cases are bilateral. In the first decade of life it is commoner on the right side, evidently due to later descent of the right testis. After the second decade, almost equally frequent on both the sides.	3. Usually bilateral. Often the patient has a poor abdominal musculature, as shown by the presence of Malgaigne's bulges. The patient is either of flabby type or of asthenic build.
4. Frequently the hernia is complete and has a pyriform shape. If it is incomplete, it is oval in shape.	4. Usually the hernia is incomplete and has a spherical shape.
5. Usually it requires straining to bring the hernia down; once down, it generally requires a little manipulation to be reduced.	5. The hernia generally appears as soon as the patient stands and disappears immediately as he lies down.
6. The hernia descends obliquely downwards and medially, and similarly, reduces upwards and laterally.	6. The hernia appears as a direct forward bulge and reduces directly backwards.
7. Invagination Test.—On coughing, the impulse is felt on the tip of the examining finger.	7. The impulse is felt on the pulp of the finger.
8. Confirmatory Test.—After the hernia is reduced, pressure is applied over the deep ring (in order to occlude it), and the patient is asked to cough. The hernia fails to appear because its door has been occluded (*deep ring occlusion test*).	8. The hernia still appears because it has nothing to do with the deep ring.

C. *According to the Nature of the Sac:*

1. CONGENITAL.—Where the. sac is congenitally present (i.e. partly or completely unobliterated processus vaginalis).

2. ACQUIRED.—Where the sac is acquired.

All direct herniae are acquired. According to many, all indirect herniae are congenital. Though the sac is present from birth, the hernia may not appear until adult life. According to others, at least some of the indirect herniae are acquired.

The clinical difference between a congenital and an acquired hernia may sometimes be made by the history. A congenital hernia becomes complete within a short period of its appearance (because the sac is preformed), whereas an acquired hernia progresses only gradually (since it has to make its own sac).

D. *According to the Nature of the Contents of the Sac:*

1. ENTEROCELE.—The sac contains intestines.

2. OMENTOCELE.—The sac contains omentum.

3. ENTERO-OMENTOCELE.—The sac contains both intestine and omentum.

4. CYSTOCELE.—A part of the bladder is in the sac. This usually occurs in a direct hernia. The history is often typical—the hernia enlarges just before micturition and diminishes in size after micturition. Pressure on the hernia causes an urge for micturition, and micturition is greatly helped if pressure is applied on the hernia during the act.

Enterocele and omentocele are, however, the two common varieties. Clinical differentiation between the two may be made by the following points:

ENTEROCELE	OMENTOCELE
1. Inspection.—Peristalsis may be seen if the coverings are thin and the hernia is big.	1. Peristalsis not seen.
2. Palpation.—Cystic, elastic feel.	2. Feels doughy and knotty.
3. Percussion.—Resonant.	3. Dull.
4. Auscultation.—Intestinal sounds may be heard in case of a big hernia.	4. Intestinal sounds not heard.
5. Reduction: (a) Reduces with a distinct gurgle. (b) Reduction is, in general, easy—there may be some difficulty in the early part of reduction, but the later part is easily reduced.	5. (a) No gurgling is heard during reduction. (b) Reduction is, in general, difficult. Even if the early part is reduced easily, the later part is always difficult to be reduced. Sometimes the hernia cannot be reduced completely.

E. *According to Reducibility:*

1. REDUCIBLE.—The contents (but not the sac) can be returned back into the abdomen.

2. IRREDUCIBLE.—The contents cannot be returned back into the abdomen. There is, however, no acute manifestation, i.e. no obstruction or strangulation. Irreducibility may be due to many factors:

a. Omentocele is very often irreducible because fat has a natural tendency to adhere to the sac. Moreover, the omentum, lying for a long time inside the hernial sac, accumulates fat and becomes too bulky to be reduced through the neck.

b. Adhesion of intestinal loops to the sac or to each other.

c. Adhesion of one part of the sac to another part.

d. Accumulation of solid faecal mass (*incarceration*) in an enterocele. This is especially like to occur when the sac contains the colon and is found most commonly in long-standing irreducible hernia in elderly people, who are habitually constipated.

e. A massive hernia (*scrotal abdomen*), whose contents are habituated in keeping themselves inside the scrotum.

F. *According to the Presence or Absence of Complications.*—This again, may be considered in two ways:

1. According to presence of other pathology in the neighbourhood, e.g. hydrocele, funiculitis, epididymoorchitis, filarial scrotum, etc.

2. According to complications developing in the hernia, e.g. obstruction, strangulation, inflammation, incarceration, etc. (see below).

When complications are present, the hernia is termed 'complicated'. Otherwise, it is called 'uncomplicated'.

Special Varieties of Inguinal Hernia

1. SLIDING HERNIA (HERNIA-EN-GLISSADE).—This occurs as a result of slipping down of the posterior parietal peritoneum on the underlying cellular tissues. The posterior wall of the hernial sac is not formed by peritoneum but by the caecum on the right side, the sigmoid colon on the left side, or the bladder on either side. It may occur both with indirect and direct herniae. It should be clearly understood that if the caecum, sigmoid colon, or the bladder are wholly within a hernial sac, the hernia is not of the sliding type. Also, inside the sac of a sliding hernia, there may be the usual contents of a hernia (i.e. small gut or omentum).

2. INTERSTITIAL HERNIA.—In this type, the hernial sac lies in between the different layers of abdominal wall. This is most commonly encountered in association with an undescended testis. The hernia is usually incomplete. According to the precise plane where the sac lies, interstitial hernia may be of the following types:

a. *Intraparietal* or *preperitoneal.*—The sac lies between the peritoneum and the fascia transversalis.

b. *Interparietal.*—The sac lies between the internal oblique muscle and external oblique aponeurosis.

c. *Extraparietal.*—The sac lies between the external oblique aponeurosis and the skin, i.e. in the subcutaneous tissue.

3. SPECIAL TYPES OF OBSTRUCTED AND STRANGULATED HERNIAE:

a. Richter's hernia.

b. Maydl's hernia.

c. Littre's hernia.

These are described under strangulated hernia (*see* below).

Etiological Factors in Inguinal Hernia

1. Presence of a preformed sac, i.e. persistence of part or whole of the processus vaginalis. Many surgeons believe that this is obligatory for an inguinal hernia. Others believe that there are some cases where the sac is acquired.
2. Weakness in the fascia transversalis:
   a. ANATOMICAL.—The fascia transversalis, which is the musculoaponeurotic continuation of the transversus abdominis muscle, forms the posterior wall of the inguinal canal. It is a weakness of this fascia which is the primary disturbance in both the types of inguinal hernia—indirect and direct. In cases of indirect hernia its gap, i.e. the deep ring, is dilated. In cases of direct hernia its aponeurotic fibres are deficient or absent in the medial part of the posterior wall of the inguinal canal.
   b. PHYSIOLOGICAL.—It is now believed by many authorities that inguinal hernia (particularly direct hernia) may be related to a defective collagen synthesis by the fibroblasts that leads to weakening of the fascia transversalis (and the rectus sheath).

Operations for Inguinal Hernia.—Three types of operation may be done:

1. HERNIOTOMY.—In this operation the sac is ligated at its neck and is excised. No repair of the inguinal canal is undertaken. This is done in infants and children in whom the hernia is just a congenital abnormality (non-obliteration of the processus vaginalis), and the muscles have not been so stretched as to weaken the inguinal canal.
2. HERNIORRHAPHY.—This means ordinary repair of the inguinal canal after excision of the sac. After excising the sac, the inguinal canal is repaired by *apposing* the conjoint tendon to the inguinal ligament. While some surgeons still prefer the old method of repair by chromicised catgut, majority prefer non-absorbable materials, e.g. prolene, silk or thread. Usually the repair is done behind the spermatic crod *(Bassini's operation)*. Herniorrhaphy is done in adult patients, who possess good muscle tone and in whom the internal ring has not been unduly stretched by a big hernia.
3. HERNIOPLASTY.—This means re-inforced repair of the inguinal canal after excision of the sac. The conjoint tendon is *not apposed* to the inguinal ligament. Instead, the gap between the two is covered up by some material, which may be heterogenous or autogenous:
   a. Heterogenous materials that are non-absorbable. Prolene or stainless steel wire is often used. Patching up the weak inguinal canal with prolene mesh or stainless steel mesh is sometimes done.
   b. Autogenous materials, which mean the patient's own tissues. The commonly used materials are:
      i. A strip of fascia lata, taken from the lateral side of the thigh. This is obtained either by a long incision on the lateral side of the thigh or by small incisions, with the help of a fasciatome. The gap in the fascia lata need not be repaired.
      ii. The excised sac, made into strips.

iii. A strip of the external oblique aponeurosis.

iv. A flap of anterior rectus sheath (which is turned down to cover up the inguinal canal).

v. An oval skin flap, which is transplanted to cover up the inguinal canal. The margins of the skin flap are tensely sutured to the margins of the canal (*dermatoplasty*). Instead of making an ordinary skin incision, for the operation, an elliptical incision is made and the skin, included within the ellipse, is taken for transplant.

vi. Skin, similarly obtained, made into a strip (as with fascia lata), i.e. *ribbon-skin* repair.

When fascia lata or the excised sac or external oblique aponeurosis are used for repair, a Gallie's needle is used. This is a wide cutting needle with a big eye. The strip is threaded on the eye and is fixed to it with a catgut or silk stitch. At each end of the strip, a piece of silk or catgut is anchored and these are used for the purpose of applying the terminal knots, thus preventing wastage of the living material. While the sutures are applied, no tension, whatsoever, is applied on them. They are simply put around the tissues loosely, as in '*darning*'.

Repair with prolene or stainless steel wire is also made by darning, i.e. the conjoint tendon and the inguinal ligament are not apposed to each other.

The *indications* for hernioplasty are:

a. All cases of direct hernia.

b. Cases of indirect hernia in patients with poor muscle tone or patients in whom the internal ring has been unduly stretched by a big hernia or when the conjoint tendon and the inguinal ligament cannot be apposed to each other without tension.

c. All cases of recurrent hernia.

d. Patients who have to continue in occupation requiring considerable physical strain.

Orchidectomy in the Operation for Inguinal Hernia.—As long as the spermatic cord has to be brought out through the deep ring, no repair of the inguinal canal is fullproof. Hence, orchidectomy should be thought of while repairing herniae in elderly patients, in patients with recurrent hernia, direct hernia or very big hernia, or in patients with very weak abdominal musculature.

Steps of Operation (Herniorrhaphy).—The incision is made on the inguinal canal, i.e. half an inch above and parallel to the medial part of the inguinal ligament, from the deep to the superficial inguinal ring. The subcutaneous tissue is cut. Here, it is made of two layers, in between which run the superficial epigastric and superficial external pudendal vessels, which are cut and ligated. The external oblique aponeurosis is cut in the same line, up to the superficial inguinal ring, and thus the inguinal canal is opened.

The cremastric muscle and fascia, which wrap up the structures of the cord and the sac, are split up in order to expose these structures.

The sac, which is a white glistening structure, has now to be dissected from the cord. This is done by starting from the fundus and proceeding towards the neck. The neck of the sac, which marks its junction with the peritoneum, is identified by the following points:

1. It is the most constricted part of the sac.
2. There is a ring of extraperitoneal fatty tissue around its outer aspect.
3. The deep epigastric vessels lie in its close relation. The vessels are medial to the sac if the hernia is indirect and lateral to it if the hernia is direct.

The contents of the sac are reduced and the sac is ligated at its neck by transfixion. The sac is then excised.

Before proceeding for repair of the inguinal canal, the most important step is to repair the stretched deep inguinal ring (*Lytle's method*). This is done by applying a few stitches of non-absorbable material, in order to plicate the fascia transversalis, in which the deep ring is located. The most lateral of these stitches displaces the spermatic cord laterally, as much as possible, and narrows the deep ring to the size of even less than the tip of the little finger.

Some surgeons stress upon repairing the weakness in the fascia transversalis (*Shouldice operation*). The fascia transversalis is dissected and displayed along the whole length of the inguinal canal. It is then divided obliquely so as to make two flaps and these two flaps are sutured to each other by double-breasting. The lower lateral flap is sutured to the undersurface of the upper medial flap and then the upper medial flap is sutured over the lower lateral flap.

The commonest form of repair of the inguinal canal is, as advocated by Bassini, behind the cord. In an ordinary repair, usually 3 to 5 interrupted stitches are applied between the conjoint tendon and the inguinal ligament. The most medial suture should include the periosteum of the pubic tubercle. While applying the middle suture, the bite on the inguinal ligament should be superficial so that the femoral vein, which lies very superficial in this situation, is not punctured. The most lateral suture should be so placed that there is neither an undue pressure on the emerging spermatic cord nor is a big gap left behind. It must be seen that approximation of the conjoint tendon and the inguinal ligament is without tension. This is possible only when the gap between the two is narrow. Where the gap is wide, a release incision has to be made on the anterior rectus sheath, so that the conjoint tendon can be drawn down and the sutures are without tension (*Tanner's sliding method*).

The external oblique aponeurosis is sutured in front of the cord, keeping open the most medial part. This is the new superficial ring, through which the cord emerges. The skin wound is closed.

Recurrence of Hernia.—About 10 per cent of inguinal herniae recur after operation. Recurrence is commoner after operations for direct hernia. However, most recurrent inguinal herniae are of the indirect variety. The causes of recurrence may be enumerated as follows:

A. FAULTS WITH THE PATIENTS:
1. Patients with very weak musculature, e.g. with presence of Malgaigne's bulge.
2. Patients with a factor of chronic straining, persisting even after the operation, e.g. chronic cough, chronic constipation, chronic straining at micturition.
3. Lifting heavy weights in early post-operative days.

B. FAULTS WITH THE HERNIA:
1. Direct herniae.
2. Very large and long-standing herniae.
3. Sliding herniae.

4. Prolonged use of truss (the musculature is weakened and is replaced by fibrous tissue).

C. FAULTS WITH THE OPERATION:
1. Failure to ligate the sac at the neck proper.
2. Failure to make the deep ring narrow by plication of the fascia transversalis.
3. Approximation of the conjoint tendon and the inguinal ligament under tension, so that the intervening muscle tissue is devitalised.
4. Use of absorbable sutures for the repair of the canal.
5. Faulty selection of operation, e.g. herniotomy in cases requiring herniorrhaphy, and herniorrhaphy in cases deserving hernioplasty.
6. Imperfect haemostasis, predisposing to infection.

D. POST-OPERATIVE COMPLICATIONS:
1. Infection of the wound. This is possibly the commonest cause of recurrence.
2. Factors causing stretching of the repair; e.g. post-operative cough, post-opertive abdominal distension, etc.

E. OCCURRENCE OF A NEW HERNIA:
A patient, who has been operated satisfactorily for an indirect hernia, may develop a direct hernia, which has nothing to do with the earlier operation.

All recurrent cases should be treated by hernioplasty and, particularly in the elderly people, with an orchiectomy added.

Complications of Hernia

1. IRREDUCIBILITY.—The contents cannot be returned back into the abdomen. There is, however, no acute manifestation. This has already been described in details.

2. OBSTRUCTION.—This denotes an acute irreducibility of a hernia, due to a constricting agent, somewhere along the course of the sac. The hernia suddenly becomes irreducible and is associated with other acute features, e.g.
   a. In an enterocele.—There is acute pain as well as acute intestinal obstruction because the lumen of the bowel is occluded by the constricting agent.
   b. In an omentocele.—There is acute pain.

3. STRANGULATION.—This is a more dangerous condition than obstruction. Here the constricting band not only causes acute irreducibility of the hernia but also interferes with the blood supply of the contents of the hernial sac, so that:
   a. In an enterocele.—There is acute pain, acute irreducibility, intestinal obstruction, and arrest of circulation in the gut.
   b. In an omentocele.—There is acute pain, acute irreducibility, and arrest of circulation in the omentum.

4. INCARCERATION.—This means accumulation of solid faecal mass in an enterocele. This is especially likely to occur if the hernia contains colon, and is found most commonly in long-standing irreducible herniae, in elderly people, who are habitually constipated.

5. INFLAMMATION.—A hernia may be inflamed in two ways:
   a. External Causes.—Pressure by an ill-fitting truss.
   b. Internal Causes.—Inflammation of the contents within the sac, e.g. acute appendicitis, acute salpingitis. The hernia becomes acutely tender but not tense (c.f. strangulation).

Certain Special Types of Strangulated Hernia

1. *Richter's Hernia.*—Only a part of the circumference of the bowel is caught in the constriction ring. This is commoner with strangulated femoral hernia. Since some part of the lumen of the gut is still open, absolute constipation may not occur during early stages.

2. *Maydl's Hernia* (retrograde strangulation).—This occurs when successive loops of the bowel pass down into the sac, come back into the abdomen, re-enter the sac, and again come up to the abdomen, thus forming a 'W'. Though the gut at all the angles of the 'W' may be strangulated, the strangulation is always more advanced in the upper angle loop, i.e. the gut inside the abdomen.

3. *Littre's Hernia.*—This is a hernia where Meckel's diverticulum is a content of the sac.

Clinical Features of Obstructed or Strangulated Hernia.—No attempt should be made to discriminate clinically between an obstructed and a strangulated hernia, and all cases should be taken as strangulated and treated as such. In general, it may be said that a case is likely to be strangulated if the history of obstruction is long and the patient is more toxic.

The clinical features of an obstructed or strangulated hernia are as follows:

1. Sudden acute pain:
   a. Over the hernia.
   b. Generalised abdominal pain, paroxysmal in character, and often located mainly at the umbilicus.
2. Sudden irreducibility of the hernia, which becomes quickly enlarged in size.
3. Vomiting and absolute constipation. These are constant features of an obstructed enterocele but may be absent in cases of omentocele or Richter's hernia.
4. The hernia is tense and extremely tender, and there is no expansile impulse on coughing and no reducibility.
5. Varying degree of toxaemia, more prominent if strangulation, has supervened.

Management of Obstructed or Strangulated Hernia.—As soon as the patient is received, arrangements should be made for immediate operation. By the time things get ready, the following measures are taken:

1. Rest, with the foot end of the bed raised (to aid reduction by gravity).
2. Local ice application to reduce congestion and oedema of the tissues; this helps spontaneous reduction.
3. A Ryle's tube is inserted, gastric suction instituted, and oral feeding stopped.
4. IV fluid transfusion started.
5. Antibiotics injected.
6. Gentle manipulations may be done to achieve reduction, with the hip flexed and internally rotated. This manoeuvre is known as *taxis*. This should, however, be done only by an expert and with utmost care since, otherwise, complications, as follows, may occur:
   a. Injury to the contents of the sac, particularly intestines, which are often friable.
   b. *Reduction-en-masse*, which means that the whole of the hernial sac, with its contents *still obstructed*, is pushed inside the abdomen by force.

c. Rupture of the hernial sac, with exit of the contents into the extra-peritoneal tissues.

Many surgeons, therefore, avoid taxis and advise operation straightway.

OPERATION FOR STRANGULATED HERNIA.—The operation may be done either under local or under general anaesthesia. The preliminary steps are the same as for an ordinary hernia. When the sac and the constriction band have been exposed, the sac should be opened up before the constriction band is cut. The dangers of cutting the constriction band, before the sac is opened, are:

a. The contents of the sac may slip inside the abdomen before they can be examined, and thus a loop of gangrenous gut or a piece of devitalised omentum may escape notice.

b. The fluid inside the sac, which is rich in toxins and sometimes bacteria, is allowed to flow inside the peritoneal cavity, from where quick absorption occurs.

The constriction band has now to be cut. For this purpose, a hernia director and a hernia bistoury may be used conveniently. In case of an inguinal hernia, this band is, in order of frequency, located:

a. At the superficial inguinal ring.
b. Midway between the superficial and the deep rings.
c. At the deep ring.
d. Anywhere along the sac.

At or near the deep ring, the deep epigastric vessels are in the danger of being damaged while the constriction band is cut. Hence, in this situation, the band should be incised parallel to the vessels, i.e. upwards and medially.

The contents of the sac should be carefully examined. The obstructed omentum, even if it is viable, should be excised since it has a notorious tendency to cause intra-abdominal adhesions. For gut, a viable loop from a non-viable one is differentiated by the following points:

VIABLE	NON-VIABLE
1. Red to reddish-blue in colour.	1. Greenish or blackish in colour.
2. Presence of pulsation in the mesentery.	2. Pulsation absent.
3. Presence of peristalsis in the loop.	3. Peristalsis absent.
4. The fluid in the sac is not offensive-smelling.	4. Foul-smelling fluid, usually red in colour.

In doubtful cases, hot towels should be applied to the loop of the gut *for at least ten minutes* to see if signs of viability set in.

If the loop of gut is viable, it is returned to the abdomen. The sac is ligated at the neck and excised. Repair of the deep ring and the inguinal canal is also done unless the patient's condition is very serious. No form of hernioplasty, however, should be attempted.

If the loop of gut is non-viable, a resection and anastomosis has to be performed. In some cases immediate resection cannot be undertaken due to poor general condition. In these cases the devitalised loop of gut is kept exteriorised on the skin surface for the time being. If this is done, absorption of toxins and bacteria, as it occurs from the serous surface, cannot occur. The indications for exteriorisation are:

1. Non-viable large gut which can later be resected by the Paul-Mikulicz technique.
2. Non-viable small gut in patients whose general condition is too low to allow immediate resection. When the patient's general condition improves with resuscitation measures after exteriorisation, the resection is undertaken at a second operation.

FEMORAL HERNIA

Surgical Anatomy.—In a femoral hernia the peritoneal sac passes through the femoral ring into the femoral canal. The femoral canal extends from the femoral ring above, to the saphenous opening below (fossa ovalis). The sac comes out of the saphenous opening into the subcutaneous tissue of the groin.

FEMORAL RING.—The boundaries of the ring are:

Anteriorly.—Inguinal ligament.
Posteriorly:

a. Fascia over the pectineus muscle.
b. (Pectineal) ligament of Cooper, which is a thickened band, running along the pectineal line of the pubis, incorporated in its periosteum.

Medially.—Concave sharp edge of the Gimbernat's (lacunar) ligament.
Laterally.—A thin septum which separates the ring from the femoral vein.

In operations for femoral hernia, the surgeon's aim is to close the mouth of the femoral canal, i.e. the femoral ring. This is done by apposing its posterior and anterior walls, i.e. the Cooper's ligament and the inguinal ligament (or the attached conjoint tendon).

FEMORAL CANAL.—This is the most medial of the three compartments of the femoral sheath (the intermediate contains the femoral vein and the lateral contains the femoral artery). The femoral sheath is a sleeve-like prolongation of the fascial lining of the abdomen, which invests the femoral vessels, to come down to the thigh. It is formed by two fascial layers. The anterior layer is the prolongation of the fascia transversalis (behind the inguinal ligament), in front of the femoral vessels. The posterior layer is the prolongation of the fascia iliac, behind the femoral vessels. Posteriorly, the femoral sheath, as a whole, rests on the pectineus medially and the psoas laterally. Thus, the femoral canal is posteriorly related to the pectineus.

The femoral canal is funnel shaped (with the wider mouth downwards) and is 2 cm long. Its upper opening is the femoral ring and the lower opening is the fossa ovalis (saphenous opening of the deep fascia). The canal is directed downwards and forwards. It contains fat, lymph vessels, and a deep inguinal node, known as the *Cloquet's node.*

The canal is closed above, at the femoral ring, by the *septum femorale,* which is a condensation of extraperitoneal fat, pierced by lymphatics. Below also, the canal is closed; this is done by the *cribriform fascia,* which fills the fossa ovalis (*see* below).

FOSSA OVALIS.—The fossa ovalis or saphenous opening is an oval opening in the deep fascia (fascia lata) of the thigh. It makes the lower end of the femoral canal. The upper margin of the opening is firm and unyielding. To its lower margin the superficial fascia of the thigh is attached. The opening is traversed by the long saphenous vein and by lymphatics which run from the superficial to the deep inguinal nodes. It is covered by loose areolar tissue, which is termed *cribriform fascia.*

FURTHER COURSE OF A FEMORAL HERNIA.—On coming out of the saphenous opening, the hernial sac lies in the loose areolar subcutaneous tissue of the groin. While it is inside the inelastic femoral canal, the hernia is narrow. Once, however, it escapes into the subcutaneous tissue, it expands, often considerably. Here it tends to progress *upwards,* often reaching at above the inguinal ligament. The tendency for the hernia to turn upwards (after its escape through the fossa ovalis) is attributed to various factors:

1. Firm attachment of the superficial fascia to the lower margin of the fossa ovalis, preventing further downward passage of the hernia.
2. Firm unyielding nature of the upper margin of the fossa ovalis, twisting the hernia upwards.
3. Forward curvature of the femoral canal.
4. Repeated flexion of the thigh.

COVERINGS OF THE SAC.—From inside outwards, the coverings are:

1. Fat and lymphatics, derived from the femoral septum.
2. Fascia transversalis, derived from the anterior wall of the canal.
3. Cribriform fascia.

Clinical Features

1. The hernia is commoner in females, in the ratio of 2:1.
2. Multiparous women are the usual sufferers.
3. The right side is more commonly affected (2:1).
4. The symptoms are less pronounced than those of inguinal hernia:
   a. Pain.—It is only occasional and is caused by adherence of greater omentum.
   b. Swelling.—This is the usual presenting feature. A femoral hernia may be differentiated from an inguinal hernia by the following points:
      i. While an inguinal hernia lies medial to the pubic spine and above the inguinal ligament, a femoral hernia lies lateral to the pubic spine and below the inguinal ligament (in the later stage, however, it may extend above the ligament).
      ii. The inguinal canal is found to be empty by the invagination test.
      iii. After reduction, when pressure is applied over the femoral canal and the patient is made to stand and cough, the hernia does not come down.
5. Strangulation is a common feature with femoral hernia because of the narrow unyielding femoral ring; also, gangrene of the strangulated loop is rapid. Richter's hernia is commonest with femoral herniae.
6. A femoral hernia can never be controlled by a truss, which tends to become displaced when the thigh is flexed.

Operations.—The hernia may be approached in three ways:

1. From above the inguinal ligament (Lotheissen's operation).

2. From below the inguinal ligament (Lockwood's operation).
3. From both above and below the inguinal ligament (McEvedy's operation).

LOTHEISSEN'S OPERATION.—The incision and the primary steps of the operation are the same as for an inguinal hernia. On exposure of the inguinal canal, the conjoint tendon is retracted upwards. The fascia transversalis is incised, in the line of skin incision, medial to the inferior epigastric vessels. The peritoneum is now seen, together with the sac, which enters through the femoral ring into the femoral canal. Sometimes the bladder is adherent to the sac and care must be taken to make it free. The sac is carefully drawn out from inside the femoral canal. If there is any content, it is reduced. The sac is transfixed at its neck (the most constricted part) and is excised.

The surgeon usually aims at obliterating the femoral ring, in order to avoid a recurrence. This is done by apposing the posterior wall (i.e. the Cooper's ligament) to the anterior wall (i.e. the inguinal ligament or the attached conjoint tendon) with two or three interrupted stitches of unabsorbable material. While doing this, care is taken not to injure or constrict the external iliac vein.

The advantages of this approach is that it allows the sac to be ligated just at its neck and also gives direct approach to the femoral ring (to perform its closure). Its disadvantage is that it involves a wide exposure and, therefore, weaken the inguinal canal.

LOCKWOOD'S OPERATION.—The incision is made 1 cm below and parallel to the medial part of the inguinal ligament. The sac, wrapped with its usual coverings, is found coming out through the saphenous opening. It is dissected out, any content reduced into the abdomen, and is ligated as high as possible. Thereafter, the sac is excised and the stump is allowed to retract through the femoral canal.

As the femoral ring cannot be reached through this approach, repair is done with a view to merely obliterate the space occupied by the hernia. This is done by two or three stitches, picking up the fasciae making the floor and the lateral margin of the saphenous opening.

McEVEDY'S OPERATION.—The incision is a vertical one, over the femoral rarely, and extended upwards above the inguinal ligament. The lower part of the sac is dissected out through the lower part of the incision. The anterior rectus sheath is incised vertically in its lowest part, a little medial to its lateral border. The rectus muscle is retracted medially. The extraperitoneal space is thus reached and here the upper part of the sac, entering through the femoral canal, is seen. The neck of the sac is transfixed and the sac is excised. Repair of the femoral ring is done as in Lotheissen's operation.

This operation is particularly advantageous in cases of strangulated femoral hernia as it gives ample room to cut the constricting band under direct vision and to perform intestinal resection, if required.

Strangulated Femoral Hernia.—As has already been stated, femoral herniae are very susceptible to strangulation because of the unyielding margins of the femoral ring. For the same reason, again, gangrene of the strangulated loop occurs rather rapidly.

Operation should, therefore, be undertaken forthwith. Since the obstruction is usually at the femoral ring, exposure of the ring is essential. For this purpose, either a Lotheissen's or a McEvedy's approach is required. On reaching the sac, it is opened. The fluid inside is sucked out and the gut carefully examined before it can slip back into the abdomen (Richter's hernia is fairly common). The constricting band has now to be cut and it is usually the sharp medial margin of the femoral ring, i.e. the Gimbernat's ligament. The margin of the ligament is cut through, in order to release the obstruction. In doing this, care has to be taken not to injure an abnormal obturator artery, which lies in this situation in about 30 per cent of subjects.

UMBILICAL HERNIA

Types.—There are two distinct types:
  I. Umbilical hernia of infants and children.
  II. Para-umbilical hernia of adults.

Umbilical Hernia of Infants and Children.—This is a true umbilical hernia, resulting from protrusion of a peritoneal sac through the organising umbilical scar, which has possibly been weakened as a result of neonatal sepsis.

TREATMENT

1. *Conservative.*—There is a tendency for spontaneous cure of the hernia (in about 90 per cent of cases it disappears during the first few months of life). Also obstruction or strangulation is extremely rare. Thus, in all the cases, treatment should be conservative, to start with. No treatment, except reassurance to the mother, is necessary. Many surgeons advocate narrowing of the opening by pulling the skin and abdominal musculature together, from the two sides, with adhesive plaster, placed as a cross, across the umbilicus. Some surgeons use the old method of putting a big coin or round piece of metal on the umbilicus, kept in position with the help of adhesive plaster; this acts as a truss, preventing the contents from coming out, thus helping obliteration of the sac.
2. *Operative.*—Where the hernia fails to disappear after the age of 18 months, operation is advocated. An earlier operation is indicated where obstruction occurs (this is rare).

The umbilicus should be preserved to save the child being teased by his friends. A small curved incision is made just below the umbilicus and the skin cicatrix is dissected upwards. This exposes the lower margin of the neck of the sac, as it comes out through the gap in the linea alba. The neck is now cleared all round the opening. Being sure that the sac is empty of contents, it is transfixed at its neck and is excised. The gap in the linea alba is repaired with two or three stitches of unabsorbable material. The umbilical cicatrix is placed back in position and the skin margins are sutured.

Para-umbilical Hernia of Adults.—In the adults, a hernia usually does not occur through the umbilical cicatrix, so it is not a true umbilical hernia. It occurs through a weak spot in the linea alba, either above (supra-umbilical) or below (infra-umbilical) the actual umbilicus; hence it is called para-umbilical. The patient is often obese, commonly a female; obesity and child-bearing are contributory factors. The hernia often becomes large in size, though its neck is usually remarkably narrow. Para-umbilical herniae are commonly irreducible. They are very prone to obstruction and strangulation because of several reasons:

1. The neck is considerably narrow, as compared to the size of the sac and the volume of its contents.
2. The contents (usually omentum, together with parts of large and small intestines) tend to become adherent to the sac and to each other.
3. The sac is very often multilocular.

TREATMENT.—The hernia, even when reducible, cannot be controlled by a belt, and operation is almost always necessary. Unless there is urgency, preliminary attempts should be made to reduce obesity. Mayo's operation is the most commonly practised procedure.

Mayo's Operation.—In this operation, after the hernial sac has been dealt with, the defect in the linea alba is repaired by overlapping the parietal tissues across a transverse axis (double-bracing). The umbilicus cannot be preserved.

A transverse elliptical incision is made, encircling the umbilicus, the size of the ellipse depending on the size of the hernial protruberance. The subcutaneous fat is dissected, till the rectus sheath is reached, and tracing it, the gap in the linea alba, through which the sac comes out, is dissected all round. The sac is now opened at its neck (because this area is usually free from adhesions). Loops of intestines, if present, are returned into the abdomen, while any adherent omentum is resected. The sac is cut all round, along its neck, and is excised, together with the adherent skin, umbilicus and fat.

No attempt is usually made to separate the peritoneal margins from the margins of the gap in the linea alba or to suture the peritoneum as a separate layer (some surgeons, however, prefer to suture the peritoneal margins separately). The opening is enlarged laterally by making a transverse incision on each side. This is required for a good overlapping across the transverse axis, and the size of the these incisions, therefore, depends on the size of the gap. The sutures, used for the overlapping, should be of non-absorbable material (nylon or silk). The first stage of overlapping is a series of three or five mattress sutures (of which one is in the midline). The sutures are so passed through the upper and the lower flaps that on tightening them, the lower flap will pass behind the upper flap for about 4 cm. In doing this, bites in the upper flap are taken about 4 cm off its margin, while those in the lower flap are taken just at its margin. The second stage of overlapping is done by suturing the free margin of the upper (now superficial) flap to the surface of the lower flap, as low down as possible. Thus, at the site of the detect, there are four layers of tissue now, i.e. two layers of peritoneum and two layers of sheath. The skin wound is closed.

EXOMPHALOS

This is a rare condition, found at birth, and is due to failure of a part or whole of the midgut to return to the coelomic cavity in the foetal life. Depending on the size, exomphalos may be of two types:
1. *Exomphalos Minor.*—The sac is small and the umbilical cord is attached to its fundus.
2. *Exomphalos Major.*—The sac is big and the umbilical cord is attached to its inferior surface.

In either case, the sac is thin and translucent, through which the contents can be seen. The sac consists of three layers. These are, from inside outwards, the peritoneum, the Wharton's jelly, and the aminotic membrane.

EPIGASTRIC HERNIA

Anatomy.—This term is applied to a hernia that occurs in the midline, through one of the diamond-shaped fissures commonly found between the interlacing fibres of the linea alba in the midline, above the umbilicus. In many of the cases (and in all the cases to start with), the hernia is just a small protrusion of the extra-peritoneal fat. Thus, it is often called *fatty hernia of the linea alba* . In some cases, however, the protruding fat may draw the peritoneum behind it as a hernial sac (and now it is a true epigastric hernia). The neck of such a sac is usually narrow and allows, if at all, only the omentum to enter it. Often the omentum gets attached to the sac.

Clinical Features.—There may be three groups of patients:

1. SYMPTOMLESS SWELLING.—The swelling is located in the midline, between the xiphoid process and umbilicus. Sometimes there may be more than one swellings. As compared to other herniae, the swelling often fails to show expansile impulse on straining and reducibility, and may be wrongly diagnosed as a lipoma. When, however, a sac is present, expansile impulse and reducibility are noticed.

2. PAINFUL SWELLING.—Sometimes the swelling is associated with local pain and tenderness. This occurs when the neck is pressed by the margins of the gap in the linea alba, causing partial strangulation.

3. REFLEX DYSPEPSIA.—Many of the patients present with features typical of duodenal ulcer, though actually there is no ulcer. In these cases the patient may or may not have noticed the swelling. It is equally important to remember that epigastric hernia and peptic ulcer may co-exist, and in all the cases, presenting with features suggestive of ulcer, the presence of an ulcer should be excluded before or during operation.

Treatment.—A long midline vertical or transverse incision should be made over the swelling. The incision should be gracious so that a good length of the linea alba can be viewed and presence of any other gap in it can be detected (often there are more than one gap). When the hernia is seen, one of the following procedures is adopted:

1. If there is just a protrusion of extra peritoneal fat, it is ligated at its pedicle and excised. The gap in the linea alba is repaired by non-absorbable sutures.
2. If there is a small hernial sac attached, the extra-peritoneal fat, together with the sac, is excised and the peritoneal opening closed. The defect in the linea alba is repaired as above.
3. If there is a big hernial sac, a Mayo's operation (overlapping) is done, as for para-umbilical hernia.

DIVARICATION OF RECTI

This is a condition usually found in elderly multiparous women. There is a wide gap between the two rectus abdominis muscles, through which the abdominal contents bulge on straining. As there is no symptom and no danger of obstruction, no active treatment is necessary. An abdominal corset is all that is required.

INCISIONAL HERNIA

An incisional hernia occurs through the weak scar of an operation (or accidental wound). It is important to note that the pathology starts during the immediate or very early postoperative period. If the main nerves, supplying the abdominal musculature, are intact, a soundly healed scar can never be the site of a hernia, whatever strain it might have to withstand.

Causes

1. OPERATIVE:
   a. Careless suturing during closure of the wound.
   b. Interference with motor nerves (injury at operation).
   c. Use of wide-bore drainage tubes.
2. POST-OPERATIVE:
   a. Infection.—This is the commonest cause. There is separation of the divided muscles and replacement of dead muscles by fibrous tissue.
   b. Post-operative Strain.—Cough, distension, etc.

Site.—A lower abdominal scar is much more commonly affected than an upper abdominal. This is because of two factors:

a. The lower abdominal parietes is anatomically weak because of the absence of the posterior rectus sheath.
b. The intra-abdominal pressure has to be borne to the maximum by the lower abdominal wall, in the erect posture (this is one of the prices that man has to pay for his erect posture, as compared to the quadrupeds).

Types.—There are two distinct types of incisional hernia:

1. The first type occurs in the midline, either in the lower or in the upper abdomen. The defect in the musculature is wide but the margins of the defect are smooth, regular, and well-defined. The hernia is reduced spontaneously as the patient lies down. Such a hernia has no real danger of strangulation and can well be controlled by an abdominal corset.
2. The second type usually occurs in the lateral part of the abdomen. The gap in the muscle is narrow but is irregular and ill-defined. The sac is usually loculated, and the contents are often adherent to it and to each other. Such a hernia carries a high risk of strangulation. An abdominal belt is not only ineffective but also dangerous in that it may aggravate the risk of strangulation.

Treatment

A. CONSERVATIVE.—In the first type of hernia, a well-fitting abdominal corset is advised.
B. OPERATIVE.—In the second type of hernia, early operation is advocated. Operation is also indicated in the first type of hernia if it cannot be effectively controlled by a corset and the patient has symptoms. Different operations have been

advocated. Some of the commonly practised procedures are mentioned below:

1. *Anatomical Restoration.*—The scar is excised. The anatomical layers are defined and mobilised. They are again sutured in layers, as is done in primary closure of an abdominal incision. The repair is preferably done with non-absorbable sutures.

2. *Mayo's Operation.*—For a midline hernia with wide gap, provided the hernia is not very close to the pubis, this operation is preferred.

3. *Keel Operation.*—In this operation *the hernial sac is not opened.* After the sac is freed from the superficial tissues, it is pushed back into the abdomen by pleating it with unabsorbable sutures, care being taken not to take bite of the underlying bowel. Subsequently a second, third or fourth layer of sutures are inserted, till the healthy margins of the aponeurosis are brought close together. The margins of the aponeurosis are then sutured to each other. This repair, when viewed in a cross-section, looks like the keel of a ship; hence the operation is so named.

4. *Approximation of Rectus Sheaths.*—This is especially suitable for midline sub-umbilical herniae. The peritoneum is sutured after excision of the sac. The anterior rectus sheath is freed from the underlying rectus muscle on each side. The sheaths from the two sides are then sutured together in the midline, preferably by overlapping.

5. *Hernioplasty* with fascial sutures or with mesh (nylon, prolene or plastic), as done for inguinal hernia.

RARE EXTERNAL HERNIA

1. INTERSTITIAL HERNIA (see under inguinal hernia).

2. SPLIGELLAN HERNIA.—This is actually an interstitial hernia. The hernia escapes through the linea semilunaris (i.e. the lower end of the posterior rectus sheath.

3. LUMBAR HERNIA:
   a. *Lower Lumbar Hernia.*—Majority of lumbar herniae belong to this group. The hernia comes out through the inferior lumbar triangle of Petit, bounded below by the crest of the ilium, anteriorly by the posterior border of external oblique, and posteriorly by the anterior border of the latissimus dorsi.
   b. *Upper Lumbar Hernia.*—Rarely a lumbar hernia may belong to this group. The hernia comes out through the upper lumbar triangle, bounded above by the twelfth rib, medially by the sacrospinalis, and laterally by the posterior border of the internal oblique.
   c. *Incisional Lumbar Hernia.*—This occurs through a lumbar scar, e.g. after kidney operations.

4. OBTURATOR HERNIA.—This occurs in elderly females who have lost much fat. The hernia passes out of the pelvis, through the obturator canal, alongside the obturator vessels and nerve.

5. GLUTEAL HERNIA.—This occurs through the greater sciatic foramen and may be:
   a. Above the pyriformis.
   b. Below the pyriformis.

6. SCIATIC HERNIA.—This occurs through the lesser sciatic foramen.

7. PERINEAL HERNIA.—The hernia occurs through the pelvic floor. It is rather common in dogs. In human beings it may occur only after excision of the rectum.

8. PUDENDAL HERNIA.—This is a hernia into the labium major.

9. ISCHIORECTAL HERNIA.—A hernia into the ischiorectal fossa.

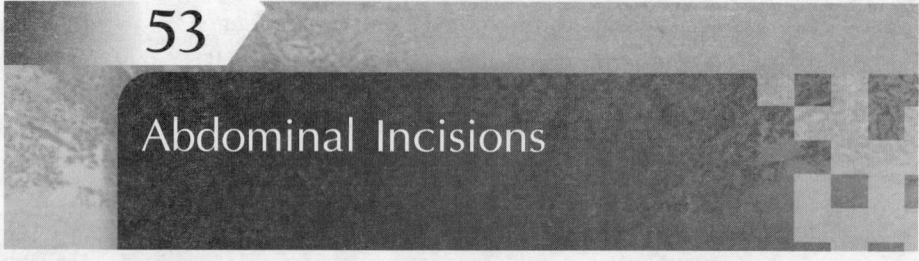

53

Abdominal Incisions

Classification

I. VERTICAL INCISIONS:

  A. Midline: 1. Upper (supra-umbilical).

                      2. Lower (infra-umbilical).

  B. Paramedian   1. Upper. Right or Left.

                      2. Lower. Right or Left.

II. TRANSVERSE INCISIONS:

  A. Upper (supra-umbilical).

  B. Lower (infra-umbilical).

III. OBLIQUE INCISIONS:

  A. Kocher s subcostal incision.

  B. Gridiron incision.

  C. Rutherford Morison s incision.

IV. OTHER INCISIONS:

  A. Mayo-Robson s incision.

  B. Lanz s incision.

  C. Battle s pararectal incision.

  D. Pfannenstiel s incision.

Midline Vertical Incisions

INDICATIONS:

A. Supra-umbilical Incision:

  1. Majority of operations on the stomach and duodenum, e.g. gastrojejunostomy with vagotomy, partial gastrectomy, etc.

  2. Upper abdominal emergencies.

B. Infra-umbilical Incision:

  For gynaecological operations.

OPENING:

1. Skin and subcutaneous tissue.

2. Linea alba.

3. Peritoneum (covered with the fascia transversalis).

CLOSURE

1. Peritoneum.

2. Linea alba.

3. Skin.

ADVANTAGES. The incision traverses the linea alba, which is more or less avascular, so that the abdomen can be quickly opened and closed. Also, it provides equal exposure of both the sides of the abdomen. This is why it is popular for upper abdominal emergencies.

DISADVANTAGE. There is no disadvantage with the supra-umbilical incision. An infra-umbilical incision, however, has the maximum possibility of developing a hernia because here the linea alba is thin as the posterior rectus sheath is absent.

Paramedian Incisions

INDICATIONS:

A. Right upper Paramedian Incision:
   1. Operations on gall bladder and common bile duct.
   2. Operations on the stomach and pylorus, e.g. enterectomy, partial gastrectomy, etc.
   3. Operations on the head of the pancreas.
B. Right Lower Paramedian Incision:
   1. Appendectomy.
   2. Operations on the terminal ileum and proximal colon, e.g. right hemicolectomy, ileo-transverse anastomosis.
C. Left Upper Paramedian Incision:
   1. Splenectomy.
   2. Gastrostomy.
D. Left Lower Paramedian Incision:
   1. Excision of the rectum.
   2. Operations on the distal colon.

In one word, the paramedian incisions are the most widely used ones for all general purposes, both in the upper and the lower abdomen.

OPENING:

1. The incision is made parallel to the midline, about one inch away from it. The skin and subcutaneous tissues are cut.
2. The anterior rectus sheath is cut along the line of the incision.
3. The rectus abdominis muscle can be dealt with in two ways:
   a. It is retracted laterally (it should not be retracted medially because this procedure severs the nerves to the muscle, which enter the muscle from its lateral side); this is the *rectos-retracting approach.*
   b. It is split vertically (along the length of its fibres), close to the medial border of the muscle; this is the *rectus-splitting approach.*
4. The posterior rectus sheath and the peritoneum (with the intervening fascia transversalis) are closely adherent to each other, and are cut as one layer.

CLOSURE:

   1. The peritoneum and posterior rectus sheath in one layer.
   2. Nothing need be done to the rectus muscle, even if it is split.
   3. The anterior rectus sheath.
   4. Skin.

ADVANTAGES:

1. It gives a wide exposure.
2. Incisional hernia practically never occurs, especially with upper para-median incisions and with rectus-retracting (instead of rectus-splitting) approach.

Transverse Incisions.—These may be employed both above and below the umbilicus (supra-umbilical or infra-umbilical).

TYPES. The transverse incisions are of two distinct types:

A. Transverse division of all the layers.
B. Vertical separation of the rectus muscles.

A. TRANSVERSE DIVISION OF ALL THE LAYERS.

Opening:

1. Skin and subcutaneous tissue.
2. Anterior rectus sheath of both the sides, transversely.
3. The rectus abdominis muscles, throughout their width and thickness, transversely.
4. The posterior rectus sheath and peritoneum (together with the intervening fascia transversalis) in one layer, transversely.

Closure:

1. The posterior rectus sheath and peritoneum in one layer.
2. Nothing need to be done to the cut rectus muscles.
3. The anterior rectus sheath.
4. Skin.

B. TRANSVERSE INCISION WITH VERTICAL SEPARATION OF THE RECTUS MUSCLES:

Opening:

1. Skin and subcutaneous tissue.
2. Anterior rectus sheath of both the sides transversely. The sheaths are then elevated from the underlying muscles, both upwards and downwards, as far as required.
3. The rectus muscle, on each side, is retracted laterally, by vertical separation in the midline.
4. The posterior rectus sheath and peritoneum (with the intervening fascia transversalis) are cut in one layer, vertically. In lower abdominal incision there is no posterior rectus sheath and this layer consists only of fascia transversalis and peritoneum.

Closure: Same as above.

Comments:

1. The first type of incision should be employed only in the upper abdomen because here the rectus muscle is adherent to the anterior rectus sheath, segmentally, by tendinous intersections. Hence, the cut muscle fibres cannot retract much, and an accurate suture of the anterior rectus sheath is all that is necessary for the repair. At the site of transection, the muscle heals with a transverse scar, making as if, an additional tendinous intersection. In the lower abdomen the recti have no tendinous intersections and so, if the muscles are cut through, the cut ends tend to retract widely. Hence, in the lower abdomen, the rectus muscles should be vertically separated (i.e. the second type of incision should be employed).
2. Division of the rectus muscles, as is done in the first type of incision, does not cause any interference with their nerve supply, since the muscles are supplied segmentally.

ADVANTAGES:

1. The scar is along the Langer s line and so,
   a. It is relatively invisible (cosmetic).
   b. There is less chance of 3 keloid developing.
2. There is minimal tension on the suture line and so,
   a. The repair is more secure.
   b. Post-operative discomfort is less (e.g. during coughing).

DISADVANTAGES:

1. The incisions cannot be extended at liberty and this may be a great handicap in obese patients.
2. They are time-consuming.
3. There may be considerable bleeding during opening.

Kocher's Subcostal Incision

INDICATIONS

1. Operations on the gall bladder.
2. Operations on the spleen.
3. Operations on the colonic flexures.
   The incision is. particularly suitable (in preference to paramedian incision) for:
   a. Obese patients with wide costal angle.
   b. Patients already having a paramedian scar.

OPENING:

1. The incision starts from just below the tip of the xiphoid process and extends downwards and laterally (as far as required), one inch below and parallel to the costal margin (right or left). Skin and subcutaneous tissues are cut.
2. The anterior rectus sheath is cut in the line of the incision and, as this is extended laterally, the external oblique and the internal oblique muscles are cut in the line of the incision.
3. The rectus muscle is cut through, along the line of the incision.
4. The posterior rectus sheath and peritoneum are cut on the medial side and, as this is extended laterally, the transversus abdominis muscle and the peritoneum are cut along the line of the incision.
5. The 8th, 9th and 10th intercostal nerves are found running between the internal oblique and the transversus. The 8th nerve has usually to be divided; the other two should be carefully preserved.

CLOSURE:

1. First Layer. Medially, the peritoneum and posterior rectus sheath together; laterally, the peritoneum, transversus abdominis and internal oblique muscles together.
2. Second Layer. Anterior rectus sheath medially, external oblique muscle laterally. No attempt is made to suture the cut rectus muscle.
3. Third Layer. Skin and subcutaneous tissue.

Gridiron Incision

1. On the Right Side. McBurney s incision, employed for appendectomy. This is the most commonly used incision for the removal of the appendix.
2. On the Left Side. For pelvic colostomy.

OPENING:

1. The incision is made along the McBurney s point, perpendicular to the line joining the anterior superior iliac spine and the umbilicus. Skin and subcutaneous tissues are cut.
2. The external oblique muscle and aponeurosis are divided along the line of the incision. There is actually splitting of their fibres since the long axis of the fibres

is along the line of the incision. In a typical Mc.Burney s incision, the exposed external oblique consists of muscular fibres in its upper part and aponeurosis in its lower part.

3. The internal oblique and transversus muscles are split together, along the line of their fibres. Therefore, in this plane, the direction of incision is perpendicular to that of the skin incision. The fascia transversalis is also cut in this line.
4. The peritoneum is incised along the line of skin incision.

CLOSURE:

1. Peritoneum.
2. The split fibres of the internal oblique and transversus are approximated by two or three interrupted stitches.
3. The external oblique.
4. Skin.

ADVANTAGES:

1. No muscle is cut; all are split along their fibres. Hence, there is practically no chance of a hernia.
2. The external oblique on one hand, and the internal oblique and transversus together on the other hand, are opened at lines perpendicular to each other (the fibres are arranged like gridiron). Hence, there is not a single point anywhere, along the line of exposure, where the musculature is completely interrupted. This further lessens the chances of incisional hernia.
3. The opening and closure are quick, easy, and practically bloodless.

DISADVANTAGE. The exposure may sometimes be inadequate in obese patients with difficult appendix. This disadvantage can, however, be overcome by enlarging the exposure in one of the following ways:

1. If an upward or downward extension is required, the fibres of the internal oblique and transversus are cut along the line of the skin incision (i.e. at right angles to their fibres) Rutherford Morison s modification.
2. If a medial extension is required, the split in the internal oblique and transversus muscles is extended medially, into the rectus sheath.

Rutherford Morison's Incision. The skin incision is the same as for McBurney s incision. Thereafter, all the muscles are divided along the line of the incision. Thus, while the fibres of the external oblique are split, those of the internal oblique and transversus muscles are cut across. This gives a more adequate exposure than a gridiron incision but is associated with more risks of development of incisional hernia. However, if the muscles are sutured properly, incisional hernia occurs only rarely.

INDICATIONS:

1. Exposure of ureter.
2. Exposure of external iliac vessels.
3. Appendectomy (usually a gridiron incision is converted into this incision in cases of difficult appendix).
4. Drainage of appendicular abscess.

Mayo-Robson's Incision.—This is actually a right paramedian incision, whose upper end is extended upwards and medially to the tip of the xiphoid process.

This provides a better exposure of the common bile duct and is, therefore, often employed for operations on the gall bladder and bile ducts. It is particularly preferred for obese patients.

Lanz's Incision.—This is a minor modification of the gridiron incision. The skin incision is made transverse and this provides a comparatively invisible scar. The other steps of the exposure are just the same as for gridiron incision.

Battle's Pararectal Incision.—This incision is only seldom employed. It is placed along the line of the fibres of the rectus abdominis, on its lateral third, in the lower part. The anterior rectus sheath is incised along the line of the incision and the rectus muscle is retracted medially. Thereafter, the peritoneum, fascia transversalis and posterior rectus sheath (if present) are cut in one layer. Since medial retraction of the rectus muscle cannot be achieved without damaging its nerve supply, the scar is likely to be weak. This is why the incision is obsolete nowadays.

Pfannenstiel's Incision.—This is actually a transverse infra-umbilical incision, with vertical separation of the recti in the midline. Its characteristics are:
1. The incision has a slight convexity downwards.
2. The peritoneum (with fascia transversalis) is incised transversely.

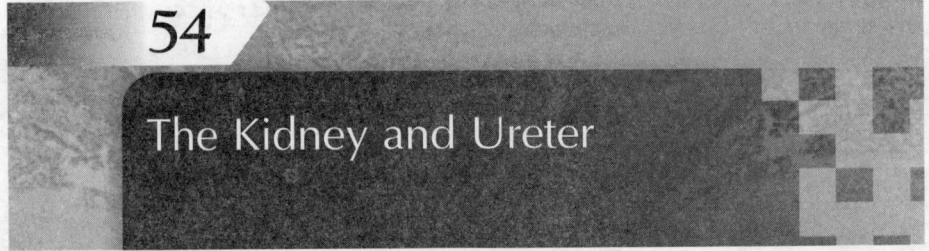

54

The Kidney and Ureter

Embryology.—The excretory part of the kidney, consisting of the renal pelvis, calyces, and straight collecting tubules, develops from the mesonephros. The secretory part, consisting of the glomeruli, convoluted tubules, and loops of Henle, develops from the metanephros. Subsequently, junction is established between the secretory and the excretory parts (failure of fusion between the two parts of the developing kidney is believed by many people to be the cause of polycystic kidney, i.e. the junction-failure theory of Hildebrandt).

In early intrauterine life three different sets of excretory apparatus appear (Fig. 54.1):

1. PRONEPHROS.—This consists of a few minute tubules, on either side of the midline, towards the cephalic segment of the embryo, opening directly into the body cavity. It disappears rapidly, leaving no trace.

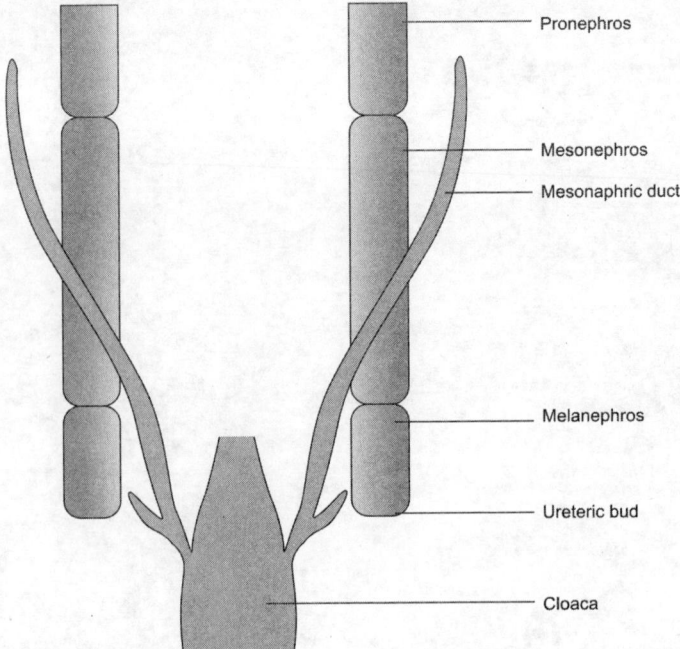

Fig. 54.1: The earliest stage in the development of the kidneys

2. MESONEPHROS.—This also consists of a number of tubules, on either side of the midline, but located towards the caudal segment of the embryo. While some of these tubules disappear, many of them persist and form a prominent longitudinal ridge, on each side of the midline, projecting into the body (coelomic) cavity. This is known as the *Wolffian body.* The tubules of Wolffian body at first open directly into the body cavity. Soon, however, a long channel develops inside the Wolffian body and this receives the openings of all the tubules. This is the *Wolffian duct* or *mesonephric duct,* which extends in a caudal direction, as far as the cloaca, into which it opens. From a *little above* the lower end of the Wolffian duct develops a small bud—the *ureteric bud.* This bud is the primitive ureter. While, the stalk of the bud gradually elongates and forms the ureter, its blind end dilates in the form of a club and forms the renal pelvis. The end of this club branches and re-branches to form the major and minor calyces, as well as the collecting tubules. The first few generations of the collecting tubules undergo cystic degeneration and disappear. Finally, a set of permanent collecting tubules develop (many authorities believe that these cystic masses of degenerated primary set of collecting tubules, if they persist, present themselves as poly- cystic kidney).

3. METANEPHROS.—This is a mass of tissue, situated near the caudal end of the Wolffian body, into which projects the ureteric bud. The tissue, which therefore covers the growing end of the ureteric bud like a cap, is called *metanephrogenic cap.* It is from this tissue that the secretory part of the kidney develops.

From what has been stated above, it is evident that each unit of the developing kidney consists of one collecting tubule and its attached secretory apparatus. All the units fuse together, and a final moulding occurs, to give the adult kidney its shape. A failure of this moulding results in *foetal lobulation.*

Ascent.—The kidneys primarily develop inside the pelvis, behind the peritoneum, just by the side of the midline, on each side. At this stage, therefore, the two kidneys are very close to each other and the two may get fused (fused kidney). Such fusion is most likely to occur at the medial surface of the two kidneys, particularly near the lower pole (horseshoe kidney). Normally each kidney ascends upwards and laterally to the loin. Failure or arrest in this ascent results in an ectopic kidney. An ectopic kidney may lie on its own side (homolateral ectopia) or may cross over, to the other side (crossed ectopia).

CONGENITAL ANOMALIES OF THE KIDNEYS AND URETERS

A. The Kidneys
1. Foetal Lobulation.
2. Supernumerary Kidney.—Some of the developing units having failed to fuse with the main mass of the developing kidney.
3. Absence or hypoplasia of one kidney, i.e. failure of development, of different degrees.
4. Ectopic Kidney:
   .a. Homolateral ectopia.
   b. Crossed ectopia.
5. Fused Kidneys:
   a. Transverse or bilateral fusion, i.e. horseshoe kidney (*see* below).
   b. Longitudinal or unilateral fusion:

     i. Congenital long kidney.—The pelves of the two kidneys are directed to the same side.

     ii. S-shaped kidney.—The two pelves are directed opposite to each other.

6. Fusion with Ectopia.
7. Cysts:
    a. Polycystic kidney—commonest.
    b. Solitary cyst.
    c. Dermoid cyst.
8. Congenital Hydronephrosis (*see* under hydronephrosis).
9. Aberrant Renal Vessels.—An aberrant vessel may be an artery or a vein, more commonly an artery. Usually the condition is unilateral and is much frequent on the left side. Normally, at the hilum of the kidney, the renal artery divides into three segmental branches—two superior and one inferior. The inferior, however, often varies in its point of origin. It may arise from the renal artery well proximal to the hilum or may even arise separately from the aorta. In such cases it enters the lower pole of the kidney separately and is in intimate contact with the pelvi-ureteric junction, where there is often a fibrous thickening around the vessel. Hydronephrosis is sometimes found in these cases and the role of the aberrant vessel in the development of the hydronephrosis is controversial (discussed under hydronephrosis).

B. The Ureters

1. Absence of one ureter (and so also the kidney), due to failure of development of the ureteric bud.
2. Double Ureter:
    a. The ureteric bud, arising from the Wolffian duct, may bifurcate and form a Y-shaped ureter (commoner). There is one ureteric orifice in the bladder.
    b. The ureteric bud may be double at its origin and form two complete ureters. In such cases the two ureters may open into the bladder, or one of them may open into the bladder and the other lower down (*see* ectopic ureteric orifice). In cases of double ureter, the rule is that the ureter, which starts higher, has its opening lower down. This means that there are two crossings between the two ureters.

    In either of the above conditions, the two components of the ureter may lead into two halves of a single kidney (but having two renal pelves) or into two separate kidneys.
3. Stenosis (narrowing) or atresia; valves or folds in the ureter.
4. Congenital Megaureter.—The ureter is dilated and its wall is also grossly thickened. However, the ureteric orifice is normal.
5. Post-caval Ureter.—The right ureter, instead of lying lateral to the inferior vena cava, lies behind it. Pressure by the vein, on the ureter, may lead to hydronephrosis.
6. Ureterocele.—This is a cystic dilation of the intramural part of the ureter, due to congenital atresia of the ureteric orifice.
7. Ureteric Diverticulum.—This is a diverticulum at the lower end of the ureter, usually due to an atresia of the ureteric orifice.
8. Ectopic Ureteric Orifice.—This condition is usually associated with complete double ureters. Developmentally, the lower opening is often located quite

low down into the Wolffian duct; also there may be an associated error in the partition of the cloaca. The ectopic opening may be located as follows:

a. In the Males:
  i. Apex of trigone.
  ii. Prostatic urethra.
  iii. Ejaculatory duct or vas deferens.
  iv. Seminal vesicle ⎫ rarely
  v. Rectum ⎭
b. In the Females:
  i. Apex of trigone.
  ii. Urethra, below the sphincter urethrae.
  iii. Vagina,
  iv. Rectum—rarely.

The clinical presentation of the condition is incontinent loss of part of the urine, together with normal bladder control of the remaining part.

SPECIAL INVESTIGATIONS FOR THE URINARY TRACT

1. URINE EXAMINATION.—As a rule, the morning midstream urine is sent for examination; catheterisation for collection of urine is usually avoided as this procedure entails the risk of introducing organisms into the bladder. A complete examination of the urine includes:
   a. Physical examination, especially the specific gravity (a low specific gravity indicates poor renal function) and reaction.
   b. Chemical examination, especially for albumin, sugar (and acetone), and blood.
   c. Microscopical examination, for casts, RBC, and pus cells.
   d. Culture and (if there is growth) sensitivity test of organisms, in particular cases.

2. BLOOD BIOCHEMISTRY.—Estimation of blood urea, NPN and creatinine gives an idea about the total renal function.

3. STRAIGHT X-RAY of the abdomen and pelvis (kidneys, ureters and bladder, i.e. KUB):
   a. To show evidence of urinary stones. Almost all urinary stones are radio-opaque. These stones are usually of irregular outline, sometimes taking the shape of the calyces or the renal pelvis. They usually have a uniform density. Renal stones on the right side may have, sometimes, to be differentiated from gall stones on the X-ray. Gall stones often have signet-ring appearance. In doubtful cases, a lateral view is helpful—a gall stone lies anterior to the vertebral bodies, while a kidney stone is superimposed on the vertebral shadow.
   The line of the ureter should be remembered while making the diagnosis of ureteric stone on the X-ray. The ureter, starting at the level between the first and the second lumbar vertebrae, passes in front of the tips of the transverse processes of the lumbar vertebrae and then in front of the sacroiliac joint. Thereafter, it runs to the ischial spine. From here it traverses upwards, forwards and medially, to the bladder.

b. The renal shadows are often evident even on the straight X-ray. An idea about the size and the position of the kidneys may be obtained.

4. INTRAVENOUS PYELOGRAPHY (IVP).—This gives an idea about:
   a. The function of the individual kidney.
   b. Pathological changes in the individual kidney.

   The dye used is sodium diatrizoate (Hypaque) and it is administered intravenously. 20 ml of the dye is injected very slowly into a vein. This dye in the blood is excreted by the kidney, if it is functioning. The first film is taken 5 minutes after injecting the dye. Thereafter, an X-ray is taken every 5 minutes, till a good picture of the bladder is obtained (usually 25 minutes). An IVP, therefore, not only shows the calyces and the pelvis but also the ureters and the bladder; a better term, therefore, is *urography*. Since the dye is excreted, the procedure is also known as *excretory pyelography*. Also, as the dye comes down along the urinary tract, it is known as *descending pyelography*.

   To prevent quick escape of the dye along the ureters, before X-rays of the kidneys are available, a tight abdominal binder is applied prior to injection of the dye (to put pressure on the ureters).

   IVP examination is contraindicated if:
   i. The renal function is poor (blood urea level above 60 mg%; urinary excretion of the dye is then insufficient to produce a reasonable film).
   ii. There is idiosyncrasy to iodine.

   In patients with a high blood urea level (e.g. 100 to 200 mg/100 ml) *infusion pyelography* may be done. Hypaque 2 ml/kg body weight is mixed with an equal volume of normal saline. This solution is infused over a period of 10 minutes and then X-rays are taken. Reasonable films may be obtained.

5. CYSTOSCOPY.—This is done with a cystoscope. It gives a good view of the bladder mucosa as well as the ureteric orifices. The cystoscope is passed along the urethra, in the same way as a bougie, and its tip enters the bladder (a local anaesthetic ointment is usually used for the purpose; some surgeons prefer general anaesthesia). The bladder is evacuated and then (about 250 ml) sterile water is pushed in, to distend the bladder. By rotating the cystoscope as well as by partially withdrawing and pushing it repeatedly, the whole of the bladder, excepting a very small area at the neck, can be visualised. When the eye of the cystoscope (indicated by a knob on the handle) looks at the 4'o'clock and 8 o'clock positions, the ureteric openings are seen. If 7 ml of a 0.4 per cent solution of indigocarmine is injected intravenously, the ureteric orifices can be easily identified, as, the dye is excreted through the kidneys (*chromocystoscopy*). The dye is usually ejected within 5 minutes of the injection. Should there be delay in excretion from one side, either the kidney is non-functioning or there is obstruction in the ureter.

   There are three types of cystoscopes:
   i. Ordinary visualising cystoscope. .
   ii. Operating cystoscope, with which biopsy, excision of a small tumour, cauterisation of tumours, etc., may be done.
   iii. Catheterising cystoscope, with arrangements for ureteric catheterisation (*see* below).

6. URETERIC CATHETERIZATION.—As has been said above, this is done with a catheterising cystoscope. The ureteric catheters are long, narrow, graduated, gum elastic tubes, with stellates. One is coloured red and the other green, to indicate the side, after introduction. Either one ureter or both may be catheterised, as desired. The catheters, passed through the cystoscope, may be negotiated into the ureteric orifices with the help of the special negotiators on the handle. Ureteric catheterisation may be performed for the following purposes:

a. To find out any obstruction in the ureter and to locate its level (the catheters are graduated).

b. To collect specimens of urine from the individual kidney.

c. To perform retrograde pyelography (*see* below).

d. To bring down stones, impacted in the lower ureter, into the bladder (the tip of the catheter is negotiated beyond the stone and lubricants are injected— *see* treatment of ureteric stones).

e. To relieve ureteric obstruction in cases of calculous anuria (*see* calculous anuria).

7. RETROGRADE PYELOGRAPHY.—This is done after the ureteric catheter is put in. Either one side or both the sides, simultaneously, may be investigated. "The dye used for the purpose is a sterile 12.5 per cent solution of sodium iodide (alternatively, Pylectan retrograde). The dye is introduced through the ureteric catheter. As soon as the renal pelvis is filled to its capacity (7 to 10 ml) the patient complains of pain in the loin and further injection is stopped. This is why this investigation should preferably be done under local anaesthesia.

The procedure is so named because the dye is injected in a dirction retrograde to the flow of urine. For the same reason, it is also called *ascending pyelography*. As this is done with cystoscope and ureteric catheters, it is also termed *instrumental pyelography*. The advantage of this procedure is that it provides a better picture of the pelvis and calyces than does an IVP and is particularly indicated in those cases where IVP produces an inconclusive picture. The disadvantage of this method, apart from the technical difficulties that it entails, is that it does not indicate the function of the kidney.

8. ULTRASONOGRAPHY.—This not only demonstrates the site and size of the kidneys but is also very useful in differentiating solid from cystic lesions.

9. RENAL ARTERIOGRAPHY.—This may be done in two ways:

a. *Translumbar Direct Approach.*—The dye is injected directly into the abdominal aorta, just above the renal arteries, i.e. plunging the needle from the back, at the L_1 level.

b. *Retrograde Indirect Approach.*—This is done by pushing a catheter, retrograde, from a femoral artery, into the aorta, up to the level of the renal arteries and then injecting the dye. For selective arteriography of one side, the catheter has to be negotiated into the particular renal artery.

An arteriography is of special help in differentiating between a renal tumour and a renal cyst, both of which appear as space-occupying lesions in the IVP in the arteriogram, while a cyst shows least vascularity, a tumour (usually malignant) is highly vascular.

10. RADIO-ISOTOPE RENOGRAPHY:—This is done with hippuran$_{131}$, injected intravenously. A scintillation counter is used for scanning the two kidneys separately. The scanning is started immediately after injection of the dye. The kidneys receive, concentrate, and then excrete the dye. The renograms, thus obtained, consist of three parts:

a. *Vascular Phase,* indicating the blood flow to the kidney.

b. *Tubular Phase,* indicating the ability of the renal tubules to excrete the hippuran.

c. *Excretory phase,* indicating the speed at which the hippuran leaves the renal pelvis.

11. CYSTOGRAPHY.—This means obtaining picture of the urinary bladder. It may be of the following types:

a. *Excretory.*—That accompanying an IVP.

b. *Retrograde.*—A rubber catheter is put in. and the bladder is evacuated. A sterile solution of 12.5 per cent sodium iodide is introduced through the catheter, till the patient feels a desire to micturate. An X-ray is taken. A filling defect suggests a neoplasm. The catheter is taken off and the patient is asked to micturate. Thereafter, another X-ray is taken (*post-evacuation film*). Presence of a diverticulum is detected when the dye is found to occupy the diverticulum while it has left the main bladder cavity.

c. *Micturating.*—This is done with X-ray image intensifiers while the patient is actually voiding urine, containing the dye. The function of the bladder neck can be well studied and any ureteric reflux detected.

12. PERI-RENAL AIR INSUFFLATION.—Air or oxygen is introduced into the perirenal space in order that the kidneys and neighbouring organs are visualised against a dark background, radiologically. Combined with a pyelography, this method is particularly valuable in differentiating cysts or tumours of the kidneys from those of. the adrenals. The air or oxygen is injected into the loose tissue of the pre-sacral space, from where it tracks upwards to the perirenal areas.

13. URETHROSCOPY.—This means visualising the urethra:

a. Anterior urethroscopy.

b. Posterior urethroscopy.

14. URETHROGRAPHY.—This is useful in the diagnosis of position and extent of a stricture or a fistula. A radio-opaque dye is injected into the urethra and X-ray taken.

HORSESHOE KIDNEY

The *points of importance* of this condition are as follows:

1. It is found once in every 1000 autopsies.

2. The connecting bridge (isthmus), lying across the front of the aorta, is usually located at the level of L$_4$. This is made either of renal parenchyma or of fibrous tissue. It usually bridges the lower poles of the kidneys, very rarely the upper poles. Often there may be an incomplete ascent, i.e. fusion with ectopia, the connecting band lying in front of the sacral promontory.

3. Hydronephrosis, infection and stone formation are much commoner in these kidneys. Either one or both the segments may be affected. This is because the ureters are angulated as they pass over the isthmus. In cases of such

complications, the bridging tissue may have to be slit in the midline or, if there is gross damage on one side, the affected half of the kidney may have to be resected.

4. The IVP findings are usually very suggestive:

   a. The shadow of the renal pelvis is superimposed on that of the calyces.

   b. The lowest calyx (and occasionally all the calyces) is found directed reverse, i.e. looking towards the vertebral column instead of laterally.

   c. The ureters are often curved like a *flower-vase*. All these findings are due to an arrest in the rotation of the kidney that normally accompanies ascent of the kidney.

POLYCYSTIC KIDNEY

This condition, in which there are multiple cysts in the kidney, is sometimes familial and may be associated with congenital cystic diseases of the liver, pancreas or lung.

Pathology.—Almost always the condition is *bilateral*. The kidneys are enlarged, sometimes enormously, though it may be that one kidney is much more affected than the other. There are numerous cysts, of different sizes, in the substance of the kidney, giving it the appearance of a: bunch of grapes. Some of the cysts are white, while others are brown due to haemorrhage inside. None of the cysts, however, communicates with the pelvis or calyces, unless there is a rupture due to tension inside. The areas of the kidney, occupied by the cysts, are non-functioning; moreover, as the cysts grow, they cause pressure-necrosis of the surrounding renal parenchyma. This results in gradual renal failure, particularly because the pathology is bilateral.

Clinical Features.—There are three distinct age groups of presentation:

A. In the foetus.—The huge abdominal lump in the foetus causes obstructed labour and results in a dead-born or still-born baby.

B. In the child.—The disease is usually evident before the age of 3 years. The child presents with bilateral renal lumps (and this has to be differentiated from Wilms' tumour, which is usually unilateral, and from congenital hydronephrosis). There may be associated renal rickets and, in a few years, death occurs due to uraemia.

C. In the adult.—The patient usually presents at about the age of 40. Thus, between the ages of 3 and 40, the condition is only rarely encountered. The different presenting features, in the adult group, may be as follows:

1. *Lump:* Bilateral renal lump is usually the presenting feature. Characteristically, there is a knobby feel due to the large cysts on the surface. Occasionally, the patient may present with unilateral lump. This, however, does not mean that the other kidney is healthy; it only suggests that the other kidney is not enlarged considerably.

Falacies of Renal Lump:

   a. When a patient presents with bilateral renal swellings, it does not necessarily mean that both the kidneys are pathological. It may be that one kidney is pathological, so much so, as to turn non-functioning, and the other kidney undergoes a compensatory hypertrophy.

b. If a kidney is palpable, usually that is the pathological kidney. However, it may rarely so happen that the pathological kidney is non-palpable and, as it has turned non-functioning, the other kidney undergoes a compensatory hypertrophy and presents itself as a renal lump.

2. *Pain:* This may be due to:
   a. Tension on the renal capsule by the enlarging cysts.
   b. Drag on the renal pedicle by the heavy organ.
   c. Repeated infection, sometimes associated with stones.
   d. Rupture of a large cyst on the surface, causing intra-abdominal pain.

3. *Haematuria:* This may occur in some cases, often profuse and sometimes repeated. This happens when a cyst ruptures into the pelvis due to over-distension.

4. *Infection:* Repeated attacks of pyelonephritis.

5. *Hypertension:* Renal hypertension occurs in the majority of cases.

6. *Uraemia:* A pre-uraemic stage, and finally uraemia, sets in, as the loss of renal tissue progresses.

Special Investigations

1. URINE EXAMINATION: High output of urine, with a low specific gravity (below 1010). There are traces of albumin but no casts or cells.

2. BLOOD BIOCHEMISTRY: There is a progressive rise in the level of serum urea, NPN and creatinine.

3. STRAIGHT X-RAY of the abdomen may show enlarged renal shadows.

4. IVP:
   a. There may be considerable delay in excretion of the dye and/or the shadows may be faint due to poor excretion by the damaged kidneys.
   b. The renal shadows may be grossly enlarged.
   c. There is bilateral generalised *spider-leg deformity* of the calyces as they are stretched over the cysts and have to traverse round them; the calyces are narrowed as well (in any space-occupying lesion of the kidney, which has no communication with the pelvis or calyces, there is a spider-leg deformity of the calyces).

5. ASCENDING PYELOGRAPHY: This may have to be done if the IVP findings are inconclusive.

Treatment

I. CONSERVATIVE: The patient is advised high intake of fluids and a low-protein diet. Urinary antiseptics are administered, as required.

II. OPERATIVE: This should be undertaken whenever possible. The standard operative treatment is *Rovsing's operation.* It is not curative but prolongs the patient's life. It consists in decompressing the cysts, so that, whatever healthy kidney tissue is still left, is saved from pressure necrosis by the enlarging cysts. The operation is done on one kidney first and, at an interval of 3 to 4 weeks, on the second kidney.

By the standard kidney exposure (extraperitoneal) the kidney is exposed. The cysts on its convex border and, thereafter, those on its posterior surface are either punctured or incised with a narrow-blade scalpel. Now the anterior surface is brought to view and the cysts therein are dealt with in a similar way.

Origin of Polycystic Kidneys.—There are several views:

1. Junction-failure theory of Hildebrandt (*see* embryology).
2. The cysts represent the cysts of degeneration of the first few generations of the collecting tubules of the developing kidneys (*see* embryology).
3. Infective origin.—The cysts are secondary to nephro-papillitis, resulting from calcium and uric acid deposits in the terminal part of the collecting tubules. This produces obstruction at the end of the collecting tubules and leads to formation of retention cysts.

It is now believed by many authorities that the condition encountered in the foetus and children on one hand, and in the adults on the other, are totally different entities. One of the first two theories explains the condition in the foetus and children. The third theory possibly explains the development of polycystic kidneys in the adults.

SOLITARY RENAL CYST

The *causes* of a solitary cyst in the kidney are:

1. CONGENITAL.—Same as for a polycystic kidney, but on a small scale and in a localised form.
2. TRAUMATIC.—A haematoma, converted into a cyst.
3. INFECTIVE.—Infection, causing blockage of tubules, that results in formation of a retention cyst.

A solitary cyst is sometimes difficult to be differentiated clinically, as well as on the IVP, from a renal neoplasm. A renal arteriogram is particularly valuable in such cases. Ultrasonography is also useful in differentiating solid from cystic lesion. *Treatment* consists in excision of the cyst, or a partial nephrectomy together with the cyst.

TYPES OF RENAL CYST

1. Polycystic kidney (discussed).
2. Solitary cyst (discussed).
3. Dermoid cyst.
4. Retention cysts.—Multiple small cysts of the granular contracted kidneys of chronic interstitial nephritis.
5. Hydatid cyst
6. Cystic degeneration in malignant tumours.

HYDRONEPHROSIS

This is an aseptic dilation of the pelvis and/or calyces, caused by intermittent and incomplete obstruction to the flow of urine.

If there is a septic dilatation, the condition is *called pyonephrosis*. There may be a pyonephrosis to start with, or there may be a hydronephrosis which undergoes secondary infection and turns into a pyonephrosis.

If there is a sudden complete obstruction to the flow of urine (e.g. ligation of the ureter, impaction of stones, etc.) the result may be:

1. Usually there is an atrophy of the obstructed kidney with compensatory hypertrophy of the opposite kidney. If, however, the other kidney is diseased

and unable to compensate, the first kidney may recover to some extent, provided the cause of obstruction is removed *(renal counterbalance).*

2. Sometimes, associated with the stoppage of function in the obstructed kidney, there is a reflex cessation of function in the opposite kidney *(reno-renal reflex).* This results in anuria, e.g. calculous anuria.

Types

A. Depending on the site of obstruction to the urinary flow, the hydronephrosis may be *unilateral* or *bilateral.* A unilateral hydronephrosis occurs when the obstruction is above the level of the bladder, i.e. located in the ureter. A bilateral hydronephrosis may result from:

1. Obstruction below the level of the bladder, i.e. located in the urethra (commoner).
2. Bilateral ureteric obstruction (rare).

B. Hydronephrosis may be *congenital* or *acquired.* The term congenital hydronephrosis is restricted by some authors to those cases where the hydronephrosis is present at birth; more people, however, apply this term to the cases where the cause of obstruction is congenital, e.g. pin-hole meatus, valves, folds, etc. Similarly, the term acquired hydronephrosis refers to those cases where the obstruction is acquired, e.g. enlarged prostate, stones, strictures, etc.

From what has been stated above, the types of hydronephrosis may be:

1. Congenital Unilateral.
2. Congenital Bilateral.
3. Acquired Unilateral.
4. Acquired Bilateral.

Etiology.—While, in many cases, the cause of obstruction is demonstrable, in others no definite cause for the obstruction is elicited. The first variety is called *secondary* (or *obstructive*) hydronephrosis while the second type is termed *primary* (or *idiopathic*) hydronephrosis.

A. CAUSES OF SECONDARY HYDRONEPHROSIS

1. Causes in the lumen *(intermural).*—Stones.
2. Causes in the wall *(intermural).*—Stricture, growth, pin-hole meatus, enlarged prostate, valves or folds, etc.
3. Causes outside the wall *(extramural).*—Pressure by rectal, uterine or ovarian tumours, gravid uterus, etc.

B. ETIOLOGY OF PRIMARY HYDRONEPHROSIS.—The cases of primary hydronephrosis may be of two types:

1. Those associated with aberrant renal vessels (see under congenital anomalies of the kidney).
2. Those not associated with aberrant vessels.

When an aberrant vessel is present, it is found to cross the pelvi-ureteric junction and there is a definite fibrous thickening around the vessel, at this site. The vessel is, thus, found sitting tightly across the lower end of the hydronephrotic sac. It may, therefore, be presumed that this vessel is the cause for the hydronephrosis. It may, however, be equally true that the hydronephrosis started for some other reason and, in the beginning, the aberrant vessel crossed the pelvi-ureteric junction without exerting any pressure on it. Subsequently, as the hydronephrotic sac did enlarge, the vessel sat tight on the sac. The role of aberrant renal vessels as a cause of hydronephrosis is, therefore, debatable. It has, however, been found that ligation and division of such a vessel often gives a lasting cure in many of these cases.

The cause of a primary hydronephrosis is now believed to be some derangement in the mechanism by which urine is normally expelled from the renal pelvis, down the ureter. There are interlacing bundles of muscle fibres, encircling the pelvis and the ureter. It is believed that rhythmic contraction of these muscles forces the urine to run from the pelvis down the ureter. There is no extrinsic nervous stimulation for this process neither is there any intrinsic nervous mechanism (because there is no myenteric plexus and no ganglion cells, c f the gut). The present idea is that contraction, starts in the renal pelvis in response to stretching of the muscle fibres, and the process of contraction spreads from one muscle cell to the next directly. Some derangement in this mechanism is believed to be the primary cause for idiopathic hydronephrosis, in which the dilatation is found to stop abruptly at the pelvi-ureteric junction. Such derangement may be either of two following patterns:

a. A spasmodic segment developing at the pelvi-ureteric junction (there is, however, no sphincter at the pelvi-ureteric junction).

b. Pelvic fibrillation, i.e. irregular contraction of the pelvic musculature.

Such a pathology, however, is not due to any derangement in sympathetic-parasympathetic balance at the renal pedicle because, as has already been said, there is no extrinsic nervous control on this process of urinary flow.

Pathology

A. There are 3 *types* of hydronephrosis:

1. PELVIC TYPE.—The renal pelvis is grossly dilated, with comparatively little distension of the calyces, and, consequently, little renal damage. This occurs when the pelvis is anatomically extra-renal (i.e. the major part of the pelvis is situated outside the kidney substance).

2. RENAL TYPE.—The calyces are dilated without much dilatation of the renal pelvis. This occurs when the pelvis is anatomically intra-renal (i.e. the major part of the pelvis is padded by the kidney substance). There is an early and gross renal damage.

3. PELVI-RENAL TYPE.——The pelvis and the calyces, both are distended. This occurs in the late stages of either of the above types.

It may be mentioned that majority of primary hydronephrosis are of the pelvic type, while majority of the secondary (obstructive) hydronephrosis are of the renal type.

B. Hydronephrosis usually progresses through 3 *stages:*

1. OPEN HYDRONEPHROSIS.—The hydronephrotic sac still communicates with the lower urinary tract because the obstruction is incomplete.

2. INTERMITTENT HYDRONEPHROSIS.—The obstruction becomes complete intermittently so that, at one stage there is oliguria with pain in the loin and enlargement of the hydronephrotic sac, and thereafter (as the obstruction passes off), there is polyuria with diminution in the size of the sac.

3. CLOSED HYDRONEPHROSIS.—Outflow from the hydronephrotic sac ceases as the obstruction becomes complete and there is no communication of the sac with the lower urinary tract.

C. The *effect of* hydronephrosis is damage to the kidney substance. This, as has been stated, is early and quickly progressive with the renal type, late and slow with the pelvic type. This damage is due to two factors:

1. The corresponding part of the kidney has a hindered drainage;
2. There is a pressure atrophy of the kidney substance, caused by the enlarging hydronephrotic sac.

D. The *fluid* in the hydronephrotic sac is never stagnant; it undergoes constant changes because of addition and reabsorption. Addition is effected by the secretion of urine and its accumulation in the sac. As regards the mechanism of reabsorption, there are several views:

1. Pyelo-venous backflow (direct absorption of the fluid by the veins in the wall of the pelvis).
2. Pyelo-lymphatic backflow (absorption by the lymphatics).
3. Pyelo-tubular backflow (the fluid flows back to the tubules, from where it is absorbed).
4. Pyelo-interstitial extravasation, followed by absorption of the fluid by veins or lymphatics.

Clinical Features.—As regards their clinical presentation, the patients of hydronephrosis may be divided into 4 broad groups:

GROUP I. Patients presenting with clinical features suggestive of the cause of the hydronephrosis but not of the hydronephrosis itself, e.g. renal colic and haematuria for renal stones, dysuria for enlarged prostate, etc.

GROUP II. Patients presenting with clinical features of the hydronephrosis itself and not with those of the cause. The presenting features are renal lump (unilateral or bilateral) and a dull aching pain in the loin (due to stretching of the renal capsule as well as drag by the heavy organ on the pedicle).

GROUP III. Patients presenting with features of the hydronephrosis itself as well as those of its cause.

GROUP IV. Hydronephrosis associated with pregnancy, usually regressing after the child-birth.

Special Investigations

1. URINE EXAMINATION.—A complete examination of the urine may reveal:
   a. The cause of the hydronephrosis.
   b. An advanced hydronephrosis (suggested by a very high output of urine with low specific gravity).

2. BLOOD BIOCHEMISTRY.—In order to assess the total renal function, the levels of serum urea, NPN and creatinine are valuable.

3. STRAIGHT X-RAY—This may show:
   a. Enlarged renal shadow.
   b. Radio-opaque stones.

4. IVP.—In the *advanced stages* of hydronephrosis, the urographic shadow may be very faint. This is partly because of poor excretion of the dye by the grossly damaged kidney and partly due to the dilution that the excreted dye undergoes as it mixes up with the huge quantity of fluid in the sac. In some cases there may not be any visible shadow.

The IVP findings in the *early stages* of hydronephrosis vary according to the type of the hydronephrosis:

a. *In the pelvic type:*
   i. Dilatation of the pelvis,
   ii. Irregular shape of the pelvis.
   iii. The pelvi-ureteric junction is no longer the lowermost part of the pelvis. It ascends a little high up, so that there is a dependant part of the pelvis, below the level of the pelvi-ureteric junction.

b. *In the renal type.*—The earliest change is seen in the minor calyx. The normal concavity at the apex of the minor calyx gets flattened and, thereafter, turns convex *(clubbing)*. Following this, there is progressive and irregular dilatation of the minor and, thereafter, the major calyces.

5. RETROGRADE PYELOGRAPHY.—This may be useful when the IVP findings are inconclusive.

GROUP A: In those cases where the hydronephrosis is secondary and the kidney has turned non-functioning, *nephrectomy* is advocated, provided the other kidney is healthy. It has, however, been found that, even in such cases, if the cause of obstruction is removed, the kidney sometimes regains function. Therefore, many surgeons advocate *conservative surgery* in such cases, i.e. simple removal of the obstruction. If the hydronephrosis is partial, i.e. limited to only one pole of the kidney, a *partial nephrectomy* is the treatment of choice.

GROUP B: In those cases where the hydronephrosis is secondary but the kidney is not grossly damaged, only the cause of the obstruction is removed. In such cases a plastic operation for the hydronephrosis itself (*see* below) may be added, provided the hydronephrosis is of the pelvic type.

GROUP C: The treatment for idiopathic hydronephrosis is still unsatisfactory, chiefly because the cause of the condition still remains obscure. The different operations that are advocated in these cases are mentioned below:

1. *Ligations and Division of an Aberrant Renal Vessel.*—It has been found that ligation and division of such a vessel often gives a lasting cure to the hydronephrosis. If it is a vein, the procedure is harmless. If, however, it is an artery, its division is immediately followed by an avascularity of the lower pole of the kidney. This is immediately detectable, as blanching occurs, and a partial nephrectomy has to be performed.

2. *Reconstructive Operation.*—*Different* types of operations are advocated, all of which include:
   a. Excision of the pelvi-ureteric junction.
   b. Adequate reduction in the size of the dilated pelvis.
   c. Provision for drainage or the remaining pelvis at its most dependant part.

Such operations are possible because almost all the cases of primary hydronephrosis are of the pelvic type. Of the different operations available, the *Anderson-Hynes operation* is the most popular. The ureter is divided just below the pelvi-ureteric junction (this is the site where the hydronephrosis stops abruptly). The redundant part of the pelvis, together with the pelvi-ureteric junction, is resected. The pelvic flaps are sutured to each other, keeping open only its lowermost part, to which the ureter is to be anastomosed. For the purpose of anastomosis, the upper end of the ureter is slit for about an inch, and the two flaps, thus made, are sutured to the two flaps left unsutured at the lowermost part of the pelvis. The anastomosis is performed on a ureteric catheter, which is withdrawn just before the anastomosis is completed.

3. *Renal Pedicle Sympathectomy.*—This operation is still advocated by some surgeons in cases of idiopathic hydronephrosis, on the belief that the spasm at the pelvi-ureteric junction or the pelvic fibrillation are due to sympathetic overactivity. The renal pedicle is exposed and, preserving the artery, the vein, and the pelvis carefully, all other soft tissues are stripped off. This procedure definitely relieves the pain associated with hydronephrosis. This may be harmful in the sense that the patient, relieved of the pain, ignores the hydronephrosis, which steadily progresses. Some authorities, however, claim that, after sympathectomy, there is also a functional improvement of the kidney and reduction of the calyceal dilatations.

URINARY STONES

Etiology.—Urinary stones are aggregations of urinary crystalloids. The urine contains huge amounts of crystalloids of different types and, as there is only a limited amount of fluid available to carry them out, they are carried in heavily super-saturated solution. This is possible because of the presence of colloids in the urine, which allow the crystalloids to be kept in solution by the process of adsorption. The urinary colloids are mucin and chondroitin-sulphuric acid. Stone formation is possible under two circumstances:

1. An imbalance in the crystalloid-colloid ratio.—Either an increase in the crystalloid level or a fall in the colloid level.
2. Modification of the colloids.—They lose their solvent action and acquire a kind of adhesive property.

With the exception of the rare types of stones (e.g. cystine, xanthine, etc.), all other urinary stones have calcium as their main ingredient. Thus, the defects, by which the calcium-containing crystalloids are allowed to be precipitated, are believed to be the main reasons for stone formation:

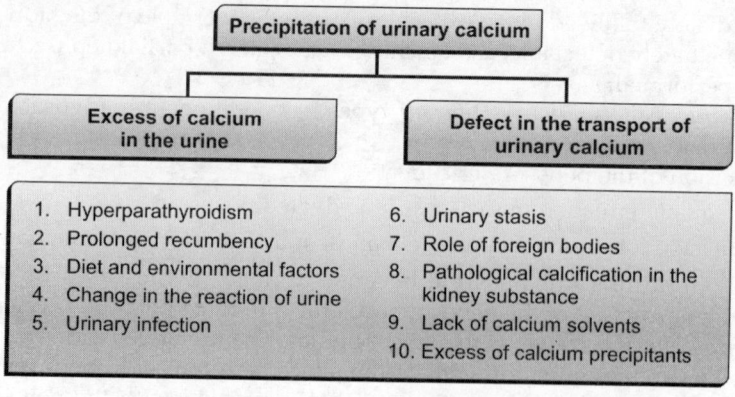

Precipitation of urinary calcium	
Excess of calcium in the urine	**Defect in the transport of urinary calcium**
1. Hyperparathyroidism	6. Urinary stasis
2. Prolonged recumbency	7. Role of foreign bodies
3. Diet and environmental factors	8. Pathological calcification in the kidney substance
4. Change in the reaction of urine	9. Lack of calcium solvents
5. Urinary infection	10. Excess of calcium precipitants

1. *Hyperparathyroidism.*—It is believed that from 2 to 10 per cent of cases of stones are due to this condition. The condition has to be suspected particularly when stones are multiple, bilateral, or recurrent.
2. *Prolonged Recumbency.*—The factors responsible are:
   a. Decalcification of the bones, resulting in excess of calcium in the blood, which is excreted in the urine.
   b. Urinary stasis, allowing the deposited calcium to aggregate.
3. *Diet and Environmental Factors:*
   a. Excess of calcium intake in the diet.
   b. Low phosphorous intake.
   c. Administration of excess of vitamin D, which allows excessive absorption of calcium from the gut.
   d. Deficiency of vitamin A, which causes desquamation of the epithelium. The desquamated epithelium forms a nidus, around which stone is deposited.
   e. Dry environment, with excess of perspiration and a low output of urine, allowing the crystalloids to be highly concentrated and deposited.
4. *Change in the Reaction of Urine.*—Only phosphate stones depend on the reaction of urine for their formation. If the urine turns alkaline, phosphate stones are likely to form. Alkalinization of urine may be brought about by:
   a. Prolonged use of antacids, as in patients of peptic ulcer.
   b. Use of alkalies.
   c. Urinary infection.—Urinary bacteria often split urea into ammonia, and the ammonium salts turn the urine alkaline.
5. *Urinary Infection.*—This is a well-established predisposing factor. Infection helps stone formation in three ways:
   a. Changing the reaction of urine to alkalinity.
   b. Bacteria, adsorbed on inorganic particles, act as nuclei for stone formation.
   e. By production of mucoprotein, which acts as a calcium precipitant.
6. *Urinary Stasis.*—This is, again, a well-recognised predisposing factor. Stasis helps stone formation in two ways:
   a. Predisposing urinary infection.
   b. Allowing the precipitated crystalloids to aggregate together.
7. *Role of Foreign Bodies.*—This is seen only in cases of bladder stones, e.g. stones deposited at the tip of self-retaining catheters (catheter-stones) or stones formed on foreign bodies, introduced into the bladder per urethra.
8. *Pathological Calcification in the Kidney Substance.*—It is believed that stone formation actually starts as a process of pathological calcification in the kidney substance itself. This is *Randall's hypothesis.* According to Randall, this process of calcification may take two forms:
   a. Type I stones of Randall, i.e. the 'primary' stones, where there is no definite cause for the formation of the stones. In these cases a plaque of calcium *(Randall's milk-patch)* is deposited within the substance of a renal papilla. The overlying surface epithelium is thereafter denuded, and this plaque is exposed to the flow of urine in the minor calyx.
   b. Type II stones of Randall, i.e. the 'secondary' stones, where there is a demonstrable cause for stone formation, e.g. hyperparathyroidism. Here, the pathological calcification starts as deposits within the collecting tubules.

In any of the above types, further crystalloids from the urine are deposited on the nuclei, formed by these pathological calcifications, and stones grow.

9. *Lack of Calcium Solvents.*—The chief calcium solvents in the urine are:

    a. Colloids.—Mucin and chondroitin-sulphuric acid.

    b. Citrates.

    c. Some organic acids.

    d. Some amino acids.

10. *Excess of Calcium Precipitants.*—Mucoprotein, which is a product of infection, is a strong calcium precipitant.

Types of Stones

Urinary stones	
Primary	**Secondary**
1. They arise in apparently healthy urinary tract.	1. They usually form in infected urine.
2. Thus, they form in acid urine.	2. They, therefore, form in alkaline urine (their development depends upon the liberation of ammonia from urea, brought about by the organisms).
3. They require no preformed nuclei and form by the process of slow precipitation of crystalloids on a colloid magma.	3. They require a preformed nucleus, e.g. a clump of bacteria, a mass of inflammatory exudate, a foreign body, or even a primary stone.
4. They are composed of substances that are present in the urine either normally (e.g. oxalate and uric acid or urate stones) or in metabolic disorders (e.g. cystine stones).	4. They are composed of substances which are not normally present in the urine, e.g. magnesium ammonium phosphate (i.e. triple phosphate), secondary stones are almost always phosphate stones.

OXALATE STONES.—These are the commonest of the urinary stones. They are made of calcium oxalate, a normal constituent of the urine. They form in healthy acid urine. There are sharp spikes on the surface of these stones. These spikes attribute some special characters to these stones:

a. Whereas small stones of other composition may rapidly pass down the ureter, into the bladder, these stones often become impacted in the ureter.

b. Wherever located, they irritate the mucous membrane and the resultant haemorrhage renders them a brown or black colour.

c. Outpour of lymph and blood, caused by the mucosal irritation, may allow secondary phosphate deposits on their surface, brought about by infection (mixed stones).

d. Because of the rough surface, the stones usually give rise to symptoms, even when they are small.

Oxalate is principally derived from food. Food, rich in oxalates, taken for long periods, may first cause oxaluria (i.e. crystals of oxalate passed in the urine) and, thereafter, formation of oxalate stones.

The calcium content of these stones is very high and, so, whatever be the size of the stones, they are radio-opaque (the size of the stones vary considerably). Very often, the spikes on the surface are evident on the X-ray.

URIC ACID AND URATE STONES.—Pure uric acid stones are rare; usually there is a combination of uric acid, urates, and calcium oxalate. In children, there may be ammonium urate stones. These stones form in healthy acid urine. They are yellowish or brown in colour. The size may vary considerably. Sometimes the stones are multiple and faceted. Usually they form in the kidneys but rarely they may originate in the bladder.

Unless there is a good calcium content, these stones may not be seen on the straight X-ray.

PHOSPHATE STONES.—They form in infected (and so, alkaline) urine. There is a central preformed nucleas (as described above). Normal urine contains phosphates but the common phosphate stones are made of triple phosphate (ammonium magnesium phosphate), of which only traces are normally present in the urine. The conversion of the normal urinary phosphates into triple phosphate probably results from liberation of ammonium carbonate from urea, brought about by the infecting organisms. Sometimes, the stones may be made of calcium phosphate or a mixture of calcium phosphate and triple phosphate.

The crystalloids of the stone are deposited in a laminated manner and these laminations are often well-seen on the cut-surface. The stones are grey to dirty-white in colour. They may form in the kidney or in the bladder but wherever located, they often attain large size. In the kidney, they often fill the renal pelvis and calyces, taking a mould thereof and forming 'stag-horn' calculi. However, the surface is smooth and this is why these stones produce only a few symptoms till they attain big size.

By reason of their size rather than their calcium content, these stones are radio-opaque. Also, the laminated appearance is often seen radiologically.

MIXED STONES.—In the centre there is an oxalate stone, on the surface there are deposits of phosphates. The oxalate stone had formed initially in non-infected acid urine but, thereafter, caused an urinary infection. The reaction of the urine had then turned alkaline, either by this infection or by the administration of an 'alkaline cure'. This resulted in the formation of phosphates, which got deposited on the surface of the oxalate stone that acted, as if, as a preformed nucleus.

CYSTINE STONES.—This rare variety of stone follows cystinuria. Cystine is an aminoacid, rich in sulphur. Normally it is excreted in the urine as sulphates. As regards cystinuria, there are two views:

a. That this is an 'inborn error in metabolism', which causes the cystine to appear in the urine unchanged (i.e. not converted into sulphates). The condition is often familial.

b. That this results simply from absence or greatly diminished reabsorption of cystine by the renal tubules.

Cystine crystals are hexagonal. The stones are soft like beeswax. They are usually multiple and of en-recurrent.

Other rare types of stones include xanthine stones, indigo stones (derived from indol), fibrin stones, bacterial stones (made of clumps of bacteria only), sulphonamide deposits, and urostealith.

RENAL STONES

Pathological Effects of Renal Stones

A. SAME KIDNEY:
1. The epithelium of the pelvis or calyces, in relation to which the stone lies, loses lustre, and becomes rough and thickened.
2. *Infection.*—Pyelitis, pyelonephritis, cystitis (descending), perinephric adhesions.
3. *Obstruction:*
   a. If intermittent and incomplete.—Hydronephrosis.
   b. If complete:
      i. Calculous anuria.
      ii. Atrophy of the kidney.
4. *Infection plus obstruction.—Pyonephrosis.*
5. *Malignancy.*—Carcinoma of the renal pelvis may occur. The lining epithelium of the renal pelvis, which is normally transitional, is converted into squamous type, by metaplasia. The resultant carcinoma may, therefore, be epidermoid in nature.

B. OPPOSITE KIDNEY:
1. Infection.—Ascending from the bladder.
2. Stone formation.
3. Compensatory hypertrophy, if the function of the affected kidney is totally lost.
4. *Calculous anuria.*—Reflex stoppage of function, in response to cessation of function in the affected kidney, due to complete obstruction caused by a stone there (reno-renal reflex).

Presenting Symptoms.—The cases may be divided into 3 groups:

I. SILENT STONES: These produce no symptoms and are discovered incidentally in an X-ray, at operation, or post-mortem.

II. HYDRONEPHROTIC GROUP: Here the patient has no complaint suggestive of stones, and presents with features of hydronephrosis, viz. a renal lump, sometimes associated with a dull aching pain in the loin.

III. THE USUAL GROUP: Majority of the patients present with pain, haematuria, and sometimes pyuria.

A. *Pain.*—There may be 3 types of pain, viz. fixed renal pain, renal colic, and referred pain.
   1. Fixed Renal Pain, which is dull aching or boring in character, occurs particularly with big-size stones, especially the jagged oxalate stones.
      The pain is felt more during exercise than at rest, and may be located:
      a. in the loin posteriorly.

    b. in the hypochondrium anteriorly,

    c. both posteriorly and anteriorly.

2. Renal Colic, which should preferably be called 'ureteric colic', occurs when a stone attempts to pass down the ureter or blocks the pelvi-ureteric junction.

    There is an acute agonising spasmodic pain, which often doubles the patient up. This may be associated with nausea and vomiting, chill and rigor, profuse sweating and a subnormal temperature.At the time of the colic, there is great rigidity of the abdominal muscles, usually marked in the lateral flat muscles and not in the rectus abdominis.

    The site and radiation of the pain are usually typical. It starts at the loin, from where it radiates to the groin and the hypogastric region, i.e. along the course of the iliohypogastric, ilioinguinal and subcostal nerves, which are closely related to the kidney. Rarely the pain is also referred, along the distribution of the genitofemoral nerve, to the inner side of the thigh and to the testis (or labium major).

    The pain persists for a variable period, often 24 hours or more, occurring intermittently. Thereafter, it passes off as suddenly as it appeared.

    After the pain passes off, one of the following features may occur:

    a. Haematuria.

    b. Compensatory polyuria.

    c. Passage of the stone in the urine.   -

    d. Strangury, i.e. passage of a little amount of urine, often blood-stained, after painful straining.

3. Referred Pain may sometimes occur, and its type is widely variable:

    a. Vague pain all over the abdomen.

    b. Pain along the inferior extremity, sometimes up to the sole.

    c. Pain in the opposite kidney (reno-renal reflex).

B. *Haematuria.*—This is a painful haematuria, the amount of which varies. Haematuria follows the pain (c f clot colic, where haematuria precedes the pain).

C. *Pyuria.*—The patient may pass opalescent urine, containing pus. This occurs when the urine is infected.

Physical Signs

1. *Tenderness:*

    a. This is usually located at the renal angle posteriorly (i.e. the angle between the lower border of the twelfth rib and the lateral border of the erector spinae).

    b. Sometimes there is tenderness at the anterior renal point (on the anterior abdominal wall, one inch below and medial to the tip of the ninth costal cartilage).

2. *Lump:* If there is an associated hydronephrosis or pyonephrosis, a renal lump may be palpable.

    [*Characters of a Renal Lump:*

    a Often reniform or oval in shape.

    b. Moving up and down with respiration.

    c. Usually, movable in both axes, unless fixed.

    d. Ballotable antero-posteriorly.

e. Fingers can be insinuated between the lump and the costal margin (c f splenic swelling).

f. Often a band of resonance may be elicited across the lump, on percussion, i.e. where the transverse colon crosses it (c f splenic swelling)].

Special Investigations

1. URINE EXAMINATION:
   a. *Physical* examination may shown
      i. Presence of blood (a three-glass test shows that the blood is present in all the glasses, i.e. intimately mixed with urine),
      ii. Presence of pus, i.e. opalescent.
   b. *Chemical* examination may show presence of blood and albumin.
   c. *Microscopic* examination may show RBC, pus cells and casts.
   d. *Bacteriological examination.*—A culture and sensitivity test may be done.

2. BLOOD BIOCHEMISTRY: Estimation of blood urea, NPN and creatinine, to assess the renal function.

3. STRAIGHT X-RAY:
   a. Almost all urinary stones are radio-opaque (c f gall stones).
   b. The renal shadow may be enlarged.
   The shadow of a renal stone may, sometimes, have to be differentiated from:
      i. Gall stone.
      ii. Calcified lymph node or calcified suprarenal gland.
      iii. Calcified tubercular lesion tin the kidney (pseudocalculous tuberculosis).
      iv. Faecolith or foreign body in the gut.
      v. Phlebolith.
      vi. Ossified tip of the twelfth rib.
      vii. Chip fracture of the tip of the transverse process of a lumbar vertebra.

4. IVP: There is great importance of doing an IVP:
   a. It determines the exact location of the stone (this may be very helpful at operation).
   b. It shows presence of any associated hydronephrosis.
   c. It reveals the function of the affected kidney as well as that of the opposite kidney.

Treatment.—The treatment is always surgical. The actual operation depends upon the location of the stone and any associated pathology. The different operations that may be performed are:

1. Pyelolithotomy.
2. Nephrolithotomy.
3. Pyelonephrolithotomy.
4. Nephrectomy.
5. Partial nephrectomy.
6. Nephrostomy.

PYELOLITHOTOMY.—This means removal of a stone by making an opening in the pelvis of the kidney. This is done when a stone is located in the pelvis and the pelvis is extrarenal. The posterior surface of the pelvis is readily available at hand with an extra-peritoneal lumbar approach (this is the usual approach for operations on kidney stones). An incision is made along the long axis of the pelvis, on its posterior surface. The stone is removed with a pyelolithotomy forceps. The pelvic wound, which heals spontaneously, need not be sutured since this may lead to stricture, A drain, put down to the renal fossa, brings out the leaked urine and blood.

NEPHROLITHOTOMY.—This denotes an operation for removal of stone by cutting through the kidney substance. This is done for:

a. Stones in the kidney substance, i.e. calyces.

b. Stones in the pelvis where the pelvis is intrarenal.

The exact location of the stone may be ascertained from the pyelogram. The stone is made prominent on the renal cortex by invaginating a finger through the pelvis. The incision, made on the kidney, may be one of the following types:

i. A radial incision (this avoids injury to big vessels, which run radially).

ii. An incision along the *Brodel's line,* which is believed to mark the lateral margin of a relatively avascular plane in the kidney. This is the plane of demarcation between the areas supplied by the anterior and the posterior branches of the renal artery and is therefore, relatively avascular. The Brodel's line is situated 5 mm behind and parallel to the actual convex border of the kidney.

After removal of the stone, the wound on the kidney must be properly sutured in order to achieve haemostasis.

PYELONEPHROLITHOTOMY.—This means making incisions on both the pelvis and the kidney substance to bring out stones. Its indications are:

a. A stone in the pelvis and another in the kidney substance, i.e. calyx.

b. A stone partially located in the pelvis and partially in a calyx.

c. A stone whose exact location in a calyx has to be ascertained by a pyelotomy incision and whose removal entails an incision on the renal parenchyma.

The renal wound must be sutured properly for perfect haemostasis.

NEPHRECTOMY.—Removal of a kidney is only practicable when the other kidney, as shown by the IVP, is healthy. The indications for nephrectomy, in cases of renal stones, are:

a. Multiple stones, scattered along the kidney substance (i.e. in different calyces).

b. Branched stones, occupying the pelvis as well as different calyces, i.e. staghorn calculi. Majority of these stones can, however, be removed by incision on the pelvis and planned incisions on the kidney substance

c. Stone with pyonephrosis.

d. Stone with gross hydronephrosis, resulting in a non-functioning kidney.

e. Stone with malignancy (epidermoid carcinoma).

Apart from the above indications, nephrectomy may have to be considered as a secondary operation:

i. In severe secondary haemorrhage following nephrolithotomy, that cannot be controlled by conservative measures.

ii. In rare cases of persistent urinary fistula following pyelolithotomy, that could not be corrected by conservative surgery.

PARTIAL NEPHRECTOMY.—This means partial resection of the renal parenchyma, usually the lower pole, sometimes the upper. Such segmental resection of the kidney is possible since the blood supply to the kidney is segmentally distributed and the calyceal drainage of the kidney segmental.

The indications of partial nephrectomy, for renal stones, are:

a. Stone associated with segmental hydronephrosis in the lower calyceal stem (usually) or the upper (occasionally). Simple removal of the stone in these cases is often followed by recurrence because of stagnation and infection of urine in the dilated calyces.

b. Irrespective of any changes in the calyceal system, some surgeons employ this operation routinely for lower calyceal stones, instead of nephrolithotomy, with the idea that the lower calyx, draining against gravity, is always prone to develop fresh stones.

A careful dissection at the renal hilum exposes the corresponding polar branch of the renal artery. This is ligated and the part of the kidney, turning pale, is noted. The capsule of the kidney is stripped off from both the surfaces of the avascular area and this avascular part is excised. Bleeding from the cut renal surface is controlled by covering it with the two layers of the stripped up capsule. The rent in the pelvis, where the calyx has been cut, is carefully sutured.

NEPHROSTOMY.—This means establishing a drainage of the renal pelvis (pyelostomy) or of renal parenchyma to the exterior, on the loin, with or without removal of the accessible calculi. This operation has to be performed only rarely in cases of renal stones, i.e. under the following circumstances:

a. Stone with pyonephrosis, when the patient is too ill to stand a nephrectomy.

b. Stone with pyonephrosis in the only functioning kidney, where the kidney must be preserved.

c. Desperate cases of calculous anuria, where ureteric catheter fails to by-pass the obstruction.

URETERIC STONES

Origin and Nature.—Stones found in the ureter always originate in the kidney. Oxalate stones, because of their jagged surface, are usually seen caught in the ureter. Stones of other compositions, because of their smooth surface, quickly pass down into the bladder and are seldom detected while they are still in the ureter.

When the stone first reaches the ureter, it has its original shape and composition. Rapidly, however, it becomes encrusted with phosphates, and becomes elongated, conforming to the shape of the ureter (*date stone*). In the majority of cases, the ureteric stone is solitary but there may be associated renal stones.

Pathological Changes.—Unless a stone quickly passes down into the bladder, it is likely to produce pathological changes, as follows:

1. IMPACTION: This usually occurs at one of the sites where the ureter has an anatomical narrowing. These sites, in order of frequency, are:

a. The intramural part of the ureter (uretero-vesical junction).

b. At the crossing of the bifurcation of common iliac vessels.

c. At the pelvi-ureteric junction.

Such impaction may cause:

   i. Incomplete Obstruction.—Hydronephrosis.

   ii. Complete Obstruction:

a. Atrophy of the kidney, with compensatory hypertrophy of the opposite kidney. If, however, the opposite kidney is diseased and unable to make for the loss, the affected kidney may regain function to some extent, provided the obstruction is removed (renal counter-balance).

b. Calculous anuria (described below).

2. ULCERATION.—Mucosal ulceration may follow impaction. Ulceration may lead to subsequent fibrosis.

3. POCKET FORMATION: Sometimes the ulcer deepens and the stone lies in a pocket within the periureteric tissues. There is no longer any obstruction to the flow of urine.

4. INFECTION: Pyelitis, pyelonephritis, and cystitis (descending) may occur. If there is an associated hydronephrosis, it may be converted into pyonephrosis.

Presenting Symptoms.—The typical presenting features are pain and haematuria.

1. PAIN: This may take two forms:

   a. *Ureteric Colic.*—As described under renal stones, this occurs when the stone tries to pass down the ureter. Stones located in the upper ureter cause colicy pain whose site and radiation are the same as for renal stones. For stones located in the lower ureter, the pain often commences anteriorly and at a lower level, and its radiation along the distribution of the genito-femoral nerve is commoner. Stones impacted in the intramural part may have referred pain to the tip of the penis.

   b. *Fixed Pain.*—This occurs when the stone gets impacted at some site. Such pain often follows a colic, when the stone descending for some distance, gets impacted at some anatomically narrow segment of the ureter (usually in the pelvic part). The pain is dull-aching in nature, its site depending on the location of the stone.

2. HAEMATURIA: This often follows a colic, and its amount and duration varies.

Physical Signs

1. *Tenderness* and, sometimes, *rigidity* may be detected along the course of the ureter, particularly after a colic. In cases of stones on the right side, there may be difficulty in making a differential diagnosis from acute appendicitis.

2. *Renal lump* may be detected, if there is an associated hydronephrosis.

Special Investigations

1. URINE EXAMINATION.—*See* renal stones.

2. BLOOD BIOCHEMISTRY.—*See* renal stones.

3. STRAIGHT X-RAY.—Typically a 'date stone' is seen somewhere along the line of the ureter. The ureter commences at the level between the first and the second

lumbar vertebra (higher on the left side) and traverses in front of the tips of the transverse processes of the lumbar vertebrae. Thereafter, it runs in front of the sacroiliac joint, and then to the ischial spine. Its further course is upwards, forwards, and medially, as it goes to enter the bladder.

4. IVP—This serves many important purposes:

   a. A stone, not visible on the straight X-ray, may be demonstrated as a *'negative shadow'* in the IVP.

   b. Hydronephrosis.—Its presence and degree may be detected. Repeated IVP may be required to find if the hydronephrosis is progressive (*see* treatment).

   c. A non-functioning kidney may be detected and the function of the opposite kidney revealed.

   d. In cases of doubtful diagnosis, if an IVP shows normal excretion after an attack of colic, the patient is not suffering from ureteric colic.

5. CYSTOSCOPY:

   a. With stones in the upper two-thirds of the ureter, the ureteric orifice is normal.

   b. When a stone is located in the lower third of the ureter, the ureteric orifice may be patulous and there may be minute petechial haemorrhages around it.

   c. When the stone is just proximal to the intramural part, the areas of haemorrhage are more definite.

   d. With stones located in the intramural part, the ureteric orifice is grossly oedematous.

   e. Sometimes the stone may be found peeping through the orifice.

6. URETERIC CATHETERIZATION.—This is more important therapeutically than for investigations (*see* below). However, if a catheter is passed in, its tip is usually arrested as it reaches the stone.

Treatment

I. CONSERVATIVE TREATMENT: In the absence of infection or other complications, calculi of small size (not larger than an orange pip) are very likely to be ejected spontaneously into the bladder and then along the urine. They may be left, as such, for long periods. Usually several attacks of colic occur and the stone advances with each colic. Conservative treatment has to be abandoned in favour of active treatment under the following circumstances:

1. The stone, when first seen, is thought to be too large to pass out spontaneously, or if there is a rapid increase in the size of the stone.

2. Recurrent attacks of colic, but without advancement of the stone along the ureter.

3. Occurrence of infection.

4. Presence of signs of progressive damage of the kidney, caused by obstruction, e.g. a progressive hydronephrosis, as demonstrated by IVP, done at intervals.

II. ACTIVE TREATMENT: There are two ways by which stones may be removed:

   A. *Instrumental Removal.*—By ureteric catheters or 'baskets', or by performing ureteric meatotomy.

   B. *Operative Removal.*—Ureterolithotomy.

A. INSTRUMENTAL REMOVAL.—This procedure is likely to be successful only in cases of small stones, no larger than an orange pip. It is particularly employed for stones impacted in the lower ureter, where the ureter is narrowest.

1. *By ureteric catheterization:* A catheter is negotiated beyond the stone and is left *in situ* for 24 to 48 hours. One ml of sterile liquid paraffin is injected through the catheter just before it is withdrawn. The stone often passes out within a few hours or days. If the catheter is arrested at the level of the stone, during introduction, a second catheter is introduced through the same ureter with the hope that the dilatation caused in the ureter may help ejection of the stone. According to some surgeons, stones in any part of the ureter may be brought out by this method.

2. *By 'baskets' or special wire loops:* These are special types of stone-dislodgers, used for removal of stones from the lower ureter, under cystoscopic view.

3. *By ureteric meatotomy:* The ureteric orifice is the narrowest part of the ureter. Enlarging the opening, by cutting in an upward and lateral direction (i.e. the line of the intramural part of the ureter), with a diathermy electrode, under cystoscopic view, may help ejection of the stone.

B. URETEROLITHOTOMY

1. *For stones in the upper third* of the ureter, the exposure is the same as the standard kidney exposure. The ureter is incised longitudinally a little above or below the site of impaction of the stone, and the stone is milked out (incision at the site of impaction is likely to cause stricture formation because the mucosa is already damaged at that site; so also, if a transverse incision is made). The ureteric wound should not be sutured as this again may result in stricture formation. A ureteric catheter should be passed down through the ureteric wound to exclude the presence of any obstruction at a lower level. A drain must be put, down to the side of the incised ureter, so that the collections of urine and blood may come out.

2. *For stones in the middle third* of the ureter, an ileal approach has to be made. The incision starts at the tip of the eleventh rib and is directed to a point midway between the umbilicus and the symphysis pubis, but stops at the lateral border of the rectus abdominis. All muscles are divided in the line of the incision and so also the fascia transversalis. The peritoneum is now pushed medially and forwards, and with the peritoneum the ureter also comes up. It is identified by its shape and peristalsis. The stone is removed in the same way as described above (this is also the exposure for lumbar sympathectomy).

3. *For stones in the lower third* of the ureter, a midline suprapubic extra-peritoneal approach is made. The incision is the same as for suprapubic cystostomy. After the rectus muscles have been retracted on each side, the posterior rectus sheath (incomplete) and the fascia transversalis are incised. The peritoneum is cautiously stripped off from the bladder and the lateral wall of the pelvis, till the bifurcation of the common iliac vessels is reached. The ureter is easily identified here, as it crosses the bifurcation. It may now be traced down to its insertion into the bladder. The stone is palpated removed.

4. *Stones in the intramural part* must be approached through the bladder:

    a. By cystoscopy and ureteric catheterization (already described).

    b. By suprapubic cystostomy and approaching the ureteric orifice directly.

CALCULOUS ANURIA

This means suppression of urine due to renal stones. Hence, it is a post-renal type of anuria. Since anuria can occur only when both the kidneys have ceased functioning, calculous anuria may occur under the following circumstances (*Swift Jolly's Classification*):

1. Stones in both the ureters, causing bilateral complete obstruction.
2. Stone in one ureter, causing complete obstruction, the other kidney being:
   a. congenitally absent, or
   b. surgically removed, or
   c. non-functioning due to pathology.
3. Stone in one ureter, causing complete obstruction, the other kidney, though healthy, ceasing to function. The exact cause of this suppression of function in the healthy kidney is obscure but it is believed to be due to a reflex (*renorenal reflex*). Urinary secretion by this kidney is restored when the obstruction on the other side is relieved.

In cases of calculous anuria, the side of recent obstruction should be found out since this is the side that has to be drained immediately. This is because, in group (1) cases this is the healthier side, in group (2) cases this is the only functioning side, and in group (3) cases both the kidneys will function when obstruction on this side is relieved. The side of recent obstruction may be detected by the following points:

    a. Pain, tenderness and rigidity on the same side.

    b. Shadow of the stone on X-ray on the same side (except in group 1 cases).

    c. A palpable (enlarged) kidney, possibly disorganised by hydro-nephrosis or pyonephrosis, on the opposite side.

Treatment

A. Medical treatment for the anuria itself.

B. Immediate relief of the obstruction:

1. Catheterization of the ureter, on the side of recent obstruction, is attempted first. If the catheter can be passed above the obstructing stone, the crisis is overcome. Attempt is then made to catheterise the other ureter. Once the catheters can be passed, they are left *in situ* for 48 to 72 hours. By this time the danger is overcome. When the catheters are removed, the stones may be spontaneously eliminated into the bladder. This process may be helped if one ml of sterile liquid paraffin is injected along the catheter just before it is removed.

2. If catheterization on the side of recent obstruction fails, open drainage of the kidney, on that side, has to be attempted. This may be done by the following procedures:
   a. If the stone is known to be in the lower ureter, proximal ureterostomy is done and drainage maintained by a T-tube.
   b. If the stone is in the upper ureter or the pelvi-ureteric junction, a pyelostomy or a nephrostomy has to be done.

If, on exploration, it is found that the kidney on the side is grossly disorganised and obviously functionless, the other kidney has to be explored for drainage.

TUBERCULOSIS OF THE URINARY TRACT

Etiology.—Urinary tuberculosis, often genitourinary tuberculosis, is always a blood-borne infection from a distant focus (usually the lung, less commonly a lymph node), and the primary lesion often remains unrecognised.

The first structure, in the genitourinary tract, to be involved is:

a. Usually the kidney.

b. Occasionally the head of the epididymis.

Spread of Tuberculosis.—The process of tuberculosis, starting in the kidney, sooner or later, comes down to affect the ureter and the bladder. Such spread is brought about by the setting in of new foci by tubercle bacilli, which are brought down by either of the following routes:

i. Along the urine

ii. Absorbed by the periureteric lymphatics.

There may be involvement of the opposite kidney. This may occur in two ways:

1. The infected urine in the bladder may ascend up along the opposite ureter due to incompetence of the uretero-vesical sphincter.

2. The second kidney, like the first, is involved by blood-borne infection.

Lower down than the bladder, there may be infection in the urethra, as well as in the genital organs. The genital organs may be involved even before there has been actual involvement of the bladder and the urethra. This is believed to occur when there is a stream of infected urine, under pressure, in the urethra. This happens when there is a severe urge for micturition but there are no immediate facilities to avoid urine. In this condition the internal sphincter opens, allowing the urine to come out into the urethra and the urine is held by voluntary contraction of the external sphincter. The urine is thus under great pressure inside the prostatic urethra and may be pushed, retrograde, along the ducts which open in the prostatic urethra, viz.

1. Along the prostatic ducts, leading to tubercular prostatitis.

2. Along the common ejaculatory duct and then:

a. To the seminal vesicles, causing tubercular vesiculitis.

b. Along the vas deferens, causing tubercular lesions in the vas deferens, and then passing further retrograde to cause lesions in the tail of the epididymis. It is to be noted that tubercular epididymitis may be caused in two ways. If the infection is primary, i.e. blood-borne, the lesion usually starts at the head of the epididymis since this is the most vascular part. On the other hand, if the infection is secondary to urinary tuberculosis, the lesion starts at the tail of the epididymis, as described here.

Pathology of Renal Tuberculosis and its Types.—With the exception of acute miliary tuberculosis; which is a part of a general tubercular process, renal tuberculosis takes a chronic course.

The first stage is one of *tubercular bacilluria*. This is the stage when the lesion is too small to be detected even by a careful retrograde pyelography. However, examination of the urine suggests presence of tubercle bacilli. If treatment is started at this stage, the results are likely to be the best.

Thereafter, the kidney may undergo different macroscopic changes. These are all detailed below:

1. TUBERCULAR PYELONEPHRITIS: This is the usual type. The lesion usually commences at one pole of the kidney. The initial lesion is either at the apex or at the base of a renal pyramid. The renal pyramid is the structure to be involved first because herein lie the ends of the collecting tubules, along which the tubercle bacilli are coming out in the urine:

   a. When the lesion starts at the apex of the pyramid, the tubercles caseate, coalesce, and then ulcerate through the covering membranae of a minor calyx. This produces an *ulcerative lesion*.

   b. When the lesion starts at the base of the pyramid; the caseating tubercles aggregate together and produce a cavity in the kidney substance. This produces a *cavernous lesion*.

   c. When such a cavity bursts open into a neighbouring calyx, an *ulcero-cavernous lesion* is produced.

   Once the lesion reaches the calyx, it spreads along the pelvis to the other parts of the kidney.

2. HYDRONEPHROSIS: If, before gross damage to the kidney has set in, there is ureteric involvement and the ureteric lesions heal by fibrosis, there is an obstruction to the flow of urine and hydronephrosis occurs. In some cases such an obstruction may occur in a calyx, causing partial (segmental) hydronephrosis.

3. PYONEPHROSIS: If a secondary infection (e.g. *B. coli*) is superimposed on such a hydronephrosis, a pyonephrosis results.

4. TUBERCULAR PYONEPHROSIS OR CASEOUS KIDNEY: A slow process of caseation spreads through the entire kidney substance and kidney is converted into a cheesy mass, divided by fibrous septa, i.e. caseous kidney. In such cases the ureter is often occluded completely by a tubercular stricture and the kidney, which has already turned functionless, is completely cut off from the urinary circulation; this process is termed *autonephrectomy*. The term tubercular pyonephrosis is rather a misnomer because all secreting tissues are destroyed, so that the pelvis is not dilated and remains small.

5. PERINEPHRIC COLD ABSCESS: In some cases, a cavernous lesion in the kidney spreads peripherally along the kidney substance and eventually reaches the capsule. Thereafter, it comes out of the capsule and forms a tubercular perinephric abscess.

6. PSEUDOCALCULOUS LESION: Occasionally the renal tubercular lesions heat by partial calcification and, on the X-ray, cast a dense irregularly mottled shadow, resembling shadows of stones (*pseudocalculous shadows*).

Clinical Features

1. FREQUENCY OF MICTURITION.—This is usually the earliest, the chief and, often, the only complaint. The frequency is noticed both in the day and at night. It is progressive. The causes of frequency, in order of sequence, are as follows:
   a. *Before actual involvement of the bladder:*
      i. Enhanced spinal reflex, caused by the inflamed kidney on the act of micturition.
      ii. Polyuria, resulting from increased blood flow through the inflamed kidney.
      iii. Irritation of the bladder, caused by the caseous debris, reaching it via the ureter.
   b. *After actual involvement of the bladder:*
      i. Tubercular cystitis (the chief cause of frequency).
      ii. Secondary cystitis, superimposed on the tubercular lesions.
      iii. Progressive diminution in the capacity of the bladder due to fibrosis in its wall (*systolic bladder or thimble bladder*).

2. PYURIA.—Presence of pus in the urine makes it opalescent.

3. HAEMATURIA.—This is not a very common symptom. Its causes may be:
   a. Bleeding from a tubercular ulcer, located on a renal papilla *(painless haematuria)*.
   b. Bleeding from ulcers in the bladder *(painful haematuria)*, occurring at the end of micturition, i.e. terminal haematuria.

4. PAINFUL MICTURITION.—This occurs only when the bladder has been involved, and may be of the following types:
   a. A suprapubic pain, when the bladder is full and cannot be emptied immediately.
   b. A burning pain in the urethra while passing urine.
   c. An agonising pain, often referred to the tip of the penis, after the act of micturition.

5. RENAL PAIN.—Pain in the loin is only occasionally complained of.

6. CONSTITUTIONAL SYMPTOMS.—Evening rise of temperature, night sweating, anorexia, loss of weight, etc. are often present.

Special Investigations

1. ROUTINE URINE EXAMINATION shows an acid urine, and presence of pus cells and RBC. The same are the findings with *B. coli* infection. If the urine is sterile on ordinary culture, the possibility of tuberculosis is more.

2. SPECIAL URINE EXAMINATION, carried out to confirm the diagnosis, may be done by two types of collections:
   a. Morning mid-stream urine.
   b. Pooled urine.—The mid-stream urine of all the acts of micturition, during 24 hours, is collected in a jar and kept in the refrigerator.
   Whatever be the method of collection, the urine is centrifuged and the deposits are subjected to:
      i. Ziehl-Neelsen's staining for AFB.

    ii. Tubercular culture in Lowenstein's medium.

    iii. Guinea-pig inoculation test.

Anti-tubercular treatment should never be instituted before the diagnosis has been confirmed bacteriologically, by these methods.

3. BLOOD EXAMINATION:—TC, DC and ESR.

4. MANTOUX TEST.

5. X-RAY CHEST.

6. STRAIGHT X-RAY: Areas of calcification may be seen on the renal shadows. These are particularly marked in the pseudocalculous type of lesion.

7. IVP:

    a. The earliest and commonest finding is a hydronephrotic change in one or more minor calyces. This is due to oedema around a tubercular lesion, at the neck of the calyx, that causes incomplete intermittent obstruction to its drainage.

    b. Ulcerative lesions in the minor calyx cause an irregularity in the outline of the calyx. When this condition is generalised in the kidney, the calyceal pattern gets what is called a *'moth-eaten appearance'*.

    c. Cavernous lesions are, usually, readily apparent as cavities.

    d. A hydronephrosis is seen in hydronephrotic type of tuberculosis.

    e. With gross damage, a non-functioning kidney may be found.

8. CYSTOSCOPY: The cystoscopic findings depend on the stage of the disease:

    a. Ejection of urine from the affected side:

        i. There may be more frequent ejection,

        ii. The ejected urine may be opalescent,

        iii. There may be delay in excretion of indigo-carmine, injected intravenously,

        iv. There may. be no ejection if the ureter has been occluded.

    b. As the lowermost part of the ureter develops tubercular lesions, its oedematous mucosa may be found pouting through the ureteric orifice.

    c. The earliest sign of vesical involvement is a pallor around the ureteric orifice on the affected side, caused by oedema. Tubercles then appear, usually first on the lateral side of the ureteric orifice. They then spread towards the dome of the same side of the bladder. These tubercles coalesce and produce multiple tubercular ulcers.

    d. The ureteric orifice now takes a typical form, called 'golf-hole' ureteric orifice, i.e. it becomes displaced upwards and its mouth remains open. This is due to two factors:

        i. The lesions in the ureter cause extensive fibrosis, which not only causes stenosis of its lumen but also a longitudinal shortening. This ureteric shortening pulls the ureteric orifice up.

        ii. The lesions in the ureteric orifice itself cause fibrosis, so that its margins become thickened and rigid. The mouth of the ureteric orifice, therefore, remains open.

    e. A secondary cystitis is then superimposed on the tubercular ulcers.

    f. The bladder wall now develops extensive fibrosis and its capacity is grossly diminished, sometimes to as low as 50 ml. This condition is known as *'systolic bladder'* or *'thimble bladder'*.

9. RETROGRADE PYELOGRAPHY: The IVP findings are so inconclusive in the early stages of the disease that a retrograde pyelography is called for. In view of the fact that cystoscopy has to be performed in all the cases, a retrograde pyelography often becomes a routine procedure.

10. BLOOD BIOCHEMISTRY: Estimation or urea, NPN and creatinine, to assess renal function.

Treatment.—Tuberculosis of the urinary tract should always be treated medically; surgery is called for only to treat complications.

MEDICAL TREATMENT.—The principles of the treatment are as follows:
1. The patient should preferably be treated in a sanatorium, at least for the first few months.
2. Good nourishing diet, with high protein and vitamins.
3. Anti-tubercular drugs, preferably a 'triple attack' either with streptomycin, ethambutol and INH or refampicin, ethambutol and INH. For details of anti-tubercular treatment *see* Chapter 36 under treatment of pulmonary tuberculosis.

SURGICAL TREATMENT.—The indications for surgical intervention are as follows:
1. A tubercular cavity, which loses all communications with the pelvis, because of fibrosis at the neck of the calyx and, therefore, cannot drain itself. A cavity, which could be seen in the earlier pyelograms but subsequently gets 'missing', belongs to this group. The wall of the cavity contains so much fibrous and necrotic tissues that the antitubercular drugs do not reach the organisms in sufficient concentration so as to kill them. In these cases a renal cavernostomy is done.
2. The kidney is largely destroyed and is also acting as a source of infection for the rest of the genitourinary tract. A nephroureterectomy is performed.
3. Renal tuberculosis is complicated by severe secondary infection. Here also a nephroureterectomy is advocated.
4. A hydronephrosis has occurred due to ureteric obstruction, and the kidney is otherwise healthy. A plastic operation for the hydronephrosis may be done.
5. The capacity of the bladder is grossly diminished, causing unbearable frequency. Some form of cystoplasty is performed.

Renal Cavernostomy.—The kidney is exposed extraperitoneally and the cavity, with the thinned out cortex covering it, is easily seen. It is first aspirated with a needle and then its roof is excised with scissors. The floor and walls of the cavity are forcefully swabbed, till healthy granulation tissue is reached. The bleeding points are secured and the wound is closed without a drain (to avoid fistula formation). Urine does not leak because the cavity has no communication with the pelvis.

Nephroureterectomy.—This is performed only when the contralateral kidney is healthy. The ureter is removed along with the kidney because it is usually diseased and, if left behind, acts as a source of infection. The ureter is ligated and divided just at its entrance into the bladder. This may be done either with a separate iliac incision or by prolonging the lumbar incision downwards.

Plastic Operation.—Where there is a pelvic type of hydronephrosis a plastic procedure, e.g. Anderson-Hynes operation, may be undertaken.

Cystoplasty.—The aim of the operation is to increase the capacity of the bladder. This is done with the help of an isolated loop of bowel, which is anastomosed to the bladder and thus made a part of it. A loop of terminal ileum or a loop of pelvic colon may be used for the purpose. Accordingly, the operation is termed *ileo-cystoplasty* or *colo-cystoplasty*. A six-inch loop of gut is isolated, with its blood supply intact. This is slit up at its antimesenteric border. The dome of the bladder is incised and the two flaps, thus made, are sutured to the two flaps of the opened-out loop of the gut.

TUMOURS OF THE KIDNEY

Classification

I. Primary tumours: Almost all kidney tumours are primary.

A. *Tumours of Epithelial Origin:*
  1. Those arising from the pelvis:
     a. Papilloma.
     b. Papillary carcinoma.
     c. Epidermoid carcinoma.
  2. Those arising from the kidney substance:
     a. Adenoma.
     b. Hypernephroma, i.e. adenocarcinoma.
     c. Alveolar carcinoma.

B. *Tumours of Connective Tissue Origin:*
  1. Fibroma.
  2. Lipoma.
  3. Myxoma.
  4. Angioma.
  5. Leiomyoma.
  6. Hamartoma.
  7. Sarcoma.

C. *Tumours of Developmental Origin:*
  Wilms' tumour.

D. *Tumours of Perinephric Tissues:*
  1. Fibroma.
  2. Lipoma.
  3. Myxoma.
  4. Hamartoma.
  5. Sarcoma.

II. Secondary tumours: These are metastatic tumours from other sites and are rare, e.g.
  Sarcoma.
  Synovioma.
  Melanoma.
  Carcinoma (e.g. thyroid).

Benign tumours of the kidney are rather infrequent and often they go unrecognised. The common tumours, encountered in the kidney, are hypernephroma, Wilms' tumour, papilloma and papillary carcinoma.

PAPILLOMA AND PAPILLARY CARCINOMA

Though called papilloma, these tumours of the kidney are, often, not as benign as their name suggests. They tend to recur after excision, and have a characteristic tendency to produce seedling (daughter) deposits in the lower urinary tract, viz., the ureter and the bladder. They are, therefore, taken as potentially malignant tumours and are considered together with papillary carcinoma.

Both papilloma and papillary carcinoma arise from the epithelium of the renal pelvis. Clinically, it is often difficult to differentiate between the two. However, the two tumours can usually be differentiated on close *macroscopic examination* of the pathological specimens:

Papilloma	Papillary Carcinoma
1. The tumour is usually pedunculated.	1. The tumour is usually sessile.
2. It is less bulky. Therefore, obstruction to the renal pelvis and resultant hydronephrosis are less frequent.	2. It is usually a bulky growth inside the renal pelvis. Hence, hydronephrosis is rather common.
3. There is no infiltration into the kidney substance	3. There is infiltration into the renal parenchyma.
4. The villi, on the surface of the tumour, are well-defined.	4. The villi are less defined and so the surface has rather a velvety appearance.
5. There is no metastasis in the regional lymph nodes or elsewhere in the body.	5. Sometimes such metastases may occur.

While these differences are important, it is equally important to note that:
a. Intermediate forms, between the two, may be recognised.
b. A tumour may be of benign appearance in one part, malignant in another.
c. A simple tumour of long duration may undergo malignant change.

Microscopically, a papilloma is composed of delicate branching processes, made of a central core of fibrous and vascular tissues, surmounted by transitional epithelium (i.e. the epithelium of the urinary tract). In cases of papillary carcinoma, the cells show characters of malignancy, and there is evidence of infiltration at the base.

Spread.—Both papilloma and papillary carcinoma have a tendency to produce deposits in the lower urinary tract, viz. the ureter and the bladder (and sometimes the opposite ureter and renal pelvis). There are two views about such deposits:

1. That these are daughters or seedling deposits from the primary tumour. Pieces of tumour tissue get detached from the parent tumour, are carried in the urine, and implanted in the lower urinary tract, to produce these deposits.

2. That all the tumours are primary, the tumour having a multicentric origin. The occurrence of such multiple tumours have been suggested by many workers to be due to some carcinogenic agent in the urine.

Clinical Features.—Typically, the patient presents with *painless haematuria*. This is because the tumour is highly vascular and bleeds readily. In some cases there may be clot colic.

On examination, often no abnormality is detected. Only when there is a secondary hydronephrosis that the kidney may be palpable.

Thus, it is not only difficult to make a diagnosis but also to decide which of the two kidneys is affected.

Special Investigations

1. Urine examination shows presence of blood. Sometimes detached villi may be seen by the naked eye.
2. Blood biochemistry, to assess renal function.
3. IVP usually shows a persistent filling defect in the pelvis. Similar filling defects may also be detected in the ureter and/or the bladder.
4. Cystoscopy is essential in that:
   a. It detects the side on which the kidney is involved—blood comes out from the ureteric orifice on the affected side. Sometimes, there is bilateral involvement.
   b. It shows whether there is any tumour in the bladder.
5. Retrograde pyelography may have to be done where the IVP findings are inconclusive.

Treatment.—Nephroureterectomy has to be performed, provided the other kidney is normal. The lower ureter is usually exposed with a separate iliac incision. While resecting the ureter, its intramural part must also be removed by doing a sleeve resection of the bladder wall.

Any associated bladder tumour must be treated simultaneously.

The patient should be kept on a periodic checkup and, if there is haematuria, immediate cystoscopy has to be advised to exclude the development of a tumour in the bladder.

Comments.—Tumours of the renal pelvis (papilloma and papillary carcinoma) differ widely in structure and behaviour from those of the kidney itself. On the other hand, they have a close resemblance to the tumours of the bladder. This is because the renal pelvis and the urinary bladder develop from same structure, i.e. the mesonephros, while the kidney substance develops from another structure, the metanephros.

HYPERNEPHROMA

This is the commonest tumour of the kidney (75 per cent).

Nomenclature.—The tumour is actually an *adenocarcinoma*, arising from the epithelial cells lining the renal tubules. It may start as an adenocarcinoma (de novo) or may be the result of a malignant change in a pre-existing adenoma. The term 'hypernephroma' is a misnomer, since it indicates that the tumour is of adrenal origin. This was the view of Von Grawitz (the tumour is also known as *Grawitz tumour)*, whose inference was based on the fact that the microscopic appearance of the tumour, at least at the first sight, closely resembles that of the zona glomerulose of the adrenal cortex. Grawitz, therefore, believed that the tumour arises from the 'adrenal cortical rests' that are sometimes present in the cortex of the kidney. This view has, however, been discarded in the present days because of the following facts:

1. Hypernephroma is never encountered in other parts of the body that are known to be rather common sites of adrenal cortical rests, e.g. broad ligament of the uterus, retroperitoneal tissues and bare area of the liver.
2. Adrenal cortical tumours, arising inside adrenal gland, are almost always associated with endocrine effects, including disturbances in sex characters. No such changes have ever been seen in any case of hypernephromas.
3. The arrangement of the cells, as seen under the microscope, though resembles that of the adrenal cortex, is actually due to the mutual pressure between the cells, which are swollen and hydropic. The cells themselves are very much like the cells of the adrenal but such cells are also encountered in other situations, like the thyroid or parathyroid. Their characteristic feature is the high content of glycogen and fat.

It is now established, beyond doubt, that this tumour is actually an adenocarcinoma arising from the renal tubules. The other variety of carcinoma that may occur in the kidney is *alveolar carcinoma*, which also arises from the tubular epithelium.

Macroscopic Features.—The tumour usually arises at one pole of the kidney (more commonly the upper), so that the shape of the kidney is preserved. It is usually oval or spherical in shape, having lobulations on the surface.

Although the tumour is highly malignant, it has a false capsule, made of condensed renal tissue and fibrous tissue. From this capsule, fibrous septa run radially, like the spokes of a wheel, inside the tumour mass, dividing it into different compartments.

The cut surface has a characteristic *variegated appearance:*

a. Over wide areas the tumour mass has a golden yellow colour. Here the cells are laden with lipid material, i.e. cholesterol and fat, and glycogen.
b. Over other areas the tumour mass is red, brown, green, or black in colour, representing different stages of haemorrhage in the tumour. These haemorrhages indicate that the tumour is highly vascular.
c. Over the rest of the areas there are cysts of degeneration of various sizes.

Microscopic Appearance

i. In contrast to the variegated macroscopic appearance, the tumour has a characteristic uniform appearance under the microscope. The cells all look alike, cuboidal or columnar. They have small, rounded, and deeply-staining nuclei. The cytoplasm is clear; the clear cytoplasm indicates that it had been laden with lipid materials that were washed away by the fat-solvents during fixing. The arrangement of the cells is also very uniform—in sheets or long columns of solid cells.
ii. There are big areas of haemorrhage.
iii. There are numerous blood vessels. Over some areas the vascular endothelium is missing and, through these gaps, tumour cells gain entrance into the vessels. This explains the quick venous spread of the tumour.

Spread

1. DIRECT SPREAD
   a. *By Continuity.*—The tumour, arising in the cortex and the adjacent parts of the medulla, is limited within its false capsule for certain length of time. Spreading peripherally, it breaks through the capsule and involves the surrounding kidney tissue. Extending centrally, it encroaches upon and ulcerates into the calyces, causing haematuria.
   b. *By Contiguity.*—Coming out of the kidney, the tumour infiltrates into the perinephric fat and fascia. Further spread may involve the neighboring organs, particularly the colon.

2. LYMPHATIC SPREAD.—This is also an important route of spread, especially when the tumour has involved the perinephric tissues. Spread occurs to the nodes at the hilum of the kidney and then to the para-aortic nodes.

3. VENOUS SPREAD.—This is the commonest and the most dangerous form of spread. Spread may occur to lungs, liver, bones, and central nervous system, in that order of frequency.

While metastases may be multiple, hypernephroma has often a tendency to cause solitary metastatic lesion. Thus, in the lung, while there may be multiple peripheral deposits, solitary central deposits (known as *cannonball metastasis)* are equally encountered. Similarly, solitary bone lesions may occur.

The venous spread may occur in two ways:
   a. *Venous Embolism.*—Cells are detatched from the tumour and float along the veins.
   b. *Venous Permeation.*—This is characteristic of hypernephroma. The tumour tissue, gaining entrance into small veins, through the gaps in their endothelial lining, grow inside the lumen of these vessels, *keeping continuity* with the parent tumour. Gradually they grow into the bigger veins and ultimately into the renal vein, progressing just as a finger advances through the gloves. In advanced cases solid columns of tumour tissue grow along the inferior vena cava into the right side of the heart. Occasionally, these solid columns of tumour tissue, inside the renal vein, may cause obstruction to the testicular vein. This results in varicocele and pain in the testis. This, however, is likely to occur only with the left-sided tumours, because it is on the left side only that the testicular vein drains into the renal vein (on the right side the testicular vein drains directly into the inferior vena cava and is obstructed only if the inferior vena cava is blocked).

Clinical Features.—The patient is usually between 30 and 50 years of age. Males suffer more frequently than the females (2 : 1). The presenting features are as follows:

1. PAINLESS HAEMATURIA.—This is the usual presenting symptom. Two-thirds of the patients present only with this symptom.

2. PAIN may be present in one-third of the cases. Even, when there is a painless haematuria, there may be clot-colic.

3. LUMP.—The patient may present with a renal lump. Lumps are palpable earlier with tumours at the lower pole of the kidney and with right sided tumours, for obvious reasons.

4. METASTATIC GROUP.—Some patients have no complaint as regards the primary tumour and present with features of metastasis only, e.g.

    a. Lung.—Pain chest, haemoptysis, cough, dyspnoea, fever.

    b. Liver.—Jaundice, ascites.

    c. Bone.—Pain, pathological fractures.

5. PYREXIA.—Some patients present with irregular and persistent pyrexia. This may be due to:

    a. Absorption of necrotic materials from the tumour.

    b. Metastasis in the lung.

6. ATYPICAL FEATURES.—Some patients may present with features like:

    a. Varicocele or pain in the testis on the left side.

    b. Anaemia, much more than that can be accounted for by the haematuria.

    c. Polycythaemia vera.

Special Investigations

1. URINE EXAMINATION.—Presence of blood.

2. BLOOD BIOCHEMISTRY, to assess renal function.

3. X-RAY CHEST for evidences of metastasis (either a solitary central cannon ball deposit or multiple peripheral deposits).

4. STRAIGHT X-RAY of the abdomen may show an enlarged kidney shadow.

5. IVP may show the following features:

    a. Absence of some minor calyces and amputation of a major calyx, because of invasion by the tumour mass. In very advanced cases the whole calyceal pattern may be lost and may be represented by only a few small irregular strips of the dye.

    b. Around the area of the tumour, the unaffected calyces may show a 'spider leg' deformity, i.e. they are elongated, narrowed and curved.

    c. When the tumour comes down to the pelvis, a filling defect is seen in the pelvis. The remaining part of the pelvis and the unaffected calyces are pushed upwards or downwards, according to the situation of the tumour at the lower pole or the upper pole of the kidney respectively.

6. CYSTOSCOPY.—Ejection of blood, from the ureteric orifice on the side on which there is a palpable kidney, is very suggestive of hypernephroma.

7. RETROGRADE PYELOGRAPHY.—This is particularly useful when the IVP findings are inconclusive.

8. ULTRASONOGRAPHY may be helpful in the diagnosis.

Treatment.—The patients may be divided into 3 groups:

GROUP A: The operable cases, i.e. cases where the kidney, with the tumour, is resectable and there is no metastases. The treatment is nephrectomy, followed by radiation.

GROUP B: The inoperable cases, i.e. either the tumour is too fixed to allow a nephrectomy or there are metastases. Treatment is only palliative, i.e. radiotherapy with or without chemotherapy.

GROUP C: The debatable group, where the primary growth is resectable and there is a solitary metastasis. This group is important since hypernephroma often produces a solitary metastasis. For these cases, many surgeons advocate nephrectomy, together with a radical surgery for the solitary metastasis, e.g. lobectomy or pneumonectomy for a lung lesion, amputation for a bone metastasis.

Nephrectomy for Hypernephroma.—As there is considerable infiltration and as the tumour is big in the majority of the cases, a standard lumbar extra-peritoneal approach usually fails to provide adequate exposure. Commonly, therefore, a transperitoneal approach is preferred (either a paramedian incision, extended as T or L, or an oblique or transverse incision).

As the tumour is mobilised, there are chances of tumour tissues being pumped along the renal vein and causing early postoperative metastases. To avoid this danger, attempts should be made to ligate the renal vein before manipulating the tumour. In practice, once exposure has been obtained and it has been ascertained that the tumour is resectable, the renal pedicle is ligated. The ureter may be cut at any convenient level but the renal vein should be ligated flush with the inferior vena cava, so that any tumour-thrombus, present in the vein, is removed along with the kidney.

While the kidney is being resected, all perinephric fat and fascia should be included in the resection, since direct spread to these tissues is as important as venous spread.

The patient must have a course of postoperative radiation for destruction of any left-out tumour tissue.

WILMS' TUMOUR

Origin.—This is a tumour of developmental origin and is also known as *nephroblastoma* or *embryoma*. As regards its origin, there are several views:
1. It arises from an aberrant sex cell.
2. It originates from some misplaced embryonic rudiment.
3. It is a remnant of the Wolffian body (i.e. arises from mesonephros).
4. It arises from the metanephros (the predominance of connective tissue in the tumour supports this view).

Incidence
1. This is a tumour of the childhood, practically never occurring after the seventh year. Probably, in most of the cases, it originates before birth.
2. Almost always the tumour is unilateral; only rarely both the kidneys are affected.

Macroscopic Appearance.—The tumour usually starts at one pole of the kidney. It has no capsule. It is greyish white in colour and not very vascular. The consistency varies—the softer the tumour the more malignant it is. Areas of haemorrhage and cystic degeneration are present.

Microscopic Appearance.—There is structure of a mixed tumour, i.e. presence of both connective tissue and epithelial tissue, the former usually predominating. Some of these elements are radiosensitive while others are radioresistant. This is why the results of radiotherapy are variable.

Spread
1. DIRECT SPREAD.—This is quick and extensive. There is rapid involvement of the renal parenchyma, so that, very early in the course of the disease, the kidney

loses its shape. The renal pelvis is encroached and obliterated but is not actually invaded till very late. On the other hand, peripheral spread is quick. The tumour comes out of the confines of the renal capsule and spreads to the peritoneum, retroperitoneal tissues and omentum. Often the major part of the abdomen is occupied by the tumour mass.

2. LYMPHATIC SPREAD is rare.

3. VENOUS SPREAD is early and important. Lungs, liver and bones may be involved.

Clinical Features

1. LUMP.—Usually the only complaint is a rapidly-growing abdominal lump. Attention to the lump is sometimes drawn after a trauma.

2. CACHEXIA.—Anorexia and loss of weight.

3. PYREXIA is often an associated feature.

4. HAEMATURIA is late and rare. It imposes a bad prognosis since it indicates that the tumour has invaded the renal pelvis.

Special Investigations

1. IVP—Though difficult to be done in a child, it usually provides the diagnosis. There is a gross irregularity of the whole calyceal pattern, and sometimes only a few calyces are seen. In advanced cases there may not be any pyelographic shadow on the affected side.

2. X-RAY CHEST, to exclude metastasis.

Treatment

1. Majority of the surgeons advocate immediate nephrectomy, followed by radiation. Operation should be undertaken as soon as the diagnosis has been made.

2. Some surgeons prefer a course of pre-operative radiation. Its advantages are:
   a. The tumour diminishes in size so that the operation becomes a little easier.
   b. The vascularity of the tumour is diminished.
   c. The diagnosis is confirmed.

The disadvantages of the procedure are:
   a. There is delay in undertaking the operation.
   b. There is often a radiation-fibrosis of the lung.

Prognosis.—This is good when the child is below one year of age—there is 80 per cent 5-year cure.

After the age of one year, there is only 30 per cent 5-year cure.

When recurrence occurs, it usually takes place within one year. Therefore, if one year has passed after the operation, chances of recurrence are remote and the child may be said to be cured.

EXPOSURE OF THE KIDNEY

As the kidney is situated deep in a recess inside a rigid cage and as it has a short pedicle, no single incision will meet all the requirements. The approach to the kidney may be as follows:

A. EXTRAPERITONEAL APPROACH.—This is the usual approach, particularly for removal of stones, since the peritoneal contents are not handled and the urine, which is often infected, cannot soil the peritoneal cavity. The extra-peritoneal approach may be:

1. Standard lumbar approach (the usual).
2. Approach through the bed of the 12th rib, i.e. excising the rib.

B. TRANSPERITONEAL APPROACH.—This is necessary for big renal swellings, particularly in malignancy.

C. THRACO-ABDOMINAL APPROACH through the 12th rib.—This is sometimes used for huge renal swellings, particularly for malignant tumours occupying the upper pole of the kidney.

Standard Lumbar Approach.—Of all the approaches to the kidney, this is the most commonly used, hence it is called standard.

The patient lies on the healthy side, with the bridge of the table between the costal margin and the iliac crest, so that when the bridge is elevated, a wider space is created between the costal margin and the iliac crest on the side to be operated. The lower limb next to the table is kept flexed at the hip and the knee, while the other lower limb is kept extended. The upper limb next to the table is kept extended, while the other upper limb, in flexion, is supported on a hand-rest and receives the infusion.

The incision starts from the renal angle and extends forwards and medially, bisecting the space between the costal margin and iliac crest. It is directed towards the anterior superior iliac spine, not necessarily reaching it. In the posterior part of the wound, the latissimus dorsi and, deep to it, the serratus posterior inferior are cut along the line of incision and, still deeper, the lumbar fascia is incised. In the anterior part, the flat muscles of the abdomen, viz. external oblique, internal oblique, and transversus abdominis are similarly cut along the line of incision. In difficult cases, the lateral border of the erector spinae may be incised a little. In cases of more difficulty, the 12th rib may be mobilised and retracted upwards. If there is still any difficulty, a subperiosteal excision of the 12th rib has to be done, care being taken not to open up the pleura (the lower reflection of the pleura usually crosses this rib horizontally in its middle third, but may be lower down).

The peritoneum is stripped forwards and medially. The pararenal fat is now seen, and a dissection through it exposes the renal fascia. Incision through the renal fascia and a little dissection of perirenal fat exposes the smooth glistening surface of the kidney. A blunt finger dissection, all round the kidney, fully mobilises the organ, which can now be brought to the surface, unless the pedicle is short. The adrenal, being located in a separated fascial compartment, is left undisturbed.

During closure, the muscles should be carefully sutured and this is done in two layers.

Transperitoneal Approach.—This has to be employed in cases of (a) large renal lumps, particularly malignancy, and (b) intraperitoneal injury causing rupture of the kidney (because the other kidney can be examined). The incison may be:

1. Paramedian, if required extended as 'T' or 'L', cutting through the rectus.
2. Oblique muscle-cutting.

3. Transverse, at the level of the umbilicus, cutting through the rectus and the lateral abdominal muscles.

On opening the abdomen, the posterior parietal peritoneum is incised along the lateral border of the colon and the corresponding flexure. The colon with the mesocolon (and the duodenum on the right side) is mobilised forwards and medially to expose the anterior surface of the kidney and its pedicle.

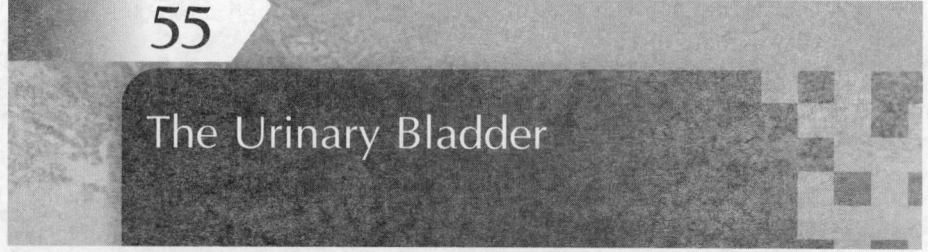

55

The Urinary Bladder

Embryology.—The bladder develops from two sources:
1. The major part of the bladder develops from the urogenital sinus, i.e. the ventral part of the cloaca.
2. The trigone develops from the Wolffian ducts.

In describing the development of the kidney (Chapter 54), it has been said that the caudal ends of the two Wolffian ducts (which develop from the mesonephros) open into the cloaca. The cloaca is divided by a transverse septum (urorectal septum) into two parts. The ventral part is called the urogenital sinus, from which the bladder develops. The Wolffian duct, on each side, opens into the urogenital sinus.

It has also been said that the ureteric bud originates from a little above the actual end of the Wolffian duct. The part of the Wolffian duct from this point up to its lowermost end is important since it is from this part that a number of structures develop:

a. The common ejaculatory duct—representing the lowermost end of the Wolffian duct on each side.
b. The trigone of the bladder.
c. The upper part of the prostatic urethra, upto the utricle.

Structures (b) and (c) develop by fusion of the terminal parts of the Wolffian ducts of the two sides (Fig. 55.1). It is for this reason that the two ureters open at the base of the trigone, one on each side, and the common ejaculatory ducts open into the prostatic urethra on either side of the utricle.

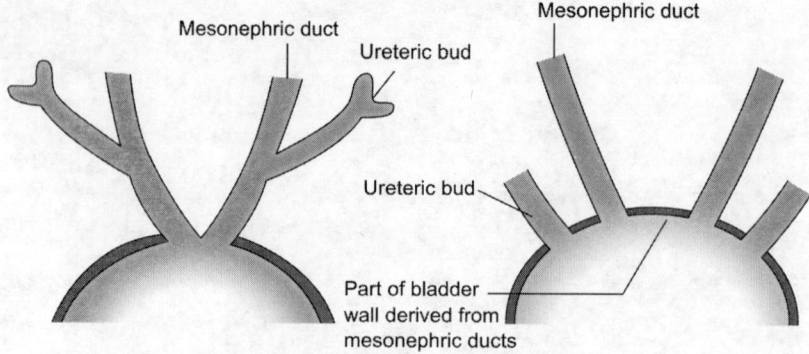

Fig. 55.1: Absorption of the mesonephric ducts. Note that the absorbed ducts (the thick line) form the trigone of the bladder and also the posterior wall of part of the urethra.

The urogenital sinus is continued cranial wards into the *urachus,* whose cavity extends as a diverticulum into the umbilical cord. Normally its lumen obliterates and it persists simply as a fibrous cord, called the *median umbilical ligament.*

Anomalies of the urachus may occur:

i. *Patent Urachus.*—The cavity of the whole length of the urachus persists, resulting in a form of umbilical fistula (which may discharge urine).

This has been described in details under umbilical fistula (Chapter 47).

ii. *Urachal Diverticulum.*—The vesical end of the urachus persists, forming a diverticulum at the apex of the bladder.

iii. *Urachal Cyst.*—The central part of the urachus persists and forms a midline, extraperitoneal, infra-umbilical cyst.

iv. *Urachal Remnants.*—At the apex of the bladder there may be remnants of the urachus, from which adenocarcinoma may originate.

ECTOPIA VESICAE

Origin.—This is a congenital malformation and is also known as *extrophy* or *extroversion* of the bladder. It is due to incomplete development of:

a. Infra-umbilical part of the anterior abdominal wall (due to failure of somatopleure to meet).

b. Anterior wall of the bladder (due to failure of the forward growth of the anterior part of the cloacal membrane).

Description.—The defect is spherical or oval, lying in the midline, below the umbilicus. Because of the intra-abdominal pressure, the posterior bladder wall is projected through the gap as a deep-red bulge, which bleeds readily. Urine is found to trickle continuously. As the exposed mucous membrane is gently pushed back:

a. The firm edges of the gap in the anterior wall is well felt.

b. The pale trigone of the bladder, located below the prolapsed part, is seen. Thus, the ureteric orifices are found situated near the lower rim of the protrusion.

Associated Anomalies

1. The symphysis pubis is absent. The pubic bones of the two sides are widely separated and kept united by a thick fibrous band. The patient, therefore, develops a waddling gait.

2. The umbilicus is either absent or is displaced downwards, and is involved in the scar tissue.

3. Genitalia:

   a. In the males:

      i. There is an epispadias (i.e. dorsal wall of urethra is absent).

      ii. The penis is drawn up and fixed to the abdominal wall.

      iii. The scrotum may be ill-developed.

      iv. The testes may be ectopic.

      v. The prostate and seminal vesicles are rudimentary or absent.

   b. In the females:

      i. The clitoris is cleft.

      ii. There may be maldevelopment of the uterus and vagina.

4. Herniae.—Umbilical and/or inguinal herniae may be present.

5. Anal sphincters may be lax.

Complications
1. Erosion and ulceration of the prolapsed mucosa, with haemorrhage.
2. Infection.—Cystitis, ascending pyelitis.
3. Neoplastic change.—Adenocarcinoma.

Treatment.—There are two principal methods of approach:
A. Diversion of the urine with excision of the bladder (or of its mucosa alone).
B. Reconstructive procedures.

A. DIVERSION OF THE URINE WITH EXCISION OF THE BLADDER:
1. *Colonic Transplantation.*—The ureters are transplanted into the colon. A few months later, the bladder (or its mucosa only) is excised. The wound is closed by plastic methods or is allowed to granulate.
2. *Ileal Conduit.*—A loop of ileum, 6 to 8 inches in length, is isolated, with its vascularity intact. Into this loop the ureters are transplanted. One end of the ileal loop is brought to the surface of the abdomen and the urine comes out through it. An ileostomy bag is fitted for collection of the urine. Later, the bladder is excised.
3. *Lowsley's Operation.*—This operation is advocated by some surgeons, provided the anal sphincters have continence. The gut is divided at the recto-sigmoid junction and the lower cut end is closed. The ureters are transplanted into this isolated lower segment, so that the rectum acts as the bladder. The upper cut end of the gut is mobilised down to the perineum and is placed just in front of the anus here. The anal sphincters, therefore, control both the original anal canal (now the outlet for the urine) and the new anal canal, made by the mobilised sigmoid colon. Later, the bladder is excised.

B. RECONSTRUCTIVE PROCEDURES:
Various procedures have been tried to reconstruct the bladder and the anterior abdominal wall. These have been successful in many cases but difficulty lies in making a sphincteric control of the reconstructed urethra. These procedures are, therefore, still in the experimental stage.

BLADDER STONES

Origin
1. The stone may be formed in the kidney and then comes down to the bladder. In the bladder, the stone increases in size.
2. The stone may originate in the bladder. Such stones are very often due to:
   a. Cystitis (often secondary to obstruction).
   b. Foreign bodies, on which the urinary crystalloids are deposited. The tip of a self-retaining catheter is one of the best examples *(catheter-stone).*

According to the nature of the urine in which the stones are formed, they may be classified as follows:

1. PRIMARY.—Where the urine is sterile. Stones coming down from the kidney usually belong to this category. Chemically, the stones are oxalate, uric acid and urate, cystine, etc.
2. SECONDARY.—Where the urine is infected. Stones originating in the bladder usually belong to this category. Chemically, these stones are usually phosphates.

Clinical Features.—The incidence is eight times commoner in the males. Some stones, particularly those located in diverticula or post-prostatic pouch, do not produce any symptom and are called *'silent stones'*. The majority, however, are associated with frequency of micturition, pain, haematuria, and sometimes dysuria.

Frequency is the commonest complaint. Often, after micturition, the patient is not fully satisfied that the bladder is empty.

Pain is felt over the hypogastrium and is often, typically, radiated to the tip of the penis (or labia majora). A child is often found screaming and pulling at the prepuce frequently, particularly after micturition. This radiation is from the sensitive trigone, where the stone lies.

Both frequency and pain tend to be exaggerated by movements and exercises, and to diminish with rest in recumbency. This is because the stone falls away from the sensitive trigone when the patient lies down (the rest of the bladder is insensitive).

Haematuria (terminal, i.e. occurring at the end of micturition) is a common complaint and is either due to cystitis or due to abrasion of the vascular trigone, caused by the stone.

Dysuria is sometimes complained of. The patient notices sudden interruption in the flow of urine during the act of micturition. This occurs when the stone comes down and blocks the internal meatus. The patient can usually start the flow again with change in posture. Acute retention is very rare.

Bimanual abdomino-vaginal or abdomino-rectal examination may sometimes reveal large bladder stones. In females, even moderate size stones may be felt per vagina.

Special Investigations

1. URINE EXAMINATION.—RBC, pus cells, and typical crystals may be found.
2. STRAIGHT X-RAY.—The stones are almost always seen on the X-ray. The abdomen must be included in the X-ray, to exclude possibilities of associated renal or ureteric stones.
3. IVP.—This may have to be done to determine normalcy of the kidneys.
4. BLADDER SOUNDING, with a bladder sound, is only rarely done nowadays.
5. CYSTOSCOPY should be done as a routine, particularly to eliminate other associated pathology, e.g. enlarged prostate, diverticula, tumours of bladder, etc.

Treatment

1. Very small stones may pass out spontaneously with the urine.
2. Usually suprapubic cystolithotomy has to be performed (see suprapubic cystolithotomy forceps, under Chapter on instruments).
3. In selected cases and with expert hands, litholapaxy may be done (see lithotrite, under Chapter on instruments).

TUMOURS OF THE BLADDER

Types.—95 per cent of bladder tumours are epithelial, originating in its mucous membrane.

5 per cent of the tumours are connective tissue growths, e.g. angioma, myoma, fibroma, sarcoma.

Classification of Epithelial Tumours

I. BENIGN, i.e. Papilloma (villous papilloma)
    1. Solitary.
    2. Multiple (papillomatosis).

II. MALIGNANT, i.e. Carcinoma
A. *Primary:*
    1. Papillary Carcinoma (commonest)
       a. De novo.
       b. Secondary to papilloma.
    2. Infiltrating Carcinoma
       a. Nodular.
       b. Ulcerative.
    3. Adenocarcinoma (rare—2%).
B. *Secondary:*
    1. From the kidneys papillary tumours (papilloma and papillary carcinoma) may spread to the bladder, by the process of implantation.
    2. From prostatic cancers a direct spread may occur.
    3. From rectum (in males), uterus (in females) and sigmoid colon (in either sex) a direct spread may occur.

VILLOUS PAPILLOMA

Nature.—As in the renal pelvis, these tumours are not as benign as their name suggests. They show a definite tendency to recur and produce *seedling deposits.*

Number.—There are two types of cases:
1. Solitary papilloma.
2. Multiple papilloma.—The condition is also known as diffuse papillomatosis as multiple growths are found scattered over a relatively wide area of the bladder.

Site.—There is a special predilection for the base of the bladder, particularly at or near a ureteric orifice.

Macroscopic Appearance.—The tumour is usually pedunculated (90 per cent) but may sometimes be sessile. The surface, however, shows well-defined villi, i.e. finger-like branching filaments (hence called villous). When there is a well-formed pedicle, the tumour has a close resemblance to a red sea anemone, with its delicate tentacles moving to and fro in the urine.

Microscopic Appearance.—There is a central fibro-vascular core, which is prolonged to the centre of all the villi. This core in the stem as well as those in the branches are surmounted by transitional epithelium (i.e. the epithelium of the urinary tract).

Clinical Features
1. Characteristically, the patient presents with haematuria—painless, profuse, but periodic. As the bleeding is from the bladder, the haematuria is usually terminal,

i.e. occurring at the end of the micturition (when the bladder actively contracts). This may be confirmed by the three-glass test.
2. If the growth obstructs the internal urethral meatus, the patient may suffer from dysuria.

BLADDER CANCERS

Etiology.—Though majority of bladder cancers originate in a previously healthy bladder, there are definitely some predisposing factors:
1. Industrial hazards.—Workers in aniline dye factories, rubber, industries, gas works and printing factories are more prone to develop bladder cancers. Particularly important are the aniline dyes and it is believed that betanaphthylamine is the chief carcinogenic agent.
2. Schistosomiasis (bilharziasis).
3. Leukoplakia.

Site
1. One-third of the tumours originate in the trigone, often near a ureteric orifice.
2. One-third of the tumours occur in the lateral wall.
3. The remaining one-third occur in:
   a. the bladder neck ⎫ in equal distribution
   b. the posterior wall ⎭
4. The dome and the anterior wall are only rarely involved.

Number.—About 25 per cent cases show multiple tumours. Such tumours are usually of the papillary type and generally show a low degree of malignancy.

Description of the Cancers

PAPILLARY CARCINOMA.—This is the commonest form of bladder cancer. It may be of two types:
a. De novo, i.e. originating primarily as a cancer.
b. Secondary malignant change in a villous papilloma.
   A papillary carcinoma differs from a villous papilloma in the following respects:
   i. The villi are stunted, closely packed, and thickened—resembling a cauliflower. They often appear to arise directly from the bladder wall.
   ii. The growth has a more sessile form.
   iii. The central and superficial parts of the tumour often undergo necrosis because of impairment of blootf supply. Hence, ulcerations are often seen on the surface.
   iv. There is usually an accompanying intractable cystitis, predisposed by the presence of the necrotic tissues.
   v. The tumour tends to spread into the depth and infiltrate the bladder wall to some extent. Thus:
      a. The bladder wall, immediately adjacent to the tumour, becomes vascular and oedematous.
      b. Submucosal nodules appear around the growth, and these may ulcerate.
      c. Fresh tumours may appear in other parts of the bladder.
      d. There may be ureteric obstruction if there is infiltration around the ureteric orifice.

INFILTRATING CARCINOMA.—These tumours are so called because, unlike papillary cancers, which tend to enlarge superficially rather than infiltrate into the depth, these growths rapidly infiltrate into the bladder wall. There are two *macroscopic types:*

a. *Ulcerative Type.*—A typical malignant ulcer, raised from the surface, having rolled out everted margins.

b. *Nodular Type.*—A sessile red nodule, often lobulated. Later, ulcerations may occur on the surface.

These tumours are sometimes called epidermoid cancers. Actually, however, there may be two *microscopic types:*

i. *Transitional cell carcinoma.*—The cells are arranged in solid masses, supported on a fibrous stroma.

ii. *Squamous cell carcinoma.*—These are believed to occur in mucous membrane that has changed to a squamous cell type, following leukoplakia.

ADENOCARCINOMA.—This is a rare tumour, occurring in less than 2 per cent of cases. It may originate in:

a. Remnants of urachus at the bladder dome.

b. Tubular glands in the trigonal mucosa at the bladder base.

c. Area of cystitis cystica.

Spread of Bladder Cancer

1. DIRECT SPREAD.—Starting in the mucosa, the tumour gradually infiltrates into the submucosa and the musculature. Thereafter, it involves the surrounding fat. Still later, the neighbouring organs may be involved, infiltrating cancers are more important in this respect than papillary growths.

2. IMPLANTATION AND CONTACT SPREAD:
   a. When the bladder is full.—Implantation or 'seedling' deposits occur.
   b. When the bladder is empty.—Contact or 'kissing' metastases occur.
   These types of spread are particularly common with papillary cancers.

3. LYMPHATIC SPREAD.—This occurs only after the muscle coat has been involved. At first the nodes on the external surface of the bladder are involved. Spread may, thereafter, occur to the internal iliac nodes.

4. VENOUS SPREAD is late and rare. Lungs and liver may be involved.

5. ALLANTOIC SPREAD.—This may rarely occur in cases of growth at the dome of the bladder; deposits may occur on the peritoneum.

Staging.—According to the extent of direct spread, *Marshall* recommended the following method of staging:

STAGE 0: Growth limited to the mucous membrane.

STAGE 1: There is no spread beyond the submucous coat.

STAGE 2: There is no extension beyond the musculature.

STAGE 3: There is involvement of perivesical fat.

STAGE 4: There is extension to neighbouring organs.

Clinical Features

1. Characteristically, the patient presents with haematuria. This is at first periodical but, thereafter, becomes continuous.

2. With the onset of cystitis, frequency of micturition and painful micturition set in. There may be strangury at the end of micturition.
3. If the growth obstructs the internal urethral meatus, dysuria may occur. Similarly, if the growth obstructs a ureteric orifice, pain in the loin (kidney) may occur.
4. Late in the course of the disease, with the involvement of the nerves, there may be referred pain to the hypogastrium, groins, perineum and thighs.

Special Investigations for Bladder Tumours

1. URINE EXAMINATION:
   a. Shows presence of blood.
   b. Demonstration of cancer cells is confirmatory.
2. CYSTOSCOPY shows the growth and permits a biopsy.
3. CYSTOGRAPHY (excretory, i.e. IVP, or retrograde) usually shows the growth as a persistent filling defect.
4. BIMANUAL EXAMINATION UNDER GENERAL ANAESTHESIA.—A recto-abdominal examination in the males and a vagino-abdominal examination in the females, performed under general anaesthesia, gives a good idea about the degree of infiltration, i.e. helps in staging.

Treatment of Bladder Tumours

A. Villous Papilloma.—These may be treated by either of the following methods:
1. CYSTODIATHERAPY.—This means destruction of the growth by fulguration, i.e. coagulation-diathermy. This may be performed by two routes:
   a. *Transurethral.*—The electrode is introduced through a cystoscope and fulguration is performed under cystoscopic vision. The procedure is repeated at intervals of 3 to 4 weeks, till all visible tumours have been destroyed.
   b. *Suprapubic.*—A suprapubic cystostomy is performed and the growth is fulgurated under direct vision. This is performed for growths which are too large, too numerous, or too inaccessible for the transurethral procedure.
2. EXCISION.—A suprapubic cystostomy is done and the growth is excised under direct vision. If the growth is pedunculated, its pedicle is divided with a diathermy knife. If the growth is sessile, it is excised together with one cm of healthy mucosa all round.

B. Carcinoma.—These may be treated by surgery, by radiation, or by a combination of the two. The nature of surgery as well as that of radiotherapy is also variable. The different methods employed are described below.

I. SURGERY:
   1. *Excision with a Resectoscope.*—This is a transurethral approach and is especially indicated for papillary carcinoma with a little infiltration. Special types of resectoscope, however, are required for the procedure to be accomplished.
   2. *Partial Cystectomy (Segmental Resection).*—This means removal of a segment of the bladder wall in its entire thickness, including the tumour and sufficient healthy tissue on all sides. It is indicated for a solitary tumour or a localised group of malignant tumours, provided the affected part is sufficiently mobile to be resected. After excision, the bladder wall is repaired. If one ureter is

involved, its lower end is included in the resection and the cut ureter is reimplanted into the bladder.

3. *Total Cystectomy.*—This means resection of the whole bladder, together with the seminal vesicles and the prostate. The ureters are transplanted into the colon or into an ileal loop. This is an extensive surgery and is only occasionally performed. It is indicated for:

   a. Infiltrating growth, involving both the ureteric openings or the internal urethral meatus.

   b. Growth too extensive to be removed by other means.

II. RADIOTHERAPY.—This may be used alone or in combination with surgery. There are three different methods of radiotherapy.

1. *Interstitial Radiation.*—This is designed to destroy a tumour without damaging the surrounding normal tissues. The radioactive materials that may be implanted are radon seeds, gold198 grains, tantalum192 wires, cobalt60 or yittrium90. This form of radiation is used in two different types of growths:

   a. In early growths. The growth is excised and the radioactive material is implanted into any residual tumour or into closely adjacent bladder wall. The implantation, again, may be made in two ways:

      i. At an open operation on the bladder

      ii. Through a cystoscope, with a special introducer.

   b. In cases of papillary carcinoma, situation near the base or neck of the bladder, a diathermy coagulation of the growth is done, combined with implantation of the radioactive material.

2. *External Radiation.*—WIth the advent of supervoltage and cobalt60 therapy, deep penetrating and concentrating radiation at the desired site is possible with sparing of the skin and surrounding tissues. This method is largely being used nowadays, more so because of the simplicity of the procedure.

3. *Intracavitary Radiation.*—Filling the bladder with colloidal solutions of gold198 or yittrium90 has been tried. Good results are being claimed because of minimal absorption and sufficient local action.

THE BLADDER MECHANISM IN LESIONS OF THE SPINAL CORD

Nerve Supply to the Bladder.—Micturition is partly a reflex and partly a voluntary act. In considering the reflex part, the sympathetic and parasympathetic supply to the bladder has to be studied, while for the voluntary part, the somatic innervation to the sphincter urethrae (i.e. the external sphincter) has to be taken into account (Fig. 55.2):

1. The *sympathetic fibres* are derived from the spinal segments T_{12}, L_1 and L_2. They pass to the hypogastric plexus, from where post-ganglionic fibres reach the bladder wall.

2. *The parasympathetic innervation* is derived from S_2, S_3 and S_4 segments of the spinal cord by way of the pelvic nerves (*nervi erigentes*). These fibres pass through the hypogastric plexus; without interruption (c.f. the sympathetic), to reach the bladder wall. In the wall of the bladder they form synapses with short post-ganglionic fibres.

3. The *somatic innervation* is to the external sphincter (and not to the bladder itself). The fibres are derived from S_2, S_3 and S_4 spinal segments. They are carried by

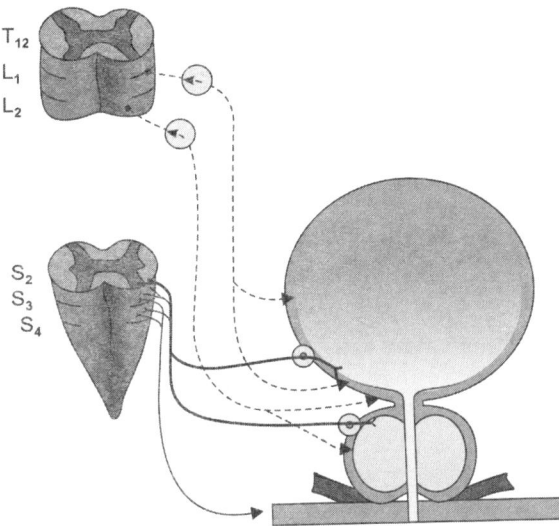

Fig. 55.2: Nervous control of the bladder. The dotted lines indicate the sympathetic (hypogastric nerve) innervation, the thick lines indicate the parasympathetic innervation (nerve erigentes), and the plain line shows the somatic innervation (pudendal nerve).

the internal pudendal nerves, which also provide sensory fibres to the posterior urethra.

The Act of Micturition.— The old belief that the sympathetic fibres are the 'filling' nerves of the bladder, and the parasympathetic fibres, the 'emptying', is no longer tenable. It is now established that it is only the parasympathetic nerves which are responsible for the bladder activity. Micturition is a reflex act, mediated through the S_2, S_3 and S_4 segments of the spinal cord.

Stretching of the bladder muscle (when the bladder is filled with about 450 ml of urine) initiates a reflex through the parasympathetic nerves that results in:

a. Contraction of the detrusor muscle with consequent rise in the intravesical pressure.

b. Simultaneous relaxation of the internal sphincter (sphincter vesicae).

c. Subsequent involuntary opening of the external sphincter (sphincter urethrae).

Once micturition starts, contraction of the detrusor is maintained, by a reflex arc, through the sacral segments of the spinal cord. This reflex is triggered by the flow of urine over the sensory nerve endings in the lining of the urethra.

The Control of Micturition

1. While the sympathetic fibres convey afferent painful stimuli of over-distension from the bladder to the brain, neither the sympathetic nor the parasympathetic convey any cortical impulse from the brain to the bladder.

2. The sphincter urethrae is the muscle concerned in the closure of the urethra. It is interesting to note that although its active contraction (i.e. stoppage of micturition) is under voluntary control (via the internal pudendal nerves), there is no corresponding voluntary power to relax it.

3. This voluntary control of micturition is established in early childhood and the pattern of the bladder behaviour from that time is described as normal. The higher centre that normally inhibits reflex micturition is located in the cerebral cortex. From here the inhibitory fibres pass down to the S_2, S_3 and S_4 segments of the spinal cord, and from there, via the internal pudendal nerves, to the sphincter urethrae.

It may thus be summarised that, while the normal act of micturition is initiated by the stretching of the detrusor and effected by the parasympathetic, it can be inhibited by cerebral control on the sphincter urethrae, if the time and place are not suitable for the act.

The Bladder Mechanism after Cord Injury.—Following complete or incomplete lesion of the spinal cord, the bladder passes through various stages of dysfunction, which may be tabulated as follows:

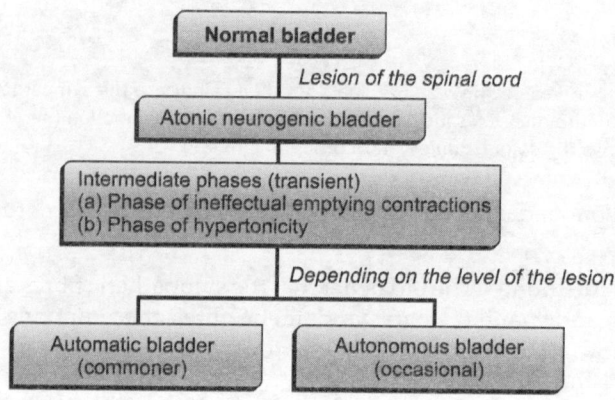

Atonic Neurogenic Bladder.—This is the condition of the bladder immediately after the injury to the spinal cord and is due to spinal shock. The detrusor muscle becomes paralysed, the internal sphincter is contracted tightly, and the external sphincter is relaxed. The only factor that allows evacuation of the bladder is the elasticity of its walls, which means that there is an overflow-incontinence as the bladder is greatly distended. As the sympathetic innervation remains intact, the patient can appreciate that the bladder is full. This phase usually lasts for some days but may be prolonged to months, and the length of this phase depends much on the treatment instituted (*see* below).

Intermediate Phases.—As the stage of spinal shock is overcome, before the bladder mechanism proceeds to the final nature of dysfunction (depending on the level of the lesion), it passes through two intermediate stages:

a. *Phase of ineffectual emptying contractions.*—There are contractions of the detrusor muscle but the internal sphincter remains in spasm. Small amounts of urine are voided frequently.

b. *Phase of hypertonicity.*—The detrusor muscle goes into spasm, and both the internal and the external sphincters relax. There is an incontinence.

The intermediate phase lasts only for a few days and ultimately the bladder becomes either an automatic bladder or an autonomous bladder, depending on the level of the spinal lesion.

Automatic Bladder.—This develops when the lesion is situated above the level of the centre of micturition in the spinal cord, i.e. above S_2 segment. The intact cord centres, though they are isolated from the cortex, assume the task of emptying the bladder at intervals. Hence the condition is known as *cord-bladder*. When the bladder fills to certain limit, the detrusor muscle contracts reflexly and the bladder empties—hence this is also known as *reflex bladder*. These automatic contractions of the bladder occur usually at intervals of one to four hours, the period being longer if infection is excluded. However, emptying is usually never complete and the amount of residual urine varies, and this by itself may invite infection.

This is the condition of the bladder, therefore, where the higher central control has been lost, i.e. a condition seen in the early childhood when the central control has not yet been established.

However, unless the lesion is very high up in the spinal cord (T_{4-6}), the sympathetic innervation remains intact and the patient can feel that the bladder is full. Thus a few minutes' warning for micturition is often available and the patient can prepare himself without wetting the bed. Sometimes there are *bizarre warnings,* e.g. flushing, sweating, etc.

That the bladder is going to take up an automatic function from the stage of atonic neurogenic bladder are indicated by:

a. Erections of the penis (i.e. return of bulbocavernous reflexes).

b. Return of anal reflexes.

c. If urine trickles by the side of the catheter when it is clamped.

Autonomous Bladder.—This occurs when the spinal lesion is situated:

a. at a level that will destroy the centre of micturition (S_{2-4}), or

b. in the cauda equina.

The internal sphincter is atonic and allows an incontinence. Contraction of the detrusor is dependant only on the nerve plexus and ganglia situated in the bladder wall, and such contractions are often inefficient.

The result, therefore, is a constant dribbling. However, the bladder can be emptied by manual compression. In any case, there is accumulation of residual urine. This results in infection as well as back pressure on the kidney, i.e. hydronephrosis.

Treatment

A. IN THE ATONIC STAGE.

1. A self-retaining soft rubber catheter (Foley's) is introduced per urethra, as early as possible, with the strictest possible asepsis. The catheter should be introduced early since over-stretching of the detrusor muscle prevents early return of its activity. Moreover, bed-wetting is avoided, which is so essential in preventing bed-sores.

2. A high fluid intake is advised.

3. Systemic alkalisers and antibiotics are administered to prevent infection.

B. IN THE STAGE OF AUTOMATICITY

1. Bladder-training is commenced. The catheter is clamped and released at regular intervals. These intervals are gradually lengthened.
2. The catheter is then removed and the patient passes urine himself, per urethra, at intervals. As has already been stated, the patient knows when the bladder is distended and thus gets sufficient time to make himself ready for the act.
3. Fluids are given only during the daytime and none after the evening.

C. IN THE STAGE OF AUTONOMY

1. If the patient can use his hands, manual expression of the bladder. If the abdominal muscles are not paralysed, their contraction is also helpful in evacuating the bladder.
2. Otherwise, the patient has to have a permanent suprapubic cystostomy or a life-long urethral catheter. Alternatively, a urinal may have to be worn permanently.

56

The Urethra and the Penis

Embryology.—The ventral wall of the cloaca, to start with, has no mesoderm in it. It consists only of two layers, ectoderm and entoderm, and this combination is known as the *cloacal membrane*. In the adult, the cloacal membrane corresponds roughly to the area between the symphysis pubis and the tip of the coccyx.

The lower margin of the urorectal septum or cloacal septum (the septum which divides the cloaca into urogenital sinus anteriorly and rectum posteriorly) reaches the cloacal membrane and divides it into two parts—an anterior *urogenital (urethral) membrane* and a posterior *anal membrane*. Subsequently, the urogenital membrane breaks down and bladder acquires an opening on the perineum.

Towards the cephalic end (i.e. the symphysis pubis end) of the cloacal membrane, there is a heaping up of the ectoderm. The elevation thus made, is primarily known as the *genital tubercle*. The tubercle gradually enlarges and is then known as the *phallus*. In the males the phallus enlarges progressively and develops into the penis, while in the females it does not enlarge so much and forms the clitoris.

By the time the urogenital membrane breaks down, the urogenital sinus extends forwards, towards the caudal aspect of the phallus. Therefore, when the urogenital membrane breaks down, the urogenital sinus (i.e. the bladder) opens not only on the perineum but also on the caudal aspect of the phallus. On the caudal aspect (i.e. the undersurface) of the phallus this opening makes a groove, which is called the *urethral groove*. The right and left margins of the groove are termed *urethral folds*. As the phallus (i.e. the penis) grows in length, the urethral groove also prolongs along its undersurface. Thus, the external opening of the urogenital sinus comes to be located on the surface, at the base of the glans penis. Simultaneously, the urethral folds of the two sides start fusing with each other. This process of fusion starts from the back and proceeds forwards. The penile part of the urethra is thus formed. A solid pencil of ectoderm grows inwards from the undersurface of the glans; subsequently it canalises and forms the terminal part of the urethra.

Hence, the male urethra develops from three sources:

1. From the internal urethral meatus to the prostatic utricle.—From the urogenital sinus (more precisely, the terminal parts of the two Wolffian duct, fused together). This represents the whole length of the female urethra.
2. From the prostatic utricle to the base of the glans penis—From the urethral groove, by fusion of the urethral folds.
3. The glandular part.—From the surface ectoderm of the glans.

HYPOSPADIAS

This is the commonest congenital anomaly of the urethra. The external urethral orifice is ectopic, and is located at some point on the undersurface of the penis or in the perineum.

Types

1. *Glandular.*—The ectopic opening is situated on the undersurface of the glans penis. There is, however, a blind depression at the site of the normal urethral opening, on the summit of the glans. Rarely there may be a channel of communication between the ectopic opening and the normal. In the commonest type of glandular hypospadias, the ectopic meatus is located on the coronary sulcus of the penis, and this is popularly known as *coronal hypospadias.*
2. *Penile.*—The urethra opens somewhere on the undersurface of the penis.
3. *Penoscrotal.*—The urethral opening is located at the junction of the penis and the scrotum, i.e. at the base of the penis.
4. *Perineal.*—The scrotum is split in the middle and the ectopic meatus is situated between the two halves.

Origin

1. The glandular type is due to failure of canalisation of the glans.
2. The other varieties are due to failure of fusion of the urethral folds, in varied degrees (*see* embryology).

Associated Abnormalities

1. In all the types, the *ectopic meatus is often narrow,* and in many cases there may be urinary obstruction of varying degrees.
2. Excepting for the glandular type (which is due to a failure of canalisation of the glans), all the other varieties may be looked upon as an absence of the urethra and the corpus spongiosum, distal to the ectopic orifice. These absent structures are represented by a fibrous cord. By the pull of this cord the penis is curved downwards, i.e. there is a bowing *(chordee).* The more proximal the ectopic meatus is, more prominent is the bowing.
3. Since the growth of the phallus and that of the urethral groove occur simultaneously, failure of the urethral groove to proceed forwards is associated with a *small penis.*
4. The inferior aspect of the *prepuce is poorly developed* (so, hypospadias and phimosis can never co-exist). The upper aspect of the prepuce looks like a hood.
5. The perineal type is sometimes associated with *bilateral undescended testes.* In these cases a male child may be mistaken for a female.

Treatment.—The coronal variety (which is the commonest type) requires no treatment except an intermittent dilatation of the meatus, if there is urinary obstruction.

In all other types, operative treatment has to be undertaken. The operation is done in two stages:

1. Straightening of the penis.
2. Construction of the urethra.

STRAIGHTENING OF THE PENIS.—This is undertaken at about the age of two years. The idea is to excise the whole length of the fibrous cord that causes bowing of the penis. A transverse incision is made on the ventral surface of the penis, about half an inch distal to the ectopic orifice. The fibrous cord is picked up and is excised in its whole length, detaching it from the corpora cavernosa. When this is done, it is found that the ectopic orifice recedes further proximally, but this is immaterial. The transverse skin wound is sutured *longitudinally.*

CONSTRUCTION OF THE URETHRA.—This should be postponed until the child is five to six years of age. Numerous operations have been described, majority of them employing some form of skin flap for the purpose of reconstruction. Of these, the *Denis Browne's operation* is the most commonly practised. A U-shaped incision is made through the skin on the ventral surface of the penis. The incision starts from the base of the glans, extends backwards a little away from the midline on one side, then carried round and behind the ectopic orifice, and thereafter continued forwards on the other side of the midline up to the base of the glans, thus isolating a strip of skin, about 1 cm wide. The lateral skin flaps, on the two sides are now widely mobilised, so that they may be apposed in the midline. They are superimposed on the isolated skin flap (which, therefore, acts as the roof of the urethra) to form the floor of the reconstructed urethra. To achieve this, without tension, a relaxing longitudinal incision is made through the skin along the whole length of the dorsum of the penis. The urethral opening is thus brought forwards to the base of the glans. Finally, an area of the glans is made raw and, through this, the terminal part of the urethra is made.

Temporary Urethrostomy.—The urine must be diverted from the reconstructed urethra till it heals, a matter of about two weeks. This is done by performing a *perineal urethrostomy,* through which a self-retaining catheter drains the bladder. The operation is done at the same stage in which the reconstruction is done. When the urethral sutures take, the catheter is withdrawn and the perineal wound heals by itself quickly.

EPISPADIAS

This is a rare condition in which the urethra opens on the dorsal surface of the penis. There may be three types:
1. Glandular.
2. Penile.
3. Total, i.e. associated with ectopia vesicae, the penis being curved upwards.

Origin.—The condition probably occurs very early in the foetal life due to a cranial shift of the cloacal membrane, so that the genital tubercle (phallus) develops on its undersurface.

Treatment.—The treatment is operative. The edges of the groove are made raw and sutured to each other over a catheter *(Duplay's operation).*

RUPTURE OF THE URETHRA

Classification.—Rupture of the urethra occurs in its two distinct parts, viz.
a. Bulbous part.
b. Membranous part.

The nature of the trauma, causing the injury, and the clinical features are widely different in these two groups. However, in either of the types, the rupture may be classified as follows:

A. The rupture may be:
 1. Incomplete,
 2. Complete,

depending on whether the whole circumference of the urethra has been torn. When the rupture is incomplete, the two cut ends cannot move away from each other, so that a catheter can be passed through. In case of complete rupture, the two ends move away from each other, so that a catheter cannot be negotiated.

B. The rupture may be:
 1. Partial,
 2. Total,

depending on whether the injury has occurred through partial thickness or the whole thickness of the urethral wall. This classification is of a little importance.

RUPTURE OF THE BULBOUS URETHRA

Trauma.—The bulbous urethra is located very superficially in the perineum, so that even a relatively minor trauma at the perineum may cause its rupture.

Effects

A. DISCONTINUITY of the urethra which causes:
 1. Retention of urine.
 2. *Extravasation of urine*, if the patient tries to pass urine. The extravasation occurs in the subcutaneous plane, where the bulbous urethra is located. The extravacated urine *cannot* pass:
    a. Beyond the midperineal point, because of the attachment of the Colles's fascia to the triangular ligament.
    b. Down the thighs, since the fascia of Scarpa blends with the fascia lata of the thigh, just below the inguinal ligament.
    c. Into the inguinal canals, because the canal is closed by the inter-columnar fibres and the external spermatic fascia, at the superficial inguinal ring.

 The fluid, therefore, extravasates in front:
  i. Into the tissues of the scrotum.
  ii. Into the superficial tissues of penis.
  iii. Into the anterior abdominal wall, between the deeper layer of the superficial fascia (Scarpa's) and the external oblique aponeurosis. In this plane it may ascend even up to the thorax.

B. HAEMORRHAGE from the cut urethra, causing:
 1. Urethral bleeding.—Blood comes out along the external urethral meatus.
 2. Perineal haematoma.

Clinical Features

1. There is a typical history of trauma on the perineum, following which the patient complains of acute pain in the perineum, retention of urine, and bleeding per urethra.

2. A perineal haematoma is seen. As the patient tries to pass urine, no urine can be voided, a few drops of blood comes out, and extravasation of urine occurs.
3. The bladder is full.

RUPTURE OF THE MEMBRANOUS URETHRA

Trauma.—The membranous urethra is located deep in the pelvis and, therefore, well-protected. Only a severe trauma can cause its rupture. Actually, such a rupture is only secondary to a much serious injury, like fracture of the pelvis or avulsion of the symphysis pubis. The rupture usually occurs at the junction of the prostatic and membranous parts, and is caused either by the splintered rami or by a drag on the perineal membrane. The rupture is usually complete. Associated with the pelvic injury, there is tear of the puboprostatic ligaments (these ligaments bind the prostate forwards to the pubis). Since the rupture is almost always complete and since the pubo-prostatic ligaments are torn, the proximal part of the urethra, together with the prostate, swings upwards and backwards, while the lower cut end is kept fixed by the perineal membrane. Thus a wide gap is created between the two ends of the urethra.

Effects
A. The major effects are those of the bigger injury, viz. fractured pelvis.
B. DISCONTINUITY of the urethra which causes:
   1. Retention of urine.
   2. Extravasation of urine, if the patient tries to pass urine. This is a deep extravasation, occurring in the pelvis and the retroperitoneal tissues, which may extend between the peritoneum and the fascia transversalis (a deep extravasation, like this, also occurs in cases of extraperitoneal rupture of the bladder).
C. HAEMORRHAGE from the cut urethra, causing:
   1. Urethral bleeding.—Blood comes out along the external urethral meatus.
   2. Periurethral haematoma, which blends with the haematoma of fracture pelvis.

Clinical Features.—The urethral injury may be primarily overlooked because of the more serious injury, i.e. fracture pelvis, unless this is kept in mind. Bleeding per urethra is an important diagnostic sign. In some cases, at least, the injury is first recognised when the patient is seen suffering from retention of urine.

Palpation of the abdomen reveals an ill-defined lump, which is due to the haematoma of the fracture pelvis. To palpate the full bladder separately through this haematoma is a difficult task. In many cases exploration is undertaken on a doubtful diagnosis either of rupture of the membranous urethra or of an extraperitoneal rupture of the bladder. If on exploration, the bladder is seen to be even moderately full, its wall must be intact and the injury is in the urethra.

A rectal examination may fail to palpate the prostate in its usual place (described above).

Special Investigations
1. *X-ray of the pelvis,* to confirm the diagnosis and to ascertain the nature of fracture.
2. *Urethrography* is often very helpful in doubtful cases.

TREATMENT OF RUPTURED URETHRA

The patient must be advised *not* to try to pass urine. If there is a painful distension of the bladder, suprapubic puncture, with a long thin needle, may be done.

Membranous urethral rupture is almost always complete and operative repair has to be undertaken.

Bulbous urethral rupture may be complete or incomplete. A soft rubber catheter should be passed, very gently, under strictest aseptic measures. Forceful introduction of a catheter damages the urethra further. Similarly, introduction of sepsis enhances the chances of stricture formation, a stricture being always apprehended after a rupture.

When the catheter can be passed in, the rupture is incomplete. The catheter is kept *in situ* for about a week, by which time the injury heals. Antibiotics must be given while the catheter is in position. Subsequently, the patient has to undergo dilatations.

In those cases of bulbous urethral rupture where a rubber catheter cannot be passed and in all cases of membranous urethral rupture (these are cases of complete rupture), operative repair has to be undertaken.

I. OPERATION FOR RUPTURE OF BULBOUS URETHRA.—A vertical incision is made on the perineum and the torn urethral ends are searched for. The distal end can easily be made out by passing a bougie from the external urethral meatus. For identification of the proximal end (if it is not available after careful searching), a suprapubic cystostomy may have to be performed to pass a retrograde bougie from the bladder. When the two ends are identified, they are sutured to each other. Suturing is not done along the whole circumference since this results in a bad stricture. Only the roof of the urethra is repaired with a few interrupted stitches, while the floor is left unsutured. This means that a complete rupture is turned into an incomplete one. The rest of the treatment is, therefore, like that of an incomplete rupture, i.e. a penile catheter is kept *in situ* for one to two weeks. If a suprapubic cystostomy has been done, this is also maintained for a few days. A course of antibiotics and postoperative dilatations are obligatory.

II. OPERATION FOR RUPTURE OF MEMBRANOUS URETHRA.—This part of the urethra is not directly accessible, so end-to-end repair is impracticable.

A suprapubic cystostomy is done and a retrograde bougie is passed down from the bladder. A urethral bougie is passed in from the external meatus. Blind attempts are made to make the tips of the two bougies touch each other at the site of the rupture. When this is possible, as the retrograde bougie is gradually withdrawn along the bladder, the urethral bougie is made to follow it, pass the rupture, into the posterior urethra. The left index finger, introduced through the internal urethral meatus, from the bladder, may be used with convenience, instead of the retrograde bougie.

A long narrow rubber tube is fitted to the tip of the urethral bougie, which is now peeping at the bladder. As the bougie is withdrawn, one end of the tube comes out at the external urethral meatus. To this end is anchored the tip of a narrow calibre Foley's catheter. As the rubber tube is drawn back into the bladder, the tip of the Foley's catheter enters the bladder. The Foley's catheter, with its balloon inflated, is kept *in situ*. This acts as a splint on which the torn urethra heals, since suturing of the torn ends is not possible. A mild traction on the catheter, in the postoperative period, brings the proximal urethral segment downwards and forwards (which has otherwise a tendency to float upwards and backwards), and keeps it in apposition with the distal segment for the purpose of healing. This method of repair is popularly known as the *rail road method.*

The Foley's catheter and a suprapubic catheter are kept for two weeks. Postoperative antibiotics and future dilatations are obligatory.

To facilitate postoperative dilatations, a long silk thread may be tied to the tip of the Foley's catheter and brought out through the suprapubic wound. At dilatation, as the Foley's catheter is withdrawn, this silk passes through the urethra. The tip of the dilator is tied to the urethral end of the silk. As the silk is pulled from the suprapubic end, the dilator easily passes in.

URETHRAL STRICTURE

Causes

I. CONGENITAL, including pin-hole meatus.

II. TRAUMATIC:
   A. *External Trauma*
      1. Bulbous part.
      2. Membranous part.
   B. *Operative Injury*
      1. Operation for filarial scrotum.
      2. Operation for rectal resection.
   C. *Post-instrumental*
      1. Prolonged use of an indwelling catheter.
      2. Forceful introduction of metal catheters, bougies, cystoscope, etc.
   D. *Postoperative*
      1. After amputation of penis, particularly partial amputation.
      2. After prostatectomy.

III. INFLAMMATORY.—Most commonly gonococcal. Very rarely due to tuberculosis or chancre.

In older days, inflammatory strictures (following gonorrhoea) were the commonest. In the present days, traumatic strictures (following urethral rupture) and strictures following amputation of penis are much the commoner.

Classifications

A. Strictures may be:
   1. Solitary.—The commonest site is the proximal part of the bulbous urethra.
   2. Multiple.—If there are multiple strictures, the deepest is the narrowest.
B. Strictures may be:
   1. Annular.
   2. 'Bridle' type.
   3. Elongated, irregular, and tortuous.

C. Strictures may be:
1. Passable
2. Impassable

depending on whether a bougie can be negotiated through the stricture or not.

D. Strictures may be:
1. Permeable
2. Impermeable

depending on whether urine is allowed to trickle through. With an impermeable stricture, therefore, there is retention of urine.

E. Strictures may be
1. Uncomplicated.
2. Complicated (*see* below)

Complications of Stricture

1. Retention of urine.
2. Periurethral abscess.
3. Urethral fistula
4. Urethral diverticulum
5. 'Back pressure' effects, e.g. hydronephrosis, infection, stone formation, etc.
6. 'Straining' effects, e.g. hernia, haemorrhoids, prolapse, etc.

Special Investigations

1. *Urethroscopy.*—To ascertain the size and situation of a stricture.
2. *Urethrography.*—In addition to the above, may show a diverticulum, false passage, fistulous tract, etc.

Treatment.—This may be discussed under two headings:
  I. Treatment for passable strictures.
  II. Treatment for impassable strictures.

Treatment for Passable Strictures

A. DILATATION OF THE URETHRA, with metal bougies, is the usual procedure. The dilatation may be (i) intermittent or (ii) continuous, the former being most commonly practised.

Intermittent dilatation means dilatation at intervals. To start with, the dilatation is done frequently but gradually the interval is increased. Finally, dilatation is advised only once a year, throughout the life of the patient, and this is popularly known as *birthday dilatation.*

In some cases, during dilatation, it may not be possible to pass bougies, excepting those with very narrow calibre. In these cases, after the maximum possible dilatation is done, a rubber catheter of corresponding size may be introduced and kept in position for a few days. This procedure often causes a 'vital' dilatation of the stricture, so that, at a subsequent dilatation, bigger size bougies may be negotiated. This procedure is called *continuous dilatation.*

In very bad cases of stricture (causing acute retention), where even narrow bougies fail, dilatation may be tried with very thin bougies made of plastic or gum-elastic. These are called 'filiform bougies'. They are passed in, with rotatory movements, one after another, and it is likely that one of them may find its way through the stricture, so that the retention is relieved.

B. INTERNAL URETHROTOMY.—This is done with an internal urethrotome. The small curved knife of the instrument can be controlled from the handle. The urethrotome is introduced along the urethra, through a passable stricture. Thereafter, as the instrument is being withdrawn, the blade is made to work, thus cutting the stricture *from inside outwards.*

Treatment for impassable Strictures.—Operative treatment has to be undertaken. The different types of operation advocated are:

A. External urethrotomy (Wheelhouse's operation).
B. Urethroplasty
C. Excision of the stricture with reconstruction of urethra

A. EXTERNAL URETHROTOMY.—This operation requires the use of two special instruments:

1. *Wheelhouse's Staff* (Fig. 56.1): This instrument is virtually a long straight director, with a groove on one of its surfaces. This groove does not reach the tip of the instrument, from where it falls short by about half an inch. On the opposite surface of the instrument, at its tip, there is a hook.

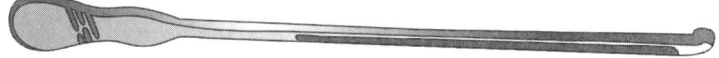

Fig. 56.1: Wheelhouse's staff

2. *Telae's Gorget* (Fig. 56.2): This is an angulated instrument. One blade has an olive-point at its tip, from which there is a groove, which gradually widens as it passes backwards.

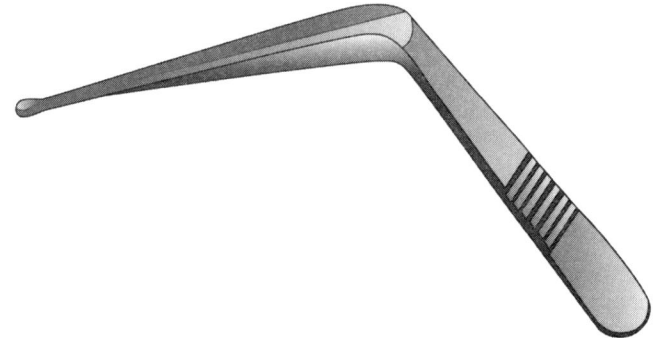

Fig 56.2: Telae's Gorget

With the patient in the lithotomy position, the lubricated Wheelhouse's staff is passed through the urethra, with the groove of the instrument towards the perineal skin. The instrument stops where its tip encounters the stricture.

A vertical incision is made over the groove of the staff near its tip. Since in the majority of cases the stricture is located in the proximal part of the bulbous urethra, the incision usually lies on .the perineum. As the knife touches the groove of the staff, the urethra has been opened. This is the part of the urethra just distal to the stricture and not the stricture itself (c.f. internal urethrotomy). The staff is withdrawn a little, and rotated by 180°, so that the hook is now used to retract the upper end of the incision. One Allis' forceps is applied to each flap of the cut urethra. Thus, a diamond-shaped space is created, at the lower end of which lies the stricture.

With a probe-pointed director an attempt is now made to find out the urethral opening in the stricture. When this is possible, the vertical urethral incision is prolonged backwards on the groove of the director. This cuts the stricture *from outside inwards* (c.f. internal urethrotomy). A Tealae's gorget is now passed, on the probe-pointed director, into the bladder. The probe-pointed director is withdrawn and urine is found coming out.

The Wheelhouse's staff is withdrawn and a rubber catheter is passed through the external urethral meatus. As its tip comes to the wound, it is guided over the groove of the Tealae's gorget, into the bladder.

The skin wound is closed but the cut urethral margins are left unsutured (to avoid further stricture formation).

In those cases where the urethral opening in the stricture cannot be made out, a suprapublic cystostomy is done. A retrograde bougie is passed down through the internal meatus and its tip is made to pass through the stricture, from inside. The stricture is cut on this bougie and then the Telae's gorget is pushed in.

Postoperatively, the patient must undergo intermittent dilatation.

This operation is gradually getting obsolete because of recurrence of stricture and is being replaced by various types of urethroplasty and reconstructive procedures (*see* below).

B. Urethroplasty.—In this operation the urethra, from the external meatus to the stricture, including the stricture itself, is slit up along its ventral surface, thus making an artificial hypospadias. At a second stage the hypospadias is repaired by the Denis Browne's method.

C Excision of the stricture with reconstruction of the urethra.—The whole length of the stricture is excised ((its two ends being identified with the help of bougies— one passed from the external meatus and the other retrograde from the bladder). Continuity is restored thereafter by one of the following methods:

1. End-to-end anastomosis, if possible (the anterior urethra with corpus spongiosum having been mobilised backwards).

2. *Pull-through operation.*—This is done when the posterior urethral segment is short. The anterior urethra is pulled through the dilated lumen of the posterior urethra and anchored to the bladder (*Badenoch's operation).*

3. Skin tubes, made to replace the gap in the urethra.

PHIMOSIS

Definition.—This is a condition in which the prepuce cannot be retracted behind the corona glandis.

Types

A. CONGENITAL.—What is commonly called a congenital phimosis is actually an acquired one, where the process of normal opening up of the prepucial sac has not occurred (in newborn babies the glans cannot be exposed but, as the child grows a little, this becomes possible). The vast majority of cases belong to this group. A true congenital phimosis is one where the prepuce balloons out at the very first micturition. The so-called congenital cases, mentioned above, are the result of either an ammoniacal dermatitis or forceful attempts to stretch, i.e. traumatic. Hence, forceful stretching should never be attempted at infancy.

B. ACQUIRED.—This is caused either by narrowing of the prepucial orifice or by adhesions developing between the prepuce and the glans penis. The causes may be:

1. *Traumatic.*—Gross trauma to the prepuce and foreskin may cause fibrosis, resulting in narrowing of the prepucial opening. Many of the so-called cases of congenital phimosis should be included in this group, these having resulted from forceful stretching.
2. *Inflammatory.*—Balanitis (inflammation of the glans) or posthitis (inflammation of the prepuce) or more commonly, balano-posthitis (a combination).
3. *Neoplastic.*—Carcinoma is often followed by phimosis.

It should be noted that:

a. An elderly patient, coming with an acquired phimosis, is either suffering from recurrent balanoposthitis (hence diabetes should be carefully investigated for) or from carcinoma of the penis.
b. Just as a congenital phimosis predisposes to carcinoma, equally, carcinoma may cause an acquired phimosis.

Complications

1. Paraphimosis.
2. Recurrent balano-posthitis.
3. Carcinoma (*see* carcinoma of penis).
4. Prepucial stone (rare).

Treatment

1. *Prophylactic.*—Forceful stretching of the prepuce, in infancy, should be avoided. A prepucial sac, which would have normally opened up, gets established as a phimosis by this over-enthusiasm.
2. *Curative.*—Operative treatment should always be undertaken. The operation is called *circumcision.* The distal part of the prepuce and the foreskin (usually the distal two-thirds) are excised all round. Adhesions between the prepuce and glans penis are carefully dissected, till the corona glandis is well exposed. The cut margins of the prepuce and the foreskin are then re-sutured to each other by interrupted stitches. The frenal artery has to be carefully ligated. Small superficial veins are also encountered and secured.

PARAPHIMOSIS

This is a complication of phimosis and results when the tight prepuce is forcefully retracted behind the glans penis. It cannot be returned back to position and remains as a constricting band behind the corona glandis. There is gross oedema and swelling of the prepuce as well as the glans. Gangrene may ensue, unless the prepuce is replaced in position. There is a great discomfort and pain.

Treatment

1. In the early cases reduction may be done, one ml of a weak solution of hyaluronidase is injected into each lateral aspect of the swollen prepuce. The swelling reduces considerably due to absorption of the oedema fluid and reduction is often possible. Alternatively, multiple punctures may be made in the oedematous prepuce, to drain the fluid out, and then reduction is done. Sometimes, anaesthesia may be necessary.

2. In the majority of cases operative treatment has to be undertaken under general anaesthesia. A narrow cuff is excised from the dorsal aspect of the constricting band. Reduction is now easily done. Circumcision may be performed immediately or at a later date.

PEYRONIE'S DISEASE

This is a condition in which there is fibrosis in one corpus cavernosum, causing a localised induration. Rarely, there may be calcification or ossification. The etiology is unknown.

The patient presents with the complaint of curving of the penis, on erection. At the onset there may be an associated pain during erection, but this usually disappears. On palpation, the indurated mass is easily made out.

Unfortunately, no treatment is available for the condition. In some cases, however, a spontaneous regression occurs after a long period. The patient should be reassured that there is no malignancy, of which he is often afraid of. Injection of hydrocortisone into the fibrous plaque and excision of the plaque are being tried. Some surgeons claim good results. Usually, however, the results are unsatisfactory.

CARCINOMA OF THE PENIS

Predisposing Factors

1. *Phimosis.*—Curiously enough, circumcision, performed soon after birth (as in the Jews), offers almost total immunity against carcinoma developing in the future. On the other hand, if the circumcision is delayed (as in the Mohammedans), there is no such immunity. Irritation by the accumulated smegma is the probable predisposing factor.

2. *Balano-posthitis.*—Recurrent attacks of balano-posthitis definitely predisposes to carcinoma.

3. *Papilloma* of the penis, if long standing, may turn into carcinoma.

4. *Leukoplakia* of the glans penis, comparable to that of the tongue, may predispose to carcinoma.

5. *Paget's disease* of the penis, a rare condition, in which there is a raw glazy glans, may lead to carcinoma.

Site of Origin.—In order of frequency, the starting points are:

1. Inner surface of the prepuce, by the side of the corona glandis.

2. Corona glandis itself.
3. Glans penis.
4. Foreskin—occasionally.
5. Skin of the body of the penis—rarely.

Microscopic types
1. Almost always the growth is a squamous-cell carcinoma, with well formed cell nests.
2. Adenocarcinoma may rarely occur; the growth arises from the smegma-secreting glands, i.e. *Tyson's glands.*
3. Anaplastic carcinoma may occur.
4. Malignant melanoma may rarely occur.
5. Basal cell carcinoma is extremely rare.

Macroscopic Types
1. Proliferative type.
2. Ulcerative type.
3. Flat infiltrating type.

In the first two varieties, which are much the commoner, the growth is raised well above the surface and usually the tumour is well-differentiated.

In the flat infiltrating type the growth is often anaplastic.

Secondary Carcinoma of the Penis.—This is a rare condition, the primary source being the prostate, bladder, or rectum. The involvement is usually by a retrograde lymphatic or retrograde venous embolism (via the dorsal vein of the penis).

Spread of Carcinoma of Penis

1. DIRECT SPREAD.—For a long lime the growth is limited locally. Whatever be the starting point, prepuce or gains, both these structures are quickly involved. Thereafter, the foreskin is infiltrated and the growth erodes out through it. Gradually, more and more of the skin is involved.

The fascial sheath of the corpora cavernosa resists infiltration for a long period, so that the growth is limited to the glans for many months. Once, however, the corpora have been involved, there is a rapid spread along the shaft of the penis.

However extensive the growth may be, it does not infiltrate into the urethra.

2. LYMPHATIC SPREAD.—Majority of the lymphatics from the glans, prepuce, foreskin, and the body of the penis drain into the superficial inguinal nodes (horizontal chain) of both the sides. Some of the lymphatics from the glans penis drain into the deep inguinal nodes. While the enlarged inguinal nodes may be metastatic, in many cases the enlargement is inflammatory, secondary to the gross infection in the fungated primary lesion.

The efferents from the inguinal nodes drain into the external iliac nodes, which may be involved but, as a rule, late.

3. VENOUS SPREAD.—This occurs only rarely and then very late in the course of the disease. The primary growth, in such cases, is often anaplastic. Involvement of distant organs is, therefore, rare.

Clinical Features.—The patient is commonly above 40, but younger people may be affected.

Either the patient has a congenital phimosis or he acquires a phimosis because of narrowing of the prepucial orifice by carcinomatous fibrosis. Thus, often, the patient does not see the growth. He just complains of an irritation inside the prepucial chamber, caused by the collection of the discharges there. A little amount of seropurulent discharges also comes out through the prepucial opening.

It is at this stage that the surgeon often performs a dorsal slit and finds the growth. Otherwise, the growth erodes through the foreskin and becomes visible by itself. There is an ugly-looking, offensive-smelling growth or ulcer, very painful, and associated with profuse purulent discharge.

Inguinal nodes show metastatic or inflammatory enlargement (sometimes difficult to judge). Only in late cases the iliac nodes are involved. Distant metastasis is very rare.

Special Investigations.—When the growth comes to the surface through the foreskin, diagnosis is established clinically. A biopsy may, however, be easily done to confirm the diagnosis and assess the degree of malignancy.

In early cases, a dorsal slit has to be performed to see the growth and to do a biopsy.

Treatment

A. FOR THE PRIMARY GROWTH

1. *Radiotherapy.*—This is indicated only in cases of small, well-differentiated growths, limited to the glans penis, particularly when the patient is young. Its *advantage* is that, while the results are comparable to those of surgery, a mutilating operation, telling on the psychology of the patient, is avoided. The *disadvantages* of radiotherapy are that it may result in a withered, shrivelled-up penis, with painful erections, and may also cause post-radiation sterility. The *contraindications* to radiotherapy are:
   i. A big growth
   ii. An anaplastic growth
   iii. A growth involving the shaft.
   iv. An elderly person who does not mind a mutilating operation.
   There are different *methods* available for radiotherapy:
      a. *Interstitial Radiation.*—Implantation of flexible radioactive tant-alam wires (total dose 6000 r in 5 to 7 days).
      b. *Surface Radiation.*—Radium mould applicators, worn intermittently or continuously (6000 r in 7 to 10 days).
      c. *Teleradiation.*—High-voltage X-ray (6000 r given, in divided doses, over 5 weeks).
   The *pre-requisite* for radiotherapy is a dorsal slit.
2. *Surgery.*—This is the choice of treatment in the majority of the cases:
   a. When the growth is limited to the glans.—Partial amputation of penis.
   b. When the growth has involved the shaft.—Total amputation of penis.

B. FOR THE INGUINAL NODES.—The treatment depends on the nature of involvement:
1. No enlarged inguinal nodes.—After the treatment for the primary growth, the patient has to be kept on a periodic check-up.
2. Significant (i.e. clinically malignant) inguinal nodes.—Bilateral inguinal block

dissection has to be performed. One of the following routines may be adopted:
   a. Bilateral block dissection is performed, together with the surgery for the primary growth, in the same operation.
   b. Dissection of the more affected side is done with the surgery for the primary growth, and dissection of the contralateral side at a later date.
   c. The block dissection operation is postponed to a later date after surgery for the primary. The two sides may then be done at the same sitting or in two, the more affected side first.
3. Inguinal nodes are enlarged but it is difficult to ascertain clinically whether the nodes are metastatic or inflammatory.—In these cases either of the following two procedures may be followed:
   a. A three-week antibiotic therapy is given after the surgery for the primary. If the nodes subside, they were possibly inflammatory and the patient is kept on a periodic check-up. If the nodes fail to disappear or enlarge further, block dissection is undertaken.
   b. A biopsy of an inguinal node may ascertain its nature of involvement, and treatment instituted accordingly.
4. Significant inguinal nodes which have become fixed or there is involvement of the external iliac nodes as well.—Surgery cannot be undertaken for the nodes. Radiotherapy is also useless, though some cases may show temporary regression. Chemotherapy may be tried.

Partial Amputation of Penis.—This is done for growths limited to the glans penis and not involving the body.

A narrow catheter, tightly applied around the base of the penis, is made to act as a tourniquet.

Usually a flap amputation is done, and the skin flaps may be designed in three ways:
   1. Equal dorsal and ventral flaps, the urethra emerging through the suture line.
   2. Longer dorsal flap and a short ventral flap, the urethra brought out through a button-hole, made in the dorsal flap.
   3. Longer ventral flap and short dorsal flap, the urethra coming out through a button-hole in the ventral flap.

The last procedure is usually preferred because the suture line is then located above the urethral opening and is not soiled by urine in the post-operative period.

Since the corpus spongiosum, with the urethra, has a tendency to recede back, when cut, it is separated from the corpora cavernosa and bisected half an inch distal to the proposed line of resection of the corpora cavernosa.

A figure-of-eight haemostatic suture, with strong catgut, is now applied around the two corpora cavernosa, together. The corpora are cut distal to the suture. The distal part of the penis thus falls off.

The big superficial vessels, including the dorsal vein, are ligated. The tourniquet is released and all bleeding points secured.

A button-hole is made in the ventral flap and the urethra is brought out through it. The skin flaps are sutured to cover the stump.

The urethral opening has a tendency to undergo stenosis because of curling in of the rnucosa. To prevent this, the end of the emerging urethra is split for about half an inch. Each flap is sutured, not to the margins of the button-hole, but to the skin beyond it.

Some surgeons advocate a catheter *in situ*, for a week, to prevent soiling by urine.

Later, the patient must undergo intermittent dilatation of the meatus, because stenosis is almost inevitable in spite of best of efforts.

Total amputation of penis—This has to be performed when the growth involves the body of the penis.

A racquet incision is made. The blade of the racquet encircles the base of the penis. The handle of the racquet starts from the ventral aspect of this incision, passes along the midline, over the scrotum, to the midperineal point.

The 'handle' part of the incision is deepened, so that the scrotum is split into two halves and these are retracted laterally. On further deepening the incision, the urethra, with the corpus spongiosum and the bulbous spongiosum, is seen (a bougie, passed along the urethra, is a useful guide). The urethra is dissected out from the muscular tissue of the bulb and is bisected in such a way that about half an inch of it hangs from the perineum.

Attention is now paid to the 'blade' part of the racquet incision, the dorsal aspect of which is deepened. The dorsal vein of the penis is ligated and divided. The suspensory ligament of penis is cut and the penis now hangs down. It is forcibly pulled downwards and backwards, so that the origin of the corpus cavernosum, from the ischiopubic ramus, on each side, is seen. These are erased off from the bone, and the penis falls off.

The skin wound is closed like a 'T', at the lower end of which, in the perineum, the urethra comes out. The end of the urethra is split and sutured to the surrounding skin margins (as in partial amputation).

A catheter is left *in situ* for about a week.

The perineal meatus functions well and seldom gets stenosed (c.f. partial amputation).

Some surgeons advocate excision of the scrotum as well, putting the testis on the medial side of the respective thigh. Apart from psychological reasons, this has also the advantage that the scrotal skin is not soiled by the urine, coming out through the perineum.

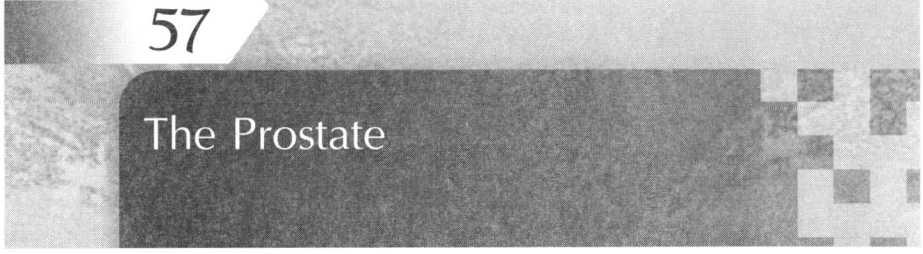

57

The Prostate

Surgical Anatomy

THE LOBES.—For the purpose of easy description, it is convenient to regard the prostate as a fibromuscular organ, permeated by glandular tubules, located around the prostatic urethra and at the neck of the bladder, with which its central part is directly continuous.

From the primitive urethra, solid columns of epithelium grow on all the sides. In a few days, these solid columns canalise, and it is from them that the glandular element of the prostate develops. The surrounding mesenchyme, into which this epithelial budding occurs, forms the fibromuscular element of the prostate. As the epithelial budding occurs in all the directions, developmentally the prostate has four lobes, viz. anterior, posterior and two lateral. The bulk of the prostatic tissue lies behind the urethra and this part is traversed by the common ejaculatory duct of the two sides, as they go to open into the prostatic urethra. Thus, there is a triangular wedge of prostatic tissue, which is bounded anteriorly by the prostatic urethra and posteriorly by the two common ejaculatory ducts. This wedge is called the *median* or *middle lobe* of the prostate (Fig. 57.1).

The upper surface of the median lobe lies under the mucous membrane of the trigone of the bladder, immediately behind the internal urethral orifice. Here it produces a little elevation which is known as the *uvula vesicae*. It also produces an elevation on the upper part of the posterior wall of the prostatic urethra and this is called the *verumontanum* or *urethral crest*. The posterior lobe lies behind the median lobe. The anterior lobe, lying in front of the urethra, contains a little glandular tissue. Thus, it is thin and is often termed *isthmus* or *anterior commissure*. The lateral lobes lie on each side of the anterior lobe, the urethra, the median lobe and the posterior lobe.

THE GLANDS.—The microscopic structure of the prostate can best be studied in the transverse section (Fig. 57.2).

In the mucosa of the prostatic urethra lie small unbranched glands, which open all round the prostatic urethra. These are called the *mucosal glands*.

External to these glands, in the submucous plane of the urethra, lie long branched glands, which open on the posterior wall of the prostatic urethra, on each side of the verumontanum. These are known as the *submucosal glands*.

Still externally, there is another set of long branched glands, which also open on the posterior wall of the urethra, on either side of the verumontanum. These are the *prostatic glands proper*.

It is found that the submucosal glands are maximum in the middle lobe and are abundant in the lateral lobes. These are the glands from which adenoma of the

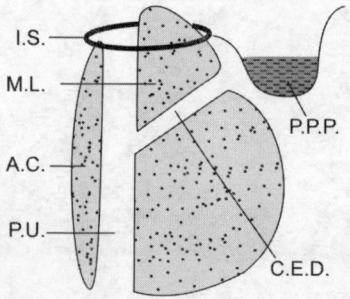
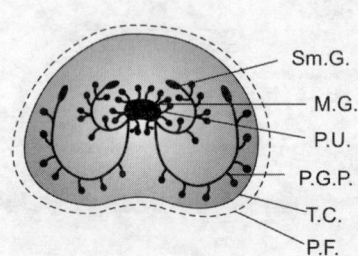

Fig. 57.1: Sagittal section of the prostate. IS = Internal sphincter. ML = Median lobe. AC = Anterior commissure (lobe). PU = Prostatic urethra. CED = Common ejaculatory duct. PPP = Postprostatic pouch.

Fig. 57.2: Schematic representation of transverse section of the prostate. PU = Prostatic urethra. MG = Mucosal glands. SmG = Submucosal glands. PGP = Prostatic glands proper. TC = True (anatomical) capsule. PF = Prostatic fascia.

prostate arises (benign or senile enlargement). The part of the prostate, which contains these glands, is called the *adenomatous zone,* i.e. the middle and lateral lobes.

The prostatic glands proper are found in abundance in the posterior lobe of the prostate. These are the glands, in which cancers of the prostate originate. Hence, the posterior lobe is called the *carcinomatous zone.*

THE COVERINGS.—The prostate has two coverings:
1. The *true capsule* of the prostate—a fibromuscular capsule.
2. External to the true capsule is the *prostatic fascia* or *sheath.* This is a part of the pelvic fascia, around the prostate.

Within the prostatic fascia lies the *prostatic venous plexus.* It lies chiefly in a deep groove between the bladder and the prostate. This plexus, in addition to the prostatic veins, receives the veins of the bladder and the dorsal vein of the penis. The prostatic veins cross the potential space between the true capsule and the prostatic fascia, to reach this venous plexus. If an attempt is made to remove the prostate, as a whole, together with its true capsule, these veins are torn, resulting in torrential haemorrhage. This procedure is, therefore, never adopted while doing a prostatectomy blindly (i.e. by Freyer's method). While doing a retropubic prostatectomy (Millin's method), however, these veins have to be divided but, since this is done under direct vision, the bleeding can well be controlled.

THE MUSCULATURE.—The muscular fibres of the trigone of the bladder converge upon the prostatic urethra and are attached at the verumontanum.

The anterior longitudinal coat of the bladder musculature becomes the muscular element in the fibromuscular true capsule of the prostate.

The inner circular muscle fibres of the bladder become condensed on the upper surface of the prostate and form the vesical (internal) sphincter.

RELATION TO THE RECTUM AND RECTAL EXAMINATION.—The posterior surface of the prostate is separated from the rectum by the prostatic fascia only, which, in this location, is called the *fascia of Denonvillier* (this fascia is formed in the foetal life by the fusion of the peritoneal flaps in the lower part of the rectovesical pouch). The posterior lobe is, therefore, easily palpable on rectal examination.

The inferolateral surface of the prostate (i.e. that of the lateral lobes) is related to the levator ani, so that this can also be palpated from the rectum.

In other words, the posterior and the lateral lobes of the prostate are palpable per rectum. It is important to realise that the median lobe, even when it is enlarged, is not palpable rectally.

STRUCTURES OPENING IN THE PROSTATIC URETHRA

1. In the centre of the verumonatanum, there is a small opening, the *prostatic utricle*. This utricle represents the uterus of the females (the Skene's tubules, opening in the female urethra, represent the prostate).
2. On each side of the verumontanum is the opening of the common ejaculatory duct.
3. On either side of the verumontanum open the multiple submucous glands of the prostatic urethra and multiple prostatic glands proper.
4. All round the prostatic urethra, there are multiple openings of the mucosal glands of the prostatic urethra.

SUBTRIGONAL AND SUBCERVICAL GLANDS.—The mucosal glands in the trigone of the bladder (called the subtrigonal glands) and those in the mucous membrane overlying the internal sphincter at the bladder neck (called the subcervical glands) are, as if, continuation upwards of the mucosal glands of the prostatic urethra.

While the mucosal glands of the prostatic urethra (in addition to the sub-mucosal glands) take share in the formation of adenoma of the prostate, the subtrigonal and subcervical glands also often participate in this hyperplasia. If this occurs, a ridge forms on the posterior wall, at this situation, and this is called the *median bar*. It is, however, to be noted that this hypertrophy occurs *outside* the prostatic capsule. Some workers believe that, in all cases of prostatic adenoma, the pathology starts in these glands.

Surgical Physiology

1. The prostate is influenced both by androgens and oestrogen. As age advances, the androgenic level falls, without a corresponding fall in the oestrogen level. It is believed by many workers that benign enlargement of the prostate, occurring in the senile age, is due to this imbalance between androgens and oestrogen.
2. The prostatic glands proper can produce considerable quantities of acid phosphatase. Only a small part of the phosphatase is excreted in the urine and the major part is absorbed in the blood. In cases of cancer of the prostate, which originates in these glands, there is usually an enormous rise in the serum acid phosphatase level, particularly when the cancer is associated with metastasis. Estimation of the serum acid phosphatase is, thus, a valuable guide in the diagnosis of carcinoma of the prostate. The normal serum level is 0–5 King Armstrong (KA) units (*see* carcinoma of the prostate).
3. *Corpora amylacea.*—This is a material found in the prostate of elderly men (and also in the Skene's tubules of women). It consists of amorphous debris and desquamated epithelium, and is deeply pigmented. Its origin is not known. Many pathologists believe that this is the forerunner of endogenous prostatic calculi.

SENILE (BENIGN) ENLARGEMENT OF THE PROSTATE

Etiology.—There are two theories:

1. Hyperplastic theory.—It is believed that the pathology is a proliferative change in the prostate, similar to that occurring in the breast of lobular hyperplasia. It results from a derangement in the normal hyperplasia-involution cycle of the prostate and this is believed to be due to an imbalance between the androgenic and oestrogenic levels, as age advances (*see* surgical physiology). In majority of the cases, hyperplasia occurs both in the glandular element and the fibromuscular stroma, resulting in *fibroadenomatous prostate*. In some cases, there is hyperplasia of the fibrous tissue at the cost of the glandular element, and this results in what is called *fibrous prostate*.

2. Neoplastic theory.—According to this theory, the pathology is actually a benign neoplasm, i.e. an adenoma in the gland. Simultaneously, neoplastic changes also occur in the incorporated fibrous tissue and muscular elements, so that the resultant tumour is an *adeno-fibro-myoma*. In some cases the fibrous tissue element may predominate, resulting in fibrous prostate.

Pathology in the Prostate Itself.—The disease may be of two types:

A. Fibroadenomatous type (fibroadenomyomatous).—This is much the commoner.

B. Fibrous type.

A. Fibroadenomatous type.—In this type, the adenomatous element is very much predominant. The prostatic enlargement may be of the following natures:

1. *Lateral lobe enlargement.*—This occurs due to:
   a. hyperplasia of the submucosal glands of the prostatic urethra, and/or
   b. hyperplasia of the mucosal glands on the lateral wall of the prostatic urethra.
2. *Median lobe enlargement.*—This occurs due to hyperplasia of the mucosal glands on the posterior wall of the prostatic urethra.
3. *Median bar.*—This is a projection from the posterior wall of the bladder neck. It occurs when there is hyperplasia of the subcervical and subtrigonal glands.

Prostatic enlargement is commonest in the median lobe and may be confined to it, but one or both lateral lobes are often involved in addition.

The unyielding nature of the sheath of the gland limits its growths in the anterior, posterior, and lateral directions. Therefore, as the gland enlarges, it first encroaches on the lumen of the prostatic urethra, which it obliterates to a varying degree. Similarly, downward enlargement of the gland is prevented by the tough triangular ligament, so that the hypertrophic prostatic tissue can only enlarge upwards, towards the bladder, because the bladder neck offers only a little resistance.

A median lobe enlargement, since it starts in the mucosal plane, will always occur deep to the musculature, i.e. it will pass through the internal sphincter into the bladder.

Similarly, when a lateral lobe enlargement is due to hyperplasia of the mucosal glands (type 1b, as described above), it will pass through the sphincter, into the bladder. On the other hand, if the enlargement is due to hyperplasia of the submucosal (type 1a), the enlargement occurs extravesically, pushing the seminal vesicles upwards. Even in the latter case, as the growth enlarges, the muscular fibres of the bladder wall are thinned out or separated, so that the gland eventually comes to lie directly beneath the mucosa of the bladder. In a case of combined median and bilateral lateral lobe enlargement of the prostate, if the internal meatus is viewed from within the bladder, it is found to be surrounded on the sides and back by an intra-vesical prostatic collar.

As the glandular hypertrophy progresses, the unaffected prostatic tissue, lying peripherally, gets compressed and condensed. This results in a *false capsule*. Thus a prostatic adenoma has three coverings. From inside outwards, these are—the false capsule, the true capsule, and the prostatic sheath. In operations for senile enlargement, the adenoma is conveniently enucleated out from within the false capsule, because this is the plane which is relatively avascular. All the three coverings are thus left behind. The false capsule, in such cases, still contains compressed prostatic element, particularly the posterior lobe, which is the carcinomatous zone. At least in some cases, therefore, a cancer of the prostate may develop even after the so-called prostatectomy for senile enlargement of the prostate.

B. FIBROUS TYPE.—There is an irregular fibrous hyperplasia at the cost of the glandular element. The hyperplasia affects the whole of the gland irregularly and no false capsule develops. The prostate adheres firmly to its investments, so that enucleation is nearly impossible. Any attempt at enucleation results in laceration of the prostatic venous plexus as well as the bladder and urethra. This type of hyperplasia is, therefore, treated in a different line from the fibroadenomatous type.

Secondary Pathological Effects

1. PROSTATIC URETHRA:
   a. The prostate enlarges upwards, pushing up the base of the bladder, so the prostatic urethra elongates (a catheter has to be introduced for a greater distance).
   b. There is an exaggeration of the normal urethral angle (requiring specially angled metallic catheters).
   c. There is a narrowing of the lumen of the prostatic urethra. In case of bilateral lateral lobe enlargement, the urethra may be converted into an anteroposterior slit only. When the prostatic enlargement is assymetric, the urethra may be pushed to one side.
   d. On the contrary, at least in some cases, the prostatic urethra is widened because of stretching of the mucous membrane over the enlarged gland.

2. URINARY BLADDER:
   a. Protrusion of the prostate inside the bladder raises the urethral opening above the level of the bladder neck. There is, thus, a dependent part of the bladder, below and behind the urethral opening. This is called the *post-prostatic pouch*. The pouch contains what is called the *residual urine*. This urine cannot be voided by the patient himself. If a catheter is introduced, after the patient has voided urine himself, the residual urine can be brought out and its quantity measured.
   b. As the bladder has to work against a continuous obstruction, its musculature undergoes hypertrophy. The hypertrophic muscle bundles are seen as criss-cross elevated ridges on the inner surface of the bladder; these are known as trabeculations. The depressed areas in between the ridges of elevations are termed *sacculations*. One or more of these sacculations may be so deepened as to form *diverticula*.

c. If the obstruction progresses unrelieved, the bladder musculature ultimately undergoes atony, resulting in distension of the organ. At this stage, the bladder cannot evacuate actively, and when it is over-distended, the intravesical pressure just forces out a few drops of urine. Thus, a stage of *overflow (paradoxical) incontinence* sets in. This atonicity also spreads to the uretero-vesical junction, whose normal sphincteric action is lost. The urine from the over-distended bladder can now have a reflux, up along the ureters.

d. *Cystitis* is a common sequela and is due to:

  i. Stagnant residual urine.

  ii. Stagnant urine in the diverticula.

  iii. Stagnant urine in the chronically over-distended bladder as a whole. Cystitis is often precipitated by catheterisation.

e. *Stones,* usually phosphatic, may form secondary to the cystitis. Most commonly, they harbour in the post-prostatic pouch.

f. The venous plexus, located between the bladder and the prostate, is pressed upon and congested. This condition is often termed *vesical piles* . Rupture of these veins may result in haematuria.

3. KIDNEYS AND URETERS:

a. Bilateral hydronephrosis with hydro-ureter may result. Rarely, a grossly enlarged lateral lobe may directly obstruct the corresponding ureteric orifice and cause a unilateral hydronephrosis.

b. Reflux of infected urine from the bladder may result in ascending infection, i.e. pyelitis, pyelonephritis.

c. A chronic inerstitial nephritis gradually sets in. This results in gradual lowering of the renal function and uraemia.

Clinical Features

1. PROSTATISM.—The features of prostatism are dysuria and frequency, sometimes associated with urgency (the term prostatism applies to a symptom-complex, occurring usually after the age of fifty years, resulting from interference with emptying of the bladder, and may be caused by senile enlargement of the prostate, prostatic fibrosis, or carcinoma of the prostate).

a. *Dysuria:* This is due to obstruction in the prostatic urethra. It is sometimes found that passage of urine becomes more difficult if the patient strains in an attempt to overcome the obstruction (c.f. stricture urethra). This is because of the following reasons:

  i. In cases of median lobe enlargement, the median lobe acts as a ball-valve, and drops on the internal meatus when the bladder actively contracts and the intravesical pressure rises.

  ii. In cases of lateral lobe enlargement (occurring intravesically) the two lateral lobes appose each other, to obstruct the meatus, when the bladder contracts.

b. *Frequency:* This is at first nocturnal, but thereafter occurs both in the daytime and at night. Earlier in the course of the disease, frequency is caused by the following factors:

  i. A part of the prostatic urethra (which is very sensitive) is exposed to the bladder urine, as the prostate enlarges intravesically.

    ii. The internal sphincter being stretched, drops of urine are allowed to come down to the prostatic urethra.

    Later, the causes of frequency are:

    iii. Cystitis.

    iv. Residual urine.

    v. Stones.

    Finally, frequency is aggravated by:

    vi. Polyuria, due to renal failure.

  c. *Urgency:* The patient cannot hold urine and has to void it as soon as there is urge for micturition. The causes of urgency are the factors i. and, ii. mentioned under frequency.

2. RETENTION OF URINE.—There may be three types of retention:
  a. Chronic retention, often associated with an overflow incontinence. The patient usually does not feel that he has a full bladder.
  b. Acute retention.
  c. Acute-on-chronic retention.

3. HAEMATURIA.—This may be caused by:
  a. Cystitis.
  b. Rupture of vesical piles.
  c. Stones.
  d. Erosion of a part of the intravesical part of the enlarged prostate.

4. HYDRONEPHROSIS.—Suggested by renal pain and/or lump, usually bilateral.

5. PAIN.—There may be different types of pain:
  a. Pain of acute retention.
  b. Pain due to cystitis—hypogastric pain, often referred to the tip of the penis.
  c. A feeling of fullness in the perineum or rectum.
  d. Loin pain due to hydronephrosis or renal infection.

6. RENAL FAILURE, as suggested by:
  a. Pre-uraemic stage, followed by uraemia.
  b. Renal hypertension.

Examination of the Patient

A. GENERAL EXAMINATION.—The following should be searched for:
  1. Features suggestive of pre-uraemia or uraemic state.
  2. Renal hypertension.
  3. Gross cardiac or other systemic lesions, due to old age.

B. ABDOMINAL EXAMINATION:
  1. A full bladder may be noticed.
  2. Renal lump due to hydronephrosis may be found.

C. RECTAL EXAMINATION OF THE PROSTATE.—This is usually done with the patient in the right lateral position, i.e. facing the surgeon, and with the knees flexed. In the absence of a full bladder, a *bimanual examination* may be more helpful with the patient in the dorsal position. By this method, even an intravesical lobe can sometimes be felt. The differentiating features between a benign enlargement and a carcinoma of the prostate, as revealed by rectal examination, are as follows:

Benign	Malignant
1. Moderate to big enlargement.	1. Enlargement usually not remarkable
2. Surface—smooth.	2. Surface—nodular.
3. Consistency—firm and elastic.	3. Consistency—hard.
4. The prostate possesses a definite degree of mobility.	4. Mobility of the prostate is restricted.
5. The midline sulcus, marking the gap between the two lateral lobes below and the two seminal vesicles above, is well felt.	5. The sulcus is often obliterated.
6. The gap between the prostate and the lateral pelvic wall, on either side, is clear.	6. This may be obliterated by malignant infiltration.
7. The rental wall is free.	7. The rectal wall may be adherent due to infiltration.

It should be noted that:

a. The findings in case of a fibrous prostate do not conform to either of the above types.

b. Enlargement of the median lobe cannot be made out by a rectal examination. Hence, if, on rectal examination, the prostate does not appear to be enlarged, it should not be declared that the patient is not suffering from an enlarged prostate. In such cases, a cystoscopy (and sometimes the bladder film of an IVP) makes the diagnosis.

c. At rectal examination, the residual urine in the post-prostatic pouch may be felt as a fluctuating swelling, above the prostate.

Special Investigations

1. URINE EXAMINATION, including culture and sensitivity test,

2. BLOOD BIOCHEMISTRY.—Estimation of serum urea, NPN and creatinine, to assess renal function.

3. STRAIGHT X-RAY of the abdomen, which may show:
   a. Stone in the bladder or kidney.
   b. Enlarged kidney shadows due to hydronephrosis.
   c. Shadow of a distended bladder.

4. IVP is of great importance and should be done in all the cases except where there are clinical signs of renal failure or where the blood urea is very high (above 60 mg%):
   a. It indicates the renal function on each side and detects presence of hydronephrotic changes.
   b. The post-evacuation bladder film gives an idea about the quantity of the residual urine.
   c. The enlarged prostate, lying intravesically, may be seen as a smooth filling defect at the bladder neck.
   d. Diverticula in the bladder can be detected.

5. CYSTOSCOPY:
   a. The residual urine can be measured.

b. Bladder changes, like trabeculations and sacculations, can be seen, and presence of diverticulum, stones (especially those not seen on X-ray), or a growth can be excluded.

c. *Marion's sign* is often positive. In a normal subject, the posterior lip of the internal urethral meatus and a ureteric orifice are not visible in the same cystoscopic field. In case of prostatic enlargement, as the urethral opening is pushed up into the bladder, this may be possible.

d. Sometimes a big intravesical enlargement may hide one or both the ureteric orifices from the cystoscopic view.

Treatment.—In considering the treatment, the patients are divided into two groups — those not presenting with acute retention, and those coming with acute retention.

GROUP A: PATIENTS NOT PRESENTING WITH ACUTE RETENTION

In this group, the treatment is prostatectomy (enucleation of the adenoma) and the only question is whether it can be undertaken immediately. The contra-indications for an immediate prostatectomy are as follows:

a. Gross impairment of renal function; a blood urea level above 60 mg% is a definite contraindication.

b. Gross urinary infection.

c. A very low general condition of the patient.

1. In the absence of the above contraindications, a prostatectomy can safely be undertaken, after routine investigations.

2. In presence of the above difficulties, the patient has to be prepared for the operation, as follows:

   a. If there is gross urinary infection, an antibiotic, to which the organisms are sensitive, has to be administered, till the infection is controlled.

   b. In the presence of gross renal impairment, continuous decompression of the bladder has to be done with a Foley's catheter, introduced per urethra, till the function recovers at least moderately.

   c. If the patient's general condition is low, this is corrected by nutritious diet and control of infection.

   Thereafter, the patient is subjected to prostatectomy.

GROUP B: PATIENTS PRESENTING WITH ACUTE RETENTION

1. The immediate aim in these cases is to relieve the retention. If a catheter can be passed, it is left *in situ*. Investigations are undertaken and the patient is prepared for prostatectomy (one-stage prostatectomy).

2. In those cases where a catheter cannot be passed, a suprapubic puncture (with a needle) and aspiration of the bladder is done. In many cases, it may be possible to pass a catheter now, as the congestion and oedema at the bladder neck (due to overdistension of the bladder) is minimised.

3. If a catheter cannot be passed in, a suprapubic cystostomy has to be done. These patients have to undergo a two-stage prostatectomy, after proper investigations.

Different Types of Prostatectomy

A. SUPRAPUBIC PROSTATECTOMY (FREYER'S). — This is the most commonly practised procedure. It may be of two types:

1. One-stage prostatectomy.

2. Two-stage prostatectomy.—This is done when the patient has to undergo an emergency suprapubic cystostomy (for acute retention). The prostatectomy is done at the second stage.

In doing a suprapubic prostatectomy, the bladder is opened by the suprapubic route. The index finger is introduced into the bladder and then, down the internal meatus, into the prostatic urethra. As the finger is moved laterally, on either side, the plane of clevage between the adenoma and the false capsule is easily reached and, by rotating the finger all round, the adenoma is enucleated. Bleeding from the prostatic bed is controlled by one of the following methods:

1. Under direct vision.—The bleeding points are ligated or cauterised. Proper illumination and wide retraction are necessary. This is possible in one-stage prostatectomy but not in a two-stage operation, where fibrosis prevents the required exposure.
2. With the help of the distended balloon of a Foley's catheter, introduced per urethra. The balloon presses on the walls of the bleeding prostatic bed (*see* Foley's catheter in Chapter on instruments).
3. Packing the prostatic cavity with roller gauze around a urethral catheter.
4. *Harris' Method.*—This consists of the following steps:
   a. The prostatic arteries are controlled by lateral stitches, inserted with a *boomerang needle*.
   b. The torn mucosa of the posterior lip of the internal meatus (i.e. the lower end of the trigone) is sutured to the torn mucosa of the posterior lip of the membranous urethra. This procedure not only achieves haemostasis but also minimises the risk of stricture formation in this part of the urethra which, otherwise, has a tendency to heal by fibrosis. The method is called *retrigonisation.*
   c. The torn mucosa of the anterior lip of the bladder is sutured to that of the anterior flap of the torn membranous urethra, around the urethral catheter (*the anterior repair*).

B. RETROPUBIC PROSTATECTOMY (MILLIN'S).—This requires the use of a self-retaining, preferably self-illuminating, retractor. The bladder, which is emptied before operation, is not opened but is pushed back, after making a suprapubic parietal incision. The pubo-prostatic ligament on each side is cut, so that space is available for dissection between the pubis and the prostate. Dissection is done under direct vision, with proper haemostasis. The prostatic fascia, the true capsule, and the false capsule are all cut, by a transverse incision, on the anterior aspect of the prostate, and the typically white adenoma is seen. The adenoma is enucleated, perfect haemostasis done, and a urethral catheter is left *in situ*.

C. PERINEAL PROSTATECTOMY (YOUNG'S).—This approach is only rarely made, and then again for operations of prostatic cancers. Its only advantage is that it allows a preliminary biopsy to be done. Apart from technical difficulties, its main disadvantage is the high incidence of incontinence.

D. TRANSURETHRAL PROSTATECTOMY.—This is done with a resectoscope, or a diathermy wire-loop, or a cold punch. Snips of prostatic tissue are resected off the wall of the prostatic urethra, with a view to making its lumen wide and prevent obstruction. Its indications are:
1. Fibrous prostate.

2. Carcinoma of the prostate.
3. Small median lobe enlargement.

Apart from the fact that it requires a trained hand, the main disadvantage is recurrence of obstruction. However, the procedure may be repeated, as and when necessary. The hospital stay of the patient is minimum.

CARCINOMA OF THE PROSTATE

This is the commonest cancer in the males above the age of 65 years. Again, in the males, this is the commonest primary for bone secondaries.

Latent and Obvious Cancers

1. LATENT CANCERS.—These do not produce any symptoms and are diagnosed only during routine post-mortem examinations. About 20 per cent of the male population above the age of 50, and above 75 per cent above the age of 90 years, show evidence of cancer in the prostate at the post-mortem examination. Usually these growths are small and it is believed that they were awaiting favourable conditions to become active, i.e. turn into obvious cancers.
2. OBVIOUS CANCERS.—These are the cases which produce symptoms.

Sites

1. The commonest site is the *carcinomatons zone*, containing the prostatic glands proper, i.e. the posterior lobe of the prostate.
2. Sometimes in one or both lateral lobes diffusely.
3. Occasionally in association with a benign enlargement.
4. As has already been stated, after prostatectomy for a benign enlargement, the false capsule, which is left behind (since it contains the posterior lobe), may be the site of cancer in some cases.

Types

1. The usual type presents as multiple nodules, which render the gland unusually hard, i.e. a hard nodular prostate. These are *spheroidal-cell adenocarcinoma.*
2. In some cases there is a small growth, which remains confined to the posterior lobe, and the prostate, on rectal examination, does not show any abnormality. However, there are widespread skeletal metastases. These are cases of *scirrhous carcinoma.*
3. Sometimes the growth is of *anaplastic type.*

Spread

1. DIRECT SPREAD.—The carcinoma, usually starting in the posterior lobe, gradually involves the whole of this lobe and then spreads to the lateral lobes. Involvement of the urethra is usually late. However, when the cancer starts in a lateral lobe, there may be early urethral involvement.
   As the growth comes out of the true capsule of the prostate, on its posterior aspect, its backward spread to the rectum is prevented for a long time by the strong fascia of Denonvilliers. It, therefore, spreads upwards, and the first structure to be involved is the seminal vesicle. A further extension upwards may cause infiltration into one or both ureters (hydronephrosis, hydro-ureter and anuria). From the lateral lobes, spread may occur to the base of the bladder, causing nodularity of its mucosal surface.

2. Lymphatic spread:
   a. Majority of the lymphatics drain posterolaterally, on either side of the rectum, into the internal iliac nodes.
   b. Some of the lymphatics drain, together with those of the seminal vesicles and the vas deferens, to the external iliac nodes on both sides.
   c. Subsequently, the para-aortic nodes may be involved.

3. Venous spread.—This is important and early, particularly with the anaplastic and the scirrhous types. This is why patients often present first with metastatic features. Spread occurs to bones, lungs and liver, in that order of frequency.

   Bone metastases from prostatic cancers are characteristic in that they are usually osteogenic (osteosclerotic), in contrast to metastases from other organs, which are generally osteolytic. The bones involved, in order of frequency, are:
   a. Pelvic bones and lumbar vertebrae.
   b. Head and neck of the femur.
   c. Skull.
   d. Sternum and ribs.
   e. Head and neck of the humerus.

While bone metastases may occur by way of the systemic circulation, it is equally true that there are extensive connections between the prostatic plexus of veins and the vertebral system of veins. It is by way of these connections that early involvement of the vertebrae may occur, as a result of retrograde flow.

Clinical Features.—The cases of carcinoma of prostate may be divided into six groups:

Group A: The latent group.— As has already been said, a large number of cases produce no symptoms and are diagnosed only postmortem.

Group B: The incidental group.—The patient is operated on the diagnosis of a senile enlargement of the prostate but histological examination of the specimen shows evidence of malignancy.

Group C: The clinically doubtful group.—The patient presents with features of prostatism (frequency, dysuria, urgency), and sometimes haematuria and/or retention. Doubt arises as to the nature of the enlargement because of the following points:
1. The history is comparatively short (the complaints are for weeks, as compared to months in senile enlargement).
2. On rectal examination, the prostate seems to be fibrotic or there is a hard nodule, or else, it appears to have an increased fixity.

Group D: The clinically obvious group.
1. There are features of prostatism, sometimes haematuria and/or retention.
2. Rectal examination reveals a typically malignant prostate—hard, nodular, little enlarged, with restricted mobility and obliteration of the mid-line sulcus (*see* clinical examination under senile enlargement of prostate).

Group E: The metastatic group.—These are the patients in whom the urinary symptoms are absent or negligible, and rectal examination may or may not reveal evidence of a prostatic carcinoma. According to the site of the metastasis, the presentation may be as follows:

1. Bones.—Pain in the bones (particularly low back and pelvic), referred pains (sciatica), and pathological fractures.
2. Lungs.—Pain in the chest, cough, haemoptysis, dyspnoea and fever.
3. Liver.—Jaundice and ascites with hard nodular liver.

GROUP F: THE UNUSUAL GROUP.—Some patients may present with unusual features, e.g.

1. Oedema of the lower limbs, external genitalia, and lower abdominal parieties, due to lymphatic obstruction (blockage of the abdominal nodes).
2. Priaprism, caused by impairment of venous return from the penis (the veins of the penis drain into the prostatic venous plexus, which is blocked by malignant cells).

Special Investigations

1. ESTIMATION OF SERUM PHOSPHATASES:
   a. *Acid phosphatase.*—This is often found to be raised, particularly when there are secondary deposits. The normal cells of the prostate as well as the prostatic cancer cells produce acid phosphatase and so also the cells in the metastatic deposits. The major part of the phosphatase, liberated by the prostatic cells, get an exit through the prostatic ducts, so that only small amounts are absorbed in the serum. However, even this may be sufficient to raise the serum acid phosphatase level in cases of prostatic cancer (normal level is 0–5 King-Armstrong units). On the other hand, the phosphatase, liberated by the metastatic deposits, are absorbed wholly in the blood and so there is an enormous rise in the serum acid phosphatase level. Thus, a high level of acid phosphatase is not only diagnostic of prostatic cancer but also suggestive of metastases.
   b. *Alkaline phosphatase.*—In case of bone metastases, there may be also an elevation in the serum alkaline phosphatase level because the deposits are usually osteosclerotic.
2. EXFOLIATIVE CYTOLOGY.—Presence ef cancer cells in the prostatic secretion, obtained by a prostatic massage, is confirmatory of diagnosis. Its disadvantages are that it may give false negative results and may cause dissemination of the cancer.
3. CYSTOSCOPY may reveal:
   a. A grating sensation, as the instrument traverses the prostatic urethra.
   b. Irregular nodularity, and sometimes ulcerations, on the base of the bladder, and puckering of the trigone.
4. VESICULOGRAPHY, i.e. X-ray of the seminal vesicles, after administration of dye, is sometimes helpful in diagnosis since distortion of the seminal vesicles, by infiltration, occurs rather early.
5. BIOPSY.—The different types of biopsy are as follows:
   a. Needle biopsy, either through the perineum or through the rectum. Special needles are used for the purpose.
   b. Transurethral biopsy, with a cystoscope.
   c. Open biopsy, done by the perineal route, as a preliminary step to perineal prostatectomy (usually freeze-section technique is used).
6. X-RAY:
   a. Pelvis and lumbar vertebrae.

b. Any other bone where a metastasis is suspected.

c. Chest.

7. BONE MARROW ASPIRATION of the sternum or ilium often reveals metastatic cancer cells.

Treatment

A. SURGERY has a little to offer in cases of prostatic carcinoma because, by the time the diagnosis is made, the cancer usually spreads beyond the capsule of the gland, making prostatectomy impossible, or produces distant metastases.

The *indications and types of surgery* are as follows:

1. Prostatectomy done on the diagnosis of a benign enlargement and revealing carcinoma on histological examination.

2. Prostatectomy done in very early cases, where the growth is till limited within the capsule and there is no distant spread. The perineal route is preferred by many surgeons as it offers the chance of a preliminary freeze-section biopsy.

3. Transurethral resection (often repeated), to overcome urinary obstruction. This is a very helpful procedure as an adjunct to hormone therapy.

B. HORMONE THERAPY.—Fortunately, majority of these cancers are hormone-sensitive, responding to oestrogen. *Oestrogen therapy*, therefore, is the main aim in treating these cases:

1. Stilboestrol is the drug most commonly used. The dose is 30 mg a day, although, to start with, higher doses (as much as 100 mg) may have to be administered. It works very well but may have some disturbing side-effects in some cases:

   a. Gynaecomastia, sometimes painful.

   b. Nausea and vomiting

   c. Oedema, often seen in the ankles, due to salt retention.

   d. Loss of libido.

   In order to overcome these side-effects of stilboestrol, other modified preparations of oestrogen are now advocated:

2. Dienoestrol, 45 mg daily.

3. TACE, 12 to 24 mg per day.

4. Honvan.—This is phosporylated oestrogen and is ineffective in the system, *as such*. Only when it reaches the prostatic cancer cells that the acid phosphatase in these cells breaks it up and releases the oestrogen locally. The oestrogen then acts directly on the cancer cells and there is no systemic ill-effect of the oestrogen. It is usually given IV to start with, and thereafter orally.

C. SURGERY FOR HORMONE TREATMENT:

1. Bilateral orchiectomy (subcapsular), to remove the main source of androgen.

2. Bilateral adrenalectomy, to remove the other source of androgen.

3. Hypophysectomy or radiation-ablation of the pituitary (by implanting yittrium90 into the pituitary), to remove the stimulation on the adrenal rests, which become active after bilateral adrenalectomy.

These operations may be tried when simple oestrogen therapy fails.

58

Testis, Epididymis, Spermatic Cord and Scrotum

Embryology.—The testis develops as an elongated mass *(germinal ridge)*, close to the medial side of the mesonephros (Wolffian body), in the lumbar region on each side. The Wolffian duct, which drains the Wolffian body, persists in its whole length, working mainly as the excretory channel of the seminal system. It gives origin to the following structures:

1. The efferent ductules of the testis.
2. The tubules of the epididymis.
3. The vas deferens.
4. The seminal vesicles.
5. The common ejaculatory duct
6. The upper part of the prostatic urethra, up to the utricle.
7. The trigone of the bladder.
8. The ureteric bud.

} belonging to the urinary system.

While the Wolffian duct persists as such the major part of the Wolffian body (i.e. mesonephros) disappears. Only traces of it persists as the *paradidymis* (organ of Garaldes).

From about the eighth week of intrauterine life, the testis begins to descend from its original lumbar position towards the groin and scrotum. The upper part of the Wolffian duct also descends with it, while the lower end of the duct remains fixed to the cloaca.

Simultaneously, the developing kidney and ureter ascend upwards from the pelvis, towards the loin. Thus, the two channels, viz. the ureter and the vas deferens, come to be hooked round each other near the base of the bladder.

The *Mullerian (paramesonephric)* duct, which lies lateral to the mesonephros, plays an important role in the development of the female genital organs. In the males it disappears almost entirely, only traces of it persisting:

1. The upper fend persists, in traces, as the *appendix testis* (sessile hydatid cyst of Morgagni), which lies on the upper pole of the testis, just in front of the epididymis.
2. The lower ends of the ducts of the two sides fuse, to form the *prostatic utricle*.

THE GUBERNACULUM TESTIS.—The testis and the mesonephros, as they lie side by side in the lumbar region, are suspended together by a common mesentery from the posterior abdominal wall. This is called the *urogenital mesentery*. The caudal end of the right and left urogenital mesenteries join each other to form a transverse bar, which is called the *genital cord*. The genital cord lies in the pelvis, transversely, between the bladder in front and the rectum behind. From each lateral end of the genital cord a fold of peritoneum passes ventrally and fuses with the anterior abdominal wall. These are called the *inguinal folds*. The mesodermal element, incorporated within each inguinal fold, differentiates into a fibromuscular band and this becomes known as the *gubernaculum testis* (gubernaculum = a rudder).

Thus, the gubernaculum is attached above to the lower pole of the testis and the mesonephric (Wolffian) duct. Below, it is attached mainly to that skin which later develops into the wall of the scrotum. In addition, strands from the lower end of the gubernaculum pass to adjacent regions. Thus, according to Lockwood, there may be *five 'tails' of the gubernaculum:*

1. The scrotal tail—which is the main one.
2. The pubic tail—attached to the pubic tubercle
3. The perineal tail—attached to the perineum;
4. The inguinal tail—attached above the inguinal ligament.
5. The femoral tail—attached to the saphenous opening.

It is believed that the gubernaculum plays the key role in drawing the testis down, from the abdomen. As the scrotal tail is the strongest, the testis normally descends to the scrotum. In case where an accessory tail becomes stronger, the testis is drawn towards the attachment of that tail and this results in an 'ectopic testis'.

THE PROCESSUS VAGINALIS.—By the time the gubernaculum develops, the peritoneal cavity extends along the inguinal canal, down to the scrotum, in the form of a tube. This prolongation is termed the processus vaginalis. The testis, which lies retroperitoneally, descends behind the processus vaginalis, to the scrotum. At birth, the connection between the processus vaginalis and the peritoneal cavity is lost by obliteration of the upper part of the tube. The process of obliteration starts at two points, viz. at the deep inguinal ring and at the upper pole of the testis. The part of the processus, which remains patent, lies in front of the testis and forms the *tunica vaginalis.*

Descent of the Testis.—From about the eighth week of the intrauterine life, the testis begins to .descend from its original lumbar position, towards the groin. It enters the scrotum at or immediately before birth.

CHRONOLOGY OF DESCENT:

At or immediately before birth	— Scrotum
Ninth month.	— Superficial inguinal ring.
Eighth month.	— Inguinal canal.
Seventh month.	— Deep inguinal ring.

FACTORS HELPING THE DECENT:

1. Pull of the gubernaculum.
2. Higher temperature inside the abdomen.
3. Relative growth of the abdominal organs and increase in the intra-abdominal pressure.
4. Influence of hormones.—Chorionic gonadotrophin, from the maternal circulation, is believed not only to stimulate the growth of the testis but also its descent.

DEFECTS IN THE DESCENT:

1. *Undescended Testis.*—The testis does not come down to the scrotum. However, it lies somewhere along its *normal path* of descent.

2. *Retractile Testis.*—This is a condition found only in children. The testis has normally developed and normally descended into the scrotum, but it is often pulled up by the contraction of the cremasters, which are very strong during childhood. Such retraction occurs in response to even minor stimuli. The retracted testis is accommodated:

a. either, in the superficial inguinal pouch, located above and lateral to the superficial inguinal ring, between the fascia of Scarpa (deep layer of superficial fascia) and the external oblique aponeurosis.

b. or, in the inguinal canal.

A retractile testis is often wrongly diagnosed as an undescended testis. However, it differs from an undescended testis in the following points:

 i. The scrotum on the side is fully developed (the scrotum is undeveloped in cases of undescended testis).

 ii. The testis is usually of normal size (an undescended testis is underdeveloped).

 iii. By manipulation, the testis can be pushed down into the scrotum, at least to its upper part (this is not possible in case of an undescended testis).

 iv. If the mother of the child says that the testis had ever been found in the scrotum, it is never an undescended testis but a retractile one.

No treatment (endocrine or operative) is necessary for retractile testis. The testis comes down to normal position as the cremasteric hyperactivity subsides, i.e. as the child reaches puberty.

3. *Ectopic Testis.*—In this condition the testis fails to descend into the scrotum and is deviated from its normal path of descent. It is believed that the main (scrotal) tail of the gubernaculum becomes ruptured and the testis is drawn towards the attachment of one of the accessory tails. Accordingly, an ectopic testis may be located, in order of frequency, in one of the following sites:

a. In the superficial inguinal pouch (the pubic tail).

b. In the perineum (the perineal tail).

c. At the root of the penis (if the inguinal tail is attached medially above the inguinal ligament).

d. Near the anterior superior iliac spine (if the inguinal tail is attached laterally above the inguinal ligament).

e. In the femoral triangle (the femoral tail).

(Vide attachments of the gubernaculum).

An ectopic testis, in contrast to an undescended testis, is usually developed well. It may, however, be associated with a congenital hernia, as is often an undescended testis. Its only danger is that it is exposed to trauma. The treatment is operative, replacing the testis in the scrotum.

UNDESCENDED TESTIS

The normal process of descent, the factors helping descent, the chronology of descent, and the abnormalities of descent have been described above.

Factors Hindering Normal Descent

1. Inefficient pull by the gubernaculum.
2. Adhesions, developing between the descending testis and/or the cord, and the neighbouring areas.

3. Short testicular vessels, particularly the veins. The vas deferens is almost always of normal length.

Pathology of an Undescended Testis

1. An undescended testis fails to develop normally.

2. After the age of six years, degenerative changes start in the testis, presumably because of the higher temperature to which it is subjected (the scrotal temperature is lower by 2 °F). By the age of sixteen years, almost the whole of the testis undergoes irreversible destruction.

3. Hence, the external secretion, i.e. spermatogenesis, gradually diminishes and ultimately ceases. If the condition is unilateral, the spermatogenetic activity is carried on by the normally descended testis. On the other hand, bilateral cases are destined to develop sterility.

4. Similarly, the internal secretion, i.e. the androgenic activity, gradually reduces. In bilateral cases the androgen level may be half the normal amount (the rest is produced by the adrenals).

5. A gap is created between the testis and the epididymis. This gap is bridged up by a *mesentery*.

Complications

1. *Trauma.*—A testis, located in the inguinal canal, is liable to repeated trauma, either by direct blow or by muscular contraction of the abdominal wall.

2. *Torsion.*—An undescended testis is vulnerable to torsion. This is because:
   a. There is absence of anchorage to the scrotum that a normally descended testis has.
   b. The mesentery, separating the testis and the epididymis, allows the testis to undergo twisting on the mesentery itself, without involving the cord.

3. *Tumour.*—Malignancy is commoner in an undescended testis. The further the testis is from the scrotum the more frequent is the incidence. The older estimation that malignancy is 20 to 30 times commoner in an undescended testis is now believed by many to be far too high. Seminoma is the commonest tumour encountered.

4. *Sterility.*—Only in bilateral cases, due to absence of spermatogenesis

5. *Congenital Hernia.*—A persistent processus vaginalis is always present and found at operation. However, hernia is clinically evident in only half of the cases.

Treatment.—There is *no scope for hormone treatment*. The treatment is always operative. The patients may be divided into 3 groups.

GROUP A: The testis is somewhere in the inguinal canal or at the external ring:

1. Orchidopexy (i.e. bringing the testis down to the scrotum and fixing it there) has to be tried. If it is not possible to bring the testis down, one of the following procedures has to be considered.

2. A two-stage operation (*see* below).

3. Orchidectomy.

4. Orchidocoelioplasty, i.e. abdominal replacement of an inguinal testis (*see* below).

GROUP B: The testis is not palpable, i.e. it is inside the abdomen.—No treatment is possible, though it is known that such a testis may undergo malignancy.

GROUP C: The patient presents only with a hernia and the testis is not palpable.—Operation for the hernia should be advised. In at least some of cases, the testis, which was not palpable clinically, is found just behind the deep inguinal ring. Attempts may then be made to bring it down.

Orchidopexy.—The optimum age for the operation is six years, after which the degenerative process in the testis usually begins. If the condition is bilateral, the operation on one side should be done six months after the other. An inguinal incision (as for the operation of inguinal hernia) is employed.

Any orchidopexy consist of three steps:

1. HERNIOTOMY—Dissection of the congenital hernial sac from the spermatic cord, ligating it at the deep ring (neck) and excising it.

2. LENGTHENING OF THE SPERMATIC CORD.—It is the short cord which is the real bar to normal descent. The measures adopted for lengthening the cord are as follows:

   a. The herniotomy itself

   b. Excision of all fibrous and fascial bands that bind the cord to the inguinal canal.

   c. If the cord is still short, a finger is introduced through the deep ring into the retroperitoneal tissues and the spermatic vessels and the vas deferense are dissected from the peritoneum, to which they are adherent. A gain in length by about an inch may be achieved by this method.

   d. If required, the fascia transversalis may be incised medial wards from the deep ring and the inferior epigastric vessels divided between ligatures. By this procedure, the structures of the cord are allowed to make a direct course to the scrotum and some increase in length is obtained.

   e. If the testis cannot still be brought down, the major part of the pampiniform plexus is divided between ligatures since these veins are sometimes short while the vas is usually of normal length.

3. FIXING THE TESTIS IN POSITION.—The testis has a notorious tendency to retract up and some method of fixation has to be employed to prevent this retraction. Depending upon the method of fixation, the operation of orchidopexy is named:

   a. *Denis Browne's Operation*—The principles of this operation are:

      i. Narrowing the neck of the scrotum (the so-called third inguinal ring) by a purse-string suture with catgut.

      ii. Anchoring the testis to the skin of the thigh by an unabsorbable suture, passing through the scrotal skin. This stitch is kept for 2 to 3 weeks and then removed.
      Some surgeons prefer to put the testis in a *subdartos pouch*.

   b. *Ombredanne's Operation.*—This is the operation usually done in the children. The testis is brought to the opposite scrotal chamber through a small opening made in the scrotal septum. The two testes lie in the same compartment.

c. *Keetley-Torek Operation.*—This operation is usually preferred in the adults. A chamber is made for the testis, the medial half of which is made by the scrotum (split up by an incision along its lateral side) and the lateral half by the subcutaneous tissue of the medial side of the thigh, adjacent to the scrotum (an incision is made through the skin of the thigh, its size being the same as that on the scrotum). The posterior flaps (of the scrotum and the thigh) are sutured together. The testis is placed on it and is anchored with a stitch to the fascia lata underneath. The anterior skin flaps are then sutured in front of the testis.

Six months later, the scrotum, with the testis, is separated from the thigh.

Two-stage Operations.—If the cord cannot be sufficiently lengthened so as to bring the testis down to the scrotum, one of the methods is to fix the testis in a position as low down as is possible without tension. At a second stage, it may be possible to lengthen the cord further and to bring the testis down to the scrotum.

Orchidectomy.—This is advocated, only when the opposite testis is normal, under the following conditions:

1. If it is impossible to bring the testis down.

2. If, at orchidopexy in an adult, the testis is found to be hopelessly atrophied

Orchido-epilioplasty.—This means abdominal replacement of an inguinal testis. This is indicated where the only remaining testis (the other testis having been removed earlier) cannot be brought down to the scrotum. The ideas behind the operation are:

1. Preserving the internal secretion of the testis, i.e. androgen

2. Protecting the gland from trauma.

TESTICULAR TUMOURS

Nearly 99 per cent of testicular tumours are malignant.

BENIGN TUMOURS

1. LEYDIG-CELL TUMOUR.—The tumour arises from the interstitial cells of Leydig:
   a. It is often termed *pre-pubertal tumour* because it usually occurs before puberty.
   b. It is a *masculanising tumour as* it causes excess output of androgen. There is sexual precocity and excessive muscular development (*infant Hercules*).

2. SERTOLI-CELL TUMOUR.—The tumour originates in the sustentacular cells that are normally found in the limiting membrane of the seminiferous tubules:—
   a. It is often termed *post-pubertal tumour* as it occurs commonly after puberty.
   b. It is a *feminising tumour* as it causes excess output of feminising hormones. There may be gynaecomastia, loss of libido, and aspermia.

MALIGNANT TESTICULAR TUMOURS

Types

1. Seminoma	40 per cent
2. Teratoma	32 per cent
3. Combination of seminoma and teratoma	14 per cent
4. Lymphoma	7 per cent
5. Other tumours	7 per cent

Pathology

I. SEMINOMA:

Origin.—There are two views:

1. It is an adenocarcinoma, arising from the lining cells of the seminiferous tubules.
2. It is a type of teratoma, arising from the primitive totipotent cells, the cells having differentiated towards the seminiferous type. According to this view, all testicular tumours arise from the primitive totipotent cells. Where the cells keep their totipotent character, a teratoma develops. Where they differentiate partly, a mixture of seminoma and teratoma is formed. When the differentiation is complete, a seminoma occurs. The fact, that there is a group where a combination of seminoma and teratoma is encountered, strongly supports this view.

Macroscopic Appearance.—The tumour arises from the mediastinum testis, causing a uniform smooth swelling of the testis. The cut surface has a very uniform homogenous appearance—cream-coloured, with a little tendency to cyst formation, i.e. degeneration. Sometimes fibrous septa divide the tumour-mass into compartments.

Microscopic Appearance.—Under the microscope, the uniformity is also well-marked. Oval cells are arranged in sheets.

II. TERATOMA:

Origin.—These tumours arise from the primitive totipotent germ cells in the developing testis. Being a teratoma, the tumour contains all the three embryological elements, viz. ectodermal, entodermal and mesodermal. However, in a particular tumour, usually one component predominates. Often it is the mesoblastic element that is preponderant, one of its important constituents being hyaline cartilage.

Macroscopic Appearance.—The testis may show uniform enlargement, but often there are lobulations on the surface. The cut surface usually shows multiple cysts of different sizes, and it is for this reason that the condition was called *fibrocystic disease* in the older days.

Types of Teratoma

A. In the past, teratoma was classified as follows:
1. *Adult Teratoma.*—The cells are of the mature type, so that the tumour is least malignant; it may be even of a benign character. *Dermoid cyst* of the testis belongs to this group.
2. *Embryonal Carcinoma.*—The cells are of the embryonal type, i.e. immature, and so the tumour is highly malignant.
3. *Teratocarcinoma.*—This is also known as *chorionepithelioma*. The tumour consists of chorionic epithelium, derived from the trophoblastic cells of

ectodermal origin. Microscopically, it shows the two features characteristic of the chorionic villi of the placenta, viz.

a. Trophoblastic cells.

b. Syncytial mass.

This is the *most malignant tumour* of the testis and, even when the primary lesion is small, widespread distant metastases occur. The tumour is usually small, having a reddish-yellow colour.

B. The present-day classification of teratoma is as follows:

1. *Teratoma Differentiated* (TD).—The cells of the tumour are mature, i.e. well-differentiated. This group represents the 'adult teratoma' of the older days, and is least malignant.

2. *Malignant Teratoma Intermediate* (MTI).—This group is of high malignancy, representing the 'embryonal carcinoma' of the older days. According to the degree of malignancy, the tumours are divided into two groups—A and B, the latter being more malignant. These are usually radioresistant.

3. *Malignant Teratoma Anaplastic* (MTA).—This consists of absolutely undifferentiated cells and is highly malignant. It is radioresistant.

4. *Malignant Teratoma Trophoblastic* (MTT).—This represents the choriocarcinoma of the older days, and is radioresistant.

Predisposing Factors to Testicular Malignancy

1. *Undescended Testis.*—Malignancy is believed to be 20 to 30 times commoner than in a normally descended testis. This figure, according to many, is exaggerated.

2. *Trauma.*—The role of trauma is doubtful. Possibly it only draws the attention of the patient to the tumour.

Spread

1. DIRECT SPREAD.—The tumour gradually destroys the whole of the testicular tissue but its spread is restricted beyond the testis, at least for some time, by the tunica albuginea. Once, however, the albuginea has been infiltrated, quick spread occurs through the scrotal tissues. Ultimately the tumour may fungate through the skin on the *anterior* aspect of the scrotum (because of the location of the testis).

2. LYMPHATIC SPREAD.—As a rule, all seminoma and majority of teratoma spread by lymphatics. Seminoma, however, has a special predilection for lymphatic spread. The important points about lymphatic spread are as follows:

a. Lymphatics from the testis have no connection with the inguinal nodes. Significant enlargement of the inguinal nodes suggests scrotal involvement since the lymphatics of the scrotum drain into the inguinal nodes.

b. The major part of the lymphatics of the testis drains into the abdominal nodes because the testis had developed inside the abdomen. The lymphatics run up along the spermatic cord, up to the deep inguinal ring. Here they leave the structures of the cord, and ascend upwards and medially, by the side of the vertebral column. They drain into the para aortic nodes, on the posterior abdominal wall, up to the level of the renal veins. Above the level of the renal veins, the lymphatics of the two sides mix up. They pass up through the diaphragm. In the chest, they have communications with the mediastinal and pulmonary (hilar) nodes. Thereafter, the lymphatics drain along the thoracic duct and, in advanced cases of testicular tumours, the left supraclavicular nodes (Virchow's) may be involved.

    c. Some of the lymphatics of the testis drain, along the vas deferens, to a few nodes situated at the bifurcation of the common iliac artery of the side.

3. VENOUS SPREAD.—All teratoma spread by veins, seminoma usually only late. Venous spread is particularly early with choriocarcinoma. Lungs, liver and bones may be involved.

Clinical Features.—The average age of the patients of teratoma is 20 to 25 years; that of seminoma is 30 to 35 years. There may be a history of trauma, at least in some cases.

The presenting features are variable, and the patients may be broadly divided into three groups—the usual group, the metastatic group, and the unusual group.

GROUP A—USUAL GROUP:

1. Though testis is an organ which is so easily palpable, the patient seldom reports before six months of the onset.
2. There is a fairly rapidly increasing swelling of the testis.
3. Pain is complained only in 30 per cent of cases, though there is often a sensation of heaviness.
4. The testicular swelling is usually smooth, sometimes lobulated (usually teratoma), firm in feel. One important point of difference from a hydrocele is that the swelling is much heavier than a hydrocele of the same size.
5. There is very early loss of testicular sensation (there are two conditions where testicular sensation is lost very early—malignancy and gumma). Tenderness is usually present, sometimes severe.
6. There is no fluctuation, and transillumination test is negative.
7. A lax secondary hydrocele may be present.
8. The epididymis is flattened behind the growth or is incorporated in it, and cannot be palpated separately.
9. The spermatic cord, in an advanced case, is grossly thickened because of cremasteric hypertrophy (the cremaster has to support the heavy organ) as well as engorgement of the testicular veins and lymphatics. The vas deferens shows no abnormality.
10. The abdomen should be carefully examined for enlarged nodes and metastatic liver.
11. A clinical examination of the chest should be done.
12. The left supraclavicular nodes should be palpated.

GROUP B.—METASTATIC GROUP:

The patient does not complain of a testicular swelling either because he ignores it as a hydrocele or because the swelling is too small to draw attention (e.g. choriocarcinoma). He presents with metastatic symptoms:

1. Abdominal and/or lumbar pain, with or without an abdominal swelling (especially in seminoma).
2. Pain in the chest, cough, haemoptysis, dyspnoea, fever (especially in teratoma).
3. Jaundice, ascites, and palpable liver (hard and nodular)—especially in teratoma.

GROUP C—UNUSUAL GROUP:

1. *Hurricane Type.*—The patient is killed within a few weeks of appearance of the tumour due to widespread metastases, e.g. MTT, MTA, and MTI—B.
2. *Slow-growing Type.*—The swelling may be present for two or three years, often ignored as a hydrocele, e.g. TD.
3. Some patients may present with features like chronic epididymoorchitis, not responding to treatment.
4. Some cases may present with gynaecomastia, e g. MTT, sertoli-cell tumour.
5. Rarely a patient may present with severe pain and an acute swelling (due to haemorrhage in the tumour).

Special Investigations

I. X-RAY:

A. X-ray Chest:
  1. To reveal pulmonary metastases.
  2. To show enlarged pulmonary and mediastinal nodes.
B. IVP.—This has two purposes:
  1. *Detection.*—Enlargement of the para-aortic nodes may be suggested by displacement of the ureter and deformity of the pelvis.
  2. *Protection.*—The exact position of the kidneys are shown, so that they may be properly shielded while radiating the abdominal nodes (to prevent nephritis and hypertension).
C. Lymphangiography.—This demonstrates the enlarged paraaortic nodes. Shrinkage of the nodes with radiation can also be studied.

II. HORMONE TEST.—A 12-hour collection of urine is assayed for human chorionic gonadotrophin (HCG) by radio-immune method. The normal levels are below 100 iu. In patients with teratoma there may be high levels of HCG:
  1. In MTT the level is always high. In some other cases of teratoma also, e.g. MTI, and MTA high levels may be encountered if chorionic tissue is present in the tumour.
  2. If, during the course of treatment, the level of HCG falls, a response to the treatment is signified.

III. BIOPSY, as such, is not performed (*see* below).

Treatment.—This consists of the following measures:

A. Simple (retrograde) orchiectomy or Exploration.
B. Radiotherapy.
C. Radical orchiectomy.
D. Chemotherapy.

SIMPLE ORCHIECTOMY (ORCHIDECTOMY).—This is the first step in the treatment of all the cases where the diagnosis is clinically certain. Its ideas are:

  a. Removing the primary tumour.
  b. Relieving pain, if any.
  c. Obtaining a biopsy specimen (any other form of biopsy, e.g. aspiration or cutting, is dangerous for a malignant testis, as these procedures allow the tumour to involve the scrotal skin and open up the way to the inguinal nodes).

The operation is done with an inguinal incision, prolonged down to the scrotum. The cord is ligated high up, *at deep inguinal ring* and orchiectomy is done (this procedure removes the major part of the lymphatics, running along the cord).

As recurrence is fairly common in the scrotal skin, following orchiectomy, many surgeons advocate hemiscrotectomy (excision of the half of the scrotum), together with simple orchiectomy.

EXPLORATION.—The procedure is reserved only for the clinically doubtful cases. It should be done only when facilities for freeze-section are available. The spermatic cord is occluded with a soft clamp. The testis is opened up with a small incision on the tunica albuginea. The suspected part is excised and the specimen is subjected to immediate biopsy. The opening in the tunica albuginea is carefully closed. If the report is positive, an immediate simple orchiectomy is done.

Biopsy (either after simple orchiectomy or after exploration) not only confirms the diagnosis but also indicates the exact nature of the tumour, and this may be of great help in deciding the future course of treatment.

RADIOTHERAPY.—Almost all seminomas are radio-sensitive, most of the teratomas are radioresistant. However, radiotherapy is the form of treatment advised in all cases, irrespective of seminoma or teratoma, after the simple orchiectomy has been done and the biopsy report obtained. With the introduction of supervoltage and cobalt radiations, there has been considerable improvement in the results. This is because of high penetration, maximum action on the tumour cells, and minimum damage to the healthy tissues.

The fields of radiation are the inguino-scrotal region, abdomen, chest, and left supraclavicular area:

i. When there is no clinical or radiological evidence of metastasis.—The inguino-scrotal region and abdomen are radiated. The average dose is 3000 rad for seminoma and 4500 rad for teratoma, given over 5 to 6 weeks.

ii. When there are evidences of metastases.—Radiation is given through one inguino-scrotal, four abdominal, two mediastinal and two left supraclavicular portals. Radiation sickness is very common with such high dosage.

RADICAL ORCHIECTOMY.—The orchiectomy part of the operation has already been done at simple orchiectomy. This operation entails *en bloc* removal of the spermatic vessels, together with all the retroperitoneal nodes, from the deep ring up to the level of the renal veins. It is indicated in those cases of teratoma which fail to respond to radiotherapy. Fixed high-up abdominal nodes is a contraindication to operation.

An iliac incision is made, continued upwards and backwards from the scar of the previous inguinal incision. The ligated end of the cord is picked up and this, together with all the retroperitoneal nodes, is dissected to as high a level as is possible. The dissected mass is left in position and the wound closed.

The patient is now turned into a lateral (kidney) position and a standard kidney incision is made. The dissected mass is picked up and further dissection done to the level of the renal veins. The whole mass is removed *en bloc*.

CHEMOTHERAPY.—This is reserved for advanced, inoperable cases of teratoma, and all recurrent cases of teratoma and seminoma. A combination chemotherapy is usually advocated.

Points of difference between Seminoma and Teratoma

SEMINOMA	TERATOMA
1. Surface usually smooth. Cut surface homogenous.	1. Surface smooth or lobulated. Cut surface usually shows marked cyst formation.
2. Microscopically, the cells show a uniform appearance.	2. Microscopically, different types of cells are seen—epidermal, mesodermal, and entodermal, although one type may predominate.
3. Prefers spread by lymphatics.	3. Prefers spread by veins.
4. Peak incidence.—30 to 35 years.	4. Peak incidence.—20 to 25 years.
5. Usually very much radiosensitive.	5. Often radioresistant.
6. Treatment.—Simple orchiectomy, followed by radiotherapy.	6. Treatment.—Simple orchiectomy after which radiation is tried. If there is no response, radical orchiectomy is advocated.
7. Prognosis after proper treatment: a. No metastasis.—80 per cent survive five years. b. With metastases.—25 per cent survive five years.	7. Prognosis, with proper treatment, varies widely according to the nature of malignancy, i.e. 1 to 40 per cent may survive for five years.

HYDROCELE

Definition.—A hydrocele is a collection of serous fluid in some part of the processus vaginalis, usually the tunica vaginalis.

Types

1. VAGINAL HYDROCELE.—This is much the commoner variety. The collection of fluid is in the tunica vaginalis. It may be of two types:

   a. *Idiopathic.*—There is no definite cause for the hydrocele. Some authorities believe that it is due to a defect in the normal process of absorption of fluid from the tunica vaginalis, possibly caused by damage to the endothelial lining by low grade infection. In this country, the majority of the cases has a background of filarial epididymoorchitis. An idiopathic or primary hydrocele is usually tense and often attains big size.

   b. *Secondary.*—The hydrocele is secondary to a local pathology, e.g. tubercular epididymitis, malignant testis, etc. It is believed to be due to excessive production of fluid within the sac. A secondary hydrocele is usually small and lax.

   The cardinal features of a vaginal hydrocele are:

   i. It is a purely scrotal swelling, i.e. it is always possible 'to get above the swelling', at the root of the scrotum.

ii. It has a cystic feel.

iii. Fluctuation test is positive.

iv. Transillumination test is positive.

2. CONGENITAL HYDROCELE.—There are two types:

a. *Complete Congenital Hydrocele.*—The whole length of the processus vaginalis is patent and there is collection of fluid in it. The defect is the same as in congenital hernia, but here the communication with the peritoneum, at the deep ring, is too narrow to allow gut or omentum to enter. Appearing on prolonged standing and disappearing during sleep, the condition is sometimes associated with tuberculous peritonitis in the children.

b. *Incomplete Congenital (or Funicular) Hydrocele.*—The processus vaginalis is shut off from the tunica vaginalis to the top of the testis. Thus, the swelling extends from the deep ring to the top of the testis. The other features are the same as in the complete variety.

3. INFANTILE HYDROCELE.—Not necessarily occurring in the infants, here the processus vaginalis is continuous with the tunica vaginalis but is shut off at the deep ring. Thus, it differs from the congenital complete variety in that its size does not alter with the patient's position.

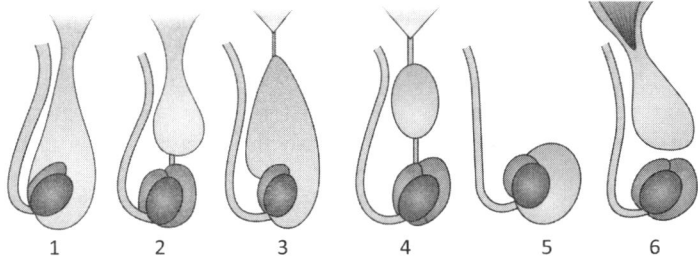

Fig. 58.1: The different types of hydrocele. 1—Congenital complete; 2—Congenital funicular; 3—Infantile; 4—Encysted hydrocele of the cord; 5—Vaginal hydrocele (commonest); 6—Hydrocele of hernial sac.

4. ENCYSTED HYDROCELE OF THE CORD.—The central part of the processus vaginalis keeps patent while its upper and lower parts obliterate. The swelling, which is localised, may be scrotal inguino-scrotal, or inguinal. It is oval in shape, cystic in feel, show fluctuation and a positive transillumination. Pulling the testis downwards brings the swelling down and fixes it *(traction test).*

5. BILOCULAR HYDROCELE.—There is an hour-glass sac, the upper part of which is inside the abdomen, and the size of the communication variable. A cross-fluctuation, between the two parts, may be elicited.

6. HYDROCELE OF THE HERNIAL SAC.—In this condition there is some stagnated fluid in a hernial sac, the opening of the sac at the internal ring having been blocked by a tag of omentum.

Operations for Vaginal Hydrocele

INCISION:

1. For a *small hydrocele,* when excision of scrotal skin is not necessary, a paramedian incision is made. This is a vertical incision, just lateral to the median raphe.

Even for unilateral hydrocele, a bilateral operation is preferable since the other vaginal sac is very likely to develop hydrocele in future. For this purpose, as well as for bilateral vaginal hydrocele, (i) either, two paramedian incisions, one on each side, is made, (ii) or, more commonly, the operation is done with only one incision. In the latter event, after operating for the hydrocele on one side, an incision is made through the median raphe and the opposite testis, with the sac, is brought out through the rent. The operation for the hydrocele on this side being done, the testis is put back to its own chamber and the opening made in the median raphe is sutured.

2. In cases of *big hydrocele*, excision of a part of the scrotal skin is necessary. For this purpose, a transverse elliptical incision is made round the lower part of the scrotum, and the skin, included in the ellipse, is excised. This incision opens up both the chambers of the scrotum. While closing, the skin wound is sutured vertically.

3. In case of a *small hydrocele associated with an inguinal hernia,* the testis, with the sac, can be pulled up to the inguinal incision for the hernia, and operated.

TYPES OF OPERATION.—Two types of operation are practised:

1. *Eversion of Sac.*—A rent is made on the anterior wall of the sac and the fluid is drained out. The testis and epididymis are pushed out through this opening and the sac is everted, inside out. The cut margins of the sac are sutured to each other, behind the testis and epididymis. The rationality of eversion, in the treatment of hydrocele, is as follows:

   a. In the early postoperative days, the secretion of the tunica vaginalis (whose secretory surface is now in contact with the subcutaneous tissue of the scrotum) is immediately absorbed by the scrotal lymphatics and veins.

   b. Later, due to constant friction with subcutaneous tissue, the secreting endothelium of the sac changes its character and gradually stops secreting.

2. *Excision of Sac.*—After the fluid is drained, the whole of the sac is excised, leaving a margin of only half an inch by the side of the testis and epididymis. Bleeding from the cut margin, which is often considerable, is controlled either by a continuous mattress suture or with diathermy.

   Excision of sac, in preference to eversion, is particularly indicated for:

   a. Thick and voluminous sac (otherwise the scrotum remains big in size).

   b. Infected sac.

   c. Haematocele.

DRAINAGE.—After any operation for hydrocele, drainage of the scrotal chamber must be provided for at least 48 hours. This is done either with corrugated rubber or with a few strands of nylon. Unless this is done, blood and secreted fluid collect inside the scrotum, and this may lead to gross secondary infection.

N.B.—While operations for vaginal hydrocele and encysted hydrocele of the cord (the latter can usually be brought down to the scrotum) are done with incision on the scrotum, the operations for the other types of hydrocele have to be undertaken with inguinal incision.

Complications of Hydrocele
1. Haematocele.—Due to trauma.
2. Suppurative hydrocele or pyocele.—Due to infection.
3. Calcification of the sac wall.
4. Atrophy of the testis in long standing cases (rare).
5. Rupture.—Due to trauma (rare).
6. Hernia of the hydrocele sac—This occurs very rarely in longstanding cases. Tension of the fluid causes herniation of the sac through the dartos muscle.

CYSTS IN CONNECTION WITH THE EPIDIDYMIS TYPES

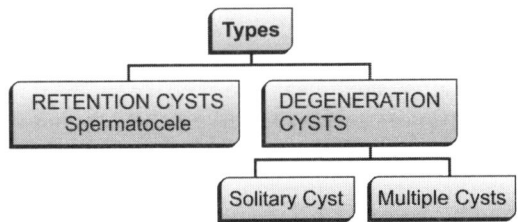

Spermatocele

ORIGIN AND PATHOLOGY.—This is a unilocular retention cyst. It is derived from some part of the sperm-conducting part of the epididymis, as a result of distal obstruction.

The cyst is located near the head of the epididymis. It is filled with fluid resembling barley water and containing spermatozoa (c.f. fluid of hydrocele, which is amber-coloured like urine, and fluid of a degenerative cyst of epididymis, which is crystal-clear).

Clinical Features:
1. The patient presents with a scrotal swelling, which is usually small. Only occasionally it may be big in size.
2. Usually there is no symptom, e.g. pain.
3. Being located at the head of the epididymis, it is always above and behind the testis (c f hydrocele).
4. The testis can be felt separately from the swelling (c.f. hydrocele). Sometimes the patient feels the swelling like a third testis.
5. The swelling is soft (c f hydrocele and degenerative cysts of epididymis).
6. The swelling is translucent.

Treatment
1. Small symptomless spermatoceles require no treatment and may be ignored.
2. If the patient is anxious about the swelling and demands treatment, either of the following two procedures may be adopted:
   a. Aspiration of the cyst.
   b. Excision of the cyst.

Degeneration Cysts of the Epididymis

MULTIPLE CYSTS.—These are usually widespread in the epididymis, but more marked at its head. The condition is often bilateral. The cysts feel like a bunch of tiny grapes, located behind the testis. They are brilliantly transilluminant (because they contain crystal-clear fluid) and, as they are multilocular, the transilluminated mass may show a latticed pattern.

Treatment is required only if the swelling is troublesome. It consists in excision of the cysts. Aspiration is useless as the mass is multilocular.

The *origin* of the cysts is debated. It is believed to be due to dilatation of the tubules of the epididymis.

SOLITARY CYSTS.—These are commoner than multiple cysts may be unilocular or multilocular, and may attain large size. They are located either outside (usually) or inside the tunica vaginalis, between the body of the testis and the head of the epididymis. They contain crystal-clear fluid and are, therefore, transilluminant.

Treatment consists in excision of the cyst.

The cyst is always degenerative in *origin* but the organ undergoing degeneration may vary. Thus, it may be a cyst of degeneration of either of the following structures:

1. The paradidymis (organ of Geralde's), which represents the remnant of the Wolffian body.
2. The vasa aberrantia, which are normal diverticula at the lower end of the vas deferens.
3. The appendix of the testis (sessile hydatid cyst of Morgagni), which represents the remnant of the müllerian duct in the males.
4. The appendix of the epididymis (pedunculated hydatid cyst of Morgagni).

(*see* embryology).

TUBERCULAR EPIDIDYMITIS

In tropical countries the commonest cause of epididymitis (or epididymoorchitis) is filaria; the next common cause is tuberculosis.

Routes of Infection

1. In the majority of cases the infection is secondary to urinary tuberculosis. From the posterior urethra the infection enters by way of the common ejaculatory duct and then flows *retrograde* along the vas deferens. In such cases the *tail* of the epididymis is involved first. Simultaneous involvement of the seminal vesicles (by way of the common ejaculatory duct) and the prostate (by way of the prostatic ducts) may occur from the posterior urethra.
2. In some cases the infection is *blood-borne* and here it is the *head* of the epididymis which is usually involved first.

Pathology.—Tubercles form in the epididymis, which becomes enlarged and nodular. Subsequently cold abscesses may form. The abscess may involve the scrotal skin and rupture on the surface, causing a persistent scrotal sinus. Because of the location of the epididymis, the sinus is usually situated on the posterior aspect of the scrotum. The testis remains normal till late in the course of the disease; however, there may be a tubercular epididymoorchitis. A lax secondary hydrocele may form.

Clinical Features

1. In two-thirds of the cases there is either an active tuberculosis of the urinary tract or a suggestive past history. Similarly, in some cases there may be history of pulmonary tuberculosis. The remaining patients show no evidence of tuberculosis elsewhere.
2. The patient's usual complaint is a dull aching pain inside the scrotum, associated with a small swelling.
3. On examination, in early cases, a discrete, slightly indurated nodule is palpable, usually in the globus minor, sometimes in the globus major. In an advanced case, the whole of the epididymis is irregularly nodular *(craggy)*, firm in feel, with little tenderness.
4. The scrotal skin may be free, may be adherent, may show evidence of a cold abscess, or may show a typical tubercular sinus or ulcer, located on the posterior surface of the scrotum (only in the rare instances of anteverted testis will the sinus be located anteriorly on the scrotum).
5. The vas deferens may be typically "beaded" due to presence of submucous tubercles.
6. A lax secondary hydrocele may be present (30 per cent of cases).
7. The testis usually feels normal.
8. Rectal examination is valuable. It may elicit an irregular indurated seminal vesicle or nodules on the prostate.
9. The kidneys should be carefully palpated.

Special Investigations

1. Blood examination.—TC, DC, and ESR.
2. Mantoux test.
3. X-ray chest.
4. Urine examination, as done for suspected cases of urinary tuberculosis (see Chapter 54).
5. IVP.
6. Cystoscopy.

Treatment

1. Where active urinary tuberculosis is present, attention is paid more in treating that. The same is true for pulmonary tuberculosis.
2. Associated or not with urinary or pulmonary tuberculosis, epididymal tuberculosis is basically treated by conservative (antitubercular) treatment, together with support to the scrotum with a suspensory bandage (this minimises the pain).
3. *Surgery* is indicated under the following circumstances:
   a. If the lesion fails to heal with antitubercular drugs.
   b. If there is a scrotal sinus.
   c. If the testis is involved.

Types of surgery:

1. *Epididymectomy.*—This is indicated when the testis is not involved (confirmed on exploration of the scrotum). The epididymis is separated from the testis and from the tunica vaginalis, the dissection starting from the lower pole of the epididymis. The vas deferens is divided opposite the upper pole of the

epididymis. If, however, the vas is involved, it is divided as high up as is possible (at the deep inguinal ring).

2. *Orchiectomy.*—The epididymis and the testis are removed together, after ligating the cord. This has to be performed if:

   a. The testis is involved in the pathology.

   b. There is troublesome bleeding during epididymectomy.

3. Excision of the scrotal sinus, together with epididymectomy or orchiectomy, has to be undertaken if a sinus is present.

VARICOCELE

This is a state of varicosity of the veins of the spermatic cord, i.e. the veins of the pampiniform plexus as well as the cremasteric veins. The veins are dilated, elongated, and tortuous.

Surgical Anatomy.—The pampiniform plexus of veins, draining the testis and epididymis, makes the major bulk of the spermatic cord. These veins gradually coalesce and, on reaching the posterior abdominal wall through the deep inguinal ring, they form the solitary (occasionally duplicated) testicular vein.

On the left side the testicular vein drains into the renal vein and the junction is a right angle. On the right side the testicular vein opens directly into the inferior vena cava and the junction is oblique.

This venous system is devoid of valves. Only near the termination of the testicular vein there may be valves, which again are often absent.

The cremasteric veins have wide communications with the veins of the pampiniform plexus. The cremasteric veins open into the inferior epigastric vein.

Thus, the pampiniform plexus, which is devoid of valves, has to carry the weight of a long column of blood. Moreover, there is no real support for these veins as they hang loose in the scrotum. They are, therefore, always in the risk of developing a state of varicosity.

As these veins undergo congestion, the channels of communication between these and the cremasteric veins open up with the idea of a collateral venous return. Soon, therefore, the cremasteric veins also undergo varicosity. According to some authorities, the main bulk of the varicocele is made by the dilated cremasteric veins.

Causes

1. Almost always the condition is *idiopathic*, no definite cause being found. It occurs almost inclusively on the left side, and there are definite anatomical explanations for such predilection (*see* below).

2. Rarely, varicocele is *secondary* to hypernephroma of the kidney. Then again, it is likely to occur on the left side, where the renal vein, being blocked by tumour tissue (venous permeation), prevents drainage of the testicular vein, which on the left side opens into the renal vein.

Causes of Predilection for the Left Side.—Various anatomical reasons have been put forward to explain why idiopathic varicocele occurs almost exclusively on the left side:

1. The left testicular vein opens at right angle (into the renal vein) while the right testicular vein opens very obliquely (into the inferior vena cava).

Thus, the outflow from the left vein is never as free as it is from the right vein.

2. The total length of the testicular vein and pampiniform plexus is always more on the left side than on the right because:
   a. The left testis hangs at a lower level.
   b. The left testicular vein opens at a higher level.
3. Blood flow along the left testicular vein may be obstructed by anatomical structures, as follows:
   a. The left testicular artery sometimes arches over the left renal vein, and may obstruct it.
   b. The descending colon, containing hard stool, may cause pressure on the termination of the testicular vein against the psoas muscle.

Varicocele and Spermatogenesis.—In some cases there may be gross interference with spermatogenesis, and oligospermia may result. This is believed to be due to the rise of temperature in the testis as a result of venous stasis. There is a natural attempt to overcome this rise of temperature by relaxation of the dartos. This relaxation results in elongation of the scrotum on the affected side.

Clinical Features

1. The patient is usually a young adult. Tall, thin and visceroptotic persons are more susceptible. The condition is more frequent (and more troublesome) in hot climates.
2. As stated, it is exclusively found on the left side.
3. Usually varicocele is painless and the only complaint of the patient is the swelling. Often, however, there is a sense of heaviness. The swelling and the sensation increase progressively towards the end of the day. They are minimum when the patient leaves the bed in the morning. If pain is present, it is due to the fact that the elongated scrotum no longer supports the testis and its weight has to be fully borne by the cord. The pain is worse on prolonged standing.
4. Some of the patients may present because of subfertility as a result of oligospermia (*see* above).
5. On examination, the dilated veins have a typical *bag of worms* feel. On coughing, there is an impulse like a fluid thrill. On making the patient recumbent and elevating the scrotum, the swelling may be made to reduce in size. Thereafter, if the external ring is pressed and the patient is asked to stand, the varicocele is found to fill from below (c f hernia).

Treatment

A. CONSERVATIVE TREATMENT.—Many of the cases can be managed by conservative methods, which include:
   1. Wearing a suspensory bandage.
   2. Reassurance to the patient.
B. OPERATIVE TREATMENT.—Operation is indicated under the following conditions:
   1. If there is pain.
   2. If there is gross oligospermia, leading to subfertility.
   3. If the testis hangs to an abnormally low level or if gross varicosity is present, and conservative treatment has failed.

The spermatic cord is exposed either with an *inguinal incision* or with a *scrotal incision*. The foot end of the table may be lowered a little to make the veins fill up, for better identification. All the coverings of the cord are carefully split. The vas deferens with its artery, and one or two veins of the pampiniform plexus are separated from the main mass of the varicocele. The affected veins are ligated and divided, preferably excising a length of 2 inches. The veins should be ligated and divided, in small bunches. This prevents slipping of ligatures, which may cause serious haemorrhage. The upper and lower cut ends of the bunches may be ligated to each other, so that the cord is shortened in length and the testis is elevated.

Some surgeons advocate simple ligature of the testicular vein above the inguinal ligament.

ELEPHANTIASIS OF THE SCROTUM

Etiology.—Elephantiasis of the scrotum is almost always due to *filariasis*, caused by infestation with the parasite *Wucheria bancrofti*, and this is limited to the tropical countries. *Nonfilarial elephantiasis*, which is encountered only rarely, is due to granuloma venereum, but in these cases the elephantiasis is never as massive as it is with filariasis.

WUCHERIA BANCROFTI.—This parasite, a nematode, passes its life cycle in two hosts— man and mosquito (Culex or Anopheles).

The *definitive host* is man, in whose lymphatic system (vessels and glands) the adult worms live and die. The worms are long and hair-like. There are male and female worms. Males and females remain coiled together and sporulate. After sporulation, female worm dies and innumerable embryos (microfilariae) are produced. These microfilariae enter the peripheral blood, where they are capable of living for a considerable time, without undergoing developmental meta-morphosis. From the peripheral blood they are sucked in by mosquitoes.

The *intermediate host* is a mosquito, in whom the microfilariae undergo further development and maturation. However, these mature microfilariae are still sexually immature.

On *entering into man again* (by the bite of the infested mosquito), these microfilariae are deposited in pairs—at first in the skin, at the site of the puncture. They then penetrate the skin and reach the lymph vessels. They settle down at some site in the lymphatic system of the upper or the lower extremity, depending on the site of the bite. The most favourite site for this settling is the inguino-scrotal region. Here they begin to grow into adult forms. After a few months they become sexually mature. The male fertilises the female, the female dies, and microfilariae are formed.

Pathogenesis.—The pathological effects caused by the Wucheria are due to the adult worms, living or dead. The microfilariae do not cause any pathology, excepting in highly reacting individuals.

The pathology can essentially be divided into two parts—lymphangitis and lymphatic obstruction.

CAUSES OF LYMPHANGITIS:

1. *Mechanical.*—Irritation, caused by the movements of the adult worm along the lymphatic system.

2. *Allergic.*—This may be due to three factors:
   a. Liberation of toxic products from the dead worms, undergoing degeneration.
   b. Liberation of toxins by the fertilised females at the time of parturition.
   c. Liberation of mild toxins by the microfilariae (this works only in the highly reacting individuals).
3. *Secondary.*—Bacterial infection usually streptococcal, is often an additional factor in causing lymphangitis.

EFFECTS OF LYMPHANGITIS:

1. *Obliterative endolymphangitis.*—There is an endothelial proliferation and inflammatory thickening of the wall of the lymph vessels, and these tend to occlude their lumen.
2. *Fibrosis* of the lymph vessels, often extensive, caused by recurrent attacks of lymphangitis.

CAUSES OF LYMPHATIC OBSTRUCTION:

1. Fibrosis:
   a. Of the lymph vessels
   b. Of the lymph nodes $\Big\}$ from recurrent infections.
2. Imprisonment of the adult worms:
   a. In the lymph vessels
   b. In the lymph nodes $\Big\}$ which have undergone fibrosis

The imprisoned worms as they die, produce further fibrosis by foreign body reaction.

Pathology of Elephantiasis Scrotum.—Elephantiasis, i.e. a solid oedema, is the end-result of filarial infestation. By the time it develops, all mature worms have practically died.

Lymphatic obstruction, brought about over a span of many years, causes exudation of lymph in the connective tissues of the scrotum. The protein in the lymph stimulates the connective tissue to excessive growth, so that the scrotum becomes enormously enlarged, sometimes to as big as a watermelon. The lymph stasis provides nourishment for luxurious growth of fibrosis tissue in the subcutaneous plane. Thus the swelling develops a tumour-like solidity, not pitting on pressure.

The scrotum is a common site for elephantiasis because of several factors:

a. The dependent position of the scrotum and the great laxity of its subcutaneous tissue, both factors allowing considerable stagnation of lymph.
b. The special predilection of the microfilariae and the adult worms for the lymphatics of the inguino-scrotal region.

The surface of the skin is rough and fissured, like the skin of an elephant (hence, the name elephantiasis). The subcutaneous tissue gets a *blubbery,* i.e. oedematous appearance *(blubber* = a jelly fish), due to the lymph-logging. The thickening commences at the most dependent part of the scrotum and extends upwards. Ultimately it involves the root of the scrotum. In at least some cases, it extends to the skin and subcutaneous tissue of the penis (*see* below). However, the thickening is always maximum towards the bottom of the scrotum.

Associated Pathology in Cases of Filarial Scrotum

1. SCROTAL SKIN:
   a. Lymph vesicles of varying size may appear, due to lymphatic obstruction.
   b. Lymphorrhagia, i.e. profuse exudation of lymph from the scrotal surface, due to rupture of the vesicles.
   c. Cellulitis, suppuration, and rarely gangrene of the scrotum, due to secondary infection of the water-logged tissues.

2. TESTIS AND EPIDIDYMIS:
   a. Epididymo-orchitis, usually due to secondary infection (streptococcal). Epididymitis is commoner and more severe than orchitis. The epididymis is tender and swollen.
   b. The lower pole of the testis gets anchored to the bottom of the scrotum by hypertrophied gubernaculum testis.
   c. Often there is an atrophy of the testis due to pressure and lack of nutrition.

3. SPERMATIC CORD.—Funiculitis, usually in association with epididymo-orchitis. The cord is tender and swollen. The lymph vessels in the cord are particularly involved. Sometimes dilatation of these vessels may produce elongated cystic swellings, which are termed *diffuse hydrocele of the cord*.

4. TUNICA VAGINALIS:
   a. Hydrocele is the commonest accompaniment and is due to an effusion into the tunica vaginalis, resulting from lymphatic obstruction.
   b. Chylocele, i.e. collection of chylous (milky) fluid in the tunica vaginalis, resulting from rupture of the obstructed lymph vessels. Hence, the fluid may contain microfilaria.

5. INGUINAL LYMPH NODES:
   a. Acute lymphadenitis.
   b. Chronic lymphadenitis.

6. PENIS:
   a. Elephantiasis of penis sometimes accompanies elephantiasis of the scrotum due to involvement of its skin and subcutaneous tissue. Only rarely elephantiasis of the penis occurs separately. In advanced cases, owing to inequal pull by the fibrous tissue deposited in the subcutaneous layer and fascia around the penis, the thickened penis is distorted. It is then termed *ram's horn penis*.
   b. More commonly, the penis is healthy but is buried either completely or partially within the elephantiatic scrotum.

7. CONSTITUTIONAL DISTURBANCES.—Filarial fever, often high (103–104 °F), usually associated with chill and rigor, and often occurring characteristically during the new-moons and full-moons. The filarial fever, epididymo orchitis, funiculitis, and acute inguinal lymphadenitis often precede the development of the elephantiasis, and thereafter usually accompany it.

8. INVOLVEMENT OF OTHER PARTS.—The lower limb in particular, the breast, etc. may show evidence of filarial involvement.

Clinical Features.—These have all been described in details under the pathology, above. The excessively thick and unyielding scrotal wall may make it impossible to palpate the contents within, viz., testis, epididymis, cord, etc. A hydrocele is usually associated, but fluctuation and transillumination cannot be elicited through the thick skin.

Special Investigations

1. *Blood Examination:*
   a. Eosinophilia is often noticed.
   b. Microfilariae may be found in thick film, drawn at night. In case of elephantiasis they are usually not seen in the blood because of lymphatic obstruction.
2. *Immunological Tests,* e.g. complement fixation test, are of a little value.

Treatment of Elephantiasis Scrotum.—This is always operative. The patient is, however, prepared pre-operatively as follows:

1. A course of specific anti-filarial drug, e.g. Hetrazan or Banocide (100 mg thrice daily, for 2 to 3 weeks).
2. A course of antibiotic, to guard against the secondary streptococcal infection. A combination of antibiotic and non-specific proteins, e.g. omnamycin, often works better.

THE OPERATION:

1. If the skin at the root of the scrotum is healthy, an elliptical incision is made on the scrotum, as for the operation of a big hydrocele, and the elephantiatic scrotal tissue is excised. In doing this, the plane of cleavage between the scrotum and the parietal layer of the tunica vaginalis should be carefully found out and dissection carried in that plane; this minimises the haemorrhage. For hydroceles, which are always present, bilateral eversion of sacs is done. If the sacs are grossly thickened, excision of the sacs is performed instead. If there is a chylocele, the sac must be excised. The remaining scrotal skin is sutured to cover the testes.

   There is, however, the risk of the remaining scrotal skin developing elephantiasis in future.

2. If the whole of the scrotum is involved, it has to be totally excised with an elliptical incision. The hydrocele or chylocele is treated, as described above. The testis, on either side, has to be accommodated in the subcutaneous tissue of the medial side of the corresponding thigh, by mobilising the skin flaps. The skin flaps of the two sides are then apposed in the midline, at the perineum. Subsequently, it is often found that this skin hangs down by the weight of the testes and takes the shape of a scrotum.

Operation for Elephantiasis Scrotum with Ram's Horn Penis.—A racket shaped incision is made. The handle of the racket is a vertical midline incision along the dorsum of the penis, extending downwards from the symphisis pubis to just above the prepuce. The blade of the racket extends on either side from the upper end of this incision, round the root of the penis and the root of the scrotum. The scrotal part is dealt with first. The whole of the scrotum is excised, as described above. Bilateral eversion of sacs (or excision) is performed. The penile skin is then excised, the excision extending up to the junction of the skin and prepuce, keeping the prepuce intact. Thus the penis is completely decorticated, as are the testes. In decorticating the penis, damage to the urethra may be prevented in two ways:

a. Continuing the dissection on the penis in the same plane as that in the scrotum.

b. Passing a catheter or bougie per urethra for its identification.

The decorticated testes are implanted in the thighs, as described above. The decorticated penis may be covered by either of the following ways:

1. By partial thickness (Thiersch's) skin grafts, taken from the thigh.
2. By drawing the prepuce back, over the raw surface of the penis, and keeping it in position with a few sutures. Fortunately, the prepuce is never involved in elephantiasis.

IDIOPATHIC (FOURNIER'S) GANGRENE OF THE SCROTUM

Etiology.—This is a quickly spreading gangrene of the scrotum, the cause of which is not definitely known. The usual explanation is that there is an obliterative arteritis of the arterioles supplying the scrotal skin, resulting from a fulminating inflammation in the subcutaneous tissue of the scrotum (usually streptococcal, sometimes staphylococcal, *B. coli, Cl. welchii*).

Clinical Features.—There is sudden appearance of inflammation in the scrotum, which quickly progresses to a stage of gangrene. This gangrene usually spreads all over the scrotum and even to the surrrounding skin. The skin sloughs out, exposing the testes covered with the tunica.

Treatment

1. An antibiotic is started after sending the discharge for culture and antibiotic-sensitivity tests. Usually chloromycetin gives the best results. The local area is covered with dressings soaked in acriflavine or by applying an antibiotic powder or ointment. In between the dressings, acriflavine bath of the scrotum is advocated.
2. If there is no response, the gangrenous skin is excised. This reduces the toxicity and provides good drainage.
3. Later, an operation is undertaken to cover up the testes. This may be done either by the remaining scrotal skin or, in its absence, by implanting the testes on the medial side of the thighs.

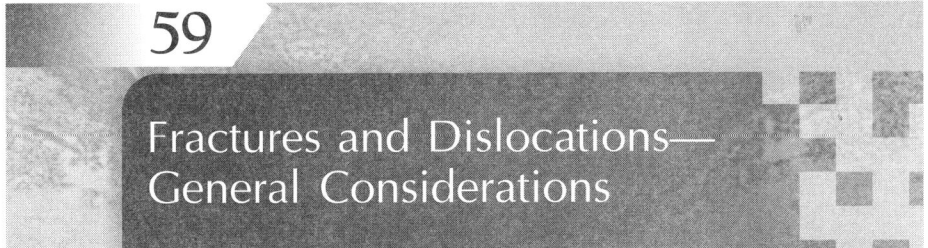

59

Fractures and Dislocations—General Considerations

Solution of continuity of a bone is called fracture.

A fracture disrupts the bone matrix, the periosteum and the endosteum, as well as the blood vessels in the cortex, medulla and periosteum. It is obvious that the force, which can break the bone, must cause considerable damage to the neighbouring soft tissues as well.

CLASSIFICATION OF FRACTURES

Fractures may be classified in different ways, as described below:

A. Fractures may be:
1. Traumatic
2. Pathological or Spontaneous } discussed below.
3. Stress or March

B. Fractures may be:
1. Simple.—There is one fracture line, i.e. two fracture fragments.
2. Comminuted.—There are more than one fracture lines, i.e. more than two fracture fragments.
3. Multiple.—There is more than one fracture either in the same bone at different levels or in different bones.
4. Compression or Crush.—The fractured bone collapses. There is, as if, a 'powdering' of the spongy bone substance, e.g. fractures of vertebra, calcaneum.

C. Fractures may be:
1. Transverse
2. Oblique } according to the disposition of the fracture line.
3. Spiral

D. Fractures may be:
1. Complete.—Here the whole thickness of the bone has been disrupted. A complete fracture may be:
   a. Impacted.—One fragment gets impacted into another.
   b. Non-impacted.—The fragments keep separate. In the majority of the cases there is a displacement between the two fragments. When displacement of a fracture is described, it is usually the position of the lower fragment, in relation to the upper, that is mentioned.
2. Incomplete.—Here some thickness of the bone still keeps intact, e.g.
a. Green-stick fractures in children. The bones, in the children, are so elastic that, when a twisting or angulating force is applied, the whole thickness of

the bone does not break. Instead, one cortex breaks while the other cortex is simply moulded.

    b. Fracture through one table of the skull, while the other table keeps intact.

E. Fractures may be:

  1. Simple or Closed.

  2. Compound or Open.—The fracture site communicates with the external air through injuries in the soft tissues, overlying the fracture. This may occur in two ways.

    a. The trauma, causing the fracture, also causes so much of soft tissue injury and break of surface that the fracture site communicates with the exterior *(external compound fracture)*.

    b. The sharp end of a fracture fragment penetrates through the overlying soft tissues and the skin *(internal compound fracture)*.

The real danger of a compound fracture is the great risk of its getting contaminated and, thereafter, infected.

Traumatic Fracture.—This means a fracture which occurs in a healthy bone, as a result of trauma. There may be three types of trauma:

1. *Direct violence.*—The bone breaks at the site where the trauma is inflicted.

2. *Indirect violence.*—*The* bone breaks at a site away from the site of the trauma. The best example is fractured clavicle in a child, as a result of fall on the outstretched hand, the trauma being conducted along the bones of the forearm and the arm.

3. *Muscular violence.*—Sudden contraction of a muscle may cause fracture of the bone to which it is attached, e.g. patella by the quadriceps femoris, olecranon process by the triceps.

Pathological or Spontaneous Fracture.—In this type, the bone, at the site of the fracture, is so weak that a rather trivial injury causes a fracture. The injury is such that it would not be able to cause a fracture, had the bone been healthy. Some common cause of weakness in the bone, that may result in pathological fractures are as follows:

GROUP A: LOCALISED BONE PATHOLOGY:

1. *Infection*

    a. Chronic pyogenic osteomyelitis, particularly when there is a large sequestrum.

    b. Syphilitic osteomyelitis of osteolytic type.

2. *Benign Tumours*

    a. Enchondroma.

    b. Osteoclastoma.

3. *Malignant Tumours*

    a. Secondary carcinoma.

    b. Ewing's tumour.

    c. Osteogenic sarcoma.

4. *Miscellaneous*

    a. Simple bone cyst.

    b. Monostotic fibrous dysplasia.

    c. Irradiated bones.

GROUP B: GENERALISED BONE DISEASES:

1. *Congenital*
   Osteogenesis imperfecta, i.e. fragile bones.
2. *Generalised Decalcification of Bones*
   a. Hyperparathyroidism.
   b. Rickets.
   c. Osteomalacia.
3. *Malignant Tumours*
   a. Multiple myeloma.
   b. Multiple secondary carcinoma.
4. *Miscellaneous*
   a. Paget's disease.
   b. Polyostotic fibrous dysplasia.
   Pathological fractures are more likely to occur in the weight-bearing bones.

Stress or Fatigue or March Fracture.—The term stress or fatigue fracture has come from cracks, occurring in the metals, over those parts which are 'fatigued' by repeated 'stress'. Bones in the body, which are similarly exposed to repeated minor trauma at the same site, may also develop such fractures, and hence they are so named. These fractures are commonest in the metatarsals (particularly the second), in the soldiers, and result from prolonged marching. So they are also known as march fractures. Rarely, such stress fractures may occur in fibula in the dancers. Still rarely, they may occur in the tibia or the neck of the femur.

One of the characteristic features of march fractures is the huge amount of callus formation that may sometimes be mistaken for tumours on the X-ray.

HEALING OF FRACTURES

For purpose of simplicity, healing of a fracture is described in 5 stages.

1. STAGE OF HAEMATOMA FORMATION.—As soon as the fracture occurs, a variable quantity of blood collects and forms a haematoma at the fracture site and around it. The blood comes from the torn vessels in the cortex, medulla and periosteum as well as the neighbouring soft tissues. It is important to note that this haematoma takes a little or no part in the repair. The haematoma is invaded by granulation tissue, whose macrophages remove the haematoma.

2. STAGE OF CELLULAR PROLIFERATION.—A cellular proliferation then occurs from either end of the fracture, along the gap in the fracture line, in an attempt to produce new tissues, to bridge up the gap. These cells develop from:
   a. Endothelial cells of the capillaries of the newly-formed granulation tissue.
   b. The periosteum and endosteum that are torn at the fracture site and are avulsed from their attachments at the surface of the bone. Cells in these structures are stimulated to proliferation either by the act of avulsion or by the action of humoral agents, originating in the medulla.
   c. Histiocytes, which possibly represent undifferentiated primitive mesen-chymal cells.
   d. Osteocytes in the fractured bone itself (doubtful).

3. STAGE OF NEW TISSUE AND CALLUS FORMATION.—A new tissue is now formed at the fracture site. The cells in the new tissue are the precursors of osteoblasts. Their

function is to lay down a loose connective tissue, composed of collagen fibres, embedded in a gel of mucopolysaccharide. This tissue is first converted into fibrous tissue and cartilage, which have very little rigidity and strength. From the third week onwards, the tissue is impregnated with calcium salt and it is called callus. Callus is hard and elastic. It has three component parts:

a. *Interstitial callus.*—It is that part of the callus which bridges the gap along the thickness of the cortical part of the bone.

b. *Internal callus.*—This is the part of the callus which is in the medullary cavity.

c. *External callus.*—It is the part which lies heaped up outside the outline of the bone.

4. STAGE OF NEW BONE FORMATION.—Eventually, the callus is replaced by fully differentiated Haversian bone. This is done by the osteoblasts, now formed from their precursors, described above.

5. STAGE OF REMODELLING.—Over the ensuing months to years, the external and the internal callus are gradually absorbed and the fracture site is remodelled to near normal.

TREATMENT OF CLOSED FRACTURES

Principles.—The principles of treatment are:

A. Reduction, if there are displacements.

B. Retention in position, i.e. immobilisation.

C. Restitution of function.

A. Reduction.—There are two methods of reduction:

1. Closed reduction.

2. Open reduction.

1. CLOSED REDUCTION.—This again may be achieved in two ways:

a. *Manipulation.*—This is the most commonly practised method. It is usually done under general anaesthesia because relaxation of the muscles is necessary to bring the fragments in position. Sometimes, however, regional or even local anaesthesia is used. Traction along the line of the bone is usually the first manoeuvre; this is done in an attempt to correct the overriding. Sometimes, this alone is sufficient to achieve reduction. Otherwise, a force, the reverse of that which caused the fracture, has to be applied.

b. *Continuous Traction.*—In those fractures, where big muscles are attached to the fragments, manipulation is incapable of reducing the fracture since the pull of the muscles is too strong to be combated by manual effort, even under general anaesthesia. In these cases a gradual reduction of the fragments is achieved by applying mechanical traction to the lower fragment. Reduction by traction is usually necessary for fractures in the big bones of the lower limb, particularly in the adults.

(For types of traction, *see* Chapter on instruments).

2. OPEN REDUCTION.—Reduction may have to be done under direct visualisation of the fragments, by operative methods. The *indications* for open reduction are as follows:

a. Where closed reduction is impossible:

    i. A small fragment is unmanageable (e.g. lateral condyle of humerus).

   ii. A small fragment is trapped in a joint (e.g. medial epicondyle of humerus).

   iii. Soft tissues are interposed between the fragments.

  b. Where closed reduction is inaccurate and the fracture demands accurate reduction, e.g. fractures involving joint surfaces.

  c. Where internal fixation is obligatory to keep the fragments in position.

B. Immobilisation.—This may be done by three methods:

  1. Plastering.

  2. Splintage.

  3. Internal fixation.

1. PLASTERING.—Immobilisation in plaster may be done in two ways:

  a. *Complete Plastering.*—The whole circumference of the limb is encased in plaster. For ordinary plastering, in any limb, the lower limit of the plaster is usually constant, as follows:

    i. For the upper limb.—Dorsally to the knuckles and ventrally to the proximal palmar crease, so that the metacarpophalangeal joints are kept free.

    ii. For the lower limb.—Covering the whole sole like a shoe and dorsally keeping the toes open.

    The exception to the above is a *tube plastering,* which does not include the hand or foot.

    The proximal extent of the plaster depends on the level of the fracture and should be such that proper immobilisation of the fragments is done. The general principle, therefore, is to include in the plaster joint proximal to the fracture.

  b. *Plaster Cast.*—Here only half the circumference of the limb is covered with the plaster, the remaining part being bandaged to keep the cast in position. The cast should be placed on that side of the limb to which the fragments have a tendency to be displaced, e.g. a dorsally placed cast for Colles' fracture.

2. SPLINTAGE.—Immobilisation in a splint, instead of plaster, is particularly suitable under the following conditions:

  a. If the fracture is such that, unless continuous traction is maintained, the fragments tend to be redisplaced (e.g. oblique or spiral fractures). While the traction prevents overlapping of the fragments, the splint gives support to the limb against angular deformity.

  b. If there is an associated wound in the limb, it can be better attended on a splint than through a plaster window.

3. INTERNAL FIXATION.—The indications and methods of internal fixation are discussed in the Chapter on instruments.

C. Restitution of Function.—While treating fractures, all attempts must be made to bring the function of the limb back to normal. It is useless to think of a fracture healing but the limb not getting back its normal function. Care must be taken to see that the movements of the joints, which have not been incorporated in the plaster or splint, are regularly practised. After the period of immobilisation is over, the immobilised area must have proper exercises. In this respect, active movements are always preferred to passive movements. Physiotherapy, in an attempt to bring back the muscle power and the movements, is very useful.

TREATMENT OF COMPOUND FRACTURES

The real danger of a compound fracture is that the wound is generally contaminated and is likely to be infected shortly. The degree of contamination varies from case to case, and depends not only on the severity of the injury but also on other factors, e.g. the place of occurrence. If the wound has not been attended for some time, contamination leads to infection, i.e. the wound is already infected. While infection may be dangerous for the soft tissue, it is equally so for the bone, as it leads to osteomyelitis and non-union.

Problems.—The problems of a compound fracture may be enumerated as follows:
1. Shock, in severe cases.
2. Infection in the bone, leading to non-union.
3. Laceration of the muscles, inviting gas gangrene.
4. Infection over a wide area leading to toxaemia and septicaemia, and also infection by spore-bearing organisms, e.g. tetanus.
5. Crushing or actual loss of skin in many cases, making a problem of wound closure.
6. Injury to important nerves, vessels and tendons.

General Principles.—All idea behind the treatment lies in removal of foreign bodies and contaminating elements, and excision of all dead tissues, leaving behind healthy well-vascularised tissues that are able to ward off infection by the organisms that inevitably remain in the wound, even after most meticulous excision. The natural healing capacity of the body can, thereafter, make for the dead tissues. In addition, treatment for the fracture has to be thought of.

Management.—This may be conveniently discussed under the following headings:
A. General treatment.
B. Treatment for the wound.
C. Problem of wound closure.
D. Treatment for the fracture.

A. General Treatment
1. Treatment for shock:
   a. Rest, including rest to the injured limb in a splint or cast.
   b. Sedatives.
   c. Fluid transfusion.
   d. Blood transfusion, if necessary.
2. Antibiotics.
3. Tetanus toxoid is to be administered in all the cases. Even if the patient is vaccinated, a booster dose should be given.
4. Serum.—The values of the ATS and AGS, as prophylactic measures, are doubtful. However, they have often to be administered, at least for medicolegal reasons.

B. Treatment of the Wound.—The wound should be attended to, as early as possible. If the patient is in severe shock, the treatment of the wound may have to be delayed for some time but it is important to note that, as long as the wound is not attended, the patient cannot completely recover from shock. The wound should be covered with sterile dressings till it is attended to.

Depending on the nature of the injury, there are two principal methods of wound management.

1. *Debridement* or *Wound Excision.*—In older days, these two terms had different meanings, but under modern concepts, they mean the same. Majority of cases of compound fractures or lacerated injuries are so grossly contaminated that they require some form of wound excision. The procedure is described below in details.

2. *Wound Toileting.*—This means opening up a wound to provide free drainage and counter-drainage. This is done for cases that arrive too late for a primary excision, so that gross infection of the wound has replaced contamination. In older days, the term 'debridement' was applied to this procedure.

WOUND EXCISION OR DEBRIDEMENT.—This should be undertaken under strict aseptic precautions *in an operation theatre.*

A general or regional block *anaesthesia* should be used (and not local anaesthesia).

A *tourniquet* should better be avoided because:

i. After the tourniquet is released, there is a chance of sudden absorption of massive quantities of toxins, from the damaged muscles.

ii. Improper use of a tourniquet may cause irremediable ischaemia of nerves.

iii. If the vessels have been injured, the use of a tourniquet further endangers the circulation of the limb.

iv. With the tourniquet on, it becomes difficult to recognise which structures are devitalised.

The advantages of a tourniquet, however, are that it conserves blood and makes identification of important structures in the wound easier. Even if a tourniquet is used, it must be released at intervals.

The *cleansing* of the wound and neighbouring skin, prior to wound excision, must be very rigid. For this purpose, the wound itself is covered up with a mop, and surrounding skin is washed with soap and water to remove all dirts and greasy substances. This cleansing must be for *five minutes by the clock.* Thereafter the skin is sterilised with spirit and other antiseptics. The mop from the wound is now removed and the wound is irrigated with some weak antiseptic solution from a syringe. The area of operation is then draped with sterilised sheets.

The structures of the wound are now separately considered for the purpose of wound excision:

1. *Skin.*—The skin may have been cut or crushed (potential skin loss) or there may be actual skin loss. All dead skin must be removed but the principle should be conservative because skin can stand ischaemia to a great extent and it is so valuable for closure of the wound. For better visualisation of the structures, the wound often requires to be extended by planned incisions on the skin. All foreign materials must be picked out.

2. *Subcutaneous Fat and Fascia.*—The subcutaneous fat is often grossly contaminated. Also, it offers very little resistance against infection and has a little power of healing. So it should be excised liberally. The fascia are divided extensively for adequate drainage.

3. *Muscles.*—Great attention must be paid and judgement exercised in excising muscles. This is because dead and contaminated muscles are not only the source of highly toxic materials but also the nidus for the growth of anaerobic

organisms, particularly those of gas gangrene. For the purpose of excision of muscles, it is best to use a dissecting forceps and a fine-pointed scissors. The dead muscles are picked up, piecemeal, with the forceps and sharply cut out. Dead muscles are identified by the following points:

   i. They are coloured beefy instead of bright red.

   ii. They do not bleed on cutting.

   iii. They do not contract when scissors work on them.

4. *Blood Vessels.*—Small vessels are safely ligated. If the main artery of the limb, is injured, reconstruction should be attempted as follows:

   a. If the two ends can be approximated without tension, end-to-end suturing is done.

   b. If there is a wide gap between the two ends, a vein graft may be used to bridge the gap. A regional big *superficial vein,* e.g. cubital or saphenous, may be used for the purpose. The vein must be grafted upside down (i.e. reversed) to overcome obstruction to the blood-flow by its valves."

   c. If reconstruction is not possible, the two ends are ligated and all measures adopted to stimulate opening up of collaterals.

5. *Nerves.*—Primary nerve suture is usually avoided, excepting for digital nerves. This is because sutures do not take in presence of infection. A delayed nerve suture, after 3 to 4 weeks or after the infection passes off (whichever is later), should be undertaken. The advantages of a delayed suture are:

   a. The neuroma, at the end of the injured nerve, gets well-localised by this time, so that the level up to which the fibres are living is well-demonstrated.

   b. The infection has passed off.

   c. As there is a thickening of the nerve-sheath by this time, sutures take well.

     For the time being, it is best to keep the two cut ends loosely approximated to each other, either with black silk or with fine wire, for ease of later identification (when wires are used, X-rays are helpful).

6. *Tendons.*—Like the nerves, cut tendons are preferably treated by delayed suture, their ends being temporarily kept approximated with black silk or wire.

7. *Bones.*—It is advisable that no piece of bone, however detached, is excised because it is only after several days that bones become infected and because they rapidly become revascularised. It is very exceptional for a piece of bone, even if completely detached, to turn into a sequestrum.

C. **The Problem of Wound Closure.**—If a contaminated wound is covered up with skin, the infecting organisms get an ideal chance to grow unnoticed below it. Also, the atmosphere becomes especially suitable for the growth of anaerobic organisms. Hence, unless there is reason to believe that the wound has not been contaminated much, immediate or *primary closure* of the wound should never be undertaken. The majority of the cases are either moderately or grossly contaminated, or are attended more than 6 hours after the injury (by which time contamination has given way to established infection). So the wound, after excision, should be left open. It is covered with dry dressings and is subsequently dressed up at intervals. As soon as it is found that the tissues are no longer infected, a *delayed primary suture* is undertaken. This is generally a matter of 5 to 7 days only. If, even after this period, infection or oedema persists, skin closure has to be postponed further. After 7 days the tissues become indurated and the epidermis grows into the edges of the wound. It is therefore necessary to freshen the skin margins while closing the skin. This is called *secondary suture* (in delayed primary suture, such freshening is not necessary).

The wound may be closed in either of the following ways:

1. By approximating the skin margins, if the gap is small.
2. By approximating the skin margins after making release incision on either side, if the gap is wider (the gaps created at the release areas may, if required, be covered with split-skin grafts).
3. By split-skin grafts.
4. By rotational flaps from neighbouring skin, the gap created by rotation being covered up with split-skin grafts.

D. **Treatment for the Fracture.**—Once the wound has been properly excised, the fracture may be regarded as a closed one and treated as such. The treatment of these fractures may be done by the following methods:

1. Majority of surgeons keep provisions for dressing the wound while the fracture is immobilised. For this purpose either (a) the limb is put on a splint with or without traction, or (b) a plaster cast is applied, or (c) a complete plastering is done with a window made at the site of the wound.
2. Some surgeons allow the wound and the fracture to heal by themselves, keeping the limb completely plastered. This is called the *Winett Orr method.* It is found that the wound, even though it is not attended, and the plaster soaks with the discharges considerably, granulates nicely, so that it can subsequently be treated easily with split-skin grafts. Sometimes, complete epithelialisation also occurs.
3. Regarding the feasibility of internal fixation for the fracture, there are two antagonising views:
   a. Internal fixation is dangerous because the metal has a notorious tendency to catch infection and this, by itself, may lead to non-union.
   b. Internal fixation is beneficial. Even without the introduction of a foreign body, a compound fracture has every possibility of developing infection in the bone. Presence of a metal definitely immobilises the fracture better than an external splintage and this enhances the chances of union even in the presence of infection. Moreover, the metal itself invites formation of more involucrum and it is certain that the newly-formed involucrum is stronger than normal bone. The principle, to be followed, however, is that the metal for internal fixation should be placed as far away as is possible from the soft tissue wound. If a sequestrum develops, it may well be removed later.

[The above description also applies to the *management of Lacerated Injuries.* Only the last item, i.e. 'treatment for the fracture' has to be omitted. However, the injured limb has to be immobilised in a splint or a plaster cast, since rest is essential for the healing of any tissue.]

COMPLICATIONS OF FRACTURES

I. General Complications

1. Shock.
2. Crush syndrome.

3. Venous thrombosis.
4. Fat embolism.

II. Local Complications

A. COMPLICATIONS RELATED to THE FRACTURE ITSELF:
1. Infection.
2. Delayed union.
3. Non-union.
4. Mal-union.
5. A vascular necrosis.
6. Shortening.

B. COMPLICATIONS ATTRIBUTABLE TO ASSOCIATED INJURY:
1. Injury to major blood vessels.
2. Injury to nerves.
3. Injury to tendons.
4. Injury to viscera.
5. Injury to joints.

C. OTHER COMPLICATIONS:
1. Skin complications.
2. Muscle complications.
3. Post-traumatic complications in neighbouring joints.
4. Post-traumatic ossification (myositis ossificans).
5. Sudeck's atrophy.

Shock.—This may be considerable in:
1. Fractures of big bones.
2. Multiple fractures.
3. Compound fractures.
4. Fractures at the extremes of ages and in the feeble.
5. Fractures associated with other injuries, e.g. head injury, visceral injury, etc.

Crush Syndrome.—This may occur if a large bulk of muscle is crushed. Acid myohaematin is released from the crushed muscles and causes extensive renal damage that leads to anuria and death. As to the cause of the renal damage, there are two views:
1. The acid myohaematin blocks the renal tubules.
2. There is a spasm of the renal artery, which causes necrosis of the tubular cells (due to anoxia).

Prevention lies in early amputation of grossly lacerated limbs and avoiding prolonged use of tourniquets. Established cases are treated in the same lines as for anuria in general.

Fat Embolism.—This signifies embolism of fat in the arterial system. There are two views as regards its origin:
a. Fat globules are derived from the bone marrow at the fracture site and enter the torn veins. They are primarily carried to the lungs. The fat, being in fluid state at normal body temperature, can pass through the pulmonary capillaries, to enter the systemic circulation.

b. The fatty deposits that occur in the system are not derived from bone marrow but result from a physical change in the fat normally present in solution in the blood plasma, so that they are precipitated in large globules.

Whatever be the origin, fat emboli may lodge in different organs and produce symptoms as follows:

1. *Lung.*—This is the commonest site. Features are pain in the chest, dyspnoea, haemoptysis, pulmonary oedema, high temperature, and presence of fat in the sputum.

2. *Heart.*—There is occlusion of small coronary vessels. Features are pain in the chest, low blood pressure, rapid and feeble pulse, cardiac irregularities, and heart failure.

3. *Skin.*—Petechial haemorrhages are seen over wide areas of the body, particularly the front of the chest.

4. *Brain.*—Headache, restlessness, delirium, convulsion, coma, vomiting, hyperthermia.

5. *Kidney.*—Presence of fat in the urine.

Many cases pass unnoticed and mild cases recover. The severe cases are fatal. No specific treatment is available.

Infection.—This complication is virtually confined to, and almost sure to occur in, compound fractures. Closed fractures may develop infection only when there is an operative interference.

As the inflammatory exudates may well drain out through the same route by which the infecting agents gain entrance, subperiosteal abscess formation does not occur and the osteomyelitis never takes an acute form (c f haematogenous osteomyelitis).

The real danger of infection lies in the possibility of a non-union.

TREATMENT:

1. Proper immobilisation of the part. Often a prolonged immobilisation is necessary.

2. Culture and sensitivity test of the discharge, and long-term administration of the specific antibiotic.

Delayed Union.—There is no hard and fast rule as to the time that a particular fracture shall take to heal. As a general rule, union is said to be delayed if the fragments are still freely mobile 3 to 4 months after the injury. The importance of delayed union is that it may eventually lead to non-union and that it should be carefully differentiated from non-union.

CAUSES.—The causes are more or less the same as for non-union but acting to a lesser extent (see below).

TREATMENT.—Masterly inactivity, continuing the immobilisation, and carefully excluding non-union.

Non-union.—A fracture is declared to have non-union when there are sure evidences that it will never heal as such, without operative interference.

These evidences are obtained radiologically, and are as follows:

1. The fracture ends become definitely rounded off.

2. The ends become dense and sclerosed, and there is absence of the medullary cavity at the ends.
3. The fracture line is very well demarcated, in contrast to this dense bone on either side.
4. There is no evidence of callus formation.

The fracture line, which looks black on the X-ray, actually contains fibrous tissue, instead of callus. Sometimes there is a gap in the fibrous tissue, so that one fragment can well be moved over the other, without much pain. This condition is called *pseudoarthrosis*.

CAUSES:
1. Infection of the bone.
2. Inadequate blood supply to one or more of the fracture fragments.
3. Inadequate immobilisation—in quality or in time.
4. Failure of proper apposition including *distraction*, which means wide separation between the fragments due to excessive traction.
5. Interposition of soft tissues between the fragments.
6. Pathological fractures associated with bone destruction.
7. Dissolution of the fracture haematoma by synovial fluid (as in fractures within joints).
8. Presence of foreign bodies, corrosive metals, etc. in the immediate vicinity of the fracture.

TREATMENT:
1. If the disability is slight, no active treatment is required. In some of these cases an external splint may permit useful function.
2. If the non-union is disabling, operative treatment has to be undertaken. The ideal treatment is bone grafting, after excision of the dense sclerosed bone ends and all intervening fibrous tissue. In some cases, where the fracture is within or near a joint, other operations, like excision of one of the fragments or its replacement by a prosthesis, is preferred.

Mal-union.—Imperfect alignment in minor degrees is rather common with majority of the fractures. This does not interfere, in any way, with normal functions and ultimately nice remodelling occurs. Sometimes, however, the lack of alignment may be so considerable that either it produces a deformity or it interferes grossly with normal functions.

There may be two types of mal-union:
1. *Gross Overlapping.*—Unless overlapping is great and causes considerable shortening, it is of little importance and is acceptable. For obvious reasons, this is more dangerous for the lower limb than the upper.
2. *Angulation.*—Even a little angulation between the fragments may be non-acceptable because of deformity, interference with function, or possibility of an osteoarthritis in the neighbouring joint.

TREATMENT.—If a mal-union is not acceptable, the treatment is refracturing or osteotomy, followed by correction and immobilisation.

Avascular Necrosis.—This means death of one (or rarely more) of the fracture fragments due to loss of its blood supply, resultant on the fracture. Though such avascular necrosis may occur with any fracture, the common sites are:

1. Head of the femur, following fracture at the neck.
2. Proximal fragment of the scaphoid, in fracture through the waist of the bone.
3. The body of the talus, following fracture through its neck.
4. The lower fourth of the tibia.
5. The whole of the lunate bone, following its dislocation.

The *effects* of avascular necrosis are:

a. Non-union.
b. As the dead bone has no elasticity, it easily crumbles under pressure, so that its articular surface becomes irregular. Moreover, with the death of the bone, the deeper layer of the covering articular cartilage (which lives on blood supply from the underlying bone) degenerates. These two factors, together, lead to osteoarthritis of the neighbouring joint.

TREATMENT:

1. Fractures at the known popular sites of avascular necrosis should be immobilised rigidly, if required with internal fixation, in an attempt to avoid non-union.
2. In the established cases, the treatment depends on the site and the disability of the patient. In many instances excision of the dead fragment, with some form of replacement, is done (e.g. replacement arthroplasty for the femoral head). In other cases, other types of arthroplasty or an arthrodesis is done.

Shortening.—This may result from:

1. Gross overriding of the fragments.
2. Actual loss of bone, e.g. gunshot injury through a bone or compression fractures, as in vertebrae, talus, or calcaneum.
3. Interference with epiphyseal growth when the fracture line involves the epiphysis. It is usually found that fracture-separation of the whole of the epiphysis is less likely to cause hindrance of growth than a fracture where the fracture line extends from the diaphysis into the epiphysis.

In the upper limb, shortening causes only a little inconvenience but in the lower limb it may be the cause of considerable difficulty. A shortening up to 1 inch can be well managed with a high-heel shoe. In cases where the shortening is more, reconstructive procedures have to be thought of.

Injury to Major Blood Vessels.—Injury to soft tissues and minor blood vessels is a constant accompaniment of all fractures. The rest given to the bone is also shared by these soft tissues and they heal. Injury to the main vessels of the limb, particularly the artery, requires special attention as it may have serious effects, which may sometimes amount to loss of the limb.

SITES.—The commonest of such injuries is that of the brachial artery in injuries around the elbow, especially supracondylar fracture. The sites at which fractures or dislocations are likely to be associated with important vascular damages are as follows:

Site	Artery	Injury
1. Temporo-parietal region	Middle meningeal	Fracture of the temporal bone.
2. Axilla	Axillary	Dislocation of the shoulder.
3. Elbow	Brachial	Supracondylar fracture
4. Knee	Popliteal	Dislocation of the knee or fracture of upper tibia.

NATURE OF INJURY.—The cases may be divided into 2 groups:

A. *Primary.*—Where the arterial injury is evident when the patient is first seen. The nature of the injury may be as follows:

1. The artery may be torn across or lacerated, either by the object which caused the injury or by the sharp end of a fracture fragment.
2. The artery may be contused, so that there is thrombosis in the lumen, resulting in its occlusion.
3. The artery may be kinked in between the fracture fragments.
4. The artery may simply go into spasm because of irritation.

B. *Secondary.*—When the arterial injury is evident after the fracture has been attended, i.e. manipulated and/or plastered or bandaged. The cause of arterial impairment in these cases may be:

1. Injury to the artery during forceful manipulation—most commonly a spasm.
2. Position of the limb—e.g. excessive flexion of the elbow in supracondylar fracture, occluding the brachial artery.
3. Tight plaster or bandage.—The artery is constricted by oedema as the tight plaster or bandage prevents the limb from swelling outwards.

EXAMINATION OF THE PATIENT:

1. In cases of compound fracture, as the wound is explored, the condition of the artery should be carefully noted.
2. In cases of closed fracture, at the sites where arterial injury is common, the circulation in the distal limb should be carefully noted. Comparison with the healthy limb should always be a guideline. Absence of pulsation, absence of nail-bed return, coldness, and a bluish discolouration are the features of arterial impairment. Of these, the first two are of considerable importance in the early cases.
3. After manipulation and plastering, the distal pulse and nail-bed return should always be noted. Also, after the fracture has been reduced and the limb immobilised, the pain should pass off; persistence of severe pain, even after the fracture has been reduced and immobilised, strongly points to arterial impairment in the limb.

EFFECTS OF ARTERIAL INJURY:

1. Traumatic aneurysm of the artery itself may occur.
2. If the arterial obstruction is complete and there is absence of significant collaterals, gangrene of the distal part of the limb results. The extent of the gangrene depends on the level and nature of obstruction.
3. If the arterial impairment is incomplete (in the majority of cases this is due to opened up collaterals), ischaemic changes are likely to supervene. The skin and the bone can stand ischaemia to a great extent so that they escape. The nerves and the muscles undergo ischaemic changes—the nerves more easily and earlier than the muscles. Hence, ischaemic paralysis of the nerves is very likely to occur. Muscles undergo ischaemic changes less commonly and later than the nerves but, while nerves can never regenerate rather easily, muscles can regenerate fully. The ischaemic muscles undergo necrosis and are replaced by granulation tissue, which eventually becomes scarred and fibrotic.

The classical example of this pathology is seen with brachial artery injury in supracondylar fractures. The muscles involved are those of the flexor group in the forearm. An elliptical mass of muscle tissue, the size and extent of which varies, undergoes necrosis *(Seddon's elliptical zone of necrosis)*. Why the flexor muscles are selectively affected is difficult to account for. It is believed that there is an associated haematoma in the aforesaid elliptical area, located in the flexor muscles. Also, swelling of the muscles adds to the tension under the deep fascia and increases the compression. The resultant fibrosis of the flexors of the forearm leads to a typical deformity—*Volkmann's ischaemic contracture.* Simultaneously, the nerves of the forearm are involved. The median and the radial are more severely affected than the ulnar, which, by reason of its peripheral situation, may escape gross damage.

MANAGEMENT.—In fractures or dislocations, where arterial injury is common, the possibility of this complication should always be borne in mind and the patient examined properly. If there is impairment of circulation, the case must be handled as an urgent emergency because the effects of ischaemia quickly become irreversible.

A. *Primary Group:*
    1 Any tight bandage or external splint that might be causing obstruction is removed. If there is any gross displacement of the fracture fragments, it is corrected by the gentlest manipulation. A maximum of half an hour's time is allowed for the circulation to return.
    2. If pulsation does not return, the artery is explored. If there is a kinking, it is carefully undone. If there is a spasm and in those cases where there was a kink, the tunica adventitia is painted with a 2.5% solution of papaverine, in an attempt to overcome the periarterial sympathetic irritation, that causes the spasm. If the artery is torn across, end-to-end suturing is done. If the artery is found to be punctured or contused (and thrombosed) or is lacerated, the damaged segment is excised. Continuity is restored either by end-to-end suturing or, if the gap is wide, by a reversed vein graft. When restoration of continuity is impossible, both the ends are ligated.
    3. Many surgeons advise internal fixation of the fracture to prevent further vascular damage from recurrent displacement.
    4. Post-operatively, attempts are made to stimulate opening up of collaterals, by heating the other healthy limbs.
B. *Secondary Group:*
    1. The plaster and all underlying dressings are split throughout their length, right down to the skin.
    2. The limb is brought to the position of ease for the artery, e.g. extension of the elbow for brachial artery.
    3. Attempts are made to stimulate collaterals by heating the other limbs.
    4. If circulation does not return in half an hour, the artery is explored and is dealt with in the same way as for the primary group.

Injury to Nerves.—Injury to nerves may be caused by:
1. The object causing the trauma, particularly in compound fractures.
2. The sharp end of a fracture fragment.

SITES.—The rather common sites of nerve injury in fractures or dislocations are as follows:

Site	Nerve	Injury
1. Cervical or thoracic spine	Spinal cord	Fracture-dislocation
2. Shoulder	Circumflex nerve	Dislocation of shoulder
3. Arm	Radial nerve	Fracture of humeral shaft
4. Elbow	Ulnar nerve	Fracture medial epicondyle
5. Elbow	Median nerve	Supracondylar fracture or dislocation of elbow
6. Lumbar spine	Cauda equina	Fracture-dislocation
7. Hip	Sciatic nerve	Posterior dislocation of hip
8. Knee	Lateral popliteal nerve	Torn lateral ligament

TIME OF NERVE INJURY:

1. *Immediate,* i.e. instantaneously with the trauma or, sometimes, a little later, by the sharp fractured ends.
2. *Late or Tardy palsy.*—This occurs much later, when the fracture is healing or has healed, and may be caused in two ways:
   a Entanglement of the nerve in the callus, e.g. radial nerve in fracture of humeral shaft, ulnar nerve in fracture of medial epicondyle.
   b. Stretching effect on the nerve as a result of deformity consequent upon a fracture, e.g. ulnar neuritis due to a cubitus valgus deformity at the elbow, following lateral condylar fracture of humerus.

NATURE OF NERVE INJURY.—There are 3 types of nerve injury:

1. *Neurapraxia* (physiological interruption).—The axons are intact, there is only a degeneration of the myelin sheaths. There is only a transient physiological block. The larger motor fibres are mainly affected, the smaller sensory fibres to a lesser extent; hence complete sensory loss is unusual. Complete and spontaneous recovery is the rule.
2. *Axonotmesis.*—The internal architecture of the nerve is preserved because the neurilemmal sheaths are undamaged. However, the axons are so badly damaged that they undergo peripheral degeneration. Following degeneration, spontaneous regeneration occurs. So, spontaneous and complete recovery may be expected. Some degree of intraneural fibrosis may, however, occur and recovery may be incomplete in these cases. Rarely, there is extensive scarring at the site of trauma and axons cannot regenerate through it, so that there is no recovery.
3. *Neurotmesis.*—The normal architecture of the nerve is lost. This may be of two types:
   a. Complete Neurotmesis.—The nerve is divided across its whole thickness, or is lacerated.
   b. Partial Neurotmesis.—The nerve is partly cut through, some portion remaining undivided.

Unless nerve suture is performed, recovery is impossible. In general, it may be assumed that nerve injuries in closed fractures are either neurapraxia or axonotmesis, and only rarely neurotmesis. On the contrary, in compound fractures, the possibilities of neurotmesis are more than the other types of nerve injury.

TREATMENT:

A. *In Closed Fractures.*—On the assumption that the injury is more likely to be neurapraxia or axonotmesis, no active treatment for the nerve is undertaken. Neurapraxia should recover in a few weeks, time, while in axonotmesis, the rate of regeneration is roughly one inch in one month. Calculated on this basis (site of injury and length to be regenerated), time is given for regeneration, without any active treatment. During this period all care should be taken to support the paralysed muscles (on splints or otherwise) in such a way that there is no undue stretching of the muscles, e.g. cock-up position of the wrist in radial nerve injury. If, after the expected period of regeneration, the paralysis does not recover, the nerve has to be explored, presuming that a neurotmesis has occurred.

B. *In Compound Fractures.*—The injury to the nerve can be ascertained during the process of wound excision. If the continuity of the nerve is intact but features of paralysis are present, there is either a neurapraxia or an axonotmesis, and no active treatment is necessary (however, in a few of these cases, a future scarring at the site of trauma may prevent regeneration). If, however, the nerve is found torn or lacerated, the ends require suturing. A delayed suture is usually undertaken, as described under management of compound fractures. (For details of nerve injuries and repair *see* Chapter 15).

Injury to Tendons

1. *Torn Tendon:*
   a. In compound fracture, a tendon may be severed by the agent causing the fracture.
   b. Injury to the quadriceps femoris and the triceps, in transverse fracture of patella and fracture of the olecranon respectively, are important, in that there is loss of continuity of the extensor mechanism of the knee and elbow.
2. *Avulsion Fractures.*—The tendon remains intact but pulls off a small flake of bone at its attachment, e.g. supraspinatus tendon, tendon of the fingers (mallet finger), etc.
3. *Late Rupture.*—The best example is rupture of the extensor pollicis longus tendon, 6 to 12 weeks after a Colles' fracture. Another example is rupture of the long head of biceps, following fracture neck of humerus.

TREATMENT:

1. In closed fractures suturing of the tendon is done.
2. In compound fractures a 'delayed suture', on the same principles as for nerve suturing, is advised.

Injury to Viscera.—Like arteries and nerves, viscera may be injured either by the agent causing the fracture or by a sharp fracture fragment. Examples of visceral injury are:

1. Lung in rib fracture.
2. Spleen, liver or kidney in fracture of the lower ribs.
3. Urethra, bladder, rectum or colon in pelvic fracture.

Injury to Joints.—Associated joint injuries are commonly found in fractures. The injury may be:

a *Dislocation.*—A joint is dislocated, i.e. 'luxated', when the articular surfaces of its component bones are wholly displaced, one from the other, so that all apposition between them is lost.

b. Subluxation.—A joint is subluxated when the articular surfaces are partly displaced but retain some contact with each other.

c. *Sprain.*—Ligamentous strain, i.e. incomplete rupture of a ligament.

Skin Complications

1. *Skin Loss.*—In compound fractures the skin may be cut or crushed (potential skin loss), or there may be actual skin loss.
2. *Fracture Blisters.*—Elevation of the superficial layers of skin due to oedema.
3. *Plaster Sores.*—Especially likely to occur where the skin is directly pressed against the bone.
4. *Bed Sores.*—Particularly likely to occur in the elderly, paralytic, and run-down patients.

Muscle Complications

1. Tear—The torn fibres tend to develop adhesions that may result in restricted movements. Active exercises and physiotherapy should be instituted as early as possible.
2. *Disuse Atrophy.*—This should also be treated by active exercises and physiotherapy.

Post-traumatic Complications in Neighbouring Joints

1. INSTABILITY.—This may occur particularly with gunshot injuries, where simultaneous loss of bone and muscles in the vicinity of a joint may lead to instability of the joint.
2. STIFFNESS.—This may be due to:
    a. Intra-articular adhesions—from organisation of blood clots, where haemarthosis has occurred.
    b. Peri-articular adhesions—from organisation of the traumatic and inflammatory oedema in the soft tissues around the joint, viz. capsule, ligaments, tendons and muscles. This is more likely to develop with prolonged immobilisation.
    Treatment of Stiffness:
    i.   Active exercises.—In the majority of cases the stiffness is overcome by proper active exercises.
    ii. Manipulation under anaesthesia.—This is undertaken when active exercises fail. Undue force should not be applied as this may worsen the stiffness or may cause fresh injuries, like fracture. It is better to perform repeated light manipulations than one forcible.
    iii Operation.—If stiffness persists, operation may have to be undertaken to release the soft tissues or to lengthen them, e.g. capsule, ligaments, tendons, etc.
3. OSTEOARTHRITIS.—The causes of osteoarthritis, as a sequela to fracture, are:
    a. Associated injuries in the joints.
    b. The fracture line extending to the joint, the resultant callus causing irregularity of the articular surface.
    c. Avascular necrosis, resulting in:

    i. Crumbling of the dead bone under pressure, causing irregularity of the articular surface.

    ii. Degeneration of the articular cartilage, resulting from loss of blood supply to the deeper layer of the cartilage (which lives on blood supply from the underlying bone).

    d. Gross mal-union, resulting in irregular pressure on the articular surfaces.

Treatment of Osteoarthritis.—This depends on the site, age, and disability of the patient. Arthroplasty, arthrodesis, or different types of osteotomy may have to be done.

Myositis Ossificans Traumatica.—This denotes ossification in a haematoma in relation to muscles and is usually the outcome of an injury—contusion, fracture or dislocation. The term myositis is a misnomer since there is no inflammation in the muscles. Equally misnomer is the term 'traumatic sub-periosteal ossification', since the ossification is not under the periosteum.

    The condition, as regards its terminology, should be differentiated from *myositis ossificans progressive,* which denotes a progressive widespread ossification in the different muscles of the body, following inflammation in these muscles, and resulting in painful hard swellings.

CAUSES.—The cause of myositis ossificans traumatica is not definitely known. Though it may occur in any muscle, following trauma, it is commonest and is of particular interest in the brachialis anticus, in front of the elbow joint, either after dislocation of the joint or after supracondylar fracture. The condition is more likely to develop:

    a. If the period of immobilisation is inadequate.

    b. If forceful passive movements are attempted after the period of immobilisation.

    c. In the children (*see* below).

PATHOLOGY.—Pathologically, the condition consists of ossification in a haematoma and appropriately called 'traumatic osteoma'. The haematoma is located more commonly *between* the muscles rather than in the muscles, so that the new bone tends to form between the muscles. Ossification is brought about by the osteoblasts, which are set to activity by the stripping of the periosteum from the underlying bone. Hence, the trauma should be such that it causes not only a haematoma but also stripping of the periosteum. Since, in children, the periosteum is loosely attached to the bone, the periosteum is stripped off easily and widely, and this is the reason why the condition is commoner in the children.

    As evidenced radiologically, the condition passes through 3 *stages:*

    i. There is a widespread area of 'wooly' irregular ossification in front of the elbow.

    ii. These conglomerate together into one big mass.

    iii. This mass gradually becomes smaller and circumscribed, till it takes a final shape and size—often spiky (known as *false exostosis).*

CLINICAL FEATURES.—In case of a dislocation of, or a fracture near, the elbow joint, after the plaster is removed, the patient complains of:

1. Pain in front of the joint.
2. Inability to extend or flex the joint fully.

Passive exercises only cause increase in the pain and decrease in the range of elbow movements.

TREATMENT:

A. *Prevention.*—In all injuries near the elbow:
1. The period of immobilisation should be adequate.
2. After removal of the plaster, forcible passive movements and massaging must be avoided.

B. *Established Cases:*
1. As soon as the condition is diagnosed, the limb is again immobilised. The immobilisation must continue up to the third stage, as seen on the X-ray.
2. After this period, as the plaster is taken off, it may be found that the pain has disappeared and the limitation of movements is tolerable. In such cases no further active treatment is advised.
3. If, however, the movements are grossly restricted, operation has to be undertaken. At operation, the newly formed bone is excised. Even after the excision, the movements may not increase (and may sometimes decrease further) because of fibrous adhesions that have formed between all the soft tissues around the elbow.

In general, some limitation of movements is always likely to occur, whichever may be the way a myositis ossificans is treated.

Sudeck's Bone Atrophy.—This signifies a painful osteoporosis of the bones, particularly seen in the short bones of the hand (and occasionally the foot), following immobilisation after fractures or other injuries. A little decalcification of the bones, in an immobilised limb, is a normal physiological process. When the decalcification is excessive, it is abnormal and produces symptoms.

CLINICAL FEATURES.—The patient complains of pain in hand (or foot), associated with stiffness of the fingers, i.e. metacarpophalangeal and interphalangeal joints ('*frozen hand*'). Sometimes there are signs of inflammation, e.g. redness and oedema, over the part.

X-ray shows gross decalcification of the bones.

TREATMENT.—No specific treatment is known and the following are often advised:
1. Encouraging active movements with prolonged physiotherapy—heat, elevation, and graduated exercises. Recovery is usually slow but steady.
2. Sometimes intra-arterial injection of novocaine accelerates recovery.
3. In obstinate cases, repeated sympathetic block or permanent sympathetic denervation by ganglionectomy (cervico-dorsal or lumbar) has to be undertaken.

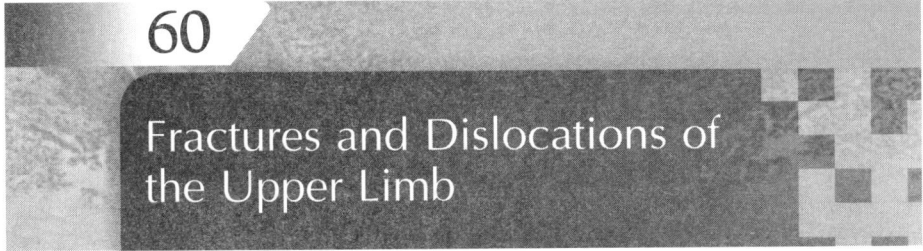

60

Fractures and Dislocations of
the Upper Limb

FRACTURED CLAVICLE

Site and Trauma

1. In the majority of cases the fracture occurs at the junction of the two curvatures in the bone, i.e. the junction of the medial two-thirds and the lateral third. The trauma is always indirect—a fall on the outstretched hand. The fracture may occur at any age but is commoner in children, and in the children the fracture is often of the *greenstick* variety. In the adults there is usually more angulation and more displacement.

2. Occasionally the fracture is at the lateral end of the clavicle—either between the conoid and trapezoid ligaments or lateral to both the ligaments. Such a fracture is caused by a direct trauma—a fall on the point of the shoulder. Almost always it occurs in the adults.

Displacements

A. In the usual variety of the fracture, i.e. at the junction of the two curvatures:
1. The lateral fragment is pulled:
   a. downwards by the weight of the limb.
   b. medially by the pectoralis major.
   c. forwards by the forward rotation of the scapula.
2. The medial fragment is not displaced much because of its strong ligamentous attachments. It may be drawn a little upwards by the pull of the sternomastoid but its upward displacement is more apparent because of the downward displacement of the lateral fragment.

B. In fractures at the lateral end, there cannot be any displacement of the fragments because of the strong ligamentous attachments.

Clinical Features

I. *In the usual type of fracture.*—The patient, most commonly a child, complains of pain over the clavicle and presents with a typical attitude. The child supports the elbow of the injured side with the other hand and bends the neck to the injured side. On examination, there is a definite tenderness at the fracture site. Often a swelling is palpated, which is subcutaneous.

II. *In fractures at the lateral end.*—The patient, usually an adult, complains of pain around the shoulder and has difficulty in raising the arm. These cases may be difficult to be diagnosed from fracture of the greater tuberosity, but the maximum tenderness is at the lateral end of the clavicle.

X-ray confirms the diagnosis.

Treatment

A. FOR THE USUAL TYPE OF FRACTURE.—Though there are so many displacements, they can all be corrected, more or less satisfactorily, by simply bracing back the shoulders. The union is usually satisfactory in 2 to 3 weeks.

A little malunion is almost inevitable but, particularly in a child, a perfect moulding occurs in course of time. Had this not been the case, the problem of deformity would be serious for a subcutaneous and visible bone like the clavicle. It is further fortunate for the clavicle that non-union is almost unknown, even with the worst type of immobilization, because the commonly practised types of immobilization, used for clavicular fracture, are never satisfactory. Another fortunate point for the clavicle is the extreme rarity of a compound fracture in the bone, though it is so superficial; this is because the overlying skin is very freely mobile (c.f. tibia). It is also fortunate that a clavicular fracture is almost never associated with injuries to the underlying big vessels.

After bracing back the shoulders, the position may be maintained by either of the following methods:

1. *Figure-of-8 Bandage.*—This is applied round both the shoulders and axillae, and as the '8' crosses on the back, the shoulders are kept braced back. The vessels and nerves in the axilla have to be protected with thick cotton pads. The bandage has to be reinforced at intervals, as it easily loosens.
2. *Use of Clavicle Rings.*—Two rings are used, one round each shoulder and axilla. They are tied together at the back and the link is tightened twice daily.
3. *Three-sling Method.*—Instead of the two clavicular rings, two slings (or handkerchieves) are used. The third sling (or handkerchief) is used for the link.
4. *Using a Clavicular Cross.*—The cross is tied to the trunk and shoulders with the help of bandages. The horizontal limb of the 'T' is on the supraspinous part of the scapulae, and the vertical limb is placed in between the two scapulae.

In any case, a sling must support the fractured limb.

All the above methods of immobilization are ineffective, unless considerable and constant pressure is exerted, which is too much uncomfortable. Consequently, many surgeons advocate only the use of a sling, which is worn for three weeks. Early shoulder movements are then instituted.

B. FOR FRACTURES AT THE LATERAL END.—The fragments may be immobilised by applying adhesive plaster round the shoulder, down the arm, round the elbow and back to the shoulder.

FRACTURED SURGICAL NECK OF HUMERUS

These fractures are caused by indirect violence, i.e. fall on the outstretched hand. It was formerly believed that, depending on the position of the limb, at the time of the fall, the fractures could be of two types:

1. *Abduction fracture,* occurring when the person falls on the abducted limb. On the X-ray, there is an abduction of the shaft in relation to the head of the humerus.
2. *Adduction fracture,* occurring when the person falls on the adducted limb. On the X-ray, the shaft of the humerus is seen in an adducted position in relation to the head.

It is now known that this differentiation, which in the older days was believed to be important, has no therapeutic or prognostic importance and is probably based upon a radiological illusion.

The upwards thrust of the trauma may cause two other changes:

i. There is a good possibility of the lower fragment (i.e. the shaft) being impacted into the head. In more than half of the cases the fracture is impacted.

ii. There may be a simultaneous fracture of the greater tuberosity.

Age of the Patient

1. In general, this is an injury of old age.
2. In the adolescents, the injury takes the form of a *fracture-separation of the upper humeral epiphysis*. On X-ray, it is found that the upper fragment consists of the head, together with a large triangular piece of the metaphysis attached to it.
3. In children, a fracture in this region is usually pathological, secondary to a solitary bone cyst.

Clinical Features.—Following the trauma, there is pain, swelling and limitation of movements in the shoulder. A definite tenderness is elicited in the region of the surgical neck. As a good amount of blood extravasates and gravitates downwards, bruising and ecchymosis may be found along the length of the arm, to a variable distance.

In cases of *impacted* fractures, a considerable range of movement is possible without much pain, while in *non-impacted* fractures, even minor movements are painful. This clinical examination is of a great importance in the treatment since, on the X-rays, it is difficult to ascertain whether the fracture is impacted or not.

X-ray confirms the diagnosis.

Treatment.—In that management of these patients, there are three *points of importance:*

1. Even with gross displacement between the fragments, a good union is possible, associated with restoration of a good range of movements of the shoulder.
2. Even after correct reduction of the fracture, it is very difficult to hold the fragments in position, except by extensive and uncomfortable plastering or splintage, or by operation.
3. A prolonged immobilization, which will be no less than 6 to 8 weeks, is very likely to cause limitation of shoulder movements in these patients, who are usually elderly.

Considering these three factors the *outline of treatment*, for these cases, may be formulated as follows:

A. Standard Treatment.—This is the treatment advocated in elderly patients, if the fracture is uncomplicated, even though there may be considerable displacements. The displacements are ignored, immobilization is discouraged, and active movements started as early as possible. This is done by putting the limb on a sling and encouraging active movements in gradually increasing ranges.

In this respect, it is important to note whether the fracture is impacted or not. This is better ascertained clinically than on X-ray.

If the fracture is impacted, the patient can start the movements early and easily.

If the fracture is non-impacted, the patient will not be able to move the shoulder because of pain. Therefore, the fracture is immobilised for 3 to 4 weeks. By this time a reasonable gluing, between the fragments, occurs and the. patient can now carry out the movements on a sling. This immobilizations is done either in adduction (by arm-trunk bandaging) or in abduction (with an abduction splint).

B. OTHER METHODS OF TREATMENT:
1. In younger patients, with gross displacement between the fragments, correct reduction of the fracture is desirable. Reduction may be done by either of the following methods:
   a. Closed manipulation under anaesthesia.
   b. Continuous traction of Thomas' humerus abduction-extension splint.
   c. Open reduction in failed cases.
After reduction, the shoulder is immobilised in abduction, for 6 to 8 weeks. This may be done either on an abduction splint or with a shoulder spica plaster.
2. When there is a fracture associated with dislocation of the shoulder, the dislocation has to be reduced first (if required by operation), and then the fracture is dealt with.

Complications
1. Fracture of the greater tuberosity.
2. Dislocation of the shoulder. In cases of fracture-dislocation, it is more commonly the anatomical, then the surgical, neck that fractures.
3. Joint Stiffness.—This is a common and important complication, particularly in the elderly, but can be minimised by early and persistent exercises.
4. Mal-union.—This is not an uncommon complication but fortunately, even with gross mal-union, shoulder movements are often restored to satisfactory ranges.
5. Nerve Injury.—Injury to the axillary nerve may occur very rarely. Treatment is expectant.

FRACTURED GREATER TUBEROSITY

Types and Trauma
A. In association with:
   1. Fracture of the surgical neck of humerus.
   2. Dislocation of shoulder.
   This is caused by fall on outstretched hand.
B. Crack fracture without separation, i.e. contusion fracture.—This may result in two ways:
   1. Direct fall on the greater tuberosity.
   2. Fall on the abducted arm, the tuberosity impinging against the acromion process.
C. Avulsion fracture with separation.—This occurs typically in a young person, trying to save himself from falling, i.e. there is a sudden resistance to a forceful abduction of the arm. The supraspinatus contracts violently, causing an avulsion of the greater tuberosity (the same trauma causes rupture of the supraspinatus tendon in middle life).

Treatment
A. In cases of *fracture without separation,* the fracture is ignored and active movements of the shoulder, on a sling, are advocated.

B. In cases of *avulsion fracture with separation,* the fragment must be reduced and held as such:

1. CLOSED REDUCTION.—The humerus can usually be brought in contact with the tuberosity, by abducting it to 90°, externally rotating by 60° and forward flexing by 40°. If this is possible, the arm is rested on an abduction frame for 6 weeks.

2. OPEN REDUCTION.—This has to be done when closed reduction fails. An abduction frame is used, as after closed reduction.

DISLOCATION OF THE SHOULDER

Incidence.—In the child, the capsule of the shoulder joint is stronger than the bond of union between the diaphysis and epiphysis of the humerus. So the common injury is fracture-separation of the epiphysis, rather than dislocation of the shoulder.

In the adults, the shoulder joint is intrinsically weak and is made strong only by virtue of its muscular support. Stability is sacrificed for mobility in the shoulder and this is the reason why shoulder dislocation is exceedingly common.

Broadly, there are two types of shoulder dislocations:

I. Acute dislocation.

II. Recurrent dislocation.

ACUTE DISLOCATION OF THE SHOULDER

Types and Mechanism.—There are three different types, of which the first is much the commoner:

A. ANTERIOR DISLOCATION.—This means that the head of the humerus is displaced anterior to the shoulder joint. This may result in two ways:

1. Due to a fall on the outstretched hand. The head forces through the anterior part of the capsule, making a tear in it. Sometimes the head makes its way through a gap created between the glenoidal labrum and the bone, i.e. avulsing the glenoidal labrum.

2. Due to a fall on the abducted arm. In this position, there is a forcible elevation of the arm, while the lateral rotation, which normally accompanies elevation, is prevented. All the thoraco-humeral muscles contract strongly in the patient's effort to save himself and the contraction of the powerful medial rotators, viz. pectoralis major, teres major, etc., prevents lateral rotation. The effect of lateral rotation, which normally accompanies elevation, is to roll the greater tuberosity out of contact of the acromion, when the humerus is being elevated. Its absence, during the forcible elevation, impinges the greater tuberosity against the acromion (this accounts for an associated fracture of greater tuberosity in many cases). The acromion now acts as a fulcrum and as the humeral shaft continues to be thrust upwards, its head is tilted downwards. The head now forces on the inferior aspect of the capsule and, since this part of the capsule is unsupported by muscles and is the weakest, the head forces through a tear in it.

The head now lies below the glenoid cavity (subglenoid), where it at once comes in relation to the circumflex nerve. The nerve is sometimes injured but usually it slips over the head and escapes injury. In this position of the humeral head, the arm is abducted completely so that it is on the head. This position is called *luxatio erecta.*

This is a very unstable position for the head and so this position is usually transient. The flexors and abductors of the shoulder draw the head upwards, forwards, and medially. The head thus rolls anteriorly, making an anterior dislocation.

In an anterior dislocation the head may lie:

a. Below the coracoid process, in front of the neck of the scapula. This is called *subcoracoid dislocation* and is much the commoner.

b. Below the clavicle, in the infraclavicular fossa. This is called *subclavicular dislocation.* The head can reach this position only after extensive laceration of the capsule and muscles. So this type is relatively uncommon.

B. SUBGLENOID DISLOCATION.—This a rare type and occurs when the head can manage to keep itself below the glenoid (usually this position is transient as has already been mentioned). The patient presents with luxatio erecta.

C. POSTERIOR DISLOCATION.—This may result from

  i. a direct backward trauma on the head, e.g. fall on the front of the shoulder, or

  ii. a forced internal rotation of the abducted arm.

Posterior dislocation of the shoulder, which is a rare entity, may be of two types:

a. *Supraspinous.*—The head rests on the posterior margin of the glenoid or on the back of the scapula, i.e. above the spinous process of scapula.

b. *Infraspinous.*—The head rests below the spinous process.

Clinical Features

1. There is pain, swelling, limitation of movements, and tenderness in the joint.

2. In cases of anterior dislocation, a fullness, due to the dislocated head, is usually found in the subcoracoid region. It appears, as if, the arm is hanging from the junction of the medial two thirds and the lateral third of the clavicle. In posterior dislocation, the coracoid process may be unduly prominent.

3. In all cases, the normal rounded contour of the shoulder, which is due to the humeral head, is lost. The shoulder is flattened and there is a prominence of the acromion process.

4. Different clinical tests are used for the confirmation of dislocation, some of which are mentioned below:

a. It is possible to make a straight ruler touch the acromial end and the lateral epicondyle simultaneously. Normally this is not possible because of the fullness of the shoulder (*Hamilton's ruler test*).

b. The patient, cannot touch the opposite shoulder, with the elbow touching the side of the body (*Duga's test*).

c. The anterior and posterior folds of axilla are at different levels (*Bryant's test*).

d. The vertical length of the axilla is increased as compared to the other side. This is measured by passing a tape round the axilla and shoulder (*Callaway's test*).

X-ray

1. Anterior dislocation is easily diagnosed in an ordinary anteroposterior view as the head, after dislocation, moves considerably medially.

2. Posterior dislocation may be missed in an ordinary anteroposterior view because the head almost always keeps just behind the joint. An axillary view may be required to display that the head is lying posterior to the glenoid.

Treatment.—The dislocation should be reduced as early as possible, preferably under anaesthesia, with full muscle relaxation. The different methods used for reduction of anterior dislocation are described below:

1. An assistant pulls on the arm *in abduction* and the surgeon presses the head, into place, with the thumbs.

2. *Kocher's Manoeuvre.*—This is the most popular method, and some surgeons do this without anaesthesia. With one hand, the surgeon presses the patient's arm firmly against his side in order to fix the distal end of the humerus, since only by this means can subsequent manipulations exert their full action on the humeral head. The elbow is flexed at a right angle. Grasping the patient's wrist with his free hand, the surgeon uses the forearm as a lever for the different steps of the manoeuvre as follows:

   a. Steady traction is applied in the line of the humerus.

   b. The arm is rotated laterally and this is effected by carrying the forearm away from the body till it is nearly in the coronal plane. If the tear is in the anterior part of the capsule, the tendon of the subcapsularis, which lies in front of the head and is tightened by this excessive lateral rotation, may press the head back, through the tear, into place.

   c. If reduction does not occur at this stage, the elbow is carried forwards and medially across the body towards the midline, the lateral rotation of the humerus being maintained. This movement stretches the capsule and so also tear in it, so that the head may enter through the tear now.

   d. Should it not do so, the arm is rotated medially so that the hand falls on the opposite shoulder, the forearm being swung over the opposite side of the chest. In this movement, the humeral head descends downwards and passes through the torn inferior part of the capsule.

3. *Hippocrates' Method.*—This is usually used where the Kocher's methods fails. The patient lies on the floor. As traction is applied by pulling firmly and steadily upon the semi-abducted and slightly medially-rotated shoulder, the surgeon's stockinged foot exerts counter-pressure on the axilla. At the same time direct backward pressure may be exerted on the dislocated head.

4. *Hanging-arm Technique.*—This may be done without anaesthesia. The patient lies prone, with the arm hanging over the edge of the table for a few minutes, to relax the muscles. Thereafter, gentle traction is combined with lateral rotation, followed by flexion and abduction. At the same time, the surgeon's other hand, in the axilla, lifts the humeral head over the glenoid rim.

After reduction, the limb should be *immobilised* in adduction and internal rotation, by arm-trunk bandaging, for three weeks.

To reduce a posterior dislocation, the arm is pulled and rotated outwards, while the head is pushed forwards into place. Thereafter, immobilization is done with the shoulder widely abducted and externally rotated, in a plaster spica, for three weeks.

Complications
1. Recurrent dislocation (vide below)
2. Associated fractures:
   a. Fracture of the greater tuberosity—as the greater tuberosity impinges against the acromion (vide mechanism of dislocation).
   b. Fracture of the neck of the humerus, i.e. fracture-dislocation. It is more often the anatomical neck, than the surgical neck, that is fractured in cases of dislocation.
   c. Compression fracture of the posterior part of the articular surface of the head, caused by the strike against the anterior margin of the glenoid.
3. Injury to nerves:
   a. Circumflex nerve (vide mechanism of dislocation). There is paralysis of the deltoid muscle, with anaesthesia over a small area on the lateral aspect of upper arm.
   b. Rarely, the brachial plexus, particularly the posterior cord.
4. Injury to axillary vessels—very rare.

RECURRENT DISLOCATION OF THE SHOULDER

In recurrent dislocation, the damage sustained by the shoulder at the first dislocation is such that it predisposes to further dislocations. These tend to occur with increasing frequency and with decreasing violence. Almost always it is an anterior dislocation, only very rarely posterior.

Pathology
1. This is a form of anterior dislocation, occurring recurrently, and is a sequela only to those cases of anterior dislocation where the head primarily came out directly through the *anterior* aspect of the joint, i.e.
   a. either through a rent in the anterior wall of the capsule,
   b. or through a gap between the glenoidal labrum and the capsule,
   c. or through a gap caused by the detachment of the glenoidal labrum from the glenoid.
   It is believed that the last injury is the commonest precursor of recurrent dislocation because the glenoidal labrum is avascular and cannot heal.
2. It is automatically believed that a recurrent dislocation is more likely to follow an acute dislocation if sufficient period of immobilizations is not allowed for the joint injury to heal itself, thus keeping the gap persistent.
3. Through the gap mentioned above, a synovial pouch protrudes forwards, and a room is made for the head, which has always a tendency to enter this room.
4. An associated constant pathology is an indentation on the posterolateral aspect of the articular surface of the humeral head, probably caused by violent impingement against the sharp anterior margin of the glenoid.

Clinical Features.—There is usually a history of an acute dislocation, which may or may not have been adequately immobilised. Following this, the patient suffers from recurrent dislocations, in increasing frequency and with trivial trauma. The dislocation is usually precipitated by movements that cause *external rotation* of the shoulder. Usually the patient can reduce the dislocation himself.

Treatment.—Operative treatment has to be undertaken. Varieties of operations have .been devised, of which the following two are most popular:

1. PUTTI-PLATT'S OPERATION.—The principle of this operation is to restrict external rotation of the shoulder, which precipitates the dislocation.

The joint is approached from the front. An incision is made along the deltopectoral groove, starting from below the clavicle and extending downwards for 5 inches. The deltoid and pectoralis major are separated and the coracoid process is exposed. This is divided near its base and is reflected downwards, together with the muscles attached to it (alternatively, the muscles, which are attached to the coracoid process, viz. the short head of biceps, coracobrachialis, and pectoralis minor, are divided half an inch below the tip of the coracoid, and are reflected downwards).

The subscapularis muscle is exposed. Behind and attached to it lies the anterior wall of the capsule of the shoulder joint. These two structures are divided together with a vertical incision, one inch away from the insertion of the subscapularis. A double-bracing (i.e. reefing) is done between these two cut flaps. This procedure rigidly restricts the external rotation of the joint.

2. BANKART'S OPERATION.—This operation is more rational in that it directly repairs the injury, but it is more difficult to be performed. The joint is approached from the front as for Putti-Platt's operation. As the subscapularis muscle is incised vertically, the joint is exposed. The rent through which the head comes out is now identified. If it is in the capsule, it is carefully repaired. If there is detachment of the capsule from the glenoidal labrum, the capsule is sutured to the labrum. If there is detachment of the glenoidal labrum from the glenoid (this is the commonest finding), the labrum is sutured to the bone, by making drill holes on the rawed anterior edge of the glenoid fossa. The subscapularis muscle is sutured, preferably with overlapping.

After any operation for recurrent dislocation, the shoulder is to be immobilized in internal rotation for 6 to 8 weeks. External rotation must be prevented during this period.

FRACTURE OF THE SHAFT OF THE HUMERUS

Mechanism and Types.—The shaft of the humerus is most commonly fractured in its middle third. The upper third is a popular site for pathological fractures—through a solitary bone cyst in the adolescents and a metastatic deposit in the elderly. In the children the fracture is often of greenstick type.

The fracture may be caused by:

1. Indirect twisting injury to the arm.—Spiral fracture.
2. Direct blow over the shaft.—Transverse, short oblique, or comminuted fractures.

Displacement.—This is variable. There may be no displacement or there may be gross overlapping, separation, or angulation. In general, the displacement depends largely on the relation of the site of the fracture to the insertion of the deltoid muscle:

1. When the fracture is *above the insertion of the deltoid.*—The proximal fragment is adducted by the latissimus dorsi, teres major and pectoralis major. The distal fragment is drawn proximally by the deltoid, triceps and biceps.

2. When the fracture is *below the insertion of the deltoid.*—The proximal fragment is abducted by the deltoid. The distal fragment is pulled upwards and adducted, a little, by the biceps and triceps.

Clinical Features.—There is pain, swelling, deformity, abnormal movements, and definite tenderness. In pathological fractures the pain may not be severe.

X-ray confirms the diagnosis.

Treatment.—Reduction of these fractures is usually unnecessary because gravity tends to correct any overlapping or angulation. Even if some angulation persists, the shoulder being a multi-axial joint, there is no interference with its function. Similarly, shortening due to uncorrected overlapping, is hardly noticeable or disadvantageous. Contact over a quarter or a third of the fractured surfaces is sufficient for union.

Equally unnecessary is rigid immobilizations because most of the fractures unite readily with a minimum of external splintage.

I. Standard Treatment.—The arm is rested in a collar and cuff (not a sling, because it supports the weight of the arm and so removes the traction-effect of gravity). The arm is bandaged with a U-cast of plaster. This runs from the shoulder, down the lateral side of the arm, then under the elbow, and up along the medial side of the arm. It has a double effect. It provides splintage to the site of fracture (thus relieving pain) and adds to the weight, producing the traction. If desired, further security may be provided by bandaging the arm (with the cast) to the trunk. This is maintained for 6 weeks.

II. Other Methods of Treatment

A. REDUCTION, if displacement is greater than can be accepted:
    1. By manipulation under general anaesthesia.
    2. By continuous traction in Thomas' Humerus abduction-extension splint.

B. IMMOBILIZATIONS
    1. *Plaster:*
        a. Complete plaster cylinder (instead of the U-cast), encircling only the upper arm, from the axilla to the elbow.
        b. Complete plaster cylinder, encircling both the arm and the forearm, with the elbow flexed to a right angle.
        c. A plaster shoulder spica, if the fragments are very unstable. The spica includes the trunk and the whole of the upper limb, with the exception of the fingers. The shoulder is held semi-abducted and the elbow flexed to a right angle.
    2. *Splint:*
        a. With traction, in Thomas' Humerus abduction-extension splint.
        b. Without traction, in an arm-splint.
    3. *Internal Fixation:*
        This is required where the fragments are very unstable. It is an alternative to a cumbersome shoulder spica, which causes gross discomfort to the patient. This may be done by:
        a. Intra-medullary nail (through greater tuberosity).
        b. Bone-plate.

Complications

1. Injury to the radial nerve.—The nerve winds round the bone in close contact to it. It may be damaged:
   a. At the time of injury.
   b. Later, by being entangled in the callus ('tardy' palsy).
2. Non-union.—Though rare, non-union may occur and, if it does, it poses a serious problem. Indeed, the mid-shaft of the humerus is recognised as a site of the most resistant cases of non-union. Treatment is by bone-grafting.

SUPRACONDYLAR FRACTURE OF HUMERUS

Types and Trauma

A. TRANSVERSE FRACTURE, usually occurring in the children. This is one of the commonest fractures of childhood. The fracture line runs transversely through the lower metaphysis of humurus, so that the injury is actually a *fracture-separation of the lower humeral epiphysis*. There may be two types of transverse fractures:

1. *Extension Type.*—This occurs as a result of fall on the outstretched hand, with the *elbow semiflexed*. The forearm is also forcefully pronated by the injury. The displacements of the lower fragment are as follows:
   a. There are backward and upward displacements, caused by the force of the trauma, passing through the upper end of the ulna.
   b. There is a backward angulation.
   c. There is usually a lateral displacement.
   d. There is pronation (i.e. internal rotation) because of the forced pronation of the forearm.
   This is the commonest type of supracondylar fracture

2. *Flexion Type.*—This occurs as a result of fall on the outstretched hand with the *elbow extended*. The lower fragment is displaced upwards and *forwards*. This is a rare injury.

B. 'T' OR 'Y' SHAPED FRACTURES, usually occurring in the adults. These occur as a result of fall on the point of the elbow, with the joint flexed. The same type of trauma produces fracture of the olecranon. Whether the humerus will break the olecranon or the olecranon will break the humerus depends on the degree of flexion of the elbow at the moment of impact.

This is a comminuted fracture, with its vertical limb extending into the elbow joint.

Clinical Features.—Except for the cases of 'T' or 'Y' fractures, which occur in the adults, the vast majority of patients are children. There is pain, progressively increasing swelling, and limitation of movements of the elbow joint. Until the swelling obscures the details, the backward shift, just above the elbow, is apparent in the common extension type of fracture. The points of difference from a posterior dislocation of the elbow joint are as follows:

   a. Age.—A child.
   b. The maximum tenderness is over the supracondylar region.
   c. Though painful, some amount of movements in the elbow joint is possible.

d. The relationship between the three bony prominences at the elbow, viz. the tip of the olecranon, the medial epicondyle, and the lateral epicondyle, keeps unaltered.

(In posterior dislocation the patient is usually an adult, the maximum tenderness is over the joint, where no movement is possible, and the relationship between the bony points is altered).

In every case of supracondylar fracture, proper examination must be made for:

1. The radial pulse (to exclude injury to the brachial artery).
2. The nerves, particularly the median.

X-ray confirms the diagnosis.

Treatment

The possibility of injury to the brachial artery, in cases of supracondylar fracture, must be paramount in the mind of the surgeon. The cases are, therefore, divided into two categories, as regards management—those uncomplicated and those complicated with arterial injury.

I. TREATMENT FOR UNCOMPLICATED CASES

1. *Reduction* must be done under general anaesthesia, with the muscles relaxed. The manipulations should be gentle and methodical if injury to the artery has to be avoided:

    a. One hand of the surgeon pulls the forearm downwards and this brings the lower fragment down. This traction is effected with the elbow still flexed. Only when the distal fragment has been brought down that the elbow should be extended. This procedure reduces the chances of injury to the brachial artery.

    b. With the traction still maintained, the forearm is supinated. This corrects the pronation (i.e. internal rotation) of the lower fragment.

    c. The lateral displacement is then corrected by the other hand of the surgeon, working on the lower fragment, pushing it inwards.

    d. This second hand of the surgeon is now so placed that the fingers are on the biceps in front of the lower end of the shaft, and the thumb is on the olecranon behind. The elbow is gently flexed and the thumb pushes the lower fragment forwards. The intact triceps prevents over-reduction.

    At every step, the radial pulse must be checked and, on completion, a check up X-ray is taken.

2. *Immobilizations.*—This may be done either with complete plastering or with a posterior cast, extending from the upper third of the arm to the hand. To keep the fragments in place, the ideal position will be maximum amount of flexion at the elbow, permitted without interfering with the radial pulse. The forearm is kept midprone. The immobilization is maintained for 4 weeks.

3. *Observation.*—After reduction and plastering, all cases must be kept under strict observation for detection of impairment of circulation. The cardinal features of vascular impairment are:

    a. Severe pain in the forearm and hand.
    b. Painful movements of the fingers.
    c. Diminished sensation in the fingers.
    d. Absence of nail-bed return.
    e. Altered colour of the fingers.

The above description of treatment applies to the commonest variety of supracondylar fracture, viz. transverse fracture of extension type. In the flexion type of fracture, reduction is achieved by pulling the arm and straightening the elbow. A posterior cast or a complete plaster is applied with the elbow *in extension,* and kept for 4 weeks. For the 'T' or 'Y' fractures, in the adults, either of the following procedures may be adopted:

a. Moulding under anaesthesia, followed by immobilizations in plaster for 6 weeks. This often results in a stiff-elbow.

b. Ignoring the fracture and encouraging movements, putting the elbow at right angle, in a colour and cuff. This minimises the chances of a stiff elbow.

c. Operative reduction and fixing the condyles with a screw.

II. TREATMENT OF CASES COMPLICATED WITH (BRACHIAL) ARTERIAL INJURY *see* Chapter 59, under 'complications of fractures'.

Complications

A. IMMEDIATE COMPLICATIONS

1. Injury to the brachial artery.—Tear, laceration, contusion (with thrombosis), kink, or spasm.

2. Injury to the median nerve.—By the protruding lower end of the proximal fragment.

3. Associated bone and joint injuries:
   a. Fracture line extending into the elbow joint, in cases of 'T' or 'Y' fractures.
   b. Fracture of the medial epicondyle.
   c. Fracture of the head of radius.
   d. Fracture of the olecranon process.

B. DELAYED COMPLICATIONS

1. Mal-union.—Little disturbance in the alignment is very common but this usually gets moulded in a child. Difficulties due to gross mal-union may be as follows:
   a. If the backward displacement and tilt are not corrected, the lower end of the upper fragment, projecting beneath the brachialis in front, will act as a mechanical obstruction to flexion.
   b. Uncorrected sideways tilt or rotation (i.e. pronation) may lead to an ugly cubitus varus deformity.
   c. Rarely, a cubitus valgus deformity may occur and this may cause late ulnar-nerve palsy by stretching the nerve.

2. Joint-stiffness.—This is fairly common. The causes may be:
   a. 'T' or 'Y' fractures in adults.
   b. Mal-union or myositis ossificans in children.

3. Median and ulnar nerve palsy.—Due to ischaemia associated with arterial injury. A late ulnar palsy may be due to cubitus valgus deformity.

4. Myositis ossificans traumatica (*see* Chapter 59).

5. Volkmann's ischaemic contracture (vide below).

VOLKMANN'S ISCHAEMIC CONTRACTURE

This denotes fibrosis of the flexor muscles of the forearm, following ischaemia, as a result of injury to the brachial artery, most commonly due to a supracondylar fracture.

Types of Arterial Damage and Pathology
See Chapter 59, under 'complications of fractures'.

Clinical Features

A. IN THE STAGE OF ISCHAEMIA:
1. Severe pain in the forearm and hand (even after the fracture has been reduced and immobilised).
2. Painful movements of the fingers.
3. Diminished sensation in the fingers.
4. Absence of nail-bed return.
5. Altered colour of the fingers.

B. IN THE DEVELOPING STAGE:
1. Inability to extend the fingers with the wrist extended (this is possible in a normal hand). Only when the wrist is flexed that the fingers can be extended.
2. Sensory and motor changes, due to ischaemic paralysis of the nerves, particularly the median, may be superimposed.

C. IN THE DEVELOPED STAGE:
1. The forearm shows wasting.
2. There is a typical deformity—the elbow is flexed, the forearm is mid-prone, the wrist shows palmar-flexion and ulnar deviation, the metacarpophalangeal joints are *extended,* and the interphalangeal joints are flexed.
3. There are often associated features of ischaemic nerve damage, particularly of the median. On the other hand, the features of nerve damage, present earlier, may disappear, because nerves can regenerate.

Treatment

I. IN THE STAGE OF ISCHAEMIA:
To diagnose the condition at this stage should be the aim in every case because the most important fact about the deformity is that its occurrence may be prevented.
For treatment in this stage *see* Chapter 59.

II. IN THE DEVELOPING STAGE:
These are the cases where the muscles have already been damaged, but an early diagnosis has been made. Physiotherapy and active movements of the fingers, aided by spring-splints, often produce good results in these cases.

III. IN THE ESTABLISHED CASES:

A. *The Older methods of Treatment*
1. Making the forearm bones shorter, in accordance to the shortened muscles.
2. Max-Page's Muscle Sliding Operation.—In this operation the common flexor origin, from the medial epicondyle, is erased off. The wrist and the finger joints are extended, and immobilised in this position. The common flexor origin thus slides down and develops a new attachment, lower down. None of the above operations prove satisfactory since they cannot provide muscle power in the flexors that has been lost because of fibrosis in the

muscles. No amount of physiotherapy can cause regeneration of the destroyed muscles.

B. *The Recent Methods of Treatment*

1. In milder cases, simply the fibrous tissues are excised, so that the contracture is released and the remaining healthy muscle mass is allowed to work. These are the cases which might be benefitted by Max-Page's operation as well.

2. In the commoner variety, i.e. the severe cases, the fibrosis is extensive. All fibrous tissue, in the muscles, is excised. To the left-behind tendons of flexor digitorum profundus and flexor policis longus are transplanted some healthy muscle (usually the wrist flexor or wrist extensor) in order to restore active flexion of the digits.

This muscle transfer may be combined with arthrodesis of the wrist in the optimum position.

If there is an associated irreparable ischaemic damage of the median nerve, nerve grafting may be added.

POSTERIOR DISLOCATION OF THE ELBOW

This is usually an injury of the adults, resulting from fall on the outstretched hand. The same trauma usually produces a supracondylar fracture, i.e. fracture-separation of the lower humeral epiphysis, in the children. This is because the capsule of the elbow joint is stronger than the bond of union between the humeral epiphysis and diaphysis in the children.

(An anterior dislocation of the elbow is rare and may occur as a complication of fracture of the olecranon)

Once posterior dislocation has taken place, lateral shift may also occur.

Associated Fractures

1. Almost always there is an associated fracture of the coronoid process.

2. Sometimes there may be an associated fracture of the radial head, capitulum, or the medial epicondyle of the humerus.

Almost always the associated fracture is a minor one.

Clinical Features.—The patient, usually an adult, presents with pain, swelling, and loss of movements of the elbow joint. The joint is held semiflexed. There is prominence posteriorly, as compared to the healthy elbow.

The differentiating features from a supracondylar fracture have been described under supracondylar fracture of the humerus.

X-ray confirms the diagnosis.

Treatment.—Reduction under general anaesthesia is usually easy. Traction is applied in the presenting position of the elbow (i.e. usually semiflexed). Thereafter, the elbow is gradually flexed to about 90°. Immobilizations in plaster is maintained for 3 weeks, in this position.

After the period of immobilizations, movements of the elbow are allowed to return spontaneously and are never forced.

Complications.—As in supracondylar fracture of humerus.

FRACTURE-SEPARATION OF LATERAL CONDYLAR EPIPHYSIS
(FRACTURED CAPITULUM)

Fracture-separation of the lateral condylar epiphysis in the children and fracture of the capitulum in the adults denote the same injury, and are caused by fall on the hand, with the elbow in slight *varus* position. The injury is much commoner in the children than in the adults.

(The medial condyle of the humerus is fractured much less frequently than the lateral condyle).

Displacements.—In severe injuries, at the moment of the fracture, the elbow is possibly dislocated postero-laterally. The fractured condyle is capsized by muscle pull and remains capsized while the elbow reduces spontaneously. This is the reason why a *gross* displacement of the condyle is usually seen. There is not only a linear displacement laterally, but also a rotational one, so much so, that often the fractured surface of the lateral condyle, instead of looking medially, looks laterally, i.e. 180° rotation.

X-ray.—Usually a gross displacement is seen, as described above. In the children, the greater part of the detached fragment is cartilagenous, so that the fragment appears much smaller radiologically than it actually is.

Treatment.—Accurate reduction is important as the fracture involves the joint surface:

1. CLOSED REDUCTION.—Under anaesthesia, the forearm is pushed postero-laterally to reproduce the elbow dislocation so as to release the capsized fragment. Thereafter, the forearm is pulled forwards again.

2. OPEN REDUCTION.—Closed manipulation often fails. The fragment is exposed, replaced in position and held with a screw. The top of the screw is left subcutaneous so that it may be easily removed subsequently.

Complications

1. Cubitus valgus, if the fragment is left unreduced.
2. Tardy ulnar nerve palsy, due to stretching of the nerve, if cubitus valgus develops.
3. Non-union sometimes occurs.
4. Osteoarthritis.—This occurs if the fracture leaves behind a permanent deformity or an irregularity of the articular surface.

SEPARATION OF MEDIAL EPICONDYLAR EPIPHYSIS
(FRACTURED MEDIAL EPICONDYLE)

This is an injury of the adolescents and is caused by fall on the hand, with the elbow extended and slightly *valgus*. Whereas condylar fractures are commoner on the lateral side, epicondylar fractures usually occur in the medial. The medial epicondyle begins to ossify by 9 years and fuses with the shaft by 16 years. Between these ages it may be separated.

Displacements

1. There may be a little displacement.
2. The epiphysis may be pulled downwards by the attached wrist flexors.

3. In severe injuries, there is often an associated momentary dislocation of the elbow and the epiphysis is pulled into the elbow. Thereafter, the dislocation reduces spontaneously but the fragment remains capsized.

Complications

1. Damage to the ulnar nerve:
   a. Immediate direct injury in displaced fractures.
   b. Tardy ulnar nerve palsy from friction against the roughened bony groove.
   In any case, the nerve has to be transposed anteriorly.
2. Elbow stiffness.—This is fairly common but usually recovers, provided the epicondyle has not been left in the joint.

Treatment.—Unless the fragment has been pulled into the joint, reduction is usually simple. Immobilizations in plaster for 3 weeks is advised.

If closed reduction fails, open reduction has to be undertaken. At the same time, anterior transposition of the ulnar nerve is done to prevent late palsy.

FRACTURE OF THE OLECRANON

Types of Fracture and Trauma

1. A simple *crack fracture without displacement.*
2. A *comminuted fracture* of the upper fragment.
3. A complete transverse fracture, the small upper fragment being pulled upwards by the strong triceps *(avulsion fracture).*

In any case, the fracture line enters the joint, near the middle of the trochlear notch.

The first two varieties result from direct trauma, e.g. fall on the point of the elbow. The third variety of fracture occurs as a result of indirect trauma, when there is a fall to the hand while the triceps is in action, i.e. sudden forcible flexion of the elbow against the action of the triceps.

Clinical Features.—There is pain, swelling, and tenderness, which is maximum over the olecranon. The movements of the elbow are painful and restricted. While in the first two varieties the elbow can be extended against resistance, in the third type it cannot be done so.

X-ray confirms the diagnosis, the nature of the fracture, as well as the amount of displacement.

Treatment

1. CRACK FRACTURE.—Simple immobilisation in plaster, from upper third of the arm, for three to four weeks, is sufficient. As the aponeurotic covering is still intact, immobilisation even *in flexion* of the elbow joint does not cause separation of the fragments. A plaster in flexion is always preferred since it is easier for the patient to carry it and also it allows functional activity of the hand and fingers.
2. TRANSVERSE FRACTURE WITH WIDE SEPARATION.—Wide separation between the fragments and interposition of the aponeurotic soft tissues prevent normal union, even though the elbow is immobilised in complete extension. Even if union results, it is a long fibrous union, which makes the elbow weak. Moreover, there

is the danger of an ankylosis of the elbow in the inconvenient position of extension because of the prolonged immobilisation.

Internal fixation is, therefore, the treatment of choice. The fixation may be done with a screw or with a combination of two pieces of Kirschner's wire and a stainless steel wire.

A vertical incision is made behind the elbow, a little lateral or medial to the midline (midline scars are exposed to pressure and are, therefore, avoided). All soft tissues down to the periosteum are cut. The periosteum is elevated with a raspatory and the fracture is reduced. The fracture may be fixed with a screw which is passed from the tip of the upper fragment into the lower (i.e. ulnar shaft). Otherwise, two small pieces of Kirschner's wire are taken and they are passed from the tip of the upper fragment into the lower fragment to fix the fracture. Thereafter, a stainless steel wire is taken. A transverse tunnel is made in the upper part of the ulnar shaft and the wire is passed through the tunnel. The ends of the wire are now circumferentially sutured along the triceps around the upper fragment and a knot is applied either medially or laterally after apposing the fragments (Fig. 60.1). This is called *tension band wiring* since the wire relieves the tension on the fracture line when the elbow is flexed.

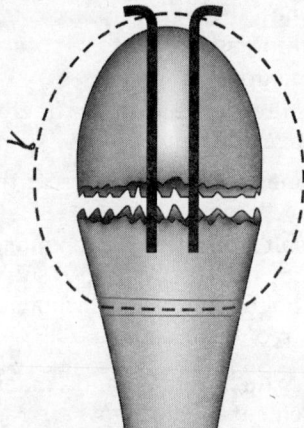

Fig. 60.1: Tension band suture for fractured olecranon

The head of the screw or the Kirschner's wires or the knot of .the circumferential wire is kept subcutaneous so that it can be removed easily, after union has occurred. The limb is plastered, *in extension,* for 6 weeks.

3. COMMINUTED FRACTURE.—Even if union occurs, the articulating surface becomes irregular and may cause painful arthritis of the elbow. Therefore, excision of the comminuted fragment is advocated. After excision, the tendon of the triceps is securely sutured to the ulnar shaft, with a stainless steel wire, passed through a tunnel made in the bone.

FRACTURED UPPER END OF RADIUS

There are two distinct types, both occurring as a result of fall on the outstretched hand while the elbow is slightly *valgus* (in this position the upper end of the radius is pushed against the capitulum and is fractured):

1. Fracture of the *neck of the radius.*—This occurs in the children. It is usually a simple transverse fracture. As a result of the upward thrust of the trauma, the fragments are often impacted.
2. Fracture of the *head of the radius.*—This occurs in the adults. There are again two types of this fracture:
   a. A simple fracture through the periphery of the head.
   b. A comminuted fracture, shattering the head.
   In addition to these fractures, the articular cartilage of the capitulum, against which the radius strikes, may be bruised or chipped. This cannot be seen on the X-ray but is important.

Clinical Features.—The symptoms of this fracture are sometimes very minor, such as a little pain, a little swelling, and a little bruising. The two distinctive physical signs are:
1. Definite tenderness over the head of the radius.
2. Pain at the radial head, on pronation and supination of the forearm.
   X-ray confirms the diagnosis.

Treatment

1. IN THE CHILDREN WITH FRACTURED NECK.—The treatment is conservative. The limb is immobilised in an above-elbow plaster for 3 weeks. The elbow is held at 90° flexion and the forearm supinated.
   If there is gross displacement (which is rare), an accurate reduction should be done. This is usually possible by closed manipulation. If this is not possible, open reduction may have to be undertaken. On no account, the head of the radius (i.e. the upper fragment) should be excised in a child. This results in severe cubitus valgus deformity. Moreover, the ulna then outgrows the radius, the inferior radioulnar joint is thereafter subluxed, and pronation and supination become grossly restricted.

2. IN THE ADULTS WITH FRACTURED HEAD:
   a. If it is a simple peripheral fracture, the treatment is conservative, as in the children.
   b. If it is a comminuted fracture, with the head shattered to pieces, *excision of the radial head* should be done, since otherwise the movements of pronation and supination are painful and restricted.

FRACTURE OF THE UPPER THIRD OF THE SHAFT OF ULNA WITH DISLOCATION OF THE SUPERIOR RADIOULNAR JOINT (MONTEGGIA FRACTURE-DISLOCATION)

Monteggia fracture-dislocation—denotes a fracture of the upper third of the shaft of the ulna, with dislocation of the radial head. Typically, there is an *anterior angulation of the ulnar shaft* and an *anterior dislocation of the radial head.* The injury may be caused in two ways:
   a. Fall on the palm with forced pronation of the forearm.
   b. Direct trauma to the back of the forearm.

   Rarely, there may be a *reverse deformity*—posterior angulation of the ulnar shaft with posterior dislocation of the radial head.

Fracture of the *lower third of the radial shaft,* with dislocation of the *inferior radio-ulnar joint* is known as *Galleazi fracture-dislocation.* This injury, which may be considered as the counterpart of Monteggia fracture-dislocation, is much less common.

Treatment

1. CONSERVATIVE TREATMENT.—Under general anaesthesia, the fracture and dislocation are simultaneously reduced by fully supinating the forearm. If reduction is possible, an above-elbow plastering is done, with the elbow flexed and the forearm supinated. A prolonged immobilisation (about 12 weeks) is required.
2. OPERATIVE TREATMENT.—This is required where closed manipulation fails. The operation is done in *two stages:*
   a. In the first stage, open reduction of the ulnar fracture, with internal fixation, is done. This may be done either with an intramedullary nail or with a bone plate.
   b. In the second stage, excision of the radial head is performed. Some surgeons advocate replacement of the radial head into the annular ligament, instead of its excision.

FRACTURE OF BOTH BONES OF THE FOREARM

While the forearm bone may be fractured singularly, fracture of both the bones is much commoner.

Trauma

1. *Indirect violence,* i.e. a twisting force, usually caused by a fall on the hand.—The bones are usually broken at different levels and the fracture lines are spiral or oblique.
2. *Direct violence,* i.e. an angulating force, e.g. direct hit by a hard object, such as a rod.—The bones fracture at the same level and the fracture lines are usually transverse.

Special Features

1. Both bone fractures are commoner in the lower two-thirds.
2. In children the fractures are almost always green-stick.
3. The radius may show rotational displacements, caused by the pull of muscles attached to it—biceps and supinator in the upper third, pronator teres in the middle third, and pronator quadratus in the lower third.

Complications

1. Delayed union and non-union.—Both bone fractures are notoriously prone to have non-union.
2. Mal-union.—Particularly angulation and rarely cross-union.

Treatment

1. IN CHILDREN WITH GREEN-STICK FRACTURES.—Reduction under general anaesthesia is usually easy and is done by simply undoing the angulation. The incomplete fracture becomes complete as the angulation is corrected. The limb is immobilised in an above-elbow plaster for 6 weeks. The elbow is held in flexion, the forearm midway between pronation and supination, and the wrist neutral.

2. IN THE ADULTS.—This is one of the most difficult fractures for closed reduction. Even after a satisfactory reduction, there is always the possibility of redisplacement of the fragments as well as movements between them inside the plaster, leading to delayed union, non-union and mal-union. The outline of treatment in the adults is as follows:
   a. *Closed reduction,* followed by immobilisation, as in the children. Spiral fractures heal in 6 weeks but transverse fractures may require 12 weeks' immobilisation.
   b. Where closed reduction fails (or where, after reduction, the fragments cannot be held in position by plastering), *open reduction with internal fixation* has to be undertaken. The radius is fixed with a bone plate and the ulna either with a bone plate or an intramedullary nail.
   c. In cases of non-union, *bone grafting* has to be done.

COLLES' FRACTURE

Definition.—This is a fracture through the lower end of the radius, within three-fourth inch of the wrist joint, associated with injury to the inferior radioulnar joint and relative displacement between the lower articulating surfaces of the radius and the ulna, with or without tear of the medial collateral ligament of the wrist, with or without avulsion of the ulnar styloid process.

This is the commonest of all fractures. However, it is a fracture of the old age, particularly of the women.

Nature of the Fracture.—The fracture is caused by a fall on the palm of the outstretched hand (possibly with an added forced supination).

The fracture line is transverse but is often comminuted in the form of a 'T', the vertical limb of which comes down to the wrist joint.

As the fracture line is transverse, as the fracture occurs through the spongy bone, and as there is an upward thrust during the fall, the lower fragment is usually impacted into the upper.

Displacements.—There are usually typical displacements of the lower fragment:

A. LINEAR DISPLACEMENTS:
   1. Upwards (usually with impaction).
   2. Backwards.
   3. Laterally.

B. ROTATIONAL DISPLACEMENTS:
   1. There is backward tilt of the lower fragment in a *transverse axis* so that the lower articular surface of the radius, instead of looking directly downwards, as in normal, looks downwards and backwards.
   2. There is supination of the lower fragment (because of the. forced supination at the time of fall), i.e. rotation along the *long axis,* so that the anterior surface of the radius, instead of looking directly forwards, looks forwards and outwards.

Points of Importance in Colles' Fracture

1. Relative displacement between the lower articulating surfaces of the radius and the ulna, due to injury to the inferior radioulnar joint (their connecting ligaments, including the triangular cartilage, are torn).

2. The backward tilt of the lower fragment, disturbing the congruity of the articular surface at the wrist joint.
3. The supination of the lower fragment.
4. The old age of the patient.
5. The tendency to redisplacement of the lower fragment, following reduction and immobilisation.

The above factors may contribute to permanent limitation of palmar flexion of the wrist, as well as supination and pronation of the forearm.

Reversed Colles' or Smith's Fracture.—This is a transverse fracture of the lower radius, with forward shift and forward tilt of the lower fragment, resulting from a fall on the back of the hand, with the wrist flexed. This is a rare fracture.

Clinical Features of Colles' Fracture.—The patient, usually elderly and more often a female, complains of pain and swelling, with limitation of movements of the wrist joint.

There is a typical *dinner fork deformity*, the teeth of the fork represented by the fingers and the curve of the fork by the posteriorly displaced lower fragment.

There is tenderness at the lower end of radius as well as on the medial side of the wrist (due to the associated injury there—*see* definition).

The radial styloid process, which is normally at a lower level than the ulnar styloid, is either at the same level with it or even at a higher level. This is because of the upward displacement of the lower fragment.

X-ray appearance is characteristic and confirmatory.

Treatment

I. REDUCTION.—Under general anaesthesia, a careful reduction is performed. The first step is disimpaction of the fragments because the lower fragment is impacted into the upper. Disimpaction is achieved by a firm traction on the hand and thumb, countertraction being effected by an assistant, holding the arm above the flexed elbow. The next step is correction of the backward displacement and tilt of the lower fragment, as well as its lateral displacement and the supination. This is best achieved with the thenar eminences of the surgeon. One thenar eminence puts a firm forward pressure on the distal fragment while the other thenar eminence puts backward pressure on the lower end of the proximal fragment. For purpose of convenience, the surgeon's right thenar eminence is used to control the distal fragment of the left radius, and vice versa.

II. IMMOBILISATION.—This may be done either with complete plaster or with a plaster cast. If a cast is used, it must be placed on the dorsal aspect because there is a tendency for the lower fragment to move backwards. The position of the limb should be—pronation of the forearm, and a little palmar flexion with ulnar deviation of the wrist. The plaster extends from *below* the elbow (keeping clear the movements of the elbow joint) down to the usual limit, i.e. knuckles on the back and proximal palmar crease in front, with the *base of the thumb free*. Immobilizations is maintained for 6 weeks.

(This plastering is called *Colles' plaster*. It should be noted that, being a below-elbow plaster, it does not control the movements of pronation and supination. This is because, in the elderly, in whom this fracture occurs, the injury to the inferior radioulnar joint results in a greater limitation of pronation and supination if these movements are restricted than if they are permitted).

III. EXERCISE.—Active movements of all the joints that have not been included in the plaster, viz. shoulder, elbow, and fingers, including the thumb. Frozen shoulder is rather frequent because of neglected shoulder movements.

Complications.—The complications are usually of *delayed type:*

1. Mal-union.—This may result in (a) an ugly deformity, (b) limitation of palmar flexion at the wrist, and (c) loss of pronation and supination of the forearm.
2. Osteoarthritis of the wrist.
3. Delayed rupture of the extensor pollicis longus tendon. This is a rare complication. Paradoxically, it is commoner with minor fractures than with fractures associated with gross displacements.
4. Sudeck's bone atrophy.
5. Restriction of movements of shoulder, elbow and fingers, if active exercises are avoided.

Treatment of Mal-united Colles' Fracture

1. If there is not much difficulty, except the deformity, it is better to leave it alone.
2. If there is difficulty in pronation and supination, excision of the lower end of ulna usually gives good results.

    If the patient is relatively young and active, a corrective osteotomy of the lower end of radius is advised, in addition to the ulnar excision.
3. If there is considerable limitation of palmar flexion, a corrective osteotomy of the lower radius is advocated.

FRACTURE OF THE SCAPHOID BONE

Important Points

1. Most commonly, the fracture occurs through the waist of the bone. This may result in an avascular necrosis of the proximal fragment because the blood supply comes from the distal side of the bone.
2. A recent fracture of the scaphoid is often missed on ordinary X-rays, i.e. antero-posterior and lateral views. Hence, diagnosis of a fractured scaphoid is better done clinically than radiologically. If there is tenderness over the anatomical snuff-box, the case should be treated as one of fracture of the scaphoid, even if X-ray reports are negative.
3. Oblique view X-rays are often helpful in showing the fracture. A fracture may sometimes become obvious radiologically after a few days, even though it was not apparent in the initial films. This is more so if the wrist was not immobilised following the trauma—the fracture line often broadening and looking like a cystic space.

Complications

1. Avascular necrosis of the proximal fragment. This is a common site for avascular necrosis.
2. Delayed union.—Fairly common.
3. Non-union.—The causes of non-union are:
    a. Imperfect immobilizations (often because the fracture is initially ignored as the X-ray reports are negative).

    b. Avascular necrosis.

    c. The fracture line being intra-articular, the fracture haematoma is washed by synovial fluid.

4. Osteoarthritis of the wrist.

Treatment

1. Reduction is usually unnecessary as there is no displacement.
2. Immobilizations in a below-elbow plaster, like Colles' plaster, but differing from it in the following respects:

    a. The proximal digit of the thumb is included in the plaster (the interphalangeal joint of the thumb and all the joints of the other fingers must be free to move).

    b. The wrist is held in dorsiflexion, with the thumb forwards, i.e. the 'glass holding' position. This is the optimum position for the wrist joint and is used for immobilizations of all fractures in the wrist and hand, except Colles fracture.

3. The immobilizations should be prolonged—a minimum of 8 weeks.

FRACTURE OF THE BASE OF THE FIRST METACARPAL

Trauma.—Usually a longitudinal violence sustained by the bone, when the patient applies a blow, as in boxing.

Types

1. A transverse or short oblique fracture, the fracture line not entering the carpometacarpal joint. The fracture shows a little displacement.
2. An oblique fracture, the fracture line entering the carpometacarpal joint at about the middle of the articular surface. There is a gross displacement between the fragments. Moreover, the shaft of the bone, containing a part of the articular surface, is dislocated from the carpal bone (trapezium). This is, therefore, a fracture-dislocation *(Bennett's fracture-dislocation)*.

Treatment

1. In the first type, simple immobilization for 3 weeks.
2. In the second type, reduction is necessary. This is done under general anaesthesia and the hand is immobilised in plaster. Often it is difficult to keep the fragments in position. In such cases an internal fixation is necessary.

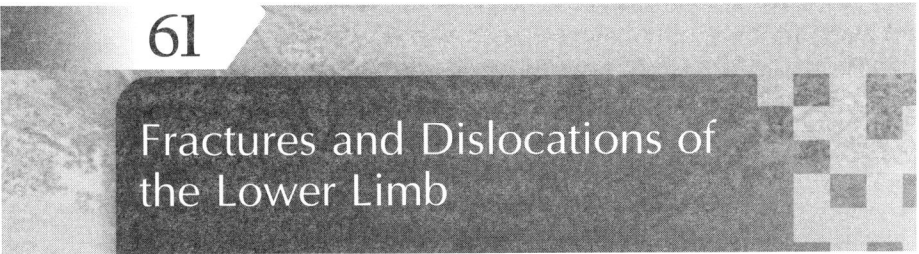

61

Fractures and Dislocations of the Lower Limb

DISLOCATION OF THE HIP

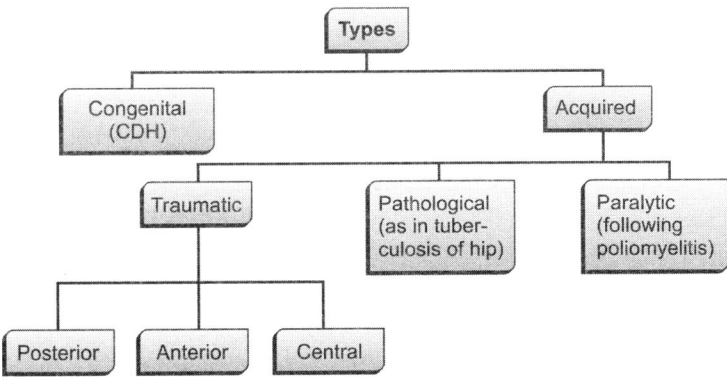

TRAUMATIC DISLOCATION OF THE HIP

Types.—There are three varieties:
1. Posterior—commonest.
2. Anterior.
3. Central.

Dislocation of hip can result only from *severe* trauma because:
a. The head of the femur is well protected in the bony socket of the acetabulum, which is further deepened by the acetabular labrum (c.f. shoulder joint).
b. Strong ligaments re-inforce the well-developed capsule of the joint.
c. Strong muscles protect the joint all round.

Types of Trauma and Injury

A. POSTERIOR DISLOCATION.—In a normal hip, the femoral head lies in a relatively unprotected position when the hip is in flexion, adduction and internal rotation. In this position, the major part of the head, instead of being covered by the socket of the acetabulum, rests on the capsule and ligaments at the back of the joint. If this position is terribly exaggerated, there is possibility of the head tearing through the capsule on the back and getting a posterior dislocation. This is typically likely to occur in a passenger in the front seat of a motor car, with one thigh resting on the other, and the car facing a head-on collision. The upper knee strikes hard against the dash board and the impact, transmitted along the femur, causes exaggeration of flexion, adduction and internal rotation at the hip.

The dislocated head may lie:

1. Above the pyriformis muscle, under cover of the glutei. This is called the *gluteal type* of dislocation.
2. Below the pyriformis muscle, in the vicinity of the greater sciatic notch. This is called the *sciatic type* of dislocation. The head may injure the sciatic nerve, lying close by.

B. ANTERIOR DISLOCATION.—The head comes out through the anterior part of the capsule, when there is a forcible abduction of the hip.

The dislocated head may lie:

1. In front of the pubis—*pubic type* of dislocation.
2. In front of the obturator foremen—*obturator type* of dislocation.

In anterior dislocation, the femoral nerve or the obturator nerve may be injured, but rarely.

C. CENTRAL DISLOCATION.—This occurs as a result of very severe trauma, with the hip midway between abduction and adduction. The head enters the pelvis through the centre of the acetabulum.

Regular and Irregular Dislocations.—The ileo-femoral ligament is a very strong bond of union between the hip bones and the femur. Even when a dislocation of the hip has occurred, this ligament often keeps intact. Those dislocations, in which the ileo-femoral ligament is still undamaged (or only its lateral limb is torn), are called 'regular' dislocations. When both the limbs of the ligament are injured (or when portions of the acetabulum of the femoral head are fractured), the dislocation is called 'irregular'. In irregular dislocations, the typical attitude of the limb, as is usually seen in different types of dislocations (*see* below), may not be found.

Clinical Features

A. POSTERIOR DISLOCATION:

1. The limb is typically in flexion, adduction and internal rotation.
2. There is a feeling of emptiness in the femoral triangle due to the absence of the femoral head, which normally occupies this position. Instead, the head may be palpable under the glutei.
3. All the movements of the hip joint are restricted and painful.
4. Measurements show:
   a. Shortening of the length from the anterior superior iliac spine to the medial side of the knee.
   b. This shortening is above the greater trochanter since the trochanter is found to lie above the *Nelaton's line*. This is an imaginary straight line joining the anterior superior iliac spine to the most prominent part of the ischial tuberosity. Normally the line just touches the tip of the greater trochanter. *X-ray* confirms the diagnosis—the *Shenton's line* is broken.

B. ANTERIOR DISLOCATION:

1. The limb is typically in flexion, abduction and external rotation.
2. There is an abnormal fullness in the femoral triangle, made by the anteriorly dislocated head.
3. There is restriction of all active and passive movements of the hip.
4. There is lengthening of the limb:

   a. Partly apparent, because of the abduction.
   b. Partly real, as measured from the anterior superior iliac spine to the medial side of the knee.
   c. The greater trochanter is below the Nelaton's line.
   X-ray confirms the diagnosis.

Treatment

Reduction under general anaesthesia has to be undertaken. With good muscle relaxation, reduction is usually not difficult. The patient lies supine and an assistant grasps the pelvis firmly at the iliac crests (countertraction). The surgeon holds the knee, with the hip and the knee flexed at right angles, so that the femur is vertical. The thigh is now steadily pulled upwards. For a posterior dislocation a gradual lateral rotation, and for an anterior dislocation a gradual medial rotation of the femur, is added. The head usually comes back into the socket.

Immobilisation may be achieved by either of the following methods:
a. Plaster spica with the hip in neutral position.
b. Limb supported from a beam with light traction.
c. Skeletal traction from the tibial tubercle in a Thomas' splint.
   The immobilisation is maintained for 6 weeks.

   In central dislocation, reduction has to be done by strong continuous skeletal traction (preferably through femoral condyles), with the hip abducted.

Complications

A. IMMEDIATE
   1. Injury to nerves:
      a. Injury to the sciatic nerve in posterior dislocation.
      b. Injury to the femoral or obturator nerve (rarely) in anterior dislocation.
   2. Associated fractures:
      a. Posterior marginal fracture of the acetabulum in posterior dislocation.
      b. Acetabulum in central dislocation.
      c. Femoral head or neck—rarely.
B. DELAYED
   1. Osteoarthritis of the hip.
   2. Avascular necrosis of the femoral head (rare).
   3. Post-traumatic ossification around the hip, i.e. myositis ossificans traumatica—rare.

FRACTURE OF THE NECK OF THE FEMUR

Fracture of the neck of the femur is common in persons above the age of 60, since the bone here gets increasingly brittle as age advances. However, the fracture may occur even in a child.

   The trauma, causing the fracture, especially in the very elderly, is often trivial—sometimes a mere stumble. Often, however, the trauma is severe; this is particularly so when the patient is young. In general, it may be stated that the older the patient, the more likely he is to sustain the fracture with trauma of lesser intensity.

   Since the neck of the femur is a rather common site of metastatic deposits (in the elderly) and of bone cysts (in the children), pathological fractures occur rather frequently. Rarely, fatigue fractures may occur in the femoral neck in young adults. Thus, fractures of the neck of the femur may be:

a. *Traumatic Fracture*—The trauma may or may not be severe but the bone is apparently healthy.

b. *Pathological Fracture.*—The trauma is trivial and the bone is pathological.

c. *Fatigue Fracture.*—There is a long-continued unusual physical activity, such as marching with full military pack.

Classification and Description.—There are various ways of classifying this fracture but the oldest of them, as described below, is the best, since it gives indications to the nature, prognosis, and management of the fracture.

According to this classification, fracture of the femoral neck may be:

I. Intracapsular.

II. Extracapsular.

INTRACAPSULAR FRACTURES.—Here, the fracture line is inside the capsule of the hip joint.

The blood supply to the head of the femur comes from three sources:

a. A small supply to the central part of the head, by way of the central vessel in the ligamentum teres femoris.

b. Terminal branches of the nutrient vessels in the substance of the bone.

c. The major part of the supply is by way of the *recurrent vessels,* running in the direction of neck to head, along the inner layers of the capsule. In case of an intracapsular fracture, the blood supply by way of (b) and (c) are interrupted, and the big femoral head has to live only on the meagre supply by way of (a). Under such precarious condition of blood supply, there is a great chance for the femoral head undergoing avascular necrosis. Even if this does not occur, there is a great risk of non-union, unless immobilisation of the fracture fragments is absolutely perfect. Unfortunately, the fracture is so deep seated and surrounded by so strong muscles, that it is impossible to achieve perfect immobilisation by external methods of plastering or splintage. Internal fixation is, therefore, the only means for rigid immobilisation of these fractures. This is done with Smith Petersen nail.

The intracapsular fractures may further be classified, according, to the exact site of the fracture line, e.g.

1. *Subcapital.*—Where the fracture line is just below the head.

2. *Transcervical.*—Where the fracture line lies at about the middle of the neck (Fig. 61.1).

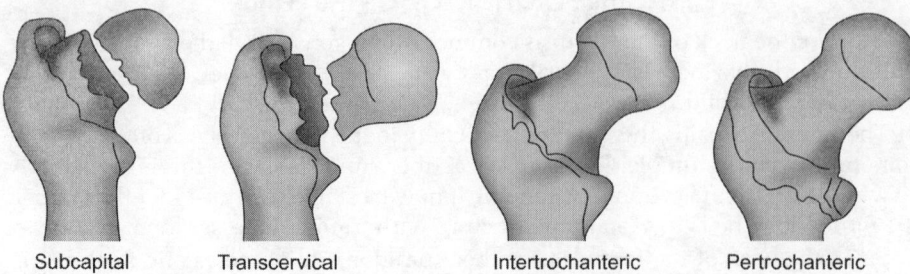

Subcapital   Transcervical   Intertrochanteric   Pertrochanteric

Fig. 61.1: Types of fracture neck of the femur according to the exact site of fracture

In older days intracapsular fractures were classified according to the disposition of the fracture line (Pauwel's classification), i.e.

1. *Adduction fracture.*—Where the fracture line is more towards vertical.
2. *Abduction fracture.*—Where the fracture line is more towards transverse.

This classification was thought to be prognostically very important. In case of an abduction fracture, as the person tries to bear weight, there is a shearing strain on the fracture line, and this may make union difficult. On the other hand, in case of an abduction fracture, as the person tries to bear weight, there is a chance of impaction between the fragments, and so possibilities of union are good (Fig. 61.2).

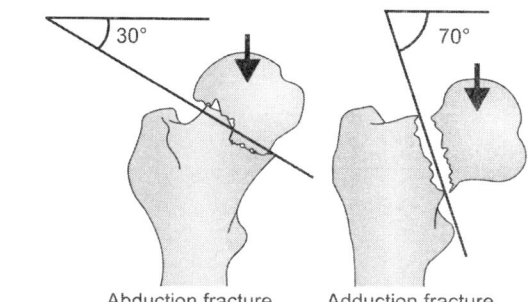

Fig. 61.2: Fracture neck of the femur—abduction and adduction types

On the X-ray the two types may be diagnosed by drawing the Pauwe's angle. This is the angle between the fracture line prolonged upwards and a transverse line drawn along the upper rim of the acetabulum. In an abduction fracture the angle is about 30°, while in an adduction fracture it is about 70° (Fig. 61.2).

It has now been made clear that this classification of femoral neck fractures into abduction and adduction types is of no importance as such—they only denote the different degrees of displacement of the fragments, being caused by the same type of trauma, which is a lateral rotation force that breaks the neck at or near the subcapital level. If the trauma is less severe, the fragments are impacted and the plane of the fractures seems more vertical. In fact, however, the plane of the fracture has been the same from the beginning.

Garden's Classification of the subcapital fractures (also applicable to transcervical fractures) gives a better idea about the fracture (Fig. 61.3):

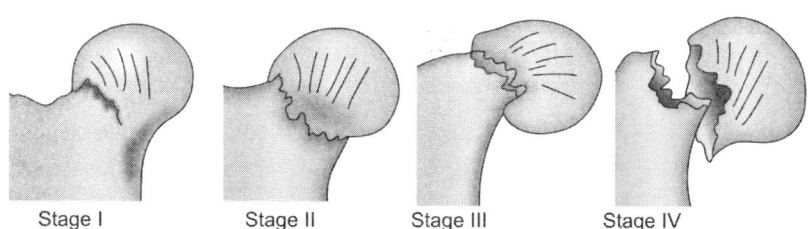

Fig. 61.3: Garden's classification of fracture neck of the femur

Stage I: Incomplete fracture. The lower cortex of the neck has not broken. These are the cases of so-called 'abducted' or 'impacted' fracture.

Stage II: Complete fracture without displacement. There is fracture through the whole thickness of the neck but the lower fragment has not been displaced. Also the head is in its normal anatomical position (as shown by the disposition of its trabeculae).

Stage III: Complete fracture with partial displacement. The distal fragment hinges against the head and the results are twofold:
a. There is no complete displacement of the distal fragment.
b. The head is tilted into abduction and medial rotation (as shown by the disposition of its trabeculae).

Stage IV: Complete fracture with full displacement. The distal fragment has undergone full lateral rotation. Intimate contact between the two fragments has been lost. The head being free, keeps its normal anatomical position (as shown- by the disposition of its trabeculae).

EXTRACAPSULAR FRACTURES.—The fracture line is outside the capsule of the hip joint. The chances of a vascular necrosis of the head are remote since the blood supplies (a) and (c) are left intact and only the supply by way of (b) is curtailed. So, these fractures may heal well even with external immobilisation by plastering or splintage. Unfortunately, however, the patients sustaining such fractures are very elderly, often 70 and above (the cancellous bone gets so brittle that even with a very minor trauma a fracture occurs). To keep such elderly patients in plaster or splint for 3 to 6 months is associated with the risks of bed sores and pressure sores, as well as pulmonary and renal complications. Arrangements have to be made so that the patient can, at least, sit up early and this can be done only by internal fixation.

From the above description, it is evident that almost all the cases of fracture of the neck of the femur (except the small percentage of impacted abduction fractures) are to be treated by internal fixation—in intracapsular fractures to avoid non-union and in extracapsular fractures to avoid the complications of old age.

According to the exact site of the fracture line, extracapsular fractures may further be divided into two groups:

1. *Basal Cervical* or *Intertrochanteric.*—The fracture is at the base of the neck, as if, uprooting the neck and the head from the shaft. The fracture line runs between the two trochanters (intertrochanteric).

2. *Pertrochanteric.*—Always a comminuted fracture, the main fracture line runs somewhere through the trochanteric mass.

Thus, *to summarise the classification of fractures of the femoral neck:*

I. The fracture may be:
  1. Traumatic.
  2. Pathological.
  3. Fatigue.

II. The fracture may be:

A. Intracapsular			Stage I
1. Subcapital	1. Adduction		Stage II
		AND	Stage III
2. Transcervical	2. Abduction		Stage IV
			(Garden's)

B. Extracapsular
1. Basal cervical (intertrochanteric).
2. Pertrochanteric.

Clinical Features.—Whatever may be the nature of the trauma, the patient cannot stand on the affected limb and complains of pain in the hip. The only exceptions to this are some cases of impacted intracapsular fracture, where the patient can walk and complains only of pain in the hip.

The attitude of the limb is diagnostic. A limb, lying helpless in the position of flexion, abduction and external rotation, is almost diagnostic of fracture of the femoral neck. Also, there is an *apparent* lengthening of the limb because of the abduction. The lower the fracture line lies along the neck, the more is the amount of external rotation; with pertrochanteric fracture it may be nearly 90°. This is because the stump of the neck, at the top of the shaft, is then smaller and the limb, with the shaft, can rotate externally without hindrance.

On examination, the movements of the hip are painful and restricted, and there is deep tenderness at the site of the femoral neck.

X-ray.—This not only diagnoses the fracture but also suggests the exact site and type of fracture. Both antero-posterior and lateral views are required, since some impacted abduction fractures are missed on ordinary antero-posterior view.

Treatment.—For reasons already discussed, majority of the fractures are treated by *internal fixation.*

The *indications for conservative treatment* are as follows:
1. In children, in whom treatment may be done:
    a. either, by manual reduction under general anaesthesia, followed by Whitman's plastering (full-pant plaster on the fractured side and half-pant on the other side).
    b. or, continuous traction on Thomas' bed knee splint.
2. In cases of impacted abduction fracture, the patient is simply put on bed with a derotation bar (to prevent external rotation) or is treated on Thomas' bed knee splint. After a month, he is allowed to sit on the bed and to move the hip. Weight-bearing, however, is allowed only when radiological signs of healing are found—usually a matter of three months.
3. Extracapsular fractures in younger patients. These may be treated either in Whitman's plaster or on Thomas' bed knee splint.
4. Extracapsular fractures in the elderly, in whom operation is contraindicated for other reasons.

The Nature of Internal Fixation
1. In cases of intracapsular fracture (subcapital or transcervical), the fixation is simply with SP nail. For details of the operation see the Chapter on instruments.
    Some surgeons prefer using 3 to 4 *Knowle's pins* instead of the SP nail. These nails are screw-headed and they get a good grip on the head. The nails are inserted at different angles and this is also beneficial. As the nails are much thinner than the SP nail, bone destruction is also less.
2. In cases of extracapsular fracture (intertrochanteric or pertrochanteric), simple SP nailing does not provide sufficient immobilisation of the lower fragment

because the nail passes only through a small thickness of the shaft. To get a better anchorage of the lower fragment, a combination of nail and plate has to be used. The nail passes through the neck like a SP nail, while the plate is fixed with screws on to the shaft, like a bone plate.

Complications of Fracture of the Neck of the Femur

A. Avascular necrosis and non-union.

B. Osteoarthritis of the hip.

A. Avascular Necrosis and Non-union.—This may occur only in cases of intra-capsular fracture. Avascular necrosis of the head will cause:

i. Failure of union between the fragments, i.e. non-union.

ii. Softening of the tissues in the femoral neck, so that the nail loosens and tends to come out, letting the upper fragment loose.

iii. Softening and inelasticity of the head, making it liable to become flattened and irregular, under pressure, so that an osteoarthritis of the hip is very likely to occur.

TREATMENT OF NON-UNION.—Non-united fracture of the femoral neck poses one of the most serious problems in fracture surgery. The treatment is difficult and the actual procedure to be followed depends on the merit and type of the particular case. However, the following methods of treatment are available:

1. *Simple Extraction of the Nail.*—This is advised in the elderly, sick, and otherwise frail patients, in whom the nail has loosened and is protruding in the thigh. As these patients are unsuitable for other drastic methods of treatment, this operation is advised. It is found that, after the nail is removed, the pain diminishes and majority of the patients can walk rather bearably, though limping. A raised heel and a stout stick are helpful.

2. *McMurray's Osteotomy* (intertrochanteric displacement osteotomy).— In this operation:

   a. The femur is divided transversely (a little oblique), from the lower margin of the greater trochanter to the upper margin of the lesser trochanter.

   b. The femoral shaft is then displaced medially, so that its top lies immediately below the femoral head (it abuts against the ischium, just below the acetabular rim).

The position is preferably maintained with a nail and plate. Alternatively, a plaster immobilisation, for 3 to 4 months, has to be done.

The rationality of this operation is that the medially displaced shaft:

   a. Gives a direct support, like a pillar, beneath the fracture line, during weight-bearing.

   b. Takes off some of the body weight from the pelvis, thus relieving the weak fractured neck from bearing the weight.

McMurray's osteotomy should only be done when the femoral head is still alive (which, however, is difficult to ascertain).

3. *Abduction Osteotomy.*—In this operation, a wedge, based laterally, is removed from the femur, just below the greater trochanter. The femoral shaft is abducted on the upper fragment, through the gap of the wedge. This position is maintained by internal fixation with nail and plate.

The rationality of this operation is to convert an adduction fracture into an abduction type. The fracture line, instead of being vertical, becomes transverse.

Thus, during the weight-bearing, instead of a shearing strain on the fracture line, there is an impacting effect. This operation, again, should only be advocated where the head is still alive.

4. *Replacement Arthroplasty:*
   a. Head Replacement.—The dead femoral head is excised and is replaced by a metal prosthesis (Austin Moore or Thompson prosthesis).
   b. Total Hip Replacement.—This is done:
      i. In those late cases where the acetabulum has also been deformed by secondary arthritic changes.
      ii. In rather younger patients in preference to head replacement because the metal head often produces osteoarthritis after several years.
   In total hip replacement the head is replaced by a metal prosthesis while an artificial socket, made of high density polythene, replaces the acetabulum and acts as a socket for the head.
5. *Excision Arthroplasty (Girdlestone's Arthroplasty).*—The dead head is excised. The acetabular cavity is made shallower by trimming off its upper margin. A mass of muscle or other soft tissue is put on the floor of the acetabular cavity. The idea is to create a false joint on this soft tissue mass, on which the femoral shaft moves rather painlessly. There is some shortening and instability.
6. *Bone Grafting and Re-nailing.*—If the reduction or primary nailing was faulty and the head is still living, the original nail is removed and a fresh nail inserted. Simultaneously, a fibular graft is passed through the fractured neck into the head.

To summarise, therefore, the treatment for non-united fractures:
   1. If the head is living.—McMurray's osteotomy or abduction osteotomy or re-nailing with fibular grafting.
   2. If the head is dead:
      a. For relatively younger patients.—Replacement arthroplasty (preferably total hip replacement).
      b. For elderly patients.—Replacement arthroplasty or Girdlestone's arthroplasty.
      c. For very elderly patients.—Simple extraction of the nail.

B. **Osteoarthritis of the Hip.**—This complication of fractured femoral neck may result from:
   1. Avascular necrosis of the head.
   2. An associated trauma to the hip joint.

FRACTURE OF THE FEMORAL SHAFT

General Characters

1. The fracture usually occurs in children and young adults.
2. It is always due to severe violence.
3. According to the nature of the trauma, the fracture may be transverse, oblique, spiral, comminuted, or greenstick (in children).
4. A transverse fracture, in a patient past middle life, may be pathological, occurring in a carcinomatous metastasis.
5. The fracture may occur at any site, almost with equal frequency in the upper, middle, and lower thirds.

The lower-third fractures have been discussed below separately under the heading of 'supracondylar fractures'.

Displacements

I. IN UPPER-THIRD FRACTURES
A. *The upper fragment is:*
1. Flexed by the iliopsoas.
2. Abducted by the glutei.
3. Everted by the external rotators (obturators).
B. *The lower fragment is:*
1. Pulled up by the hamstrings and quadriceps.
2. Adducted by the adductors.
3. Everted by the weight of the limb.

II. IN MIDDLE-THIRD FRACTURES.—The displacements are variable, according to the trauma. Usually:
A. *The upper fragment* is adducted by the adductors.
B. *The lower fragment* is pulled up by the hamstrings and the quadriceps, and the hamstrings being stronger, pull the lower fragment *behind* the upper fragment.

Principles of Treatment

1. Treatment for shock.—The amount of extravasation may be considerable and blood transfusion is usually required.
2. Restoration of alignment.—In absence of proper alignment, i.e. mal-union, there is an abnormal strain on the knee, which may lead to osteoarthritis.
3. Restoration of length.—There is often a gross overlapping due to the strong pull on the lower fragment by the quadriceps and hamstrings.
4. Immobilisation.
5. Prevention of stiffness of knee (which is due to scarring in the thigh muscles, adhesion formation in the joint, and prolonged immobilisation).

Treatment in Adults

A. CONSERVATIVE TREATMENT.—This may be done by either of the following methods:
1. Balanced traction in Thomas' bed knee splint, till the fracture heals (usually 12 weeks). Either a skin traction or a skeletal traction (through the tibial tubercle) may be used, but a skeletal traction is preferred for the adults (this is more comfortable for the patient).
2. Reduction under general anaesthesia and then a fixed traction on Thomas' bed knee splint. A fixed traction cannot usually reduce the fracture by itself (as a balanced traction can) because the skin of the perineum cannot stand a countertraction force as great as is required to reduce the fracture. The fixed traction is continued till the fracture heals.
3. Balanced traction without a splint. Weights are attached and hung over pulleys fitted at the foot-end of the bed, which is raised. It should be appreciated that a Thomas' bed knee splint does, in no way, immobilise the fracture. It is just a device for the attachment of the slings (which prevent backwards sagging of the bones) and the strings. If a splint is not used, the strong muscles themselves splint the fracture and pillows are placed in position to prevent backward sagging of the bones.

4. Alternatively, when X-rays show that the displacements have been corrected and the fragments are maintained in position, the traction may be taken off and the limb put in a Whitman's plaster, till healing occurs.
(For description of different types of traction *see* Chapter on instruments).

B. INTERNAL FIXATION.—Femoral shaft is the commonest site where a fracture is treated by internal fixation and that with an intramedullary nail. This has become more popular with the introduction of the 'closed', i.e. 'blind' method of IM nailing, which overcomes the disadvantages of the open method of the operation (viz. avascularity of the fragments and infection).

The *special indications* for internal fixation, in preference to conservative treatment, are as follows:
1. When satisfactory reduction cannot be secured and maintained by the closed methods:
   a. Mid-shaft fractures, sometimes, cannot be properly reduced.
   b. Upper-third fractures cannot often be maintained in position.
   c. Most commonly reduction is hindered by interposition of soft tissues.
2. Elderly patients, who should not be kept confined to bed for long period because of the fear of:
   a. Lung complications.
   b. Renal complications.
   c. Stiffness of knee.
3. If there are multiple injuries in the lower limb, internal fixation facilitates the management of the other injuries.
4. For socio-economic reasons, where a young patient should be made ambulatory early.
5. For pathological fractures.
   It should be noted, however, that even after IM nailing, the patient has to be in bed for a considerable period. An early ambulation almost invariably leads to bending of the nail and refracturing. The real value of IM nailing, therefore, lies in the maintenance of the fragments in position.

Treatment in Children.—Operative treatment is never necessary in children. They may be treated by either of the following methods:
1. Reduction under general anaesthesia, followed by Whitman's plastering.
2. Treatment by traction, as in the adults. Balanced traction without a splint is particularly suitable for children.
3. *Gallows* or *Bryant's traction.*—This is the best method for children, below 4 years of age. With adhesive skin strapping to the legs, the child's lower limbs are suspended from an overhead beam, so that the buttocks are clear off the mattress. The child's weight acts as countertraction. A four-week regime is usually sufficient for the children of this age. If required, a Whitman's plastering may be done for a few weeks more.

SUPRACONDYLAR FRACTURE OF THE FEMUR

The fracture is usually more or less transverse, but it may be comminuted.
Displacements
1. There may not be any displacement between the fragments.

2. Usually there is an anterior tilting (flexion) of the lower fragment, i.e. the convexity of the condyles is drawn forwards. This is caused by the pull of the gastrocnemius (from below), effected on the back of the upper end of the lower fragment. There is, however, not much loss of end-to-end apposition.
3. In a severe case, in addition to the above, there is a gross overlapping between the fragments.

Complications
1. Injury to the popliteal artery by the upper end of the lower fragment.
2. Injury to a major nerve trunk.
3. Stiffness of the knee—fairly common.
4. Non-union.—This may rarely occur if movements of the knee are started early.

Treatment

I. STANDARD TREATMENT.—The key to correction of the flexion displacement of the lower fragment lies in flexing the knee. This has a two-fold effect:
a. The gastrocnemius muscle is relaxed.
b. The quadriceps, as it is stretched, pushes the lower fragment, from the front, into position.
   The fracture is, therefore, treated either
   i. in a Bohler's modification of Braun's splint, or
   ii. in a Thomas' bed knee splint with a flexion piece attached to it. On the splint, a skeletal traction is applied through the tibial tubercle and maintained for 12 weeks, by which time the fracture usually heals.

II. PLASTER SPICA.—If there is no displacement, the fracture may be treated in a hip spica.

III. OPERATIVE REDUCTION AND INTERNAL FIXATION.—This may be required, on some rare occasions, where the fracture cannot be reduced satisfactorily by the closed method or cannot be held in position by ordinary methods.

FRACTURED PATELLA

Trauma and Types.—There are two distinct types of the fracture, according to the nature of the trauma:

1. DIRECT TRAUMA
   a. A direct hit on the patella.
   b. A fall on the patella, with the knee fully flexed, when the patella strikes the ground.
   Depending on the severity of the violence, the fracture may be:
   i. A simple transverse crack fracture.
   ii. A stellate fracture, i.e. a comminuted fracture, with the fracture lines running radially.
   Since the aponeurotic covering of the patella (derived from the quadriceps) remains intact, the fracture fragments cannot move away from each other and keep in contact. The quadriceps expansion, on each side of the patella, also remains intact.
2. INDIRECT TRAUMA.—Here the fracture of the patella is only a component of a bigger injury, i.e. a transverse injury along the whole breadth of the extension apparatus

of the knee joint, including the patella itself. This extension apparatus consists of the quadriceps femoris and its insertion, viz. the ligamentum patellae, the patella, and the aponeurotic expansion of the quadriceps on either side of the patella.

This occurs when a person slips on one leg (say for example, the right leg), the injury occurring in the other knee, i.e. the left knee. As the right leg slips forwards, the left knee is in a semiflexed position, with the extension apparatus of the knee joint stretched in a convex manner and the patella at the summit of the convexity, lying in front of the femoral condyles. As the person slips forwards, the centre of gravity of the body moves forwards and the person is just to fall. His fall can only be prevented by a forcible contraction of the quadriceps. This sudden and violent contraction of the quadriceps in the stretched position of its extension apparatus causes a transverse injury along the whole breadth of the apparatus at the level of the maximum convexity, i.e. at the level of the centre of the patella. So (a) the inelastic patella is fractured transversely, and (b) the quadriceps expansion, on either side of the patella, is torn transversely.

As there is a strong pull on the upper fragment by the quadriceps, there is a wide separation between the two fractured fragments.

This transverse fracture of the patella may be:

a. At the centre of the patella (usually).
b. Near the upper pole.
c. Near the lower pole.

In any type of patellar fracture, there is collection of blood in the knee (haemarthrosis).

Clinical Features
1. The knee is swollen. The normal depression on either side of the patella is obliterated. The outline of the patella cannot be seen.
2. The knee is held in a flexed position (this makes more space in the joint, to accommodate the effused blood).
3. There is tenderness in the knee as a whole, but the maximum point of tenderness is on the patella.
4. In fractures with separation, the gap in the bone can usually be made out because patella is a subcutaneous bone.
5. There is presence of fluid (blood) in the knee joint.
6. The patient is usually unable to lift the straight leg. In case of simple crack fracture, however, he may be able to lift the straight leg.

X-ray.—This confirms the diagnosis of the fracture as well as its nature. A lateral view is more helpful.

While looking at the X-ray, the condition of *congenital bipartite patella* should be kept in mind. It differs from a fractured patella in the following points:

a. The margins of the gap are smooth.
b. Each margin has a rim of cortical bone.
c. The gap is at a site unusual for a fracture, i.e. the superolateral corner.
d. X-ray of the other knee shows the same anomaly because the condition is usually bilateral.

Treatment
A. SIMPLE CRACK FRACTURES.—A conservative treatment is sufficient. The knee is kept

in plaster immobilisation for 3 weeks. The plaster extends from the upper third of the thigh to the malleoli, the knee being kept in 5° flexion.

If there is considerable haemarthrosis, the joint is aspirated prior to plastering.

B. TRANSVERSE FRACTURES.—The treatment depends mainly on the age of the patient.

1. If the patient is *below* 40, *internal fixation* of the fracture is advisable. This may be done by one of the following methods:

   a. With Screws.—Two screws are passed from the lower pole of the patella, through the fracture, into the upper fragment—one on the medial side and another on the lateral side.

   b. With Wire.—A stainless steel wire is used for fixation of the fragments. The wiring may be done in two ways:

      i. The wire is passed through a transverse tunnel made in each fragment, and the knot is placed on one side of the patella.

      ii. The wire is placed like a purse-string suture through the soft tissues all round the patella, the knot is tightened, and is placed on one side of the patella. This is called *circumferential wiring* or *tension band* suturing (Fig. 61.4).

   Whatever be the method of internal fixation, the limb must be kept in plaster for 2 months, with the knee in 5° flexion.

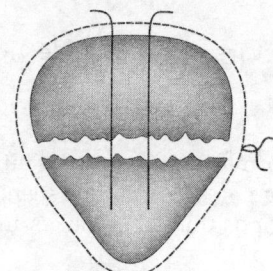

Fig. 61.4: Tension band suturing of the patella. Two small pieces of Kirschner's wire have been passed from the upper into the lower fragment. A circumferential wiring has been done

2. In patients *above* 40, internal fixation, followed by two months, immobilisation, is very likely to restrict the joint movements. In the elderly patients, therefore, *excision of the patella* is the treatment of choice.

   A transverse incision is usually employed. *Vertical*, J-shaped or U-shaped incision are preferred by some surgeons. Whatever be the nature of the incision, the exposure must be wide, since the operation not only entails excision of the patella but also includes repair of the torn quadriceps expansion on each side of the patella. On opening, all blood clots from inside the joint, are removed. The patellar fragments are shelled out from the extensor aponeurotic covering. Thereafter, the transverse tear in the quadriceps aponeurosis, all along its width, is repaired with interrupted catgut stitches.

3. Even in the younger age group, excision of the patella, instead of internal fixation, has to be undertaken under certain circumstances:

   a. If the gap between the fragments is too wide to be bridged up.

   b. If, after apposition of the fragments, the posterior surface of the fracture line appears to be so irregular that it is likely to traumatise the femoral articular cartilage and cause osteoarthritis.

    c. If either of the fragments is comminuted.

4. Instead of total excision, a *partial excision of the patella* may be considered if one of the fragments is very small. Only the small fragment is excised. The remaining major part of the patella is sutured securely to either the quadriceps or the ligamentum patellae, depending on which fragment is excised, upper or lower respectively.

C. STELLATE FRACTURES.—Here the fragments are in good apposition and union is likely to be perfect. But the gross irregularity that is likely to occur on the articular surface of the patella will cause repeated trauma to the femoral articular cartilage and lead to osteoarthritis of the knee. Hence, *excision of the patella* has to be undertaken.

FRACTURE OF THE SHAFTS OF THE TIBIA AND FIBULA

Trauma and Types

1. DIRECT VIOLENCE, i.e. a direct hit locally:
   a. The fractures tend to be *transverse* (or short oblique).
   b. The two bones are usually fractured at the *same level.*
2. INDIRECT VIOLENCE, i.e. a twisting force:
   a. The fractures tend to be *spiral.*
   b. The two bones are fractured at *different levels.* Most commonly the tibia fractures at the junction of the lower and middle thirds, while the fibula breaks at the junction of the middle and upper thirds.

Certain Points of Importance

1. As a rule, there is considerable displacement of the fragments.
2. The tibia or the fibula may be fractured alone, but this is relatively uncommon. Displacements are relatively slight then. A fibular fracture requires a little or no treatment. Fracture of the tibia alone has to be treated in the same lines as for both-bone fracture. While an intact fibula prevents much displacement between the tibial fragments, it may sometimes cause difficulty in treatment. Thus, it may prevent the fracture surfaces from coming in close apposition (delayed union) or hinder restoration of normal alignment (mal-union). This is what is called the *strut-like effect* of the intact fibula.
3. Tibia being a subcutaneous bone, many of its fractures are compound. In fact, this is the commonest site for a compound fracture. Moreover, skin closure is difficult in these cases because the bone is subcutaneous.

Outline of Treatment.—The treatment may be done by either of the following three methods:

1. Reduction under general anaesthesia, followed by plaster immobilisation. This is practicable for:
   a. Children (usually below the age of 16).
   b. Adults in whom stable reduction can be obtained.
   An above-knee plaster, with the knee a little flexed, has to be applied. The immobilisation has to be continued for 12 to 16 weeks. Spiral fractures heal much earlier than transverse fractures.

2. Skeletal traction.—This is applied through the calcaneum or the lower end of the tibia, with the limb supported on a Braun's splint. This is the usual form of treatment in the adults and is particularly necessary if stable reduction cannot be maintained by plaster alone. After traction for 4 to 6 weeks, the fracture usually becomes stable and the limb may be plastered as above.

3. Internal fixation.—This is sometimes used as an alternative to skeletal traction for fractures that cannot be reduced properly by closed method or cannot be maintained in position. Only the tibia needs fixation. The following methods may be used:

    a. Screws.—Spiral fractures may be stabilised with two screws.

    b. Plate and screws.

    c. Intramedullary nail.

FRACTURES AROUND THE ANKLE

Different varieties of fractures and fracture-dislocations occur around the ankle, and these are collectively known as *Pott's fracture.*

Mechanism

A. Most commonly these injuries occur as a result of forcible movements of the foot in relation to the tibia—the foot being forcibly inverted, everted, externally rotated, or internally rotated. Though it is described that the foot moves on a fixed tibia and the injuries are named so, in practice these injuries almost always occur with the foot fixed (anchored to the ground) while the momentum of the body makes the tibia forcibly move on the fixed foot:

    1. The foot is inherently more stable in eversion than in inversion. So, injuries due to inversion (i.e. adduction) are commoner than those due to eversion (i.e. abduction) of the foot.

    2. During walking, the foot is placed a little externally rotated. So, injuries due to external rotation are far more common than those due to forcible internal rotation. In fact, the latter type of injury is almost unknown.

    Therefore, adduction injuries and external rotation injuries are the commoner types of ankle injuries, the external rotation variety being the commonest.

B. Sometimes, as a result of fall from a height, the talus is driven up into the distal tibia. These are called *vertical compression injuries.*

C. Very rarely, the ankle may be injured by a force which shears the talus transversely across the tibia. These are known as *transverse shear injuries.*

The Ankle Mortice.—The most important singular factor to consider in these injuries is whether the tibio-fibular mortice, which accommodates the talus, is stable. This means that no abnormal movement is possible between the tibia and the talus, and there is no talar shift or tilt. With a stable mortice, the prognosis is good and treatment easy. On the other hand, an unstable mortice requires reconstruction either by closed or by open method, i.e. a proper reduction has to be achieved.

External Rotation Injuries.—The foot is forcibly externally rotated in relation to the tibia. According to the force, there are three degrees of injury:

1st Degree: There is a twisting force to the lateral malleolus, which suffers a spiral fracture (shearing fracture). The lower fragment is still attached to the tibia by the intact tibio-fibular ligament, i.e. the mortice is stable (Fig. 61.5A).

2nd Degree: Further force tears the tibio-fibular ligament and allows the talus to continue to move laterally. This results in:

a. Either, rupture of the medial (deltoid) ligament (Fig. 61.5B).
b. Or, a low transverse fracture (i.e. avulsion fracture) of the medial malleolus (Fig. 61.5C).

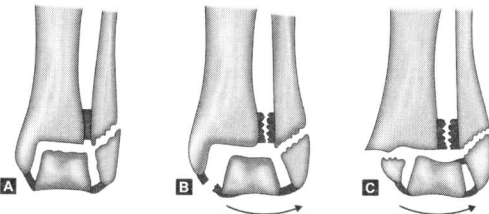

Fig. 61.5: External rotation injuries of the ankle

In either case, the mortice is unstable and the talus shifts laterally with the injuring force.

3rd Degree: There is an additional injury if the momentum of the body weight drives the tibia forwards. Once the mortice is broken, the talus is free to slide beneath the posterior margin of the tibia (which is often called the 'third malleolus'). As a result, there is a posterior marginal fracture of the tibial articular surface. This allows a posterior shift of the talus (Fig. 61.6).

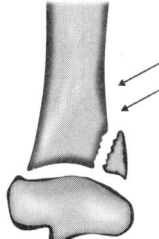

Fig. 61.6: Fracture of the 'third malleolus'

Adduction (Inversion) Injuries

1st Degree: When the ankle is forcibly inverted (adducted), there is injury to the lateral ligament—partial tear (sprain) or complete tear (rupture). *These are the commonest ankle injuries,* loosely termed 'sprained ankle' (Fig. 61.7A). The mortice is stable but, with a complete tear, the talus may be tilted medially.

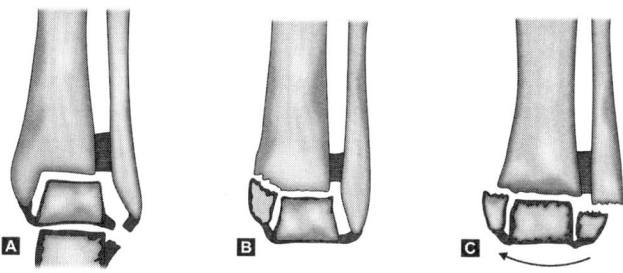

Fig. 61.7: Adduction (inversion) injuries of the ankle

2nd Degree:

a. With further forcible adduction, the medial malleolus may be fractured obliquely (shearing fracture—Fig. 61.7B).
b. With still further force, there may be an added low transverse fracture (avulsion fracture) of the lateral malleolus. The mortice is now unstable and the injuring force causes medial shift of the talus (Fig. 61.7C).

3rd Degree: Same as with external rotation injury. Due to the forward movement of the tibia with the momentum of the body weight, there may be a posterior marginal fracture of the tibial articular surface with posterior shift of the talus (Fig. 61.6).

Abduction (Eversion) Injuries.—Forcible eversion (abduction) of the talus levers the lateral malleolus outwards:

1. If the tibio-fibular ligament is intact, the fibula fractures high-up, in the calf region.
2. If the tibio-fibular ligament ruptures, the mortice springs open and the fibula moves away from the tibia. This is called *diastasis of the inferior tibio-fibular joint.* There is lateral shift of the talus.

Internal Rotation Injuries.—Very rare and same as adduction injuries.

Vertical Compression Injuries

1. If the violence is moderate, there is anterior marginal fracture of the tibia, with anterior shift of the talus.
2. With severe violence, the .talus is forcibly driven up into the tibia, resulting in a comminuted fracture of the tibial articular surface and a fracture of the fibular shaft as well (Fig. 61.8).

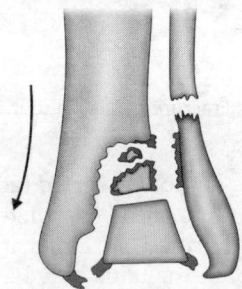

Fig. 61.8: Vertical compression injury of the ankle

Transverse Shear Injuries.—There are transverse fractures of both medial and lateral malleoli, at the level of the top of the talus. The mortice is absolutely unstable.

X-ray Appearance

A. The first point to note is whether the ankle mortice is stable because this decides the prognosis and treatment.
B. The appearance of the *fibular* fracture is often diagnostic of the mechanism (and so, the type) of the injury, as follows:
    1. External rotation.—Spiral (shearing) fracture of the malleolus at the level of the tibio-fibular joint.

2. Inversion.—Low transverse (avulsion) fracture.
3. Internal rotation.—Low transverse (avulsion) fracture.
4. Eversion.—High fracture in the shaft.
5. Transverse shear.—Transverse fracture at the level of the dome of the talus.

Treatment

A. INJURIES WITH STABLE MORTICE:
   1. Ligament (lateral) injury.—Compression bandage, early movements, and exercises.
   2. Fracture of lateral malleolus.—Plastering with a walking iron for 4 weeks.
   3. Fracture of medial malleolus.—Complete plastering for 6 weeks.

B. INJURIES WITH UNSTABLE MORTICE:
These require perfect reduction to reconstruct the mortice and to hold it in position:
   1. *Closed Method.*—This is tried first. General anaesthesia is used. Manual traction is applied first and then a force reverse of that which caused the injury. 6 to 12 weeks' below-knee plaster immobilisation is required, according to the nature of the fracture.
   2. *Operative Treatment.*—This is required when closed reduction fails or the position cannot be maintained by external plastering. The usual technique is to secure the fragments in perfect position with one or more screws. Thus, the medial malleolus or the lateral malleolus or both may have to be screwed.
   For tibio-fibular diastasis, a screw is passed through the fibula into the tibia.
   The additional protection of a below-knee plaster, for 8 to 12 weeks, is always advised.

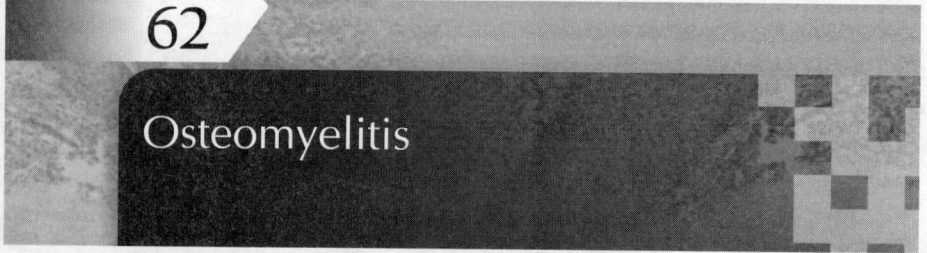

62

Osteomyelitis

Definition.—Osteomyelitis means infection of bone with all its components, viz. cortex, medulla and periosteum.

Types

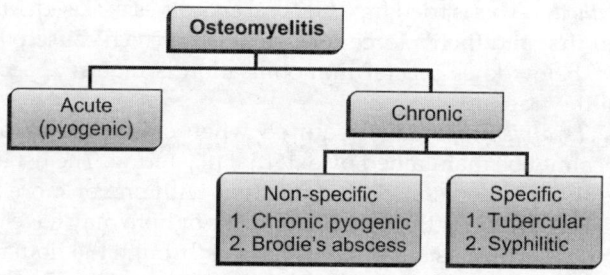

ACUTE PYOGENIC OSTEOMYELITIS

This is an acute inflammatory process in the bone, involving all its elements, namely the cortex, medulla, and periosteum, resulting from infection by pyogenic organisms.

Etiology

A. ORGANISMS.—The commonest organism is *Staphylococcus aureus*, and this is often penicillin resistant. The next common is *Staph. albus*.

   Other infecting organisms may be *Strept. hemolyticus*, Pneumococcus, or *B. typhosus*.

B. ROUTES OF INFECTION.—There are two main routes:

   1. Hematogenous.—The commoner route. The source of infection is a septic focus, e.g. infected umbilicus, infected tonsils, middle ear suppuration, infected skin, etc. It should be remembered that an osteomyelitis is always preceded by a septicaemia, and a number of bones may sometimes be affected.

   2. *Exogenous*.—The infection in the bone is by implantation, e.g. (a) compound fractures, (b) operations on bones, particularly open reduction of fractures and internal fixation, (c) amputation stumps. This type of infection may occur in any part of the bone, depending on where the organisms are implanted. Since the route of entry of the infecting organisms also provides the path of drainage for the inflammatory exudates, the condition never presents in an acute form.

C. How AND WHERE THE INFECTION STARTS.—The start of an acute osteomyelitis varies in a child (juvenile type) and an adult (adult type), as follows:

JUVENILE	ADULT
1. Almost always starts in the metaphysis.	1. Since there is no metaphysis, it may start anywhere in the bone.
2. Always starts very acute, and there may be a fulminating type that often ends fatally.	2. Never starts so acute.
3. Always starts as an osteomyelitis; any periostitis is secondary.	3. Always starts as a primary periostitis.

Since the juvenile type is much the commoner, this will be described here in details. There are some predisposing and some precipitating factors:

Predisposing Factors:
a. A septic focus, acting as a source of infection (vide above).
b. Lowered general resistance.

Precipitating Factors:
Usually a trauma, often minor, near the end of a long bone.

The disease almost always starts in the metaphysis, since this part of the bone suffers most in twisting injuries of the joint. Being the growing part of the bone, it is highly vascular, so that even a minor injury may cause a small haematoma. A haematoma at the metaphysis is again very prone to infection because:

a. Blood vessels being numerous, quantitatively more bacteria have an access here.

b. At the metaphysis, the blood vessels make an acute hair-pin bend, so that there is a slowing down of circulation and the organisms get a chance to settle here.

c. The cells of the reticulo-endothelial system, which harbour bacteria, are preponderant in the metaphysis.

Thus, the haematoma in the metaphysis gets infected and turns into a small abscess.

Pathology

STAGE I: SUPPURATION.—The pathology starts as a small abscess in the metaphysis. The future of the disease depends on how this abscess behaves. Unless the patient has a good resistance or has been subjected to early and efficient treatment, this abscess spreads very quickly through the metaphysis, which being rich in cancellous bone, favours this spread.

As a rule, the abscess:

a. has no tendency to spread directly into the medullary cavity;

b. has no capacity to pierce through the overlying epiphyseal cartilage, epiphysis, and the articular cartilage; to gain direct access into the neighbouring joint.

The abscess commonly spreads *only* towards the surface, along the metaphysis. On coming out of the cortex here, it comes under the periosteum and forms a subperiosteal abscess (if the metaphysis is intracapsular in this situation, an acute suppurative arthritis results). This abscess, unless drained quickly, spreads subperiosteally, both around the bone and along the shaft. The abscess may then re-enter the bone at another level along the Volkmann canals or may burst into the surrounding soft tissues.

STAGE II: NECROSIS.—As a secondary process, part of the diaphysis is now in the danger of losing its blood supply as follows:

1. As the subperiosteal abscess enlarges, the periosteum is stripped off the bone. The subperiosteal blood vessels run transversely in this space, from the periosteum to the cortex, to supply it. With the accumulation of pus in this space, these vessels are lengthened and narrowed, as well as pressed upon, so that they are obliterated. A part of the cortex is, therefore, devascularised and necrosed.
2. The subperiosteal abscess trickles through the Volkmann canals in the diaphysis and causes tension within the rigid bony canals, causing necrosis of the bone.
3. Inflammatory thrombosis of blood vessels may occur and cause necrosis of bone.

The above factors lead to the formation of a dead piece of bone, which is called *sequestrum*. Thus, a sequestrum is a dead piece of bone, formed by a process of aseptic necrosis, though the contributory process itself is a septic process in the bone. In those cases where a main branch of the nutrient artery, or the nutrient artery itself, undergoes infective thrombosis, the sequestrum may be very big in size and this is called *massive sequestrum*.

The sequestrum being a dead piece of bone, cannot live in direct contact with living bone, from which it is demarcated by newly forming granulation tissue. When the growth of the granulation tissue is complete, usually a matter of 6 to 10 weeks, the sequestrum gets separated or detached from the bone, and lies free. A sequestrum has two surfaces. The outer surface is polished because this was being bathed in the osteomyelitic pus. The inner surface is irregular having an eaten-up appearance, as this was the surface in contact with the granulation tissue.

The causes of death of the bone, leading to the formation of sequestrum, are, however, more than one:

a. Cutting off the blood supply (as already described).
b. Effect of bacterial toxins.
c. An anoxia of stagnant type.

Once a sequestrum has formed, the process of osteomyelitis has become chronic.

While presence of sequestrum denotes a chronic osteomyelitis, the nature of the sequestrum varies according to the type of infection:

a. In pyogenic infection (much the commoner), the sequestrum is usually moderate to big in size, with one surface smooth and the other having an irregular eaten-up appearance (*coralliform*, i.e. like corals).
b. In tuberculosis, sequestrum formation is rare. If they form at all, they are very small and thin (*feathery*).
c. In syphilis (nowadays syphilitic osteomyelitis is very rare), the sequestrum is big, thick, hard and dense (*ivory*).

There are two types of sequestra which deserve special mention:

1. *Coloured Sequestrum.*—If a sequestrum, while being formed, is exposed to the atmosphere (e.g. at the subcutaneous surface of tibia or ulna), it often takes a black colour. Iron, derived from hemoglobin of disintegrating RBC, combines

with H$_2$S, present in atmospheric air, and forms ferrous sulphide. This gets deposited on the bone and accounts for the black colour.

2. *Ring Sequestrum.*—This term is applied to a sequestrum formed at the end of an amputation stump, if the bone here is exposed or is infected otherwise. It is so named because its distal end is like a smooth ring—smooth because it was cut with a saw at amputation, and ring because it has the medullary cavity at the centre. The proximal end, which is separated from the living bone by granulation tissue, is, however, irregular and conical. The sequestrum is made of the whole thickness of the bone (c.f. an ordinary sequestrum) because of excessive stripping of the periosteum, all round the bone, prior to cutting the bone at amputation.

STAGE III: NEW BONE FORMATION.—As the periosteum is stripped off from the underlying bone by the subperiosteal pus, the osteoblasts in its inner layer are stimulated to form new bone. Usually the new bone formation is extensive, forming a complete encasing for the osteomyelitic cavity, and this is known as *involucrum*. The pus, under tension, may make multiple openings in the involucrum. These openings are called *cloaca*. Through the cloacae, pus and small pieces of sequestrum may be eliminated.

STAGE IV: SOFT TISSUE INVOLVEMENT.—Either a subperiosteal abscess ruptures into the soft tissues or pus gains entrance into the soft tissues through the cloacae, forming surface abscesses. These may point and rupture on the skin, forming persistent sinus or fistula, through which pus and, sometimes, pieces of sequestrum come out.

Complications of Acute Osteomyelitis

A. GENERAL COMPLICATIONS:

1. Toxaemia.—Very common because of circulation of toxins, absorbed from the osteomyelitic abscess.
2. Septicaemia.—Due to circulation of septic materials, absorbed from the osteomyelitic focus.
3. Bacteriaemia.—This may be preceding or following the process of osteomyelitis.
4. Pyaemia.—Leading to pyaemic abscesses at different sites, including the brain.
5. Amyloid degeneration.—A late complication of *chronic* osteomyelitis, resulting from long standing discharge of pus through sinuses.

B. LOCAL COMPLICATIONS:

1. Subperiosteal abscess, soft tissue abscess, discharging sinus on the skin, and rarely malignant change at the opening of the discharging sinus.
2. Neighbouring Joint:
   a. A sympathetic effusion is common.
   b. Acute suppurative arthritis
      i. if the metaphysis is intra-articular, or
      ii. rarely, by rupture of a metaphyseal abscess through the epiphyseal cartilage, epiphysis and articular cartilage, or
      iii. by metastatic infection.
   c. Pathological dislocation following (b).

    d. Stiffness of joint either due to prolonged immobilisation or as a sequela to acute suppurative arthritis.

3. Pathological Fracture.—Particularly after separation of a big sequestrum, and in the weight-bearing bones.

4. Deformity.—This is rare and may be due to:

    a. Arrest of growth in the bone end due to destruction of epiphyseal cartilage.

    b. Arrest of growth due to prolonged immobilisation.

    c. Occasionally, exaggerated growth at the epiphysis because of hyperaemia.

5. Chronic Osteomyelitis.—As a sequela to acute osteomyelitis. *This is the commonest complication.*

6. Bordie's Abscess (vide below).

Clinical Features.—Except for the cases where osteomyelitis is as a result of exogenous infection, children are the usual sufferers. The history of trauma may or may not be significant. Boys suffer more often than girls.

There is often a high rise of temperature, associated with gross constitutional symptoms, e.g. headache, backache, chill, rigor, etc. These are due to toxaemia, septicaemia and bacteriaemia.

Locally, the child complains of severe pain near a joint and does not move it. The local findings depend on whether the bone is deep or superficial. In case of a deep bone, only a little swelling and an acute tenderness may be noticed. In case of superficial bone, like tibia, all features of acute inflammation, viz., redness, oedema, swelling, and severe tenderness, are elicited. Diagnosis from an acute suppurative arthritis may often be difficult. The suggestive points of difference are as follows:—

    a. If the joint can be moved, even a little, it is not an arthritis.

    b. In arthritis the maximum tenderness is on the joint line and the epiphysis, while in osteomyelitis it is on the metaphysis.

Special Investigations

1. Blood Count.—A high polymorphonuclear leucocytosis is a constant feature.

2. X-ray *does not help* in acute cases.

Treatment

A. General treatment:

    1. Rest.

    2. Analgesics and antipyretics.

    3. Blood culture and sensitivity test for the organisms.

    4. Antibiotics.—By the time the sensitivity report is received, an antibiotic is started. As the organisms are usually penicillin-resistant, a broad spectrum antibiotic is administered. Erythromycin works well.

B. Local treatment:

    1. *Rest.*—Immediate absolute rest to the part is essential. Either a splint or a strong plaster cast may be used for the purpose. A *traction* is often helpful and, for the upper femur, it is essential in order to prevent dislocation of the hip.

    2. *Drainage.*—If, even with a suitable antibiotic, the pyrexia and the local tenderness do not decline after 24 hours, drainage of the subperiosteal abscess

has to be undertaken. Incision is better than aspiration and must be adequate. The pus must be sent for culture and sensitivity test.

Some surgeons, in addition to the above, recommend drainage of the metaphyseal abscess and, to do so, they advocate *multiple drilling of the metaphysis.*

CHRONIC PYOGENIC OSTEOMYELITIS

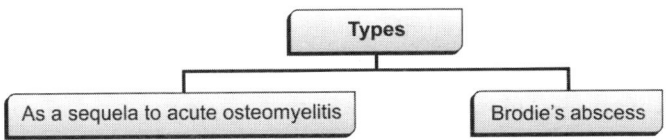

Chronic Pyogenic Osteomyelitis as a Sequela to Acute Osteomyelitis

TYPES.—Pathologically, there may be two types.

a. With sequestrum (commoner).

b. Without sequestrum.—In these cases the chronicity may be due to a foreign body or, more commonly, due to resistant organisms or haphazard antibiotic treatment.

CLINICAL FEATURES.—In both the above conditions, the presenting features are the same. The patient presents with pain, swelling, and persistent discharging sinuses, through which sequestra may be expelled. There is one variety where the patient suffers from recurrent acute exacerbations.

On examination, thickening of the bone is usually elicited, particularly when the bone is superficial, The sinuses are fixed to the bone. Often the scar of a previous operation or incision is seen. The openings of the sinuses are often covered by spouting granulation tissue, and this indicates the presence of a sequestrum.

X-RAY APPEARANCE.—The sequestrum appears as dense white bone. This is because of absence of the normal process of calcium reabsorption from the bone, as the blood supply to the bone has been cut off. The space between the sequestrum and the healthy bone looks black and this is the area occupied by granulation tissue. The involucrum is usually well seen on the outer aspect of the sequestrum and the space between the involucrum and the sequestrum, looking black, contains the osteomyelitic pus. The adjacent parts of the bone may show gross osteosclerosis and thickening.

TREATMENT

1. *If there is no sequestrum:*
   a. Some surgeons advocate conservative treatment. This consists of long-continued immobilisation and a long-term antibiotic therapy, the antibiotic being selected on culture and sensitivity test of the discharge.
   b. Others advocate an operative treatment, as is done in the presence of a sequestrum (*see* below).
2. *If there is a sequestrum,* operation has to be undertaken and the operation is called *sequestrectomy.* The incision is made according to the position of the sequestrum and the osteomyelitic cavity, as seen on the X-ray. All soft tissues and periosteum are incised in the same .line (taking care of important structures). The periosteum is elevated from the outer surface of the involucrum, with a raspatory. The

involucrum is removed piecemeal with a chisel or gouge. The pus from the cavity is swabbed out and the sequestrum (or sequestra) is removed with a sequestrum forceps. Care must be taken that no sequestrum is left behind. The granulation tissues on the wall of the bone is scooped out with a Volkmann's spoon. The osteomyelitic cavity has now to be obliterated. This is done by removing the ridge of bone from the wall on either side of the cavity, with a chisel or gouge. This process is called *saucerisation*. Unless this is done, blood and pus will reaccumulate in the cavity, resulting in recurrence. The muscles and skin are sutured, with a drain down to the bone.

Brodie's Abscess.—This is a small chronic pyogenic osteomyelitic abscess, occurring insidiously in a bone, i.e. not being preceded by an attack of acute osteomyelitis (c.f. chronic osteomyelitis resulting from acute osteomyelitis). Such an abscess may occur, only if:

a. The virulence of the infecting organisms is low.
b. There is a quick control of an acute infection either by the patient's resistance or by antibiotic treatment, and the organisms are kept localised and dormant, but not killed.

PATHOLOGY.—There is a small abscess in the metaphysis of a long bone, the commonest being the upper end of tibia. The lower end of femur, upper end of humerus, or any other bone may be affected. A small sequestrum may occasionally be present. The cavity is surrounded by a ring of dense bone. As regards the fluid inside, it is clear, serous and sterile during the periods of quiescence, but purulent (from which staphylococci can often be cultured) during the period of flares.

CLINICAL FEATURES.—The patient usually complains of recurrent attacks of pain at the end of a long bone, where tenderness and sometimes, swelling are elicited.

SPECIAL INVESTIGATIONS
1. *X-ray*—There is a small cavity, surrounded by a ring of dense bone, in the metaphyseal region. A small sequestrum may be seen.
2. *Excisional Biopsy.*

TREATMENT.—The abscess is opened and its wall, together with the ring of sclerosed bone, is excised. Sequestrum, if any, is removed. Biopsy of the material confirms the diagnosis.

63

Bone Tumours

Classification—The World Health Organisation's (WHO) classification (1972) may be summarised as follows:

1. *Bone-forming Tumours.*—Osteoma, osteoblastoma, osteosarcoma.
2. *Cartilage-forming Tumours.*—Chondroma, chondroblastoma, chondrosarcoma.
3. *Giant-cell tumours.*—Origin debated.
4. *Marrow Tumours.*—Ewing's tumour, myeloma.
5. *Vascular Tumours.*—Haemangioma, angiosarcoma, glomus tumours.
6. *Other Connective Tissue Tumours.*—Lipoma, liposarcoma, fibrosarcoma, etc.
7. *Other Tumours.*—Adamantinoma, neurilemmoma, neurofibroma, etc.
8. *Tumour-like Lesions.*—Bone cyst, fibrous dysplasia, eosinophilic granuloma.

OSTEOMA

Types

1. Cancellous osteoma.
2. Compact osteoma.
3. Osteoid osteoma.

Cancellous Osteoma.—This is also called *exostosis* since it is just a minor disorder of growth of a bone, a part of which grows outside the shaft. In other words, it is not believed to be a tumour but a variant form of diaphysial aclasis (vide below), only one bone being affected in the pathology.

The tumour is typically conical in shape, with a broad base, by which it is primarily attached to the epiphysis of the *growing end* of a long bone, the commonest bones being those at the knee joint. As the mother bone grows in length, the tumour is 'left behind' so that, as age advances, the tumour appears more and more to arise from the shaft (diaphysis) of the bone. The tumour has a cortex and a medulla which are continuous along its base with those of the mother bone. There is a cartilagenous cap at the tip (which is probably a displaced portion of the epiphyseal cartilage), from which the tumour grows in size, and its growth ceases with cessation of skeletal growth. Even after that, the cartilagenous cap may persist. There is often a bursa at the tip. The tumour *points away* from the growing end of the bone.

The patient usually presents with a symptomless bony lump. Occasionally there may be symptoms, e.g.

a. Interference with tendon action.
b. Pressure on a nerve.
c. Inflammation of the bursa at the tip.

The tumour never turns malignant. It may have to be excised:
  i. For psychological reasons.
  ii. If it produces symptoms.

Compact Osteoma.—This is so called because it consists only of compact bone. Typically, it arises from the flat bones, notably the skull (especially frontal or parietal). There is just a bony swelling, with a sessile base. Rarely it may arise from the inner table of the skull and then it may indent the brain.

No treatment is essential. Only for cosmetic reasons or when pressing on the brain, the tumour has to be excised.

Osteoid Osteoma.—This is so named because, microscopically, the tumour has the structure of osteoid tissue, i.e. newly formed bone, in a vascular connective tissue stroma. The tumour may occur in any bone except the skull, but most commonly it occurs in the tibia and the femur. It is usually small, less than 1 cm in diameter. It is surrounded by dense bone.

The patient, usually aged between 10 and 25, and more commonly a male, complains of severe pain inside the bone. Only when the tumour is near the surface of the bone that a swelling may be palpable. It is to be noted that the pain is often much too severe in proportion to the size of the lesion and a patient, with a deep-seated lesion, having no suggestive physical signs, is often wrongly taken as a neurotic.

On the X-ray, the most characteristic feature is a small area of dense sclerosis. If the tumour is near the surface of the bone, the periosteum is visibly raised and is often sclerosed as well. A careful examination often reveals a small translucent area in the centre.

The condition is often difficult to be diagnosed from Brodie's abscess, in which the central translucent area is usually much more prominent than the sclerosis. Sometimes only biopsy reveals the real nature of the lesion.

Treatment consists in excision of the osteoma.

CHONDROMA

These are tumours containing normal cartilage, originating from the precartilaginous cells of the bone. The tumour may arise from short bones, long bones or flat bones.

A. SHORT BONE CHONDROMA.—The commonest sites for chondroma are the short pipe bones, i.e. metacarpals, metatarsals and proximal phalanges. There are two varieties—echochondroma and ecchondroma.
1. *Enchondroma.*—This is the commoner type. The chondroma is located entirely inside the bone, covered by the cortex of the bone all round.
   The patient, usually an adolescent or young adult, presents with a painless swelling or, more commonly, with a pathological fracture.
   X-ray shows that the cortex is expanded and thinned out over a central rarefied area. Characteristically, there are irregular specks of calcification in the rarefied area (c.f. fibrous dysplasia and bone cyst, where such calcification is not seen).
   Treatment consists in scraping out the tumour from inside the cortex and, if required, a few chip grafts.

2. *Ecchondroma.*—When the chondroma is partially or completely on to the surface of the bone, it is called ecchondroma. In the short bones it is much rare than enchondroma.

The patient presents with a painless swelling on the bone

X-ray shows a rarefied area on the cortex, with a very clear outline.

Treatment consists in scraping out the tumour.

B. LONG BONE CHONDROMA.—Though not commonly, long bones may be the site of chondroma. These are usually ecchondroma.

The patient, an adolescent, complains of persistent ache.

X-ray shows a well-defined rarefied area, with irregular specks of calcification.

Treatment is excision.

C. FLAT BONE CHONDROMA.—Ecchondroma may arise from the pelvic bones or scapula, but these are usually indistinguishable from the more common types of cartilagenous tumours, viz. benign chondroblastoma and osteochondroma.

Treatment is excision.

CHONDROBLASTOMA

This tumour differs from chondroma in that, while in chondroma the cells are mature chondrocytes, in chondroblastoma they are chondroblasts, which are the precursors of chondrocyte. However, the tumour is benign though it is more prone to turn malignant than chondroma.

The tumour may occur in the long bones at the epiphysis (especially upper end of humerus and femur), or in the flat bones (pelvis or scapula).

The patient, an adolescent or young adult, presents with a constant aching pain.

X-ray shows an area of bone destruction, whose margins are very well-defined. There is no reaction in the surrounding bone.

Treatment is simple curettage.

OSTEOCHONDROMA

This is a fairly common tumour, arising from the precartilagenous cells of the bone and consisting of both bone and cartilage (as the name suggests).

It arises from the metaphyseal region of a long bone, the commonest site being the bones at the knee joint. Occasionally the tumour may occur in the flat bones, like pelvis or scapula.

The tumour consists of a big tabulated mass, with a wide base. It has a big cartilagenous cap and often a bursa at the top (an osteochondroma differs from a cancellous osteoma in three respects— it is more sessile, it is more lobulated, and its cartilagenous cap is massive).

The patient, usually between 10 and 25 years of age, usually presents with a large but painless lump, which is attached to the bone but is free from all soft tissues. Sometimes there may be symptoms, e.g.

a. Aching pain.

b. Interference with tendon action.

c. Pressure on a nerve.

d. Inflammation of the bursa.

e. If the tumour is intrapelvic, it may cause pressure symptoms.

X-ray shows the tumour to arise from the medulla. It has a broad base, it is tabulated, and it shows irregular areas of calcification. It does not show the clear outlines of the cortex and medulla, as seen in a cancellous osteoma.

Unlike cancellous osteoma, the tumour may occasionally turn malignant (osteosarcoma), and so it should be excised.

GIANT CELL TUMOUR

Origin.—The origin of the tumour is debated and there are principally two views:
1. That it is a fibrous dysplasia, resulting from derangement in the normal process of bone formation by osteoblasts and bone removal by osteoclasts.
2. That it is actually a tumour. However, from which cells the tumour originates, is a matter of controversy. There are two views:
   a. That the tumour arises from cells .in the supporting connective tissue of the bone marrow, which do not take part in the formation of bone.
   b. That the tumour arises from the spindle cells of the bone.

One point is certain that the tumour does not arise from the osteoclasts. Hence the term 'osteoclastoma' is a misnomer. The other name for the tumour, i.e. *giant-cell tumour* is more appropriate because giant cells are constant constituents of the tumour.

Incidence.—The tumour almost always occurs between the ages of 20 and 30, that is when epiphyseal growth has just been completed. Hence, the view that it arises from the epiphysis is not tenable (some pathologists believe that it arises from the metaphysis and quickly comes down to the epiphysis). However, as the tumour is almost always situated at the end of a long bone, it may be said that it arises from that part of the bone where the epiphysis was located. The bones commonly affected, in order of frequency, are the lower end of femur, upper end of tibia, lower end of radius, and lower end of ulna. Apart from long bones, osteoclastoma may occur in the scapula, pelvis and mandible.

Pathology

A. MACROSCOPIC FEATURES.—The tumour is well-localised, tabulated, and has characteristically a maroon colour because of haemorrhage within. A tumour occurring at the lower end of the radius may have a white colour and is known as *osteodastoma alba*. While the tumour grows inside the bone, it causes an expansion and thinning of the cortex. This thinning occurs because there is no new bone formation. Clinically, this may be elicited as *egg-shell crackling*, if the bone is pressed upon (this, however, should not be tried). This, again, is the cause for pathological fractures, which may occur especially in the weight-bearing bones. As the tumour grows inside the bone and destroys bone tissue, some of the bony trabeculae, still keeping intact traverse the tumour mass. On the X-ray, these give a *soap-bubble appearance,* which, though diagnostic of osteodastoma, is not necessarily a constant feature.

B. MICROSCOPIC FEATURES
1. There are two types of cells:
   a. Spindle cells, which are the basic mononuclear cells but the exact nature of which is still unknown.

b. Giant cells of 'foreign body' type, i.e. big and multi-nucleated. There are several views about the origin of these giant cells:
  i. That they are the products of the basic mononuclear cells.
  ii. That they are derived from the osteoclasts.
  iii. That they are modified megakaryocytes.
2. The tumour is vascular and there are big areas of haemorrhage

Gradation. — In older days, depending on the cell types and the cytology of the basic mononuclear cells, giant cell tumours were divided into 3 grades:

Grade I: Definitely benign.

Grade II: Usually benign, but there are chances of malignancy.

Grade III: Malignant, behaving like osteosarcoma.

In the present days, this gradation is not relied upon. All the tumours are believed to be potentially malignant. In fact, about one-third of the tumours remain benign, one-third become locally invasive, and one-third metastatise.

Clinical Features.— A patient, usually between 20 and 30 years, presents with a *painless* swelling at the end of a long bone. Only when the osteoclastoma is big that a dull aching pain may occur. Pathological fracture may occur and, then again, the condition becomes painful. On examination, there is a localised bony swelling, free from the soft tissues, and only a little tender. Egg-shell crackling should not be attempted.

Some cases may present with all features of osteosarcoma, viz. pain, rapidly increasing swelling, extreme tenderness, loss of localisation and even metastases.

Special Investigations

I. LOCAL X-RAY.—The suggestive features of giant cell tumour are:
  1. It occurs at the end of a long bone.
  2. The tumour is usually eccentric in situation.
  3. The long axis of the tumour is along the transverse axis of the bone.
  4. There is a definite line of demarcation from the healthy bone.
  5. There is destruction of bone substance and no new bone formation, so that the cortex is expanded and thinned out over the tumour.
  6. There is often a soap-bubble appearance.
  7. There is no soft tissue shadow.
  When malignancy supervenes, the following features may be noted:
  a. The clear line of demarcation from healthy bone is lost.
  b. The outline of the thin expanded cortex is lost.
  c. There is a soft tissue shadow.
  [Radiologically, a solitary bone cyst differs from a giant cell tumour in the following points:
  i. It occurs at an earlier age.
  ii. The metaphysis is involved.
  iii. The long axis of the cyst is along the long axis of the bone
  iv. It is situated centrally, i.e. not eccentric.
II. BIOPSY.—This must be done in all the cases.
III. X-RAY CHEST.

Management

A. SURGERY.—Simple curettage of the tumour, from inside the bone, is not justified for fear of recurrence (this is why the tumour is described as locally malignant). Depending upon the case, three types of surgery are advised:

1. *Simple Excision.*—The tumour, with a part of adjacent healthy bone, is excised. This is possible only when excision of the bone does not interfere seriously with the anatomy and function of the neighbouring joint. Thus, it may be undertaken for growths in the
   a. upper end of fibula.
   b. lower end of ulna.
   c. rib.
   d. mandible.

2. *Excision with Prosthetic Replacement or Arthrodesis of the Neighbouring Joint.*— Since giant cell tumour most commonly occurs at bone-end, which is a constituent part of a joint, excision of the bone makes the joint useless. Therefore, either the excised segment has to be replaced by specialty designed prosthesis or arthrodesis of the joint has to be undertaken with excision of the tumour-bearing part of the bone, e.g.
   a. Lower end of femur,
   b. Upper end of tibia.
   c. Lower end of radius.

3. *Amputation.*—This is indicated for:
   a. Tumours which recur with increasing evidence of malignancy.
   b. Tumours which are frankly malignant.

B. RADIOTHERAPY.—The tumour is moderately radiosensitive and radiation may be the treatment of choice under the following circumstances:

1. A growth in a rather inaccessible bone, e.g. vertebra, pelvis, etc.
2. A small growth in a long bone.

A dose of 2000r is advocated. The disadvantages of radiotherapy are:

a. The results are uncertain.
b. There are chances of recurrence.
c. The tumour may turn malignant.

ANEURYSMAL BONE CYST

Pathology.—The origin is not known. Vascular, sponge-like tissue, having a bluish black colour and a honey-comb appearance on cut surface, is found inside the bone. The ends and shafts of long bones are most commonly affected. Vertebrae are also rather common sites.

The presenting feature is like a giant-cell tumour, from which the condition is difficult to be diagnosed clinically as well as radiologically. Often biopsy only provides the accurate diagnosis.

X-ray

1. There is expansion of the bone, without any new bone formation and, therefore, thinning of the cortex (like giant cell tumour).
2. The expansion is eccentric (like giant cell tumour).
3. There may be soap-bubble appearance (like giant cell tumour).

4. The long axis of the lesion is along the lung axis of the bone *(unlike* giant cell tumour).

Treatment

1. SURGERY.—This is done for the long bones. Curettage of the cyst, with cancellous bone grafting of the cavity, is the treatment. The scraped-out material must be sent for histological examination.
2. RADIOTHERAPY.—This is advised for inaccessible bones, e.g. vertebrae.

HAEMANGIOMA

This is most commonly found in the vertebrae, where it causes rarefaction. Haemangioma of long bones may cause elongation of the bone and usually presents as pathological fracture.

OSTEOSARCOMA

This tumour is often called osteogenic sarcoma not because it produces bone but because it arises from the cells which produce bone, i.e. osteoblasts. Though majority of the tumours show evidence of new bone formation, there are many where there is no evidence of bone formation; instead, there is more evidence of bone destruction. Accordingly, there is a tendency to classify these tumours into two broad groups:

I. Osteogenic.
II. Osteolytic.
A non-committal name is *osteosarcoma.*

Incidence.—Typically, the tumour occurs between the ages of 10 and 20, and its frequency quickly diminishes with age. The earlier the onset of the tumour, the worse is the prognosis. Characteristically, it starts in the metaphysis of a long bone. The bones affected, in order of frequency are the lower end of femur, upper end of tibia, and upper end of humerus. While any long bone may be affected, those at the wrist and at the ankle are relatively immune. On the other hand, the tumour may occur in the pelvic bones, scapula, and jaw bones.

Pathology.—Many workers classify the tumours pathologically into four broad groups:

1. PERIOSTEAL.—This is the commoner variety. The tumour is believed to arise from the inner layer of the periosteum and from the connective tissue that attaches the periosteum to the bone. Early onset of pain and presence of Codman's triangle *(see* below) are in support of this view. In the majority of cases, therefore, the tumour mass is seen, in its major part, as a swelling *outside* the confines of the bone (hence the tumour is also known as *parosteal).* However, there is an extensive infiltration into the cortex and medulla, but the defines of the cortex and the medulla are still maintained to some extent.
2. ENDOSTEAL.—In this variety, the central part of the bone, i.e. the medullary canal, shows the major part of the tumour mass, which infiltrates outwards through the cortex and the periosteum. This variety is, therefore, also known as *central.* It arises from the endosteum.

3. SCLEROSING.—In this type, an extensive sclerosis of the bone is seen, presumably because of less vascularity and more bone formation. However, it is as malignant as the other varieties.

4. TELANGIECTATIC.—Though all osteogenic sarcoma are highly vascular, in this variety the vessels, in their number and size, are out of proportion to the tumour mass. Understandably, this is the worst type.

In all varieties of osteogenic sarcoma, the tumour is usually a highly vascular fleshy mass. On the whole, it has a soft to firm feel, and the amount of bone in the tumour is variable. The capacity to form new bone lies with the spindle cells, from which the tumour arises. As the tumour gets more and more malignant, these cells lose their capacity to form new bone.

Microscopic Appearance

I. CELLS.—Varieties of cells are seen (i.e. *pleomorphism):*
1. The spindle cells from which the tumour originates.
2. Tumour giant cells or malignant giant cells—containing few nuclei, which are oval or indented, or joined together.
3. Foreign body giant cells—big, multinucleated.

II. INTERCELLULAR SUBSTANCE.—This, again, is highly variable and, even in the same tumour, different types may be seen:

Hyaline	Myxomatous
Fibrous	Osteoid
Cartilagenous	Osseous

III. VESSELS.—These are numerous and thin-walled. Over some areas the endothelial lining of the vessels may be missing, so that the tumour mass gains direct entry into the vessels (this accounts for the quick vascular spread).

Spread

1. DIRECT SPREAD.—Usually starting under the periosteum, the tumour raises the periosteum from the bone surface and continues to grow under it for a considerable period. During this period, the periosteum resists its outward spread. Thereafter, the periosteum is infiltrated and the surrounding soft tissues are involved. The overlying skin becomes tense, glistening, red and vascular but, unless it has been traumatised (e.g. biopsy), fungation is rare.

   Going in the depth, the tumour extensively infiltrates into the cortex and the medulla, though the architecture of the bone is maintained, While a variable amount of spread occurs longitudinally along the cortex, the medullary spread up and down is usually extensive. Small lesions in the medulla, well away from the original growth, are so frequent that, when amputation is performed, the bone should not be cut anywhere along its length; the amputation is always somewhere above the upper end of the bone.

2. LYMPHATIC SPREAD.—The lymphatic spread is as important as the venous spread. Thus, the inguinal nodes are very often involved and should be carefully examined in cases of femoral or tibial growths.

3. VENOUS SPREAD.—Common and very early to occur. The lung is most frequently involved. Less commonly, or in the later stages, other viscera or other bones may be affected.

New Bone Formation.—Though not always, this tumour usually shows a variable amount of new bone formation. This takes two forms:

1. SUN-RAY SPICULES.—As the tumour is usually of periosteal type and elevates the periosteum from the bone, the small transverse subperiosteal blood vessels stand out. Tumour cells are deposited along their walls (extravascularly). These cells, usually having the capacity to form new bone, lay down bone along these vessels. On the X-ray, the new bone has the appearance of transverse sun-rays. Even in the pathological specimens, the sun-ray spicules are seen. They, thus, represent *tumour bone.*

2. CODMAN'S TRIANGLE.—In the usual periosteal type the tumour gets massive under the periosteum and elevates the periosteum considerably. The periosteum rejoins the bone a little away from the diaphyseal end of the tumour. Stripping of the periosteum from the rather healthy diaphysis of the bone, beyond the extent of the tumour, causes new bone formation under the periosteum, in the gap there. This new bone, thus, takes the form of a triangle, the base of which is on the diaphyseal end of the tumour and the apex at the site where the periosteum rejoins the shaft. This is called Codman's triangle and this represents *reactive bone.*

Clinical Features.—The patient is usually between 10 and 20 years, and more commonly a male. There may be a history of trauma but that only draws the attention of the patient to the pathology.

The presenting features are pain and swelling. Usually pain precedes the appearance of the swelling by a few months. This is because of the irritation of the sensitive periosteum in the commoner periosteal type of growth. The swelling rapidly increases in size and the pain intensifies.

The swelling is in the metaphyseal region of a long bone. It is usually firm to soft in feel, and is highly tender. There is a local rise of temperature due to excessive vascularity of the tumour; occasionally the swelling may be pulsatile. The skin is usually red, tense and glistening, with prominent veins on it.

The regional nodes, the lungs, and the liver should be clinically examined.

1. LOCAL X-RAY.—The characteristic features are:
   a. The growth is at the metaphysis.
   b. Usually the outer aspect (periosteal type) and occasionally the inner aspect (endosteal type) of the bone is more involved. Though there is evidence of extensive infiltration through the cortex and the medulla, their outlines can usually be made out.
   c. There is no clear line of demarcation from the healthy bone.
   d. Usually, but not always, there is evidence of new bone formation—sun-ray spicules and Codman's triangle.
   e. There is a big soft tissue shadow.

2. X-RAY CHEST.—Metastases may take the form of multiple deposits or a solitary 'cannon-ball' deposit.

3. BIOPSY.

Treatment

1. AMPUTATION.—This is imperative in all the cases, be there any chest metastasis or not.

The advantages of amputation are:
  i. The bulk of the tumour is removed, making chemotherapy effective.
  ii. Pain is relieved.

The amputation should always be somewhere above the upper end of the affected bone (see spread of the tumour), e.g.

a. Upper third thigh for the upper tibia.
b. Disarticulation at the hip for the lower femur.
c. Hind-quarter amputation for the upper femur.
d. Disarticulation at the shoulder or a fore-quarter amputation for upper humerus.

The older method of Standford Cade in the form of preliminary radiotherapy and amputation only if there is no chest metastasis after six months is no longer advocated.

2. CHEMOTHERAPY.—This aims at destroying the minute undetectable metastases. It should be started within a week of amputation. Combination chemotherapy is advocated. Methotrexate and vincristine, and methotrexate and adriamycin are used alternately at 3 weeks' intervals. A few hours after the administration of the drugs, citrovorum factor is administered to restore the patient's normal cellular activity.

3. RADIOTHERAPY.—This is reserved for:
    a. Tumours at inaccessible sites, e.g. pelvis jaw.
    b. Patients refusing amputation.

4. IMMUNOTHERAPY.—This is being tried in some centres, with:
    a. Infusion of processed lymphocytes.
    b. Interferon.

EWING'S TUMOUR

Origin.—There is much controversy about the origin of this tumour:

1. Ewing believed that the tumour arises from the vascular endothelium in the bone marrow. This view is now obsolete.
2. Majority of workers believe that the tumour arises from the reticulum cells of the bone marrow. Hence it is also called *reticulocytoma.*
3. Some pathologists believe that the tumour arises from the primitive mesenchymal cells of bone.
4. The microscopic appearance of the tumour sometimes closely resembles that of the neuroblastoma of the adrenal. So, it is believed by some workers that the tumour is a metastatic growth from an unrecognised neuroblastoma of the adrenal.
5. There are some evidences that the tumour is sometimes a metastatic growth from an unrecognised bronchial carcinoma.

Pathology.—The essential features of this tumour are:

1. It arises from the diaphysis of long bones. The bones affected, in order of frequency, are tibia, humerus, femur, fibula, clavicle and calcaneum. Other bones may be affected, but usually the skull is never involved.
2. It occurs most frequently in ages between 5 and 15.
3. It has a notorious tendency to spread to other bones as well as to viscera.
4. The tumour cells have no capacity to form new bone.

Macroscopic Appearance.—The tumour is usually big in size and has the colour either of the brain or, if there is haemorrhage, of red currant jelly. It causes expansion of the medulla, with extensive destruction of the cortical bone, but the periosteum has a tendency to resist infiltration. As the periosteum is raised by the tumour mass, a layer of *reactive* new bone is formed on its deeper surface. The tumour cells gradually infiltrate through this layer of bone and again raise the periosteum, which further produces another layer of bone, and this process may continue. This gives, on the X-ray, the characteristic *onion-scale appearance,* the white layers representing the reactive new bone and the black layers, in between, representing the areas occupied by the tumour cells. It should be noted that there is *no tumour bone formation.*

Microscopic Appearance.—A characteristic uniformity of cells is seen, the cells being large polyhedral with very faint nuclei. There is practically no intercellular substance. Sometimes the cells are arranged in the form of *pseudorossettes,* and this is why the tumour is believed, by some workers, to be a metastatic lesion from unrecognised adrenal neuroblastoma.

Spread

1. DIRECT SPREAD.—There is extensive spread through the medulla and the cortex, both in vertical and transverse axes. The periosteum resists spread for sometime, but ultimately the tumour comes out and involves the overlying soft tissues. Fungation through the skin is rare, unless there is interference, e.g. biopsy.

2. LYMPHATIC SPREAD.—Rare.

3. VENOUS SPREAD.—Early and common: Other bones, as well as the viscera, may be involved, e.g. lung, liver.

Clinical Features.—The patient is usually between 5 and 15 years, and more commonly a male. Sometimes there is a history of trauma, following which there is pain, swelling, and fever.

These clinical features may lead to a wrong diagnosis of osteomyelitis. Moreover, incision on the swelling, on this diagnosis, often brings out semi-solid grey material, looking like pus, and this further confuses the diagnosis. If this is done, fungation occurs and then X-ray shows that a wrong diagnosis was made.

Pain and swelling in other bones, as well as clinical features suggestive of visceral metastases, may be evident.

Special Investigations

1. LOCAL X-RAY:
   a. Involvement of the diaphysis.
   b. Extensive destruction of the bone, as shown by widening of the medulla as well as gross rarefaction of the cortex.
   c. There may or may not be evidence of new bone formation, which, when present, may take the form of onion-scale appearance, i.e. as if the shaft has been lamellated.
2. X-RAY OF OTHER BONES, if there are symptoms.
3. X-RAY CHEST.
4. BIOPSY in doubtful cases.

Treatment.—Fortunately, the tumour is highly radiosensitive—as if it melts away with radiation. Hence *radiation* is the treatment.

Unfortunately, recurrences and metastases almost always occur and these are progressively radio-resistant. Here lies the difficulty in treating these cases and also the bad prognosis.

If a growth fungates or is unbearably painful, *amputation* may have to be performed.

RETICULUM CELL SARCOMA

This is a variant form of Ewing's tumour, having the following features:

1. The tumour is usually solitary and is commoner in the metaphysis of long bones.
2. It is locally less malignant than Ewing's tumour and also distant metastases are less frequent.

    Characteristically, however, it has a tendency to cause extensive lymph node metastasis, which Ewing's tumour usually does not.
3. Microscopically, reticulum fibres, occupying the intercellular spaces, may be demonstrated by special silver staining.
4. Prognosis is better than Ewing's tumour after amputation and radiation to the stump.

CHONDROSARCOMA

Types and Origin

1. *Primary Chondrosarcoma.*—This is actually an osteogenic sarcoma, in which the intercellular substance is mainly cartilagenous.
2. *Secondary Chondrosarcoma.*—This results from malignant change in:
    a. Long bone chondroma.
    b. Osteochondroma.
    c. One of the bony outgrowths in diaphyseal sclasis.

Pathology.—The pelvis, scapula, ribs, and ends of long bones are the most frequently affected. The tumour is characteristically slow-growing, with a lobulated surface. The affected bone shows a varying amount of destruction. The tumour gradually invades the neighbouring soft tissues and may produce distant blood-borne metastases.

Special Investigations

1. *Local X-ray.*
    a. Huge soft tissue shadow.
    b. Areas of patchy calcification.
    c. Irregular destruction of bone.
2. *Biopsy*

Treatment

1. The early cases may be treated by wide excision.
2. The late cases have to be treated by amputation. A chondrosarcoma, arising from the scapula, may require a forequarter amputation.

The tumour is radio resistant.

PAROSTEAL FIBROSARCOMA

Origin.—The tumour is so called because it may arise from:

a. Fibrous layer of periosteum.

b. Extraperiosteal connective tissue.

Pathology.—The ends of long bones (usually those at the knee) are commonly affected. The tumour is large but slow-growing, and *encapsulated*. It slowly erodes the cortex from outside. It may be difficult, in a particular case, to suggest whether the tumour is arising from the parosteal region or from the neighbouring soft tissues.

This tumour has the *best prognosis* of all primary malignant tumours of the bone, because it has less chances of local recurrence and causes late, if ever, distant metastases.

Special Investigations

1. *Local X-ray:*

   a. Huge soft tissue shadow.

   b. Erosion of the adjacent cortex.

2. *Biopsy.*

Treatment

1. Wide excision, with post-operative high-dose radiation, gives good results. Simple radiation is useless as the tumour is usually radio-resistant.

2. Amputation, if the tumour is suitably placed.

MULTIPLE MYELOMA

Origin.—The tumour arises from the plasma cells of the bone marrow. Hence it is also known as *plasmacytoma*.

Pathology.—The tumour almost always occurs after the age of 40, and is characterised by multiple bony lesions and presence of excess of protein in the system.

The tumour has a multicentric origin, appearing simultaneously in several bones. The most commonly affected are those containing red bones marrow in the adult life. In this respect, the skull and the bones of the chest wall, viz., sternum, ribs and vertebrae, are most commonly involved. The pelvic bones, mandible and clavicle are the next popular sites. However, the long bones may also be involved.

The tumours are usually small, multiple, and greyish or reddish in colour. They cause destruction of bone, which however is very well localised, giving on the X-ray a typical punched-out appearance. There is no evidence of new bone formation. These features may sometimes make the condition difficult to be diagnosed from secondary carcinoma of bones. However, failure to find out the primary growth, the different laboratory tests, and sternal puncture examination usually confirm the diagnosis.

Microscopically, there is a striking uniformity of the cells. The cells are round, i.e. the plasma cells or myeloma cells. There are big hyperchromatic nuclei, which are sometimes multiple. There is no intercellular substance.

The other characteristic feature in the pathology is an excess of protein in the system. There is hyperproteinemia, with an increase in the globulin fraction, as shown by electrophoresis. The source of this extra protein is believed to be the bone marrow, where there is a widespread destruction by the tumour.

The urine also contains an abnormal protein known as *Bence Jone's proteose*. In its presence, the urine gets cloudy when heated to 55°C but the opacity disappears on further heating to 85°C and reappears on cooling. The cause of this protein in the urine is believed to be the hyperproteinemia. The proteose may be deposited in the renal tubules. In the elderly people, this may cause chronic nephritis and renal failure, rather easily.

Another characteristic feature is the deposition of protein in the form of amyloids. Characteristically, such amyloid deposits are not found at sites where they commonly occur in amyloid degeneration, i.e. liver, spleen and kidneys. In contrast, they occur in rather abnormal sites, such as intestinal wall, voluntary muscles, bones, and even in the tumours themselves.

Clinical Features.—The patient, usually above the age of 40, presents with the following features:
1. Painful lumps, usually multiple, in relation to the bones mentioned above.
2. Back pain, referred root pains, and occasionally paraplegia due to vertebral deposits.
3. Occasionally, pathological fractures.
4. General weakness, anaemia and cachexia.
5. Polyuria and other features of renal failure, including pre-uraemic state.
6. Pulmonary complications, e.g. emphysema.

Special Investigations
1. *Blood Examination:*
   a. Progressive anaemia due to destruction of bone marrow.
   b. High ESR.
   c. Increased tendency of rouleaux formation by the R.B.C.
2. *Blood Biochemistry:*
   a. Increased plasma protein, particularly the globulin.
   b. Electrophoresis shows excess of proteins, related to gamma-globulin fraction.
3. *Urine Examination:*
   a. Bence-Jone's proteose may be present.
   b. Casts and other elements, suggestive of chronic nephritis, may also be found.
4. *Sternal Puncture.*—This is the best method of confirming the diagnosis. There is an abundance of plasma cells.
5. *Local X-ray.*—There are multiple punched-out areas of destruction, with clear margins and with no evidence of new bone formation.
6. *Biopsy* from a lump in doubtful cases.

Treatment.—Multiplicity of the lesions makes curative treatment impossible. The main line of treatment is chemotherapy. A very painful lump, or one growing very rapidly, may be treated additionally by radiation.

SOLITARY PLASMACYTOMA

In contrast to multiple myeloma, this tumour is solitary, without any evidence of metastasis for long periods. It can, therefore, be treated by amputation, with postoperative radiation. Even radiotherapy alone is often curative.

SECONDARY CARCINOMA OF BONE

These account for the majority of malignant bone tumours and are far more commoner than primary malignant tumours of bone.

Sources

1. In two-thirds of the cases, the primary is either in the breast or in the prostate.
2. In half of the remaining one-thirds, i.e. one-sixth of the total cases, the primary lies in the kidney, bronchus, thyroid, gastrointestinal tract, urinary bladder, etc.
3. In the remaining one-sixth, the primary cannot be found out in spite of all endeavours (obscure primary).

Those carcinoma, which have predilections for metastasis in the bones, are called ossophile tumours, e.g. breast, prostate, kidney, bronchus, thyroid, etc.

On the other hand, bone metastasis is rare in certain cancers, e.g. those in the gastrointestinal tract, urinary bladder, skin etc. These are called ossophobe tumours.

Types of Bone Lesion

1. In the majority of cases the secondary lesion causes destruction of bone, i.e. they are osteolytic.
2. In some cases there may be new bone formation and these lesions are called osteosclerotic. The commonest of .this type is a secondary from prostatic carcinoma, presumably because, in carcinoma of the prostate, there is an increase in the phosphatase level.

Routes of Involvement

1. Most commonly the spread to the bone, from the primary, occurs by way of systematic circulation. The cells, gaining entrance into the veins, travel through the vena cava to the heart. They then reach the lung, where they multiply. Thereafter, possibly they penetrate the lung capillaries, enter the systemic circulation, and reach the bones.
2. There is a direct communication between the pelvic venous plexus and the vertebral veins. Carcinoma from pelvic organs may, thus, directly reach the pelvic bones and vertebrae.
3. Tumours of the oral cavity may involve the jaw bones and those of the rectum may involve the sacrum, by direct contiguity.

Onset.—The lesion may start:
1. While the primary has already been diagnosed.
2. Before the primary has been diagnosed.
3. After, sometimes long after, removal of the primary.

Incidence.—Secondary tumours are often multiple and the bones commonly involved are those which contain red bone marrow in adult life, viz.
a. Skull.
b. Trunk Bones.—Vertebrae, ribs, sternum, and pelvis, i.e. bones forming the trunk.
c. Root Bones.—Head of femur, head of humerus, i.e. bones at the root of a limb.

Certain tumours have predilection for certain bones, usually those in relatively close proximity to the parent growth. Thus, breast cancers metastatise most often to spine, ribs and sternum; prostatic cancers often spread to pelvic bones and lumbar spines.

Special Features of Certain Metastases

1. Hypernephroma.—The bone metastasis is often solitary.
2. Thyroid Carcinoma:
   a. The metastasis is often solitary as in hypernephroma.
   b. The secondary growth often secretes thyroxin.
   c. Whatever be the histological type of the primary tumour, the metastatic lesion is always of the follicular variety.

In general, the macroscopic and microscopic appearances of bone secondaries correspond to those of the primary tumour.

Clinical Features

1. Pain, sometimes swelling, and often a pathological fracture, are the usual-presenting features.
2. A vertebral metastasis may present with back pain, compression fracture, root pain, or paraplegia.

Special Investigations

1. *Local X-ray* usually shows evidence of bone destruction, with no definite outline (osteolytic), and sometimes there is a pathological fracture. Metastases from prostate may show osteosclerosis and this may have to be differentiated from Paget's disease.
2. *Biopsy* in doubtful cases.
3. *Bone-scanning* with isotopes is nowadays being used to detect early lesions. Short-lived isotopes, e.g. fluorine18 are preferred.
4. All investigations with regard to the *primary tumour* or to find out the primary tumour has to be undertaken. The breast, prostate, kidney, bronchus and thyroid should be specially investigated.

Treatment

I. CURATIVE.—This is more or less out of question excepting when the primary growth is suitable for radical surgery and there is a solitary bone metastasis, which may be treated by amputation. Hypernephroma and thyroid cancers may occasionally present such chances.

II. PALLIATIVE.—This is the usual aim, and the treatment may be outlined as follows:
A. *Drugs:*
   1. Analgesics for relief of pain. Habit-forming drugs should be avoided as far as practicable.
   2. Chemotherapy.—Combination chemotherapy is preferred.
   3. Endocrine treatment in certain tumours:
      a. Prostatic cancers.—Oestrogen treatment.
      b. Breast cancers.—Anti-oestrogenic treatment in the premenopausal age group, and oestrogenic treatment in patients past menopause.
      c. Thyroid cancers.—Thyroxin administration.

B. *Radiation:*   .

This is one of the best ways of palliation.

C. *Surgery:*

1. A fungating growth from a bone secondary may require amputation.
2. For relief of pain, excision of nerve roots, spinothalamic tractotomy, etc. may have to be considered.
3. Endocrine surgery, e.g. oophrectomy, adrenalectomy hypophysectomy, etc., breast and prostatic cancers.
4. For pathological fractures, internal fixation provides good results.

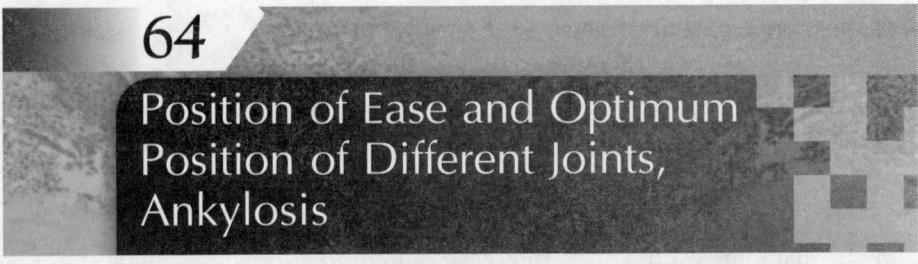

Position of Ease.—In this position the joint has maximum space within it. So, this is the position that the joint assumes when there is effusion within.

HIP.—Flexion, abduction and external rotation.

KNEE.—Flexion.

ANKLE.—Slight plantar flexion (with a little inversion of foot).

SHOULDER.—Adduction.

ELBOW.—Flexion (with the forearm pronated).

WRIST.—Little palmar flexion.

Optimum Position.—This is the position of maximum function of the joint. So, if for any reason, the joint is fixed, this is the position that the patient will like to have. Hence, arthrodesis of a joint should be done in this position. Similarly, where ankylosis is apprehended, following immobilisation for a disease (e.g. tuberculosis), the limb should be plastered with the joint in this position. The optimum position for the major joints are as follows:

HIP:	20° flexion (this permits sitting).
	10° abduction (if there is shortening, this is increased).
	Neutral rotation.
KNEE: ANKLE:	5 to 10° flexion.
	Neutral as regards dorsal or plantar flexion (with the foot in neutral position as regards abduction or adduction).
SHOULDER:	70° abduction.
	30° in front of coronal plane.
	Rotation in such a manner that the hand can reach the mouth.
ELBOW:	Depends on the occupation—90° for a clerk, 160° for a labourer. Pronation and supination of the forearm also depend on the occupation; usually a mid-prone position is preferred (more pronation in clerks to help writing).
	When both the elbows are fixed, one is kept at 90° and the other at 160°.
WRIST:	15 to 20° dorsiflexion.

ANKYLOSIS

Definition.—This denotes limitation of movements of a joint.

Classification

I. TRUE ANKYLOSIS.—This is caused by infra-articular lesions. This may again be of two types:

    A. *Fibrous Ankylosis.*—Here the constituent bones of the joint are held together by fibrous tissue, grown abnormally. This may result from:

        1. Organisation of haemorrhage inside the joint.

        2. Tubercular arthritis.

        3. Rheumatoid arthritis.

        4. Gonococcal arthritis.

    In a fibrous ankylosis some movements, however minor, are still possible in the joint. When these movements are painless, the fibrous ankylosis is said to be *sound.* If the movements are painful, the ankylosis is termed *unsound.*

    B. *Bony Ankylosis:*—Here the constituent bones are held together by a bony bond. As compared to fibrous ankylosis, no movement, whatsoever, is possible in the joint, and so the joint is painless. A bony ankylosis may result from:

        1. Fractures involving articular surfaces.

        2. Pyogenic arthritis.

        3. Tubercular arthritis when secondarily infected.

II. FALSE ANKYLOSIS.—This is caused by contracture of periarticular soft tissues or by bony block in the periarticular structures:

    1. *Skin and Subcutaneous Tissues:* Contracture following burn.

    2. *Muscles and Tendons:*

        a. Adhesion to bones following trauma.

        b. Adhesion to bones following inflammation.

        c. Volkmann's ischaemic contracture.

    3. *Fascia:*

        a. Dupuytren's contracture.

        b. Inflammatory fibrofascitis.

    4. *Ligaments and Capsule:*

    Long-continued immobilisation.

    5. *Bone:*

        a. Displaced fracture fragment.

        b. Excess of callus.

        c. Myositis ossificans.

        d. Ankylosing spondylitis.

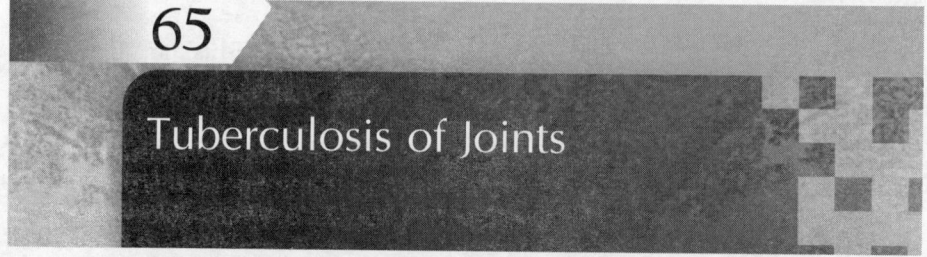

65

Tuberculosis of Joints

PATHOLOGY IN GENERAL

Joint tuberculosis may occur at any age but most commonly the children suffer. The joints affected, in order of frequency, are the hip, knee, elbow, shoulder, ankle and wrist.

In the children, the incidence of hip tuberculosis alone exceeds tuberculosis of all other joints taken together (excepting spine). Wrist tuberculosis occurs exclusively in the adults. Bone and joint tuberculosis are always secondary.

Onset.—There are two distinct types:

1. SYNOVIAL OR PRIMARY TYPE: Here the process of tuberculosis starts in the synovial membrane. Since synovial membrane is a component of the joint itself, this variety is called the 'primary' type. This type is commoner in the adults. It is commoner in the knee than in the hip.

2. OSSEOUS OR SECONDARY TYPE: Here the process of tuberculosis starts in the constituent bone of a joint and then secondarily involves the synovial membrane. This type is commoner in the children. The hip is more commonly affected in this way than the knee.

In the osseous type, the lesion usually starts in the metaphysis and only rarely in the epiphysis. From the metaphysis, the tubercular lesion reaches the synovial membrane, almost always by way of the *circulus vasculosus*. Only rarely does a metaphyseal lesion pierce through the epiphyseal cartilage to reach the synovial membrane.

Stages.—Irrespective of the nature of its onset, the disease runs in three stages:

1. STAGE OF SYNOVITIS.—Whatever be the type of lesion, the first pathological state of the joint is one of synovitis. The synovial membrane is oedematous and grossly hypertrophied. Tubercles are deposited on both its surfaces, particularly the inner. There is only a little increase in the synovial fluid, and the gross swelling of the joint, clinically seen, is not much due to the fluid as it is due to the hypertrophic synovial membrane. However, the fluid is very rich in fibrin, and deposits of fibrin may present as loose bodies, termed 'melon-seed bodies'.

2. STAGE OF ARTHRITIS.—This stage starts with the process of erosion of the articular cartilage. The tubercular granulation tissue, on the outer wall of the synovial membrane, erodes into the *outer* surface of the articular cartilage. At a later stage, reactive granulation tissue, from the underlying bone, grows into the *inner* surface of the articular cartilage, in an attempt to separate it from the bone.

Thus, there is gross destruction of both the surfaces of the articular cartilage by granulation tissue.

3. STAGE OF BONE DESTRUCTION AND FURTHER PROGRESS.—Over wide areas, the articular surface of the bones becomes rare, since the covering articular cartilage is destroyed by erosion. The process of tuberculosis now causes destruction of the underlying bones, which become the seat of a 'rarefying osteitis'.

By this time, the capsule and the ligaments of the joint undergo gelatinous degeneration, resulting in softening, so that a pathological dislocation sets in. In the meantime, tubercular cold abscess from the joint often makes way through the overlying muscles and may come to the surface. If the joint is superficial and not covered by muscles (e.g. knee), oedema of the skin occurs and the fluid causes capillary emptying of the skin, making the skin look white. This is what is typically called *white swollen knee,* in contrast to a red swelling of the knee that occurs in pyogenic arthritis.

In contrast to the typical description above, two *special forms* of joint tuberculosis may be seen:

a. *Hydrops.*—In these cases the synovial membrane is not much hypertrophied but there is an excess of synovial fluid.

b. *Caries Sicca, i.e. Dry Tuberculosis.*—Typically seen in the shoulder (however, the commoner type of tuberculosis, as described above, is commoner in the shoulder). In this rare form, all the tissues of the joint, particularly the overlying muscles, undergo atrophy.

TUBERCULOSIS OF THE HIP

Though the disease may occur at any age, children below 10 years are the usual sufferers. The disease is blood-borne from a distant focus, usually the lungs or lymph nodes.

In the hip, tuberculosis is only rarely synovial in onset. In the majority of cases it is osseous in type. The starting point in the bone may be as follows:

1. Most commonly it is a triangular area on the postero-inferior surface of the neck of the femur (this is called *Babcock's triangle).*
2. The acetabular rim.
3. The head of the femur.

Rarely, tuberculosis may start in the greater trochanter, and in these cases the lesion is extracapsular (i.e. outside the hip joint).

Pathology.—As in all other joints, the disease runs in 3 stages:
1. Stage of synovitis.
2. Stage of arthritis.
3. Stage of bone destruction and further progress. (Vide pathology above).

Clinical Features.—The patient is usually a child and sometimes there is a history of trauma preceding the onset. Typically, the presenting features are:
1. Pain:
   a. Aggravated by movements
   b. Sometimes radiated to the knee joint (by way of the genicular branch of the obturator nerve).
2. Limping.

3. Constitutional symptoms.—Fever, loss of weight, night-sweating, etc.

The exact clinical features vary according to the pathological stage of the disease, as described below.

I. STAGE OF SYNOVITIS.—In this stage the hypertrophic synovial membrane has to be accommodated inside the joint and, to make this possible, the joint must assume a position in which there is maximum space inside the joint. Hence the attitude of the limb in this stage is:

   a. Flexion, abduction and external rotation, and

   b. Because there is abduction, there is an *apparent lengthening* of the limb.

   As a secondary effect of this attitude:

      i. There is a tilting down of the pelvis towards the *affected side*.

      ii. There is a lumbar scoliosis, with the convexity towards the *affected side*.

      iii. There is an increased lumbar lordosis.

   Active and passive movements in *all directions* are restricted and painful.

II. STAGE OF ARTHRITIS.—In this stage, as the articular cartilages get eroded, the underlying bones get exposed over wide areas. A friction between the opposing surfaces of the naked bones is likely to cause severe pain and, in order to prevent this, the surrounding muscles go into spasm. At night, when the child is asleep, this voluntary spasm passes off and the raw bones get in touch with each other, waking the patient up in pain, i.e. *night cry*.

The attitude of the limb in this stage is typically:

   a. Flexion adduction and internal rotation, and

   b. Because there is adduction, there is an *apparent shortening* of the limb.

   As a secondary effect of this attitude:

      i. There is a tilting down of the pelvis towards the *opposite side*.

      ii. There is a lumbar scoliosis, with the convexity towards the *opposite side*.

      iii. There is a lumbar lordosis.

The typical position of the limb at this stage is due to two factors:

1. There is a protective muscle spasm of all the muscles around the joint. However, the adductors and the flexors are always more powerful, hence the attitude.

2. As the joint becomes more and more painful, the patient prefers to lie on the sound hip. Naturally, the affected hip is kept permanently in the above position (this is the position that the hip normally assumes when a person lies on the opposite side).

III. STAGE OF BONE DESTRUCTION AND FURTHER PROGRESS.—Rarefying osteitis of the constituent bones of the joint makes the bones soft, so that the head and neck of the femur on one hand, and the acetabulum on the other, get softened and undergo gradual destruction.

When the hip is in the neutral position or in abduction, the muscle pull makes the head of the femur strike against the centre of the acetabular cavity. But when the hip is flexed and adducted (as these patients have), the muscle pull (i.e. the muscle spasm in these patients) makes the femoral head strike against the posterior roof of the acetabulum. The acetabulum having been softened by this time, the head crushes through the posterior acetabular rim, towards the dorsum ili, i.e. tends to get a posterior dislocation. In the meantime, there is a gelatinous degeneration of the capsule and ligaments of the joint and this makes *posterior dislocation* of the head possible. In this new position, the head makes its own room in the form of a depression in the softened dorsum ili, i.e. as if a new acetabulum has been made. This condition is called *wandering acetabulum* (i.e. travelling or false acetabulum).

In this stage, in addition to the already existing deformities of flexion, adduction and internal rotation, a *true shortening* of the limb occurs. The causes for this true shortening are:

1. Destruction of the femoral head.
2. Softening and shortening of the femoral neck.
3. Pathological (posterior) dislocation of the hip.
4. Sometimes, impaired growth at the lower femoral epiphysis, due to prolonged immobilisation.

A *cold abscess* or a *tubercular sinus* may be found in this stage. In the majority of cases these are seen on the glutei, but sometimes they may occur in the thigh.

Special Investigations

1. Local X-ray:
   a. In the stage of synovitis, no radiological abnormality may be seen. Sometimes, however, the primary focus in the bone may be seen as an area of rarefied osteitis.
   b. In an established case, the findings are:
      i. Diminution of the joint space (because of destruction of the articular cartilages which make the joint space on the X-ray).
      ii. Variable amount of rarefaction and destruction of the femoral head and acetabulum.
      iii. Rarefaction in the femoral neck, sometimes associated with broadening of the neck, diminution of the neck-shaft angle (i.e. coxa vara), and increased anteversion of the neck.
   c. In a late case, evidence of posterior dislocation, i.e. wandering acetabulum.
2. X-ray Chest.
3. Mantoux Test.
4. Blood Examination.—TC, DC, and ESR.
5. If there is a cold abscess, aspiration of the abscess, and bacteriological and culture examination of the pus (tubercular pus is sterile on ordinary culture).

Treatment

Stage I: Stage of recumbency, rigid immobilisation, and active antitubercular treatment

A. *General Antitubercular Treatment.*—Same as in caries spine (*see* Chapter 24).

B. *Local Treatment.*—With the patient recumbent, a rigid immobilisation of the joint has to be done. To start with, there is usually a deformity. Hence, along with immobilisation, the muscle spasm has to be overcome in order to correct the deformity. This is done by *traction* in a Thomas' bed knee splint. After the deformity has been corrected, a Whitman's plaster may replace the splint, for the purpose of more rigid immobilisation. Alternatively, treatment may be continued on the splint.

This rigid immobilisation has to be continued till the progress of the disease has been arrested, i.e. the *stage of quiescence* has been reached (this does not, however, mean that healing has started). Apart from improvement in the general condition, resolution of cold abscesses, and improvement in the clinical condition, the local X-ray is the main criterion to ascertain that the stage of quiescence has been reached. Three consecutive monthly X-rays should show that there is no further bone destruction.

As an auxiliary part of treatment in this stage, cold abscess, if any, has to be repeatedly aspirated together with local installation of INH solution.

STAGE II: STAGE OF AMBULATION WITH SUPPORT

The patient is allowed to move the hip gradually, and then to walk, but is not allowed to bear weight on the limb. Various appliances are available with which the patient can walk, without bearing weight on the affected limb. All of these are made on the principles of walking callipers.

The patient has to use these till local X-rays show active signs of healing.

STAGE III: PERMANENT TREATMENT IN THE HEALED STAGE

A. In the absence of secondary infection (gaining entrance through a sinus), a tubercular joint always heals by fibrous ankylosis (if secondary infection occurs, healing may occur by bony ankylosis). With fibrous ankylosis, the hip is never sound. The difficulties of fibrous ankylosis are:
   a. Some movements, however small, are still left in the joint, and these are really painful.
   b. Tubercular bacilli often lie in a dormant state inside the joint, even after healing has occurred, and movements of the joint may cause flaring up of these bacilli any time at a subsequent date.

To overcome these difficulties, arthrodesis (i.e. fixing of the joint) has to be advised in almost all the cases.

Another problem in these cases is the permanent deformity of flexion, adduction and internal rotation. This has often to be corrected.

With a view to correcting the hip deformity and fixing the hip joint, the following types of surgery may be considered:
   1. *Subtrochanteric Osteotomy:*
      The femur is cut through, below the trochanters, and the adduction deformity is corrected.
   2. *Arthrodesis:*
      a. In older days, a tubercular joint would never be opened up and, while thinking of fixing a joint, *extra-articular arthrodesis* would always be deemed ideal. This means fixing the joint from outside, without opening it. The types of extra-articular arthrodesis in the hip are:
         i. *Iliofemoral arthrodesis.*—A tibial cortical bone block is taken. Its two ends are fitted into the two sloughts made—one in the dorsum ili and another in the greater trochanter.
         ii. *Ischiofemoral arthrodesis.*—The bone block is placed in sloughts made in ischium and the femoral shaft.
      b. In recent days, with the wide use of effective antitubercular drugs, *intra-articular arthrodesis* is being more frequently practised. The joint is opened up, all tubercular tissues (particularly the synovial membrane) are scraped

out, and the joint is fixed from inside. One of the easy means of fixing is to pass in a long SP nail, from the femoral neck through the joint, into the acetabulum.

3. *Combined Osteotomy and Arthrodesis:*
   This is the most popular method in a case where there is a persistent deformity. A subtrochanteric osteotomy is performed to correct the deformity. An extra-articular ischiofemoral arthrodesis is now performed—the graft on the femoral side being fitted in the gap of the osteotomy. This is called *Brittain's arthrodesis.*

B. As an alternative procedure to arthrodesis, as the permanent treatment, the following methods of treatment may have to be thought of:
   1. In this country, the patients' life is often difficult with arthrodesis because they cannot squat and the females cannot carry out the routine domestic activities easily. For these people, therefore, some form of *arthroplasty* is often preferred. In this respect, *'Girdlestone's arthroplasty'* is very useful. In this operation, the head and the neck of the femur are excised (thus removing the major diseased area), and the acetabular rim is trimmed. The gluteus muscles are put on the floor of the acetabulum, and the upper end of the femur is allowed to move on this floor, thus making a *pseudoarthrosis.*
   2. If the disease is arrested very early, i.e. at the stage of synovitis, a normal range of movements may be expected because the articular cartilages are still intact. In these cases, after rigid immobilisation for six months, active movements of the joint are encouraged.

TUBERCULOSIS OF THE KNEE

In contrast to hip tuberculosis, tuberculosis of knee is:
1. A little more frequent in the adults.
2. Synovial in type to start with (sometimes, however, it may be osseous).

As with the hip joint, the disease is always secondary to tuberculosis elsewhere, particularly the lung and lymph nodes, though the primary lesion may not be demonstrable.   ' -

Pathology.—As in the other joints, the disease runs in 3 stages:
1. Stage of synovitis.
2. Stage of arthritis.
3. Stage of bone destruction and further progress.
                    (Vide pathology in general, described earlier)

Clinical Features.—The patient presents with pain and swelling in the joint, and the movements are painful. There may be a history of trauma. Constitutional symptoms like fever, loss of weight, night-sweating, etc. may be present.

On examination, the following features may be seen:
1. The swelling in the knee is prominent. This swelling is:
   a. Partially real, resulting from hypertrophy of the synovial membrane (having a typical doughy feel) and a little increase in synovial fluid.
   b. Partially apparent, due to wasting of the quadriceps femoris.
2. All movements of the knee are painful and restricted.
3. The knee may have a characteristic white appearance and this is due to oedema of the skin with resultant emptying of the skin capillaries. This is

known as *white swollen knee,* as compared to a red swelling seen in pyogenic arthritis.

4. At a later stage, cold abscesses and sinuses are frequently seen because the joint is superficial.

5. When the disease has progressed considerably, degeneration of the cruciate ligaments, together with the muscle spasms, results in a typical deformity, i.e. flexion, external rotation and posterior subluxation. This is popularly known as the *triple displacement.*

Special Investigations

1. Local X-ray shows early diminution of the joint space. The neighbouring bones show variable amount of rarefaction and destruction. As a later stage, posterior subluxation may be evident.

2. Aspiration of synovial fluid for bacteriological and culture examination (tubercular pus is usually sterile on ordinary culture).

3. Synovial biopsy in doubtful cases. This is easily done as the joint is superficial.

4. X-ray chest.

5. Blood examination.—TC, DC, and ESR.

6. Mantoux test.

Treatment

STAGE I: STAGE OF RECUMBENCY, RIGID IMMOBILISATION, AND ACTIVE ANTITUBERCULAR TREATMENT

A. *General Antitubercular Treatment.*—Same as in caries spine (*see* Chapter 24):

B. *Local Treatment.*—The patient should not bear weight on the limb and the knee must be completely immobilised. To start with, usually there is a muscle spasm. So, immobilisation is done primarily in a Thomas' bed knee splint with skin *traction.* After the muscle spasm is overcome, immobilisation is continued in complete plaster. The plaster extends from the upper third of the thigh to the sole, with the knee in 5 to 10 degrees flexion, which is the optimum position for the joint. This immobilisation has to be continued till the progress of the disease is arrested, i.e. the *stage of quiescence* is reached. Apart from improvement in the general condition, resolution of cold abscesses, and improvement in local clinical condition, the local X-ray is the main criterion to ascertain that the stage of quiescence has been reached. Three consecutive monthly X-rays should show that there is no further bone destruction.

[If the disease is diagnosed very early in its course, i.e. at the stage of synovitis, when the articular cartilages have not been destroyed, a normal range of movements may be expected. In these cases either of the following two procedures may be adopted:

a. After the limb has been immobilised for six months, active movements of the knee are started, provided there is no evidence of involvement of the articular cartilages or bones during this period.

b. A *synovectomy,* i.e. excision of the synovial membrane, is done, with the idea of removing the focus of infection. The joint is closed without a drain and the limb is immobilised in plaster.

In any case, full antitubercular treatment must be instituted.]

STAGE II: STAGE OF AMBULATION WITH SUPPORT

The patient is allowed to walk without bearing weight through the knee. To achieve this, a walking calliper is used. This has to be continued till X-rays show definite signs of healing.

STAGE III: PERMANENT TREATMENT IN HEALED STAGE

As healing occurs by fibrous ankylosis (unless there is a secondary infection through sinuses), the joint is unsound. The difficulties of a fibrous ankylosis are:

a. Some movements, however small, are still left in the joint, and these are really painful.

b. Tubercle bacilli often lie in a dormant state inside the joint, even after healing has occurred, and movements of the joint may cause flaring up of these bacilli any time at a subsequent date.

To overcome these difficulties, arthrodesis (i.e. fixing) of the joint has to be advised in almost all the cases. For this purpose, *Charnley's arthrodesis* is most commonly practised.

In this operation, all soft tissues from inside the joint, including the synovial membrane, are removed. The patella is excised. The diseased articular cartilages, on the femur and the tibia, are excised. Parts of the femoral and tibial condyles, including all diseased areas, are excised, so that the contiguous femoral and tibial surfaces are flat. Two Bohler's pins are taken. One is passed transversely through the femur and the other through the tibia, each a little away from the cut surface. A charnley's compression damp is now fitted to these pins. The idea of the clamp is to achieve close apposition, as well as rigid compression, between the raw ends of the femur and the tibia, so that there is early union and complete arthrodesis. The limb, with the compression clamp in position, is kept in immobilisation, either in a Thomas' bed knee splint or in plaster, for about 3 months. By this time union occurs. During immobilisation, the knee is kept at 5 to 10° flexion, which is the optimum position for the joint.

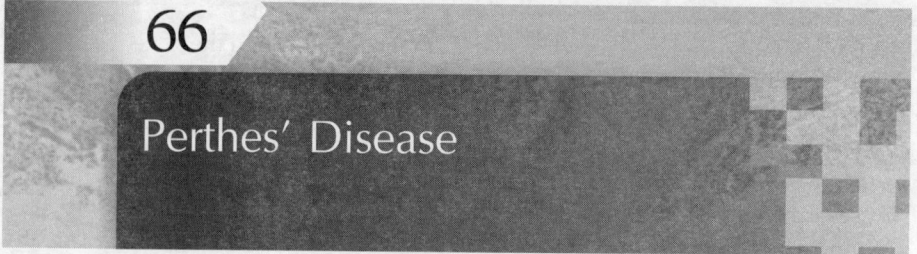

66

Perthes' Disease

This is also known as "Legg-Calvé-Perthes' disease". This is a form of *crushing osteochondritis* and here the condition affects the ossific nucleus of the femoral head. [The different types of osteochondritis are described later in this Chapter.]

Etiology.—The disease typically occurs between 5 and 10 years of age, and is at least 2 times commoner in the males. The condition is definitely due to an *avascular necrosis* of the ossific nucleus of the femoral head, resulting from an obliteration of blood supply to the head. This obliteration is due to two factors—an already existing deficient blood flow due to anatomical reasons and a precipitating factor which cuts off even this deficient flow:

1. DEFICIENT BLOOD SUPPLY.—(Fig. 66.1). Up to the age of 3 to 4 years, the epiphysis of the femoral head is mainly supplied by blood vessels coming from the metaphysis; only a little supply comes from the lateral epiphyseal vessels. At about the age of 7 to 8 years, the blood vessels in the ligamentum teres femoris develop. Between the ages of 4 and 7 years, the blood supply from the metaphysis is curtailed because the femoral neck is developing at this stage and the major part of the blood is exhausted in it. At this age, till the vessel in the ligamentum teres develops, the epiphysis is nourished only by the lateral epiphyseal vessels. These lateral epiphyseal vessels are located in the retinacula and they are, therefore, susceptible to obliteration by pressure from within e.g. an effusion in the joint.

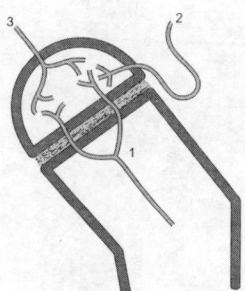

Fig. 66.1: Blood supply of the head of the femur. 1. Metaphyseal vessels; 2. Lateral epiphyseal vessels; 3. Vessels in the ligamentum teres femoris.

2. PRECIPITATING FACTOR.—The aforesaid obliteration of the lateral epiphyseal vessels may be caused by:
   a. *Traumatic Effusion.*—There is often a history of trauma and the disease is commoner in the boys. One type of trauma is forceful reduction of CDH, of which Perthes' disease is sometimes a sequela.

b. *Infection.*—According to some authorities, staphylococcal infection is the cause. Occurrence of temperature, at the onset, in many cases (suggesting transient synovitis), supports this view.

c. *Dysplasia.*—Minor developmental errors may subject the capsule to undue strain and expose the epiphyseal blood vessels to repeated trauma. Such errors are often demonstrable in these cases, in the form of either a sloping acetabular roof or a subluxation of the joint, resulting in a much lateral situation of the femoral head inside the joint.

Pathology

1. STAGE OF AVASCULAR NECROSIS.:—The ossific nucleus undergoes avascular necrosis. So, the head of the femur fails to grow and on the X-ray, looks smaller than that of the opposite side. However, the cartilagenous, part of the head continues to grow and, since the bony part of the head is smaller in size, the cartilagenous part grows to a size bigger than normal. Hence, on the X-ray, the joint space is found to be wider than that of the opposite side (c.f. tuberculosis).

   As the bone is dead, it looks sclerosed on X-ray (c.f. tuberculosis, where rarefaction is found).

   As the dead bone is inelastic, it becomes flat and fragmented on weight-bearing, and these are evident on the X-ray.

2. STAGE OF REGENERATION BY CREEPING SUBSTITUTION.—New blood vessels from the neck of the femur begin to grow into the dead head, to cause its regeneration. As new blood vessels are creeping into the dead head, the process is called *regeneration by creeping substitution.*

   To achieve this, the neck has to become hypervascular. As a result, it looks rarefied with evidence of small cysts, on the X-ray. The neck becomes soft and, as it bears weight, it becomes wider and depressed down, so that the neck-shaft angle diminishes and a coxa vara results.

   The new blood vessels, growing into the head, produce patchy areas of regeneration, which are evident on the X-ray as rarefied patches in the sclerosed bone. The process of regeneration starts at the periphery and proceeds to the centre, and ultimately the whole of the bony head is regenerated. Since the head had failed to develop and had become flat earlier, it can never have the full size and the spherical shape of a normal head and it keeps permanently flat.

3. LATE EFFECT.—Perthes' disease, as such, is therefore, rather harmless because complete regeneration of the head occurs (in about 3 to 4 years' time). But the permanent flattening of the head will definitely cause an early osteoarthritis of the hip, in the future life of the patient, and here lies the real danger of the disease.

Clinical Features.—The disease occurs most commonly between 5 and 10 years of age, and is at least twice commoner in the boys. There may be a history of trauma. The earlier the disease starts, the better is the prognosis, and cases occurring after 10 years are destined to have poor results.

The typical presenting features are *pain* and *limping*. Often there is a little *rise of temperature* for the first few days.

For the first few days, i.e. about a week, the hip is irritable and all the movements are restricted. The age of the patient, pain, limp, rise of temperature, and limitation of all movements at this stage make, in all probabilities, a diagnosis of a tubercular hip. If, however, the hip is put on rest, preferably in traction, for a week, the phase of irritation passes off. If the joint is now re-examined, a marked range of painless movements may be possible, in contrast to what is seen in tubercular hip. In Perthes' disease, flexion and extension are always possible to the full ranges, so also adduction.

As the head has become flattened, rotations (both internal and external) are grossly restricted.

Because there is a coxa vara deformity, abduction is restricted. This is best seen when abduction in flexion is tried.

X-ray

A. In the stage of avascular necrosis:
1. The bony head is smaller.
2. The joint space is wider.
3. The bony head is sclerosed.
4. The bony head is flattened.
5. The bony head is fragmented.

B. In the stage of regeneration:
1. The neck is rarefied.
2. The neck is widened.
3. There is a coxa vara.
4. The head shows sclerosis, in which there are patchy areas of rarefaction, the extent of which depends on the stage of regeneration.
5. The head is still flat.
6. The acetabulum may show areas of altered density (which is probably secondary).

C. At later age:
1. The head is flat.
2. There are evidences of osteoarthritis, e.g. diminution of joint space and presence of osteophytes.

Differential Diagnosis from Tuberculosis of Hip.—As has already been stated, this disease may be wrongly diagnosed as tuberculosis of hip and hence the other name for the disease is *pseudocoxalgia* (i.e. hip pain, giving a false impression of tuberculosis). The points of difference from tuberculosis are as follows:
1. The disease is restricted to the age group of 5 to 10 years, while tuberculosis may occur at any age, though commonly in childhood.
2. It is at least two times commoner in males; tuberculosis has no such sex discrimination.
3. The child is healthy.
4. Constitutional symptoms of tuberculosis, e.g. evening temperature, anorexia, loss of weight, night-sweating, etc. are absent. For the first few days, however, there may be a little temperature in some cases.
5. The stage of irritability, i.e. painful movements and muscle spasm, subside quickly with rest, as compared to tuberculosis.
6. Excepting during the phase of irritation (when all movements are restricted and painful as in tuberculosis), demonstration of different movements usually establishes the diagnosis. Flexion, extension and adduction are possible through

full ranges. Only the rotations (internal and external) and abduction (particularly abduction in flexion) are restricted. In tuberculosis all the movements are restricted.

7. X-ray findings are confirmatory. The most important distinguishing features are:
   a. Increase in the joint space.
   b. Sclerosis of the femoral head.
   c. Diminution in size, with fragmentation and flattening of the head.
   In tuberculosis, the joint space is diminished, the head is rarefied but its shape and size remain unaltered.
8. Manotoux test is negative.
9. ESR is not raised.

Treatment.—As the disease is self-limiting, the whole idea behind the treatment is to keep the flattening and distortion of the head to the minimum, and thereby prevent early, and severe osteoarthritis.

The cases are divided into two groups, according to the radiographic appearance of the femoral head:

1. If the lateral X-ray shows that less than half of the head is affected by the disease, the prognosis is good, irrespective of the nature of treatment. In these cases the patient is put in recumbency during the initial phase to allow the symptoms to settle down and thereafter allowed to move free with periodic X-ray check-up.
2. If the X-rays show that:
   a. More than half of the head is involved in the disease and/or
   b. The lateral part of the head is bulging out of the acetabulum, the prognosis is poor and these cases are destined to develop osteoarthritis in future unless promptly and actively treated now (the head as well as the acetabulum are likely to get deformed).

The idea behind the treatment in these cases is to hold the upper femur in such an abducted position that the head is totally contained in the acetabulum, which acts as a mould to preserve the shape of the femoral head till revascularisation has occurred. This abduction may be achieved in two ways:

   i. By holding the hips abducted to 20–30 degrees, in plaster or a removable splint, for one year. Splint is preferred because the patient can be ambulatory (though awkward).
   ii. By doing a *varus osteotomy* of the femur. The femur is divided just below the greater trochanter and the shaft is so angled that it is adducted about 20 degrees in relation to the proximal fragment. The fragments are fixed with a metal nail-plate and screws. Union occurs in 5 to 6 weeks. Thus, with the leg in the neutral position, the head and the neck of the femur are abducted and the head is pushed into the acetabulum.

OSTEOCHONDRITIS

The term osteochondritis is used to describe certain obscure affections of the developing ossific nuclei in children and adolescents. The term is nowadays, broadly used to include certain conditions, where the affection is very likely to be traumatic in origin, e.g. the 'pulling osteochondritis' group.

In general, osteochondritis may be divided into three broad groups:
 I. 'Crushing' osteochondritis.
 II. 'Splitting' osteochondritis.
 III. 'Pulling' osteochondritis.

Crushing Osteochondritis.—This is also known as *juvenile osteochondritis*. The ossific nucleus, which undergoes avascular necrosis, is crushed under pressure. The examples are as follows:
1. The epiphysis of femoral head.—Perthes' disease.
2. The head of the second metatarsal.—Freiberg's disease.
3. The 'ring' epiphysis of the vertebral bodies.—Schuermann's disease.
4. The central epiphysis of a vertebral body.—Calve's disease.
5. The nucleus of the navicular bone.—Köhler's disease.
6. The nucleus of the lunate bone.—Kienböck's disease.

Splitting Osteochondritis.—This is also known as *osteochondritis dissecans*. An ovoid piece of bone, about 1/3 to 1 inch in diameter and less in height, becomes separated, possibly because it is avascular. The commonest site is at the femoral condyle, where the separated piece acts as a loose body in the joint. Other rare examples are capitulum in the elbow, talus in the ankle, etc.

Pulling Osteochondritis.—This is also known as *traction osteochondritis*. It is almost certain that these are traumatic in origin, resulting from strong traction on the apophysis, by the tendon attached to it. The examples are:
1. The tibial apophysis (tubercle), where the ligamentum patellae is attached.—Osgood-Schlatter's disease in the knee.
2. The calcanean apophysis, where the tendo Achillis is inserted.— Sever's disease in the heel.

67

Congenital Dislocation of Hip

Pathology—This may be discussed under two headings:
 I. Changes in the bones.
 II. Changes in the soft tissues.

I. Changes in the Bones

A. THE PELVIS:
1. The pelvis is smaller in size on the affected side.
2. In bilateral cases there is considerable forward tilting of the pelvis.

B. THE ACETABULUM:
1. The acetabular cavity is shallow and triangular in shape.
2. The ossific centre for the roof of the acetabulum is late to develop. The postero-superior quadrant of the acetabular margin (i.e. shelf) is, therefore, poorly developed.
3. This shelf slopes upwards at a steep angle, instead of forming a nearly horizontal roof for the acetabulum. Thus, there is a change in the direction of the acetabulum, which instead of being directed downwards, is directed anterolaterally.
4. The cavity of the acetabulum is filled up considerably with fibrofatty tissues.
5. The head of the femur, being dislocated upwards and backwards, may make a new acetabulum in this situation, in the long-standing cases.

C. THE FEMORAL HEAD:
1. The bony head of the femur appears late, looks smaller, and sometimes becomes wedge-shaped.
2. The cartilagenous head grows normally and may even be bigger than normal.

D. THE FEMORAL NECK:
1. It is shortened.
2. It is anteverted (beyond the normal angle for infants, which is 25 degrees). This anteversion is of great importance while considering treatment of the disease.

II. Changes in the Soft Tissues

1. The acetabular labrum is often increased in size, sometimes considerably, so that it is folded and pushed into the acetabular cavity. This folded portion, which is called 'limbus', may sometimes hinder reduction of the dislocation.
2. The capsule of the hip joint, in contrast to traumatic dislocations, keeps intact. So, for the dislocation to occur, the capsule is elongated considerably. Anteriorly, where the psoas major crosses the capsule, there is a constriction in the capsule, so that it has an hour-glass shape. This again may be an obstacle to reduction.

3. The ligamentum teres femoris is often hypertrophied, sometimes considerably, and this also may be a hindrance to reduction.
4. The muscles are adaptively shortened:
   a. The adductors and the psoas major are shortened, and these (particularly the adductors) may be causing difficulty in reduction.
   b. The hamstrings, being shortened, may hinder complete extension of the knee after reduction has been done (and this is a confirmatory test for successful reduction).
5. The hip abductors, originating on the ilium and getting inserted into the greater trochanter,—particularly the gluteus medius, which is the strongest abductor— cannot work efficiently because the origin and insertion of these muscles have come close to each other. This is manifested as positive Trendelenburg's sign and a Trendelenburg's gait.

[A positive *Trendelenburg's sign* (and a Trendelenburg's gait) indicates defect in the abduction mechanism of the hip. In eliciting this test, it should be remembered that the limb, on which the patient is asked to stand, has the hip which is being tested, though the observations are based on the level of the opposite hip.

When a person stands on one leg, the weight of the opposite lower limb is transmitted to the standing limb by way of the pelvis, which must be raised on that side in which the limb is off the ground. This is done by drawing the pelvis downwards, towards the greater trochanter, on the standing side. This again is made possible by the contraction of the abductors, particularly the gluteus medius, of this side—the insertion of the muscles being fixed at the greater trochanter, the contraction of the muscles draws the ilium downwards, towards the greater trochanter.

When the abduction mechanism on the standing side is inefficient, the pelvis on the other side, instead of being elevated, sinks down. This is positive Trendelenburg's test.

The conditions under which such failure of abduction mechanism may occur are:—
a. Paralysis of the abductors.—Anterior poliomyelitis, muscular dystrophy.
b. Conditions in which the origin and insertion of the abductors, i.e. the pelvis and the greater trochanter, are approximated to each other, so that the greater trochanter touches the pelvis early in the process of abduction, making no further abduction possible.—Coxa vara and conditions producing a coxa vara deformity.
c. Deficiency of the fulcrum on which abduction occurs.— Dislocation of the hip, congenital or acquired.
d. Discontinuity of the lever on which abduction occurs.—Fracture of the femoral neck.
e. Painful condition in the abductors.—Any inflammatory condition, acute or chronic].

Etiology.—The disease is commoner 7 to 9 times in the *females.*

About one-third of the cases are *bilateral* and girls are 9 times common sufferers than boys in the bilateral cases.

In 20 per cent of cases there is a *familial* history.

The cause of the condition is still unknown. The one constant feature in the pathology is a shallow acetabulum with a steep roof. Controversy exists as to whether this is primary and is the cause of the dislocation or this is secondary to the dislocation because pressure of the head is important in making the depth of the acetabulum and here this pressure is absent. The following theories are put forward as to the cause of the disease:

1. *Genetically determined joint laxity.*—The patient's relatives may have either dislocated hips or other types of hypermobile joints (in 20 per cent of cases there is a familial history of CDH).

2. *Hormonal joint laxity.*—A ligament-relaxing hormone called 'relaxin', secreted by the gravid uterus, crosses the placental barrier to enter the foetus. If the hormonal environment of the foetus is also female, relaxin acts on the joints of the foetus in the same way as it does on those of the mother, to produce joint laxity (the disease is commoner, 7 to 9 times, in the females).

3. *Genetically determined dysplasia of the hip.*—There is a defect in the development of the acetabulum, particularly the roof. This view is largely discarded now because, in the newborn infant with CDH, both the acetabulum and the femoral head are found to be of normal shape and size. Moreover, an adequate roof almost always forms after reduction of CDH.

4. *Breech malposition of the foetus.*—The infant is either delivered in the breech position or spends the major part of the last 2 months in utero in breech presentation. In this position the uterine pressure tends to rotate the limbs in such a way that favours dislocation, particularly if the hip ligaments are already lax (as in 1 or 2).

Clinical Features.—Since very early diagnosis (i.e. immediately after birth) gives an excellent prospect of cure and since the prognosis worsens progressively with delay in starting treatment, all infants should be routinely examined, immediately after birth, for presence of CDH. This is particularly so for infants in whom there is a family history of the disease, and more so in the girls.

Symptoms

I. Unilateral case:

1. Asymmetry of the skin creases, particularly those at the groins and the thighs, together with asymmetry of the gluteal folds. Commonly these are the features that draw the first attention of the parents.

2. One leg looks shorter than the other.

3. As abduction is restricted, the mother may experience difficulties in putting the baby's napkins.

4. The mother may notice the hip-clicks on movements.

5. Sometimes late walking is complained of.

6. After walking starts, the dipping gait (i.e. Trendelenburg's gait) is noticed—there is a painless limp.

II. Bilateral cases:

These cases often pass unnoticed because the only presenting feature is a 'waddling gait', which is often mistaken by the parents as normal toddling.

Physical Signs

I. UNILATERAL CASES:

A. *Inspection*
1. A Trendelenburg's gait is seen and Trendelenburg's test is positive.
2. Asymmetry of the skin creases—the groin crease is most significant.
3. The pelvis looks a little wider on the affected side.
4. The affected lower limb looks slightly short and may be rotated outwards a little.
5. The normal fullness of the femoral triangle is missing because of absence of the femoral head in the normal position.

B. *Palpation*
1. The head cannot be felt in its socket.
2. A bony lump, possibly the head, may be felt in the buttock, under cover of the glutei.

C. *Movements*
1. A telescopic movement may be elicited in the hip.
2. Abduction, particularly abduction in flexion, is restricted. Normally this is possible up to 90 degrees in an infant. In CDH it stops halfway, and a little pressure may make the remaining abduction possible after a click is heard. The click is due to the re-entry of the dislocated head into the acetabulum and is called *Ortolani's click of entry*. This is diagnostic.
3. *Barlow's Sign (von Rosen's Sign):* This sign is of particular value in diagnosing the disease in the newborn, when no other symptom or sign is detectable. The surgeon holds the upper femur, between the middle finger placed on the greater trochanter and the thumb placed in the groin. By levering the femoral head in and out of the acetabulum, the examining hand experiences of peculiar sensation of an abnormal posterior movement plus a distinct 'click', as the femoral head leaves the acetabulum.

   This test is demonstrable only when the hip is 'dislocatable' and is not actually 'dislocated'. When 'dislocation' has already occurred, the Ortolani's test, as described above, can be elicited.

D. *Measurements*
1. There is a true shortening .of the limb.
2. The tip of the greater trochanter is above the 'Nelaton's line'. This is a straight line drawn from the most prominent point of the ischial tuberosity to the anterior superior iliac spine. Normally the tip of the greater trochanter just touches this line.

II. BILATERAL CASES:

The physical signs may be difficult to be demonstrated because comparison with the normal cannot be made. However, the following points are suggestive:
1. A wide perineal gap.
2. The pelvis is abnormally wide on both sides.
3. The normal fullness of the femoral triangle on both the sides is missing because of absence of the femoral heads in position.
4. The femoral heads may be felt in the buttocks, under the glutei.
5. The movement of abduction in flexion on both the sides is restricted. Ortolani's test or Barlow's test may be positive on both the sides.

°

6. Telescopic movement may be elicited in both the hips.

7. The greater trochanter is above the Nelaton's line on both the sides.

X-ray

1. The head of the femur appears smaller and is sometimes deformed.

2. In older children the dislocation is obvious—the epiphysis of the head is displaced upwards and outwards.

3. The 'Shenton's line' is interrupted (this line consists of a continuous curve, produced by the inferior margin of the superior pubic ramus and the medial cortex of the femoral neck and shaft).

4. Till the ossific nucleus of the head is well-developed, diagnosis on the X-ray may be difficult. The following signs are useful:

   a. *Perkin's Line or Perkin's Square.*—On each side a line is dropped vertically downwards from the upper outer end of the acetabulum. A transverse line is now drawn, joining the central points of the triradiate cartilage of the two sides and this is prolonged outwards. In a normal case, the epiphysis of the femoral head lies medial to the vertical line and below the transverse line. In cases of CDH:

      i. In earlier cases, the head lies lateral to the vertical line but still below the transverse line.

      ii. In more advanced cases, the head lies lateral to the vertical line and above the transverse line.

   b. *Wiberg's Angle or Acetabular Angle.*—The angle between the roof of the acetabulum and a transverse line passing through the centre of the triradiate cartilage is normally 20°. In CDH, where the acetabular roof is steep, the angle increases to about 45°.

   c. *Von Rosen's Lines.*—These are the best guide for the newborn babies. An X-ray is taken with both the hips abducted to 45° and internally rotated. The line of the femoral shaft is prolonged upwards on both the sides. On the normal side the line passes through the hollow of the acetabulum, while on the dislocated side it strikes the pelvis above the top of the acetabulum.

5. A lateral view of the hip may be helpful in determining anteversion of the neck.

6. An arthrogram may be useful in suggesting obstacles to reduction (vide below).

Treatment.—The earlier the treatment is started, the better is the prognosis and easier the management. Best results are obtained if treatment is started immediately after birth. The cases may be considered under three headings:

1. *Before the age of weight-bearing.*—It should be remembered that weight-bearing starts right when the child begins to crawl (i.e. at about 6 months) and not when it begins walking (i.e. about 12 to 18 months). So this group includes cases from immediately after birth to the age of 6 months.

2. *From the age of weight-bearing to the age limit (see below).*

3. *After the age limit.*—This is the age after which not only reduction is extremely difficult but also attempts to reduce merely worsens the condition. The age limit is 7 years for the unilateral cases. Manipulation after this age makes a painless condition painful. Hence the patient should be allowed to keep as such,

till he develops pain due to osteoarthritis, which is seldom below the age of 30 years (this means that he has only a limp but that is painless during the period of 7 to 30 years).

In bilateral cases the age limit is still lower, i.e. 4 years, which means that after the age of 4 years, the child should be left as such. The age limit is lower in the bilateral cases because:

a. The deformity is less apparent. Instead of the dipping gait found in the unilateral cases, there is simply a waddling gait, which is more tolerable.

b. Pain develops much later in the bilateral cases—rarely before the age of 45 years—so that the patient can spend a long painless life. Even at this age the pain is not in the hip but in the back, and this is moderately controllable by a corset and physiotherapy.

c. There is a chance that treatment may be more successful in one hip than in the other so that a bilateral dislocation is converted into an unilateral one (which is less tolerable).

I. Treatment Before the Age of Weight-Bearing

Close manipulation, without anaesthesia, is usually successful. This can easily be done by abducting the affected leg. After reduction, the limb has to be kept in abduction and there are various devices by which abduction can be maintained, e.g. Putti's diverticular, Denis Browne splint, von Rosen's aluminium splint, etc. Abduction has to be maintained till X-ray shows the formation of a good acetabular roof, usually a matter of 6 to 9 months.

II. Treatment After the Age of Weight-Bearing but Before the Age Limit

A. Closed reduction, under anaesthesia, is tried first. To achieve reduction, the hip is widely abducted (to stretch the abductors), and then flexed. Thereafter, the thigh is pushed upwards in an attempt to put the head in the socket, and this is conveniently assisted by manipulation of the head from the buttock. The procedure requires considerable manipulations that may cause damage of blood supply to the femoral head. This results in Perthes' disease, which occurs in 25 per cent of these cases.

To minimise this complication, a preliminary traction is applied to the limb, in gradually-increasing abduction, for about 4 weeks. Thereafter, reduction by close manipulation is usually easy.

After reduction, immobilisation in plaster has to be done with both the hips abducted to 90° and the thighs brought to the coronal plane of the body, i.e. the *frog position*. X-ray check-up is done every three months and the plaster has to be kept till X-ray shows that the acetabular roof has been well-formed. During X-ray, everytime, the plaster is changed, reducing the abduction to some extent. Since such a plaster is troublesome, some surgeons advocate plaster immobilisation for only 6 weeks, after which the plaster is replaced by special splints, which keep the hips in the coronal plane but allow considerable movements. This latter method is gaining fast popularity.

B. Operative treatment has to be undertaken where closed reduction fails. Failure to reduce by closed methods may be due to:

a. The limbus.

b. The hour-glass contracture of the capsule.

c. The hypertrophied ligamentum teres femoris and the fibrofatty tissue that fills up the acetabulum.

d. Contracture of the psoas and the adductors. The different operative procedures are as follows:

1. *Open reduction.*

2. *Rotation osteotomy of the femur.*—At open reduction, it may be found that, unless the hip is kept in considerable internal rotation, the head tends to come out. In these cases, either at the operation of open reduction or at a subsequent stage, a rotation osteotomy has to be done. An intertrochanteric osteotomy is done. Above the level of the osteotomy the hip is allowed to remain internally rotated but below the osteotomy the femur is externally rotated, till the toes look forwards. The position is maintained by internal fixation.

3. *Shelf operation.*— If it is found during open reduction, or subsequently, that the acetabular roof is not well-formed, this operation may be undertaken (either during open reduction or subsequently). The ilium is cut through, a little above the acetabulum, and then levered down to form the acetabular roof. The gap in the ilium, thus made, is filled by bone chips.

4. *Pelvic osteotomy.*—This gives a better acetabular roof than the shelf operation. The innominate bone is cut through above the acetabulum, up to the sciatic notch. The lower fragment is levered down, to form the acetabular roof. A tibial graft is put in the gap of the osteotomy.

III. Treatment After the Age Limit

A. ORTHODOX TREATMENT.—No active treatment is advocated till symptoms of osteoarthritis set in:

1. For unilateral cases arthrodesis, arthroplasty or osteotomy has to be undertaken for the painful osteoarthritis.

2. In bilateral cases the low back pain is usually amenable to spinal braces and physiotherapy.

B. MODERN TREATMENT.—In recent days arthroplasty of different types (e.g. Colonna's operation) are being tried in patients who are above the age limit but have not yet developed pain, i.e. before the onset of osteoarthritis.

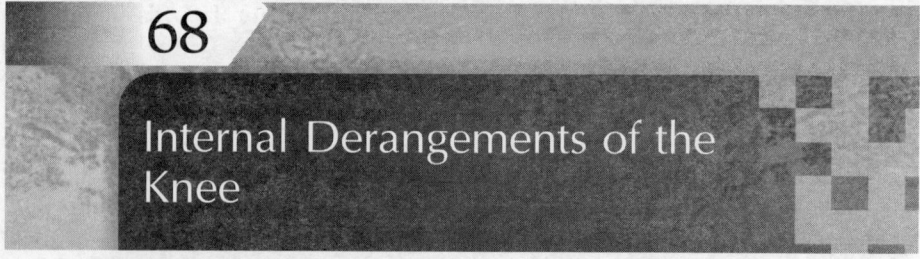

68

Internal Derangements of the Knee

These include the different intra-articular lesions in the knee, resulting from trauma.

I. LIGAMENTS:
A. Injury to the collateral ligaments:
  1. Medial.
  2. Lateral.
B. Injury to the cruciate ligaments:
  1. Anterior.
  2. Posterior.
II. CARTILAGE: Injury to the semilunar cartilages:
  1. Medial.
  2. Lateral.
III. FAT: Injury to the infra-patellar pad of fat.
IV. SYNOVIAL MEMBRANE: Traumatic synovitis (with thickening of the synovial fringes).
V. BONE: Fracture of the tibial spine.
VI. LOOSE BODIES of traumatic origin.

INJURY TO THE COLLATERAL LIGAMENTS

Trauma
1. The *lateral ligament* is torn by forcible adduction of the tibia on the femur.
2. Injury of the *medial ligament* may occur as follows:
  a. The superficial fibres are torn by forcible abduction of the extended knee, the ligament being usually torn at its bony attachment on the femur.
  b. The deeper fibres are torn as a result of rotational strain on the flexed knee (usually with an associated injury to the medial semilunar cartilage, which is attached to this part of the ligament).

Medial collateral ligament is much more frequently injured than the lateral because the knee is more commonly struck on its lateral than on its medial aspect.

Types
1. Sprain or partial rupture.
2. Complete rupture.

Clinical Features
1. *Swelling* of the knee, due to effusion.
2. *Pain*:
  a. Passive abduction causes pain on the medial side of the knee in cases of medial collateral ligament injury.

b. Passive adduction similarly produces pain on the lateral side of the knee in lateral ligament injury.

3. *Tenderness:*

   a. In ordinary medial ligament injury, the exact point of tenderness is at the femoral attachment of the ligament.

   b. In cases of injury only to the deeper fibres of the medial collateral ligament, the tenderness is on the ligament at the level of the joint, without any tenderness at its bony attachment. (In such cases there is often an associated injury to the medial semilunar cartilage).

   c. In cases of injury to the lateral collateral ligament, the tenderness is somewhere along the ligament, more commonly towards its fibular attachment.

4. *Instability* of the joint in the extended position may sometimes be complained of in cases of complete rupture.

Treatment

1. CONSERVATIVE TREATMENT.—This is the usual method. This consists of:

   a. Aspiration of the haemarthrosis (i.e. collection of blood in the joint).

   b. Immobilisation in a tube cast for 6 weeks. This means a complete plastering, extending from the upper thigh to just above the ankle, with the knee in 10° flexion. The patient walks but the knee is supported by the plaster.

   c. Active quadriceps exercises thereafter.

2. OPERATIVE TREATMENT.—Repair of the ligament, followed by immobilization, is advocated:

   a. If there is gross instability,

   b. If associated lesions in the joint are suspected.

   c. As a matter of preference by some surgeons.

PELLEGRINI—STIEDA'S DISEASE

This is a condition in which irregular ossification occurs in a haematoma between the medial collateral ligament and its femoral attachment, resulting from incomplete avulsion of the ligament. Diagnosis is made on X-ray.

Treatment consists of active exercises.

INJURY TO THE CRUCIATE LIGAMENTS

Trauma.—The violence must be severe. The injury may be as follows:

1. *In association with injuries to the collateral ligaments.*—Wide abduction or adduction of the knee that is required to cause complete rupture of the medial or lateral collateral ligament of the knee cannot occur as long as the cruciate ligaments are intact. Therefore, many of the cases of collateral ligament injury (medial or lateral) are associated with injury to the cruciate ligaments.

2. *Isolated injuries of the cruciate ligaments:*

   a. The *anterior* cruciate ligament is torn by a force driving the upper end of the tibia *forwards* relative to the femur (forcible hyperextension of the knee).

   b. The *posterior* ligament is torn by a force driving the upper end of the tibia *backwards* (tibia stuck with the knee flexed).

Clinical Diagnosis

1. In anterior cruciate ligament tear there is an abnormal *forward* mobility of the tibia on the femur.

2. In posterior ligament tear there is an abnormal *backward* mobility.

Treatment.—This is usually conservative because operative reconstruction seldom produces better results. The lines of treatment are:

1. Aspiration of haemarthrosis.

2. Plaster immobilisation for 6 weeks.

3. Active quadriceps exercises thereafter. The laxity of the joint is easily overcome by powerful muscles.

FRACTURE (AVULSION) OF THE TIBIAL SPINE

The tibial spine may be avulsed, instead of the cruciate ligaments being injured, in some cases. The bone fragment may be displaced upwards from its bed. The characteristic physical signs are:

1. Tenderness beneath the ligamentum patellae.

2. Bony-block to complete extension of the knee (c.f. elastic block found in tears of semilunar cartilage).

   Diagnosis is confirmed by *X-ray*.

Anatomy.—The attachments at the top of the tibia, *from before backwards*, are:—

1. Medial meniscus (anterior horn).

2. Anterior cruciate ligament.

3. Lateral meniscus (anterior horn).

4. Lateral meniscus (posterior horn).

5. Medial meniscus (posterior horn).

6. Posterior cruciate ligament.

INJURY TO THE SEMILUNAR CARTILAGES (MENISCI)

The medial semilunar cartilage is injured much more commonly than the lateral (20 : 1), because it is attached to the medial collateral ligament (the lateral meniscus is free). The medial cartilage is semilunar in shape, with the ends separated from one another. The lateral cartilage is nearly circular in outline, with the ends close to each other.

Mechanism—A meniscus is torn by a rotational force, grinding it between the femur and the tibia:

1. The knee must be flexed since rotation cannot occur when the knee is extended.

2. The knee must be weight-bearing.

3. The injury is caused by a rotational strain on this flexed, weight-bearing knee:

   a. The medial meniscus is injured if the femur is internally rotated on the tibia or the tibia externally rotated on the femur.

b. The lateral meniscus is injured by external rotation of the femur on the tibia or internal rotation of the tibia on the femur.

Thus, these injuries usually occur in footballers, but they may also occur in people who work in a squatting position, e.g. coal-miners.

4. A forcible abduction during the rotational strain helps in causing injury to the medial meniscus. The inner side of the joint is opened up and this exerts a suction influence on the cartilage (due to negative pressure). The cartilage is drawn inwards between the condyles of the tibia and femur, which injure it.

5. Occasionally a cartilage (particularly the lateral) is discoid in shape instead of being semilunar. Such cartilages are more prone to injury.

6. Tears can occur with less force in middle life when fibrosis has limited the normal mobility of the cartilage.

Types of Tear.—There are 3 types, but all begin as a longitudinal split (a transverse tear is always artefact):

1. If the longitudinal tear extends along the whole length of the meniscus it is a *bucket-handle tear*.
2. If the initial longitudinal tear emerges at the concave border of the cartilage, there is formation of a pedunculated tag:
   a. In *posterior horn* tear the tag or fragment remains attached at the posterior horn.
   b. In *anterior horn* tear it remains attached at the anterior horn.

Progress and Effects

1. Following the original tear, progressive damage to the meniscus is common.
2. The torn portion, if displaced, may become jammed between the femur and the tibia. Since the femoral condyle is so shaped that it requires maximum space when the knee is straight, the chief ill-effect of the displaced fragment is that it limits full extension (i.e. *locking*). Such displacement and locking is particularly likely to occur with a 'bucket-handle' tear.
3. The knee may subsequently be prone to *giving way*. This denotes a condition in which the knee suddenly flexes under the patient. Its causes are:
   a. The torn meniscus.
   b. Damage to the 'mechano-receptors' in the capsule of the knee, upon whose normal activity the co-ordination of the thigh muscles depends.
   c. Quadriceps weakness due to wasting.
4. A meniscus is avascular and hence incapable of repair (unless the tear is peripheral). After excision, partial regeneration may occur but the new meniscus has a blood supply.
5. A meniscus is avascular and so, when it is torn, there is no haemarthrosis. However, a synovial effusion occurs, and this results in swelling of the knee.
6. Recurrent displacement of the torn fragment may lead to osteoarthritis of the joint.

Symptoms

1. Following a typical rotational strain, the patient:
   a. Falls.

b. Gets an acute pain at the antero-medial aspect of the knee, and is unable to continue with what he was doing.

c. Is unable to straighten the knee, i.e. there is 'locking'. This occurs particularly with bucket-handle tear. By 'locking' is meant inability to extend the knee fully. It is not a 'jamming' because flexion is unrestricted.

d. Gets a swelling in the knee after a few hours.

2. The pain and the swelling gradually disappear. But, within weeks or months, the knee suddenly 'gives way' again during a twisting strain, and symptoms appear as before. Similar incidents occur repeatedly and with relatively little force.

3. Between the acute phases, the knees may either be normal or be prone to two sequelae:

a. Locking.

b. Giving way.

Physical Signs of Torn Medial Meniscus

1. Swelling.—Only in the acute phase.

2. Tenderness:

a. At a definite point at the joint level, midway between the ligamentum patellae and the medial collateral ligament—in case of anterior horn tear.

b. At a point posterior to the medial collateral ligament—in case of posterior horn tear.

c. On the medial collateral ligament—in cases of central or 'bucket-handle' tear.

The best way of eliciting tenderness is to exert gentle pressure at the above points with the knee flexed. If the joint is now slowly extended, the patient feels pain because the torn cartilage comes in contact with the pressing finger.

3. Limitation of last few degrees of extension in many cases of 'bucket-handle' tear.

4. Wasting of the quadriceps.—This may be the only feature in the 'silent' phase.

5. *Mc Murray's Test.*—The patient lies recumbent. The surgeon holds the foot firmly with the knee completely flexed (so that the heel touches the buttock), and does the following movements:

a. The foot is externally rotated.

b. The leg is abducted at the knee.

c. The knee is slowly extended.

With these movements if (i) there is a definite click and (ii) the patient complains of a pain similar to what he experiences every time the knee gives way, the diagnosis is certain. The more anteriorly located the tear is, the click will occur in the more extended position of the knee.

6. *Apley's Grinding Test.*—The patient lies prone. The surgeon puts his own knee on the patient's thigh to fix the femur. He now applies compression and lateral rotation to the leg from the foot (i.e. grinding). If this causes pain, there is a tear of the medial meniscus.

Physical Signs of Torn Lateral Meniscus

The signs are less clearly defined. Tenderness is on the lateral side. While the Mc Murray's test is elicited, the foot should be internally rotated.

X-ray.—There is no abnormality.

Treatment
1. If the diagnosis is certain, meniscectomy, i.e. excision of the meniscus, has to be undertaken. Otherwise recurrent attacks occur and also osteoarthritis supervenes.
2. If the diagnosis cannot be made with certainty, quadriceps exercises, in order to build up the thigh muscles, are advocated. If symptoms suggestive of cartilage injury persist, the knee is explored.
3. If the knee is locked, manipulation under anaesthesia is the standard practice. Later, meniscectomy is undertaken.

DISCOID MENISCUS

This is a true congenital condition and is found almost entirely in the lateral meniscus, very rarely in the medial. Its importances are:
1. It may produce pain on the lateral side of the knee.
2. It is more prone to undergo tear than a normal shaped semilunar cartilage. This is because the meniscus is constantly grinded between the femur and the tibia.
3. It may cause a peculiar loud 'click', which can be felt and heard during the terminal phase of active extension of the knee.
4. It may require excision when producing symptoms.

CYSTS OF SEMILUNAR CARTILAGE

Pathology.—These result from myxomatous degeneration occurring in the substance of the cartilage itself. The lateral meniscus is involved much more frequently than the medial (20 : 1).

Cause.—The cause is unknown but there is often a history of direct injury at the site of the cyst.

Clinical Features
1. The swelling is located at the level of the joint, usually anterior to the lateral (or medial) collateral ligament.
2. The swelling is somewhat more prominent when the knee is held slightly flexed.
3. It is so tense that fluctuation cannot be elicited. Often it has a bony hard consistency.
4. It is tender on pressure and may cause pain, worse at night.
5. It is a self-limiting condition and may undergo spontaneous regression after a number of years.

Treatment.—Excision of the cyst together with the meniscus. Simple excision of the cyst almost invariably results in recurrence.

INJURY TO INFRAPATELLAR PAD OF FAT

A hypertrophic pad of fat may be nipped between the femur and the tibia during extension of the knee. The characteristic features are:
1. Sudden pain and locking *without* being followed by so sudden unlocking (c.f. loose body and cartilage injury).
2. Tenderness on both the sides of ligamentum patellae.

LOOSE BODIES IN THE KNEE JOINT

Causes and Origin

A. INJURY:

1. Piece of bone or cartilage, broken off by a single definite trauma (including avulsed tibial spine).

2. Portion of torn meniscus.

3. Osteochondritis dissecans (i.e. transchondral fracture), in which the fracture line runs entirely in the articular bone (i.e. bone covered by articular cartilage). In this condition the overlying cartilage, all round the fracture, also breaks and the osteocartilagenous piece makes a loose body.

4. Chipped off articular cartilage.

5. Fibrinous loose bodies, following haemarthrosis.

B. DEGENERATION:

1. In osteoarthritis
   a. Osteophytes.
   b. Synovial villi.
   c. Flakes of articular cartilage.

2. In Charcot's disease large loose bodies may form.

C. INFLAMMATION.—Melon-seed bodies in tubercular synovitis.

D. IDIOPATHIC.—A synovial villus may undergo hypertrophy and get pedunculated. A cartilagenous nodule forms at its bulbous tip. A wide area of the synovium may be affected this way and the cartilagenous nodules may get detached to lie in the joint. This condition is called *chondromatosis*. When these nodules are calcified, the condition is known as *osteochondromatosis.* These are the conditions in which innumerable loose bodies (as many as 700) may form.

Presenting Features

1. Locking of the joint (recurrent). The angle at which locking occurs may differ from time to tome.

2. Severe pain during locking.

3. The patient may sometimes point out the loose body.

X-ray.—Only osseous loose bodies can be diagnosed on X-ray. These may have to be differentiated from:

a. Fabella.—A sesamoid bone in the lateral head of the gastrocnemius (slightly above the joint line, well posterolateral to femur, oval in shape with long axis vertical).

b. Pellegrini-Stieda's disease (*see* above).

Treatment.—A loose body, causing symptoms, should be removed, unless the joint is severely osteoarthritic.

CHRONICALLY SWOLLEN KNEE

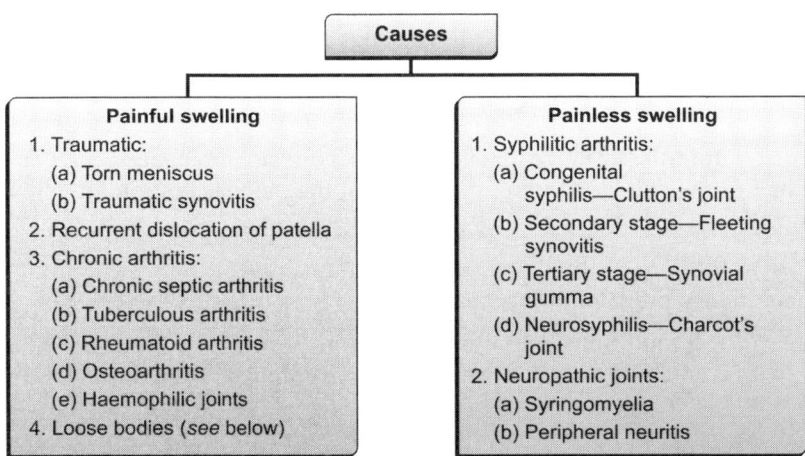

Causes

Painful swelling	Painless swelling
1. Traumatic:	1. Syphilitic arthritis:
(a) Torn meniscus	(a) Congenital syphilis—Clutton's joint
(b) Traumatic synovitis	(b) Secondary stage—Fleeting synovitis
2. Recurrent dislocation of patella	(c) Tertiary stage—Synovial gumma
3. Chronic arthritis:	(d) Neurosyphilis—Charcot's joint
(a) Chronic septic arthritis	2. Neuropathic joints:
(b) Tuberculous arthritis	(a) Syringomyelia
(c) Rheumatoid arthritis	(b) Peripheral neuritis
(d) Osteoarthritis	
(e) Haemophilic joints	
4. Loose bodies (*see below*)	

BURSAE AROUND THE KNEE

Anatomy .—Numerous bursae, some of which communicate with the interior of the joint, lie in relation to the tendons around the knee. They are as follows:

A. *Anterior.*
1. Suprapatellar bursa.
2. (Subcutaneous) prepatellar bursa.
3. Subcutaneous infrapatellar bursa.
4. Deep infrapatellar bursa.

B. *Posterolateral:*
1. Bursa between the lateral head of the gastrocnemius and the capsule of the joint.
2. Bursa between the biceps femoris tendon and the lateral collateral ligament of the knee.
3. Popliteal recess—A protrusion of synovial membrane of the knee, situated between the popliteus tendon and the lateral condyle of tibia.

C. *Posteromedial:*
1. Bursa between the medial head of gastrocnemius and the capsule of the joint (frequently communicating with the joint).
2. Bursa (frequently communicating with the above bursa) situated between the medial head of the gastrocnemius and the semimembranosus tendon.
3. 'Anserine' bursa—This is a bursa of irregular form, separating the tendons of sartorius, gracilis and semitendinosus, from one another as well as from the medial collateral ligament of the knee.

Involvement.—Many of the above bursae may give rise to swellings around the knee joint, as follows:
1. Suprapatellar Bursa, which always communicates with the joint, may become distended in case of any effusion in the joint.
2. Subcutaneous Prepatellar Bursa may undergo inflammation (bursitis), i.e. *Housemaid's knee.*

3. Subcutaneous Infrapatellar Bursa may undergo inflammation, i.e. *Clergyman's knee.*

4. Semimembranous Bursa, i.e. the bursa situated between the medial head of the gastrocnemius and the semimembranosus tendon, may become distended.

5. Anserine Bursa may sometimes get distended.

Prepatellar Bursitis.—The prepatellar bursa, lying subcutaneous, in front of the lower half of the patella and the upper part of the patellar tendon, may undergo inflammation. The bursitis may be of two types:

1. Irritative prepatellar bursitis.

2. Inflammatory prepatellar bursitis.

Either of the conditions commonly occurs in people who do much kneeling, e.g. carpet layers, miners and housemaids (hence the condition is also known as housemaid's knee).

IRRITATIVE PREPATELLAR BURSITIS.—This is caused by continuous friction of the bursa between the skin and the patella. The swelling is circumscribed and fluctuant. The joint is normal.

TREATMENT:
a. Conservative Treatment.—Aspiration, firm bandaging, and avoiding kneeling.
b. Operative Treatment.—Excision of the bursa may have to be done in recurrent cases.

INFLAMMATORY PREPATELLAR BURSITIS.—This results from infection with pyogenic organisms (possibly due to foreign body implantation).

Treatment consists in administration of antibiotics and, if there is suppuration, incision for drainage.

Subcutaneous Infrapatellar Bursitis.—The infrapatellar bursa is located at a lower level than the prepatellar bursa, i.e. superficial to the patellar ligament. Irritative bursitis of this bursa results from kneeling, as in clergymen (hence called Clergyman's knee). In clergymen this bursa is involved rather than the prepatellar bursa (as in the housemaids) because one who prays kneels more uprightly than one who scrubs.

Rarely the bursa is affected in gout or syphilis.

Treatment is the same as for irritative prepatellar bursitis.

Semimembranous Bursitis.—This bursa lies between the medial head of the gastrocnemius and the semimembranosus tendon.

It may become distended with fluid in children or adults, and present as a swelling.

CLINICAL FEATURES
1. The swelling is painless.
2. It is situated behind the knee, close to the medial condyle of the femur (the sac bulges backwards between the muscle planes).
3. It is more prominent with the knee straight.
4. It is fluctuant.

5. The swelling is irreducible. The fluid cannot be pushed into the joint, though the bursa communicates with the joint, presumably because the muscles compress and obstruct the normal communication.
6. The knee joint is normal.

TREATMENT
1. Often no treatment is required. The condition is self-limiting and the swelling may spontaneously regress after a few years.
2. Aspiration, followed by firm bandaging, may be helpful.
3. Excision of the swelling may have to be undertaken:
   a. If the swelling becomes uncomfortably large.
   b. If it aches.
   The excision is done with a transverse incision.

Morrant Baker's Cyst.—A Baker's cyst is simply a herniation of the synovial cavity of the knee. It is not a primary condition and is always secondary to persistent effusion in the knee, the commonest condition being osteoarthritis. The sac extends backwards and downwards and, in a long-standing case, may extend for a considerable distance downwards—even to the calf.

CLINICAL FEATURES
1. There is a swelling, near the midline, behind the knee (or in the upper calf).
2. It is fluctuant.
3. The condition is often bilateral.
4. The underlying abnormality in the knee (e.g. osteoarthritis), with the effusion, is usually obvious.

TREATMENT
1. Usually the primary treatment is the treatment for the underlying pathology, e.g. osteoarthritis.
2. If the cyst is very large, it should be excised.

GENU VALGUM (KNOCK-KNEE) AND GENU VARUM (BOW-LEG)

These two deformities occur most commonly in childhood. Of the two, knock-knee is a little more commoner.

In genu valgum the knee is angled inwards, the tibia being abducted in relation to the femur. With the knee straight, the two medial malleoli cannot be made to touch each other. The amount of deformity may be measured by noting the distance between the two malleoli.

In genu varum the knee and the leg are bowed outwards. The deformity may be measured by noting the distance between the two medial femoral condyles.

Causes

A. IDIOPATHIC OR PRIMARY—Majority of the cases belong to this group. The patient is a child and almost invariably the condition is bilateral. Almost always a spontaneous correction occurs.

B. SECONDARY:
   1. Trauma.—Malunited fracture of the lower part of the femur or upper part of the tibia.
   2. Bone softening.—Rickets, osteomalacia, Paget's disease.
   3. Stretched ligaments.—Charcot's disease, paralytic deformities.

4. Uneven growth of epiphyseal plates in children.—Following injury, osteomyelitis, dyschondroplasia.

Treatment

1. Spontaneous recovery almost always occurs by the age of 6 years, and simple reassurance to the parents is all that is necessary. No splintage or adjustment of footwear is of any value. If deformity persists after this age, active treatment has to be thought of.

2. Active treatment in persistent cases before the cessation of epiphyseal growth:
   a. Placing staples across the epiphyseal plates at the knee, on the convex side of the deformity, to retard growth on that side.
   b. *Epiphyseodesis.*—Excising the epiphysis on the convex side of the deformity and fusing the epiphysis to the metaphysis with a bone block.

3. Active treatment in persistent cases after growth is complete.— Correction can only be achieved by wedge osteotomy. The base of the wedge is placed towards the convex side of the deformity. A supracondylar osteotomy is done for genu valgum and an upper tibial osteotomy for genu varum.

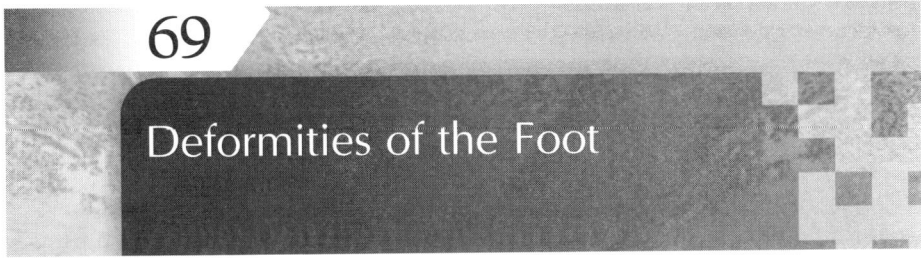

69

Deformities of the Foot

CLUB FOOT (TALIPES)

Nomenclature.—The term 'club foot' or 'talipes' applies to any abnormality in the shape of the foot. According to the nature of the deformity, the talipes is qualified as follows:

Equinus.—The foot is fixed in plantar flexion (and cannot be fully dorsiflexed).

Calcaneus.—The foot is fixed in the dorsiflexion (and cannot be fully plantar flexed).

Varus.—The foot is inverted (and cannot be fully everted). In addition, there is an adduction at the midtarsal joint.

Valgus.—The foot is everted (and cannot be fully inverted). In addition, there is an abduction at the midtarsal joint.

    In congenital club foot the deformities only rarely occur singly; usually they are found in combinations of *equinovarus* or *calcaneovalgus*. Talipes equinovarus is much the commoner variety of club foot. Talipes calcaneo-valgus is much easier to be corrected but, unfortunately, it is much less frequent than equinovarus.

TALIPES EQUINOVARUS

Causes

A. CONGENITAL.—The majority of the cases are congenital. The etiology of congenital talipes equinovarus is discussed below in details.

B. ACQUIRED:
    1. *Paralytic*
       a. Anterior poliomyelitis.
       b. Injury to the lateral popliteal nerve.
    2. *Muscular*
       a. Spastic.
       b. Dystrophy of peroneal muscles.
    3. *Traumatic*
       a. Due to scarring.
       b. Injury to lower tibial epiphysis.

Etiology of Congenital Talipes Equinovarus.—There are different views as to the etiology of congenital talipes equinovarus:

1. *Genetic Factor.*—There may be a genetic factor, at least in some cases, because the condition is occasionally familial.

2. *Dysplasia:*
    a. Majority of workers believe that the primary disturbance is a developmental

defect of the soft tissues, particularly affecting the ligaments on the concave side of the foot.

   b. Some workers believe that the primary disturbance is a developmental defect of the neck of the talus.

3. *Ischaemia.*—According to some authorities, the primary disturbance is in the muscles of the calf, which undergo some form of contractors, possibly due to ischaemia.

4. *Mechanical Factors.*—It is believed that the intrauterine pressure forces the lower limbs of the foetus against the uterine wall abnormally, moulding the feet in the position of deformity.

5. *Non-mechanical Factors.*—Certain drugs (e.g. thalidomide), taken by the mother, early in pregnancy, may cause multiple deformities in the foetus, including talipes.

Pathology

A. THE DEFORMITIES:

   1. *Equinus,* i.e. plantar flexion, occurs in all the bones of the foot, including the talus. Contrary to the popular belief, the talus is less plantar flexed than the other bones, and so the head of the talus dislocates progressively from the midtarsal joint in a dorsal and lateral direction.

   2. *Varus,* i.e. inversion of the calcaneum and the navicular on the talus.

   3. *Adduction.*—This occurs at the midtarsal and tarso metatarsal joints.

   4. *External rotation* of the bones of the forefoot is produced by torsion of the shafts of the metatarsals.

B. CHANGES IN THE BONES:

   1. The foot, as a whole, is smaller in size, i.e. less developed.

   2. The talus has a long neck, which is angulated, so that the head of the talus is displaced downwards and medially.

   3. The calcaneum is small, so that the heel is small.

   4. The navicular is articulated to the medial side of the talus.

   5. The metatarsal shafts are externally rotated.

C. CHANGES IN THE SOFT TISSUES:

   1. *Skin*:

      a. Callositis develop on the pressure points, particularly on the lateral margin of the dorsum, in front of the lateral malleolus.

      b. There is a deep crease on the plantar aspect, at the site of maximum angulation.

      c. Adaptive shortening on the concave side of the curve. This may cause difficulty in skin closure during operative treatment.

   2. *Muscles.*—The muscles on the concave side of the deformity are adoptively shortened but they .are histologically normal:

      a. The flexors of the foot, i.e. calf muscles with tendo Achilles.

      b. The inverters, viz. tibialis anterior and posterior.

      c. The flexors of the toes.

   3. *Ligaments and Capsule* on the concave side of the deformity, i.e. medial sides of the foot, and to some extent, those of the sole, are shortened.

   4. *Vessels and Nerves* under the flexor retinaculum are shortened.

Treatment

A. The Orthodox Principle of Treatment.— The principle of the treatment is to overcorrect the deformity and to hold the foot in she overcorrected position, till it is stable. The earlier the treatment is started, the easier it is to correct the deformity and the more are the chances of making it stable. The best results are obtained if treatment is started immediately after birth. The method of correction and holding depends largely on the age at which treatment is started:

1. MANIPULATION AND STRAPPING.—Up to the age of 2 months, correction can be achieved without anaesthesia. By manipulation, the deformity is corrected or, better, overcorrected. The position is maintained with the help of adhesive plasters, protecting the skin with felt (some surgeons incorporate a padded aluminium splint within the adhesive plaster to make immobilisation more perfect). The position is checked up every week and the strappings are changed. A long-continued treatment (at least for one year, better till the child begins to walk) is required since the foot has a notorious tendency to go back to the deformity. After the age of one year, if further immobilisation is required, the foot may be conveniently placed in reverse boot, i.e. the boot for a right foot is fitted to the left and vice versa. This reversion, by itself, corrects the deformity. Alternatively, after the age of one year, if further immobilisation is necessary, the foot may be fitted to a Denis Browne splint. Even when the child begins to walk, and strapping and immobilisation discarded, it is better that the feet are fitted to the Denis Browne splint at night.

2. WRENCHING AND PLASTERING.—After the age of two months, correction is not possible without anaesthesia; even with anaesthesia, full correction may not be possible at the first attempt. In these cases correction, as far as is practicable, is done under anaesthesia and the position is maintained in a plaster. The plaster should extend from above knee, with the knee bent (in children the plaster has otherwise a tendency to slip off the foot). Subsequently, every fortnight, a wedge of the plaster is removed from the convex side of the deformity, and the deformity is further corrected. These manipulations are done without anaesthesia and after each manipulation the plaster is reinforced. After several such manipulations a complete correction (or better, overcorrection) is achieved and, in this position, the plaster immobilisation is maintained for six months. Subsequently, a Denis Browne splint is used day and night, till the child begins to walk, and thereafter only at night. Alternatively, a 'reverse boot' may be advocated.

3. SOFT TISSUE OPERATIONS.—These are undertaken when correction by manipulation fails. Results are better if the operations are undertaken below the age of 5 years because, after this age, the structural bone deformities progress too far to be corrected by these operations, and bone operations have to be done. Different types of soft tissue operations are practised, the principles of which are detailed below:

   a. To correct the equinus deformity:
      i. The tendo Achilles is elongated by Z-plasty or other plastic procedures.
      ii. If, with the elongation of tendo Achilles as above, the equinus is not fully corrected, the posterior capsule of the ankle joint is divided.

b. To correct the varus and adduction deformities:

    i. *Perkin's Operation.*—Two parallel incisions are made on the medial side of the foot, below the medial malleolus, one on each side of the neurovascular bundle there. Through each incision all soft tissues, down to the bone (on the concave side of the deformity), are divided under direct vision. When the foot falls into a corrected position the wound is closed and an above-knee plaster applied for 6 months.

    ii. *Medial Release.*—As in Perkin's operation, all the soft tissues on the concave side of the deformity are cut through under direct vision. Simultaneously, the tendons of tibialis anterior, tibialis posterior, flexor hallucis longus and flexor digitorum longus are elongated by Z-plasty.

    iii. *Tendon Transplantation.*—The tendon of tibialis posterior is erased off from its insertion at the medial side of the foot and is transferred through the interosseous membrane to the lateral side, where it is transplanted at the base of the fifth metatarsal. The muscle now supplements the action of the evertors.

    iv. While Perkin's operation or the 'medial release' operation is being undertaken, the tarsal bones are restored to their normal relationship, as far as practicable, particular attention being paid to the talus and the navicular.

4. Bone operations.—After the age of 5 years, *in addition to elongation of the soft tissues*, bone carpentry is essential because of the gross structural changes in the bones:

a. With the Perkin's operation or 'medial release' operation, excision of a lateral segment, including the calcaneocuboid joint, is done.

b. When the varus deformity is marked, osteotomy of the calcaneum is performed and a bone wedge is inserted on the medial side through the osteotomy.

c. After the age of 12 years, a tarsectomy has to be undertaken. The detailed anatomy of the foot is ignored and a wedge of bone of appropriate size, with its base dorsolaterally, is removed from the tarsus, so that when the resulting gap is closed by moulding, the foot becomes plantigrade.

B. **The New Approach to Treatment.**—According to recent thoughts, cases of talipes equinovarus belong to two distinct groups—'easy' and 'resistant'.

1. The 'easy' group.—These are the cases where:

a The calf muscles are well-developed.

b. The heel is neither very small nor very high.

c Within three weeks of starting the manipulation, overcorrection can be achieved.

In these cases manipulation and strapping, as advocated under the orthodox treatment, almost always produce fair results.

2. The 'resistant' group.—These are the cases where:

a. The calf muscles are wasted.

b. The heel is very small and/or very high.

c. Overcorrection cannot be achieved within three weeks of starting of manipulation.

These are the cases where The deformity is difficult to be corrected or it tends to recur even after correction and prolonged immobilisation. In these cases early soft tissue operations are advocated, before adaptive shortening of soft tissues and structural changes in the bone set in. Such operations are advised by the age of 3 to 6 weeks.

With a medial incision, the tendo Achilles is lengthened. Through the incision it is found out which soft tissues are causing obstacle to the correction of the foot. These tissues are either divided or (if they are tendons) elongated, the commonest structure being the tibialis posterior. The foot is held in plaster, in the overcorrected position, for 6 weeks.

FLATFOOT (PES PLANUS)

This is a condition in which there is flattening of the *longitudinal arch* of the foot. It is usually associated with a valgus deformity of the foot (i.e. twisting outwards).

At birth, the foot is always flat. The arches of the foot develop only when the child stands. The arches are maintained by:

 a. Shape of the bones.
 b. Ligaments.
 c. Muscles of the sole and the calf muscles.

Types

1. CONGENITAL FLATFOOT.—The arches have failed to develop.
2. INFANTILE FLATFOOT.—This is usually physiological. All infants have flatfoot for a year or two, which gets corrected spontaneously.
3. TRAUMATIC FLATFOOT.—This is caused by fractures which abolish the arch, e.g. Pott's fracture, fracture of the calcaneum.
4. IDIOPATHIC ADULT FLATFOOT.—This is the commonest type to cause symptoms (*see* below). The cause is unknown but is often believed to be due to repeated 'foot strain'. This is also known as *'relaxed flatfoot'*.
5. SPASTIC FLATFOOT.—This is caused by spasmodic contraction of the peroneal muscles.

Effects.—Simple presence of anatomical 'flatness' is of no importance. It is only when its harmful effects set in, that the condition demands correction. The effects of a fully established flatfoot may be as follows:

1. Loss of spring in the foot.—A shuffling gait.
2. Loss of shock-absorbing function, which leads to:
   a. Increased liability to trauma.
   b. Development of tarsal osteoarthritis.
3. Loss of space in the sole of the foot, leading to:
   a. Compression of the nerves.—Neuralgic pain.
   b. Compression of the vessels.—Coldness and vascular disturbances, in the toes.

Treatment

1. Arch-supports, moulded to the corrected shape of foot, are worn.
2. Exercises, to improve function of the muscles of sole and calf, are advised.

SPLAY FOOT

This is a condition of transverse flatfoot, which means that the *transverse arch* of the forefoot is dropped. Callosities tend to develop on the metatarsal heads, which are exposed to pressure.

CLAWFOOT (PES CAVUS)

In this condition there is an increased concavity of the arch of the foot, i.e. accentuation of the longitudinal arch. Thus, it is the reverse of flatfoot, and so known as *hollow foot*.

The condition is homologous to clawhand, and is similarly caused by paralysis of the interossei and lumbrical muscles, as in poliomyelitis, Friedreich's ataxia, etc. Many cases, however, are idiopathic.

HALLUX VALGUS

In hallux valgus the great toe is deviated laterally at the metatarsophalangeal joint.

Cause.—Not definitely known. The following factors are held responsible:
1. Congenital varus position of the first metatarsal.
2. Acquired.—Wearing narrow-pointed shoes, which force the great toe laterally (hence commoner in women, who usually wear narrow-pointed shoes).

Pathology.—As the condition progresses, the following secondary changes set in:
1. An exostosis develops on the medial side of the metatarsal head (possibly caused by pressure on the periosteum).
2. A "bunion" (inflamed adventitious bursa) forms over the medial prominence of the joint. This may become inflamed, occasionally suppurated. The bursa is the result of pressure and friction.

   Sometimes a similar lesion, called a 'bunionette', develops on the lateral side of the head of the fifth metatarsal.
3. Over-riding or under-riding of the second toe by the first.
4. Later, there is an osteoarthritis of the first metatarsophalangeal joint, consequent upon mal-alignment.
5. Once the valgus deformity has developed, the long tendons of the hallux are shifted laterally. As this shift occurs, the direction of pull of these tendons causes a 'bow-string' effect, increasing the deformity progressively.

Treatment

1. EXCISION ARTHROPLASTY.—This is the standard procedure. There are two varieties of operation:
   a. *Keller's Operation.*—This is the most widely practised procedure. An excision arthoplasty of the first metatarsophalangeal joint is performed by excising the proximal two-thirds of the proximal phalanx. The prominent portion of the metatarsal head is also trimmed.
   b. *Mayo's Operation.*—This is also an excision arthroplasly, in which the head of the first metatarsal is excised instead of the base of the proximal phalanx. The prominent portion of the proximal phalanx is trimmed.

2. ARTHRODESIS of the metatarsophalangeal joint is preferred by some surgeons to anthroplasty.

3. DISPLACEMENT OSTEOTOMY of the neck of the first metatarsal, in an attempt to correct the deformity and prevent its recurrence, is sometimes done for younger patients with relatively mild deformity.

4. CONSERVATIVE OPERATIONS:

   a. *Bunionectomy.*—Excising the bunion with the underlying knob of bone.

   b. Trimming of the exostosis.

   These conservative operations are unsatisfactory as recurrence is almost inevitable.

HALLUX RIGIDUS

The metatarsophalangeal joint of the great toe is stiff and painful. There are two distinct types:

1. ADOLESCENT TYPE.—Due to traumatic synovitis in the joint.

2. ADULT TYPE.—Due to osteoarthritis of the joint.

   The complaint of the patient is pain at the base of the great toe on walking.

Treatment

1. *Conservative:*

   a. Fitting a metatarsal bar beneath the sole of the shoe.

   b. Short-wave diathermy applied to the joint.

2. *Operative.*—Excision arthroplasty or arthrodesis (as in hallux valgus).

HAMMER TOE

This condition usually affects the second toe, but sometimes the third or fourth.

Deformity

1. Hyperextension of the metatarsophalangeal joint.

2. Hyperflexion of the proximal interphalangeal joint.

3. Hyperextension of the distal interphalangeal joint.

   Callosities or adventitious bursa may develop over the dorsum of the flexed joint, from pressure against shoes.

Treatment

1. *Mild Cases.*—Conservative treatment with protective felt pads.

2. *Severe Cases.*—Operative treatment is necessary. The joint surfaces (proximal interphalangeal) are excised, the deformity is corrected, and the joint is arthrodeses.

INGROWING TOE NAIL

The condition is common only in the big toe.

Causes

1. Many cases are idiopathic. Some persons have toes that are more prone to have ingrowing nails.

2. Encasing sweat feet in tight shoes.

3. Cutting the nail short and convexly.

Pathology and Clinical Features—A sharp anterior corner of the nail impinges against the soft skin-fold. At first there is a mechanical irritation, and this is followed by bacterial infection of the skin-fold. There is a local chronic suppuration and a granulating fleshy mass appears at the side of the nail. This is associated with pain and discharge. The lesion may be at the medial or the lateral border of the nail, or both.

Treatment
1. *Mild cases* may be treated conservatively:
   a. Keeping the feet clean and dry.
   b. Avoiding tight shoes.
   c. Cutting the nails square.
   d. Tucking pledgets of gauge, soaked in alcohol, beneath the corner of the nail.
2. *Long-standing cases* are treated by partial or complete excision of the nail, together with the margin of the skin-fold. The germinal envelope of the part of the nail must be removed with the nail since, otherwise, there is recurrence of a nail-spike.
3. *In recurrent cases* permanent ablation of the nail, by excision of the nail bed, has to be undertaken.

ONCHOGRYPHOSIS

This is a Greek term which means *hooked nail*. The big toe is usually affected. The nail is thickened, hard and curved, ultimately resembling a miniature ram's horn. It is more prone to occur in elderly people, especially if bed-ridden. Fungal infection often supervenes and trauma may occur.

Treatment
1. Temporary relief may be obtained by cutting the excess of the nail with a Gigli's wire saw.
2. For permanent cure, the nail, *with its bed,* has to be excised.

SUBUNGUAL EXOSTOSIS

The exostosis grows from the dorsal surface of the distal phalanx. The great toe is usually affected. The exostosis grows between the tip of the nail and the terminal pulp. The nail is undergrown, deformed and raised. A granulating fleshy mass protrudes forwards from under the nail. The condition is acutely painful.

Treatment consists in excision of the exostosis through an incision made just beyond the tip of the nail.

70

Deformities of the Hand and Fingers

I. Congenital Deformities

1. POLYDACTYLISM OR SUPERNUMERARY FINGERS.—The extra finger may be excised for reason of cosmesis. Sometimes there may be difficulty in deciding which of the fingers is additional. X-ray is helpful in these cases.

2. ECTRODACTYLISM, i.e. absence of a finger. There is a rare condition, called *lobster hand'* where there is absence of the middle three fingers.

3. SYNDACTYLISM OR WEBBED FINGERS.—This may be of the following types:
   a. *Congenital:*
      i. Primary.—Here not only does the skin cover the two fingers together but also the bones of the fingers are fused. The condition is often familial and no treatment is available.
      ii. Secondary.—Here the two fingers are bridged by skin only. This is possibly due to amniotic adhesions. The fingers can be separated by plastic operations.
   b. *Acquired:* These are cases following burn. The fingers can be separated by plastic procedures.

4. MACRODACTYLISM.—Overgrowth of fingers.

5. MICRODACTYLISM.—Undergrown fingers.

6. CONGENITAL CONTRACTURE OF LITTLE FINGER.—The proximal interphalangeal joint is fixed in the flexed position. The condition is often bilateral.

7. MADELUNG'S DEFORMITY.—This is due to a congenital subluxation or dislocation of the inferior radioulnar joint. A fully established case consists of:
   a. Relatively short radius.
   b. Radial deviation of hand.
   c. Prominent head of ulna.
   d. Contracture of the little finger.

8. CLUB HAND.—There is absence of the radius, with gross radial deviation of the wrist and hand.

II. Acquired Deformities

A. DEFORMITIES FOLLOWING TRAUMA:
   1. *Skin.*—Contracture (Post-burn and post-injury).
   2. *Arteries:*
      a. Volkmann's ischaemic contracture (*see* Chapter 59).
      b. Bunnell's ischaemic contracture of the hand (*see* below).

3. *Nerves.*—Ulnar, median, or musculospiral nerve; brachial plexus (*see* Chapter 15).
4. *Tendons.*—Mallet finger is the commonest (*see* below).
5. *Joints.*—Finger stiffness.

B. DEFORMITIES FOLLOWING INFLAMMATION:
   1. *Tendon sheaths.*—Trigger finger (*see* Chapter 18).
   2. *Bones.*—Tubercular dactylitis (*see* below).
   3. *Joints:*
      a. Rheumatoid arthritis.
      b. Gout

C. OTHER CONDITIONS:
   1. Claw hand (*see* Chapter 15),
   2. Dupuytren's contracture.

BUNNELL'S ISCHAEMIC CONTRACTURE OF THE HAND

This condition sometimes follows forearm injuries, particularly after tight plaster or bandages. The intrinsic muscles of the hand are fibrosed and shortened. This results in flexion of the metacarpophalangeal joints, while the interphalangeal joints remain straight. The thumb is typically adducted across the palm (Bunnell's *'intrinsic-plus'* position).

MALLET FINGER

This is a condition of persistent flexion of the distal interphalangeal joint. This is caused by rupture of the extensor tendon at its insertion into the terminal phalanx or by avulsion of a small fragment of the bone with the tendon. It results from forced flexion of the finger tip during active extension—as in making bed or catching a ball *(baseball finger).*

Immediately after the injury, there is pain and swelling. From then on, the terminal joint is held flexed and the patient cannot actively extend it, though passive extension is possible.

A recent case sometimes shows an avulsion fracture on the X-ray.

Treatment
1. Immediately after the injury, the finger is immobilised in a splint for 3 weeks, with the distal joint fully extended and the proximal interphalangeal joint flexed to 90 degrees. This is a position in which the distal part of the extensor expansion is relaxed and is allowed to heal.
2. If the deformity persists or if early treatment had been neglected, the choice lies between accepting the disability (which is slight) and undergoing an operation. The disability is due to the lengthening that the extensor tendon undergoes. Hence, at operation, the tendon is shortened by excising a small segment at the level of the middle phalanx.

TUBERCULAR DACTYLITIS (SPINA VENTOSA)

This means tubercular infection of the metacarpals, metatarsals or phalanges. The infection is blood-borne, reaching the bone by way of the nutrient artery. Hence, the middle of the bone is typically affected.

The spongy bone in the shaft is replaced by tubercular granulation tissue, which thereafter destroys the cortex. Simultaneously, the periosteum is raised and new bone is deposited under it, at the middle of the phalanx. This produces a characteristic spindle-shaped deformity (normally the middle of the phalanx is its most constricted part). There may be a sequestrum within.

The patient is typically a child.

X-ray shows the above changes characteristically. Because of the ballooning of the phalanx, the condition is known as 'spina ventosa' (spina = projection, ventos = air; blown out, as if, with air).

The condition closely resembles an enchondroma. However, enchondroma is rare in the children.

Treatment
1. Immobilisation and antitubercular treatment.
2. If there is a sequestrum.—Sequestrectomy with scraping of the cavity, followed by immobilisation.

DUPUYTREN'S CONTRACTURE

Pathology.—This is an affection of the palmar aponeurosis (palmar fascia), which gets thickened and contracted. The palmar fascia is normally a thin and tough membrane. Its fibres radiate from the termination of the palmaris longus tendon in front of the wrist and, running along the palm, get inserted into the proximal and middle phalanges of the fingers. It lies immediately deep to the skin. In Dupuytren's contracture, there is thickening and contraction of the palmar aponeurosis, and the overlying skin gets adherent to it. The contraction leads to flexion of the proximal and middle phalanges but the terminal phalanx remains unaffected because the palmar fascia does not extend to that phalanx. Usually the disease affects only a part of the aponeurosis, more commonly the medial half. Hence, serious deformity is usually confined to the little and ring fingers, the middle and the index fingers being either spared or only moderately deformed.

The joints of the finger, which are normal at first, may undergo secondary capsular contractures in long-standing cases.

A similar pathology rarely occurs in the plantar fascia of the foot but there it usually takes the form of a firm nodule.

Etiology.—Not known. Trauma is sometimes believed to be the cause. A familial history in some of the cases and frequent bilateral occurrence are points against traumatic origin.

Clinical Features.—The condition is much commoner in the males and is often bilateral. The patient is usually middle-aged. To start with, there is a nodule in the mid-palm, opposite the base of the ring finger. This nodule, which represents the thickened aponeurosis, gradually increases in size and takes the form of cord-like band, extending into the affected fingers. The joint movements are gradually restricted, till fully established fixed flexion deformity develops. The finger cannot be extended, either actively or passively, even with the wrist flexed (c.f. Volkmann's ischaemic contracture). The condition differs from congenital contracture of the little finger, in which the proximal phalanx is hyperextended while the other two phalanges are flexed.

Treatment

1. Early cases may be treated by night splintage and gentle stretching by the patient himself.
2. A contracture, not progressing, particularly in an elderly person, should better be left alone.
3. Advanced and progressive cases require *operative treatment.* This entails excision of the affected segment of the palmar fascia by careful dissection. Simple transverse division of the bands invariably results in recurrence. The results are good, provided permanent joint stiffness, due to capsular contracture, have not developed.

71

Basic Techniques in Anaesthesia

It was on 16th October, 1846 that William Thomas Green Morton first demonstrated clinical anaesthesia with diethyl ether. Since then various anaesthetic drugs and techniques had been discovered which helped the development of surgery to its modern state.

Diethyl Ether.—It is a volatile anaesthetic agent and is highly inflammable. It must not be used in a room where there is an open fire. It is highly potent and provides optimal muscular relaxation. It has however, some disadvantages, e.g. post-operative vomiting, stormy induction and stimulation of pituitary-adrenal axis during anaesthesia.

METHODS OF ADMINISTRATION

1. *Open Drop Method.*—The face is covered with a face-pad having a hole cut in the centre to give access to the nose and mouth. This is to prevent conjunctivitis (sometimes with corneal ulceration).

   A Schimmelbusch mask (which is covered with 12–16 layers of gauze) is now placed on the face-pad. With the help of a dropper (Bellamy Gardner), ether is dropped on the mask as regularly and evenly as possible. The process must never be hurried, but the concentration of ether on the mask should be kept as high as will be tolerated by the patient. In the beginning, the respirations may be irregular and this is the stage of excitation. As the depth of anaesthesia increases, the respiration becomes quite and abdominothoracic in type. This is the surgical plane of anaesthesia (third stage) and operation can be done now. The maximum vapour concentration achieved by this method is about 14 per cent.

2. *Semi-open Method.*—Towels may be draped around the mask to hasten induction by increasing concentration of ether vapour. A flow of oxygen by a nasal catheter under the mask may be used.

3. *By Boyle Anaesthetic Machine.*—There is a vaporizing bottle where ether is poured, and along with nitrous oxide and oxygen it may be used in graded concentration.

Fluothane (Halothane).—Among the other volatile anaesthetic agents like methoxyflurane, englurane, etc., fluothane is commonly used in our country. It has several advantages. It is highly potent, causes pleasant induction and quick recovery, is non-inflammable at ordinary room temperature and does not produce postoperative vomiting. Its disadvantages are high cost, fall in blood pressure and likelihood of producing liver damage.

Fluothane is used with nitrous oxide and oxygen by means of anaesthetic machine. There are special types of vaporizing bottle (Goldman or fluotec), to be attached with the machine. Due to its high cost and high boiling point, open drop or semi-open methods are not used.

Nitrous Oxide.—It is the only inorganic gas used in anaesthesia. It is non-inflammable, but supports the combustion of other agents. Nitrous oxide is carried in solution in the plasma and, probably by displacing oxygen from the cerebral cells, produces anaesthesia. It is fifty times more potent analgesic than pethidine. Nitrous oxide is supplied in blue-coloured cylinders. With the help of pressure-reducing valve, attached to the Boyle anaesthetic machine, it can be delivered in required concentration.

Cyclopropane.—It is another highly potent but inflammable anaesthetic gas. It is supplied in small orange coloured cylinders. Its use is limited nowadays. It is not readily available in our country.

Oxygen.—Though it is not an anaesthetic gas yet it must be supplemented in the anaesthetic gas and vapour mixture. This is to meet up the basal oxygen consumption of the tissues and to avoid hypoxia. Under general anaesthesia, there is always a type of intrapulmonary shunting and alteration in the ventilation-perfusion ratio. A concentration of 33 per cent oxygen in the inspired gases will compensate for the ill-effects of anaesthesia (c.f. normal air which contains 20.9 per cent oxygen). It is supplied in cylinders, compressed at a pressure of about 2500 lb per square inch. Oxygen cylinders are coloured black with white shoulders. With the help of pressure-reducing valve, attached to the Boyle anaesthetic machine, it can be delivered in required concentration.

BALANCED ANAESTHESIA

In modern times, anaesthetists do not depend on a single anaesthetic agent. By using several drugs, a balance is secured which provides varying degrees of analgesia and muscular relaxation in the presence of light anaesthesia. Thus the disadvantages of deep general anaesthesia are avoided. The balanced anaesthesia consists of three components—hypnosis, analgesia and muscular relaxation. Avoidance of explosive anaesthetic mixture is the additional advantage which permits the use of diathermy or other electrical gadgets during surgery.

HYPNOTICS.—The commonly used drugs are thiopentone sodium, methohexitone, propanidid, althesin, ketamine and diazepam. The intravenous use of any of the above-mentioned drugs induces and maintains sleep. Thus the induction is very pleasant and smooth.

ANALGESICS.—Nitrous oxide, ether, small dose of intravenous pethidine, etc., are sufficient to maintain analgesia during anaesthesia.

MUSCLE RELAXANTS.—These drugs not only facilitate endotracheal intubation but also provide excellent working condition for surgery. There are two types of drugs:

Depolarizing Group.—Suxamethonium belongs to this group. These drugs have very quick onset of action (30–40 seconds) but their action is short-lasting.

Non-depolarizing Group.—Tubocurarine, gallamine, pancuronium, etc., belong to this group. Their onset of action is not so fast like suxamethonium (1.5 to 2 minutes) but their action lasts for 30 to 40 minutes. There are various factors which influence their neuromuscular blocking effect. There is no specific *antidote* of depolarizers but non-depolarizers can be easily reversed by anticholinesterase drugs, e.g. neostigmine, edrophonium, etc.

Balanced anaesthesia requires the service of a specialist anaesthesiologist, a Boyle anaesthetic machine with fully-charged cylinders, laryngoscope, endotracheal tube and the connection pieces. Following premedication with atropine and a narcotic analgesic, anaesthesia is induced with a sleep dose of thiopentone (or any other hypnotic) and a relaxant intravenously. The patient is ventilated with 100 per cent oxygen by the face mask of the anaesthetic machine. When the jaws are relaxed, a cuffed endotracheal tube is placed inside the trachea under direct vision laryngoscopy. The tube is then connected with the anaesthetic machine and artificial ventilation started with the help of a reservoir bag. A light plain of anaesthesia is maintained by nitrous oxide and 33 per cent oxygen. Trace ether, fluothane or fractional doses of pethidine may be used. Additional doses of muscle relaxants are administered when needed. Intermittent positive pressure ventilation (IPPV) is mandatory although the operation. At the end of the operation the patient is ventilated with 100 per cent oxygen. The residual muscle relaxant effect is reversed with neostigmine, preceded by atropine. The rubber tubing attached to the needle of the intravenous drip will facilitate administration of drugs as and when required and repeated venepuncture can be avoided.

Boyle Anaesthetic Machine.—It is a continuous-flow type of machine used in anaesthesia. It was discovered in 1917 by Henry Boyle and underwent various modifications afterwards. Nitrous oxide and oxygen are delivered from separate cylinders which are fitted in yoke assembly. The colour of the cylinders are protected by international law and cannot be changed. The preset pressure-reducing valves reduce the pressure to about 60 lb per square inch and the flow of individual gases are controlled by a flowmeter. There are two vaporizing bottles (one for ether and the other for triline) and the gases can be diverted through them by means of a rotating tap. The mixture of gases now goes to the patient via a corrugated antistatic delivery tube. In case of close circuit, the exhaled gases are passed through soda lime (placed in a canister) to get rid of CO_2.

Laryngoscope.—Macintosh laryngoscope is commonly used for direct vision laryngoscopy. It has detachable blades of varying sizes with a light source in front. When the patient is under anaesthesia and the jaws are relaxed, the tip of the blade is introduced inside the mouth. The concavity of the blade fits the tongue and pushes it laterally so that a clear vision of the interior is obtained. The tip is now placed in the glosso-epiglottic fold and the lower jaw is lifted up

Uses of Laryngoscope. — Introduction of endotracheal tube, removal of foreign body, visualisation of rima glottidis and insertion of Ryle's tube in an unconscious patient.

Endotracheal Tube.—The commonly used endotracheal tubes are made of synthetic rubber or polyvinyl chloride (PVC). These are used both for the naso-tracheal and the orotracheal routes. The endotracheal tubes which are passed through oral routes have an annular inflatable cuff at the distal end. The cuff can be inflated via a 'pilot' balloon attached to the tubes. When inflated, it will provide a leak-proof anaesthetic circuit and prevent any chance of aspiration under anaesthesia.

INDICATIONS FOR ENDOTRACHEAL INTUBATION

1. Any operation where the respiration is controlled or assisted.
2. Cases where anaesthesia without encroaching upon the surgical field is difficult, e.g. facio-maxillary surgery, operations on head and neck, etc.
3. When there are possibilities of obstruction of the patient's airway:
   a. Tracheal deviation.
   b. Awkward posturing of the patient (e.g. prone position).
   c. Loaded stomach or cases of intestinal obstruction where there is a possibility of blockage of the airway by vomitus.
   d. When long-continued ventilation is required, e.g. cases of poisoning, prolonged unconsciousness following head injury, cardiac arrest, tetanus, poliomyelitis, etc. Here endotracheal intubation has multifaceted advantages, i.e. isolation of the airway from food passage, tracheo-bronchial toileting, etc. Service of a ventilator is needed.

DANGERS OF ENDOTRACHEAL INTUBATION

1. *Trauma* of the tracheal mucous membrane, avascular pressure necrosis by the inflated cuff, damage of rima glottis if extubation is tried without deflating the cuff.
2. *Infection.*—Tracheitis, laryngitis, tracheobronchitis, etc.
3. *Reflex.*—The tube may itself precipitate laryngospasm, bronchospasm, cardiac dysrrhythmia and even cardiac arrest.

It should be borne in mind that during endotracheal anaesthesia the endo-tracheal tube may be termed as extended trachea. Hence any kinking or biting of the tube will lead to severe airway obstruction. Similarly a too small tube may lead to respiratory obstruction. Accidentally the tube may enter into the right bronchus and thus precipitate hypoxia and subsequent collapse of the left lung. Hence immediately after intubation auscultation of both the lungs should be done as a routine. Before use, the tubes should be washed with soap and water, both outside and inside, with a test-tube brush. They may be sterilised by 1–1000 biniodide solution or by weak cetavlon solution.

REGIONAL ANAESTHESIA

This is done by application of a local anaesthetic drug to a nerve cell or fibre or ganglion and blocking the efferent and afferent conductions from the site of application of the drug. It is preferable to use the term analgesia and not anaesthesia in this regard because consciousness is retained during regional analgesia.

Types of Regional Anaesthesia

1. TOPICAL.—The drug is applied to a mucous surface and then it penetrates the tissues to the nerve endings. One should be cautious during topical application of local analgesic drug to pharynx and inflamed urethra because it is quickly absorbed.
2. INFILTRATION.—The drug is injected into tissues at the nerve endings, usually along the line of incision.
3. FIELD BLOCK.—The drug is injected not along the line of incision but at the site of major branches of the nerves to the area, usually encircling the line of incision.

4. NERVE BLOCK.—The drug is injected directly to a nerve or plexus to block the corresponding dermatomes, e.g. brachial plexus block, radial nerve block etc.

5. SPINAL OR SUBARACHNOID BLOCK.—The drug is deposited in the subarachnoid space and acts on the anterior and posterior nerve roots as they emerge from the cord. The reflex arc is interrupted.

6. EPIDURAL OR EXTRADURAL BLOCK.—The drug is deposited extradurally (outside the dura). There are several postulations regarding its mechanism of action:

   a. It diffuses across the dura into the subarachnoid space.

   b. It passes along the nerves into the paravertebral space.

   c. There is a neuraxial spread.

   For details of spinal anaesthesia *see* lumbar puncture needle under Chapter 72.

PRE-ANAESTHETIC MEDICATION

Some drugs or measures are used in the pre-operative period which help the patient to undertake anaesthesia smoothly and safely.

The *aims* of pre-medication are:

1. To allay anxiety and tension.
2. To reduce secretions specially of mouth and respiratory tract.
3. To reduce reflex irritability of the vagus.
4. To reduce the metabolic rate.
5. To potentiate the subsequent anaesthetic drugs.
6. To overcome the undesirable side effects of anaesthesia.
7. To prevent the toxicity of anaesthetic drugs which are going to be used.

Classification of Pre-medicants

1. *Narcotic analgesics.*—Morphine, pethidine, pentazocine, etc.
2. *Tranquilizers.*—Chlorpromazine, promethazine, trifluopromazine, diazepam, chlordiazepoxide, nitrazepam, etc.
3. *Anticholinergic drugs.*—Atropine, hyoscine, glycopyrrolate.
4. *Sedative or hypnotic drugs.*—Phenobarbitone, quinalbarbitone.
5. *Neuroleptic drugs.*—Haloperidol, droperidol.

At bed time on the night before operation, the patient should get a sedative or major tranquilizer orally, to have a peaceful night. On the day of operation, at least 45 minutes before anaesthesia, he should get an intramuscular injection of a narcotic analgesic and an anticholinergic drug. But the best premedicant is pre-operative assurance by the anaesthetists, surgeons and house-officers. It reminds the famous line of Kipling—'Words are the most powerful drugs known to mankind'.

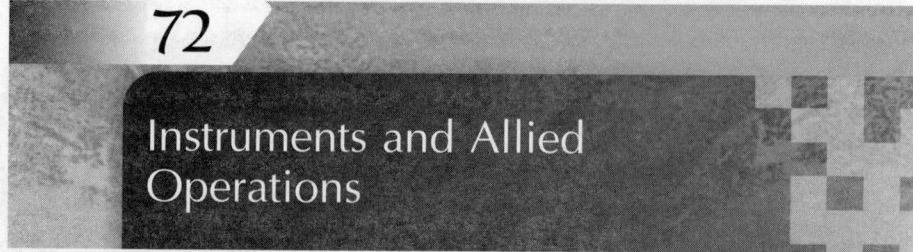

72

Instruments and Allied Operations

STERILISATION OF INSTRUMENTS

Blunt Instruments.—These are sterilised by either of the following methods:

1. *Boiling* in boiling water for at least half an hour. Boiling for such a long period is necessary in order to kill the spores of the spore-bearing organisms. Addition of a little sodium carbonate (making a 2% solution) minimises corrosion of the instruments.

2. *Autoclaving,* i.e. sterilisation with steam under pressure. Usually a heat of 120°C and a pressure of 15 lb/sq. inch, for half an hour, are necessary to kill the spores.

   Autoclaving is a better method of sterilisation than boiling, but requires the use of autoclaves, i.e. pressure-sterilisers, which are not available everywhere.

3. When an instrument is very urgently required to be sterilised, it may be exposed to direct heat, i.e. *flaming* (by pouring spirit on it and then putting fire).

Sharp Instruments.—These are sterilised with chemicals, e.g. lysol, carbolic acid, iodine, etc. These chemicals cause necrosis of the protoplasm of the bacteria. In hospital-practice, the commonest method is to put the sharp instruments in concentrated lysol for at least half an hour. If diluted lysol is used, the instrument should be immersed for at least 24 hours.

Sharp instruments should not be boiled since their sharpness is lost on boiling. If they are required to be boiled at all, their sharp parts are wrapped with cotton and then they are boiled; this minimises the loss of sharpness.

Rubber Goods and Other Articles.—Catheters, rubber drains, rubber tubes, etc. are sterilised by boiling.

Draping sheets, gowns, dressings, etc. are sterilised by autoclaving. Gloves are better sterilised by autoclaving (dry gloves) than by boiling (wet gloves).

HAEMOSTATIC FORCEPS (HAEMOSTATS)

The name 'haemostatic forceps' is more accurate than 'artery forceps' because these forceps are used for both arteries and veins. However, the term 'artery forceps' is very commonly used.

Types.—There are four common varieties:

1. Ordinary (Spencer Wells')
2. Kocher's

3. Lane's
4. Mosquito

Sterilisation.—Boiling or autoclaving.

SPENCER WELLS' ARTERY FORCEPS

This is the most commonly used type. There are two varieties:
a. Straight.
b. Curved (Fig. 72.1).

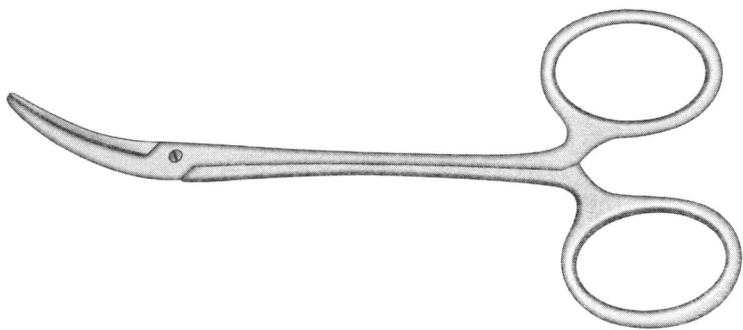

Fig. 72.1: Spencer Wells' artery forceps (curved)

These are used to catch hold of ordinary bleeding vessels. The transverse serrations on the blades prevent slipping of the tissues held between them. The catches in the handles crush the vessel held by the instrument. When the vessel is crushed, the tunica intima curls into the lumen and plugs it; the tunica media and adventitia are crushed and they obliterate the lumen. Thus haemostasis is achieved.

The Natural Method of Haemostasis.—When a blood vessel is cut, there is often a spontaneous haemostasis. This is achieved by two component factors:
1. *Vascular Component.*—The injured vessel undergoes some changes. The tunica intima curls in and plugs the lumen. The tunica media, with the adventitia, goes into spasm. Partially injured vessels tend to bleed more because this natural process fails to occur.
2. *Blood Phenomenon.*—Coagulation of blood.

Removal of the Haemostatic Forceps
1. Crushing.—The vessel may simply be crushed and the forceps, with the vessel, twisted. This may be sufficient for small bleeding points.
2. Ligation.—This is the most commonly practised procedure. Catgut, silk or thread may be used for the purpose.
3. Cautery with a diathermy.

Other Uses of Haemostatic Forceps
1. May be used to hold the end of ligatures.
2. Often used as a tissue forceps for holding peritoneum, sheath, aponeurosis, etc. (but not skin or nerves, which are grossly damaged on crushing).

3. In absence of proper instruments, may be used as catheter clamp, appendix crusher, sinus forceps, needle holder, sequestrum forceps, dressing forceps, etc.
4. To open an abscess by *Hilton's method.* In this method a small incision is made over the most fluctuant part of the abscess. The opening is dilated immediately by inserting the closed blades of the forceps and then separating the blades. As the instrument is withdrawn with its blades still separated, the opening gets further dilated. This method is of particular value where the abscess overlies important structures, e.g. blood vessels, nerves, etc., which may be damaged if a free incision is employed.

TYPES OF HAEMORRHAGE

ARTERIAL BLEEDING	VENOUS BLEEDING
1. More forceful, requires more pressure to be controlled.	1. Less severe, controlled by less pressure or by simple elevation of the limb.
2. Bright red in colour.	2. Bluish red.
3. Occurs in jerks, synchronous with heart beats (spurting).	3. Occurs as a continuous flow.
4. More bleeding occurs from the proximal cut end.	4. More bleeding occurs from the distal cut end.

A. Haemorrhage may be:
  1. Arterial
  2. Venous
  3. Capillary
Capillary bleeding is in the form of oozing. The blood is a little bluish but gets red as soon as it comes out.
B. Haemorrhage may be:
  1. External.
  2. Internal:
     a. Injury to internal organs.—Liver, spleen, kidney, mesentery, lung, etc.
     b. Bleeding from ulcers or growth in the gut.—Peptic ulcer haemorrhage, haemorrhage from malignant growths, etc.
     c. Bleeding in the lumen and the wall of a loop of strangulated gut.
C. Haemorrhage may be:
  1. Primary.
  2. Reactionary.
  3. Secondary.

1. PRIMARY OR IMMEDIATE.—Occurring instantaneously with the injury to the vessel.
2. REACTIONARY.—This occurs usually within 48 hours of the injury to the vessel, and is caused by the rise of pressure after an operation or injury. At the time of operation or immediately after a major injury, the blood pressure may be low. The vessels not bleeding then or the vessels insecurely ligated may start bleeding when the pressure subsequently rises to normal.

3. SECONDARY.—This results from interference with the natural process of repair of an injured vessel. It may be caused by:

a. *Infection*, most commonly. As the bleeding is secondary to infection, it is called 'secondary'. Normally the clot at the cut end of the vessel undergoes fibrosis. When infection occurs (either from the wound itself or by blood stream along the vessel), the clot undergoes suppuration and liquefaction, and then gives way under pressure of the blood stream behind. Also, the infection spreads to the vessel wall, which becomes friable and undergoes erosion.

b. *Malignant infiltration* into a blood vessel. Rather common examples are malignant nodes in the neck, infiltrating into the big vessels in the neck, or nodes in the inguinal region, infiltrating into the femoral vessels. In these cases, the severe haemorrhage is the terminal event in the patient. The best examples are carcinoma of the tongue and carcinoma of the penis.

Secondary haemorrhage, therefore, may occur at any interval from the time of injury, but it is commonest between the 7th and 14th day. The haemorrhage may be very severe. It is often preceded by a little soakage of the dressings with fresh blood. This is called *warning haemorrhage.*

Treatment of Secondary Haemorrhage

A. GENERAL TREATMENT

1. Treatment for Shock:
   a. Absolute rest.
   b. Sedation.—Inj. morphine, pethidine, etc.
   c. Fluid transfusion in suitable dosage. In all cases of secondary haemorrhage, blood samples must be grouped and cross-matched since any time.
   d. Blood transfusion may have to be started.
2. Control of Infection.—Antibiotics are administered, preferably an antibiotic to which the organisms, in the wound, are sensitive. For all infected wounds a culture and antibiotic-sensitivity test of the organisms should be done beforehand. If this has not been done, a swab is taken from the wound and, by the time reports are obtained, a broad spectrum antibiotic is started.

B. LOCAL TREATMENT

1. Absolute rest to the limb, preferably in a splint or cast, and the limb is kept elevated.
2. Pressure bandaging of the wound. In the majority of cases a pressure bandage arrests the haemorrhage.
3. If bleeding continues, the wound is opened up at the operation theatre and the clots carefully removed. The main bleeding points are gently picked up with haemostatic forceps and ligated. The vessels often become so friable by infection that it is impossible to catch the bleeding points with forceps, and such attempts simply cause more injury to the vessels and more bleeding. Under-running the vessels with sutures, without applying artery forceps, may be possible.
4. In uncontrolled cases proximal ligature of the main vessel of the limb (e.g. brachial, popliteal) has to be done. If collaterals develop (as is usual in the upper limb) the limb survives, but the bleeding may start again. On the other

hand, if adequate collaterals fail to develop (as is often in the lower limb), gangrene supervenes.

5. If gangrene sets in as above, or if bleeding continues even after proximal ligation, amputation of the limb has to be undertaken.

KOCHER'S ARTERY FORCEPS

This may be:

a. Straight (Fig. 72.2).

b. Curved.

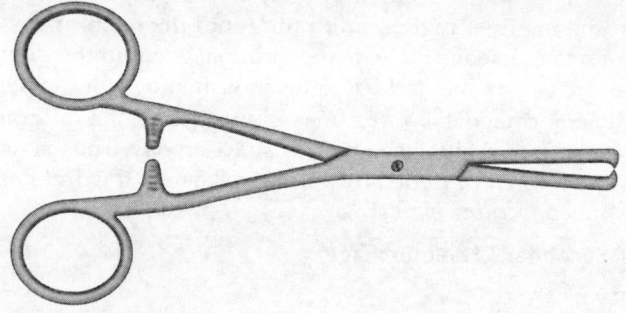

Fig. 72.2: Kocher's artery forceps (straight)

The forceps differs from an ordinary artery forceps in that it has a tooth at the tip of the blades. It is, therefore, used to hold:

1. Bleeding vessels in a tough or fibrous background, from where an ordinary artery forceps would slip, e.g. scalp, palm, sole, periosteal vessels, etc.

2. Vessels having a tendency to retract, e.g. perforating vessels at radical mastectomy.

3. Superior thyroid vessels.—Kocher originally used this instrument to catch hold of the superior thyroid vessels in the substance of the thyroid, before ligating them. Ligation of the superior thyroid vessels in the substance of the thyroid is advised so as to avoid injury to the superior laryngeal nerve, which lies just a little away from the upper pole of the thyroid. While the superior thyroid artery and the vein run together and are included in the same ligature, the inferior thyroid artery and the corresponding veins run separately. The veins are situated at the lower pole of the thyroid, where they are ligated. The artery enters the posteromedial border of the gland. The inferior thyroid artery should be ligated as far away from the thyroid as is possible in order to avoid injury to the recurrent laryngeal nerve, which lies very close to the thyroid at that point. Moreover, if the ligature is applied close to the thyroid, only one branch of the artery may be ligated and not the main trunk, which may have divided a little away from the thyroid.

Other Uses

1. As an appendix crusher. The tooth at the tip prevents slipping of the appendix, out of the blades of the instrument.

2. As a pile clamp.

3. As a tissue forceps, to hold a semilunar cartilage during its excision.

LANE'S ARTERY FORCEPS

This is a long instrument. All instruments devised by Lane are long since Lane was a surgeon of the time when asepsis, instead of antisepsis, was the weapon against infection. If the instruments are long, there is less chance of infection of the wound from the surgeon's hands. While the handles of this instrument are long, its blades are very short. Each blade has:

a. transverse serrations,
b. a fenestration at the centre,
c. a tooth at the tip.

It is usually used to catch bleeding periosteal vessels.

MOSQUITO FORCEPS

This is a small artery forceps. Mosquito forceps may be:
 a. Straight (Fig. 72.3).
 b. Curved.

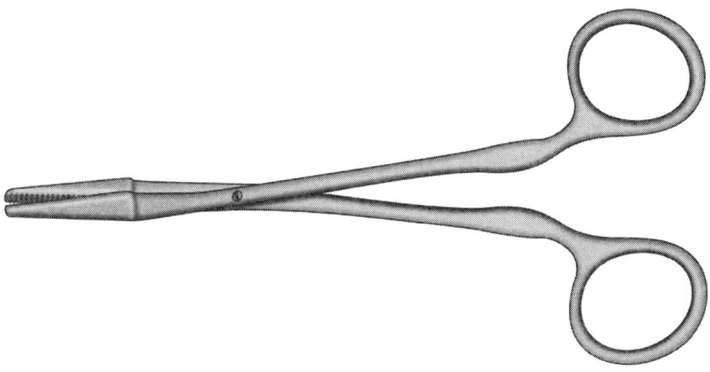

Fig. 72.3: Mosquito forceps (straight)

Uses

1. To catch small bleeding vessels, as in operations of cleft lip, cleft palate, phimosis, etc.
2. It is often used in the operation of appendectomy:
    a. To perforate the mesoappendix in order to pass a ligature around the appendicular artery.
    b. To invaginate the stump of the appendix within the purse-string suture on the caecal wall (*see* below).

Appendicectomy and Use of Mosquito Forceps.—The incisions for appendicectomy (or appendectomy) are:

1. McBurney's incision.
2. Right lower paramedian incision.
3. Lanz's incision.—This is a cosmetic, small, transverse incision on the skin, the remaining steps being the same as in McBurney's incision.
4. Rutherford Morison's muscle-cutting incision (usually not employed).
5. Battle's pararectal incision.—An incision just medial to the outer border of rectus and parallel to it (obsolete).

For details of these incisions *see* Chapter 53.

On opening the abdomen, the caecum is picked up. On following the *Taenia coli* downwards, the base of the appendix is reached.

The appendicular artery, lying in the mesoappendix, near its free margin, has to be ligated. This may be done with a needle and catgut or with the help of a *mosquito forceps*. The forceps perforates the mesoappendix and brings out the ligature through it, around the artery. After ligating the artery, the mesoappendix is separated from the appendix.

A purse-string suture is applied on the caecal wall, a little away from the base of the appendix. An atraumatic needle with catgut is often used for the purpose.

The base of the appendix has now to be ligated. For efficient closure of its lumen:

a. The base is crushed with an appendix crusher (Fig. 72.92) or with a Kocher's artery forceps. Ligature on the crushed area is usually airtight and water-tight since, on crushing, the muscle and the mucosa curl inwards, obliterating the lumen, and also the suture sits tightly over the crushed area.

b. A transfixion suture is applied on the crushed area (ordinary ligature may slip out because of intracaecal pressure).

The appendix is cut distal to the suture and removed. The stump of the appendix is carbolised in order to kill the bacteria, left on the mucosa, distal to the suture.

The stump is now held with a *mosquito forceps* and invaginated into the caecal wall by tightening the purse-string around it.

Crushing of the base of the appendix has to be avoided if:

a. The appendicular wall is gangrenous.

b. The appendix is turgid and any pressure is likely to cause its rupture.

c. The caecal wall is grossly oedematous and friable.

TISSUE FORCEPS

These forceps are used to hold tissues—either tissues to be left in the body or tissues to be excised. The commonly used varieties are:

1. Allis' tissue forceps (Fig. 72.4).
2. Lane's tissue forceps (Fig. 72.5).
3. Babcock's tissue forceps (Fig. 72.6).
4. Rutherford Morison's tissue forceps (Fig. 72.7).

Sterilisation.—Boiling or autoclaving.

ALLIS' AND LANE'S TISSUE FORCEPS

ALLIS' FORCEPS	LANE'S FORCEPS
1. Delicate and short.	1. Stout and long (Lane's instruments are all long).
2. The teeth on the blades are delicate, so that this instrument is used to hold delicate tissues, e.g. peritoneum, aponeurosis, soft muscles, intestines, etc. Tough structures	2. The teeth on the blades are sharp and stout, so that tough structures, e.g. skin, coarse muscles, etc., are held with it. Intestines should never be held with

tend to slip out of the blades and hence it is not used to hold them.

3. There is little gap between the blades which are solid. So little amount of tissues can be accommodated between the blades.

it as the teeth will injure them. Glands, tumours, etc., which are going to be excised, may be held during dissection, for better grip.

3. There is wide gap between the blades that can accommodate a bulk of tissue. Moreover, there is a big fenestration in each blade, through which, part of the tissues held may bulge out; hence a bigger quantity of tissue may be grasped.

Allis' tissue forceps is often used to hold the stomach and the intestines during anastomosis by the *open method* (c f anastomosis by *close method*, in which occlusion clamps are used). Altogether 4 forceps are applied, two to each loop, and these are held by the assistants. They keep the loops steady and in apposition while the anastomosis is being performed.

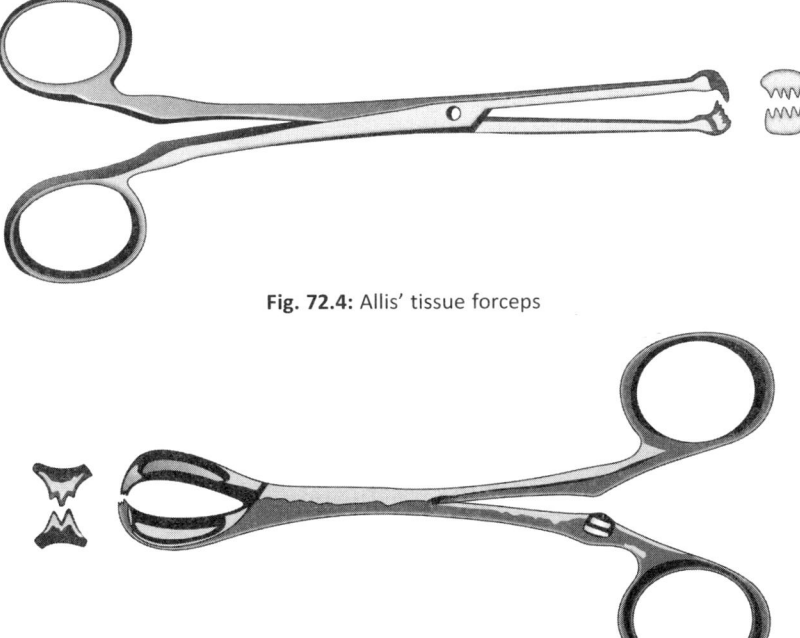

Fig. 72.4: Allis' tissue forceps

Fig. 72.5: Lane's tissue forceps

BABCOCK'S TISSUE FORCEPS

The blades are fenestrated (and so, light) and there is no tooth on the blades. They are designed to hold the intestines. They may also be used to hold delicate structures like peritoneum, fascia, delicate muscles, etc. This forceps is especially used to hold the appendix, the organ being accommodated in the gap between the blades, so that it is not injured.

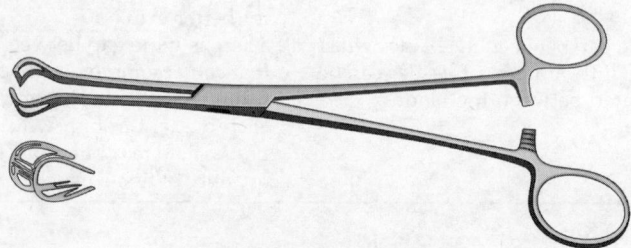

Fig. 72.6: Babcock's tissue forceps

RUTHERFORD MORISON'S TISSUE FORCEPS

This was originally used to hold the peritoneum (hence called peritoneum forceps). Its use are the same as Allis' tissue forceps but, as its teeth are sharp, the forceps should not be applied on the intestines.

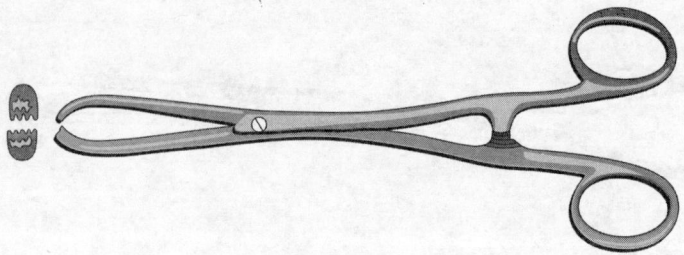

Fig. 72.7: Rutherford Morison's tissue forceps.

DISSECTING FORCEPS

There are two varieties:
1. Plain (Fig. 72.8).
2. Toothed (Fig. 72.9).

These are used to hold the tissues during the process of dissection or suturing.

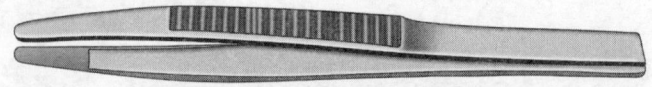

Fig. 72.8: Plain Dissecting Forceps

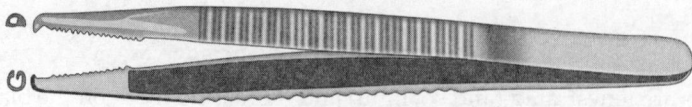

Fig. 72.9: Toothed dissecting forceps

The plain dissecting forceps, having no tooth at the tip, are used to hold delicate structures, e.g. peritoneum, fascia, delicate muscles, etc. They are also used to hold the intestines, blood vessels, nerve sheaths, etc. Tough structures are not held with them since they tend to slip out of the instrument.

The toothed forceps are used to hold tough structures like skin, aponeurosis, rectus sheath, coarse muscles, etc. Delicate structures, e.g. intestines, blood vessels, nerve sheaths, etc., should never be held by them for fear of injury.

Sterilisation.—Boiling or autoclaving.

SWAB HOLDER

This is a long instrument with the blades expanded at their ends, where there are transverse serrations and a central fenestration (through and through)—Fig. 72.10.

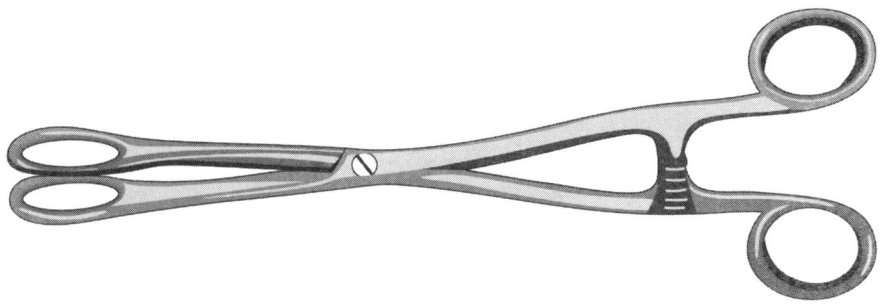

Fig. 72.10: Swab holder

Uses
1. To hold a swab in order to cleanse the field of operation in the depth (the length of the instrument facilitates its work).
2. To hold a swab and clean the area of operation (skin or mucosa) before starting the operation. Cleaning starts along the proposed line of incision and then proceeds peripherally. If the reverse is done, dirt and bacteria, from the periphery, are carried on the swab towards the line of incision. Different antiseptics are used for the purpose, e.g. spirit, iodine, cetavlon, mertheolate, etc. A popular method is spirit, iodine, and then followed by spirit.
3. To swab the throat when there are profuse secretions, which the patient cannot swallow himself, e.g. during anaesthesia and in unconscious patients.
4. To press on the tonsillar bed to arrest haemorrhage.
5. To hold the fundus of the gall bladder during cholecystectomy.

Sterilisation.—Boiling or autoclaving.

DRESSING FORCEPS

This is a short instrument and the tips of the blades are spoon-shaped, having transverse serrations and a central groove. There are no catches on the handles (Fig. 72.11).

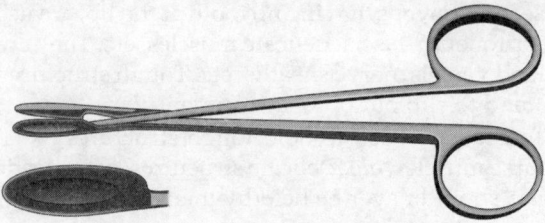

Fig. 72.11: Dressing forceps

Use.—To hold a swab while dressing wounds.

Sterilisation.—Boiling or autoclaving.

TOWEL CLIP

There are two types:
1. The pinchter type (Fig. 72.12).
2. The forceps type (Fig. 72.13).

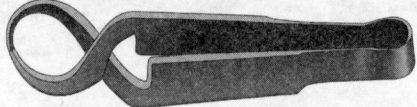

Fig. 72.12: Towel clip (pinchter type)

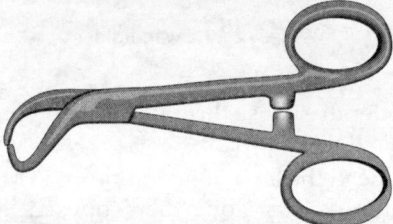

Fig. 72.13: Towel clip (forceps type)

Uses
1. To hold the corners of the draping sheets at operation (hence called *corner clips*).
2. The forceps type may be used as a tongue-holding forceps (the pointed tips of the blades are applied to the sides of the tongue).

Sterilisation.—Boiling or autoclaving.

MOYNIHAN'S TETRA FORCEPS

This is so called because there are 4 teeth in the forceps, two in each blade (Fig. 72.14).

Use.—To fix the tetra towels to the skin flap, on either side of an incision. This is necessary to prevent bacteria from the skin surface gaining entry into the wound across the cut skin margin. Though the surface skin is sterilised with antiseptics at the start of an operation, bacteria still harbour in the deeper layers of the skin, e.g. in sweat glands, hair follicles, etc.

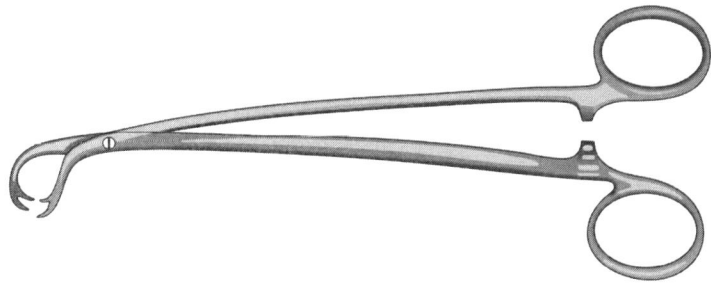

Fig. 72.14: Moynihan's tetra forceps

As time passes during the operation, these bacteria move on to the surface of the skin and then topple over the cut skin margin to gain entry into the wound. The tetra towels prevent this.

These tetra towels and forceps may be used in any operation, including those on the limbs, but they are specially used in abdominal operations. The curvature of the instrument is so made that it fits to the abdominal contour, where it lies flat and does not stand in the way of the surgeon's working.

To apply the tetra towel, the towel is first placed across the wound with one of its margins applied to one cut skin margin. After it has been fixed with the tetra forceps, the towel is everted away from the wound on the skin surface, over the forceps.

In absence of the tetra forceps, the towels may be fixed to the skin with temporary stitches.

Sterilisation.—Boiling or autoclaving.

TONGUE FORCEPS

There are two common varieties:

1. SWAB HOLDER TYPE.—It differs from a swab holder in that the fenestration on the blade is triangular and the transverse serrations are very coarse. This is a bad instrument since it is likely to cause damage to the tongue. Hence it is seldom used (Fig. 72.15).

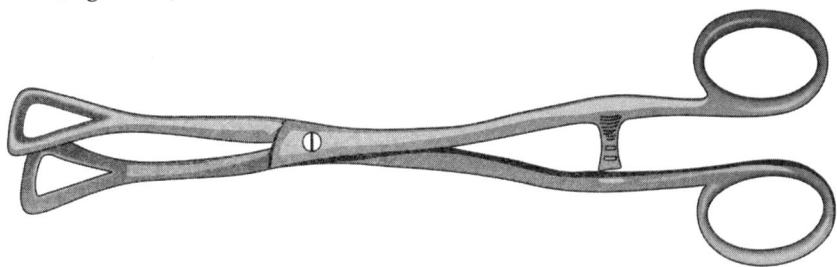

Fig. 72.15: Tongue forceps (swab holder type)

2. TOWEL CLIP TYPE.—It differs from the forceps variety of towel clip in that the tip of one of the blades is expanded, into which the tip of the other blade may fit. This is a much better instrument than the preceding variety of tongue forceps since it pricks the tongue only at one point (the other tip being blunt)—Fig. 72.16.

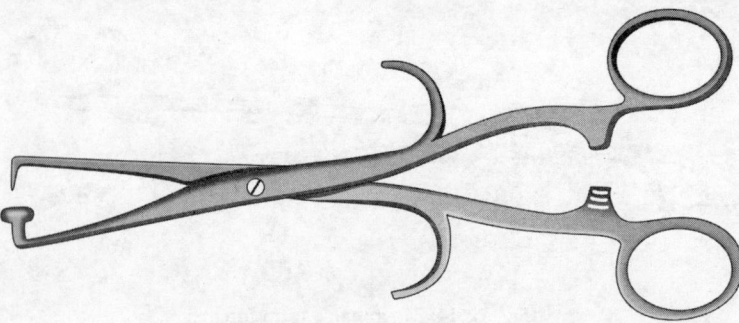

Fig. 72.16: Tongue forceps (towel clip type)

Use.—To hold the tongue in order to pull it out. This may be required:

1. During any operation on the tongue.

2. To arrest haemorrhage from the tongue (when the tongue is drawn forwards, the lingual arteries are compressed between the lower teeth and the tongue itself).

3. During the third stage of anaesthesia, when the tongue has a tendency to fall back and obstruct the air passage (this is usually done with an airway tube instead of this instrument).

A better way of pulling the tongue out (instead of using these forceps) is to pass a thick silk with the help of a needle, through the substance of the tongue, from one margin of the tongue to the other, and to apply traction on this silk.

Sterilisation.—Boiling or autoclaving.

GLAND HOLDING FORCEPS

There are two varieties:

1. SWAB HOLDER VARIETY.—This instrument differs from a swab holder or tongue forceps in that there are no serrations on the blades. It differs from a pile forceps in that there are no grooves on the blades (Fig. 72.17).

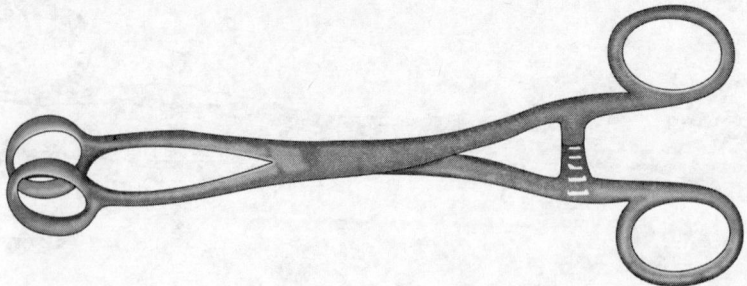

Fig. 72.17: Gland holding forceps

2. KOCHER'S VARIETY.—There are two spikes in each blade, which are typically curved (Fig. 72.18).

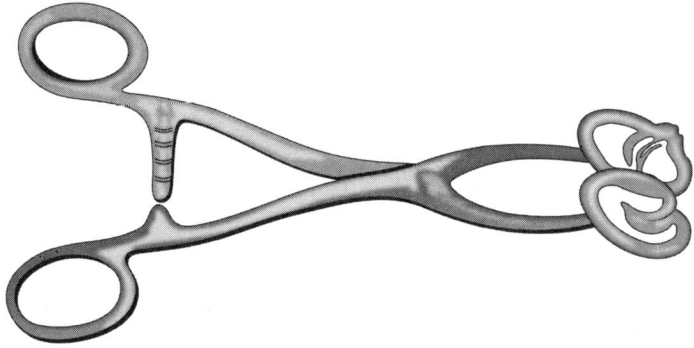

Fig. 72.18: Kocher's gland holding forceps

Use.—To hold glands or tumours during the process of dissection. The Kocher's variety is much the better since the spikes cut into the tissues and prevent slipping out of the structures during the course of dissection.

Sterilisation.—Boiling or autoclaving.

PILE FORCEPS

There is a circular groove along the inner side of each blade, around the fenestration in the blade (thus it differs from a swab holder, a tongue forceps, or a gland holding forceps)—Fig. 72.19.

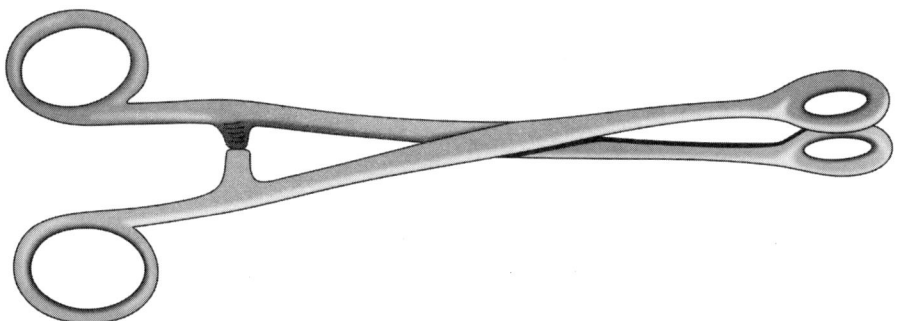

Fig. 72.19: Pile forceps

Use.—To draw the piles down, through the anal opening, before ligating their pedicles. Allis' tissue forceps is better for the purpose.

Sterilisation.—Boiling or autoclaving.

PROBE

(Metallic malleable olive-pointed probe, usually with an eye). (Fig. 72.20)

Use.—To probe into a sinus or a fistula to know its direction and length. The instrument had been made malleable, otherwise it might make false passage while passing through a curve track. For the same reason, the tip is olive-pointed, instead of being sharp. The eye at the other end may be used:

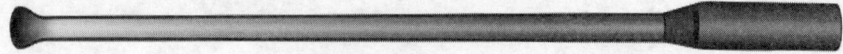

Fig. 72.20: Probe

1. To thread a small piece of gauze, medicated with some antiseptic ointment or powder, and to pass it through a fistula (as was done in older days).
2. To thread a stainless steel wire or a stout silk, as is sometimes done in operations for high anal fistulae.

Sterilisation.—Concentrated lysol or boiling or autoclaving.

SINUS AND FISTULA

A fistula is a track, lined by unhealthy granulation tissue or epithelium, having an opening at each end. One of the ends, opens into an organ while the other end opens either into another organ or on the skin. When the opening is on the skin the fistula is called 'external fistula'. When both the openings are in the viscera, the fistula is called 'internal fistula'.

Examples of *external fistula* are anal fistula (commonest), umbilical fistula, parotid fistula, etc.

Examples of *internal fistula* are vesico-vaginal fistula, gastro-colic fistula, cholecysto-duodenal fistula, etc.

A sinus is a blind track, lined by unhealthy granulation tissue or epithelium. It has, therefore, only one opening.

DIRECTOR

This is a narrow metal strip, having a groove along its length on one of its, surfaces.

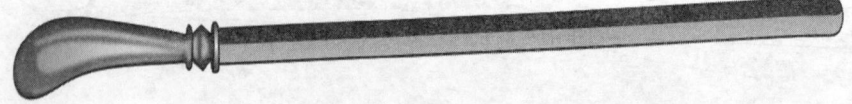

Fig. 72.21: Director with Spoon

Use.—To open up the track of a fistula. The groove of the director directs the blade of the knife when a fistula is being cut open (hence the name). The director is introduced into the track with the groove facing the overlying skin. When the knife works down from the skin, as its blade touches the groove of the director, the track of the fistula is opened along its length.

Sterilisation.—Concentrated lysol or boiling or autoclaving.

DIRECTOR WITH SPOON

At one end of a director, a spoon (or blunt scoop) is attached (Fig. 72.21). The spoon may serve two purposes:

1. Contents of an abscess cavity, sinus, or fistula may be collected on it for the purpose of examination.

2. Some antiseptic powder may be taken on it to be sprinkled into the track of a fistula or sinus or into an abscess cavity.

PROBE-POINTED DIRECTOR WITH FRENUM-SLIT

This is a combination of a probe and a director, serving dual purposes (Fig. 72.22).

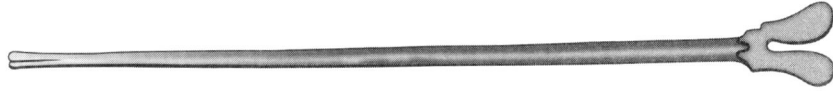

Fig. 72.22: Probe-pointed director with frenum-slit

It has a special use in Wheelhouse's operation (Chapter 56).

The *frenum-slit* is used in the operation for tongue-tie. This is a congenital condition, in which the tongue is too fixed to the floor of the mouth because of a wide frenum. The patient cannot protrude the tip of the tongue and cannot articulate properly during speech. The treatment is operative and consists of a minor operation in which the anterior part of the frenum is incised, thereby separating it from the floor of the mouth. The margins of the cut frenum and those of the mucosa of the floor of the mouth are then sutured separately. While cutting the frenum, the frenum-slit is applied to it (the frenum being accommodated in the slit) and the frenum is cut above it. Thus, the instrument protects the structures on the floor of the mouth. The frenum should not be cut too much, otherwise the extra-mobile tongue may fall back over the larynx during sleep.

Sterilisation.—Boiling or autoclaving.

SINUS FORCEPS

This instrument has long narrow blades; which are serrated transversely for only half an inch at their tip. There are no catches on the handles (Fig. 72.23).

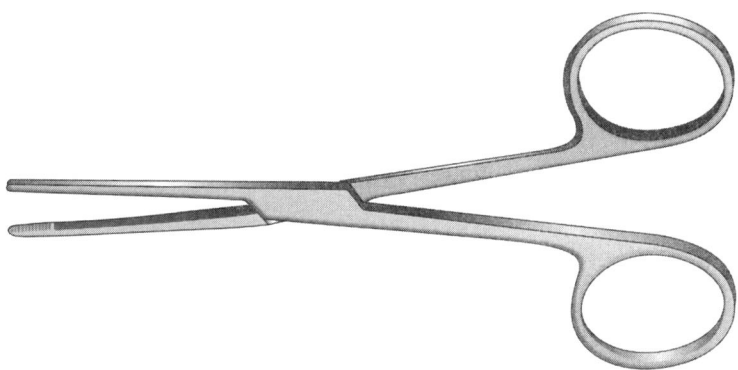

Fig. 72.23: Sinus forceps

Uses
1. To open an abscess by Hilton's method (see haemostatic forceps).
2. To hold a small piece of gauze between the blades in order to clean the cavity of an abscess or fistula.

Sterilisation.—Boiling or autoclaving.

PILE CLAMP

This instrument looks like the sinus forceps but differs from it in that the serrations on the blades are longitudinal and that there are catches in the handles (Fig. 72.24).

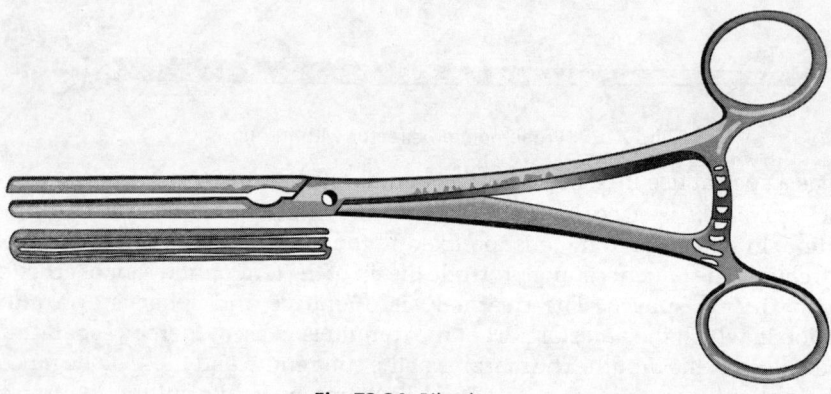

Fig. 72.24: Pile clamp

Use.—To clamp the base of the piles before applying ligature on it.

Sterilisation.—Boiling or autoclaving.

VOLKMANN'S SPOON (OR SCOOP)

Uses

1. *As a scoop,* to scrape:
   a. Sinus, fistula, chronic abscess cavity, chronic ulcer, etc.
   b. Cavity in the bone, e.g. osteomyelitis, bone cyst, osteoclastoma, etc.

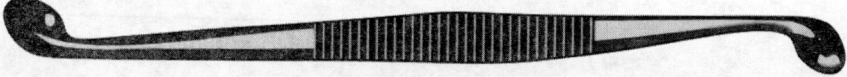

Fig. 72.25: Volkmann's spoon (scoop).

2. *As a spoon:*
   a. To collect contents from inside a cavity for the purpose of examination.
   b. To put some antiseptic powder into a cavity or wound.

Sterilisation.—Boiling or autoclaving (Fig. 72.25).

ANAL SPECULUM

This instrument is 3-inch long. The lighting has to be done from outside (e.g. with a torch). Since the anal canal is directed downwards and backwards, the (lubricated) instrument has to be pushed upwards and forwards, i.e. directed towards umbilicus. As the anal canal is only 1½-inch long, the instrument reaches the lower part of the rectum. But the direction of the instrument has to be changed after it has traversed the anal canal—it has now to be pushed towards the sacral hollow.

On removal of the obturator, the lower rectal mucosa is seen. As the speculum is gradually withdrawn, the anal mucosa is seen (Fig. 72.26).

The patient is put either in the left lateral position or in the knee-elbow position, the former being preferred.

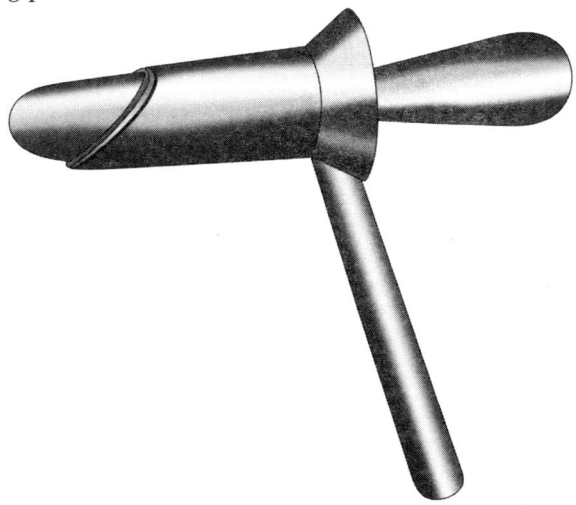

Fig. 72.26: Anal speculum

Uses
1. To visualise the anal canal for purpose of examination, e.g. piles, polyp, etc.
2. For injection of piles.

RECTAL SPECULUM (SIM'S)

This has fenestrated wide blades that can be apposed or separated by moving the handles. With the blades apposed, the instrument is passed in. The rectum is opened up as much as is required by separating the blades (done by compressing the handles). The position of the blades is maintained by tightening the screw on the handle (Fig. 72.27).

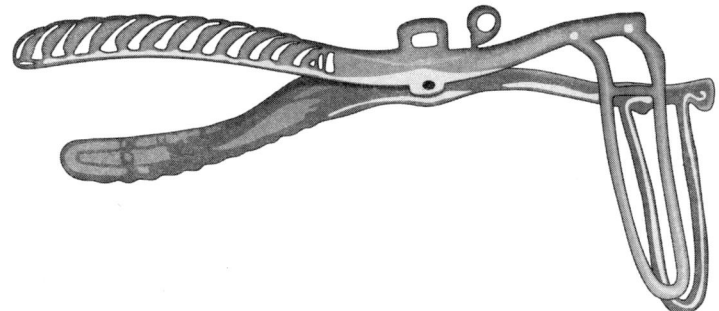

Fig. 72.27: Sim's rectal speculum

Sterilisation.—Boiling or autoclaving.

PROCTOSCOPE

This looks like the anal speculum but is much longer (about 8 inches). Both the rectum and the anal canal can be seen with it. The rectum is 5 inches long and the anal canal 1½ inches. The lighting arrangement is with a long rod, bearing a lamp at its tip. This rod is introduced after withdrawing the obturator of the instrument.

While introducing a proctoscope, the normal curvatures of the rectum and the anal canal should be borne in mind. At first the instrument is passed upwards and forwards (i.e. directed towards the umbilicus), to negotiate through the anal canal. When it reaches the lower end of the rectum, it is directed upwards and backwards (towards the sacrum) to pass into the rectum. The patient is put either in the left lateral position or in the knee-elbow position. (See surgical anatomy of the rectum and anal canal, Chapter 50).

Sterilisation.—-Boiling or autoclaving.

SIGMOIDOSCOPE

This instrument, with which the anal canal, the whole of the rectum, and the major part of the pelvic colon can be seen, is about 14 inches long. There is a glass eye-piece to which the light-carrier is attached. This can be fitted to the instrument after the obturator of the instrument is withdrawn. There are also arrangements for inflating the gut with air. This is done with the help of a rubber bulb, as the instrument is passed in. This process facilitates introduction of the instrument, diminishes risks of injury to the gut by the instrument, and also helps better visualisation (Fig. 72.28).

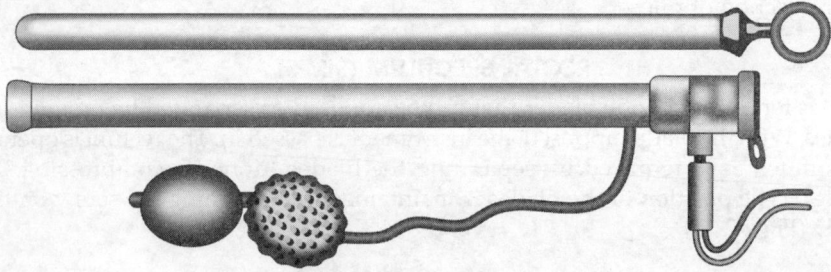

Fig. 72.28: Sigmoidoscope

The patient is put either in knee-elbow position (males usually) or in left lateral position (females usually). The introduction is done with the help of a local anaesthetic ointment, with which the sigmoidoscope is smeared. As with the protoscope, the instrument (with the obturator fitted) is first directed towards the umbilicus and, when the anal canal is passed, the direction is changed towards the hollow of the sacrum. At this stage, the obturator is withdrawn and the eye piece as well as the inflating balloon are fitted, so that further introduction is carried under direct vision. As the rectum is being passed, the instrument is again directed anteriorly so as to reach the pelvi-rectal junction. At this level obstruction is encountered, and this is the level where great care should be taken so that the pelvi-rectal junction is traversed without injuring the gut. Further negotiation of the instrument is usually easy.

While the gut is examined when the instrument is going in, better observations are made as it is being slowly withdrawn. Some surgeons introduce the whole length of the instrument with the obturator in position and visualise the gut only while withdrawing the instrument. This minimises the risk of injury to the gut by the tip of the instrument, during its introduction.

RUBBER CATHETER

Uses

1. To relieve retention of urine.
2. To obtain a specimen of urine from an unconscious patient for purpose of examination.
3. To diagnose injuries of the urinary tract.
4. To ascertain whether absence of micturition is due to retention or suppression (see below).

Before a catheter is introduced, the following measures are often helpful in relieving retention:

1. Change of posture from recumbency to sitting or standing (particularly in post-operative patients).
2. Application of heat and cold, alternately, over the hypogastrium.
3. Injection of drugs—either atropine group or carbachol group.

Introduction.—The parts are washed with soap and water. A weak solution of dettol or savlon may be used for cleaning. The catheter is sterilised by boiling. The sterilised catheter is lubricated with glycerine or olive oil, or better, with an analgesic ointment. It is then introduced slowly along the urethra. As the bladder neck is reached a resistance is felt, and a little force pushes the catheter into the bladder. If any obstruction is felt in the passage, a little holding of the catheter in the same spot often overcomes the obstruction, if it is due to spasm. When urine starts ejecting, it must be made to come out slowly, since rapid evacuation of the bladder may lead to the following complications:

1. Cardiac Embarrassment.—Due to sudden release of intra-abdominal tension.
2. Haematuria.—Sudden evacuation of the bladder causes negative pressure in its lumen and a sucking effect on its wall. As a result, the dilated thin-walled submucous veins of the bladder may rupture, sometimes causing torrential haemorrhage.
3. Reflex Anuria.—Cessation of renal function reflexly.

After the urine has been evacuated:

a. The catheter may be withdrawn, if retention is unlikely to recur, or
b. The catheter is kept in position with the help of adhesive plasters, if retention is likely to recur (repeated introduction of catheter causes severe infection). For purpose of continuous catheterisation, catheters made of latex are preferable since they are softer and cause less damage to the urethral wall (Foley's self-retaining catheter of narrow calibre is the best for this purpose).

When a catheter has entered the bladder but urine is not coming out, the possibilities are:

a. The catheter is blocked.
b. The eye of the catheter has been passed above the level of the urine in the bladder. In these cases, a little withdrawal of the catheter brings out urine.

c. The patient is suffering from suppression of urine and not retention. Suppression means that urine is not being excreted by the kidneys. If the quantity of urine is less than 300 ml in 24 hours, the condition is called *oliguria*. If there is no urinary output for 12 hours, the condition is termed *anuria*.

RETENTION	SUPPRESSION
1. The patient usually complains of severe urge for micturition (excepting some patients of chronic retention).	1. Usually there is no urge for micturition.
2. On inspection.—The hypogastriun appears to be full. In thin-built persons the distended bladder can often be seen.	2. Nil.
3. On palpation.—A distended bladder may be made out.	3. Nil.
4. On percussion.—The dull note of a distended bladder is evident.	4. Nil.
5. Introduction of a catheter brings out urine.	5. Little or no urine is brought out by the catheter.

Other Uses of Catheter
1. For administration of nasal oxygen.
2. For administration of enema.
3. As a drainage tube.
4. As a Ryle's tube in children.
5. As a tourniquet.

Complications
1. Shock.—Rare, unless rapid evacuation is made.
2. Sepsis.—Urethritis, cystitis, and ascending infection.
3. Haemorrhage.—This may be due to:
   a. Trauma to urethra.
   b. Infection, e.g. urethritis, cystitis.
   c. Rapid evacuation of the bladder.
4. Catheter fever.

If a rubber catheter cannot be negotiated:
1. A rubber catheter of smaller calibre may be tried.

2. Catheters made of stiffer materials (e.g. plastic, gum elastic) may be tried. Catheters with angled tip *(coudie)* or with both angled and tapering tip are often successful when ordinary catheters fail.

3. Dilatation of the urethra with a bougie, followed by introduction of the catheter is sometimes helpful.

4. If this fails, there must be some obstruction at the bladder neck (e.g. enlarged prostate) or urethra (e.g. stricture). The site of obstruction is ascertained from the level of arrest of the catheter.

Accordingly, a metallic catheter (either male metallic or prostatic) is tried. Alternatively, a rubber catheter, mounted on a wire stretcher, which has been angled like a metallic catheter, may be tried and, if the catheter goes in, the stretcher is carefully withdrawn.

5. When this fails, *suprapubic puncture* of the bladder may be done with a thin-bore long needle and the bladder carefully aspirated. After evacuation of the bladder, the spasm and oedema at the bladder neck or at a stricture often pass off, and a rubber catheter may then be negotiated.

6. If this fails or if retention recurs after withdrawal of a male metallic catheter, suprapubic cystomy has to be undertaken.

METAL CATHETERS

There are three types:

1. Female metallic catheter (Fig. 72.29).
2. Male metallic catheter (Fig. 72.30).
3. Prostatic catheter (Fig. 72.31).

FEMALE METALLIC CATHETER

This is short and straight because the urethra is short in length and straight in the females. There are multiple holes at the tip because some of these may get blocked.

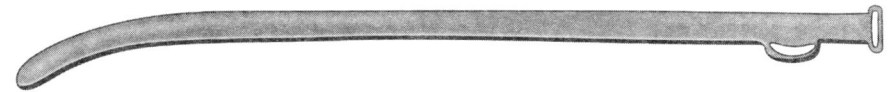

Fig. 72.29: Female metallic catheter

Uses

1. To relieve retention of urine in the females where rubber catheter fails. This is rare. In fact, retention of urine is rather infrequent in females.
2. As a routine, gynaecologists use this catheter to evacuate the bladder before any uterine or vaginal operation.

MALE METALLIC CATHETER AND PROSTATIC CATHETER

Use.—To relieve retention of urine when rubber catheter fails (see under rubber catheter).

With the help of the rubber catheter or a bougie, the level and nature of obstruction is noted, and accordingly, a male metallic catheter (for stricture urethra) or a prostatic catheter (for enlarged prostate) is chosen.

MALE METALLIC CATHETER

1. Shorter in length.

2. The angle is narrower.

3. The eyes are situated laterally.

PROSTATIC CATHETER

1. Longer, since in cases of enlarged prostate, there is an increase in length of the prostatic urethra.

2. The angle is wider, since in cases of enlarged prostate, the urethral angle is exaggerated.

3. The eyes are located anteroposteriorly. In cases of enlarged prostate, the lateral lobes often enlarge into the bladder and the lobes themselves might block the eyes of the catheter, had they been situated laterally.

Fig. 72.30: Male metallic catheter

The metal catheters (and all metallic instruments meant for introduction along the urethra) are curved because the male urethra is curved along its length.

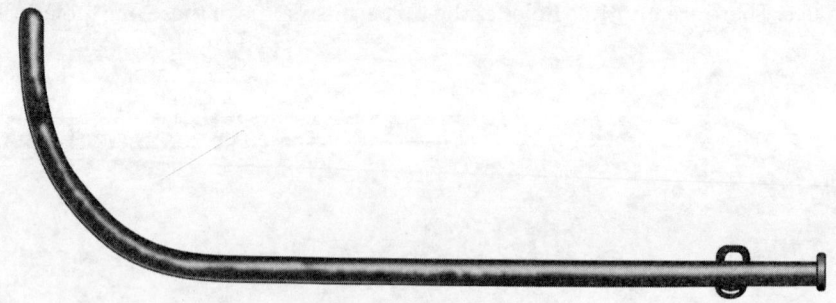

Fig. 72.31: Prostatic catheter

The two eyes of the catheter are not located at the same level since this would make the catheter weaker at that spot.

The two rings on the handle of the catheter are meant for attachment of threads that are used to fix the catheter in position. The other end of the threads is tied to the thigh of the patient on either side.

Sterilisation.—Boiling or autoclaving.

Introduction.—The parts are sterilised (*see* rubber catheter). An analgesic ointment is introduced into the urethra with the help of a nozzle (fitted to the tube of the ointment) or with a syringe (without needle). Five minutes' time is given for the ointment to produce its effect and during this period, escape of the ointment is prevented by digital pressure on the urethra. The sterilised catheter is lubricated with the ointment and is introduced.

The surgeon stands on the left side of the patient and holds the penis elevated with his left hand. With the right hand he holds the catheter, parallel to the left inguinal ligament, with the convexity of the catheter forwards and 'with its tip backwards, placed on the external urethral meatus. The instrument is allowed to go in by its own weight and, as it moves in, the handle of the instrument gradually comes to the midline on the abdomen. A resistance is then felt, and at this stage the tip of the catheter has reached the base of the triangular ligament that marks the junction of the penile and membranous parts of the urethra, which is the site of its maximum curvature. The handle of the catheter is now gently depressed between the two thighs of the patient, in an attempt to make the tip of the catheter follow the curvature of the posterior urethra and enter the bladder.

When the catheter goes into the bladder:
1. A sudden loss of resistance is felt and the handle can be depressed between the two thighs easily.
2. The instrument is strictly in the midline.
3. The catheter can be rotated freely on either side.
4. The patient complains of very little pain, if at all.
5. Urine comes out.
6. Little or no blood comes out.

In case the catheter has made a false passage:
a. There is a continuous sense of resistance and the handle cannot be gently depressed between the two thighs.
b. The catheter deviates from the midline.
c. The instrument cannot be freely rotated.
d. The patient complains of severe pain (hence, urethral instrumentation should preferably be done under local anaesthesia, instead of general).
e. No urine comes out.
f. There is bleeding, sometimes severe.

Complications.—These are much more frequent and more serious than with a rubber catheter:
1. Shock.
2. Sepsis.
3. Haemorrhage, particularly from false passage.
4. Catheter fever.
5. False passage.

When a metal catheter can be passed, it is usually not taken out immediately. It is fixed in position by tying threads from the rings on the handle to the thighs of the patient. The catheter should not be kept for more than 48 hours because there is the risk of gross damage to the delicate urethral mucosa, inviting infection and stricture formation. After 48 hours, as the catheter is withdrawn:
   a. The patient may be able to void urine himself (rare).
   b. A rubber catheter may now be made to pass.
   c. If a rubber catheter fails, or if the urethra is grossly damaged or infected, a suprapubic cystostomy has to be performed.

SELF-RETAINING CATHETERS

Types.—The common varieties, in use, are:
1. Malecot's catheter (Fig. 72.32).
2. De Pezzer's catheter (Fig. 72.33).
3. Foley's catheter.

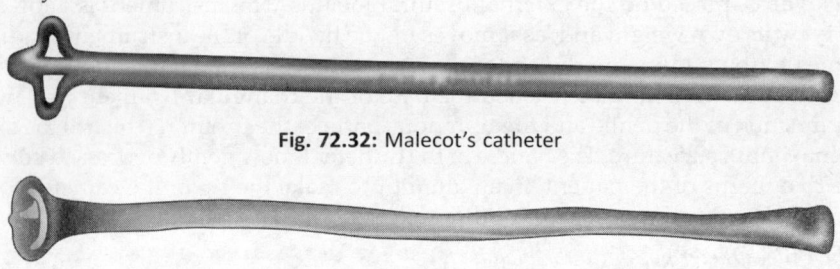

Fig. 72.32: Malecot's catheter

Fig. 72.33: De Pezzer's catheter

These catheters are called 'self-retaining' because they can retain themselves into the bladder without external anchorage. The self-retaining mechanism is the same with the Malecot's and De Pezzer's varieties, but is different with the Foley's catheter.

MALECOT'S & DE PEZZER'S SELF-RETAINING CATHETERS AND SELF-RETAINING CATHETER INTRODUCER

The self-retaining mechanism, in these two varieties of catheters, lies in their expanded tip. During introduction, the tip is stretched with the help of a self-retaining catheter introducer. It is thus made narrow and the catheter can well be introduced, through a small suprapubic opening, into the bladder. Thereafter, as the introducer is withdrawn, the tip re-expands and so the catheter cannot come out (Fig. 72.34).

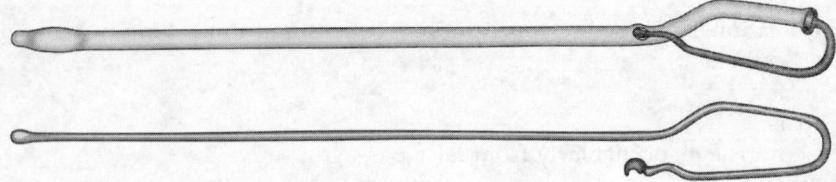

Fig. 72.34: Self-retaining catheter introducer (a stretched Malecot's catheter is shown)

These catheters are only meant for the suprapubic route and hence they are usually used in suprapubic cystostomy. However, narrow-calibre catheters, of these varieties, may be introduced per urethra in females, since in females the urethra is straight and short (rarely used).

A suprapubic self-retaining catheter must be changed regularly, at about one month's interval, since phosphates get deposited at the expanded tip of the catheter as well as in its lumen. The results are that:

a. The catheter is blocked.

b. There is infection in the bladder (cystitis).

c. The tip gets inelastic, so that it becomes very difficult to bring the catheter out.

The catheter may be withdrawn either with the help of the introducer, stretching its tip, or (since blind introduction of the introducer may damage the bladder wall by coming out through the gaps at the tip of the catheter), by drawing it out with a sharp pull (the resultant trauma to the tissues is negligible).

Sterilisation.—The catheters are sterilised by boiling, and the introducer either by boiling or by autoclaving.

FOLEY'S SELF-RETAINING CATHETER

The self-retaining mechanism of this catheter is in the balloon near its tip. At the other end of the catheter there are two tubes. The wider tube communicates with the eyes of the catheter and is meant for draining urine. The narrower tube communicates with the balloon. Through the narrower tube water is to be injected after the catheter has been passed into the bladder. The balloon distends and prevents the catheter from coming out. The amount of water to be injected (the capacity of the balloon) is written on the catheter. Also, the calibre of the catheter is mentioned on it. When the catheter has to be withdrawn, the water is aspirated out with a syringe from the narrower tube.

Sterilisation.—By boiling.

Uses

1. Via a suprapubic cystostomy to drain the bladder.
2. Via the urethra in either sex. A narrow-calibre catheter may be passed per urethra, in either sex, for continuous catheterisation of the bladder. Apart from its self-retaining capacity, it is preferred to an ordinary rubber catheter because it causes less damage to the urethra as it is made of softer material (latex).
3. Via the urethra in the males to arrest haemorrhage from the prostatic bed after prostatectomy. In these cases the eyes of the catheter lie in the bladder but the balloon is kept in the prostatic cavity. As the balloon is inflated, it puts pressure on the prostatic bed and stops bleeding (a mild traction on the catheter works more efficiently in arresting haemorrhage).
4. Via the urethra in the males to act as a splint after repair of membranous urethral rupture by the 'rail-road method'.

Methods of Arresting Haemorrhage after Prostatectomy

A. DIRECT METHOD.—With proper exposure, retraction and illumination, the bleeding points are seen, and ligated and/or cauterised under direct vision.

B. INDIRECT METHODS:

1. Pressure on the prostatic bed with the balloon of a Foley's catheter.
2. Plugging the prostatic bed with roller gauge around a urethral catheter. through a circuit.

3. Continuous irrigation of the prostatic bed with ice cold water through a urethral catheter → prostatic bed → bladder → suprapubic catheter.

SUPRAPUBIC CYSTOSTOMY

This means making an opening in the bladder via the suprapubic route. If the bladder is closed immediately after opening, the operation should be called *cystostomy*.

Indications

1. Cases of retention of urine where catheterisation fails.

2. As a preliminary to two-stage prostatectomy (here the suprapubic cystostomy makes the first stage of the operation).

3. For removal of bladder stones and foreign bodies.

4. Sometimes in the operations for rupture urethra, stricture urethra, etc.

Pre-operative Preparation.—The most important pre-requisite for the operation is that the bladder must be full. In those cases where the bladder is empty it must be filled up with sterile water through a urethral catheter; alternatively, the patient should be advised not to void urine for a few hours before the operation. Unless the operation is done on a full bladder:

1. It is really difficult to find out the empty bladder that sinks inside the pelvis.

2. The operation becomes intraperitoneal since, when the bladder is empty, the anterior parietal peritoneum comes down to cover its anterior wall so that the approach via the suprapubic route becomes intraperitoneal. When the bladder is full, the parietal peritoneum is reflected directly on to the fundus of the bladder, without covering the anterior wall, so that there is direct approach to the bladder, without opening up the peritoneal cavity.

Operation.—The operation is usually done with local infiltration anaesthesia. Spinal (or epidural) or general anaesthesia may also be employed.

A midline suprapubic incision is made. The anterior rectus sheath is cut in the midline (linea alba). The rectus abdominis and pyramidalis muscles of the two sides are retracted from the midline. The extraperitoneal fat is dissected and the peritoneal fold, seen in the upper part of the incision is gently rubbed off the wall of the bladder. The anterior wall of the bladder is identified by:

1. Typical colour of its musculature.

2. Big longitudinal veins running on its surface.

3. Aspiration with a syringe and needle (bringing out urine) in cases of doubt.

The bladder wall is now steadied either with two tissue forceps or with two stay-knots—one applied on each side of the proposed line of incision on the bladder. These stay-knots (or forceps) will control the evacuation of the bladder (which should not be rapid) and will also prevent sinking down of the bladder into the pelvis.

The incision on the bladder is usually vertical, in order to avoid injury to the longitudinally-running big veins. A self-retaining catheter is introduced through the opening. The excess of the opening, around the catheter, is sutured. A drain is put into the retropubic space (cave of Retzius), and the wound is closed in layers. This drain is removed after 48 hours.

KIDD'S TROCAR AND CANULA

This is a two-way trocar and canula. It is used in performing suprapubic cystostomy by the blind method, in relieving acute retention of urine (Fig. 72.35).

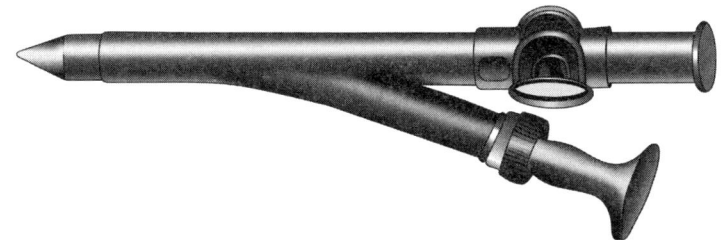

Fig. 72.35: Kidd's trocar and canula

A small incision, only skin-deep, is made in the midline, above the pubis. The tip of the instrument is pushed through this incision, till the bladder is entered. The trocar is then withdrawn. A self-retaining catheter is introduced through the canula. A Foley's catheter can be introduced as such. If a Malecot's or De Pezzer's catheter is used, it is passed in with the help of a self-retaining catheter introducer. Once the catheter goes into the bladder, the canula is taken out over it.

It is always preferable to do a suprapubic cystostomy by the open operative method than by this blind method because:

1. There may be injury to the big veins on the bladder wall, causing troublesome haemorrhage.
2. Collections are apt to occur in the cave of Retzius (retropubic space) because of leakage of urine and blood, and these remain undrained.
3. Rarely, there may be injury to the peritoneum or intestines (this is usually unlikely to occur since the peritoneum moves up with the fundus of the bladder as the latter gets distended).

Sterilisation.—Boiling or autoclaving.

SUPRAPUBIC CYSTOLITHOTOMY FORCEPS

This forceps is used for the removal of bladder stones by the suprapubic route (Fig. 72.36).

The knobs or pins on the inner side of the blades are meant for good grip on the stone, which might otherwise slip out. Of the two handles, one has a ring, meant for the thumb. The other handle has a wide hook, meant for the other fingers. There are no catches on the handles since the stones should never be crushed.

The preliminary steps of the operation (suprapubic cystolithotomy) are the same as for suprapubic cystostomy. After the bladder is opened, the stones are brought out with this forceps.

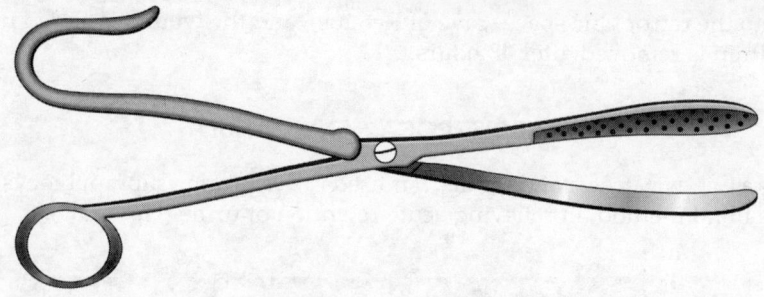

Fig. 72.36: Suprapubic cystolithotomy forceps

Whether a primary closure of the bladder wound should be done or a temporary suprapubic cystostomy should be maintained is a matter of decision, and depends on two factors:

1. Whether the stone is primary, i.e. not due to urinary obstruction. If there is obstruction and it is believed that the stone is secondary to it, a suprapubic cystostomy is maintained.

2. Whether the urine is infected or not. In presence of infected urine (as suggested by preliminary urine examination and by the smell and appearance of the urine at operation), a cystostomy is maintained.

If a primary closure of the bladder is done, a urethral catheter is kept for a few days for continuous drainage of the bladder, so that there is no tension on the suture line that would prevent healing. If a suprapubic cystostomy is done, removal of the self-retaining catheter is followed by spontaneous healing of the wound, provided the infection or the distal obstruction has been overcome.

LITHOTRITE

This is an instrument used for crushing bladder stones (Fig. 72.37). The operation is called 'lithotrity'. After the stones are crushed, the particles are. washed out by irrigating the bladder with the help of an evacuating canula (Fig. 72.38). The combined process of crushing the stones and flushing the bladder is called 'litholapaxy'.

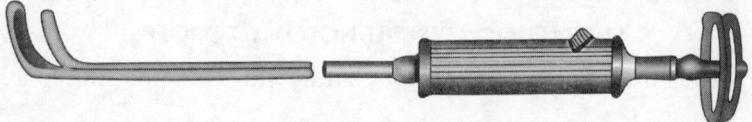

Fig. 72.37: Lithotrite

Sterilisation:—Autoclave or concentrated lysol.

Litholapaxy.—The bladder must be full. An analgesic ointment is introduced into the urethra. A preliminary cystoscopy is performed to ascertain the number and size of the stones. The lithotrite, with its blades apposed, is introduced per urethra (in the same way as a metal catheter). The first use of the instrument is as a bladder sound, to locate the stone. The blades are now opened by rotating the ring on the handle of the instrument and the stone is caught blindly between the blades. The instrument is then rotated by 90° on either side to be sure that bladder wall has not been incorporated between the blades. The stone is now crushed by apposing the blades. All stones, and big fragments thereof, are dealt with in the same way.

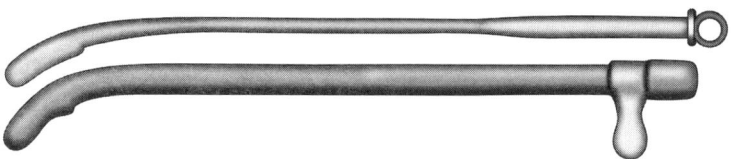

Fig. 72.38: Evacuating canula (the stellate is shown above)

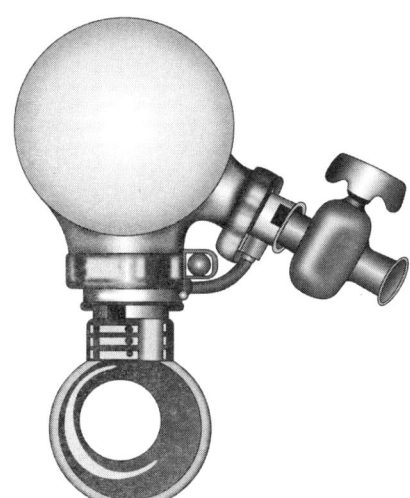

Fig. 72.38A: Evacuating pump

The instrument is withdrawn, with its blades closed. An evacuating canula (Fig. 72.38) is introduced per urethra to evacuate the fluid from the bladder (with the stone fragments). This is usually done with the help of an aspirator (Fig. 72.38A), which is fitted to the evacuating canula. The aspirator has a rubber ball, communicating with a glass bulb at its bottom. The ball is filled with sterile water and is compressed and released alternately, so that, with a to and fro movement, the fluid inside the bladder is brought out into the glass bulb. The process is repeated, till the return fluid from the bladder is clear.

The *advantage* of the operation is that it avoids cutting and, if required, can be repeated. But the disadvantages are many and are as follows:

1 It requires a very expert to perform the operation.
2. It has many centra-indications:
   a. Type of stones:
      i. Too big a stone (bladder wall may be grasped with the stone).

    ii. Too small a stone (cannot be caught blindly).

    iii. Too hard a stone, e.g. oxalate (cannot be crushed).

    iv. Too soft a stone, e.g. cystine (moulded and not crushed).

    v. Stone in a diverticulum or in the post-prostatic pouch.

    vi. Stone encrusting a foreign body.

  b. Presence of infection.

  c. Presence of obstruction (the instrument cannot be passed).

CYSTOSCOPE

Figure 72.39 shows the different parts of the cystoscope. The types of cystoscope and their use have been described in details in Chapter 55.

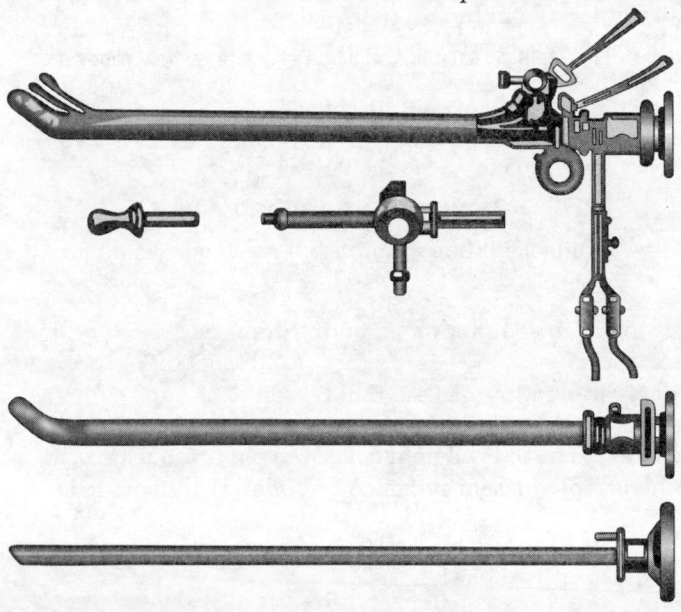

Fig. 72.39: Cystoscope (in the middle is seen the visualising cystoscope and, below it, the inner sheath. The catheterising cystoscope, with two ureteric catheters, is seen above)

BLADDER SOUND

This is a long instrument, right-angled just near the tip (Fig. 72.40).

It is used to 'sound' a stone in the bladder and is introduced per urethra in the same way as a metal catheter, with the help of local analgesic ointment.

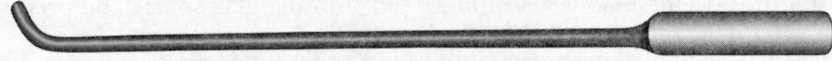

Fig. 72.40: Bladder sound

Sterilisation.—Boiling or autoclaving.

BOUGIE OR URETHRAL DILATOR

Types.—There are two common varieties:

1. Lister's bougie (Fig. 72.41).

2. Clutton's bougie (Fig. 72.42).

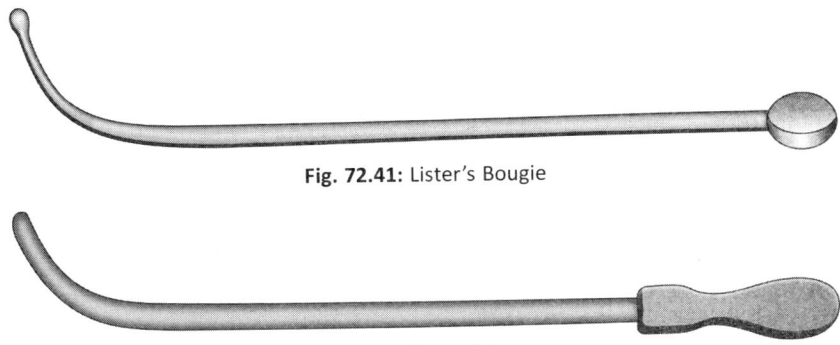

Fig. 72.41: Lister's Bougie

Fig. 72.42: Clutton's Bougie

LISTER'S	CLUTTON'S
1. The tip is olive-pointed.	1. The tip is plain.
2. The end of the handle is round.	2. The end of the handle is trapezoid.
3. The figures on the handle indicate the minimum and maximum *diameter* of the instrument. The difference between the two figures is 3.	3. These figures indicate the minimum and maximum *circumference* of the instrument. The difference between the two figures is 4.
4. The maximum size is 9/12.	4. The maximum size is 24/28. It is of much bigger calibre than the highest size Lister's bougie.

Uses
1. For intermittent dilatation in cases of stricture urethra.
2. For preliminary dilatation of the urethra to facilitate introduction of rubber catheters, cystoscopes, lithotrites, etc. in difficult cases.

Introduction.—Same as metal catheters.

Complications.—Same as metal catheters.

Sterilisation.—Boiling or autoclaving.

RETROGRADE BOUGIE

This is so called because it traverses in a direction opposite to that of an ordinary bougie, i.e. it goes down from the bladder into the urethra. Hence, suprapubic cystostomy is a preliminary step for its use. The bougie is passed through the suprapubic opening in the bladder and its tip is passed through the internal meatus into the urethra, with the guidance of a finger in the bladder. The curvature of the instrument is so made that it passes clear of the symphysis pubis.

Uses
1. In the repair of ruptured urethra by the 'rail-road method' (*see* Chapter 56).

2. To identify the upper end of the urethra while operating for stricture urethra (*see* Chapter 56).

Sterilisation.—Boiling or autoclaving.

URETHRAL FORCEPS

This is a delicate forceps with crocodile jaws. It may be used for removal of foreign bodies or impacted stones from the urethra (Fig. 72.43).

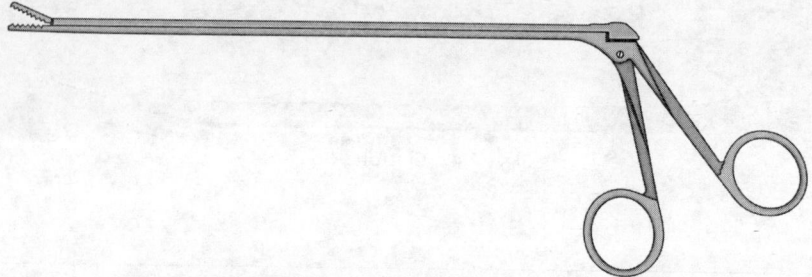

Fig. 72.43: Urethral forceps

Sterilisation.—Concentrated lysol or autoclave.

PHIMOSIS FORCEPS

This forceps has light slender blades. The blades are straight and have longitudinal serrations (Fig. 72.44).

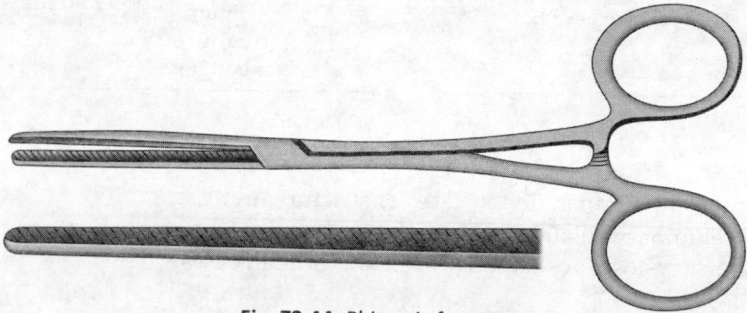

Fig. 72.44: Phimosis forceps

The forceps is sometimes used in the operation of circumcision for phimosis in the children, in whom the foreskin is usually considerably long. The foreskin and the prepuce are drawn forwards and the forceps is applied on them, distal to the glans penis. The excess of foreskin and prepuce, distal to the forceps, is excised. The forceps is thereafter removed, all bleeding points secured, and the cut margin of the foreskin is sutured to the cut margin of the prepuce with interrupted stitches.

Sterilisation.—Boiling or autoclaving.

CHEEK RETRACTOR

This is meant for retraction of the cheek which may be necessary for:

1. Examination of the inner side of the cheek, the lateral parts of the gingio-labial folds, and the retromolar area.

2. Operations on the said areas.
3. Examination and probing of the opening of the parotid duct. The parotid ducts open on the inner side of the cheek, opposite the crown of the upper second molar teeth (the submandibular ducts open on the floor of the mouth on either side of the frenum linguae; the sublingual ducts, multiple and small, open on the floor of the mouth under the tongue or into the submandibular ducts).
The groove of the retractor fits into the angle of the mouth (Fig. 72.45).

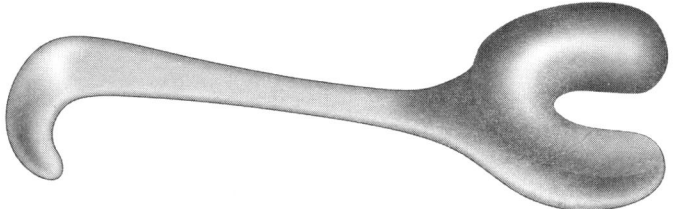

Fig. 72.45: Check retractor

Sterilisation.—Boiling or autoclaving.

DOYEN'S MOUTH GAG

This instrument is used to keep the mouth open. It is, therefore, used in operation's inside the mouth and on the tongue, tonsils and pharynx (Fig. 72.46).

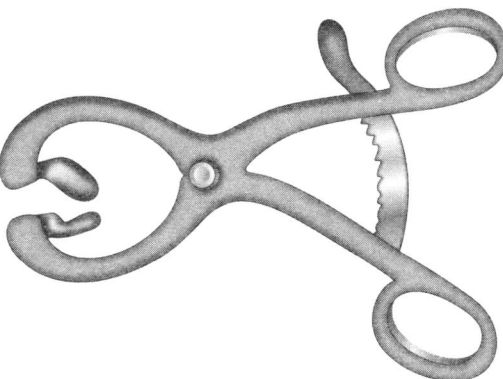

Fig. 72.46: Doyen's mouth gag

The instrument is passed between the upper and the lower teeth, with the blades apposed. Thereafter, as the handles are apposed, the blades diverge and the mouth is opened. When this has been done, the handles lock by themselves and the mouth cannot close. To withdraw the instrument, the lock at the handle is released, so that the handles can now be diverged and the blades apposed.

Sterilisation.—Boiling or autoclaving.

BOYLE DAVIS GAG

This is a bigger gag than the Doyen's variety and is particularly used in operations for cleft palate and tonsils (by the dissection method)—Fig. 72.47.

Sterilisation.—Boiling or autoclaving.

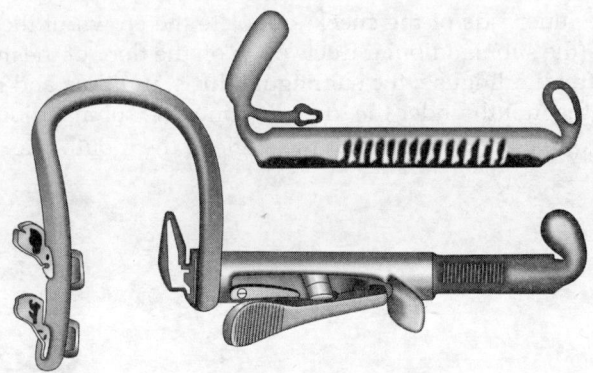

Fig. 72.47: Boyle davis mouth gag

AIRWAY TUBE

Types.—These may be made of:

a. Metal (Fig. 72.48).

b. Rubber (Fig. 72.49).

These are called airway tube because they help entry of air into the air-passages. They are used in unconscious patients or patients under anaesthesia:

a. In whom the tongue may roll back and cause complete obstruction of the air passage; the curvature of the tube is so made that, when it is put in, it draws the tongue forwards;

b. In whom the tongue may be bitten by the teeth. The instrument separates the upper row of teeth from the lower. During anaesthesia, they also prevent the endotracheal tube being bitten by the patient.

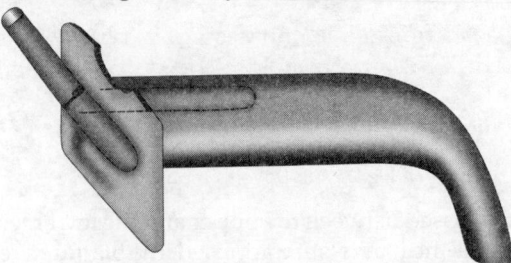

Fig. 72.48: Metal airway tube

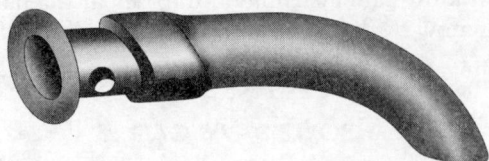

Fig. 72.49: Rubber airway tube

The narrow tube, attached at the outer end, is meant for fixing an oxygen tube, if necessary. There are multiple openings at the inner end because some of these openings may be blocked by mucus-plugs.

As soon as the patient's cough reflex returns, he tries to cough the tube out. The tube is then withdrawn.

Sterilisation.—Boiling or autoclaving.

LOGAN'S BOW

This is sometimes used to overcome tension on the suture line after repair of cleft lip. However, if mobilisation of the flaps is adequate, there is seldom any necessity for these appliances to be used (Fig. 72.50).

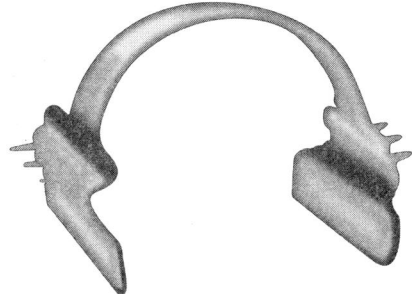

Fig. 72.50: Logan's bow

Sterilisation.—Concentrated lysol or autoclave.

CLEFT PALATE RASPATORY

This raspatory, i.e. periosteum elevator, is designed especially for the purpose of elevating the mucoperiosteum from the hard palate, while mobilising the flaps for repair of cleft palate (Fig. 72.51).

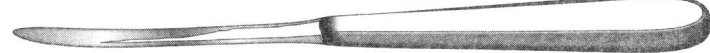

Fig. 72.51: Cleft palate raspatory

Sterilisation.—Concentrated lysol.

METAL TRACHEOSTOMY TUBE

This is meant for air entry into the trachea, along a tracheostomy wound. There are two component tubes—an outer and an inner. If the inner tube gets blocked with mucus, it may be taken out, keeping the outer tube in position. The inner tube, cleansed, can be reinserted (Fig. 72.52).

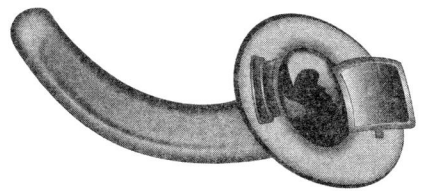

Fig. 72.52: Metal tracheostomy tube

The curvature of the tube is so made that the tip does not cause trauma to the trachea.

There is a special variety, where the outer tube is bivalved. Its advantage is that it can be introduced through the stab wound on the trachea without the help of a tracheal dilator because it, itself, dilates the opening during introduction.

The rings at the base of the inner tube may be used:

a. for withdrawal of the inner tube,

b. for fixation of the tube to the neck with the help of tapes, tied loosely around the neck.

With the tracheostomy tube in position, oxygen has often to be administered. This may be done with an oxygen funnel, placed on the tube, or with an oxygen catheter, the tip of which is introduced into the tube. The wound is covered with a thin layer of acriflavine-soaked gauge, so that air enters into the tube through this layer of gauge.

After tracheostomy, there is often a profuse secretion, which tends to block the tube. This has to be cleansed either with mild suction or with a feather.

The metal tracheostomy tube should not be kept for more than 48 hours because it causes damage to the delicate mucosa. After 48 hours, the metal tube has to be replaced by a rubber or polythene tube.

Sterilisation.—Boiling or autoclaving.

RUBBER OR POLYTHENE TRACHEOSTOMY TUBE

These are used to replace a metal tracheostomy tube, which should not be kept for more than 48 hours after the operation. They can be kept for indefinite periods. When it is evident that there is no further obstruction to the upper air passage, the tube is withdrawn (this can be ascertained by occluding the lumen of the tube with an adhesive plaster). The wound heals spontaneously (Fig. 72.53).

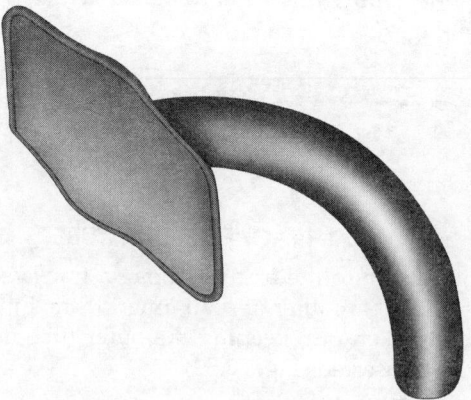

Fig. 72.53: Polythene tracheostomy tube

TRACHEAL DILATOR

This is meant to dilate the stab wound made on the trachea in the operation of tracheostomy, so that the metal tracheostomy tube can be introduced.

Sterilisation.—By boiling.

The working mechanism of this instrument differs from an ordinary forceps in that the blades open up when the handles are apposed and vice versa. This facilitates the purpose for which it is used (Fig. 72.54).

Sterilisation.—Boiling or autoclaving.

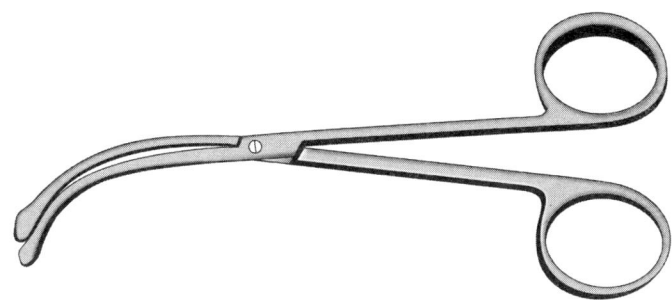

Fig. 72.54: Tracheal dilator

BLUNT HOOK

This is used as a retractor to pull the isthmus of the thyroid upwards, while performing a low tracheostomy (Fig. 72.55).

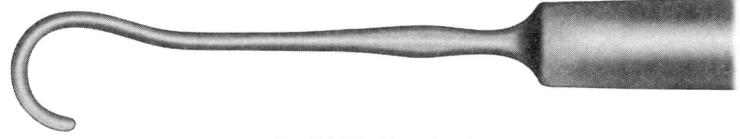

Fig. 72.55: Blunt hook

The isthmus of the thyroid overlaps the 2nd, 3rd and 4th tracheal rings and, in a low tracheostomy, the trachea is opened up at this level. Hence, the isthmus has either to be retracted up or to be split in the midline.

Sterilisation.—Boiling or autoclaving.

SHARP HOOK

In contrast to a blunt hook, the end is sharp. This is used to steady the trachea while making the stab wound on it, in the operation of tracheostomy. During respiratory obstruction (and it is in this condition that a tracheostomy is usually performed), the trachea moves very quickly up and down. Hence, it must be steadied while being stabbed. The sharp hook, inserted just below the cricoid cartilage, steadies the trachea (Fig. 72.56).

Sterilisation.—Concentrated lysol.

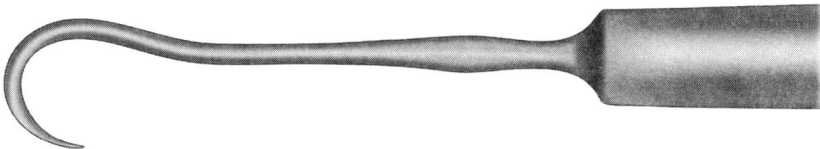

Fig. 72.56: Sharp hook

TRACHEOSTOMY

This means making a fistulous opening in the trachea.

Indications

A. AS AN EMERGENCY PROCEDURE

1. In cases of acute respiratory obstruction:
   a. By diphtheric membrane.
   b. By foreign body.
   c. In carcinoma of larynx or carcinoma of the posterior third of the tongue, particularly when the patient is undergoing radiotherapy.
   d. Oedema of the glottis.
   e. Bilateral recurrent laryngeal nerve injury at thyroidectomy.
2. When there is prolonged unconsciousness, e.g. in head injuries, poisonings, etc. In these conditions it is beneficial since:
   a. The dead space is obliterated.
   b. Toileting of the respiratory passage is made easier.

B. AS A PLANNED OPERATION

1. After repairing laryngeal injuries, and in laryngeal diseases, including malignancy, in order to give rest to the part.
2. In operations on the mandible, when there is a tendency for the tongue to fall back in the post-operative period.
3. As a preliminary procedure, e.g. in repair of laryngeal fistula, laryngectomy, etc.

Types.—In older days the classification was:

1. High
2. Median
3. Low

Depending on whether the trachea was opened above, behind, or below the isthmus of the thyroid.

A high tracheostomy was often followed by infection of the laryngeal cartilages, leading to permanent laryngeal stenosis. Again, too low a tracheostomy is associated with the risk of damaging the engorged inferior thyroid veins or even the innominate veins, which are grossly dilated and often peep into the neck during respiratory obstructions.

The standard procedure, nowadays, is to perform a median tracheostomy—the trachea being opened behind the isthmus of the thyroid, which is either split in the midline or is retracted upwards.

Under local infiltration anaesthesia (without anaesthesia in severe emergencies), *with the neck extended,* a vertical incision is made in the midline over the trachea. The infrahyoid strap muscles are split in the midline and retracted on either side. The isthmus of the thyroid is drawn up with a blunt retractor or a blunt hook. Alternatively, the isthmus is cut through in the midline. The trachea is steadied with a sharp hook, inserted just below the cricoid cartilage, and stabbed. The opening is dilated with a tracheal dilator and a metal tracheostomy tube of suitable size is introduced. The troublesome oozing that occurs during the operation is due to venous congestion from respiratory obstruction. As soon as the obstruction is relieved, the oozing stops. The excess of the skin wound is closed round the tube. The tube is fixed in position with tapes, loosely tied around the neck. The tube, together with the wound, is covered with a thin layer of gauge soaked with acriflavine, so that air is freely strained-in through the layers of the gauge.

KOCHER'S THYROID DISSECTOR

This dissector is meant to dissect the superior pole of the thyroid before ligating the superior thyroid vessels in the substance of the thyroid (see Kocher's artery forceps).

Sterilisation.—Boiling or autoclaving (Fig. 72.57).

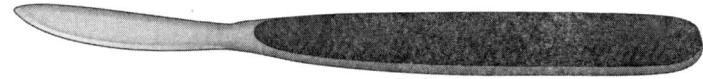

Fig. 72.57: Kocher's thyroid dissector

CORD FORCEPS

This forceps has a wide ring at one end, which is made into two halves—one attached to each blade. The ring can accommodate the spermatic cord, without causing pressure on it. It is used to retract the cord forwards while repairing the posterior wall of the inguinal canal *behind* the spermatic cord (Bassini's herniorrhaphy)—Fig. 72.58.

Sterilisation.—Boiling or autoclaving.

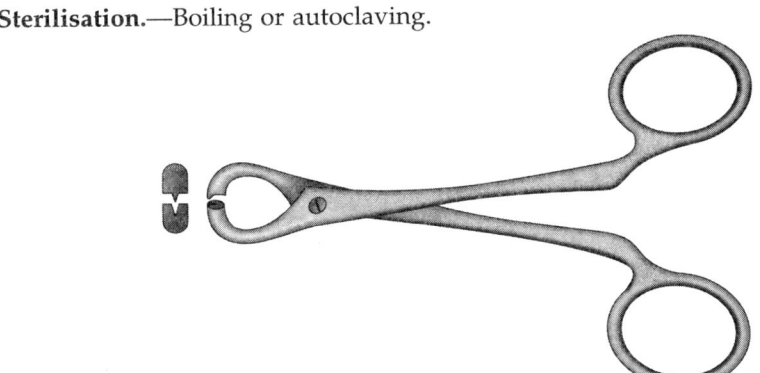

Fig. 72.58: Cord forceps

CHILDE'S HERNIA DIRECTOR

This instrument is wider at the centre and is grooved on one surface, to act as a director. It is used in cutting the constriction band while operating for an obstructed or strangulated hernia. The instrument is carefully passed behind the constriction band, with the groove towards the surface, till the central expanded part is under the constriction band. The broad blade protects the underlying structures (in the sac) while the band is cut on the groove of the director (Fig. 72.59).

Sterilisation.—Boiling or autoclaving.

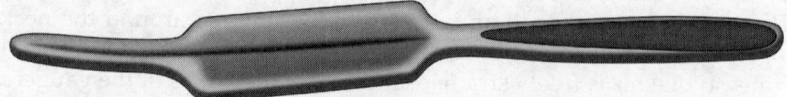

Fig. 72.59: Childe's hernia director

KAY'S HERNIA DIRECTOR

This instrument is grooved on one of its surfaces and acts as a director. Its use is the same as for the Childe's hernia director, i.e. cutting the constriction band of an obstructed or strangulated hernia. As the blade of this instrument is narrower than that of the Childe's -variety, it can be passed more easily behind the constriction band but cannot afford the same degree of protection to the underlying structures which the broad blade of a Childe's director can (Fig. 72.60).

Sterilisation.—Boiling or autoclaving.

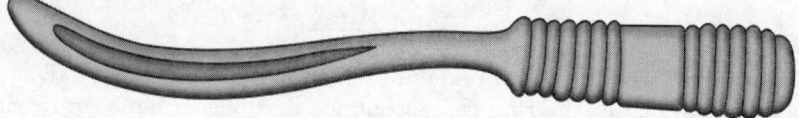

Fig. 72.60: Kay's hernia director

HERNIA BISTOURY

This is used in conjunction with a hernia director (Childe's or Kay's) to cut the constriction band of an obstructed or strangulated hernia. The tip of the instrument is passed along the groove of the director *behind* the constriction band, with its blade facing outwards. The constriction band is cut *from inside outwards* by the blade. The tip of the instrument is made blunt so that it can be passed blindly along the groove of the. director, without causing any damage (Fig. 72.61).

Sterilisation.—Concentrated lysol.

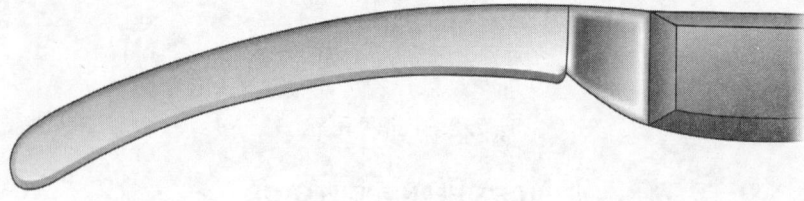

Fig. 72.61: Hernia bistoury

TROCAR AND CANULA

This is a combination of a trocar (the inner sharp-pointed part) and a canula (the outer sheath) and is used for tapping of hydrocele (Fig. 72.62). A lumbar puncture needle may be used instead.

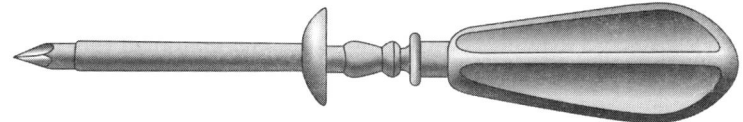

Fig. 72.62: Trocar and canula

The position of the testis is first ascertained by palpation and transillumination. Tapping must be done under strict aseptic conditions. It is performed through the lower part of the anterior aspect of the scrotum. The skin of the scrotum, over this part is made tense by grasping the scrotal skin at the upper part of the scrotum. A local anaesthetic agent is infiltrated into this skin, avoiding any visible blood vessel. The trocar and canula, together, are carefully thrust in, taking care that they do not go in too far as to injure the testis (particular care should be taken for a small hydrocele). The trocar is withdrawn and the fluid is allowed to evacuate through the canula. Thereafter, the canula is taken out. The wound is sealed with benzoin and a suspensory bandage is applied to support the scrotum.

Tapping should not be ordinarily advised because of the following dangers and disadvantages:

1. Injury to the testis.
2. Bleeding inside the sac (haematocele).
3. Infection in the sac (suppurative hydrocele).
4. Recurrence of hydrocele—occurs in almost all the cases.
5. A persistent discharging sinus through the opening.

Hence, for a hydrocele, an operation should always be advised, and not tapping.

RUBBER DRAINS

Types.—There are three common types in use:
1. Rubber Tubes or Catheters (including self-retaining catheters).
2. Corrugated Rubber Sheet (Fig. 72.63).

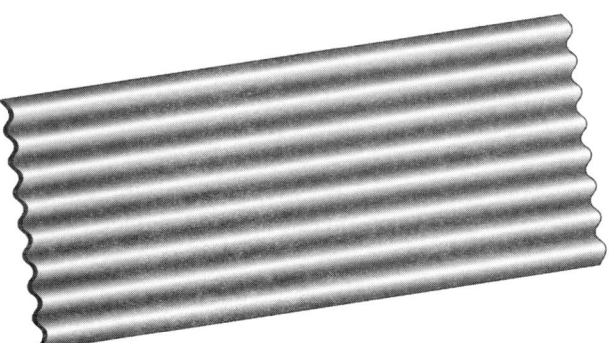

Fig. 72.63: Corrugated rubber drain

3. Cigarette Drain.—There is a rubber tube, through the lumen of which a strip of gauge is passed (as if the gauge is the tobacco and the rubber, the paper of a cigarette).

Gauge is inferior to rubber, for the purpose of drainage, in the following respects:

i. When the soaked exudates dry up, the gauge can no longer serve as a drain.

ii. The inner end of the gauge may get attached to the wall of a cavity and withdrawal of the gauge may cause bleeding from the wall.

iii. If gauge drains are used for the abdominal cavity, they may adhere to the omentum and sometimes the viscera, making withdrawal difficult.

However, rubber tubes have the disadvantage that their inner end, because of stiffness, may cause damage to the wall of the cavity drained, or to the abdominal organs when used in the abdomen. In this respect, corrugated rubber sheets are much less dangerous.

A cigarette drain provides the advantage of two drains. If necessary, the gauge may be withdrawn first and the rubber tube kept in position for a few hours or days more. Cigarette drains are very commonly used for draining the abdominal cavity, e.g. the Morison's pouch after cholecystectomy.

Corrugated rubber sheets (narrow strips) are most commonly used in the operation of hydrocele.

Catheter drains (including self-retaining catheters) are most commonly used for the pleural cavity.

Sterilisation.—Boiling or autoclaving.

SUTURE OR LIGATURE MATERIALS

Ligation means tying a structure, e.g. artery, vein, etc. with a ligature material.

Suturing means apposition of two structures, and this requires a needle and a ligature material.

Ligature materials may be divided into two broad groups:

GROUP A: Absorbable materials, i.e. materials which get absorbed in the tissues, e.g. catgut, kangaroo tendon.

GROUP B: Non-absorbable materials, i.e. materials which keep as such within the tissues, e.g. silk, cotton or linen thread, stainless steel wire, etc.

CATGUT

Though called catgut, it is made from the submucous coat of sheep's intestine (the word catgut has possibly come from kit-gut which means the strings of the violin—kitten meaning cat).

The submucous coat is obtained by stripping the muscle and the mucous membrane from its two surfaces. Thereafter, it is subjected to the following processes:

1. It has to be washed with ether to dissolve the fat.

2. It has to be immersed in carbolic acid for 8 days, so that the spores of the spore-bearing organisms are destroyed.

3. Ordinarily catgut is absorbed in the tissues within a week. Hence, if its presence in the tissues is necessary for a longer period, it has to be specially hardened. This is done by processing the catgut in salts of chromic acid for a

variable period and the longer they are processed, the harder they become. These types of catgut are called chromic or chromicised catgut and they stay in the tissues for 10 to 40 days. Thus, catgut may be;

a. Plain.

b. Chromicised.

Catgut is supplied in glass spools, which are air-tight. Inside the spool there is 70% alcohol; which acts as a preservative, and 5% glycerine that keeps the catgut soft. At operation, when the spools are supplied, their outer surface should be sterilised by immersing them either in 20% lysol for 24 hours or in cases of emergency, in concentrated lysol for half an hour.

The size of the catgut is according to its thickness, e.g. 6/0, 5/0, 4/0, 3/0, 2/0, 0, 1, 2, 3 and 4 from the finest to the thickest varieties.

The maximum *advantage of* catgut, as a suture material, is that it is absorbed in the tissues and, therefore, can be used even in presence of infection, where non-absorbable sutures should not be used.

The *disadvantages* of catgut are:

1. The foreign protein in the catgut is likely to cause tissue irritation and this may result in necrosis and infection in the tissues. This is manifested as 'catgut indigestion' or 'stitch abscess'. Its incidence can be minimised by the use of catgut of the finer calibres. So, at operations, the finest catgut, with which the tissues concerned may be sutured, should be used.

2. The tensile strength of the catgut diminishes in the tissues after 3–4 days and so, if suturing is done under tension, it is likely to give way.

3. As catgut swells inside the tissues, the knots are likely to open up later.

4. Catgut is costly.

KANGAROO TENDON

These are strips made from the tendon present in the tail of a kangaroo. This is a type of absorbable suture, each piece being about twelve inches in length. It is seldom used nowadays.

THREAD (COTTON OR LINEN)

As a non-absorbable suture, thread is gaining fast popularity, since it costs little and causes minimum complications. In fact, all tissues, excepting usually the mucous membrane, may be sutured with thread. It is commonly used for blood vessels, peritoneum, sheaths and aponeuroses, and also the skin.

Sterilisation.—Boiling or autoclaving.

SILK

The disadvantage of silk, in comparison to thread, is that it has the power of absorption and so it catches infection, rather easily. However, silk is frequently used as a ligature material for many tissues, including blood vessels, nerves, intestines, peritoneum, sheaths and aponeuroses, and the skin. Repair of herniae is also commonly done with silk. Silk, anchored to atrumatic needles, is known as 'anacap silk' and this is often used in suturing intestines, blood vessels, nerves, etc. and in plastic operations.

Sterilisation.—Boiling or autoclaving.

NYLON

This is a synthetic material and is a non-absorbable suture. It is most commonly used for the skin but is often used for repair of herniae.

Sterilisation.—Boiling or autoclaving.

STAINLESS STEEL WIRE

This is mainly used for:
1. Suturing of bones, e.g. olecranon, patella, etc.
2. Repair of herniae.

Sterilisation.—Boiling or autoclaving.

NEEDLES

Needles may be:
1. Straight, or
2. Curved, and the curvature may be half-circle, 3/8th or 5/8th of a circle. In general, the straight needles are used while working on the surface, and the curved needles at the depth.
   According to the cross-section, a needle may be:
   a. Round bodied.
   b. Triangular (triangular cutting).
   c. Flat (Hagedorn).
   While differentiating between a round bodied and a triangular cutting needle, the cross-section towards the tip should be considered, since all these needles are round bodied towards the eye.
   In addition to the above, there are some special types of needles:

1. INTESTINAL NEEDLES.—These are, in fact, slender round bodied needles. Sometimes they have 'spring-eye' which cause less damage to the intestines while passing through them.

2. ATRAUMATIC NEEDLES.—These have no eye (eyeless needles) and the suture material is fixed to the base of the needle. With an ordinary needle, the maximum trauma on the tissues is inflicted by the passage of the eye, because the eye is the thickest part of the needle and also because there is a doubling up of the suture material at the eye. With an eyeless needle, this trauma is minimised and so this is called 'atraumatic'. The suture material attached to the needle is either catgut or silk. When silk is attached to an eyeless needle, it is popularly termed 'anacap'. Atraumatic needles are used for the intestines, nerves, blood vessels, eyes, as well as in plastic operations. Their main disadvantage is that they are costly since the needle has to be discarded when the suture material has been used up.

3. GALLIE'S NEEDLE.—This is a very stout, triangular cutting, curved needle, used for hernioplasty with autogenous material (*see* hernioplasty—Chapter 52).— Fig. 72.64.

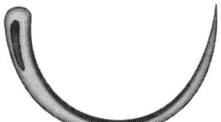

Fig. 72.64: Gallie's needle

4. LIVER SUTURE NEEDLE.—This is a long, curved, flat needle with a blunt tip. A sharp tip causes more damage to the liver, so the tip is made blunt. While suturing the liver, thick catgut should be used since finer catgut tends to tear through the liver substance when the knots are tightened (Fig. 72.65).

Fig. 72.65: Liver suture needle

Round Bodied Needles.—These are used for suturing delicate structures, e.g. peritoneum, muscles, intestines, etc. For the intestines, the intestinal needles (round bodied needles, which are slender and usually with spring eye) or, better, atraumatic needles should be used.

Triangular Cutting and Hagedorn Needles.—These are used to suture tough structures, e.g. skin, rectus sheath, aponeurosis, etc. They should not be used in suturing delicate structures particularly the intestines.

Sterilisation.—All needles are sterilised in concentrated lysol.

NEEDLE HOLDER

These may be:
1. Straight
2. Curved

The straight needle holders are used on the surface and the curved holders are conveniently used in the depth. The curvature of a curved needle holder is so made that it fits into the curvature of the palm, so that it can be used to work in the depth even through a small exposure (Fig. 72.66).

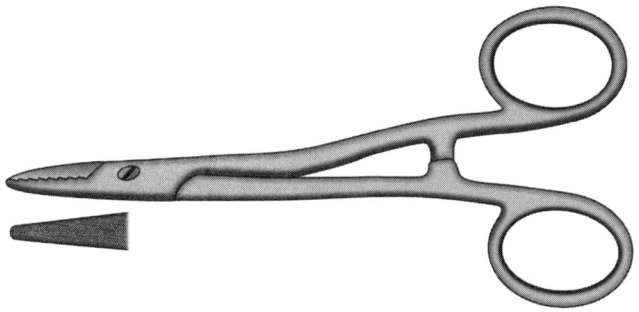

Fig. 72.66: Needle holder (curved)

The handle of a needle holder is long while the blade is short. The serrations on the inner side of the blades prevent slipping and turning of the needle. These needle holders may be used for all needles excepting the Hagedorn variety, which tends to turn inside the blades since it is flat. There is a special type of needle holder for the Hagedorn needle.

Sterilisation.—Boiling or autoclaving.

MICHEL CLIPS

These consist of small metal strips, at each end of which there is a sharp spike. These soused for apposition of skin margins, i.e. as substitutes for silk or nylon (Fig. 72.67).

The spikes pierce through the skin to get fixed there, while the elastic clip is pressed to bring the two ends closer, so that the skin margins are approximated.

A series of these clips, mounted on a wire-cabinet, is available. The wire-cabinet is conveniently mounted on a toothed dissecting forceps, and the same dissecting forceps is used to hold the skin margins while applying the clips. The application is done with the help of a special applicator. There is a special extractor for removal of the clips.

Sterilisation.—Concentrated lysol or autoclave.

MICHEL CLIP APPLICATOR

This instrument looks like a dissecting forceps but has a transverse groove in each blade, near the tip. These grooves accommodate the expanded ends of the michel clips. Pressure on the blades flexes the clip, held between them, and the skin margins are approximated (Fig. 72.67).

Sterilisation.—Boiling or autoclaving.

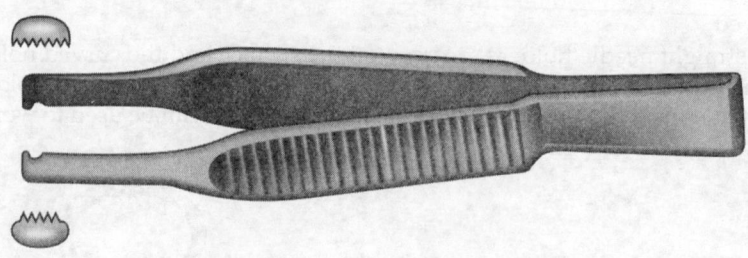

Fig. 72.67: Michel clip applicator

MICHEL CLIP EXTRACTOR

This instrument is like a forceps, having two small blades, one of which receives the other in its groove. The narrower blade is passed between the skin surface and the concave surface at the apex of the applied clip, while the wider blade is put on the convex surface of the apex. Apposition of the two blades re-straightens the clip and makes it loose from the skin, that it can be removed (Fig. 72.68).

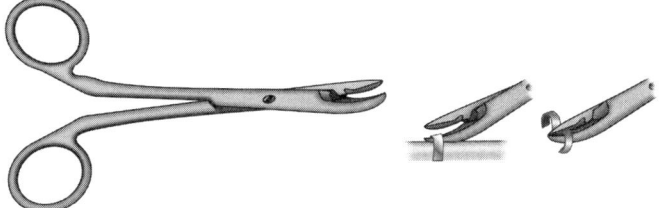

Fig. 72.68: Michel clip extractor (figure shows how the clips are removed)

Sometimes the Michel clip applicator and the extractor are incorporated in one instrument.

Sterilisation.—Boiling or autoclaving.

BOOMERANG NEEDLE WITH HOLDER

These are specially meant for suturing the bleeding prostatic bed, after prostatectomy. The holder is so made that pressure on the tip of the handle causes a sweeping movement of the needle. The needle is detachable from the holder (as shown in Fig. 72.69).

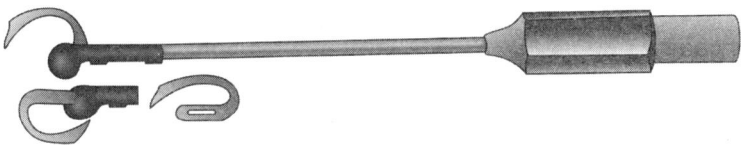

Fig. 72.69: Boomerang needle with holder

Sterilisation.—Concentrated lysol.

ANEURYSM NEEDLE

This instrument looks like a 'sign of interrogation having an eye at the tip. The tip is blunt (c f pedicle needle, where the tip is sharp). The eye is meant for threading ligature material (Fig. 72.70).

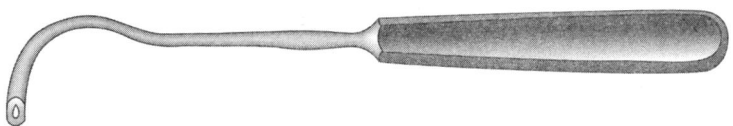

Fig. 72.70: Aneurysm needle

Uses

1. To pass a ligature round a structure while ligating it, e.g. artery, vein, pedicle of an organ, duct (e.g. cystic duct) or tubular organ (e.g. ureter). In doing so, either the needle is threaded and then passed round the structure, or it is passed round the structure and then threaded, while still in position.
2. To isolate a vein for the purpose of fluid transfusion by venesection.
3. The original use of this instrument was for ligation of an aneurysm. The five classical methods of ligation, widely used in older days, are shown in Fig. 72.71.

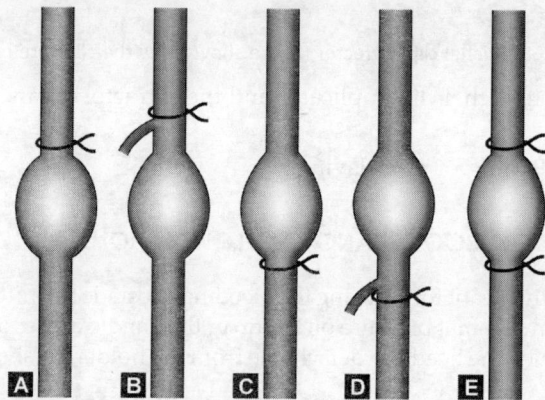

Fig. 72.71: The time-old methods of ligature of aneurysms. A. Anel's. B. Hunter's. C. Brasdor's. D. Wardrop's. E. Antylus'.

While passing the needle round an artery, the following principles should be followed:

a. It should be passed from the side of the accompanying vein. If the reverse is done, the vein is likely to be injured by the emerging tip.
b. It should be passed between the artery and its overlying sheath.

Sterilisation.—Boiling or autoclaving.

PEDICLE NEEDLE

This looks like an aneurysm needle but differs from it in that the tip is sharp (Fig. 72.72). This is because the instrument is used to pierce through the pedicle of a tumour (or an organ), while ligating it by transfixion. Simple ligature of a pedicle is dangerous as it tends to slip under pressure from behind. So, transfixion should always be employed.

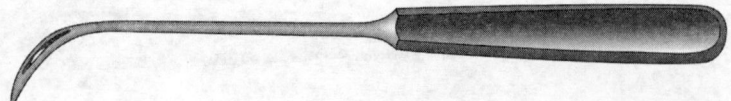

Fig. 72.72: Pedicle needle

In ligating a pedicle, the pedicle needle is only seldom used because it ligates the pedicle en masse. It is always desirable to dissect the individual structures at the pedicle and to ligate them separately. The principles to be followed, while ligating a pedicle, are as follows:

1. Wherever possible, the artery and the vein should be ligated separately, since ligature of these structures together (mass ligature) is associated with the grave risk of slipping under pressure.
2. While ligating the pedicle of a vascular organ (e.g. a huge spleen), the artery should be ligated first and the vein a little later, thus allowing the organ to pump out the excess of blood along the vein. This conserves a good amount of blood.
3. Reversely, while ligating the pedicle of a malignant tumour that has a tendency to spread by veins (e.g. hypernephroma), the vein should be ligated early, before manipulations are attempted. This prevents venous dissemination during manipulations.
4. Two structures, running at an angle to each other at the pedicle (i.e. not parallel, e.g. cystic duct and cystic artery), should not be included in the same ligature since the ligature may slip off the angle.

Sterilisation.—Concentrated lysol.

PEDICLE CLAMP

These are stout clamps, applied on the pedicle of an organ or tumour, before ligating it, while removing the organ or the tumour. Clamps of different angles are available, and the particular type suitable for the depth and the organ is used (Figs 72.73 and 72.74). They are commonly used for:

1. Nephrectomy.
2. Splenectomy.
3. Oophorectomy for big cysts.
4. Excision of any big tumour.

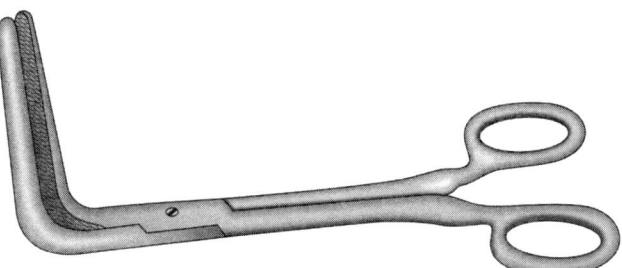

Fig. 72.73: Pedicle clamp

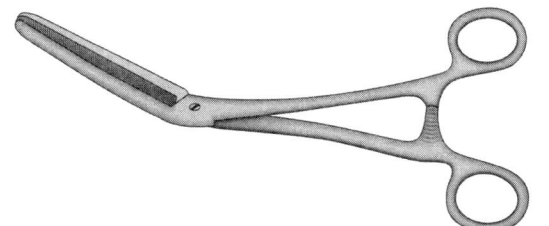

Fig. 72.74: Pedicle clamp

While removing an organ or a big tumour, three clamps are applied and, the pedicle is cut between the middle and the distal clamp. The pedicle is then sutured by transfixion, either with a pedicle needle or an ordinary needle. The first suture is put in the groove made by the proximal clamp with the middle clamp still in position. The middle clamp is then removed and a second suture is applied in the groove made by it. Thereafter, the arteries and the veins should be ligated separately for purpose of security.

This procedure is followed when the individual structures at the pedicle cannot be dissected out and ligated separately. Wherever possible, this latter procedure, without the use of pedicle clamps, should be adopted because it obviates the risk of slipping of ligature.

Sterilisation.—Boiling or autoclaving.

CHOLECYSTECTOMY FORCEPS

These stout forceps are used in the operation of cholecystectomy, i.e. removal of the gall bladder.

Types. — There are two types:

1. Moynihan's cholecystectomy forceps (Fig. 72.75).
2. Henry Gray's cholecystectomy forceps (Fig. 72.76).

The essential difference between the two is that the curvature at the tip of the blades is gradual in the Moynihan's variety whereas it is a right angle in the Gray's forceps. However, in none of these varieties the blade is straight, since it is difficult to pass a ligature beyond the tip of a straight forceps while ligating a structure held by it at the depth, e.g. cystic duct and cystic artery. In this respect, again, the Gray's forceps is disadvantageous in comparison to the Moynihan's variety because it is equally difficult to pass a ligature beyond the tip of a right angled forceps.

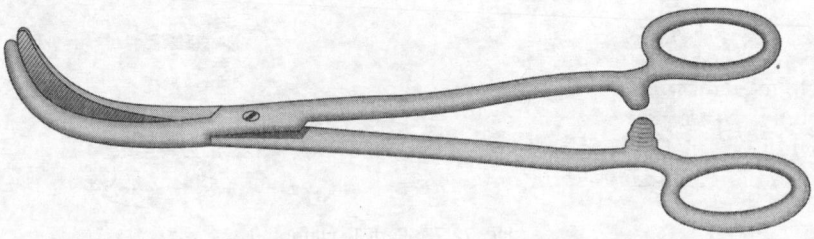

Fig. 72.75: Moynihan's cholecystectomy forceps

The Gray's forceps is, however, advantageous than the Moynihan's variety in the following respects:

a. Dissection of the structures at the neck of the gall bladder, if it is done with the help of a forceps, is better achieved with a right-angled forceps.
b. If the forceps is used in place of an aneurysm needle to pass a ligature around the cystic artery or cystic duct, the purpose is better served with a right-angled forceps.

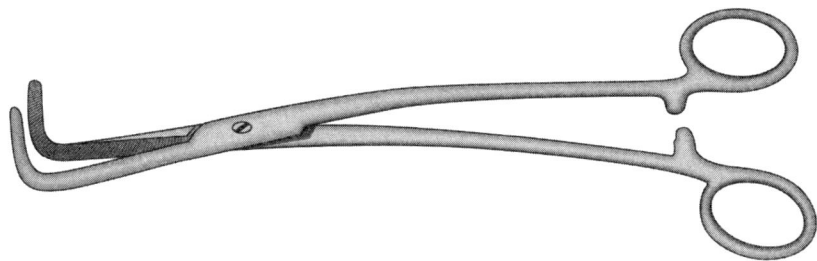

Fig. 72.76: Henry Gray's cholecystectomy forceps

Use of Cholecystectomy Forceps
1. The first forceps is used to hold the fundus of the gall bladder and draw it outwards to have a view of the region of the neck.
2. A second forceps is now applied to the Hartmann's pouch in order to draw it outwards to have a better view of the neck.
3. A forceps may be used for the purpose of blunt dissection and isolation of the cystic duct and the cystic artery, after the anterior layer of the lesser omentum, at its free margin, has been incised and reflected.
4. The forceps may be used to clamp the cystic artery and the cystic duct before cutting these structures. Ligatures are then applied on these forceps.
5. As an alternative to (4), the forceps may be used as an aneurysm needle to pass ligatures around the artery and the duct (separately), and the structures are cut after the ligatures are applied.
6. Whatever method, (4) or (5), is employed, if the gall bladder ends of the artery and the duct are clamped by a forceps each before cutting these structures so as to avoid spillage.

Thus, in an ordinary operation of cholecystectomy, 4 cholecystectomy forceps are required—one for the fundus, one for the Hartman's pouch, and one each for the cystic duct and the cystic artery.

Sterilisation.—Boiling or autoclaving.

CHOLECYSTECTOMY

The abdomen is opened by either of the following incisions:
1. Right upper paramedian incision.
2. A modification of the above, by extending the upper end of the incision to the tip of the xiphisternum in the midline (Mayo-Robson's incision). A better exposure of the common bile duct is obtained by this incision.
3. Kocher's subcostal incision which runs half an inch below the right costal margin and parallel to it. This incision is particularly suitable for:
   a. Short obese patients with a wide costal angle, in whom a paramedian incision does not provide an adequate exposure.
   b. Where there is a right paramedian scan on the abdomen from a previous operation.
4. Upper midline incision.
   On opening the abdomen, the following points are to be used:
   A. Whether the gall bladder is pathological and should be removed. This is ascertained by the following points:

1. There is a change in the size of the gall bladder—either it becomes small and fibrotic (as in chronic cholecystitis) or it is enlarged (as in mucocele or empyema).
2. The wall is thickened, except in cases of mucocele.
3. The colour of the gall bladder, normally greenish, has changed to white or yellowish white. This is because of subserous deposit of fat as well as presence of fibrous tissue in the wall.
4. Adhesions with the surrounding structures, viz. greater omentum, duodenum, stomach, colon, etc. are usually seen.
5. Stones are usually palpable inside the gall bladder.

B. Whether there are stones in the common bile duct and/or whether the common bile duct should be explored (exploration of the common bile duct is called choledochostomy and removal of stones from the duct is termed choledocholithotomy.

Only the supraduodenal part of the common bile duct is palpable. This is done by passing the left index finger through the foramen of Winslow, behind the duct, at the right free margin of the lesser omentum. The thumb is kept in front of the duct, and the duct is palpated between the index finger and the thumb to detect presence of stones.

Even when a stone is not palpable by this process, the common bile duct has to be explored under some circumstances. *The indications for exploration of the common bile duct are:*

1. If stones are palpable in the duct.
2. If the duct is dilated.
3. If the duct wall is thickened.
4. If the gall bladder contains multiple small stones, or biliary sand, or biliary mud, some of which are very likely to have passed down to the duct.
5. If there is a definite history of obstructive jaundice or if the patient is still jaundiced.
6. If there is a history of recurrent attacks of cholangitis, as suggested by 'Charcot's triad', i.e. pain, jaundice and fever.

C. Whether there is any other gross pathology in the abdomen (i.e. general exploration of the abdomen). The appendix, stomach, duodenum, pancreas, and (in the females) the uterus and its appendages should be particularly examined.

The operation of cholecystectomy may be done by two methods of dissection:

1. Neck to fundus dissection ('duct-first' method), which is preferred by majority of the surgeons. The cystic artery and cystic duct are first ligated and cut, and then the gall bladder is dissected out from the liver bed.
2. Fundus to neck dissection ('fundus-first' method), which is done if there are too many adhesions at the neck or if the structures at the neck cannot be identified properly in the beginning. The gall bladder is dissected out from the liver bed, starting from the fundus. As the neck is reached, the cystic artery and the cystic duct are properly identified and dealt with.

In the usually performed 'duct-first' method, the gall bladder is pulled outwards with two cholecystectomy forceps, one applied to the fundus and the other to the Hartmann's pouch. A fold of peritoneum now stands up at the neck of the gall bladder and this extends to the anterior layer of the lesser omentum. This fold is incised and the incision is prolonged on to the anterior layer of the lesser omentum A careful dissection at this stage identifies the structures at the right free margin of the lesser omentum, particularly the duct system.

The cystic artery and the cystic duct are to be ligated now. As these two structures run at an angle to each other, they should be ligated separately.

The cystic duct makes a loop in its course since the cystic artery is shorter in length than the cystic duct. Unless this loop is undone, it is difficult to find out the actual site of junction of the cystic duct with the common bile duct, which is the exact site where the cystic duct has to be ligated. If the duct is ligated encroaching on the common bile duct, there is the danger of stricture formation in the common duct. Again, if a portion of the cystic duct is left behind, this may dilate in future, making a 'secondary' gall bladder that may produce post-cholecystectomy syndrome. The undoing of the loop in the cystic duct can only be achieved by cutting the cystic artery. Hence, in the operation of cholecystectomy, the cystic artery has to be cut first and then the cystic duct.

An oval incision is now made on the peritoneum, on the undersurface of the gall bladder, and the gall bladder is dissected out, subperitoneally, from the liver bed. Oozing of blood and bile from the liver bed is stopped by apposing the peritoneal flaps, left behind, on the two sides, after removal of the gall bladder. The little oozing that may still occur tends to collect in the (hepato-renal) pouch of Morison. This is brought out by putting a cigarette drain or a corrugated rubber drain down to this pouch. The other end of the drain is brought to the surface either through a stab wound in the loin or through the original line of incision.

DESJARDIN'S CHOLEDOCHOLITHOTOMY FORCEPS

This is a long slender forceps, with no catches on the handles. It has long curved blades, each blade having a fenestration at its end (Fig. 72.77).

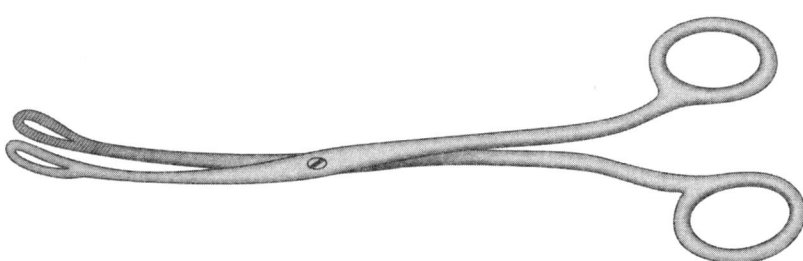

Fig. 72.77: Desjardin's choledocholithotomy forceps

It is used for removal of stones from the bile ducts, viz. common bile duct, common hepatic duct, right or left hepatic duct. There are no catches as the stones should never be crushed. The fenestrations on the blades apply only a light pressure on the stone while giving a good grip.

Sterilisation.—Boiling or autoclaving.

GALL STONE SCOOP (MOYNIHAN'S)

This is used for removing stones from the gall bladder or bile duct. A choledocholithotomy forceps is better for the purpose (Fig. 72.78).

Sterilisation.—Boiling or autoclaving.

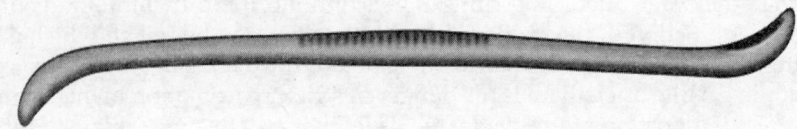

Fig. 72.78: Gall stone scoop

CHOLEDOCHOLITHOTOMY AND CHOLEDOCHOSTOMY

Indications.—*See* cholecystectomy forceps.

Operation.— Stones may be situated in the supraduodenal, retroduodenal, or intramural part of the common bile duct. In the majority of cases, the stones are located in the supraduodenal part. Even when a stone lies in the other parts of the duct, it may often be brought out by passing down a Desjardin's forceps from a supraduodenal opening in the common bile duct. Hence, in all the cases, it is the supraduodenal part that should be opened first. Only when a stone, located lower down, cannot be brought out by this route that a lower part of the duct has to be opened up. Accordingly, choledocholithotomy may be:

1. Supraduodenal (most commonly done)
2. Retroduodenal.
3. Transduodenal.

SUPRADUODENAL CHOLEDOCHOLITHOTOMY.— Before opening the common bile duct, it must be firmly at hand and must be properly identified. The duct is situated at the right free margin of the lesser omentum. In cases of doubt, aspiration with a fine needle should be done. In order to get a good grip on the duct and to draw it towards the anterior abdominal incision, two stay-knots are applied on it, one on each side of the proposed line of incision on the duct.

The incision is placed vertically, along the long axis of the duct (to avoid future stricture). If it is found that the stone is impacted somewhere in the duct, the incision on the duct should be made a little above or below the site of impaction and the stone should be milked towards the incision. This is because the stone might have produced considerable fibrosis at the site of impaction, and the fibrosis is exaggerated if an incision is made right at this site.

The stones are now brought out with a Desjardin's forceps or with a Moynihan's scoop. A urethral, bougie is then passed upwards along the two hepatic ducts and thereafter, downwards along the common bile duct, till its tip is felt inside the second part of the duodenum. This is necessary in order to ascertain that no stone or other obstruction has been left behind. With a catheter inserted through the opening, the duct is washed off possible gravely or mud.

A primary closure of the duct is usually avoided for the following reasons:

1. The duct wall is thin and sutures placed on it are likely to yield under intraductal pressure. After handling of the common bile duct, there is a temporary spasm of the sphincter of Oddi and the pressure inside the duct usually rises. This may result in leakage of bile.
2. In cases of impacted stones, the bile in the liver is stagnated and infected, and it is not desirable that this bile enters the gut.

For these reasons, the duct is temporarily drained. This drainage is performed by insertion of a rubber catheter or a T-tube (*see* below). The excess of the opening, the duct, by the side of the tube, is sutured.

RETRODUODENAL CHOLEDOCHOLITHOTOMY.—This is performed for a stone so impacted in the retroduodenal part of the common bile duct that it cannot be brought out through a supraduodenal opening in the duct.

In these cases, the retroduodenal part of the duct is brought to view by mobilising the duodenum. This is done by making a vertical incision on the posterior parietal peritoneum, just lateral to the second part of the duodenum (Kocherisation). The retroduodenal part of the duct is then opened and the stones are brought out. The wound in the duct here is closed, and a T-tube drainage is maintained through the supraduodenal opening.

TRANSDUODENAL CHOLEDOCHOLITHOTOMY.—This is done for stones impacted in the intramural part of the common bile duct.

A urethral bougie is passed down through the supraduodenal opening in the duct and its tip is made to project against the anterior wall of the second part of the duodenum, opposite the sphincter of Oddi, through which the bougie passes. A vertical incision is now made on the anterior duodenal wall, over the tip of the bougie, and the duodenum is opened up. The next incision is made to cut through the posterior duodenal wall, the sphincter of Oddi, and the terminal part of the common bile duct. Thus, a sphincterotomy has been done, and the stone is taken out.

For better drainage of the bile, the posterior wound is not sutured. The opening on the anterior duodenal wall is closed transversely and this prevents a duodenal stricture. A T-tube drainage is maintained through the supraduodenal opening in the duct.

T-TUBE (KEHR'S)

This is a flexible tube, made of latex or rubber, having two limbs, connected to each other in the form of 'T'. The horizontal limb of the T, which is cut short to a desirable size, is inserted vertically along the long axis of the common bile duct. The other limb is brought out, through the opening in the common bile duct, on to the surface, either through a stab wound or through the original incision (described above, in the operation of choledocholithotomy).

Withdrawal of the T-tube.—The principle is that the tube must be in position:
a. as long as the bile is infected.
b. Till normal passage of bile to the gut is established.
That the tube can be withdrawn is ascertained by the following points:
  i. The drained bile looks healthy.

ii. The quantity of bile, drained out, is greatly diminished.

iii. The stools are normal-coloured (i.e. contain bile).

iv. As a confirmatory test, the tube is clamped for 24 hours. If symptoms, suggestive of bile-stagnation in the liver, e.g. epigastric discomfort, nausea and vomiting, do not set in during this period, the tube may be safely withdrawn.

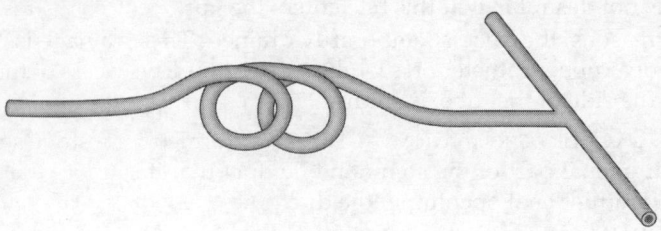

Fig. 72.79: Kehr's t-tube

Before withdrawing the tube, a T-tube cholangiography may be done with advantage. 20 ml of diodone is pushed along the tube and X-rays taken. This ascertains absence of any further obstruction or 'left-behind' stones in the duct.

The tube is withdrawn just by a smart pull. The resultant fistula heals spontaneously, provided there is no distal obstruction in the duct.

Sterilisation.—By boiling.

GASTROINTESTINAL CLAMPS

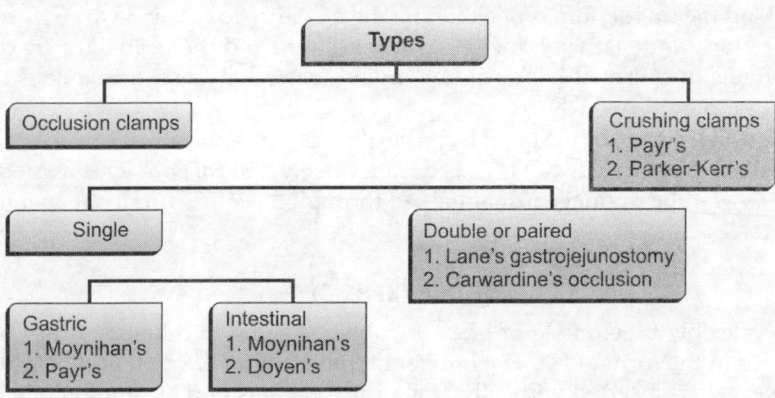

Occlusion Clamps.—These clamps are used in performing anastomosis of the gut, e.g. gastrojejunostomy, intestinal anastomosis, etc. When applied to the gut, they serve the following purposes:

1. They occlude the lumen of the gut, so that the contents cannot soil the field of operation and the peritoneal cavity.

2. They cause temporary haemostasis during anastomosis.

3. They help in holding the loops of gut in apposition while anastomosis is being performed.

Anastomosis, performed with the help of occlusion clamps, is called *closed method* of anastomosis. Some surgeons discourage the use of these clamps, during anastomosis, because:

a. Even though it is believed that these clamps do not cause crushing of the wall, some damage to the mucosa is very likely to occur and this may predispose to the formation of anastomotic ulcers.

b. Because of the temporary haemostasis, produced by the clamps, some bleeding vessels at the cut margins of the gut may be overlooked during the anastomosis, and these may bleed seriously in the post-operative period.

When occlusion clamps are not used, anastomosis may be done with the help of four Allis' or Babcock's tissue forceps—two applied to each loop of gut in order to steady and hold it. This is known as the *open method* of anastomosis.

While doing an anastomosis, four layers of suture are required. When clamps or forceps have been applied, each loop of gut makes, in itself, an anterior and a posterior flap, between which the gut is cut. Actual anastomosis is made with through and through sutures between the two loops of the gut; this means that the sutures take bite of all the layers of the gut. Thus, for the two flaps (anterior and posterior) there are two through and through sutures—one anterior and one posterior. To minimise the risk of leakage occurring through these sutures, they are covered up by another layer of suture. This suture picks up only the outer thickness of the gut wall (seromuscular), drawn from either side. For each through and through suture, there should be a protective seromuscular suture. Thus, there is an anterior and posterior seromuscular suture. Hence, in an anastomosis, four layers of suture are necessary. The sequence of these sutures are:

1. Posterior seromuscular (this should be applied first because, after application of the posterior through and through suture, its back cannot be seen).
2. Posterior through and through.
3. Anterior through and through.
4. Anterior seromuscular.

In practice, two atraumatic sutures are used for anastomosis—one for the two seromuscular sutures and the other for the two through and through sutures.

Crushing Clamps.—These clamps, when applied to the gut, not only occlude its lumen but also crush its walls. These are used when the gut has to be closed, i.e. stumps are made, e.g.:

1. Duodenal stump, in Polya gastrectomy.
2. Gastric stump towards the lesser curvature side, in different types of gastrectomy.
3. Intestinal stump, in intestinal resection and anastomosis by side-to-side, end-to-side, or side-to-end methods.

These stumps must be air-proof and water-proof, and crushing clamps help in achieving this:

a. Crushing of the gut wall causes the mucosa to curl inwards and plug the lumen.

b. Sutures sit tightly on the crushed muscle coat (which they do not when the muscles are fleshy).

In making stumps also, two layers of suture are required—one through and through, followed by a protective seromuscular.

MOYNIHAN'S GASTRIC OCCLUSION
AND INTESTINAL OCCLUSION CLAMPS

The difference between the two is only in size—the gastric clamp is bigger. The clamps may be:
a. Straight (Fig. 72.80).
b. Curved.

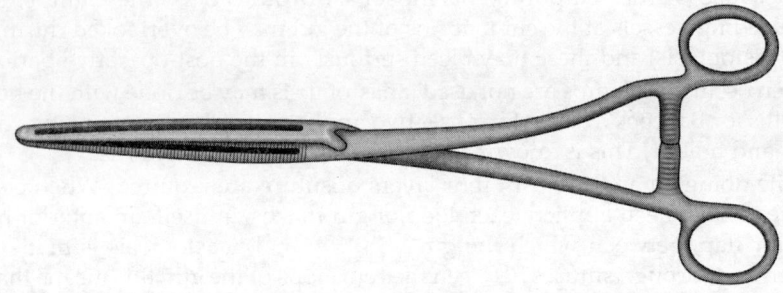

Fig. 72.80: Moynihan's gastric occlusion clamp (straight)

There are transverse serrations on the blades and these prevent slipping out of the gut. Each blade has a central longitudinal fenestration; this increases its elasticity and makes it lighter, thus causing minimum trauma to the gut wall. To minimise chances of trauma further, rubber tubings are usually fitted to the blades, during use.

Use

A. Gastric occlusion clamp:
1. In gastrojejunostomy.
2. In performing anastomosis after partial gastrectomy, either by the Billroth I or by the Polya method.

B. Intestinal occlusion clamp:
1. In intestinal anastomosis.
2. In performing intestinal anastomosis after resection.

Sterilisation.—Boiling or autoclaving. The rubber tubes should be sterilised separately and fitted at operation.

LANE'S GASTROJEJUNOSTOMY CLAMP

This is a double or paired clamp, consisting of the two long occlusion clamps. The clamps can be detached from each other. Provisions are so made with two rings and a screw that the clamps can be attached together either with their handles on the same side or with handles opposite to each other, according to convenience (Fig. 72.81).

The are used in gastrojejunostomy. The two clamps are separated and one is applied to each loop of gut. Thereafter, the two are fitted together as is convenient. The fitting arrangement is advantageous in that the two clamps need not be held together by external support.

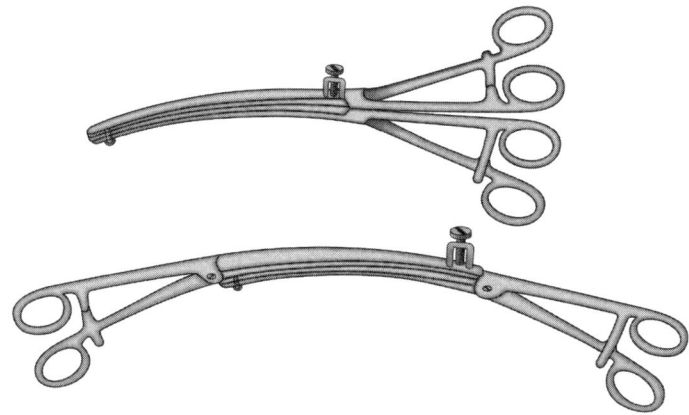

Fig. 72.81: Lane's Gastrojejunostomy clamp (the figure shows how the clamp can be applied in two different ways)

Sterilisation.—Boiling or autoclaving.

PAYR'S GASTRIC OCCLUSION CLAMP

There are two types:

1. Straight
2. Curved

These clamps are characterised by the presence of small balls along one edge of the blades, with corresponding holes on the opposite blade to receive them. Thus the blades exert very little pressure on the stomach, causing minimal damage to its wall. They are used without rubber tubings wall.

Use.—Same as Moynihan's gastric occlusion clamp.

Sterilisation.—Boiling or autoclaving.

DOYEN'S INTESTINAL OCCLUSION CLAMP

There are two types:

1. Straight (Fig. 72.82).
2. Curved.

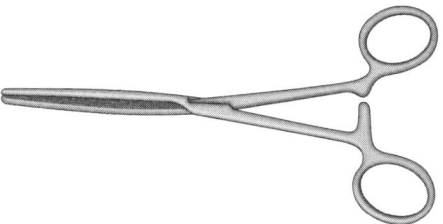

Fig. 72.82: Doyen's intestinal occlusion clamp

There are fine longitudinal serrations on the blades.

Use.—Same as Moynihan's intestinal occlusion clamp.

Sterilisation.—Boiling or autoclaving.

CARWARDINE'S DOUBLE INTESTINAL CLAMP

The two clamps, in this instrument, are small and meant for intestinal anastomosis. The fitting arrangement is with a screw on the handle, which allows the clamps to be fitted with their handles in the same direction only (c f Lane's gastrojejunostomy clamp)—Fig. 72.83.

Sterilisation.—Boiling or autoclaving.

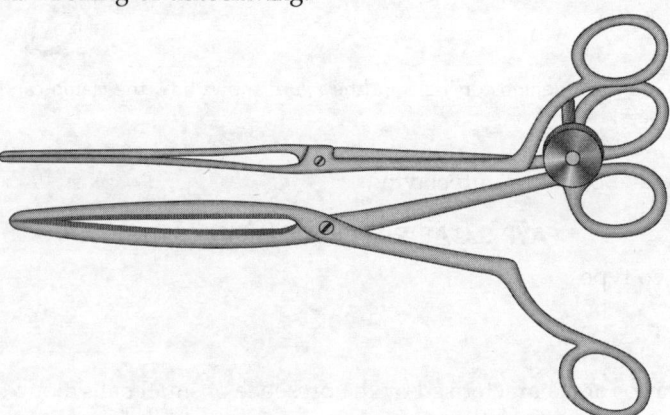

Fig. 72.83: Carwardine's double intestinal clamp

PAYR'S CRUSHING CLAMP

This is a heavy instrument and it exerts a great crushing effect by virtue of a double lever action. There are longitudinal serrations on the blades (Fig. 72.84). The clamp may be:

a. Short.
b. Long.

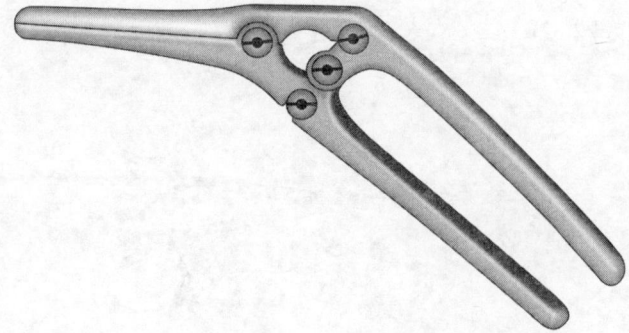

Fig. 72.84: Payr's crushing clamp

The short clamp is meant for the intestine, e.g. duodenal stump (in Polya gastrectomy), intestinal stump (as in interstinal resection and anastomosis by side-to-side, end-to-side, or side-to-end method).

The long clamp is used for the stomach, e.g. in closing the lesser curvature side of the transected stomach either in Polya or in Billroth I gastrectomy.

Sterilisation.—Boiling or autoclaving.

PARKER-KERR'S CRUSHING CLAMP

This is a heavy instrument, looking like a big artery forceps, but is stouter in comparison and has *longitudinal* serrations on the blades (Fig. 72.85). It is used in making duodenal and intestinal stumps (*see* Payr's clamp).

Sterilisation.—Boiling or autoclaving.

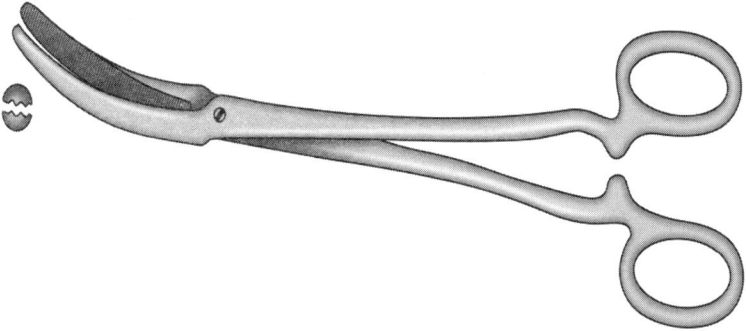

Fig. 72.85: Parker-kerr's crushing clamp

OPERATIONS ON THE STOMACH

GASTROSTOMY

This operation implies making a fistulous opening in the stomach. The patient is fed through a tube, inserted along this opening.

It is employed to by-pass obstructions in the pharynx, oesophagus or cardiac end of the stomach:

a. When the obstruction is acute inflammatory or traumatic, the gastrostomy is *temporary.*

b. When the obstruction is due to an inoperable carcinoma, the gastrostomy is *permanent.* The value of gastrostomy in these cases is doubtful and this procedure is quickly going out of practice.

Considering the poor general condition of the patient, the operation is usually done under local infiltration anaesthesia. A left upper paramedian incision is made. The stomach, which is usually empty and contracted is pulled down. The opening in the stomach is made on its anterior wall, midway between the lesser and greater curvatures, and just below the level of the costal margin. This area is picked up with two tissue forceps, and a small incision is made, through which a self-retaining catheter is passed in, for about two inches. The catheter is secured in position with a catgut stitch, transfixing it to the stomach wall. To be sure that the catheter is in the lumen of the stomach, some water should be pushed in through it.

While this part of the operation is the same in all the cases, an attempt is made to make a valvular track into the stomach in order to prevent leakage of acid gastric juice, which is highly irritant to the skin. According to the method of making this valvular process, the operation of gastrotomy varies. There are two common procedures:

1. KADER-SENN'S (STAMM'S) METHOD.—A seromuscular purse-string suture is applied on the stomach wall, about 1 cm away from the tube, and the tube is invaginated into the purse-string. A second purse-string suture (and sometimes another) is then applied round this area of invagination in order to get further invagination. Thus, a cone is produced in the stomach wall around the tube, its apex making the opening of the gastrostomy inside the stomach.

2. WITZEL'S METHOD.—After the tube has been passed into the stomach, a part of the tube, just outside the opening is buried in a short tunnel, made over the stomach wall, by bringing the wall over the tube, from either side, with seromuscular stitches.

In any case, before the abdomen is closed, the stomach wall, adjacent to the opening, is anchored, by a few stitches, to the parietal peritoneum.

GASTROJEJUNOSTOMY

This means an anastomosis between the stomach and the jejunum.

Indications

1. The operation is most commonly done as an adjunct to vagotomy, in the treatment of chronic duodenal ulcer.
2. Gastrojejunostomy, alone, is indicated in those cases of pyloric stenosis where the patient is elderly. In these cases there is an atrophic gastritis, so that the acid secretion of the stomach will never reach a high level to cause stomal ulcer.
3. Occasionally, the operation is done as a palliative measure for carcinoma of the stomach.

Types

A. Gastrojejunostomy may be
   1. Anterior
   2. Posterior,

   depending on whether the anastomosis is made on the anterior or the posterior wall of the stomach. Anterior gastrojejunostomy is technically easier but it is discouraged by many surgeons as it is associated with more risks of complications, including stomal ulceration.

   For a posterior gastrojejunostomy to be done, the posterior wall of the stomach has to be drawn out of the lesser sac into the greater sac of peritoneum where the jejunal loops lie. This is done by making an opening in a relatively avascular area of the transverse mesocolon. Hence, a posterior gastrojejunostomy is also known as *retrocolic,* while the anterior one is called *antecolic.* After a retrocolic anastomosis has been done, the margins of the cut transverse mesocolon are sutured to the stomach wall, just by the side of the anastomosis, in order to prevent herniation of the coils of small intestine into the lesser sac.

B. Gastrojejunostomy should be no-loop, no-tension. This means that, between the duodenojejunal flexure and the stoma, there should neither be a redundant loop of jejunum (causing stagnation) nor a very short loop (causing tension on the stoma). On an average, a loop of 3 to 5 inches is kept.

C. Gastrojejunostomy may be
   1. Vertical
   2. Transverse
   3. Oblique,
   depending on the type of incision on the stomach wall.

D. Gastrojejunostomy may be
   1. Isoperistaltic
   2. Antiperistaltic,

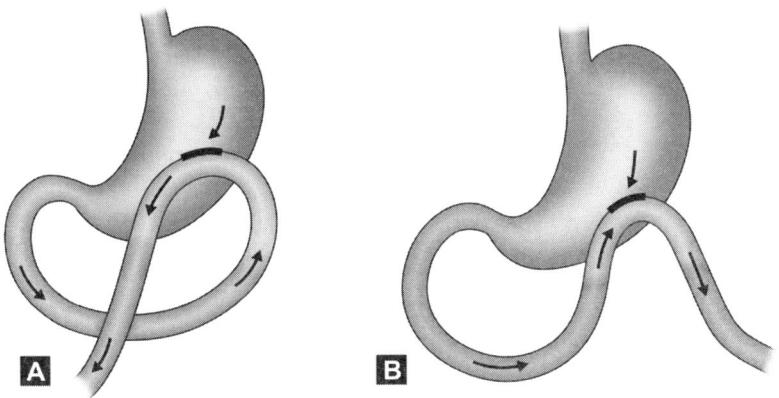

Fig. 72.86: Gastrojejunostomy: A. isoperistaltic, B. antiperistaltic

according to the direction of jejunal loop in relation to the stomach (Fig. 72.86). An isoperistaltic anastomosis is usually performed and, to do so, the affarent side of the jejunal loop is approximated to the lesser curvature side of the stomach, during the anastomosis.

GASTRECTOMY (RESECTION OF STOMACH)

Types

1. PARTIAL GASTRECTOMY.—This means resection of the distal 3/5th of the stomach, including the pylorus. This is usually done for gastric ulcer.

2. SUBTOTAL GASTRECTOMY.—This means resection of the distal 7/8th of the stomach, including the pylorus. This is a type of surgery for duodenal ulcer.

3. TOTAL GASTRECTOMY.—The whole stomach, including the pylorus, is resected. After the resection, the duodenum is closed and the jejunum is anastomosed to the oesophagus, by the Roux-Y method (Fig. 72.87).

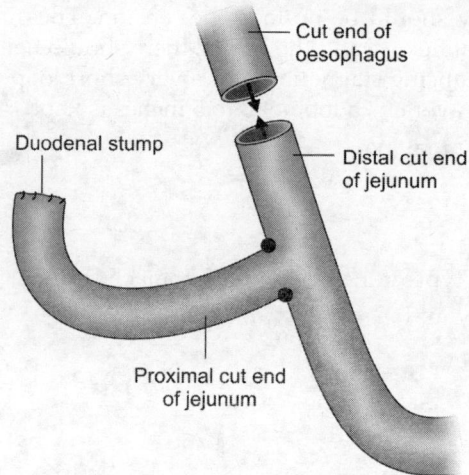

Fig. 72.87: Roux-Y method of anastomosis

4. RADICAL GASTRECTOMY.—This is done for resectable cases of gastric carcinoma. The operation removes, en bloc, the cancer-bearing area of the stomach, with sufficient healthy wall proximally and distally, together with all the nodes draining the stomach. Depending on the site of the growth, the operation may be:

a. *Lower Radical Gastrectomy.*—for growths in the lower part of the stomach.

b. *Upper Radical Gastrectomy.*—for growths in the upper part.

c. *Total Radical Gastrectomy.*—The whole of the stomach is removed for a growth infiltrating widely along the wall of the stomach.

Anastomosis after Gastric Resection.—There are two principal types of anastomosis after a partial or subtotal gastrectomy, and the gastrectomy is named accordingly:

1. BILLROTH I GASTRECTOMY.—The cut end of the duodenum is directly anastomosed to the cut end of the stomach. To make for the disparity in size between the two, the lesser curvature side of the stomach is closed in the form of a stump, and the duodenum is anastomosed, end-to-end, with the gastric opening, left towards the greater curvature side (Fig. 72.88).

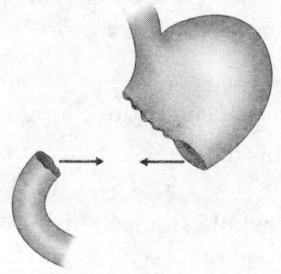

Fig. 72.88: Billroth I gastrectomy

This anastomosis is preferable in that it restores a physiological continuity. However, in those cases where the gap between the duodenum and the cut stomach is too wide to allow suture without tension or where the duodenum is fixed by adhesions, this anastomosis cannot be performed. In subtotal gastrectomy for a duodenal ulcer, therefore, this anastomosis is seldom practicable.

2. POLYA GASTRECTOMY.—The cut end of the duodenum is closed (duodenal stump) and the cut end of the stomach is anastomosed to the first jejunal loop, end-to-side, by making an opening on the side of the jejunal loop.

Since the stoma with such a simple anastomosis is wide, it allows food to pass into both affarent and efferent jejunal loops (Fig. 72.89A). Entry of food into the affarent loop is undesirable as it produces symptoms. The technique of small stoma or valvular stoma, therefore, came in. The valve, known as Finsterer's or Hoffmeister's valve, consists of the closed lesser curvature side of the gastric opening, to which the affarent jejunal loop is anchored by a few stitches (Fig. 72.89B).

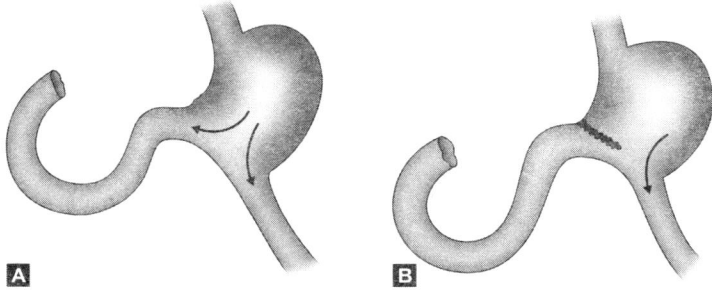

Fig. 72.89: Polya gastrectomy: A. shows the difficulty of a wide stoma, B. shows a valvular small stoma

INTESTINAL ANASTOMOSIS

A simple anastomosis between two loops of intestine is sometimes necessary to by-pass:

a. A stricture (usually tubercular).

b. An obstruction, caused by a complicated mass of adhesions (e.g. caseated mesenteric glands).

A side-to-side anastomosis is performed.

An ileo-transverse anastomosis is an anastomosis made between the terminal loop of the ileum and the transverse colon. This is done:

A. As an anastomosis after a right hemicolectomy.

B. By itself:

    1. In inoperable cases of carcinoma of the right colon, as a palliative procedure.

    2. In pathological conditions of the right colon or terminal ileum, causing intestinal obstruction, where it is not absolutely necessary (as in hyperplastic ileo-caecal tuberculosis) or is not desirable (as in Crohn's disease) to resect the pathological segment.

    3. As a preliminary drainage operation in carcinoma of the right colon:

        a. Where the patient's condition is too low to undergo resection straightway.

b. When the patient presents with acute intestinal obstruction. When simple ileo-transverse anastomosis is done without resection of the gut, the anastomosis is usually made side-to-side. Ileo-transverse anastomosis, associated with a right hemicolectomy is usually made end-to-end.

INTESTINAL RESECTION AND ANASTOMOSIS

Resection of a part of the small intestine is usually technically easy. The common indications are:

1. Gangrenous change, following strangulation in a hernial sac (most commonly inguinal hernia).
2. Irreparable injury.
3. Isolated pathology, affecting a short segment (e.g. tubercular ulcer).

After resection, anastomosis may be done in four ways, as shown in Fig. 72.90.

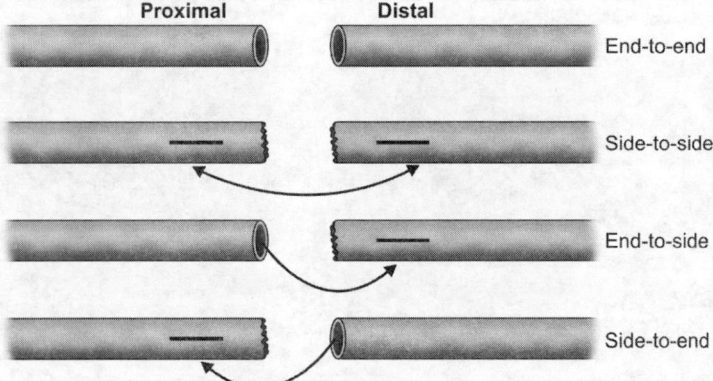

Fig. 72.90: Different Methods of intestinal anastomosis after resection

RESECTION OF LARGE INTESTINE

In comparison to small gut resection, resection of the large intestine, limited to the extent that the pathology deserves, is seldom practicable. This is because of the following factors:

1. The large gut has poor blood supply, and vessels supplying it, viz. ileocolic, right colic, middle colic, left colic and the sigmoids, end in the marginal artery, which runs along the inner border of the colon and supplies it. Resection of the large gut is usually undertaken for malignancy and, in these cases, it is imperative that all the nodes, draining the corresponding area, is resected with the loop of the diseased colon, en masse. These nodes are situated along the blood vessels, supplying the colon, and some of them (intermediate nodes) are located by the side of the big vessels, named above. Excision of these nodes require ligation of these big vessels (e.g. the ileocolic and right colic vessels have to be ligated for growths in the right side of colon). This makes a wide area of the colon avascular, making its resection imperative, though the growth by itself did not demand such a wide resection.

2. After resection, it is desirable that the anastomosis is performed between two mobile loops of gut, because anastomosis between fixed loops tends to give way under tension. Hence, excision of only a part of the length of right or left colon cannot be performed.

3. At its fixed parts, the large gut has no peritoneal covering posteriorly. Anastomosis, made between the areas devoid of peritoneum, is associated with the grave risk of leakage. From this point of view, again, it is desirable that an anastomosis is done between two mobile parts of the gut.

In view of the above factors, large gut resections have to be planned as follows:

1. RIGHT HEMICOLECTOMY.—This means excision of the terminal 6 to 8 inches of the ileum, the caecum, appendix, ascending colon, hepatic flexure and the proximal half of transverse colon, i.e. the area supplied by the ileo-colic and right colic arteries. This operation is usually done for:

a. Carcinoma of the right side of the colon.

b. Hyperplastic ileo-caecal tuberculosis.

After resection, anastomosis is done between the terminal ileum and the transverse colon.

2. LEFT HEMICOLECTOMY.—This is usually done for carcinoma on the left side of the colon. This operation removes the distal half of the transverse colon, splenic flexure, descending colon, and the fixed upper part of the pelvic colon.

Anastomosis is done, thereafter, between the transverse colon and the pelvic colon.

3. WEDGE RESECTION OF TRANSVERSE COLON WITH A V-SHAPED AREA OF THE ATTACHED MESOCOLON.—This is usually done for carcinoma of the transverse colon. The resection must include three inches of healthy gut on either side of the growth.

4. WEDGE RESECTION OF THE PELVIC COLON.—This is usually done for:

a. Carcinoma of the pelvic colon.

b. Volvulus, which usually occurs in the pelvic colon. After resection, anastomosis is done between the remaining upper part of the pelvic colon and the rectum.

Difficulties of Large Gut Resection.—As compared to the small gut, resection of the large gut is more difficult and associated with more risks as follows:

1. Extensive mobilisation is necessary as the gut is fixed to the posterior abdominal wall (excepting transverse and pelvic colon).

2. As already stated, because of (a) characteristic blood supply; (b) fixity of the loops to the posterior abdominal wall, and (c) absence of peritoneum on the posterior surface of the gut over the fixed areas, wider resection, than the pathology actually demands, has to be undertaken.

3. The anastomosis, following the resection, is difficult because of:
   a. lack of complete peritoneal covering,
   b. presence of appendices epiploic,
   c. presence of sacculations,
   d. irregular thickness of the wall.

4. The anastomosis has a greater tendency to leak because of:
   a. precarious blood supply,
   b. lack of complete peritoneal covering,

c. great strain on the suture line by forceful peristalsis, demanded by the solid and semisolid contents,

d. infection from the colonic contents, which are highly infective.

5. The patients are usually old, with lowered general resistance, because of malnutrition and toxic absorption.

COLOSTOMY

Types

A. Colostomy may be:

1. TERMINAL COLOSTOMY.—This means bringing out the terminal end of the colon on the abdomen, after resecting the rectum and anal canal, as in cases of carcinoma of the rectum. There is a single stoma.

2. LOOP COLOSTOMY.—This means bringing out a loop of colon on the abdominal surface and opening it. There is a double stoma, one communicating with the proximal loop and the other with the distal. If provisions are so made that the colonic contents cannot enter the distal loop, the colostomy is called defunctioning.

B. Colostomy may be:

1. PELVIC COLOSTOMY.—The opening is in the pelvic colon, and this may be either a terminal or a loop colostomy.

2. TRANSVERSE COLOSTOMY.—An opening in the transverse colon; this is always a loop colostomy.

C. Colostomy may be:

1. TEMPORARY, which is done:
   a. For immediate relief, in cases of acute obstruction.
   b. In preparing for resection of distal tumours.
   c. In defunctioning inflamed areas, as in diverticulitis or intractable anal fistula.

2. PERMANENT, which means making an abdominal anus and is imperative:
   a. In cases of non-resectable tumours.
   b. After resection of rectum and anal canal for carcinoma.

Indications

1. *Congenital.*—A temporary colostomy is indicated:
   a. In cases of high imperforate anus.
   b. In bad cases of rectovaginal or rectovesical fistula.

2. *Traumatic*
   a. Injuries of the rectum.
   b. Injuries of the colon.

   In these cases, after the injury is repaired, it is desirable that the colonic contents do not pass through the repaired gut and interfere with its healing. Hence, a temporary proximal colostomy is done along with the repair.

3. *Inflammatory:*
   a. Intractable stricture (permanent colostomy).
   b. Multiple fistula-in-ano, in these cases, unless the stools are diverted by a temporary colostomy, the fistulae do not heal.

4. *Neoplastic.*—In cases of carcinoma of the left colon or rectum:
   a. Permanent terminal colostomy, following resection of rectum and anal canal.
   b. Palliative permanent loop colostomy, for inoperable cancers of rectum or left colon (for inoperable growths of the right colon, the palliative procedure is ileo-transverse anastomosis).
   c. Temporary loop colostomy, as a preparatory procedure, prior to resection of the left colon or rectum, for carcinoma.

5. *Other Causes.*—Some cases of volvulus, after de-rotation has been done. A temporary loop colostomy in these cases:
   a. drains the obstructed gut,
   b. fixes the pelvic colon to the abdominal wall and helps prevention of recurrence.

The Operation of Loop Colostomy.—The operation may be done either on the pelvic colon or on the transverse. For a pelvic colostomy, the incision may be:
a. A gridiron incision on the left side, similar to McBurney's incision on the right.
b. An infraumbilical midline incision, retracting the rectus on either side.

With these incisions, the patient gets the benefit of controlling the stoma by the abdominal musculature. The incision should be as small as practicable because infection in the muscles, resulting from leakage of stool, may lead to the development of incisional hernia.

On opening the abdomen, the index finger is passed through the incision and, as it sweeps on the iliac bone, the iliac colon is hooked forward. A pull on the iliac colon brings out the pelvic colon.

The opening on the pelvic colon should be done in its uppermost part since, otherwise, the mobile redundant loop of the pelvic colon, above the stoma, may prolapse through the colostomy during straining, which the fixed iliac colon cannot. This loop is kept outside the abdomen with the help of a glass rod, which is passed through an avascular part of the mesocolon. This rod is kept on the surface of the abdomen and, to keep the rod in position, a piece of rubber tube connects its ends. While closing the wound, the following points are to be observed:—

1. The cut peritoneal margin is sutured to the exteriorised loop by several interrupted stitches.

2. The lateral space, i.e. the space between the left lateral abdominal wall and the emerging colonic loop, should be obliterated; otherwise, there may be herniation of small intestinal coils into this space. This is done simply by putting a few stitches between the lateral peritoneal flap and the emerging loop.

3. The excess of the abdominal opening, by the side of the exteriorised loop, should be closed neither too tight nor too loose—the index finger should pass freely between the loop and the sutured wound margins.

The exteriorised loop is covered with vaseline gauge.

For a transverse colostomy, the site selected should be in its proximal half, on the right of the middle colic artery, because the distal part may eventually have to survive on this vessel. For this purpose, a right paramedian incision is preferred.

Opening of the Colostomy.—As a rule, the colostomy should be opened after 48 hours of exteriorisation of the loop. Immediate opening is associated with the danger of leakage of stool into the peritoneal cavity. After 48 hours, complete peritoneal sealing occurs.

Where there is a gross distension, and immediate relief is obligatory, either of the following procedures may be adopted:

1. A long rubber tube is passed through an opening made in the proximal loop. The tube is secured in position with a purse-string suture, applied around the opening. This long tube drains the stool well away from the wound. A Paul's tube (Fig. 72.91), connected with a long rubber tubing, may be used instead of the rubber tube.

2. A purse-string suture is applied on the loop and a needle is inserted through the purse-string to aspirate and deflate the gut. As the needle is withdrawn, the purse-string is tightened. Final opening of the colostomy can then be delayed for 48 hours.

Terminal Colostomy.—After resection of the rectum and anal canal, the cut end of the colon makes a permanent opening on the abdominal wall (abdominal anus). The colon is usually brought out through a separate muscle-splitting incision on the left iliac fossa (as for loop colostomy). The original operative incision is closed.

Defunctioning Colostomy.—This is done when it is desired that no stool should enter the distal limb of a colostomy loop. In other words, the distal loop actually becomes defunct (in an ordinary loop colostomy, some stool passes across the colostomy into the distal stoma and the distal loop). A defunctioning colostomy is usually done only in the transverse colon.

The desired colonic loop is pulled forwards and, keeping a small length at the summit of the loop free, its proximal and distal limbs are approximated to each other, with a few interrupted seromuscular stitches. Two additional parietal incisions are made, one on each side of, and parallel to, the main incision, one inch away from it. Through each of these openings, the blades of an occlusion clamp are passed into the abdomen. One of these clamps the proximal loop and the other the distal, a little away from the summit of the loop. The loop is completely cut through between the two clamps. One cut loop, with the clamp on it, is drawn out of the abdomen through each of the side openings. The main incision is closed. The clamps are removed after 48 hours and the colostomy starts working. Since a gap of 2 inches has been established between the two openings, no stool from the proximal loop can enter the distal.

PAUL'S TUBE

This is a glass tube, bent as 'L', i.e. at a right angle, at its middle. It is used when a colostomy has to be opened immediately because of gross distension of the gut, e.g. acute obstruction. At one end of the tube there are two rims and this end has to be tied to the colonic opening. To the other end, where there is only one rim, a long rubber tubing is attached so that the colostomy drains well away from the wound (Fig. 72.91).

Sterilisation.—Boiling.

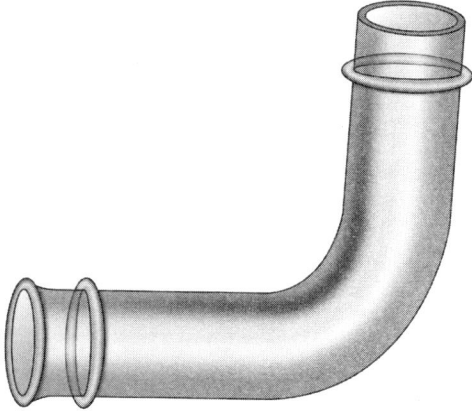

Fig. 72.91: Paul's tube

CORNER'S APPENDIX CRUSHER

This instrument is occasionally used for crushing the base of the appendix in appendectomy (Fig. 72.92). The hook at the end of one blade serves two purposes:

a. It prevents the appendix from slipping off the clamp.

b. It prevents the inclusion of the wall of the caecum within the blades of the forceps.

The instrument is very heavy and is, therefore, not liked by the surgeons. A Kocher's artery forceps, which has a tooth at its tip (comparable to the hook of the crusher), is usually used for the purpose.

Crushing is done prior to applying the transfixion suture at the base of the appendix. This is necessary for making the stump water-tight and air-tight, which helps crushing in the following ways:

1. The proximal end of the crushed mucosa and muscles curl inwards and plug the lumen.

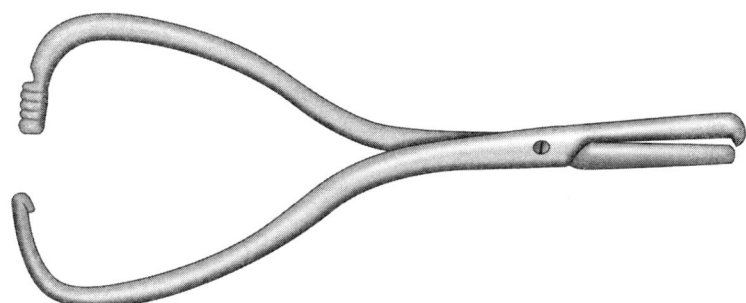

Fig. 72.92: Corner's appendix crusher

2. Sutures sit tightly on the crushed muscles (which they do not when the muscles are fleshy).

3. Crushing is haemostatic. Crushing should be avoided if:

a. The wall of the appendix is gangrenous.

b. The appendix is turgid, and any pressure on it is likely to cause its rupture.

c. The caecal wall is grossly oedematous and friable.

Sterilisation.—Boiling or autoclaving.

PYELOLITHOTOMY (NEPHROLITHOTOMY) FORCEPS

This is a straight forceps, having an angulation just at the tip of its blades. It is used to remove renal stones. The serrations at the tip of the blades provide good grip on the stone. The fenestrations on the blades accommodate part of the stone and also hold it tight. The handles have no catches since the stones should never be crushed (Fig. 72.93). For details of the operation *see* Chapter 54.

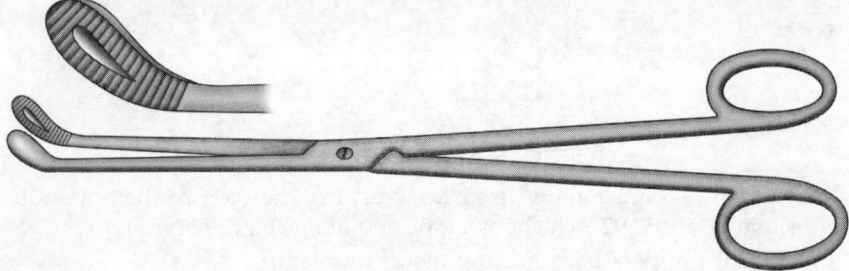

Fig. 72.93: Pyelolithotomy forceps

Sterilisation.—Boiling or autoclaving.

PERIOSTEUM ELEVATOR

These are also known as *'raspatory'* or *'rugine'*. Various types are available, of which the Faraboeuf's raspatory is popular. This is because it has a 'thumb rest' near the tip, which gives a good grip and better control on the instrument (Fig. 72.94).

For any operation on the bones, the periosteum has to be elevated because:

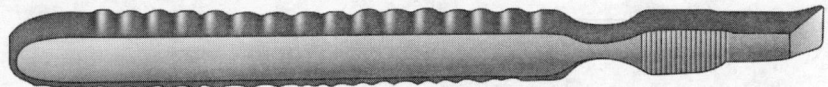

Fig. 72.94: Faraboeuf's periosteum elevator

a. Unless the periosteum is elevated, cutting instruments cannot work on the bone, as they tend to slip off.

b. As the periosteum is elevated from the bone, all soft tissues, including the important structures, are kept away from the bone, on which the operation is being performed.

Thus, periosteum elevators are used in the operations of sequestrectomy, amputation, SP nailing, IM nailing, bone plating, etc.

The periosteum itself is incised with a scalpel and its flaps are elevated from the bone by the periosteum elevator, working between the bone and the periosteum.

Sterilisation.—Concentrated lysol or autoclave.

CHISEL

The cutting edge of this instrument has one surface bevelled while the other surface is flat (c f osteotome, in which both the surfaces are bevelled). When a chisel is used, it cuts out irregular pieces of bone because one surface of the cutting edge is blunt (c f osteotome, which makes a clean cut through the bone). Some of the common uses of the instrument are—removal of chips from the iliac crest, saucerisation of the wall of osteomyelitic cavity, removal of the involucrum in sequestrectomy, removal of the upper femoral cortex at the site of introduction of SP nail, excision of exostosis, etc.

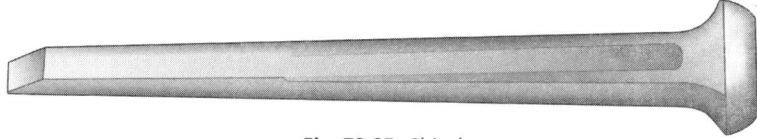

Fig. 72.95: Chisel

While cutting, when the flat surface of the instrument is placed on the bone, a thick chunk of bone is chiselled out; when the bevelled surface is in contact with the bone, a thin slice is removed (Fig. 72.95).

Sterilisation.—Concentrated lysol or autoclave.

OSTEOTOME

This instrument differs from a chisel in that both the surfaces, at its cutting edge, are bevelled; so that it makes a clean cut through the bone (Fig. 72.96). It is used for osteotomy, which means operative division of a bone. An osteotomy may also be done with a saw or by multiple drilling along the proposed line of division and then fracturing it by force.

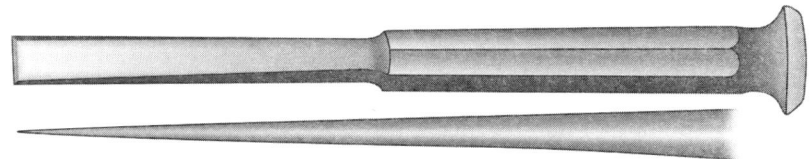

Fig. 72.96: Osteotome

Types of Osteotomy.—Principally, there are two types:

1. Linear osteotomy.—One straight cut is made through the bone. This is commonly done for correction of malunited fractures (a) for corrective reasons, or (b) to relieve abnormal strain on the joints above and below, or (c) to relieve stretching effects on nerves. The bone is cut across at the fracture site, brought to correct alignment, and fixed up. Another important example is McMurray's osteotomy, done in cases of non-united fractures of neck of the femur. Subtrochanteric osteotomy for correcting flexion-adduction deformities of the hip, and transtrochanteric osteotomy for coxa vara are other examples.

2. Wedge osteotomy.—This is done for correction of deformities, congenital or acquired. Two cuts are made through the bone, at an angle to each other. The

bone is cut through 3/4th of its thickness, the remaining 1/4th being forcibly broken. Thus a wedge of bone is removed, the base of which is on the longer side of the bone. When the bone is moulded to obliterate the gap, the deformity is corrected.

One example of wedge osteotomy is Macwen's osteotomy for correction of genu valgum (knock-knee). In this operation, an incision is made on the medial side of the thigh, just above the knee. A wedge from the lower femur is removed, with the base of the wedge on the medial side. The bone is moulded over the gap and the deformity is corrected.

Another example of wedge osteotomy is that performed for advanced cases of talipes equinovarus. A wedge is removed from the trasus, the base of the wedge being on the convex aspect of the deformity, i.e.. the superolateral aspect of the foot. The foot is moulded over the gap and the deformity is corrected.

Sterilisation.—Concentrated lysol or autoclave.

BONE GOUGE

This is used like a chisel, to cut out small irregular pieces of bones (Fig. 72.97).

Sterilisation.—Concentrated lysol or autoclave.

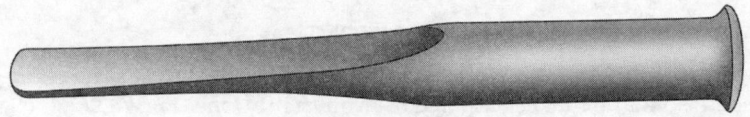

Fig. 72.97: Bone gouge

MALLET

This may be made of steel, lead, wood, etc. It is used to hammer cutting instruments like chisel, osteotome, gouge, etc. (Fig. 72.98).

Sterilisation.—Boiling or autoclaving.

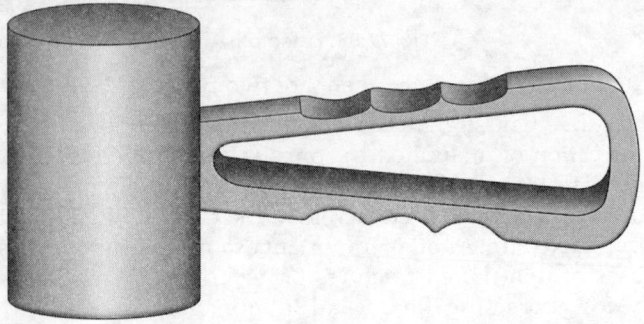

Fig. 72.98: Mallet

BONE HOLDING FORCEPS

Types.—There are three common types:

1. Ferguson's 'lion-toothed' bone holding forceps.—From the side, the teeth look like the teeth of a lion (Fig. 72.99).

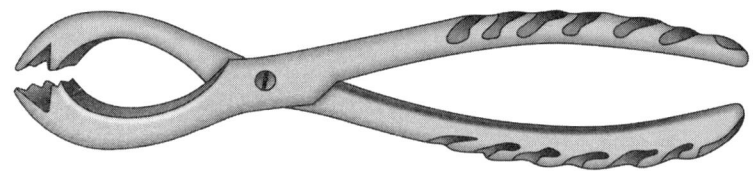

Fig. 72.99: Ferguson's bone holding forceps

2. Faraboeuf's bone holding forceps (Fig. 72.100).

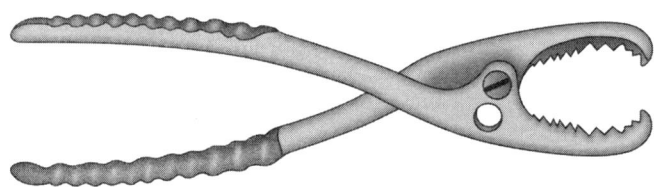

Fig. 72.100: Faraboeuf's bone holding forceps

3. Lane's bone holding forceps.—Like other instruments designed by Lane, this instrument is also a long one (Fig. 72.101).

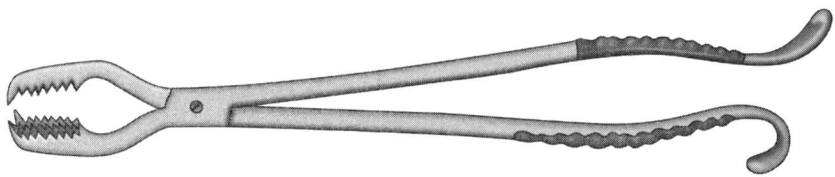

Fig. 72.101: Lane's bone holding forceps

These forceps are used to hold the bones steadily while operating on them, e.g. IM nailing, bone plating, etc.

Sterilisation.—Concentrated lysol or autoclave.

BONE NIBBLER OR GOUGE FORCEPS

This is used to nibble out small pieces of bone:

a. In making the sharp margin of a cut bone-end blunt, as in an amputation stump.
b. Enlarging a trephine opening in the skull.
c. Enlarging a laminectomy opening.

Sterilisation.—Concentrated lysol or autoclave. (Fig. 72.102).

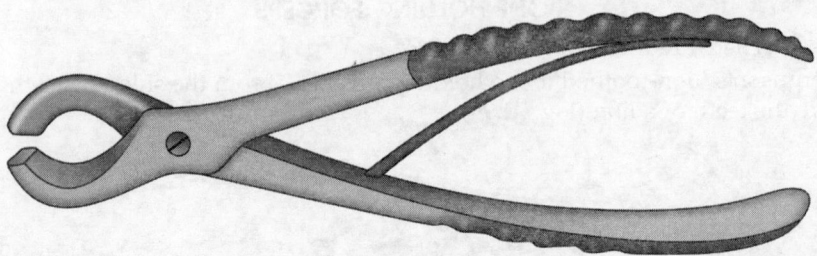

Fig. 72.102: Bone nibbler

SEQUESTRUM FORCEPS (NECROSIS FORCEPS)

This forceps is used to remove sequestrum from a chronic osteomyelitic cavity. A sequestrum is a piece of dead bone formed as a result of an aseptic necrosis, which, however, is a sequela to an inflammatory process in the bone, in the majority of cases such inflammation being pyogenic.

The transverse serrations on the blades of the instrument give a good grip on the sequestrum. The fenestration in each blade accommodates the sequestrum in addition to giving it a good grip. There are no catches on the handle since the sequestrum should not be crushed while being held (Fig. 72.103).

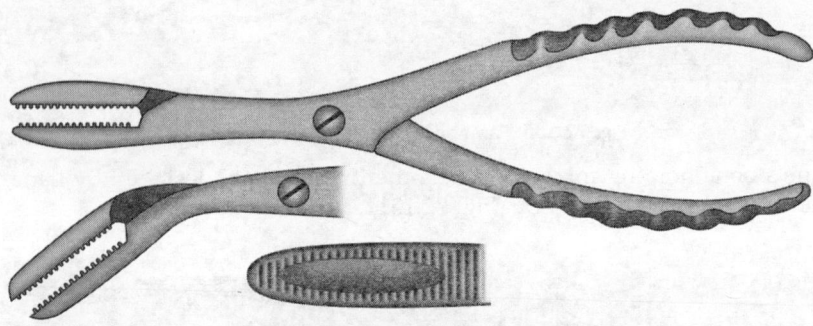

Fig. 72.103: Sequestrum forceps

Sterilisation.—Concentrated lysol or autoclave.

BONE CUTTING FORCEPS

These are used to cut small and weaker bones, e.g. phalanges, metacarpals, metatarsals, ribs, etc. (Fig. 72.104). Bigger bones are cut with saw.

Sterilisation.—Concentrated lysol or autoclave.

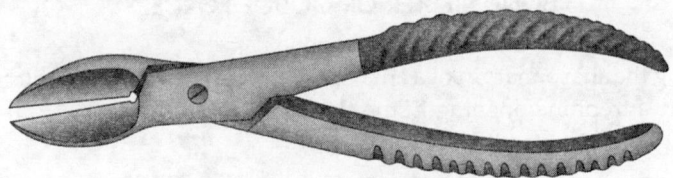

Fig. 72.104: Bone Cutting forceps

GIGLI'S WIRE SAW AND ACCESSORIES

Pars

1. Gigli's wire saw.
2. Two handles.
3. Introducer.
4. Guide.

Figure 72.105 shows the Gigli's wire saw with the handles. Figure 72.106 .shows the wire saw introducer, on the groove of which the wire saw guide has been made to pass.

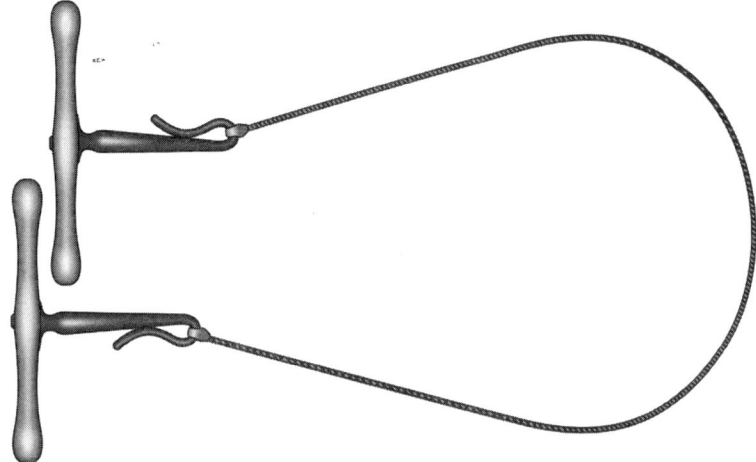

Fig. 72.105: Gigli's wire saw

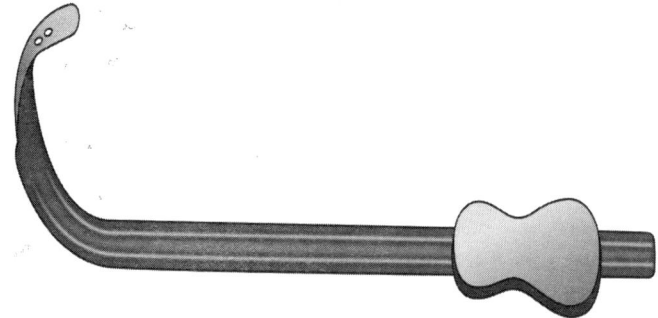

Fig. 72.106: Wire saw introducer (on the groove of which the wire saw director has been passed)

The Gigli's wire saw is made by twisting a few pieces of wire together, that gives it a cutting property when moved to and fro along its long axis. At either end there is a ring, to which the hook of the handle can be fitted (if handles are not used, the wire saw will cut the gloves). While cutting, bone particles collect in the crevices of the saw and the saw loses its cutting property. This difficulty is overcome by putting drops of water on the saw while it works.

The original use of the saw was to make osteoplastic flaps for exposure of any part of the cerebral hemispheres. The saw is often used to cut the mandible.

OSTEOPLASTIC FLAPS

The flap may be on the parietal, fronto-parietal, or occipito-parietal regions of the skull, as per necessity. A flap of skull is cut and turned down, together with the adherent scalp. This piece of bone has to live on the accessory blood supply that it receives from the vessels of the scalp, particularly on those which enter the bone at muscular attachments. Such flaps are usually based on the temporalis muscle. The scalp flap is made by a U-incision and, underneath this, the skull flap is made as a ∩, with a narrow base, that can be fractured easily. The skull flap is made by 5 or more trephine holes, the intervening bone between the adjacent holes being cut, thereafter, with the help of Gigli's wire saw. For this purpose, one end of the wire saw is passed in from one hole and brought out through the adjacent hole. As the saw is moved to and fro, the skull is cut from inside outwards. The process is repeated between all the holes, excepting those two at the base, the bone between which is fractured by force. For details *see* Chapter 24.

Thus, while an ordinary saw cuts a bone from outside inwards, the wire saw cuts it from inside outwards.

When the wire saw is introduced into the skull, it may cause injury to the underlying dura and the brain. In order to avoid this, the Gigli's wire saw introducer is used. This is a plate of metal, having a groove on one of its surfaces, that acts as a director. This is passed carefully from one trephine hole to the adjacent, being sure that it lies between the skull and the dura; thus it protects the dura.

On the groove of the introducer, the wire saw guide is now passed between the adjacent trephine holes. This is an elastic piece of metal, which is made to glide along the groove of the introducer. The guide has a hole at its end and to this hole is attached the ring of the wire saw. As the guide is drawn out through one trephine hole, the end of the wire saw, passing on the surface of the introducer, comes out.

Sterilisation.—The wire saw is sterilised in concentrated lysol or autoclave. The other accessories may be sterilised by boiling or autoclaving.

RESECTION OF THE MANDIBLE

Common Indications

1. Locally malignant tumours, e.g. admantinoma (commoner), osteoclastoma (rare).
2. Malignant tumours, e.g. oral, lingual and cheek cancers, involving the mandible (commoner), sarcoma of the mandible (rare).
3. Recurrent obstinate cases of chronic osteomyelitis.

Principles.—Wherever the pathology admits, the symphysis menti should be preserved, since preservation of the symphysis:

a. limits the deformity to the minimum (there is a gross deformity if the symphysis is excised).

b. preserves movements of the tongue and normal speech. After resection; the gap is filled up:

   i. either, by a prosthesis (the cut piece of mandible is sent to the maker to prepare the mould for the prosthesis).

ii. or, by a 12th rib graft (the curvature of the rib fits nicely with that of the jaw). If the 12th rib is very narrow, the 11th may be used instead, for better cosmesis.

In either case, the replacement operation has to be done at a second stage. In the interval between the two stages, the two cut ends of the bone have a tendency to be apposed to each other by contraction of the soft tissues, thereby causing a deformity. This may be prevented by either of the following procedures:

a. By doing an interdental wiring between the tooth at the cut end of the mandible and the corresponding tooth in the maxilla, on either side of the resection.

b. By placing a piece of thick wire, e.g. Kirschner's wire, in the gap. The ends of the wire are plunged into the cut medulla of the two sides.

Operation.—To minimise bleeding, the external carotid artery of the side may be primarily ligated through a separate incision in the neck.

The incision for the mandibular resection is made on the skin, along the lower border of the mandible. The scar gets hidden behind the fold there.

All structures, down to the periosteum, are cut, care being taken to ligate the facial vessels. The periosteum from either surface of the mandible is elevated with a raspatory. On the outer surface, this process separates all soft tissues of the cheek, including the masseter. Similarly, on the inner surface, structures at the floor of the mouth and the internal pterygoid muscle are detached from the bone. The bone is cut on the medial side with a Gigli's wire saw. On the lateral side also it may be cut in the same way or, if desired, it may be disarticulated from the temporo-mandibular joint. In the latter case, the attachment of the temporalis muscle has to be erased from the coronoid process, or the coronoid has to be cut through. While closing the wound, care should be taken to suture the floor of the mouth to the inner side of the cheek. The skin margins are sutured, keeping a drain.

ESMARCH'S OPERATION

This operation is often advocated for periarticular ankylosis of the jaw. The idea is to make a pseudoarthrosis (a false joint) near the affected temporo-mandibular joint.

The incision is made on the skin over the lower border of the mandible, towards the lateral side. The bone is made bare, as for resection of the mandible. A wedge osteotomy is now performed, with the base of the wedge (measuring 1½ inches) at the lower border of mandible, and the apex (measuring ¾ th inch) at the upper border. This is done with a Gigli's wire saw. A flap of the masseter muscle may be interposed between the cut bone surfaces. Early movements, active and passive, are started.

Intra-articular ankylosis of the jaw is treated by excision of the head and neck of mandible.

EXCISION OF THE MAXILLA

This is most commonly performed for sarcoma or carcinoma of the maxilla. The external carotid artery of the side is ligated at the neck, as a preliminary measure, to reduce haemorrhage.

The incision splits the upper lip in the midline, and then proceeds along the margin of the nose to the inner canthus of the eye. It is then continued along the inner side of the lower eyelid to the outer canthus of the eye and then a little downwards and outwards. The periosteum on the orbital floor is gently elevated and a spatula is put between the elevated periosteum and the bone to protect the orbital contents. The whole of the cheek is then mobilised from the outer surface of the maxilla, which now lies bare.

The maxilla is disconnected as follows:
1. Its nasal process is cut at its junction with the nasal bone.
2. The above division of the bone is continued backwards to the inferior orbital fissure by cutting through the lacrimal and ethmoid bones.
3. The zygomatic process is cut.
4. The alveolus and the hard palate are cut through in the midline (taking care not to injure the soft palate).

The bone is held with a bone holding forceps and is removed with a little force, care being taken to ligate the maxillary nerve and artery white being cut. The cheek flap is replaced in position and sutured. The deformity is astonishingly minimum.

HEY'S SAW

This is a small saw, having two cutting margins of different curvatures. It is used to cut the jaw, laminae, and skull bones (Fig. 72.107).

Sterilisation.—Concentrated lysol or autoclave.

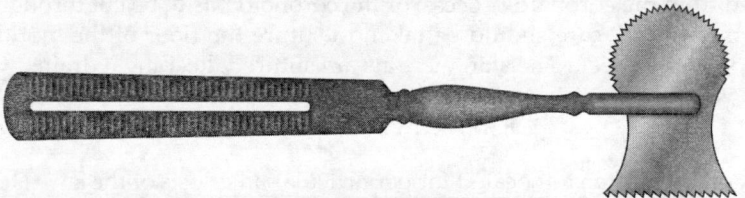

Fig. 72.107: Hey's saw

LAMINECTOMY SAW

This is a small saw, having an elliptical blade. It is used for laminectomy (Fig. 72.108).

Sterilisation.—Concentrated lysol or autoclave.

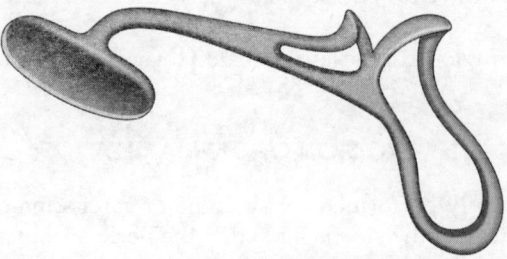

Fig. 72.108: Laminectomy saw

LAMINECTOMY FORCEPS (HORSLEY'S)

This is used to cut the spinous processes and laminae, in the operation of laminectomy. The narrow tip of the blade facilitates its introduction under the lamina, before cutting the bone (Fig. 72.109).

Sterilisation.—Concentrated lysol or autoclave.

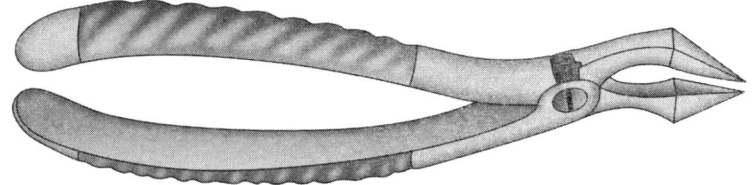

Fig. 72.109: Horsley's laminectomy forceps

LAMINECTOMY

Indications

1. In cases of fracture-dislocation of the spine with paraplegia (in these cases the paralysis recovers to certain extent with conservative methods and then becomes static or deteriorates).
2. In cases of caries spine with Pott's paraplegia, where the paralysis fails to recover under conservative treatment (with immobilisation). It has been found that laminectomy is of little value in these cases and a costo-transversectomy or an antero-laterai decompression is preferred.
3. For removal of tumours of the spinal and meninges.
4. For removal of foreign bodies.
5. For excision of the nucleus pulposus in cases of prolapsed intervertebral disc (the nucleus prolapses backwards into the vertebral canal, usually to one side of the midline, through a gap in the annulus fibrosus).
6. For spinothalamic tractotomy in relieving pain of an irremovable malignant growth.

Operation.—A vertical incision, 6 to 8 inches, is made, a little to one or other side of the midline, with its centre at the level of the lesion. The muscles, attached to the side of the spinous process and the back of the lamina, are erased off from these bones, on one side first and then on the other side. The supraspinous and interspinous ligaments are cut. The spinous process is nibbled out with a bone nibbler. The ligamentum flavum, attached to the upper and lower borders of the lamina, on each side, is divided. The laminae on both the sides are now excised carefully with a laminectomy forceps or a bone nibbler (the laminectomy saw or the Hey's saw is usually not used). Whatever instrument is used, great care must be taken not to injure the dura. Some surgeons, therefore, advocate that a small trephine hole be first made over some part of the lamina. Once the lamina has been cut through over some area, the rest of it can easily by excised with a laminectomy forceps or a bone nibbler

If pulsation can now be demonstrated in the dura, there is no abnormality higher up. If the dural pulsation is absent, the lamina above is exposed and excised. If required, laminae still higher have to be excised.

In those cases where wider exposure of the vertebral canal is required, e.g. spinal tumours, 3 to 4 laminae may have to be excised. The overlying muscles are carefully sutured and the skin wound is closed.

COSTO-TRANSVERSECTOMY

Since it has been found that laminectomy cannot drain a paravertebral cold abscess properly, this operation (costo-transversectomy) is employed for evacuation of abscesses, resulting from caries spine, in the thoracic region. An incision, about 3 inches long, is made along the posterior part of an appropriate rib, in relation to the abscess. The rib is cleared of its periosteum and is divided 2 inches away from its medial end. The medial part of the rib is then avulsed away. The related transverse process is chiselled off. The abscess is now opened, evacuated and medicated with streptomycin. The wound is closed without a drain.

While this operation drains all liquid caseous material, it is insufficient for removal of necrotic materials of more solid consistency. For this purpose, a wider exposure, in the form of anterolateral decompression, is necessary.

ANTERO-LATERAL DECOMPRESSION

This operation is more radical in the sense that it gives direct access to the local focus of the disease in caries spine. A vertical incision is made a little to one or other side of the midline. The posterior ends of several ribs are removed, together with the related transverse processes, as in the operation of costo-transversectomy. Thereafter, the pedicle and the adjacent anterolateral part of the vertebral bodies are also excised. Care must be taken not to injure the laminae and the articular processes in order to prevent lateral subluxation of the spine. All tubercular caseous material, sequestra, degenerated disc, etc. are removed. 'Internal gibbus', if any, is smoothened. The wound is sprinkled with streptomycin powder and is closed without a drain.

Nowadays an anterior approach (trans-pleural or trans-abdominal) is being made for a more direct access to the antero-lateral region of the vertebrae.

AMPUTATION SAW

This is used to cut the bone in amputations. The ridge on the blunt margin of the blade is jointed so that it can be pulled up from the blade when necessary. Had the ridge been fixed, it would come in the way of the instrument while it would work in the depth of the muscle mass. Had there been no ridge, the blade might break (Fig. 72.110).

Sterilisation.—Concentrated lysol or autoclave.

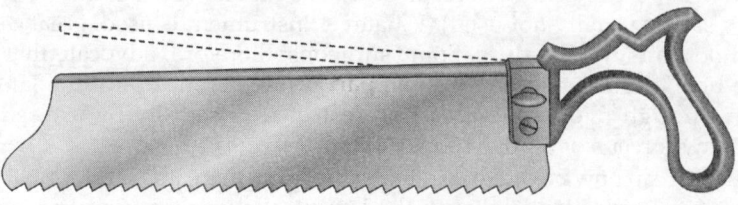

Fig. 72.110: Amputation saw

SYME'S AMPUTATION KNIFE

This is used to cut all soft tissues, down to the periosteum, in amputations. In practice, the skin is incised with a scalpel and all other soft tissues are cut with the amputation knife. The advantage of this knife, over an ordinary scalpel, is that it has a long blade, which makes a clean cut through the muscle mass (the blade of an ordinary scalpel being small, the blunt handle, going in, causes laceration of the muscles)—Fig. 72.111.

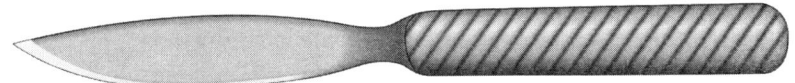

Fig. 72.111: Syme's amputation knife

The instrument is held in the 'grasping' position, with the whole of the hand, and the tissues are cut in one sweeping movement.

Sterilisation.—Concentrated lysol or autoclave.

SYME'S AMPUTATION

This amputation is performed near the ankle and offers a very satisfactory stump. The patient can walk directly on the stump or can use the cheapest and easiest variety of artificial limbs, e.g. 'elephant boot', as the stump is covered by the fatty heel flap.

The incision starts from below the tip of the lateral malleolus and passing along the sole, ends at a point little below the medial malleolus. These two points are joined by another incision just in front of the ankle.

Both the incisions are deepened to the bone so that:

a. Anteriorly, all the extensor tendons and the anterior tibial vessels and nerve are cut.

b. Medially, all the flexor tendons and the posterior tibial vessels and nerve are cut.

c. Laterally, the peroneal tendons are cut.

The foot is now forcibly plantar-flexed and the ankle joint is opened up. The knife passes through the joint and the whole foot is separated from the calcaneum.

The malleoli, together with about 3/4" of the lower ends of tibia and fibula, are cut, so that the cut bone surfaces are at the same level. The heel flap is brought to cover the stump and is sutured to the dorsal skin.

The sole effort in the operation is to keep the vitality of the heel flap. This is achieved by:

1. Avoiding bringing up the first incision too much forwards at the medial malleolus. Otherwise, the medial calcanean artery is cut and this is the sole supply to the flap.

2. Making the heel flap thick, instead of thin—the knife should be kept closely applied to the bone while separating the tendo Achillis from the calcaneum.

AWL AND BRADAWL

An awl is used to make a hole or a tunnel through a bone, either for a screw or for a wire. Introduction of the wire through a tunnel, thus made, may be difficult. To overcome this difficulty, a bradawl may be used. This is like an awl but has an eye near the tip. The wire is threaded on the eye after the instrument has passed through the bone. The wire traverses the tunnel as the instrument is withdrawn. Thus an awl or a bradawl may have to be used:

1. While screwing a bone.
2. In bone suturing, e.g. olecranon suture, patella suture, etc.

Sterilisation.—Concentrated lysol or autoclave (Fig. 72.112).

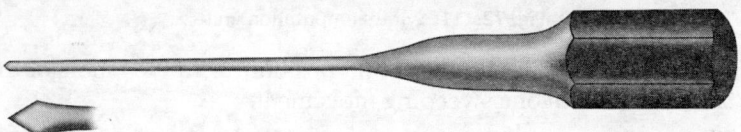

Fig. 72.112: Awl

WIRE GUIDE

This is a thin canula, with a cutting end, and having an oblique handle. There is a stellate inside the canula (Fig. 72.113).

The instrument works as a guide for wires, to be introduced through bones. The wire guide, with its stellate, makes a tunnel in the bone and the stellate is then withdrawn. The wire is now passed through the canula and the wire guide is taken out. The instrument may be used in operations like olecranon suturing, patella suturing, etc.

Sterilisation.—Concentrated lysol or autoclave.

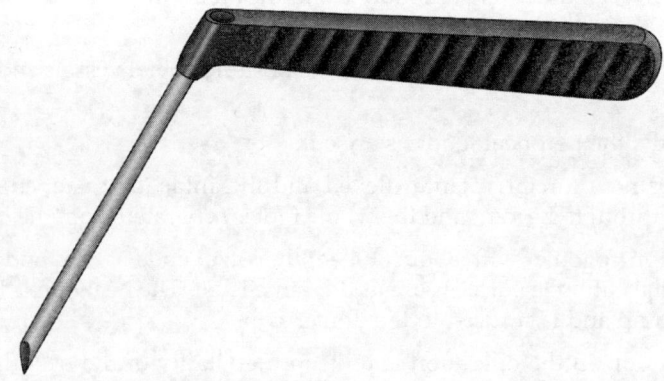

Fig. 72.113: Wire guide

INTERNAL FIXATION IN FRACTURES

Indications.—Internal fixation, in preference to external immobilisation, is indicated under the following circumstances:

1. If, after reduction, it is not possible to keep the fragments in acceptable position,

even with the best of plastering or splintage, e.g. avulsion fracture of the olecranon process.

2. When an open reduction has to be done. As the bone is exposed, advantage of an internal fixation is taken of.
3. As a method of choice in certain fractures, where a rigid immobilisation is obligatory to effect a union and such immobilisation is not secured by external means, e.g. intra-capsular fracture of the femoral neck.
4. As a method of choice, again, in certain fractures, where early ambulation of the patient is desired, e.g. extra-capsular fracture of the femoral neck.

Methods
1. Bone Plating.—The plate is fixed with the help of screws.
2. Bone Grafting.—Slab grafts, fixed with screws (see below).
3. Intramedullary Nailing, including special types of nails, e.g. Smith Petersen nail.
4. Screwing.—As in fractures of olecranon, patella, etc. or in oblique fractures of long bones, where two or more screws are passed transversely along the bone, across the fracture site.
5. Wiring.—The different methods of wiring are as follows:
   a. The wire is passed through tunnels made in the fragments, e.g. fractures of olecranon or patella.
   b. Two wires are wrapped around the bone in oblique or spiral fractures (circumferential wiring).
   c. Interdental wiring.

Advantages
1. The time spent in the hospital and away from work is reduced considerably.
2. The function of the limb, particularly those of the joints included in the immobilisation, can be restored early.
3. Complications, like delayed union or non-union, are less likely to occur because of the rigid immobilisation.

Disadvantages
1. Wound infection, which is otherwise absent in closed fractures, is fairly common and the metals catch infection notoriously.
2. Excessive stripping of soft tissues from the bone may:
   a. Jeopardise blood supply to the fragments, thereby hindering union.
   b. Lead to adhesions, causing restriction of joint movements.
3. Operative mortality, though rare, may occur.

BONE GRAFTING

Indications
1. For Bones:
   a. In the treatment of non-union.
   b. In filling up cavities in the bone, e.g. after curettage of bone cysts, chondroma, etc.
2. For Joints.—In performing arthrodesis.

Types

A. According to the donor, a graft may be:

1. Autogenous.

2. Homogenous.

3. Heterogenous.

B. According to the nature of the graft itself, it may be:

1. Slab or Cortical.

2. Sliver.

3. Chip.

AUTOGENOUS GRAFT.—This means a graft taken from the patient himself. This is the type of graft usually used, as it 'takes' most rapidly. Although every graft dies, and, thereafter, merely acts as a scaffolding, on which new bone grows, the cells on the surface of an autogenous graft possibly survive.

The disadvantage of an autogenous grafting is that an additional operative procedure on the patient is necessary and the donor site may get an infected haematoma.

HOMOGENOUS GRAFT.—This means a graft taken from another individual of the same species, i.e. human being. The source of such graft may be:

a. Fresh dead body.

b. Ribs removed at thoracoplasty.

Bone-banks are nowadays working, where such grafts are stored.

While the advantage of homogenous graft is that an ample supply (often prefabricated so as to fit the host site) are available, its main disadvantage is that it 'takes' far more slowly than an autogenous graft.

HETEROGENOUS GRAFT.—This means a graft taken from another species. These are now commercially prepared from calf-bones, e.g. 'Kiel bone'.

While the main advantage is an unlimited supply (as per necessary texture), the disadvantages are:

a. The rate of 'taking' is slow and 'taking' is often uncertain.

b. They often contain foreign proteins and infective materials.

SLAB OR CORTICAL GRAFT.—This is a thick graft, mainly containing the cortex, and is usually taken from the subcutaneous surface of tibia. It is put over the host area (receiving area) by either of the following methods:

1. *As an Onlay Graft.*—The graft is placed on the surface of the bone (made raw), and fixed with the help of screws.

2. *As an Inlay Graft:*

   a. A trench is made on the surface of the host bone and the graft, made to the size of the trench, is placed in it. If it is tightly fitting, no fixation is necessary. Otherwise, it is fixed in position with screws.

   b. Another method is to drive the graft into the host medulla, e.g. a fibular graft passed through the neck of the femur, in the treatment of non-united fracture of the femoral neck.

SLIVER GRAFTS.—These are long but thin slices of bone, usually taken from the posterior part of the iliac crest. Several such pieces are put over the host site and kept in position by suturing the periosteum and other soft tissues over them.

CHIP GRAFTS.—These are small pieces of spongy bone, taken from the iliac crest. They are used either alone (as in filling cavities in bones) or in conjunction with slab or sliver grafts. They are fixed in position, if necessary, by suturing the periosteum and soft tissues over them.

SMITH PETERSEN NAIL

This is a triflanged metallic nail, one end of which is cutting and the other end is blunt. There is a central canal, about 2 mm wide, and this is meant for the guide-wire on which the nail is hammered into the bone (this central canal is Watson-Jone's modification). The size of the nail should be so chosen that, after its introduction, the lateral end abuts against the outer cortex of the femur, while the inner end is just short of the articular cartilage at the femoral head (Fig. 72.114).

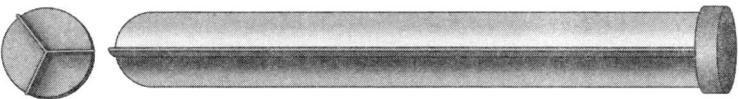

Fig. 72.114: SP nail

It is used for internal fixation in cases of intra-capsular fractures of the femoral neck (for extra-capsular fractures, a combination of nail and plate is used).

The nail has to be made triflanged, instead of round, in order to prevent rotatory movements between the fragments while causing minimum damage to the cancellous bone through which it passes. It is made of stainless steel or other non-ionisable metal.

The nail is removed (there is a special extractor for the purpose) when the fracture has united, but seldom before six months. Other indications for its removal are:

1. If there is gross infection with sinus formation.
2. If there is avascular necrosis of the head, resulting in non-union.
3. If there is gross osteoarthritis of the hip joint.

Sterilisation.—Concentrated lysol or autoclave.

SP NAIL GUIDEWIRE

This is called guidewire as it guides an SP nail, which is threaded on it. One end of the wire is sharp and the other end blunt. The wire is graduated, (cf Kirschner's wire, which has no graduation). The graduations help in determining the exact size of the SP nail, required for the particular patient (Fig. 72.115).

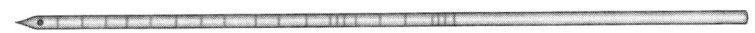

Fig. 72.115: SP Nail guidewire

In practice, 2 to 3 guidewires are introduced through the femoral neck in different directions, as per discretion. This is done either by manual pressure or by drilling.

X-rays are taken. The one which appears to be more or less central (both antero-posteriorly and from above downwards) is kept, and the others are removed. The SP nail is threaded on this wire.

Sterilisation.—Concentrated lysol or autoclave.

PUNCH

This is simply a piece of metal pipe. It is threaded on the projecting part of the guide-wire, after the SP nail has been threaded on the latter, so that the nail can be hammered (otherwise, because of the projecting guide-wire, the mallet cannot hammer on the nail)—Fig. 72.116.

Sterilisation.—Boiling or autoclaving.

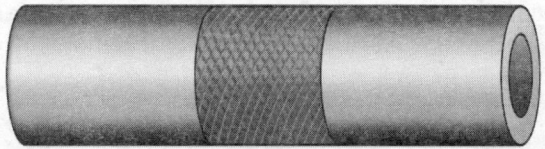

Fig. 72.116: Punch

IMPACTING PUNCH

This is also a metallic pipe but is a little expanded at either end. The side with the smaller expansion is to be hammered, while that with the wider expansion fits clear of the head of the SP nail and touches the bone surface (Fig. 72.117).

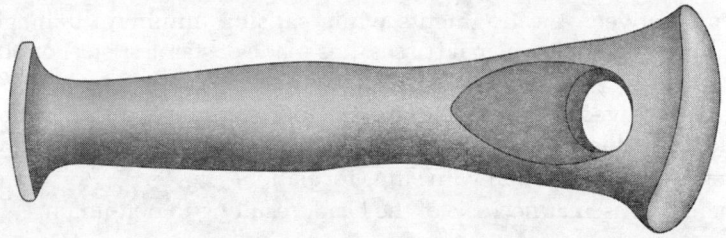

Fig. 72.117: Impacting punch

As the SP nail is hammered in with the ordinary punch, there is a little separation between the two fracture fragments. Thereafter, this impacting punch is used and, because the hit of the hammer is directly on the bone at the base of the nail, apposition between two fragments occurs (hence it is called impacting).

Sterilisation.—Boiling or autoclaving.

THE OPERATION OF SP NAILING

This is done for internal fixation in intra-capsular fractures of the femoral neck. The operation should be done as early as possible, after the injury.

Under general anaesthesia, reduction of the fracture is achieved on a specially equipped orthopaedic table (orthopaedic horse). Flexion, adduction and internal rotation of the hip effects a reduction, which is confirmed by a portable X-ray.

A Michel clip, placed 2 cm below the mid-inguinal point, marks the position of the femoral head and helps directing the guide-wires through the neck.

A vertical incision is made downwards from the tip of the greater trochanter. All soft tissues, including the periosteum, are divided, and the periosteum is elevated. A search is now made for the transverse ridge, which marks the junction of the greater trochanter with the shaft. The guide-wires are to be introduced through a point about 3/4th inch below this line. The cortical bone around this point is chiselled off with a chisel or a gouge. Two or three guide-wires are now pushed in through the said point (by manual pressure or by drilling). These are directed towards the Michel clip, marking the head. X-rays (antero-posterior and lateral views) are taken. The wire, which is more or less central in position, is kept, and the others are removed.

An SP nail, whose length is indicated by the graduations on the guide-wire, is threaded on the wire. A punch is threaded on the projecting part of the wire and the nail is hammered in. Thereafter, final impact is achieved by putting the impacting punch over the projecting part of the nail and hammering the impacting punch on the bone. The final position of the nail is checked again by portable X-rays (both antero-posterior and lateral views). The soft tissues and the skin are sutured.

No plaster immobilisation is necessary but external rotation of the limb must be prevented in the post-operative period. This is achieved by fitting a de-rotation bar (wooden) to the sole of the foot, with the help of plaster bandage.

This bar is maintained for about four weeks, after which movements of the hip are allowed. The patient thereafter sits on the bed, but weight-bearing is allowed only after X-rays show healing of the fracture, and never before three months.

INTRAMEDULLARY NAIL

This nail is meant for plunging into the medullary cavity of long bones. It is used for internal fixation of fractures in the shaft of long bones. The commonest use of this nail is in fractures of the shaft of the femur but it may also be used for the humerus, tibia and ulna. The points of exit and entrance of the nail, in the different bones, are as follows:

Femur.—Greater trochanter.

Tibia.—Tibial tuberosity.

Humerus.—Greater tuberosity.

Ulna.—Olecranon process.

Both the ends of the nail are pointed so that each end can pass through the bone, and this is required to suit with the technique of the operation (see below). A little away from each end, there is a constricted part, i.e. the neck, and this is utilised during extraction of the nail (the extractor fits on the neck to have a good grip while the nail is being drawn out).

There are two measurements for the nail—one the calibre, and the other the length. The nail is made of non-ionisable metal. Various types are available, e.g. triangular nail, Küntscher nail, etc.

Sterilisation.—Concentrated lysol or autoclave.

THE OPERATION OF INTRAMEDULLARY NAILING

With an appropriate incision, the fracture site is exposed. The fracture ends are made fresh and smooth, and are lifted up from the muscle bed with bone levers. An intramedullary nail of suitable size and calibre is now drilled in, through the medulla at the lower end of the upper fragment. The direction is so kept that the nail travels towards the point of exit of the specific bone, as mentioned above (e.g. greater trochanter in case of femur). As the end of the nail points under the skin, a small incision is made on it, so that the nail, pushed from below, can escape through it. It is pushed further up, till its lower end comes to the level of the fracture. The two fracture fragments are now brought into alignment and the nail is hammered in, from above, into the medullary cavity of the lower fragment. Thus, an internal fixation is achieved.

The upper end of the nail, with its neck, is kept under the skin, so that the nail can be easily withdrawn later. Both the wounds are closed.

Even with the internal fixation, an external immobilisation is essential— otherwise the nail bends under pressure.

Extraction of the Nail.—The nail is removed with an extractor:

1. When there is radiological evidence of union of the fracture.
2. If there is gross infection with sinus formation.
3. If the nail bends under pressure (it is then really difficult to extract the nail).

BONE PLATE

These are made of non-ionisable metals and are used for internal fixation in fractures of long bones. They are most commonly used for the radius and ulna. The holes in the plate are meant for screws, which fix the plate in position. The minimum number of screws is four, two on either side of the fracture (Fig. 72.118). For bigger plates, the number of screws is more. The screws should be long enough to pass through the nearer cortex, the medulla, and part of the distal cortex. If there is no anchorage with the distal cortex, there is a tendency for the screw to loosen.

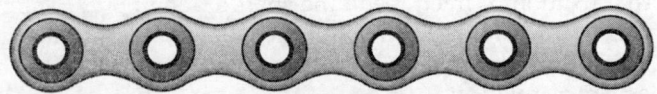

Fig. 72.118: Bone plate

The plates may be kept permanently. They are taken out:

1. If there is gross infection and sinus formation.
2. If there is non-union and another operation is required.

Sterilisation.—Boiling or autoclaving or in concentrated lysol.

SCREWS

These are used:

1. With bone plates, to fix the plate.
2. With cortical bone grafts, to fix the graft.
3. For internal fixation by themselves:

a. In fractures of olecranon and patella.
b. In oblique fractures of long bones.

Sterilisation.—Concentrated lysol or autoclave.

BONE LEVER

This is used to keep a bone elevated from the muscle mass (after stripping the periosteum), while operating on it, e.g. bone-plating, bone-grafting, intramedullary nailing, etc. (Fig. 72.119).

Sterilisation.—Boiling or autoclaving.

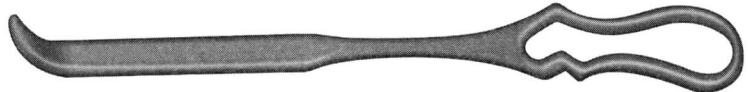

Fig. 72.119: Bone lever

KIRSCHNER'S WIRE

This is used for the purpose of skeletal traction. One end of the wire is sharp and is meant to be drilled through the bone. The other end, which is blunt, is fitted to the drill. The wire can be introduced with local infiltration anaesthesia.

The bones, in which skeletal traction is commonly employed, in the treatment of fractures, are:

1. Femur.—Through the tibial tuberosity in the adults and the femoral condyles in the children.
2. Tibia.—Through the lower end of tibia or posterior tuberosity of calcaneum.
3. Ulna.—Through the olecranon.

Simple traction from the ends of the wire will result in bending of the wire, without efficient traction. To overcome this difficulty, a stirrup with a stretcher is fitted to the protruding ends of the wire.

The stirrup, which is a stout metallic 'U' is so made that, when the Kirschner's wire is fitted to it, it keeps the wire straight and does not allow it to be bent under traction. On the curve of the stirrup there are several holes, to any of which a hook may be fitted. The traction cord is tied to this hook. Since the hook can swivel freely on the stirrup, the pin does not move with the movements of the cord (Fig. 72.120).

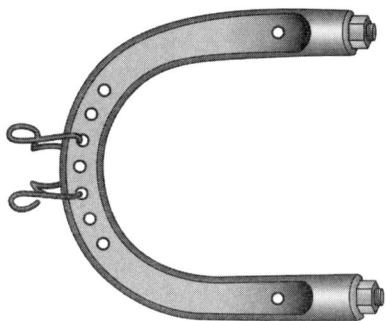

Fig. 72.120: Stirrup

Stienmann's pin is like a Kirschner's wire, used for the same purpose.

Bohler's pin is a much stouter wire, also used for skeletal traction. It does not bend under traction. So, it may be used with the help of a rotatory stirrup, i.e. without a stretcher. The advantage of a rotatory stirrup is that, when it moves, the pin does not move with it. So, there is no pain with the movements of the stirrup (Fig. 72.121). The disadvantage of a Bohler's pin, however, is that it is very thick and, therefore, causes more necrosis and infection in the bone than a Kirschner's wire of Stienmann's pin.

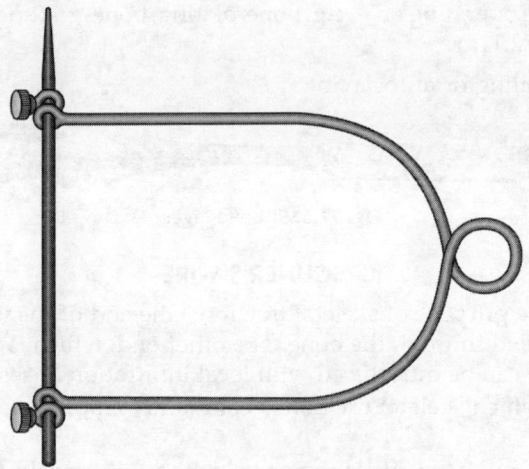

Fig. 72.121: Bohler's pin with rotatory stirrup

Sterilisation.—These wires and pins are sterilised either in concentrated lysol or in autoclave.

TRACTION

Indications

1. In the treatment of fractures:
    a. To achieve a gradual reduction.—Where reduction by manipulation is not possible because of strong muscular attachments of the displaced fragments, e.g. fractures of the long bones of the lower limbs in the adults.
    b. To hold the fragments in alignment.—Where there is a tendency for the fragments to be redisplaced (spiral fractures of the long bones, especially, have this tendency).

    In the majority of cases, traction is applied to serve both the above purposes. Most commonly this is required for fractures of the long bones of the lower limbs in adults, though it may have to be employed for fractures in the upper limbs or fractures in children.

2. To overcome muscle spasms, particularly in arthritis—traumatic, pyogenic, or tubercular.

3. To prevent deformities and contractures.

4. To cause extension of the spine, as in spondylosis, prolapsed disc, etc.

Distraction.—In transverse fractures, an overtraction may lead to wide separation between the fragments and this may hinder union. This is called distraction. This can be minimised by regular exercises of the longitudinal muscles running across the fracture.

Methods of Traction

1. SKIN TRACTION (SURFACE TRACTION).—This is done with adhesive plaster, applied to the shaved skin of the limb. The plaster is pasted to the skin, starting from one side of the limb (say, lateral). It is brought down to the end of the limb (say, the sole), and then, leaving some gap between it and the sole, it is taken up along the opposite side of the limb (i.e. medial). In case of a femoral shaft fracture, where this type of traction is commonly applied, the plaster should start and end at a level as high as possible in the upper part of the thigh (irrespective of the level of the fracture). To the curve of the 'U' of the adhesive plaster, below the sole, a wooden spreader is attached. There is a central hole in the spreader, through which the traction cord passes (Fig. 72.122).

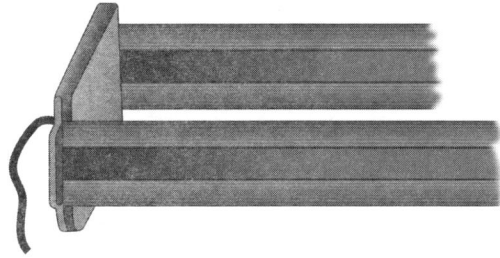

Fig. 72.122: Spreader for surface traction (the wooden spreader is parted to the adhesive plaster. The traction rope is attached to the spreader)

2. SKELETAL TRACTION.—The traction is applied directly to the bone, by means of a Kirschner's wire, Stienmann's pin, or Bohler's pin. Skeletal traction is more efficient than skin traction. Its disadvantages, however, are the risks of bone necrosis and infection.

3. TRACTION BY GRAVITY ALONE.—This is used especially for the humerus. An overriding of the fragments is easily undone by holding the limb adequately in a wrist sling. The weight of the arm provides a continuous traction.

Mechanism of Traction.—For every traction, there must be a balancing countertraction. Otherwise, the traction will simply pull the limb and the patient downwards, towards the traction. According to the nature of the countertraction, traction may be of the following types:

1. FIXED TRACTION.—Here the traction is achieved against a fixed point, e.g. traction exerted by tying the traction cord to the cross-piece of a Thomas' splint, after pulling the limb down, till the ring of the splint presses against the ischial tuberosity.

2. BALANCED TRACTION.—Here the countertraction is effected by the body weight, the foot end of the bed being raised. The traction in these cases may be:

   a. Fixed.—When the traction tape is tied on the rail at the foot end of the bed.

   b. Mobile.—When the traction tape is passed over a pulley and weights are attached to its end.

3. COMBINED TRACTION.—Here a combination of (1) and (2) is used. The traction tape is tied to the cross-piece of the Thomas' splint, the splint is tied to the foot end of the bed, and the foot end of the bed is raised.

DOYEN'S RASPATORY

This raspatory is specially meant for elevation of periosteum from the inner side of the rib (Fig. 72.123). Periosteum from the outer surface of the rib is elevated by an ordinary periosteum elevator.

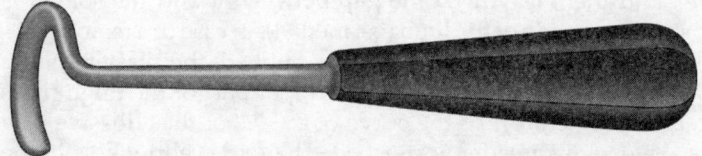

Fig. 72.123: Doyen's raspatory

Periosteum has to be elevated from both the surfaces of the rib during excision of a rib or part of it. Elevation of periosteum from the inner surface of the rib is necessary because:

1. With the periosteum, the intercostal vessels and nerve are raised from the rib, so that these structures are not injured while cutting the rib.
2. The periosteum on the inner side of the rib is closely adherent to the parietal pleura, which is shifted with it, and thus, avoids injury.
3. Unless the periosteum is elevated, the rib cannot be cut with a cutting instrument, which then tends to slip.

The periostenum on the outer surface of the rib is incised along is long axis, midway between the upper and lower borders of the rib, at the desired site. At each end of this incision, a vertical incision is made on the periosteum. With an ordinary raspatory, the flaps of the outer periosteum are elevated up and down so as to reach the upper and lower borders of the rib. The Doyen's raspatory is now inserted between the elevated flap of periosteum and the upper border of the rib, so that the blade of the raspatory reaches the inner surface of the rib, between it and the periosteum. As the raspatory is drawn along the rib, the periosteum on the inner side of the rib is elevated. If necessary, the Doyen's raspatory may be introduced along the lower border of the rib as well, for further elevation of the periosteum.

While drawing the Doyen's raspatory along the rib, it should be drawn from behind forwards at the upper border of the rib, and from before backwards at the lower border. This procedure avoids laceration of the intercostal muscles and makes the movements of the raspatory easier.

During resection of the rib, the intercostal vessels may be injured and the bleeding may be difficult to be controlled, as the vessels tend to retract to an inaccessible position and they are often friable (as in empyema). To avoid bleeding from the intercostal vessels, the vessels should be ligated primarily, proximal and distal to the site of rib resection. This is best done by passing a ligature around the rib, so that, when the ligature is tightened, the vessels are compressed against the rib.

Resection of rib or ribs may be necessary for:

1. Open drainage of empyema.
2. Thoracotomy, i.e. opening the chest for some operation inside. Resection of a rib gives better exposure than that obtained by an approach made through an intercostal space.

3. Thoracoplasty for pulmonary tuberculosis.

For details of rib resection and intercostal drainage *see* Chapter 35.

COMBINED RASPATORY AND RIB SHEAR

This instrument, with its two handles fitted, is a bone cutting forceps and can be used for cutting a rib, i.e. it works as a rib shear. Its handle are detachable and, when they are detached, one of them looks like a Doyen's raspatory and may be used for it. Thus, the instrument is a combination of a raspatory and a rib shear (Fig. 72.124).

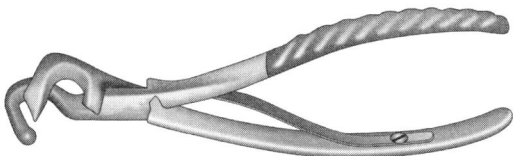

Fig. 72.124: Combined raspatory and rib shear

Use.—In rib resection.

Sterilisation.—Concentrated lysol or autoclave.

TREPHINE

This is a hollow circular saw which, when working on the skull bones, brings out a circular piece of bone and thus provides entry into the cavity of the skull. The operation is known as 'trephining'. At the centre of the saw there is a pin, that can be manipulated up and down from the handle of the instrument. This pin is brought down below the level of the saw during the first stage of working of the trephine. The pin fixes the trephine on the skull, otherwise the trephine would slip off the skull instead of cutting, through it. After the trephine has cut through some thickness of the bone, the central pin is drawn up and the rest of the trephining is done. If the pin is not withdrawn, it enters the skull cavity earlier than the saw and may injure the contents there (Fig. 72.125).

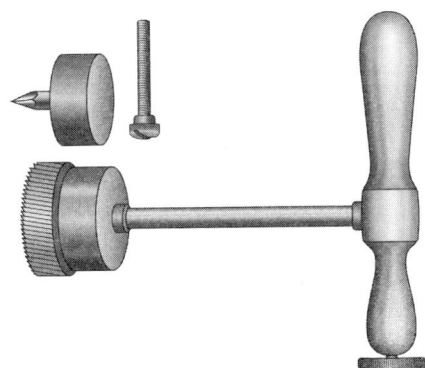

Fig. 72.125: Trephine

Sterilisation.—Concentrated lysol or autoclave.

Indications for Trephining

1. In cases of head injury:
   a. To arrest bleeding and evacuate clots in extradural and subdural haemorrhages.—A parietal trephining is done.

   b. To decompress the brain in cases of cerebral compression due to oedema, where conservative methods have failed.—Bitemporal trephining may have to be done.

2. While raising an osteoplastic flap.—Several trephine holes are made and a Gigli's wire saw, working in between the holes, raises up the flap (see Gigli's wire saw).

BURR

This is used, like a trephine, in making an opening in the skull (burr-holing). Burrs of different diameters are available. Also, they are available in two shapes—spherical (the head is round) and cylindrospherical (the head is round on cross-section but its height is long). The long heavy drilling instrument, on which a burr is fitted, is called 'brace' (Fig. 72.126).

Burrs are often preferred to trephines because they are less likely to damage the underlying dura or brain.

The indications for burr-holing are the same as those for trephining (see trephine).

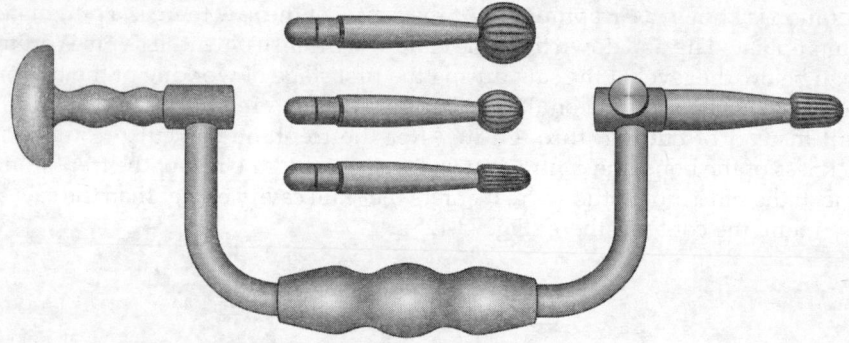

Fig. 72.126: Brace with burr (burrs of different types are shown)

Sterilisation.—The brace and the burrs are sterilised by autoclaving. The burrs only may be sterilised in concentrated lysol.

DE VILBISS' SKULL-CUTTING FORCEPS

This is a special type of bone cutting forceps, used for cutting the skull bone, in between two trephine holes, while making osteoplastic flaps. A Gigli's wire saw is better for the purpose (see Gigli's wire saw).

Sterilisation.—Concentrated lysol or autoclave (Fig. 72.127).

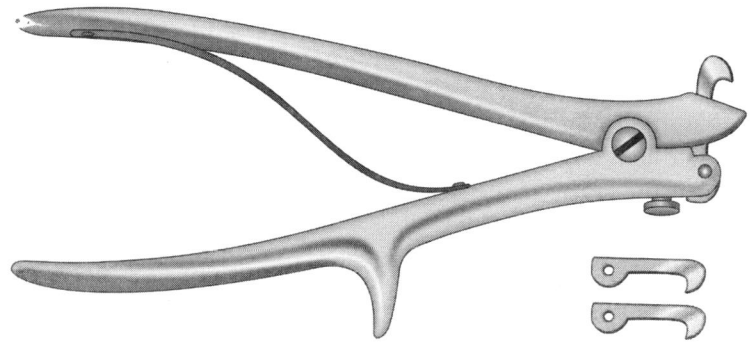

Fig. 72.127: De Vilbiss' skull-cutting forceps

LUMBAR PUNCTURE NEEDLE

This is a long needle with a stillette. The tip of the needle is meant for introduction into the subarachnoid space in the lumbar region, hence it is so named. The needle is fairly malleable; otherwise it might break if the patient strains during its introduction. The bevel, at the tip of the needle, is purposely made short (as compared to other injecting needles), so that a part of the opening may not remain outside the subarachnoid space while the tip has entered the space. The needle is not very sharp—had it been so, it might cause injury to the nerves of the cauda equina.

Site of Puncture.—The lower part of the sheath, formed by the arachnoid and the, dura mater, contains only the cauda equina (formed by the lumbar and sacral nerve roots) and the thread-like continuation of the piamater (called the filum terminate). The spinal cord, in an adult, ends at the level of the second lumbar vertebra, while the subarachnoid space, mentioned above, extends down to the level of the second sacral vertebra. In lumbar puncture advantage is taken of the absence of the spinal cord in the lumbar part of the vertebral canal, so that a needle can be introduced safely into the subarachnoid space without fear of damaging the cord. A space of 2.5 mm, in width, exists between the nerve roots of the two sides, so that, if the needle is kept strictly in the midline it will avoid injury to these roots.

The space between the adjoining vertebral laminae is greatest in the *lower* lumbar region. It is for this reason that either the interval between the third and fourth or that between the fourth and fifth lumbar vertebrae is selected for the introduction of the needle. Also, the patient is placed with the trunk strongly flexed; this procedure further increases the said space. The line joining the highest points of the two iliac crests passes over the fourth lumbar spine. The interspace above or below this line is selected for the puncture.

Technique of Puncture.—The patient must be so placed that there is maximum flexion of the lumbar spine. This may be done in two ways:

1. He lies on his side, curled up as much as practicable, attempting to approximate the head and the knees. This is the usual position.

2. He sits on the operating table, bending forwards to the maximum. This is the position when a low spinal anaesthesia has to be administered (*see* below).

The site of puncture is made out and the skin is properly sterilised. The skin and the underlying soft tissues, including the interspinous ligaments, through which the lumbar puncture needle has to traverse, are anaesthetised with 1% novocaine solution. This is done with an ordinary needle.

The lumbar puncture needle is introduced at right angles to the skin. As it is thrust forwards, care must be taken to see that it does not slope to one side. The needle is slanted slightly towards the patient's head, so that it enters obliquely beneath the spinous process of the upper vertebra. As the needle encounters the tough ligamentum flavum (which stretches between the adjacent laminae), there is a feeling of resistance. As soon as this resistance is overcome, the vertebral canal has been entered. With a little more travel, the needle pierces the dura and the arachnoid, to reach the subarachnoid space. Withdrawal of the stillette is now followed by escape of CSF. In some cases the patient has to be rolled a little towards the surgeon, aiding flow of the CSF by gravity. If the needle strikes the bone during its introduction, it has to be withdrawn to the subcutaneous plane and reinserted in a different direction.

Indications for Lumbar Puncture

A. DIAGNOSTIC PURPOSES

1. *To study the CSF:*
   a. The pressure of the CSF—A manometer is attached to the needle. The normal pressure is 120 mm of water in the recumbent posture. The rate of flow from a puncture is roughly one drop per second. A raised pressure may be encountered in meningitis and in many cases of head injury. In head injuries, associated with severe brain stem lesion, the pressure may be abnormally low.
   b. Tie naked-eye character of the CSF in meningitis of different types and in head injuries.—In head injuries, with haemorrhage outside the membranes, the fluid is crystal clear. In cerebral contusion or laceration it is blood stained.
   c. The bacteriological and other character of the CSF:
      i. Microscopical
      ii. Culture
      iii. WR or gold test, for syphilis.
   d. Chemical test.—To assess the protein content, if a tumour is suspected. In neurofibroma the protein is raised from the normal of 20–40 mg per cent to 200–400 mg per cent. When a tumour causes complete spinal block, the CSF, below the block, is encysted, and protein and pigments diffuse into it from the blood vessels. In such cases, the fluid becomes yellow and may clot spontaneously (Froin's syndrome),

2. *To test for spinal block:*

   a. Queckenstedt's Test.—Compression of the jugular vein in the neck, is normally associated with a rise in the pressure of the CSF. When there is a block in the vertebral canal (e.g. by a spinal tumour) this phenomenon is absent.
   b. Froin's syndrome.—Described above.

c. If there is a spinal block, the pressure of the CSF (determined by lumbar puncture) is lower than that of the fluid in the cistern (determined by cisternal puncture).

3. *To perform myelography:*

This is often done for the diagnosis of spinal cord conditions (e.g. a tumour). A radio-opaque dye, e.g. Pantopaque, is injected through the lumbar puncture and the patient is placed in the Trendelenburg position. The heavy dye gravitates up the canal and demarcates the lower limit of the obstruction. The method may be combined with a similar injection through a cisternal puncture which demonstrates the upper limit of the obstruction.

B. THERAPEUTIC PURPOSES

1. For injection of antibiotics in meningitis, e.g. penicillin.
2. To reduce intracranial pressure.—4 to 5 ml of heavily blood-strained fluid may be removed every alternate day in cases of cerebral laceration with gross extravasation.
3. For relief of intractable pain, e.g. advanced carcinoma, etc.—Phenol or absolute alcohol may be injected.

C. ANAESTHETIC PURPOSES

For spinal anaesthesia (described below).

SPINAL ANAESTHESIA

This method aims at putting a local anaesthetic agent into the subarachnoid space, in order to block the sensory nerve roots. The drug is introduced at the level of the lumbar spine, i.e. by a lumbar puncture (for details of lumbar puncture; see above).

The drugs used are Procaine (Novocaine), Lignocaine, Cinchocaine (Nupercaine), etc. Each has its individual supporters. However, there are two kinds such solutions:

a. Light or hypobaric
b. Heavy or hyperbaric,

depending on whether the solution is lighter or heavier than CSF, the specific gravity of which varies between 1004 and 1010.

Methods of Spinal Anaesthesia

1. *Standardly:*

a. For bilateral blocks.—The patient is placed in the left lateral position, with the foot end of the table raised (15° Trendelenburg). 12 to 14 ml of a *light* local anaesthetic solution is injected by lumbar puncture and the patient is quickly turned to a prone position. This allows the light solution to float up dorsally and act on the sensory nerve roots, which are located at the posterior aspect of the spinal cord. After about 10 minutes, the patient is made supine and the operation started.

b. For unilateral blocks.—The patient is made to lie on the side opposite to which the operation has to be performed, i.e. the affected side up. After injecting a *light* solution, as above, he is kept in this position for about 10 minutes. The drug floats up and paralyses the sensory nerve roots on the desired side. The patient is then turned on his back and the operation started.

Abdominal operations and operations in the lower extremities may be performed with bilateral blocks. Unilateral blocks are of special value in operations for hernia.

2. *Low Spinal.*—With the patient sitting on the operating table, bending forwards to his maximum, a lumbar puncture is made between L_3 and L_4 vertebrae. 1 ml of a *heavy* local anaesthetic solution is injected, after which the patient is kept sitting for 2 minutes. Thereafter, he is made to lie down, with the head end of the table raised, so that the anaesthetic agent remains at the lower part of the spine. This method is useful for all operations in the perineum.

3. *High Spinal.*—The puncture is made as in the standard method, and 15 ml of a *light* local anaesthetic solution is injected. The patient is now made prone and is placed in such a manner that the highest point of the spine is at the level of the T_4 vertebra. This position may be obtained by raising the bridge of the table or by placing pillows under the chest. The position is maintained for about 10 minutes. Thereafter, the patient is turned on his back and the operation started.

This type of anaesthesia is useful for upper abdominal and lower thoracic operations.

Advantages of Spinal Anaesthesia.—In older days, (a) when knowledge of general anaesthesia was not so perfect as it is now and was associated with risks of pulmonary complications and complications related to the. heart, kidneys and liver, and (b) when muscle relaxants were not available, spinal anaesthesia was popular because of its following advantages:

1. Excellent muscular relaxation, so useful for abdominal surgery.
2. Absence of post-operative pulmonary complications.
3. Non-interference with the work of the heart, kidneys and liver.

Disadvantages

1. Fall of blood pressure as a result of paralysis of the vasomotor nerves (unilateral block is beneficial in this respect since only half the number of vasomotor nerves are impaired).
2. Infection, i.e. meningitis, may occur/though rarely.
3. The patient may suffer from apprehension during the operation.

It is because of these disadvantages, particularly the fall in blood pressure, the spinal anaesthesia is nowadays largely avoided. This is more so because of the vast improvement in the field of general anaesthesia. However, epidural anaesthesia is quickly gaining popularity and has almost completely replaced spinal anaesthesia.

Indications

A. For anaesthetic purpose:
1. All operations below the diaphragm, particularly the lower abdominal operations, operations on perineum, repair of hernia, and operations on the lower extremities.
2. Sometimes lower thoracic operations (with high spinal anaesthesia).

B. For diagnostic purpose.—In Buerger's disease, a spinal anaesthesia removes temporarily, the spasmodic factor of the arterial obstruction. The amount of circulatory improvement, following spinal anaesthesia is therefore, a good guide to decide how much benefit may be afforded to the patient by performing lumbar sympathectomy.

C. FOR THERAPEUTIC PURPOSE.—In achalasia gastrica, a high spinal anaesthesia paralyses the sympathetic supply to the cardiac sphincter. Usually the patient remains free for about six months and, if it is so, the injection may be repeated at intervals.

Contraindications

1. Low blood pressure (e.g. below 100 mm of Hg), presence of shock, advanced myocardial degeneration.
2. Diseases of the vertebral column (e.g. osteoarthritis, caries) and local sepsis in the soft tissues at. the proposed site of puncture.
3. Apprehensive patients and children.
4. Diseases of the central nervous system.

73
Splints

Uses.—These are appliances meant for supporting limb that has been injured, inflamed, deformed, or paralysed.

1. *Injury.*—This is the commonest indication for the use of splints. The purpose of splintage, in injury, are as follows:
   a. Rest is an essential requirement for the healing of any injured tissue. While all fractures require some form of splintage for union to occur, soft tissues also need protection against unnecessary movements for healing to progress.
   b. Correct splintage relieves pain.
2. *Inflammation.*—Splintage helps in two ways:
   a. Controls spread of infection by minimising movements.
   b. Relieves pain.
3. *Deformity.*—Splints are helpful in two ways:
   a. Arrest progress of the deformity.
   b. Corrective splints may help correcting the deformity, e.g. talipes, scoliosis, contracture, etc.
4. *Paralysis.*—Splints support the paralysed muscles, thereby preventing their undue stretching, so that the muscles can work efficiently if the paralysis is overcome.

Classification.—There are various ways of classifying splints:

A. Splints may be:
   1. Ambulatory.—The patient can move about with the splint.
   2. Non-ambulatory.—The patient cannot move about.

B. Splints may be:
   1. Adjustable.—The parts can be adjusted to each other so that the angles, bends, and sizes may be altered.
   2. Fixed.

C. Splints may be:
   1. Unilateral.—It can be used on one side only, right or left.
   2. Universal.—It can be used on both the sides.

D. Splints may be:
   1. Fixation splints.—These are used only for fixation, e.g. plaster of Paris, straight wooden splint, etc.
   2. Traction splints.—These may be used for applying traction.

E. Splints may be:
   1. Splints for general purposes.
   2. Splints for the upper limb.
   3. Splints for the lower limb.

SPLINTS FOR GENERAL PURPOSES

STRAIGHT WOODEN SPLINT

These are pieces of thin and light pine wood, made to different length and width. The size is chosen according to the length and breadth of the limb. In doing this, it must be remembered that the splint should be wider than the limb in order to give an adequate support. The splint is fixed to the limb with bandages.

Advantages

1. Easily available and cheap.
2. Can be carried easily.

Disadvantages

1. The surface, being flat, cannot adopt itself accurately to the contour of the limb, so that immobilisation is never perfect.
2. The bony points of the limb may be pressed upon by the splint. This disadvantage may be overcome by padding the splint generously with cotton.

Uses

1. First aid for any fracture of the extremities.
2. Fixing the limb during intravenous transfusion.
3. Fixing the limbs of an infant during operation under local anaesthesia.
4. A short splint may be applied transversely across the back of the shoulder and fixed by a figure-of-eight bandage, in treating fractured clavicle (Hey Grove's method).

CRAMMER'S WIRE

Made of aluminium alloy, this splint consists of two long, parallel, rather thick wires, connected to each other at intervals of short length by a number of short and relatively thin pieces of wire (Fig. 73.1). The advantage of the splint is that it may be made into many types of splint, e.g. abduction splint, cock-up splint, etc. The splints are available in 1 to 4 inches width, and these may be cut to any length as required.

Fig. 73.1: Crammer's wire

Uses

1. Keeping it straight and padding with cotton, it may be used just like a straight wooden splint (see above).
2. Bending as desired, it may be made into different forms of splint, e.g. abduction splint, cock-up splint, etc.
3. It may be used to re-inforce a plaster cast, and in this respect it is particularly suitable for an abduction plastering (spica) of the shoulder.

GOOCH'S SPLINTING

This consists of a backing of canvas, to one surface of which strips of soft wood are glued. Thus the splint is malleable. Sheets of different length and width are available and these are supplied rolled. It may however be cut to shape, as desired, with a strong knife (Fig. 73.2).

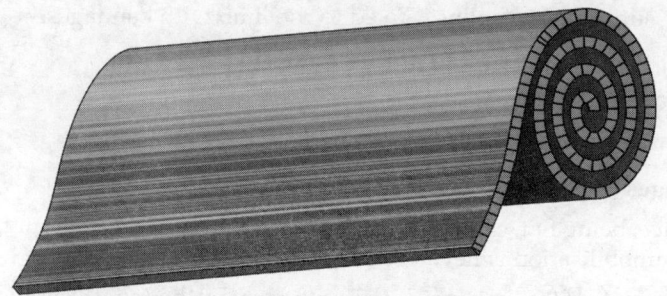

Fig. 73.2: Gooch's splinting

Methods of Application

1. With the canvas side next to the skin or the wooden side next to the skin.
2. Rolled to the limb with the long axis of the wood pieces either along the long axis of the limb or across the long axis of the limb.

Mode of Action

1. When applied with the canvas side next to the skin and the wood pieces transversely round the limb, it affords rigidity in the long axis of the limb and flexibility across.
2. When applied with the woods next to the skin, it affords rigidity in both the axes of the limb.

SPLINTS FOR THE UPPERLIMB

CLAVICULAR CROSS

This is a T-shaped wooden splint; with its arms 4 inches wide.

Use.—It is sometimes used for treating fracture of the clavicle in combination with a figure-of-eight bandage. The horizontal bar extends from one acromion process to the other, across the back. The vertical bar extends downwards along the midline of the back, to just below the level of the iliac crests. After bracing back the shoulders (to reduce the fracture), the splint is applied and is held in position with a figure-of-eight bandage. The axillae must be padded generously with cotton to prevent pressure on the axillary vessels.

Disadvantage.—Since ordinary figure-of-eight bandaging is sufficient for the treatment of fractured clavicle, this splint is rarely used, especially because it causes inconvenience to the patient in lying supine.

THOMAS' ARM SPLINT

This splint is made of iron rod. It is a traction splint, i.e. it may be used to apply traction (Fig. 73.3).

Parts
1. A circular ring to fit round the axilla and shoulder.
2. Two long side bars, one end of each of these being attached to the ring.

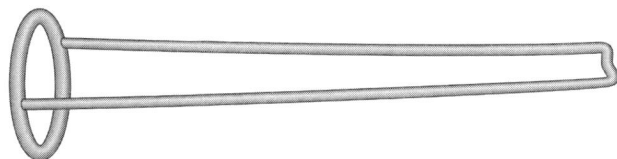

Fig. 73.3: Thomas' arm splint

3. A cross bar, uniting the two side bars at their other end. The cross bar is notched at its middle, so that it has the shape of a W. This notch is meant for tying the traction cord.

Measurements
1. The ring should be a little wider than the girth of the axilla and the shoulder so that it can be padded generously before application. This padding is essential to prevent pressure on the axillary vessels and chest wall.
2. The side bars should extend from the ring to about 6 inches beyond the tip of the middle finger. This space of 6 inches is required for traction (with spreader and cord) to be applied, especially because the adhesive plaster, with which traction is applied, tends to slip down a little in course of time.

Side Determination.—As the side bars divide the ring into two equal halves, the same splint may be used on either side, i.e. the splint is universal.

Uses
A. *Without Traction:*
    1. First aid and transport in any injury of the upper limb.
    2. Compound fractures of the bones of the arm and the forearm.
    3. Avulsion of the greater tuberosity of humerus or rupture of the supraspinatus tendon.
B. *With or Without Traction.*—Adduction fracture of the surgical neck of the humerus.
C. *With Traction.*—After excision of the elbow joint.

Disadvantages
1. The splint is non-ambulatory.
2. Pressure sores on the axilla and chest wall, on which the countertraction is effected.
3. Stiffness of the elbow.
4. Disturbance of the carrying angle of the elbow.
5. Imperfect reduction of the fracture fragments while treating fractures of the surgical neck of the humerus.

SINCLAIR'S MODIFICATION OF THOMAS' ARM SPLINT

The modification lies only in the attachment of the side bars to the circular ring. They are not fixed to the ring. Instead, they are so attached, that the ring swivels on the side bars. The advantage is that the arm may be adducted with the splint on during transport of the patient on a stretcher.

ROBERT JONES' HUMERUS EXTENSION SPLINT

This is a splint made of iron rod. It is so made that traction can be applied on the humerus and so it is called 'extension' splint (Fig. 73.4).

Parts

1. An axillary ring, the lower half of which is well-padded. This padding is essential because the pressure of counter-traction falls on the axilla.

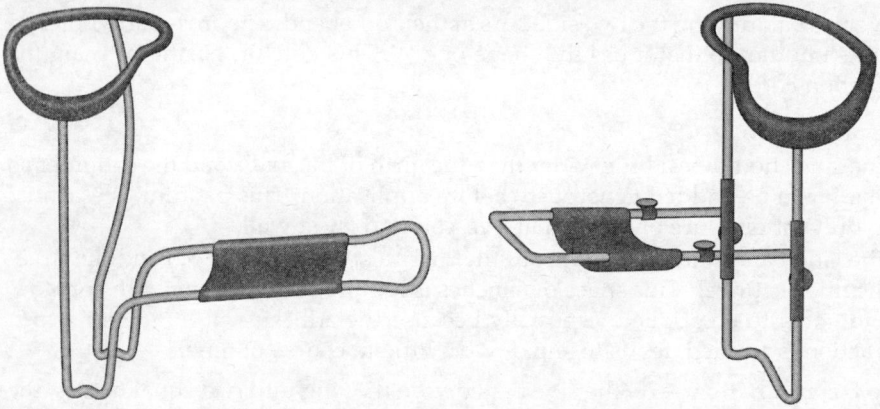

Fig. 73.4: Robert Jones' humerus extension splint

Fig. 73.5: Robert Jones' humerus extension splint (universal type)

2. Two side bars, attached at their upper end to the axillary ring. The bars are bent at a right-angle at a site that corresponds to a little below the elbow joint. At the angle, the bars are notched (like the letter W). To these notches are tied the lower ends of the adhesive plasters, applied on the medial and lateral sides of the arm, for the purpose of surface traction on the humerus. The angle of the side bars has to extend to a little below the elbow for traction to be effective, especially so because the adhesive plasters tend to slip down a little in course of time. The forearm parts of the side bars are connected to each other with a leather sling, which supports the forearm.

Use.—The practical use of this splint is in the treatment of fractures of the shaft of the humerus that require active traction (especially those below the insertion of the deltoid). In this respect, it has the advantage over the Thomas' splint in that the patient can move about with the splint.

Measurements

1. The ring should be a little wider than the girth of the axilla and shoulder, to make space for adequate padding under the axilla.
2. The arm part of the side bars should extend to at least 4 inches below the elbow. Therefore, the measurement of the lateral bar, in this part, should be the distance from the tip of the acromion to the lateral epicondyle plus 4 inches.
3. The forearm bars should extend to a little distal to the wrist.

Side Determination.—The splint is held with the forearm bars anteriorly. The lateral side bar of the arm, which is longer than the medial, indicates the side.

ROBERT JONES' HUMERUS EXTENSION SPLINT (UNIVERSAL TYPE)

This is a modification of the ordinary Robert Jones' splint in the following respects:
1. It may be used on either arm, right or left.
2. The arm bars as well as the forearm bars may be adjusted to different lengths, as required. Thus, the same splint may be used for many patients.
   It is for these reasons that the splint is called 'universal' (Fig. 73.5).

ABDUCTION SPLINT (AEROPLANE SPLINT)

This splint is especially used for the purpose of keeping the shoulder in abduction (Fig. 73.6).

Parts
1. Metal pieces:
   a. Chest piece.
   b. Arm piece.
   c. Forearm piece.
   d. Wrist piece.
2. Leather straps are attached to the metal pieces at different levels. They keep the heavy splint in position.
3. Arrangements for traction are often added.
4. The splint is so heavy that, in addition to the leather straps, cotton bandages (8 to 10) are required to keep it in position.

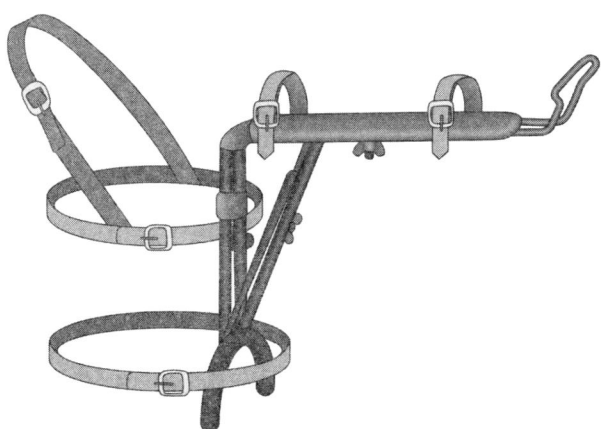

Fig. 73.6: Aeroplane splint

Adjustment.—The chest, arm, forearm, and wrist pieces are joined to each other almost at right angles. However, the pieces are so screwed, that the height of the splint and the length of its limbs can be altered according to necessity.

Alternative.—If a splint like this is not available, several pieces of Crammer's wire may be combined to prepare one like this. In such cases, plaster-of-Paris casts may be re-inforced, if required.

Uses
1. Abduction fracture of the neck of the humerus.
2. Avulsion fracture of the greater tuberosity of the humerus.
3. Rupture of the supraspinatus tendon (or support after operative repair of the tendon).
4. Fracture of the neck of the scapula.
5. Paralysis of the deltoid (or abductors of the shoulder).
6. Arthritis of the shoulder, particularly tubercular.
7. Following arthrodesis of the shoulder.

Advantages
1. It is ambulatory.
2. It keeps the shoulder in the optimum position (70° abduction and 30° in front of coronal plane).

Disadvantages
1. The heavy splint tends to slide down.
2. It is cumbersome.
3. It is particularly uncomfortable during sleep.

COCK-UP SPLINTS

These splints are used to keep the wrist in dorsiflexion. The optimum position for the wrist is 15° to 20° dorsiflexion, and these splints achieve this.

Types.—There are two varieties:
1. Short Cock-up Splint.—Here the fingers are left free (Fig. 73.7).

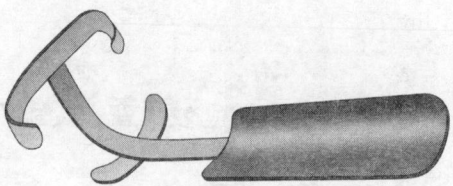

Fig. 73.7: Short cock-up splint

2. Long Cock-up Splint.—Here the fingers are incorporated in the splint and are kept in extension (Fig. 73.8).

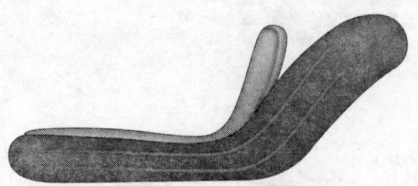

Fig. 73.8: Long cock-up splint

Indications.—These splints are widely used and are indicated in a number of conditions:

A. *Traumatic:*
   1. All fractures of the carpal and metacarpal bones (Colles' fracture, however, should not be treated with this splint because dorsiflexion of the wrist tends to cause further dorsal displacement of the lower fragment).
   2. Injuries of extensor tendons of the fingers.
   3. After operations on extensor tendons of the fingers.

B. *Inflammatory:*
   1. Arthritis of the wrist, including tubercular.
   2. Tenosynovitis of the extensor tendons of the fingers.

C. *Deformity:*
   1. To prevent contractures during healing of burns.
   2. Following release operations for contractures.

D. *Paralysis.*—Wrist drop due to radial nerve injury.

SPLINTS FOR THE LOWER LIMB

THOMAS' HIP SPLINT

Types
1. Single—for one hip.
2. Double—for both hips.

Use.—These splints are sometimes used in the treatment of tuberculosis of the hip joint:

1. *Single Hip Splint.*—This is used during the quiescent stage of the disease, when the patient is allowed to work, but without bearing weight on the limb. The splint is applied to the affected side and kept in position with leather straps at the leg, thigh, trunk and shoulders. An iron ring, called 'patten' is fitted to the shoe of the healthy limb in order to lengthen that limb, so that the affected limb is off the ground and does not take weight. The patient walks with the help of crutches. Thus, the splint is ambulatory.
2. *Double Hip Splint.*—This splint immobilises both the hip joints. It is used during the active stage of tuberculosis. The patient lies in bed with the hip joints abducted. Thus, the splint is non-ambulatory.

THOMAS' BED KNEE SPLINT

This splint, like a Thomas' arm splint, is made of iron rods, and is a traction splint, i.e. it may be used for applying traction (Fig. 73.9).

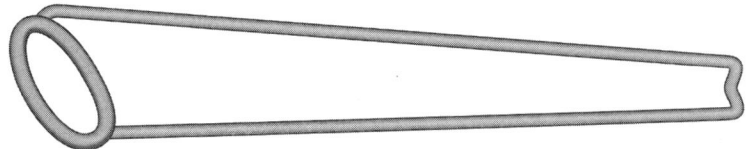

Fig. 73.9: Thomas' Bed knee splint

The splint is so named because it was introduced by Thomas for immobilising the knee joint in tubercular arthritis, the patient being confined to bed.

Parts

1. Two long side bars, one bar being longer than the other.

2. A ring to which the side bars are welded. The ring is set to the bars obliquely, at an angle of 120°. The ring is not uniformly circular and the bars are so attached to the ring that they divide it into a narrower and a wider segment. The narrower segment is meant for the anterior aspect and the wider segment for the posterior aspect, where it accommodates the buttock.

3. A cross bar, uniting the side bars at the other end. The cross bar is notched at the middle, so that it has the shape of a W. This notch is meant for tying the traction cord.

4. Two leather slings, fixed between the side bars, at different levels, for the support of the limb. The sling under the thigh is so tightened as to keep two-thirds of the thigh in front and one-third behind the side bars.

Differences from a Thomas' Arm Splint

1. The two side bars are inequal in size.

2. The side bars are not attached at right angles to the ring but obliquely at an angle of 120°.

3. The ring is not uniformly circular, it has bends on its own axis.

4. The side bars divide the ring into two inequal segments.

Side Determination.—The narrower segment of the ring is placed anteriorly. The longer side bar (which corresponds to the lateral side of the limb), indicates the side.

Universal Type.—For reason of economy, in the hospitals, the side bars are attached to the ring at its middle, on either side, so that the ring is divided into two equal halves. Thus, the same splint may be used for either limb. Hence, it is called 'universal type', i.e. with no choice of side.

Measurement

1. The size of the ring should be such that it fits round the upper thigh, with the posterior part of the ring against the ischial tuberosity. Measurement is taken circularly from the ischiopubic ramus to a point midway between the highest point of the iliac crest and the tip of the greater trochanter, thence to the ischial tuberosity, back to the point of starting at the ischiopubic ramus. To this must be added the provision of padding. Since all the pressure is borne by the postero-internal part of the ring, this part should be padded more generously than the rest of the ring.

2. For the medial bar, the length from the uppermost part of the medial side of the thigh to the medial side of the sole (with the knee in full extension) should be measured.

3. For the lateral bar, the length from the midpoint between the highest point of the iliac crest and the greater tuberosity to the lateral side of the sole is measured. The knee must be in full extension.

To both these lengths, a length of about 8 inches is added. This length, clear off the limb, is required for the traction to be applied, especially because the adhesive plaster, with which traction is applied, tends to slip down a little in course of time.

Accessories or Additional Attachments

1. *Foot Piece:* This may be attached towards the lower end of the splint to prevent:
   a. foot drop,
   b. eversion of the limb.

   In all cases of prolonged immobilisation, there is a tendency for foot drop to develop. In fractures of the femur, there is also a tendency for the limb to get everted. These two difficulties may be overcome by using a foot piece (Fig. 73.10).

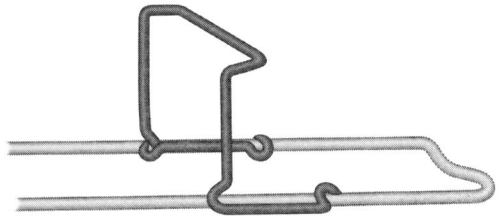

Fig. 73.10: Foot piece for attachment to Thomas' bed knee splint

2. *Flexion Piece:* This is attached towards the middle of the side bars and is useful where it is necessary to flex the knee (in an ordinary Thomas' splint, the knee is kept almost extended). It is, therefore, of special value in treating supracondylar fractures of the femur, where the posterior tilting of the lower fragment cannot be corrected without attaching a flexion piece. Supra-condylar fractures are better treated in Bohler-Braun splint. As with the Bohler-Braun splint, it is the upper end of the lower fragment (and not the knee joint) which should correspond to the site of attachment of the flexion piece (Fig. 73.11).

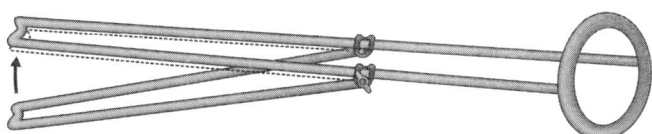

Fig. 73.11: Thomas' bed knee splint with flexion piece

Uses

1. The chief use of the splint is as a first aid for all injuries of the lower limb, for the purpose of transport. It is of particular use in this respect in cases of fractures of the neck and shaft of the femur.
2. It is used for treating (with traction) fractures of the shaft of the femur.
3. It may be used for treating supracondylar fractures of the femur, provided a flexion piece is attached.
4. In fractures of the neck of the femur, the splint may be used for the following purposes:
   a. Ordinarily, for keeping the limb in rest, pending internal fixation, i.e. SP nailing.

    b. Immobilisation and prevention of rotation, where a conservative treatment is instituted, e.g. impacted abduction fractures, extracapsular fractures.

    c. Continuous traction in children.

5. Posterior dislocation of the hip with fracture of the upper rim of the acetabulum (traction is necessary till the acetabular fracture is united).

6. Tuberculosis of the hip joint. Here traction is at first applied in the direction of the deformity. Thereafter, as the muscle spasm gradually passes off, the limb is gradually brought to the optimum position of the hip joint, which is 10° abduction, 20° flexion, and neutral rotation.

7. Tuberculosis of the knee joint, as originally advocated by Thomas. Thomas' main aim was immobilisation of the knee. In the present days, the splint is used for better purposes, with the attachment of a flexion piece. These patients often present with flexion deformity at the knee. Traction is applied on the attached flexion piece, which is gradually elevated towards the main splint (i.e. the angle is diminished), as the muscle spasm is relieved. Thus, the deformity is corrected.

8. In treating all wounds of the lower limb—dressing is easy, pressure on the injured area (if it is located posteriorly) is avoided, and there is immobilisation, which is so essential for healing.

Preparation of the Limb for Traction.—As has already been said, this is a traction splint, which means that traction may be applied with the help of this splint.

A surface traction is employed with the help of adhesive plasters, applied to the skin. For femoral fractures (where the splint is most commonly used), adhesive plaster 3″ wide is applied on the medial and lateral sides of the limb with hairs shaved. This should start from as high as possible in the upper part of the thigh (irrespective of the level of the femoral fracture) and come down to just above the level of the ankle. The two malleoli are protected with cotton pads to prevent development of sores. Attempts, are made to re-inforce the attachment of the adhesive plaster to the skin, by applying cotton bandages around the limb, over the adhesive plaster, upto a level of 2 inches above the ankle. The limb is now prepared to wear the splint, which is carefully guided up from below.

FIXED TRACTION.—This may be effected in two ways:

a. The lower end of each adhesive plaster (i.e. on each side), which is kept long to come down to a little below the level of the foot, is brought round the lowest end of the respective side bar and tied tightly to the notch of the crossbar.

b. A continuous length of adhesive plaster is used from one side of the limb to the other, turning like a U, a few inches below the sole. In the gap of the U, is applied a wooden spreader (*see* Fig. 72.122). A traction cord is attached to the centre of the wooden spreader and this cord is tightly tied to the notch of the crossbar.

MOBILE TRACTION.—This has to be applied with a spreader and traction cord, as described above. The cord is passed over a pulley, which is fitted to the rail at the foot end of the bed. To the end of the cord, weights of desired quantities are tied.

COUNTERTRACTION.—There are two types of countertraction:

1. *Fixed:* A fixed traction, as described above, is applied and countertraction is afforded by the ring, pressing against the ischial tuberosity, which is carefully padded to prevent pressure sores.
2. *Balanced:* The traction cord is tied to the rail at the foot end of the bed. The foot end of the bed is raised by 12 to 18 inches. The tendency for the patient to slide upwards, by gravity, acts as a countertraction. The advantage of this method is that the chances of pressure sores on the ischial tuberosity are minimised, as the patient moves away from the ring of the splint, by weight. The patient unknowingly regulates, i.e. balances the amount of traction.

Complications and their Preventions
1. Pressure sores at the ischial tuberosity may be prevented by:
    a. Proper padding of the ring at this site.
    b. Use of balanced countertraction, i.e. raising the foot end of the patient, thus relieving pressure at the buttock.
2. Knee complications: The knee tends to get stiff, as it is hyperextended. Also, there is a possibility of developing genu recurvatum because of over-stretching of the posterior ligaments of the knee joint. These may be prevented by the following precautions:
    a. The knee is kept a little flexed, by putting a thick pad of cotton behind it.
    b. Alternatively, a flexion piece may be attached to the splint, to keep the knee flexed.
3. Foot drop: This may be prevented by:
    a. Regular ankle exercises.
    b. Use of a foot piece.
4. Eversion of the limb, which often tends to occur during traction. This may be prevented by the following method:
    The adhesive plaster strip on the lateral side of the limb is affixed a little behind the midlateral line and that on the medial side of the limb a little towards the front.

BRAUN'S SPLINT

This splint, made of iron rods, has only one pulley for application of mobile traction (Fig. 73.12).

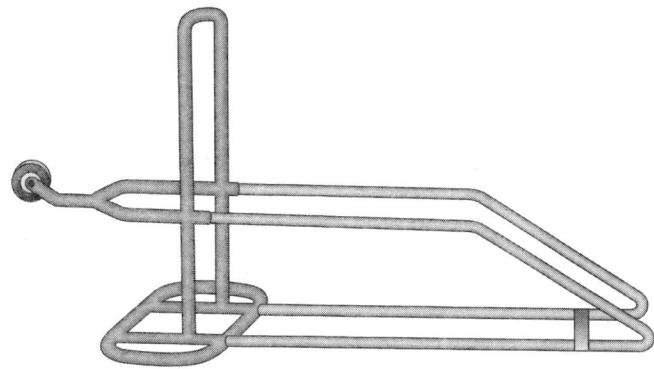

Fig. 73.12: Braun's splint

Uses

1. *With Traction.*—*The* splint is especially intended for applying skeletal traction, in cases of fracture of both bones of the leg, with overlapping of the fragments. Skeletal traction is applied with help of a Kirschner's wire, Stienmann's pin, or Bohler's pin, through the calcaneal tuberosity (or, occasionally, through the lower third of the tibia). To the wire or pin is attached a stirrup, and to the stirrup is tied one end of the traction cord. The traction cord passes over the pulley and weights are attached to it to effect a mobile traction. The foot end of the bed may be raised for effecting countertraction.

2. *Without Traction:*
   a. Compound fracture, without overlapping, in the long bones.— Immobilisation is achieved while dressing can be done.
   b. Lacerated injury in the leg.—The part is kept at rest and, as the limb is kept elevated, oedema is prevented. Both these factors play an important role in the healing of wound.

BOHLER'S MODIFICATION OF BRAUN'S SPLINT

The modification lies in the addition of the upper three pulleys, making a total of four (as compared to one pulley, i.e. the lowest, in the original Braun's splint)— Fig. 73.13.

It is chiefly a traction splint, meant for skeletal traction, in cases of:
a. Fractures (with overlapping) of both bones of the leg.
b. Fractures in the lower two-thirds of the femur, particularly supracondylar fracture.

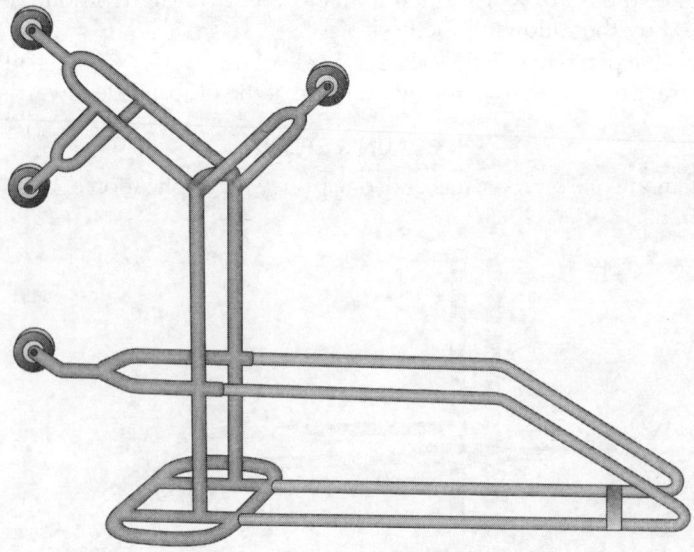

Fig. 73.13: Bohler's modification of Braun's splint

The four pulleys, on either of which the traction cord may be passed, are for the following purposes:

1. The lowermost for tibia and fibula.
2. The second from bottom for supracondylar fractures of femur.
3. The third for fractures of the femoral shaft in the middle third.
4. The uppermost for prevention of foot drop. It is worth noting that this pulley is directed towards the head end of the splint because the foot has to be drawn towards the head in order to prevent a foot drop.

Skeletal traction is applied with Kirschner's wire, Stienmann's pin, or Bohler's pin, to which a stirrup is fitted. The traction cord is tied to the stirrup and it passes over the corresponding pulley. Weights are tied to it, so that a mobile traction is applied.

The foot end of the bed is raised by 12 to 18 inches and this achieves counter-traction.

The traction pin, in cases of leg bone fractures, is usually passed through the calcanean tuberosity but occasionally through the lower third of the tibia. In cases of femoral fracture, the traction pin passes either through the tibial tuberosity (in adults) or through the femur itself, just above the condyles (in children).

In treating supracondylar fractures, with this splint, three points are to be carefully remembered:

1. There is a posterior tilting of the lower fragment, caused by the pull of the gastrocnemius. To correct this, flexion of the knee is essential because it serves two purposes:
   a. The gastrocnemius muscles are relaxed.
   b. The quadriceps, as it is stretched, pushes the lower fragment, from the front, into position.

2. The fracture line and not the knee should correspond to the angle of the splint. It is only by this process that the upper end of the lower fragment, which is tilted back, is forced forwards to position.

3. The traction should be applied in a line, considerably lower than that of the femur. This helps in correcting the backward tilt.

BACK SPLINT WITH MOVABLE FOOT PIECE

This is a straight wooden splint, at the distal end of which a foot piece is attached at a right angle (Fig. 73.14). There is a hollow in the main splint, just proximal to the foot piece. This hollow serves two purposes:

1. The foot piece can be moved along the hollow, upwards and downwards, as desired.
2. The hollow accommodates the heel, thereby preventing pressure sores.

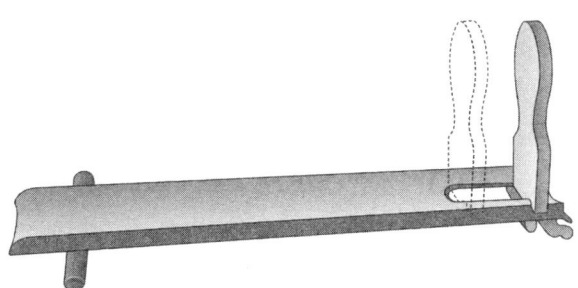

Fig. 73.14: Back Splint with movable foot piece

Uses.—This is essentially a leg splint and may be used for:
1. First aid and transport in fractures of tibia and fibula.
2. Wounds in the leg.—Dressings can be done and rest afforded.
3. Compound fractures of the leg bones without overlapping.—Dressings can be done and rest afforded.
4. Inflammatory conditions of the leg.
5. Before and after operation for fractured patella.

Measurement.—The splint should extend upto the upper third of the thigh. The size can be adjusted to some extent by moving the foot piece up or down.

Modifications
1. It may be converted into a box splint if two side splints (wooden bars) are used in addition.
2. A special type of the splint is available, where there is a hinge at the site of the knee. By adjusting the hinge, the knee may be flexed to the desired angle (Fig. 73.15).

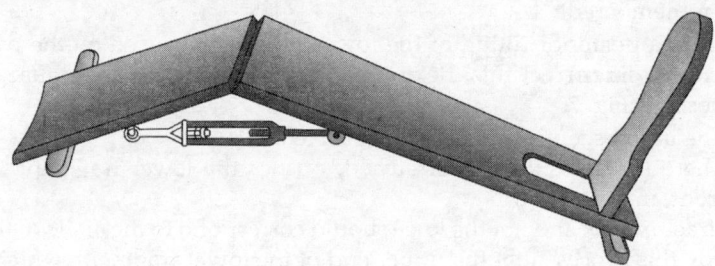

Fig. 73.15: Hinged back splint

Method of Application.—The splint is well padded with cotton, excepting at the hollow for the heel. In other words, the heel should be free to the air through the hollow. The maximum pressure point is the tendo Achillis above the heel and it is at this place that maximum cotton padding should be done. The splint is fixed to the limb with cotton bandages. Bandaging starts from the foot, fixing the foot to the foot piece; and then proceeds upwards to the thigh.

The foot end of the splint should be placed on a sandbag, so that gravity prevents oedema in the limb. After the foot and the limb have been fixed to the splint with bandages, if the splint is pushed downwards, some amount of traction may be effected. However, this is negligible.

LISTON'S LONG SPLINT

The splint is really long, measuring about 5 feet, meant to extend from the axilla to beyond the foot. Its width is 4 inches and it is usually ½ inch thick (Fig. 73.16).

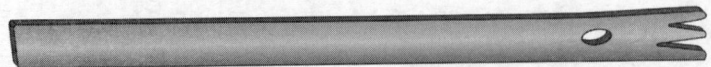

Fig. 73.16: Liston's long splint

Method of Application.—This splint is fixed to the lower limb and the trunk with the help of cotton bandages. The spikes at the lower end of the splint are meant for application of bandages that fix the splint to the ankle. There are usually two holes towards the upper end of the splint and these are meant for tying the perineal bands. The hole towards the lower end of the splint is to accommodate the lateral malleolus.

Uses

1. It is also known as Listen's thigh splint because, in older days, it was used for treating all fractures in the femur. Traction could be applied by fixing the splint firmly to the ankle and then pushing it downwards. Simultaneously, the perineal bands would be tightened to effect countertraction.
2. Presently, however, the splint is used almost exclusively for the purpose of first aid and transport in fractures of the lower limb.

MARSH'S KNEE CAGE

This splint essentially consists of two lateral bars, which are hinged opposite the knee. There are two circular leather bands, well padded, which fix the splint in position. One of these is for the thigh and the other for the calf. The hinges on the bar allow flexion and extension of the knee but the bars themselves prevent any abnormal movement such as lateral movement, rotational movement, and hyperextension (Fig. 73.17). The splint is therefore of use in:

1. Cartilage injuries.
2. Ligament injuries.

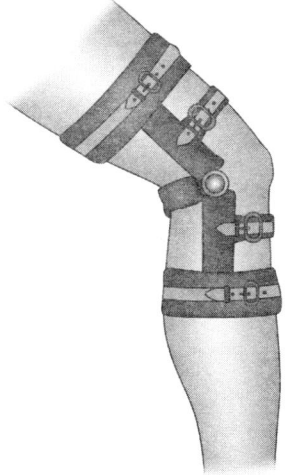

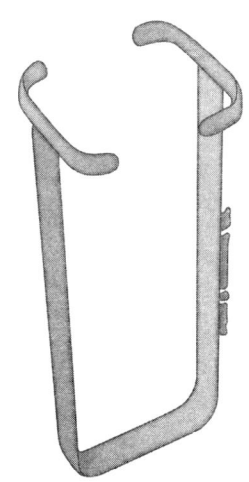

Fig. 73.17: Marsh's knee cage   **Fig. 73.18:** Bohler's walking iron

BOHLER'S WALKING IRON

This is a U-shaped metal bar. At the upper end of each limb there is a malleable metallic plate. These plates are so bent as to fit to the convexity of the calf. The bend of U is to touch the ground when the patient walks, with the splint on. It is often re-inforced with a piece of leather, resembling the half-sole of a shoe, so that the patient can walk with greater confidence (Fig. 73.18).

The walking iron is of particular value in the treatment of minor fractures in the foot (most commonly that of a metatarsal, particularly the base of the fifth metatarsal), where immobilisation is as important as prevention of weight-bearing. If an ordinary plastering is done, the patient cannot walk because:

a. The sole-piece of the plaster is broken and worn out.

b. Weight-bearing is not prevented.

The walking iron is incorporated in the plaster of the foot and leg in such a way that the sole is about 2 inches above the bend of the iron. Thus, while immobilisation is achieved by the plaster, weight from the limb is carried along the limbs of the iron directly to the sole-piece. Therefore, weight is taken off the fractured bone and the sole-piece of the plaster is protected from damage.

The patient has to walk with the aid of a stick.

In those cases where the patient may be allowed to walk with the plaster, a *plaster rocker* may be incorporated in the sole-piece of the plaster, so that the plaster is not damaged on bearing weight. This is used in place of an walking iron.

DENIS BROWNE'S TALIPES SPLINT

This splint is used in the treatment of talipes equinorvarus.

Parts.—The splint consists of 3 parts, all made of aluminium—two L-shaped splints and a cross bar. Each L-shaped splint is meant for one foot and the cross bar connects the two, with the idea of keeping the two lower limbs in abduction.

Each L-shaped splint has a horizontal plate and a vertical plate. The horizontal plate receives the sole of the foot. The vertical plate is meant to be applied against the lateral side of the leg. It has an outward curvature that accommodates the lateral malleolus (Fig. 73.19).

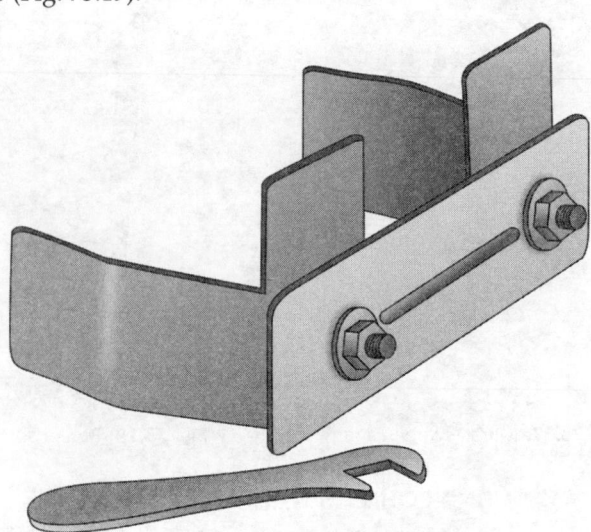

Fig. 73.19: Denis Browne's talipes splint

Mode of Use.—These splints are usually used in early infancy, when, following reduction, the foot is kept in the corrected position with adhesive plasters. The L-splints help in re-inforcing the adhesive plaster immobilization. Upto the age of two months, corrective manipulation can be done without anaesthesia. The sole of the foot is placed on the horizontal plate of the L-splint and the deformity is corrected by manipulation. Adhesive plaster, 1" wide, is used to fix the foot to the splint, the tender skin being protected with felt. The vertical plate of the splint is then applied on the lateral side of the lower leg and similarly fixed in position after full correction of the deformity. Another L-splint is applied to the opposite foot even when this is normal (if this foot is also deformed, manipulative reduction is done simultaneously as above).

The cross bar is now fixed to the two L-splints, by tightening the nuts below. In cases of bilateral talipes, the two feet are kept in abduction (i.e. pointing lateralwards) as much as possible. In unilateral cases, the normal foot is kept only in 20° abduction.

Advantages.—Denis Browne claimed that the splint is advantageous over plaster-immobilisation in two ways:
1. Plastering in infants has to be done upto the thigh and not below knee since otherwise the plaster tends to slip out of the limb.
2. Plastering is followed by disuse wasting of the muscles. If the splint is used, muscular wasting is prevented because the child resorts to kicking about.

After-treatment.—Every week or fortnight the position is checked up and the strappings are changed. A long-continued treatment (at least for one year, better till the child begins to walk) is required because the foot has a notorious tendency to go back to the deformed state. At the age of one year, if further immobilisation is required, the foot may be conveniently placed in a 'reverse boot', i.e. the boot for a right foot is fitted to the left and vice versa. This reversion, by itself, corrects the deformity.

TRUSS

Truss is used in the conservative management of inguinal hernia. It prevents the descent of a hernia by pressing over the *deep* inguinal ring. A truss should never press on the superficial inguinal ring because of the risk of pressure on the spermatic vessels.

Truss should never be used for a femoral hernia because here the hernia comes out through the femoral ring in a downward direction and pressure cannot be applied on the ring effectively. Moreover, as the course of a femoral hernia is angulated and tortuous, truss should not be placed over it.

In cases of umbilical hernia in infants and children, a modified form of truss is used. A metal disc or a big coin is placed over the umbilicus (with the hernia reduced), and this is pressed in position with adhesive plasters, that are changed every week.

Types
1. *Single Truss.*—Used for unilateral hernia (Fig. 73.20).
2. *Double Truss.*—Used for bilateral hernia (Fig. 73.21).

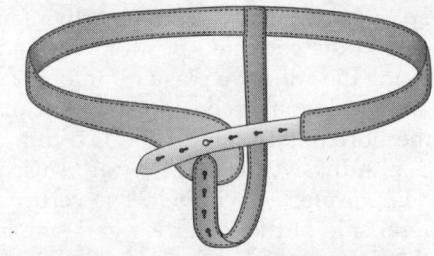

Fig. 73.20: Hernia truss for the right side

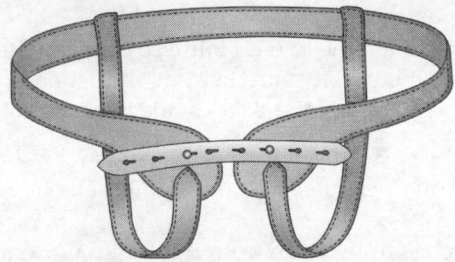

Fig. 73.21: Bilateral hernia truss

Parts

A. Single truss consists of the following parts:
1. A steel spring (covered with leather), to one end of which is attached a pad and to the other end (which extends upto the anterior superior iliac spine of the opposite side) is fixed the leather abdominal strap.
2. A pad attached to one end of the spring. Its skeleton is a piece of soft iron, which on its inner surface, is well-padded with cork or foam and is covered with leather. The pad is ovoid, with its medial side (which is free) wider than the lateral side (to which the steel spring is attached). The medial side points downwards. The pad is about 3 inches is in length and 2 inches wide. On its outer surface there are two studs.
3. A leather abdominal strap, one end of which is attached to the steel spring while the other end is free and has several holes, into any one of which the upper stud on the pad may be inserted.
4. A leather perineal strap, also with several holes. One end of the strap is fixed to about the middle of the spring and the other end is free, to be fitted with the help of one of the holes to the lower stud on the pad.

B. Double truss consists of the following parts:
1. A steel spring.
2. Two pads, each attached to one end of the spring, there being no abdominal leather strap.
3. Two perineal straps, each fitting to the lower stud on the pad of the corresponding side.
4. Sometimes an additional leather strap that joins the two pads in front. This strap is meant to be attached to the upper stud of the pad on either side.

Wearing.—With the hernia reduced, the pad is placed over the inguinal canal. The abdominal strap is tightened. The perineal strap is brought across the perineum and is tightened. The purpose of the perineal strap is to prevent the truss from slipping upwards, which it has a tendency to do.

Clear Instructions for Use

1. The hernia must be reduced completely before the truss is fitted.
2. The patient should use it throughout the day. It may have to be worn also during night if the patient suffers from cough at night.
3. The patient should never be on his feet without the truss. This means that he should take off the truss only after lying down and put it on, again, before he gets up.

Determination of Side in Unilateral Truss.—The truss is held with the perineal strap hanging downwards. The pad lies anteriorly with its free medial end pointing downwards. The truss belongs to the side on which the pad is located.

Measurement

1. For single truss, measurement is taken from the pubic spine, the measuring tape passing midway between the iliac crest and the greater trochanter and coming back to the same pubic spine.
2. For double truss, measurement is taken from one pubic spine to the other, the measuring tape passing round the pelvis as above.

Criteria for a Well-fitting Truss.—With the truss on:

1. The patient is asked to cough—the hernia should not come out.
2. The patient is asked to squat—the hernia should not come out and the truss should not be displaced.
3. The patient is asked to walk—the truss should not be displaced and the perineal strap should cause no friction.

Disadvantages of Using Truss

1. The patient has a false sense of security—obstruction and strangulation cannot be prevented:
   a. If the hernia is big.
   b. If the truss cannot apply pressure properly.
2. Majority of the patients do not use the truss regularly as per instructions. Moreover, if the hernia is not properly reduced before wearing the truss, or if the truss is not well-fitting (leaving a gap), the truss, by itself, causes obstruction or strangulation.
3. The underlying muscles undergo pressure atrophy, so that, if operation is undertaken, the repair of the canal has to be done with atrophied and fibrosed muscles and this is never satisfactory.
4. The skin over the area is devitalised by pressure so that primary union may not occur after operation.
5. Truss encourages development of adhesions, which:
   a. may cause difficulty in dissecting the sac from the structures of the cord at operation.
   b. may invite obstruction or strangulation.

Indication for Use.—As a routine, therefore, for disadvantages, mentioned above, use of a truss should be strongly discouraged. Its only indication is in a elderly feeble patient, who, for reasons otherwise (e.g. cardiac), is unfit to undergo anaesthesia or operation. Even in these patients, operation may be done with local anaesthesia or regional nerve block.

Contraindications
1. The absolute contraindication is an irreducible hernia. The cold irreducible hernia is converted into an acute obstructed one by the use of a truss.
2. If there is chronic strain, e.g. chronic cough, constipation, dysuria, etc.
3. If the patient has to do strenuous job, e.g. a labourer.
4. If there is an associated undescended testis.

BANDAGE SMEARED WITH PLASTER-OF-PARIS

Plaster-of-Paris is dehydrated calcium sulphate. It is a white powder that absorbs water and, thereafter as it dries up, it turns into a hard mass.

Preparation of Bandages.—Ordinary cotton bandages are taken. The bandage is opened part by part, a thin layer of plaster-of-Paris powder is put on it, and it is re-rolled. This rolling should be neither too loose nor too tight. If it is loose, the plaster powder falls out and also the central core of the bandage tends to slide out during use. If it is tight, water fails to penetrate into the central core of the bandage. According to necessity, bandages of different sizes are used, e.g. 3 inches, 4 inches, 6 inches, etc.

Prepared bandages of finer quality, e.g. Gypsona, are also available, ready for use.

Application.—These bandages may be used in two ways—complete plastering and plaster casts,

COMPLETE PLASTERING.—The bandage is placed in a bucket of water, with its tail a little opened out (otherwise, when the bandage is wet, the tail may be difficult to be made out). It is preferable that the water is a little warm since it affords a longer time for the bandage to be applied before the plaster settles, i.e. dries up. The bandage should be immersed in water till bubbles cease to rise; this indicates that the central core has also absorbed water. Thereafter, it is taken out of water, grasped by the two sides, and squeezed towards the middle, so that the excess of water is expressed. It is now applied around the limb or trunk. One after another bandage is used, till the plastering is sufficiently extensive so as to immobilise the part for which it is intended. Also, it should be sufficiently thick so as to afford the rigidity for immobilisation. There should not be any thick cotton pad between the skin and the plaster—immobilisation cannot be perfect then. This is because the plaster shell tends to shrink on drying, making the space between the skin and the plaster wider. Also, when plastering is done for fractures, the oedema around the fracture site tends to disappear within a few days, making the plaster loose. It is, therefore, advisable that the plaster bandages are applied direct to the skin, i.e. unpadded. This, however, has the disadvantage that the hairs tend to adhere to the plaster. It is wise to use a thin layer of cotton between the skin and the plaster. In any case, it is very important to protect all the bony prominences with cotton. The application should be rapid before the plaster can settle, i.e. dry up.

When a plaster extends from the trunk to a limb it is called plaster spica, e.g. shoulder spica, hip spica.

In the region of big joints, the plastering should be re-inforced with plaster casts, Crammer's wire, etc.

PLASTER CASTS.—These are slabs made from plaster-of-Paris bandages. They are applied on one surface of a limb and held in position with cotton bandages.

To prepare a cast, the size is first determined by measuring the two points between which the cast is meant to extend. Plaster-of-Paris bandages are unrolled, spread, and made to the size, layer after layer, in continuity. The number of layers depends on the strength of the limb on which the cast is meant to be used. For the upper limb 6 to 8 layers and for the lower limb 8 to 10 layers are usually advised. The two ends are now held with two hands and the whole mass is immersed in water, till bubbles cease to rise. The excess of water in squeezed out. The cast is kept on a flat surface and both its surface may be used, and the cast is moulded over the limb along its curvatures, and is fixed in position with cotton bandages.

Plaster casts are used for the following purposes:
   a. Temporary immbolisation, as an emergency measure, pending reduction and complete plastering, for fracture and dislocations.
   b. Final immobilisation in some cases, in preference to complete plastering.
   c. Re-inforcement at the big joints in extensive complete plasterings, e.g. hip spica, shoulder spica, etc.

Advice After Plastering
1. The limb should be kept elevated, otherwise oedema occurs.
2. The limb must be examined a few hours later to find out any evidence of vascular insufficiency. The fingers and toes should be examined carefully—whether they are cold and discoloured, or show absence of nail-bed return. If there is any such indication, the plaster should either be slit open longitudinally or be removed completely.
3. The joints that are not incorporated in the plaster (e.g. fingers, shoulder, toes) must be subjected to active exercises, during the period of immobilisation, in order to prevent stiffness.

Complication of Plastering
1. Oedema of the limb distal to the plaster. This is very common and the only means to prevent it are elevation of the limb and active movements of the fingers or toes.
2. Plaster blisters may occur in the skin distal to the plaster. The cause is oedema, the fluid collecting under the cuticle presenting as blisters.
3. Plaster sores occur in the skin over the area incorporated within the plaster, particularly at the pressure points. Their occurrence is indicated by persistent localized pain and, sometimes, offensive smell due to purulent discharges.
4. Impairment of blood supply to the distal part of the limb. This may be caused either by a tight plastering or by rough manipulations during reduction. If there is complete obstruction to blood flow, gangrene occurs. In cases of partial obstruction ischaemic necrosis of the nerves and the muscles may set in, the

commonest example Volkmann's ischaemic contracture in supracondylar fracture of humerus. If a patient complains of persistent pain in the limb even after plaster immobilisation, vascular impairment has to be thought of (ordinarily, the pain of a fracture subsides after reduction and immobilisation), and immediate action taken.

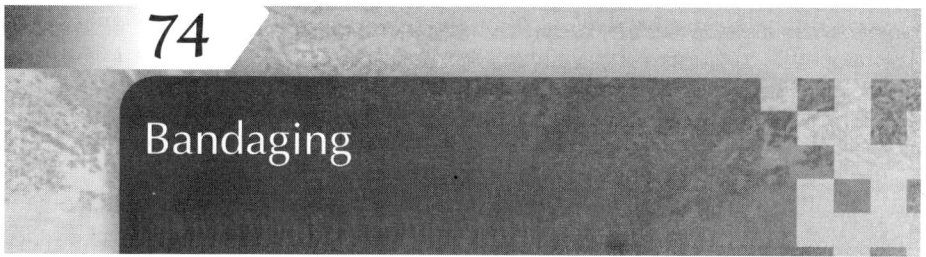

74

Bandaging

Types of Bandages

1. The commonly used bandages are made of cotton. They are cheap and may be washed as well as sterilised. They are called 'roller bandage' as the bandaging material is kept rolled. The open end of the bandage is called its 'tail', while the rolled part is called the 'head'.
2. Cotton-crepe, i.e. elastocrepe bandage, provides greater compression and support because of its elasticity. Elastoweb bandages, which have strong rubber threads incorporated, provide even greater compression and support.
3. Adhesive bandages, made of cotton. These may be inelastic (e.g. leukoplast) or elastic (e.g. elastoplast). These are gaining fast popularity and are replacing ordinary bandages widely.
4. Plaster-of-Paris bandages are invaluable in the treatment of fractures and dislocations.
5. Bandages impregnated with medicaments, e.g. hydrocortisone/zinc oxide, etc. are used to protect and soothe the skin as well as to promote healing in chronic conditions, such as varicose ulcers.
6. Esmarch's bandage, made of flat 3" rubber, is used as a tourniquet.

Use of Ordinary Bandages

1. To hold the surgical dressings.
2. To hold splints and plaster casts.
3. To afford first-aid to the injured.
4. To control bleeding by pressure.
5. To prevent or reduce oedema or swelling.
6. To immobilise a part or to correct deformities (plaster bandages).

Special Types of Bandages

1. Many-tailed abdominal binder.
2. T-bandage, mainly used for the perineum and anus.
3. Moorfield's bandage for fixing dressings over both eyes.
4. Four-tailed bandage used for fracture of the mandible.
5. Triangular bandage, used for slinging the forearm or bandaging an amputation stump.
6. Suspensory bandage for the scrotum.

Principles of Bandaging

1. A bandage of the correct size should be chosen:

Toe or finger	—	1"
Head and neck	—	3"
Upper limb	—	2 to 3"
Lower limb	—	3 to 4"
Trunk	—	4 to 6"

2. The limb to be bandaged is placed in the position in which it is to remain after bandaging. Otherwise, the bandage gets too tight or too loose as the position of the joint is subsequently altered.
3. Absorbent cotton wool should be placed between two skin surfaces that are bandaged together. This absorbs the sweat and prevents friction (otherwise blisters may form).

   Similarly, all prominences should be well padded with cotton, to prevent ulceration.
4. The bandage should be applied with uniform pressure throughout. The amount of pressure varies according to the necessity (e.g. tight bandaging for haemostasis). Ordinarily, the bandage should neither be too tight (interfering with circulation) nor too loose (gets displaced). When tight bandaging, to control haemorrhage, is done, more pressure should be applied distally and less proximally, in order to avoid venous and lymphatic congestion. Such tight bandages should be loosened after 24 hours.
5. The outer surface of the bandage is placed next to the skin for easy unrolling. The bandage should be applied from below upwards, wherever possible. Also, in the limbs, it should run from the medial to the lateral aspect across the front (i.e. from within outwards).
6. A firm start is made by fixing the bandage with at least two turns at the same level. These are called 'fixation turns'. During the process of bandaging, each succeeding turn overlaps two-thirds of the width of the preceding turn. The margins are kept parallel as far as practicable. The bandaging should be finished with a complete turn and fixed securely. The fixation may be done by either of the following procedures:
   a. With strips of adhesive plaster pasted.
   b. With the end of the bandage split and tied.
   c. With a safety-pin, taking care that it does not cause trauma (the pin should lie parallel to the cut edge of the bandage).
   d. By stitching the end with thread.
7. The tips of the fingers and toes should be kept exposed wherever possible (to watch the circulation).
8. Wet bandages should not be used as they carry infection and also tend to shrink when they get dry. Use of too much bandages should be avoided because it is cumbersome as well as expensive.
9. A sling should always be used with a bandage for the upper extremity.

Standard Turns of Bandaging
1. *Circular.*—The bandage is carried horizontally around the part. It is used for:
   a. Head.
   b. Trunk.
   c. Fixation turns at the beginning and end of bandaging in the limbs. Ordinarily, circular turns should not be used around the limb all along the length since they may interfere with circulation.
2. *Spiral.*—The bandage is carried up spirally. It is used over parts having uniform circumference:
   a. Fingers.
   b. Limbs in children.
   c. Upper arm.

3. *Reverse Spiral.*—This is used along with spiral turns to make the bandaging uniform over parts of inequal dimension, e.g. forearm. When spiral turns are continuously applied over these parts it is found that, after a few turns, the head of the bandage hangs on one side. To make for this, the turn is reversed, i.e. the bandage is folded on itself, so that its upper margin now becomes the lower and the outer surface becomes the inner.

4. *Figure-of-Eight.*—This consists of spiral turns, but the turns are carried alternately up and down, so that two successive turns, together, make a figure-of-eight. It is used for:

   a. Unflexed joints—the crossing of the bandage should take place on the flexor aspect.

   b. Limbs of inequal dimension—as an alternative to reverse spiral turns.

   c. Fracture of the clavicle.

5. *Spica.*—This is so named because the finished bandaging has the appearance of an ear of barley. It is actually a figure-of-eight bandage, applied across a joint, whose upper and lower components have gross dissimilarity of dimension, e.g. hip, shoulder, etc. In other words, one loop of each figure-of-eight is much wider than the other.

   Spica may be of three types:

   a. Ascending Spica.—The crossing of the first figure-of-eight turn is at the lowest level (Figs 74.6 and 74.23).

   b. Descending Spica.—The first crossing is at the highest level (Figs 74.7 and 74.24).

   c. Divergent Spica.—Here the bandage converges towards the crossing of the figure-of-eight and diverges on the opposite side of the limb. This is used for the flexed joints (Figs 74.5, 74.19 and 74.22).

6. *Recurrent.*—This is used for:

   a. Amputation stump (Fig. 74.26).

   b. Finger-tip.

   c. Head.

The bandage is applied over the end of the stump or finger-tip or head, by forward and backward turns, and these are fixed by spiral turns.

In addition to the above standard turns, special turns have to be used, according to necessity, as in the head, eye, ear, breast, scrotum, etc.

INDIVIDUAL BANDAGES

In a limb the bandage is always started across the anterior surface; beginning from the medial side and going laterally. A sling is applied for support in the upper limb.

FINGER

1. When the tip may be kept uncovered.—An 1" bandage is taken, A couple of turns are applied round the wrist for fixation. The bandage is then brought across the back of the hand, from the lateral to the medial side, upto the lateral border of the base of the finger. Thereafter, the bandage is carried straight towards the tip of the finger (but short of it), with one or two oblique turns.

Then it is brought back to the root of the finger by several spiral turns. Now the bandage crosses the former turn on the back of the hand, to reach the wrist at its medial border. A few final fixation turns are applied around the wrist and the end is secured (Fig. 74.1).

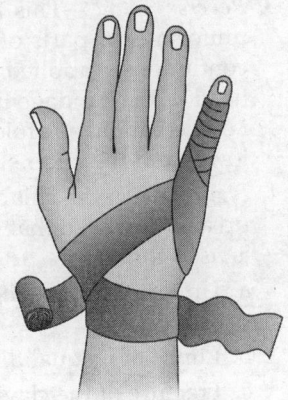

2. *When the tip has to be covered.*—This is required after incision of a whitlow and after amputation. The starting process is the same as in (1). As the bandage reaches the tip of the finger, several recurrent turns are applied across the tip over its dorsal and palmar surfaces. The recurrent turns are fixed by spiral turns. Subsequently, spiral turns are applied to bring the bandage back to the root of the finger. Thereafter, the process is the same as in (1).

Fig. 74.1: Bandage for a finger

3. *When more than one finger have to be bandaged.*—Each finger should be bandaged separately, starting with the little finger.

THUMB

An 1" bandage, applied as spica, is the best, particularly to arrest haemorrhage from the ball of the thumb, by pressure. The bandage is fixed at the wrist with a couple of turns. From the anterolateral aspect of the wrist it is carried across the back of the thumb, between the thumb and the index finger, to the tip of the thumb. It makes a loop there. Thereafter, it is brought back across the back of the hand to the medial side of the wrist and a loop is applied round the wrist. The bandage is again taken towards the tip of the thumb, as above, covering two-thirds of the previous thumb turn. Subsequently, alternate wrist and thumb turns are applied and the bandaging is completed at the wrist. The bandaging actually consists of figure-of-eight turns (Fig. 74.2).

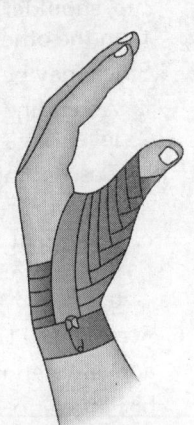

Fig. 74.2: Bandage for the thumb

HAND AND PALM

1. *Ordinary Bandaging.*—A *figure-of-eight* bandage is advised. A 2" bandage is selected. A couple of fixation turns is applied round the wrist. From the anterolateral aspect of the wrist the bandage is carried obliquely across the back of the hand to the base of the little finger. It crosses the palm, to reach between the thumb and the index finger. It is then continued over the dorsum of the hand, across the previous hand turn, to reach the posteromedial aspect of the wrist. It is again carried obliquely across the dorsum of the hand to the lateral side, covering the proximal two-thirds of the previous turn, and the process of figure-of-eight is repeated. The bandage is completed with fixation turns at the wrist (Fig. 74.3).

2. *For a Bleeding Palm.*—A *closed-fist* bandage, applied tightly, for the purpose of haemostasis, is required. The patient is advised to grasp a pad of cotton (or, better gauge) tightly. A couple of fixation turns are applied on the wrist as usual. From the anterolateral aspect of the wrist the bandage is carried obliquely across

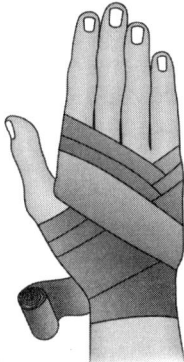

Fig. 74.3: Bandage for the hand and palm (figure-of-eight)

the back of the hand. It then covers the knuckles at the medial side of the closed fist to come to the palmar surface. A turn is now made round the wrist and then again across the back of the hand, to cover the knuckles of the fist. This covers the lateral two-thirds of the previous knuckle-turn. The process is repeated till the knuckle of the index finger is covered. The bandage is completed with fixation turns round the wrist. The essentiality of the bandage is that it must be tight in order to achieve haemostasis, and if the bandage is applied properly, the patient cannot open up the closed fist (Fig. 74.4).

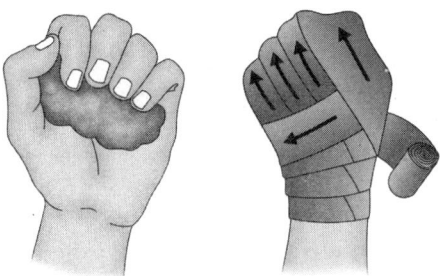

Fig. 74.4: Pressure bandage for bleeding palm (closed-fist bandage)

Bleeding Palm.—Ordinary bleeding from the palm is easily controllable. Bleeding from the palmar arches, however, may be difficult to control. These are the cases where a closed-fist bandage is helpful.

There are two palmar arches:

1. *Superficial Palmar Arch.*—This is formed by the termination of the ulnar artery and completed by the superficial palmar branch of the radial artery. It is very superficial in the palm, therefore, very prone to injury. It lies only deep to the skin, palmar aponeurosis, and palmaris brevis muscle. It is superficial to the flexor tendons. It lies at the level of the *distal* border of the outstretched thumb. It gives off four palmar digital branches.

2. *Deep Palmar Arch.*—This is formed by the termination of the radial artery and is completed by the deep branch of the ulnar artery. It lies deep to the flexor tendons, at the level of the *proximal* border of the outstretched thumb. It gives

off three palmar metacarpal arteries, which anastomose with the digital branches from the superficial palmar arch, in the region of the metacarpal heads.

FOREARM

Two types of bandages may be applied:
1. Reversal spiral.
2. Figure-of-eight.

If any case, a 2½" bandage is used and the bandaging starts from below and proceeds upwards.

ELBOW (FLEXED)

Unless otherwise indicated, the elbow is bandaged in the position of 90° flexion.

A divergent spica is applied with a 2½" bandage. Two fixation turns are applied round the elbow, so that the point of the elbow rests on the middle of them; Thereafter, figure-of-eight turns are applied, working alternately above and below the elbow, crossing in front of the joint (Fig. 74.5).

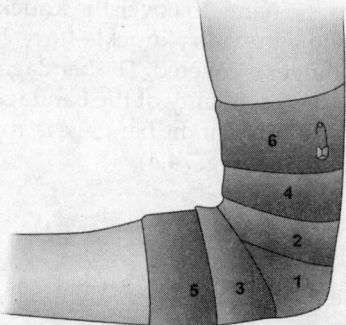

Fig. 74.5: Bandage for the flexed elbow (divergent spica)

UPPER ARM

Simple and reverse spiral turns are applied, starting from below and proceeding upwards. A 3" bandage is used.

WHOLE UPPER LIMB

A 2½" bandage is used:
1. To start with, the bandage is applied as for hand, starting from the wrist (figure-of-eight).
2. Reverse spiral or figure-of-eight turns are applied on the forearm.
3. The elbow is flexed at 90° and a divergent spica is applied.
4. The upper arm is bandaged with simple and reverse spiral turns.

AXILLA OR SHOULDER

A 3" bandage is used and a cotton pad is applied to each axilla. Either an ascending or a descending spica is applied:

1. ASCENDING SPICA.—The bandage is started at the upper part of the arm with a couple of fixation turns. Thereafter, simple or reverse spiral turns are applied to

take the bandage to the level of the axilla. From behind the arm, the bandage is carried across the back, to under the opposite axilla and then across the chest to the top of the bandage round the arm. A complete turn is applied round the arm and then the bandage is taken (below the trunk turn) on the anterolateral aspect of the arm again, to its back. Thereafter, it is continued to the back, opposite axilla, chest, and back to the arm again. The process is continued till the shoulder is completely covered. Each turn of the bandage (both on the trunk and on the arm) covers the upper two-thirds of the preceding turn. The bandage ends on the chest (Fig. 74.6).

2. DESCENDING SPICA.—The bandage is the same as above, but the figure-of-eight turns start on the upper aspect of the shoulder and gradually work downwards, i.e. the successive turns are applied to cover the lower two-thirds of the preceding turns. The bandage ends on the arm (Fig. 74.7).

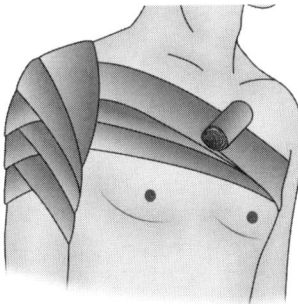

Fig. 74.6: Ascending spica for the axilla and shoulder

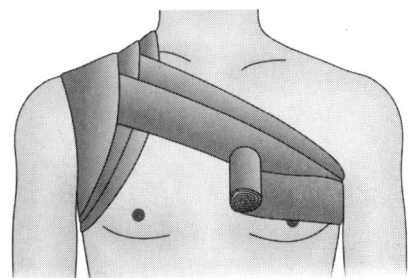

Fig. 74.7: Descending spica for the axilla and shoulder

FRACTURED CLAVICLE

A 4" bandage is used. The patient is sitted and the shoulders are braced back, with the hands resting on the hips. The surgeon stands behind the patient.

Large cotton pads are put over the shoulder and under the axilla (these prevent compression of the axillary vessels and nerves).

The bandaging is started from the front of the sound shoulder and crosses obliquely across the back to under the axilla on the fractured side and then in front of the shoulder on that side. It then crosses the back obliquely again to reach under the axilla on the sound side and then in front of the shoulder, thus completing a figure-of-eight turn. These turns are repeated, till the shoulders are well braced back. A sling is applied on the fractured side.

The bandage gets loose and has to be repeated every 3–4 days. It is kept for a period of 3 weeks.

BREAST

1. FOR THE SUPPORT OF THE BREAST (AND AFTER INCISION FOR BREAST ABSCESS).—4" to 6" bandages are used. The bandaging is started from below the affected breast and crosses horizontally across the chest, to the back. Two such horizontal turns are applied round the body, for fixation. Thereafter, the bandage is carried obliquely, over the lower part of the affected breast, to the opposite shoulder. It then crosses the back obliquely downwards, to reach the starting point of the oblique turn. Then a horizontal turn is applied round the body. Another oblique turn is then applied, covering the upper two-thirds of the preceding oblique turn. Then again a horizontal turn, to the body, is applied. This process is continued till:

a. The breast is well-supported (where only support to the breast is required).

b. The dressings are covered (after incision of breast abscess). The bandage is secured in front of the chest (Fig. 74.8).

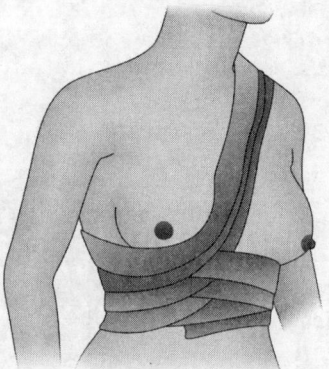

Fig. 74.8: Bandage to support the breast

2. AFTER RADICAL MASTECTOMY.—4" to 6" bandages are used. Adequate cotton pads are applied on the operated breast, axilla and upper arm.

The bandaging is started from below the operated breast but proceeds immediately under the same axilla, to the back (i.e. in the reverse direction of the previous bandaging). One or two such horizontal turns are applied for fixation. It is then carried obliquely over the lower part of the operated breast to the shoulder, and then round the arm (covering the lower margin of the dressings in the axilla and arm). As the bandage comes back to over the shoulder again, it is carried obliquely downwards, across the back, to under the opposite axilla. A horizontal turn is now applied round the body, covering the upper two-thirds of the previous turn. Another oblique turn on the breast, then the shoulder, and the turn round the arm are applied. The turns on the breast and the arm cover the upper two thirds of the respective preceding turns, i.e. the bandage gradually proceeds upwards. The process is repeated till the dressings have been completely covered. The bandage is completed in the front (Fig. 74.9).

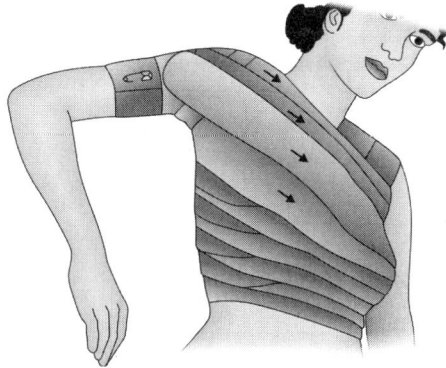

Fig. 74.9: Bandage after radical mastectomy

NECK

1. FRONT OF NECK (AFTER THYROIDECTOMY).—A 3" bandage is taken. A pad of cotton is placed under each axilla.

A couple of fixation turns are applied round the neck. From one side of the front of the neck, the bandage is carried obliquely across the upper chest, to under the opposite axilla. It is then carried horizontally across the back, to under the opposite axilla. It then proceeds obliquely upwards, across the chest (crossing the previous oblique turn at the centre of the chest), to the neck. Thereafter, it passes round the back of the neck, to reach the side of the neck, from where the oblique turn had started. This figure-of-eight bandaging is continued till the dressings are covered (Fig. 74.10).

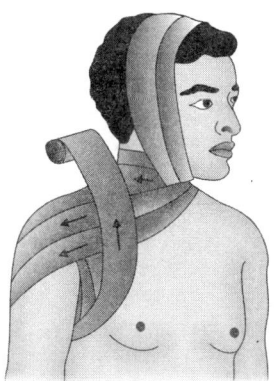

Fig. 74.10: Bandage after thyroidectomy

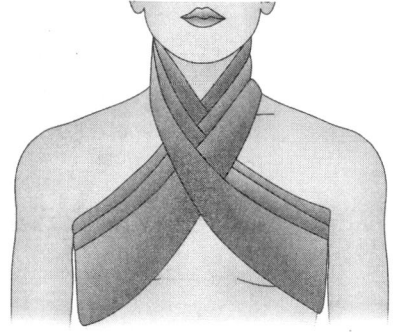

Fig. 74.11: Bandage after block dissection of the cervical nodes

2. BACK OF NECK (CARBUNCLE).—A 3" bandage is taken. The bandaging is started on the forehead, applying horizontal turn round the head. It is then taken backwards above the ear, obliquely across the neck, to reach below the other ear. Thereafter, it crosses the front of the neck to the other side. It then proceeds obliquely upwards (crossing the previous oblique turn at the centre of the back of the neck) to above the ear, and then cross the forehead to the starting of the first

oblique turn. This process is repeated, but the bandage is taken lower down each time it crosses the back of the neck.

3. AFTER BLOCK DISSECTION OF THE CERVICAL NODES.—A 3" bandage is taken. A pad of cotton is placed in the axilla on the operated side.

Supposing the bandage is for an operation on the right side, a couple of fixation turn is put round the neck, starting in front of the neck, running from left to right. It then ascends from beneath the right jaw in front of the ear to the top of the head and, thereafter, down behind the ear on the left side. After a turn round the neck; the bandage descends obliquely to the upper-most part of the anterolateral aspect of the right arm. Then it passes backwards to under the axilla on the back. It comes forwards from under the axilla and proceeds to the back of the neck and makes a turn round the neck. Then, again, it ascends from beneath the right jaw in front of the ear to the top of the head. The process is repeated. Thus, the bandage alternately passes round the head and the axilla in between the neck turns (Fig. 74.11).

FRACTURED MANDIBLE

Two types of bandaging may be done, of which the second type is the simpler:

1. FOUR-TAILED BANDAGE.—A long piece (about 2 feet) of a 4" bandage is taken. Just at its centre a 3" longitudinal slit is made (this is for the chin). The bandage is also longitudinally slit at each end, and this slit reaches to within 6" of the centre.

The bandage is so placed that the chin passes through the central slit. The upper strip on either side is taken horizontally to behind the neck, where the two are tied together. The lower strip from either side is taken upwards, in front of the ear, and the two are tied on the top of the head. Last of all, the four ends at the two knots are tied together by another piece of roller bandage (Fig. 74.12).

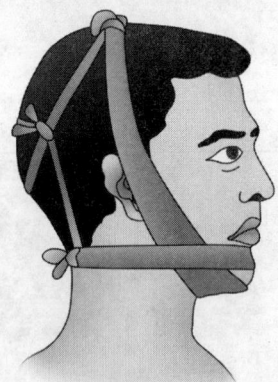

Fig. 74.12: Four-tailed bandage for the lower jaw

2. BARREL BANDAGE.—A 5 feet long, 3" bandage is taken. The centre of the bandage is placed on the chin and the ends are carried to the top of the head where the first loop of a reef knot is applied. The loop, making the knot, is loosened and separated. One half is slipped forwards to be placed over the forehead while the other half is slipped backwards to be placed just below the occipital protuberance. The two ends of the bandage are now pulled tight and taken to the top of the head, where they are secured with a knot (Fig. 74.13).

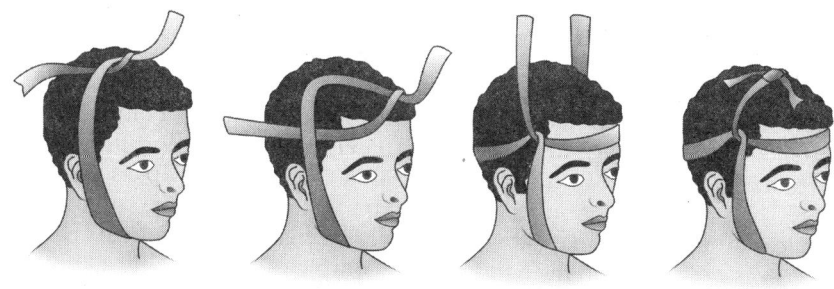

Fig. 74.13: Barrel bandage for the lower jaw

HEAD

Two types of bandaging are commonly used:

1. TWISTED BANDAGE.—This is applied under ordinary circumstances, e.g. keeping the dressings in position. A 3″ bandage is taken. About one foot of the free end is allowed to remain loose and the bandaging starts from below the left ear. A horizontal turn is applied round the forehead, running below the level of the occipital protuberance. As the roller comes back to the starting point, it is twisted round the free end of the bandage and carried to the top of the head, down the right side of the face, under the mandible, back to the starting point. It is twisted round the free end and then it passes over the head, comes to below the right occiput, and then back to the starting point, where it is twisted again. This process is repeated, twisting the bandage over its free end, every time it crosses the starting point, till the scalp is covered (Fig. 74.14).

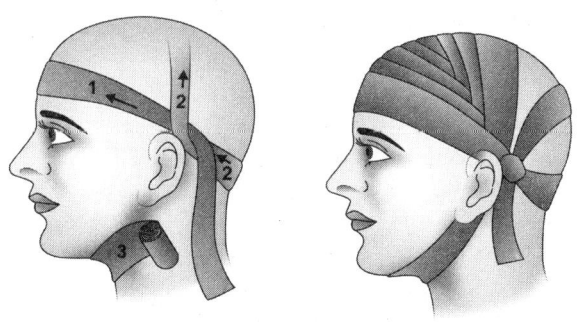

Fig. 74.14: Twisted bandage for the head

2. CAPELINE BANDAGE.—This is especially meant for controlling haemorrhage from the scalp, since it works more or less as a pressure bandage. Two bandages are taken, one 2″ and the other 3″. The ends of the two are tied together with a knot. The surgeon stands behind the patient, holding the 2″ bandage with the left hand and the 3″ bandage with the right hand. The central knot is placed on the forehead and each bandage is taken horizontally, above the ear, to the back of the head, well below the occiput, where they are made to twist each other. The 3″ bandage now crosses the summit of the head in the centre, from the back to the forehead, in the midline. In the meantime, the 2″ bandage passes horizontally to the front of the forehead. Here it is made to cross in front of the 3″ bandage, which has by this time

reached the front of the forehead. The 3" bandage is now made to pass alternately backwards and forwards on the top of the head and, each time it reaches the forehead and the occiput, it is crossed superficially by the 2" bandage which is simultaneously running horizontally round the head, at the level of the forehead. The turns of the 3" bandage are placed alternately to the right and the left of the first turn, that was placed in the midline, so that they gradually pass laterally on the head. The process is continued, till the loops of the 3" bandage come down to more or less a horizontal level, above the ear. The two bandages then cross each other below the occiput and the bandaging is completed by applying a knot in the centre of the forehead (Fig. 74.15).

It is important to note that:

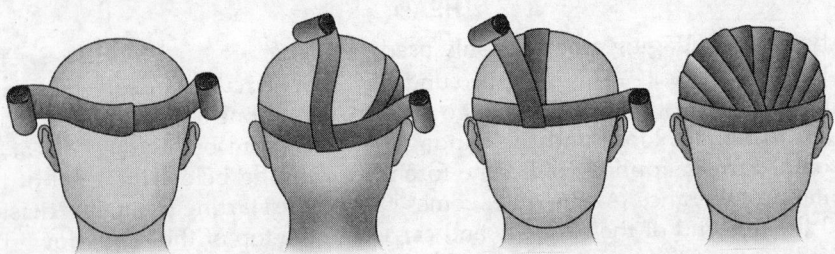

Fig. 74.15: Capeline bandage for the head

1. The knots have to be put on the forehead and not on the back, otherwise the patient cannot lie on the occiput.
2. The bandage is applied tightly for haemostasis and this may cause headache. If this is unbearable, the bandage has to be loosened.

The Layers of the Scalp.—There are five layers:

S—Skin.

Cn—Connective tissue.

A—Aponeurosis of the occipito-frontalis (galea aponeurotica).

L—Loose connective tissue.

P—Pericranium.

CONNECTIVE TISSUE.—This is dense and provides a firm bond of union between the skin above and the galea aponeurotica below. The blood vessels in the layer are firmly anchored by the connective tissue and so, when they are torn, they are prevented from normal retraction. This is why scalp wounds bleed so profusely. However:

a. Bleeding can always be arrested by pressure against the underlying bone and so pressure bandages (e.g. capeline bandage) are useful.

b. At operation, if artery forceps are applied to the galea aponeurotica and are everted, haemostasis is achieved.

Because the fibrous tissue is so dense, subcutaneous haematoma (in this layer) can never be extensive. On the other hand, inflammatory collections (abscesses) cause severe pain because they are under tension.

The blood supply to the scalp being profuse, wounds of the scalp, however damaging, heal perfectly.

GALEA APONEUROTICA.—This is a strong membrane, to which two muscles gain attachment, viz. the frontalis in front and the occipitalis behind. Laterally, on each side, it becomes thin and is attached to the zygomatic arch. Since it is connected to the underlying pericranium by loose connective tissues, blood and pus can collect extensively between it and the pericranium. A subaponeurotic collection, therefore, can extend posteriorly to the superior nuchal line (from where the occipitalis originates) and laterally to the zygomatic arches. Anteriorly, it extends to the root of the nose and the eyelids (because the frontalis has no bony origin; it arises from the skin and subcutaneous tissues in the region of eyebrows and root of the nose, and blends with the orbicularis occuli).

LOOSE CONNECTIVE TISSUE.—It contains some emissary veins, which communicate with the intracranial venous sinuses. Inflammatory collections in this layer may, therefore, cause thrombosis of the venous sinuses. Hence, this layer of the scalp is called 'the dangerous area of the scalp'.

PERICRANIUM.—This represents the periosteum on the outer surface of the skull. It is loosely attached to the bones, except at the sutures, where it is continuous with the periosteum on the inner surface of the skull (endosteum). So, blood and inflammatory collections can easily strip it up from the bone but then the swelling will be limited by the suture lines, giving it the size and shape of the underlying bone.

Blood Supply of the Scalp

1. Superficial temporal (anterior and posterior branches).—Terminal branch of external carotid.
2. Supratrochlear and supraorbital.—Both are branches of the ophthalmic artery (branch of internal carotid).
3. Posterior auricular.—Branch of external carotid.
4. Occipital.—Branch of external carotid.

Black Eye.—This is caused by subcutaneous extravasation of blood in the eyelids. It may be caused by:

1. Local violence.—The extravasation appears within an hour after the trauma and appears simultaneously in the upper and lower lids.
2. Blow on the skull, causing subaponeurotic haemorrhage.—Since the blood slowly gravitates downwards under the origin of the frontalis (vide galea aponeurotica, described above), the black eye appears after a day or two. Also, it is first seen in the upper lid and only later in the lower lid.

Subconjunctival haemorrhage, i.e. haemorrhage just under the conjunctiva, is the result of a direct trauma on the eye. The posterior limit of the haemorrhage can be seen.

Haemorrhage into the orbit results from fracture of the orbital plate of the frontal bone. The blood tracts forwards, under the conjunctiva, appearing in a triangular shape, the apex being at the margin of the cornea. This is, therefore, known as 'flame-shaped' haemorrhage. While the posterior limit of the haemorrhage can be seen in an ordinary subconjunctival haemorrhage, it cannot be seen in orbital haemorrhage.

GREAT TOE

1. When the tip can be kept uncovered.—An 1" bandage is taken. Two circular fixation turns are put round the lower part of the leg, just above the ankle. From

the anteromedial side of the leg the bandage crosses obliquely the proximal part of the dorsum of the foot, to reach the sole. It then crosses the sole obliquely forwards, to reach the medial border of the foot, just proximal to the ball of the great toe. It is now carried obliquely across the dorsum of the great toe, to reach near its tip, at the lateral border. Several spiral turns are applied, bringing the bandage gradually back towards the base of the toe. On reaching the medial border of the base, the bandage crosses the dorsum of the foot obliquely to the lateral border of the foot. Then it is carried obliquely backwards, across the sole, to the medial side of the foot. Finally, it ascends to the leg, where it is completed with a couple of fixation turns (Fig. 74.16).

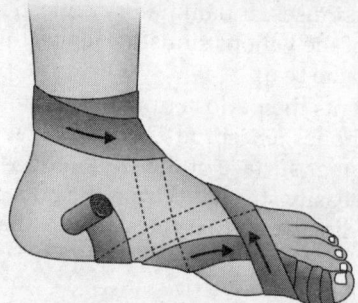

Fig. 74.16: Bandage for the great toe

2. When the tip has to be covered (e.g. after incision for whitlow or after amputation).—As the bandage reaches the tip of the toe, a few recurrent turns are applied antero-posteriorly, across the tip, and these are covered by spiral turns as usual. The rest of the bandaging is as in (1).

FOOT

A 3" bandage is taken. A figure-of-eight fixation turn is put round the ankle and the foot. Thereafter, from the anteromedial aspect of the ankle, the bandage is carried obliquely to the lateral border of the distal part of the foot. The distal part of the foot is covered with several spiral turns, gradually proceeding backwards. The proximal part of the foot is covered with reverse spiral turns, the reverses taking place near the lateral border of the dorsum. Finally, two figure-of-eight turns are applied around the ankle and the heel, before the bandage is completed at the ankle (Fig. 74.17).

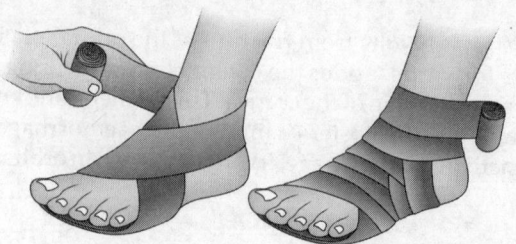

Fig. 74.17: Bandage for the foot

HEEL OR ANKLE

A 3" bandage is used. Two types of bandaging may be done:

1. LOOPED BANDAGE (SEVEN-TURN BANDAGE).—A couple of fixation turns are applied round the lower part of the leg (Fig. 74.18). Then:

First turn.—The bandage is carried downwards and laterally, covering the lateral malleolus, to the lateral border of the foot. It then passes across the sole, to under the medial malleolus at its back.

Second turn.—The bandage passes behind the ankle and then round its lateral border, to come to the front of the ankle. Then it passes downwards and inwards, to the sole, which it crosses, to reach under the lateral malleolus. Thereafter, it is taken to cover the tendo Achillis, to bring it back to under the medial malleolus. The bandage is carried in front of the ankle to cover the lateral malleolus (as in the beginning of the first turn).

Subsequently, the third, fifth and seventh turns are like the first turn, while the fourth and sixth turns are like the second turn.

2. DIVERGENT SPICA.—a. The bandaging starts from the lateral malleolus, and then across the dorsum, back to the starting point. This makes the fixation turn (Fig. 74.19).

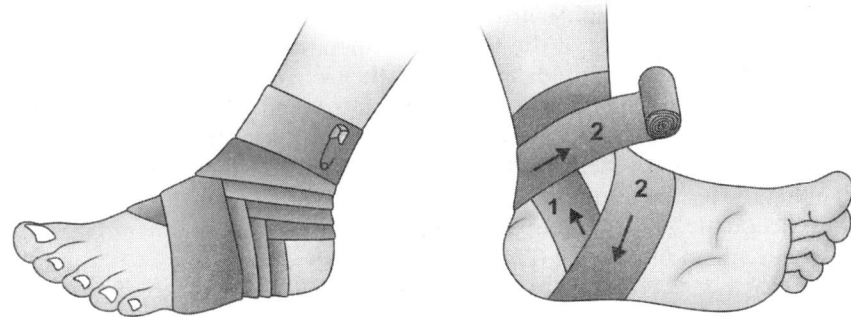

Fig. 74.18: Seven-turn bandage for the heel   Fig. 74.19: Divergent spica for the heel

b. The bandage is carried over the point of the heel. The tense middle part of the loop covers the heel, while the margins of the loop lie loose.

c. Two turns are applied, one above and the other below the previous turn (b), to fix the loose margins.

d. The bandage is applied-alternately round the foot and the lower part of the leg (gradually proceeding forwards on the foot and upwards along the leg).

LEG

A couple of figure-of-eight fixation turns are applied round the foot and ankle (as in bandaging for the foot). The lower part of the leg is covered with few spiral turns. The upper part of the leg is bandaged with reverse spiral turns, the reverses occurring on the anterolateral aspect of the leg (Fig. 74.20).

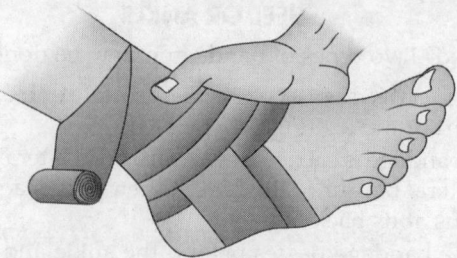

Fig. 74.20: Start of a bandage for the leg

KNEE

A 3" bandage is used. Two types of bandaging are practised, according to the necessity:

1. FIGURE-OF-EIGHT.—This bandage, applied firmly, grossly restricts the movements of the knee as well as controls and reduces its swelling. It is, therefore, useful in post-traumatic and post-operative conditions.

A pad of cotton is put around the knee. A 3" bandage is selected. The bandaging starts from just below the patella and proceeds laterally, and then along the back of the knee to the medial side. It then passes on the tail of the bandage to the lateral aspect of the knee and, thereafter, obliquely upwards, across the back of the knee, to the medial side of the thigh, a little above the knee. It is taken in a little upward direction to the lateral side of the thigh, and then, across the back, it descends along the medial side of the thigh and knee to the front of the leg. Thus, it makes a loop along the thigh. From the front of the leg it is taken to the lateral side of the leg in a downward direction, and then, across the back of the leg, to its medial side. It ascends along the medial side of the leg and knee, to the thigh, thus making a loop along the leg. Thus it forms a figure-of-eight, making one loop on the thigh and the other on the leg. These loops are repeated, gradually in an upward direction, both in the thigh and in the leg (Fig. 74.21).

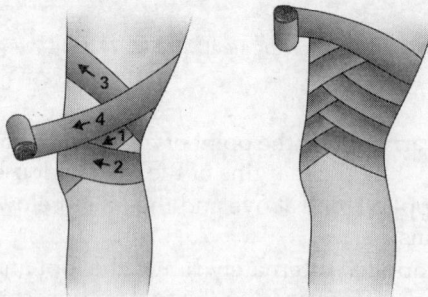

Fig. 74.21: Figure-of-eight bandage for the knee

2. DIVERGENT SPICA.—This allows certain amount of movements in the joint. The knee must be slightly flexed. A 3" bandage is used.

The bandaging starts at the level of the patella, starting on the medial side and passing anterolaterally, and then, round the knee, back to the starting point. The next turn is similarly applied but at a slightly higher level, covering the loose upper margin of the first turn. It comes back to the starting point on the medial side of the knee. The third turn is applied at a slightly lower level than the first turn, so as to cover its loose lower margin, and again comes back to the starting point. Thereafter, alternate layers are applied above and below the knee, ascending and descending slightly than the respective previous turns, but coming back each time to the starting point on the medial side of the knee. This means that the bandage diverges on the lateral side and converges on the medial side of the limb (Fig. 74.22).

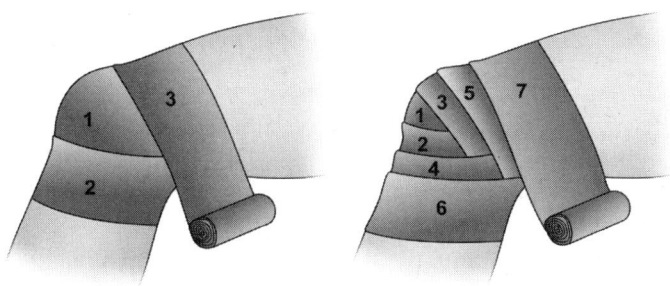

Fig. 74.22: Divergent spica for the knee

THIGH

A 4" bandage is used. The bandaging starts below and proceeds upwards. To start with, spiral turns are applied. In the upper part, reverse spiral turns are applied, the reverses occurring on the anterolateral aspect of the thigh.

WHOLE LOWER LIMB

3" bandages are used. The bandaging starts from the distal part of the foot:
1. Foot.—Spiral turns in the forefoot and reverse spirals in the proximal part of the foot.
2. Ankle and heel.—Divergent spica or looped bandage.
3. Leg.—Spiral turns in the lower part and reverse spirals in the upper part of the leg.
4. Knee.—Figure-of-eight turns.
5. Thigh.—Spiral turns in the lower part and reverse spirals in the upper part.

HIP OR GROIN

4" bandages are used. For facility of bandaging, the pelvis of the patient is raised on a 'pelvic rest'. The two thighs are kept moderately flexed and abducted. Spica bandages are applied and these may be of the following types:

1. Ascending spica.—A spiral turn is applied at about the middle of the thigh, starting from the medial side and passing laterally, across, the front. Thereafter, two reverse spiral turns are applied, the reverse occurring on the anterolateral aspect of the thigh. The bandage is then carried obliquely, laterally and upwards, in front of the groin, to behind the hip. It then encircles the pelvis, midway between

the greater trochanter and the iliac crest. As it comes to the front of the body, it is carried downwards and medially, crossing the last turn and leaving its lower one-third uncovered. A turn is now taken round the thigh and then the bandage is taken across the groin, again, for a pelvic turn. These thigh and pelvic turns are repeated alternately, each successive turn being at a higher level, i.e. covering the upper two-thirds of the respective preceding turn. The bandaging is completed on the abdomen (Fig. 74.23).

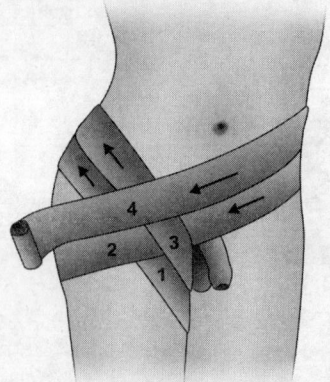 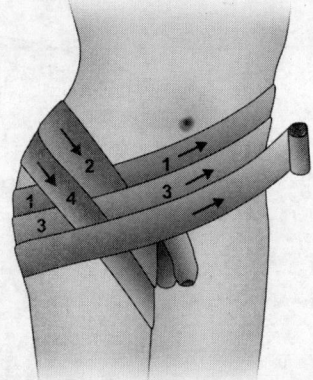

Fig. 74.23: Ascending spica for the hip or groin   **Fig. 74.24:** Descending spica for the hip or groin

2. DESCENDING SPICA.—The bandaging is started on the thigh, below the groin. The first turn in the pelvis is similarly applied at a higher level. The figure-of-eight turns are applied in the same way as for an ascending spica, but they work gradually downwards, i.e. each successive turn covers the lower two-thirds of the preceding turn. The bandage ends on the thigh (Fig. 74.24).

3. DOUBLE SPICA.—This is rarely applied, where both the hips or groins have to be covered. In between the pelvic turns, the groin turns are applied alternately on the right and the left.

SCROTUM

1. LOOPED BANDAGE.—A 4" bandage is used and the pelvis of the patient is raised on a 'pelvic rest'. Cotton pads are put on the scrotum as well as on the lower abdomen.

A couple of fixation turns are applied round the pelvis, midway between the greater trochanter and the iliac crest. From the front, the bandage is taken obliquely downwards across a groin (say, right) to cover the scrotal dressings and reach the perineum, in front of the anus. It then ascends obliquely along the opposite gluteal fold (i.e. left), to reach the pelvis. On the pelvis, a complete turn is taken. Thereafter, the bandage is taken obliquely downwards, across the opposite groin (i.e. right) on to the scrotum and perineum. It then ascends obliquely along the (left) gluteal fold. A pelvic turn is again applied. Thus, in between the pelvic turns, the bandage makes loops on the right and left groins, alternately, to cover the scrotum (Fig. 74.25).

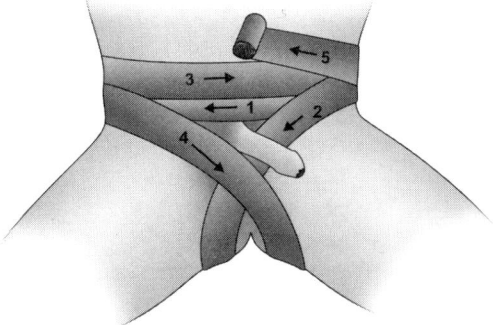

Fig. 74.25: Looped bandage for the scrotum

This bandage, which applies considerable pressure on the scrotum, is commonly used:

a. After operation for hydrocele.

b. After operation for large inguinal hernia (to limit collections in the scrotum).

2. COCONUT BANDAGE.—A 4" bandage is used. A cotton pad is put on the scrotum.

A turn is applied round the lower abdomen, above the level of the iliac crest, and a knot is put. The bandage is then brought along one side of the scrotum to cover its under surface and taken up along the other side of the scrotum to reach the fixation turn on the abdomen. It takes a twist round the fixation turn and is brought back on to the scrotum. Thereafter, several turns are applied tightly round the scrotum (if required, the bandage is twisted on itself, just above the scrotum). Finally, a knot is applied on the bandage by twisting it above the level of the scrotum.

This is only a supportive bandage for the scrotum and is useful for:

a. Relief of pain in the testis, epididymis or spermatic cord.

b. After operation for small-size hydrocele.

c. After operation for small-size hernia.

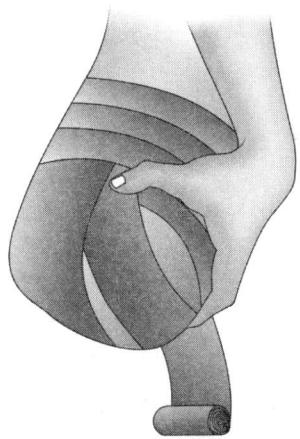

Fig. 74.26: Recurrent bandage for an amputation stump

Index